76.50

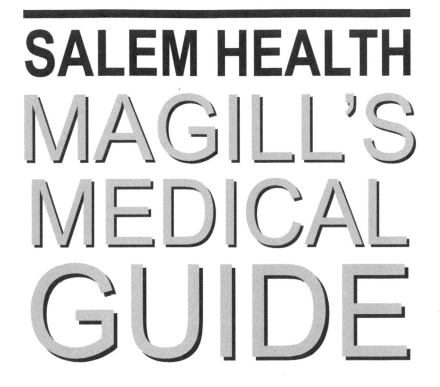

SALEM HEALTH
MAGILL'S
MEDICAL
GUIDE

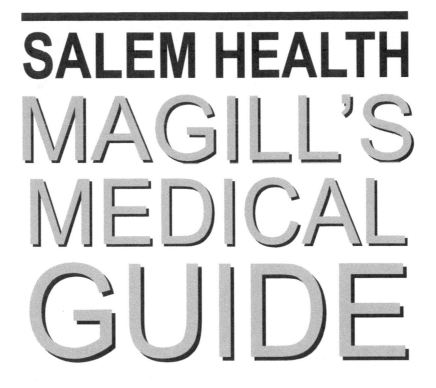

SALEM HEALTH

MAGILL'S MEDICAL GUIDE

Seventh Edition

Volume II

Chyme – Gram staining

Medical Editors

Bryan C. Auday, Ph.D.
Gordon College

Michael A. Buratovich, Ph.D.
Spring Arbor University

Geraldine F. Marrocco, Ed.D., APRN, CNS, ANP-BC
Yale University School of Nursing

Paul Moglia, Ph.D.
South Nassau Communities Hospital

SALEM PRESS
A Division of EBSCO Information Services, Inc.
Ipswich, Massachusetts

GREY HOUSE PUBLISHING

Magill's Medical Guide: Health and Illness, 1995
Supplement, 1996
Magill's Medical Guide, revised edition, 1998
Second revised edition, 2002
Third revised edition, 2005
Fourth revised edition, 2008
Sixth edition, 2011
Seventh edition, 2014

∞ The paper used in these volumes conforms to the American National Standard for Permanence of Paper for Printed Library Materials, Z39.48-1992 (R1997).

Note to Readers

The material presented in *Magill's Medical Guide* is intended for broad informational and educational purposes. Readers who suspect that they suffer from any of the physical or psychological disorders, diseases, or conditions described in this set should contact a physician without delay; this work should not be used as a substitute for professional medical diagnosis or treatment. This set is not to be considered definitive on the covered topics, and readers should remember that the field of health care is characterized by a diversity of medical opinions and constant expansion in knowledge and understanding.

Library of Congress Cataloging-in-Publication Data

Magill's medical guide / medical editors: Bryan C. Auday, Ph.D., Gordon College [and three others].
— Seventh Edition.

5 volumes : illustrations ; cm. — (Salem health)

Title page verso indicates: Seventh Revised Edition, 2014.
Includes bibliographical references and index.
ISBN: 978-1-61925-214-1 (set)
ISBN: 978-1-61925-503-6 (v.1)
ISBN: 978-1-61925-504-3 (v.2)
ISBN: 978-1-61925-505-0 (v.3)
ISBN: 978-1-61925-506-7 (v.4)
ISBN: 978-1-61925-507-4 (v.5)

1. Medicine--Encyclopedias. I. Auday, Bryan C., editor. II. Series: Salem health (Pasadena, Calif.)

RC41 .M345 2014
610.3

First Printing

COMPLETE TABLE OF CONTENTS

VOLUME I

VOLUME II

Shading indicates current volume.

Shading indicates current volume.

Shading indicates current volume.

VOLUME III

VOLUME IV

VOLUME V

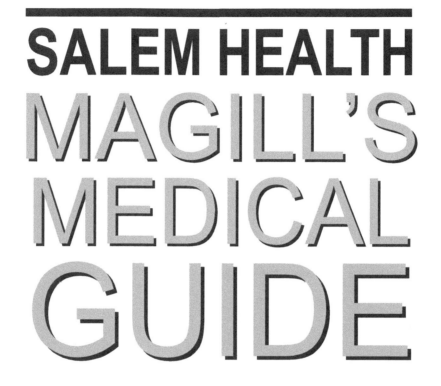

SALEM HEALTH

MAGILL'S MEDICAL GUIDE

CHYME

Biology

Also known as: Chymus

Anatomy or system affected: Gallbladder, gastrointestinal system, intestines, liver, pancreas, stomach

Specialties and related fields: Gastroenterology, internal medicine

Definition: The slurry-like mixture of food and digestive juices produced in the digestive tract.

Structure and Functions

Chewing and swallowing produces a bolus of food that descends through the esophagus into the stomach. There, the stomach walls secrete hydrochloric acid while waves of muscular contraction called peristalsis mix the stomach contents. The gastric juices break the bolus into small food particles, producing a thick fluid called chyme. Peristalsis causes the chyme to collect in the antrum, the lowest section of the stomach. The pyloric sphincter passes small portions of chyme into the duodenum at regular intervals.

Chyme is highly acidic because of the stomach acid. To protect the membrane lining the duodenum, the pancreas releases bicarbonate to neutralize the acid. In the duodenum, digestion continues. Bile produced in the liver is added to the chyme to emulsify fats into small globules. The pancreas contributes enzymes that break down fats, proteins, and carbohydrates so that nutrients, minerals, and salts can be absorbed through the membrane of the small intestine and into the bloodstream.

Over a period of three to five hours, peristalsis pushes the chyme through the small intestine and into the colon. There, bacteria convert some ingredients of the chyme into vitamin K and vitamin B, which the colon extracts along with excess water. Bacteria also produce various gases. These gases are mixed with the remaining waste matter, or feces.

Disorders and Diseases

Most disorders relating to chyme come from excessive food or water intake. When too much is eaten, the stomach distends and presses on the diaphragm. Peristalsis and the sheer bulk of the chyme can make breathing difficult and uncomfortable. When food contains a high proportion of fat, spices, or fibers and is eaten too quickly, the stomach can be overburdened. The churning of peristalsis may force some of the chyme back up the esophagus, causing a burning sensation there known as acid reflux or heartburn. This indigestion of the chyme, or dyspepsia, can make the stomach feel sour and achy and can lead to stomach ulcers. The stomach also may react to psychological stress by producing too much acid.

When the pancreas fails to produce enough bicarbonate to neutralize the acid in chyme after it enters the duodenum, the acid may burn through the mucosa in its wall and into tissue, producing a duodenal ulcer. Too much bile added to the chyme, if not reabsorbed in the distal small intestine, can lead to diarrhea, whereas too little bile can contribute to malabsorption of nutrients. Similarly, excessive water intake

may leach sodium from the body or cause the intestine to process the chyme too quickly for all the nutrients to be removed from it.

—Roger Smith, Ph.D.

See also Acid-base chemistry; Acid reflux disease; Bile; Diarrhea and dysentery; Digestion; Enzymes; Food biochemistry; Gastroenterology; Gastroenterology, pediatric; Gastrointestinal disorders; Gastrointestinal system; Heartburn; Indigestion; Intestines; Malabsorption; Metabolism; Nutrition; Peristalsis; Ulcers; Vitamins and minerals.

For Further Information:

Corcoran, Mary K., and Jef Czekaj. *The Quest to Digest.* Watertown, Mass.: Charlesbridge, 2006.

Lipski, Elizabeth. Digestive Wellness. 4th ed. New York: McGraw-Hill, 2012.

Parker, Steve. *The Human Body Book.* New York: DK Adult, 2001.

Seymour, Simon. *Guts: Our Digestive System.* New York: HarperCollins, 2005.

CIRCULATION

Biology

Anatomy or system affected: Blood, blood vessels, circulatory system, liver

Specialties and related fields: Cardiology, hematology, vascular medicine

Definition: The flow of blood throughout the body; the circulatory system consists of the heart, lungs, arteries, and veins.

Key terms:

aneurysm: a localized enlargement of a vessel, usually an artery

atherosclerosis: accumulation of plaque within the arteries

calcification: the deposit of lime salts in organic tissue, leading to calcium in the arterial wall

capillaries: hairlike vessels that connect the ends of the smallest arteries to the beginnings of the smallest veins

claudication: muscle cramps that occur when arterial blood flow does not meet the muscles' demand for oxygen

diastole: the period of relaxation in the cardiac cycle

hypertension: a blood pressure higher than what is considered to be normal

lumen: the space within an artery, vein, or other tube

stenosis: the constriction or narrowing of a passage

systole: the period of contraction in the cardiac cycle

thrombus: a blood clot that, commonly, obstructs a vein but may also occur in an artery or the heart

vasoconstriction: a decrease in the diameter of a blood vessel

vasodilation: an increase in the diameter of a blood vessel

Structure and Functions

The cardiovascular system is made up of the heart, arteries, veins, capillaries, and lungs. The heart serves as a pump to deliver blood to the arteries for distribution throughout the body. The veins bring the blood back to the heart, and the lungs oxygenate the blood before returning it to the arterial system.

Contraction of the heart muscle forces blood out of the

heart. This period of contraction is known as systole. The heart muscle relaxes after each contraction, which allows blood flow into the heart. This period of relaxation is known as diastole. A typical blood pressure taken at the upper arm provides a pressure reading during two phases of the cardiac cycle. The first number is known as the systolic pressure and represents the pressure of the heart during peak contraction. The second number is known as the diastolic pressure and represents the pressure while the heart is at rest. A typical pressure reading for a young adult would be 120/80. When blood pressure is abnormally elevated, it is commonly referred to as high blood pressure, or hypertension.

The heart is separated into two halves by a wall of muscle known as the septum. The two halves are known as the left and right heart. The left side of the heart is responsible for high-pressure arterial distribution and is larger and stronger than the right side. The right side of the heart is responsible for accepting low-pressure venous return and redirecting it to the lungs.

Because of these pressure differences from one side of the heart to the other, the vessel wall constructions of the arteries and the veins differ. Strong construction of the arterial wall allows tolerance of significant pressure elevations from the left heart. The arterial wall is made up of three major tissue layers, known as tunics. Secondary layers of tissue that provide strength and elasticity to the artery are known as elastic and connective tissues. As with the artery, the wall of the vein is made up of three distinct tissue layers. Compared to that of an artery, the wall of a vein is thinner and less elastic, which allows the wall to be easily compressed by surrounding muscle during contraction.

While the heart is at rest, between contractions, newly oxygenated arterial blood passes from the lungs and enters the left heart. Each time the heart contracts, blood is forced from the left heart into a major artery known as the aorta. From the aorta, blood is distributed throughout the body. Once depleted of nutrients and oxygen, arterial blood passes through an extensive array of minute vessels known as capillaries. A significant pressure drop occurs as blood is dispersed throughout the immense network of capillaries. The capillaries empty into the venous system, which carries the blood back to the heart.

The primary responsibility of the venous system is to return deoxygenated blood to the lungs and heart. Much more energy is required from the body to move venous flow compared to arterial flow. Unlike the artery, the vein does not depend on the heart or gravity for energy to move blood. The venous system has a unique means of blood transportation known as the "venous pump," which moves blood toward the heart.

The components making up the venous pump include muscle contraction against the venous wall, intra-abdominal pressure changes, and one-way venous valves. Compression against the walls of a vein induces movement of blood. Muscle contraction against a vein wall occurs throughout the body during periods of activity. Activity includes every movement, from breathing to running. Variations in respiration cause fluctuations in the pressure within the abdomen, which produces a siphonlike effect on the veins, pulling venous blood upward. Valves are located within the veins of the extremities and pelvis. A venous valve has two leaflets, which protrude inward from opposite sides of the vein wall and meet one another in the center. Valves are necessary to prevent blood from flowing backward, away from the heart.

The venous system is divided into two groups known as the deep and superficial veins. The deep veins are located parallel to the arteries, while the superficial veins are located just beneath the skin surface and are often visible through the skin.

The Circulatory System

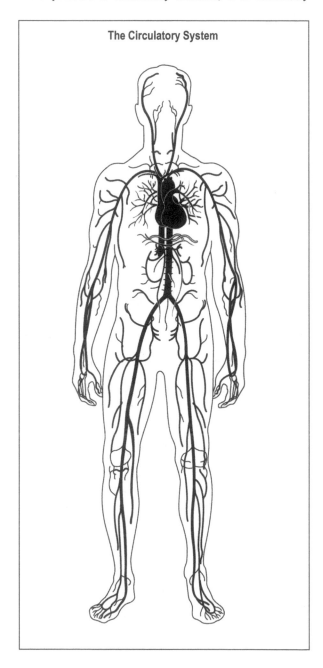

Disorders and Diseases

Numerous variables may affect the flow of blood. The autonomic nervous system is connected to muscle within the wall of the artery by way of neurological pathways known as sympathetic branches. Various drugs and/or conditions can trigger responses in the sympathetic branches and produce constriction of the smooth muscle in the arterial wall (vasoconstriction) or relaxation of the arterial wall (vasodilation). Alcohol consumption and a hot bath are examples of conditions that produce vasodilation. Exposure to cold and cigarette smoking are examples of conditions that produce vasoconstriction. Various drugs used in the medical environment are capable of producing similar effects. The diameter of the lumen of an artery influences the pressure and the flow of blood through it.

Another condition that alters the arterial diameter is atherosclerosis, a disease primarily of the large arteries, which allows the formation of fat (lipid) deposits to build on the inner layer of the artery. Lipid deposits are more commonly known as atherosclerotic plaque. Plaque accumulation reduces the diameter of the arterial lumen, causing various degrees of flow restriction. Plaque is similar to rust accumulation within a pipe that restricts the flow of water. A restriction of flow is referred to as a stenosis. The majority of stenotic lesions occur at the places where arteries divide into branches, also known as bifurcations. In advanced stages of plaque development, plaque may become calcified. Calcified plaque is hard and may become irregular, ulcerate, or hemorrhage, providing an environment for new clot formation and/or release of small pieces of plaque debris downstream. When pieces of plaque break off, they may move downstream into smaller blood vessels, causing a blockage and restricting the flow of oxygenated blood; this can cause tissue death, stroke, and heart attack.

An arterial wall may become very hard and rigid, a condition commonly known as hardening of the arteries. Hardened arteries may eventually become twisted, kinked, or dilated as a result of the hardening process of the arterial wall. A hardened artery which has become dilated is known as an aneurysm.

Normal arterial flow is undisturbed. When blood cells travel freely, they move together at a similar speed with very little variance. This is known as laminar flow. Nonlaminar (turbulent) flow is seen when irregular plaque or kinks in the arterial wall disrupt the smooth flow of cells. Plaque with an irregular surface may produce mild turbulence, while a narrow stenosis produces significant turbulence immediately downstream from the stenosis.

Many moderate or severe stenoses can be heard with the use of a standard stethoscope over the vessel of interest. A high-pitched sound can be heard consequent to the increased velocity of the blood cells moving through a narrow space. (A similar effect is produced when a standard garden hose is kinked to create a spray and a hissing sound is heard.) Medically, this sound is often referred to as a bruit. *Bruit* (pronounced "broo-ee") is a French word meaning noise.

Patients with significant lower extremity arterial disease will consistently experience calf pain and occasionally experience thigh discomfort with exercise. The discomfort is relieved when the patient stands still for a few moments. This is known as vascular claudication and occurs from a pressure drop as a consequence of a severely stenotic (reduced in diameter by greater than 75 percent) or occluded artery. If the muscle cannot get enough oxygen as a result of reduced blood flow, it will cramp, forcing the patient to stop and rest until blood supply has caught up to muscle demand. Alternate pathways around an obstruction prevent pain at rest, when muscle demand is low. Alternate pathways are also referred to as collateral pathways. Small, otherwise insignificant branches from a main artery become important vessels when the body uses them as collateral pathways around an obstruction. Time and exercise help to collateralize arterial branches into larger, more prominent arterial pathways. If collateral pathways do not provide enough flow to prevent the patient from experiencing painful muscle cramps while performing a daily exercise routine or to heal a wound on the foot, it may be necessary to perform either a surgical bypass around the obstruction or another interventional procedure such as angioplasty, atherectomy, or laser surgery.

Claudication may also occur in the heart. The main coronary arteries lie on the surface of the heart and distribute blood to the heart muscle. Patients suffering from coronary artery disease (CAD) may experience tightness, heaviness, or pain in the chest subsequent to flow restriction to the heart muscle as a result of atherosclerotic plaque within the coronary arteries. These symptoms are known as angina pectoris, or simply angina, usually occurring with exercise and relieved by rest. Intensity of the symptoms is relative to the extent of disease. A myocardial infarction (heart attack) is the result of a coronary artery occlusion.

Unlike the arteries, the venous system is not affected by atherosclerosis. The primary diseases of the veins include blood clot formation and varicose veins. A varicose vein is an enlarged and meandering vein with poorly functioning valves. A varicosity typically involves the veins near the skin surface, the superficial veins, and is often visualized as an irregular and/or raised segment through the skin surface. Varicosities are most common in the lower legs.

Valve leaflets are common sites for development of a thrombus. Thrombosis is the formation of a clot within a vein, which occurs when blood flow is delayed or obstructed for many hours. Several conditions that may induce venous clotting include prolonged bed rest (postoperative patients), prolonged sitting (long airplane or automobile rides), and the use of oral contraceptives. Cancer patients are at high risk of clot formation secondary to a metabolic disorder that affects the natural blood-thinning process.

Because numerous tributaries are connected to the superficial system, it is easy for the body to compensate for a clot in this system by rerouting blood through other branches. The deep venous system, however, has fewer branches, which promotes the progression of a thrombus toward the heart. A thrombus in the deep venous system is more serious because the risk of pulmonary emboli, commonly known as blood clots in the lungs, is much higher than superficial vein thrombosis. The further a thrombus propagates, the higher the risk to the patient.

Lower extremity venous return must take an alternate route via the superficial venous system when the deep system is obstructed by a thrombus. This is known as compensatory flow around an obstruction.

Perspective and Prospects

Historically, the vasculature of the human body was evaluated by placing one's fingers on the skin, palpating for the presence or absence of a pulse, and making note of the patient's symptoms. Prior to the 1960s, treatment of the circulatory system was very limited or nonexistent, resulting in a high death rate and large numbers of amputations, strokes, and heart attacks. The development of arteriography (the angiogram), a procedure in which dye is injected into the vessels while x-rays are obtained, revealed more about the vasculature and the nature of disease involving it. In conjunction with arteriography came corrective bypass surgery.

This period of development was followed by vast improvements in diagnostics, treatment, and knowledge of preventive maintenance. Today, synthetic bypass grafts are commonplace and are used to reroute flow around an obstruction. In many cases, procedures such as atherectomy and angioplasty, in which plaque or a thrombus is removed through a catheter inserted into the vessel, are often performed as outpatient procedures. In cases where an artery been seriously narrowed or weakened, a stent, a small mesh tube, may be inserted into the blood vessel to keep it open and unobstructed following the angioplasty procedure.

Diagnostic imaging of the cardiovascular system and the study of hemodynamics with the use of ultrasound have been useful for patient screening, the monitoring of disease progression, and the postoperative evaluation of surgical/interventional procedures. Ultrasound is a particularly valuable diagnostic tool because, compared to x-rays or arteriography, it is less expensive; it is also quick, painless, and noninvasive (no radiation, needle, or dye is required).

In addition to technological advances, new medications have been made available to reduce the risk of graft rejection, hypertension, and clotting, and to lower blood cholesterol. Preventive measures such as a healthy diet, weight maintenance, and regular exercise, however, constitute the most effective approach to good cardiovascular health. Much new information has been made available to improve the knowledge of the general public regarding diet, exercise, and the avoidance of unhealthy habits such as cigarette smoking as the way to create and maintain a healthier cardiovascular system.

—*Bonnie L. Wolff*

See also Aneurysmectomy; Aneurysms; Angina; Angiography; Angioplasty; Arteriosclerosis; Biofeedback; Bleeding; Blood and blood disorders; Blood testing; Blood vessels; Bypass surgery; Cardiopulmonary resuscitation (CPR); Catheterization; Chest; Cholesterol; Claudication; Coronary artery bypass graft; Cyanosis; Diabetes mellitus; Dialysis; Disseminated intravascular coagulation (DIC); Echocardiography; Edema; Embolism; Endarterectomy; Exercise physiology; Heart; Heart disease; Heat exhaustion and heatstroke; Hematology; Hematology, pediatric; Hemorrhoid banding and removal; Hemorrhoids; Hormones; Hypercholesterolemia; Hypertension; Ischemia; Kidneys; Lymphatic system; Phlebitis; Phlebotomy; Preeclampsia and eclampsia; Pulmonary hypertension; Shock; Shunts; Stents; Strokes; Systems and organs; Thrombolytic therapy and TPA; Thrombosis and thrombus; Transfusion; Transient ischemic attacks (TIAs); Varicose vein removal; Varicose veins; Vascular medicine; Vascular system; Vasculitis; Venous insufficiency.

For Further Information:

Ford, Earl S. "Combined Television Viewing and Computer Use and Mortality from All-Causes and Diseases of the Circulatory System among Adults in the United States." *BMC Public Health* 12.1 (2012): 70-79.

Guyton, Arthur C., and John E. Hall. *Human Physiology and Mechanisms of Disease.* 6th ed. Philadelphia: W. B. Saunders, 1997.

Marder, Victor J., et al., eds. *Disorders of Thrombosis and Hemostasis: Basic Principles and Clinical Practice.* 6th ed. Philadelphia: Lippincott Williams & Wilkins, 2012.

Marieb, Elaine N., and Katja Hoehn. *Human Anatomy and Physiology.* 9th ed. San Francisco: Pearson/Benjamin Cummings, 2012.

Saltin, Bengt, et al., eds. *Exercise and Circulation in Health and Disease.* Champaign, Ill.: Human Kinetics, 2000.

Strandness, D. Eugene, Jr. *Duplex Scanning in Vascular Disorders.* 4th ed. London: Lippincott Williams & Wilkins, 2009.

CIRCUMCISION, FEMALE, AND GENITAL MUTILATION

Procedure

Anatomy or system affected: Genitals, reproductive system

Specialties and related fields: General surgery, gynecology, plastic surgery, psychiatry

Definition: The partial or complete surgical removal of the clitoris, labia minora, or labia majora (or all) for cultural reasons. Often performed without anesthesia or sterilized instruments, and often performed on young females without assent or understanding.

Key terms:

clitoridectomy: the removal of the entire clitoris, the prepuce, and adjacent labia

deinfibulation: an anterior episiotomy

episiotomy: the incision of the labia

infibulation: a clitoridectomy followed by the sewing up of the vulva

pharaonic circumcision: another term for infibulation

prepuce: the covering of the clitoris

sunna circumcision: the removal of the tip of the clitoris and/or the prepuce

Indications and Procedures

The various forms of female circumcision and female genital mutilation, although not universal to all cultures, have been practiced in numerous societies of the world for nearly two thousand years. Recorded evidence cites that female circumcision predates the advent of both Christianity and Islam and that early Christians, Muslims, and the Jewish group Falashas practiced circumcision on young girls. Historically, during the nineteenth century and until the 1940s, clitoridectomies were performed in Europe and America as a procedure to "cure" female masturbation, nervousness, and other specific types of perceived psychological dysfunction.

The 1989-1990 Demographic Health Survey of Circumcision stated that circumcision is still performed annually on an estimated 80 to 114 million women; 85 percent of these procedures involve clitoridectomy, while approximately 15 percent involve infibulation. Infibulation, or pharaonic circumcision, is the removal of the clitoris, the labia minora, and much of the labia majora, on occasion, the remaining sides of the vulva are stitched together to close up the vagina, except for a small opening maintained for the passage of blood and urine.

Certain contemporary cultures of Africa, the Middle East, and parts of Yemen, India, and Malaysia continue these practices. Contemporary Middle Eastern countries practicing female circumcision and genital mutilation are Jordan, Iraq, Yemen, Syria, and southern Algeria. In Africa, it is practiced in the majority of the countries, including Egypt, the Ivory Coast, Kenya, Mali, Mozambique, Sudan, and Upper Volta. It has been estimated that 99 percent of northern Sudanese women aged fifteen to forty-nine are circumcised. In and around Alexandria, Egypt, 99 percent of rural and lower-income urban women are circumcised. The World Health Organization estimates that as of 2013, approximately 140 million women worldwide have been circumsized during their childhood, with 101 million of these women in Africa.

Cross-culturally, there are essentially four types of female genital circumcision and female genital mutilation. Circumcision, or sunna circumcision, is removal of the prepuce or hood of the clitoris, with the body of the clitoris remaining intact. Sunna means "tradition" in Arabic. Excision circumcision, or clitoridectomy, is the removal of the entire clitoris (both prepuce and glans) and all or part of the adjacent labia majora and the labia minora. Intermediate circumcision is the removal of the clitoris, all or part of the labia minora, and sometimes part of the labia majora.

All types of female genital mutilation frequently may create severe, long-term effects, such as pelvic infections that usually lead to infertility, chronic recurrent urinary tract infections, painful intercourse, obstetrical complications, and in some cases, surgically induced scars that can cause tearing of the tissue and even hemorrhaging during childbirth. In fact, it is not unusual for women who have been infibulated to require surgical enlargement of the vagina on their wedding night or when delivering children. Unfortunately, babies born to infibulated women may frequently suffer brain damage because of oxygen deprivation (hypoxia) caused by a prolonged and obstructed delivery. Babies may die during the painful birthing process because of a damaged birth canal. Other physical and psychological difficulties for the circumcised woman may be sexual dysfunction, delayed menarche, and genital malformation.

From a cultural perspective, there are numerous reasons or justifications given for these procedures. They are often described as rites of passage and proof of adulthood, and it is of-

ten argued that the procedures raise a woman's status in her community, because of both the added purity that circumcision brings and the bravery that initiates are called upon to demonstrate. The procedure also is believed to confer maturity and inculcate positive character traits, such as the ability to endure pain and to be submissive. In some cultures, the circumcision ritual is considered to be positive because the girl is the center of attention. She receives presents and moral instruction from her elders, creating a bond between the generations, as all women in the society must undergo the procedure; they thus share an important experience.

Furthermore, it is thought that a girl who has been circumcised will not be troubled by lustful thoughts or sensations or by physical temptations such as masturbation. Therefore, there is less risk of premarital relationships that can end in the stigma and social difficulties of illegitimate birth. The bond between husband and wife may be closer because one or both of them will never have had sex with anyone else. The relationship may be motivated by love rather than lust because there will be no physical drive for the wife, only an emotional one. There is little incentive for extramarital sex for the wife; hence, the marriage may be more secure. Children may be better cared for because the husband can be more confident that he is their father. Generally, a girl who is not circumcised is considered unclean by local villagers and therefore unmarriageable. In some societies, a girl who is not circumcised is believed to be dangerous, even deadly, if her clitoris touches a man's penis.

All of these arguments for female genital mutilation and female circumcision must be weighed against the pain and terror, the lack of consent, and the subjugation of girls and women that is inherent in the practice. The practice must also be weighed against the medical risks.

Female genital circumcision and female genital mutilation surgeries are invariably conducted in unsanitary conditions in which a midwife or close female relative uses unsterile sharp instruments, such as pieces of glass, razor blades, kitchen knives, or scissors. The induction of tetanus, septicemia, hemorrhaging, and even shock are not uncommon. Human immunodeficiency virus (HIV) can be transmitted. No anesthesia is used. These procedures usually are experienced by the girl at approximately three years of age, although the actual age depends upon the customs of the particular society or village. To minimize the risk of the transmission of viruses, countries such as Egypt have made it illegal for female genital mutilation to be practiced by anyone other than trained doctors and nurses in hospitals.

Treatment and Therapy

There is no information regarding the surgical restoration of severed or damaged genitals. Because of severe cultural sanctions by the participating groups, which continue to hold tenaciously to such practices, female genital circumcision is seldom discussed with outsiders. Those who follow these customs do not report their occurrence. Consequently, there are few data concerning the frequency of female genital circumcision and female genital mutilation within the United

States, despite the knowledge that some immigrant groups from Africa, the Middle East, and Asia continue to practice these surgeries. Health care workers estimate that, within the United States, approximately ten thousand girls undergo these surgical procedures each year. Usually, the procedure is conducted in the home. Those who can pay physicians to perform the surgery may do so; in these cases, local anesthesia is used and the risk of infection is less.

Perspective and Prospects

Because of the high number of female genital mutilations and the deaths that this procedure has caused, it is now prohibited in some communities in the United States, Great Britain, France, Sweden, and Switzerland, and in some countries of Africa, such as Egypt, Kenya, and Senegal. The National Organization of Circumcision Information Resource Centers (NOCIRC) is opposed to the procedures, as well as to male circumcision. The United Nations Children's Fund (UNICEF) and the World Health Organization (WHO) consider female genital mutilation to be a violation of human rights and recommend its eradication. In the United States, former representative Patricia Schroeder had introduced a bill that would outlaw female genital mutilation. The bill, called the Federal Prohibition of Female Genital Mutilation Act of 1995, was passed in 1996. The Canadian Criminal Code was enacted to protect children who are ordinarily residents in Canada from being removed from the country and subjected to female genital mutilation.

Both female genital circumcision and female genital mutilation perpetuate customs that seek to control female bodies and sexuality. It is hoped that with increasing legislation and attitude changes regarding bioethical issues, fewer girls and young women will undergo these mutilating surgical procedures. One problem in this campaign is the conflict between cultural self-determination and basic human rights. Feminists, physicians, and ethicists must work respectfully with, and not independently of, local resources for cultural self-examination and change.

—John Alan Ross, Ph.D.

See also Bleeding; Childbirth; Childbirth complications; Circumcision, male; Episiotomy; Ethics; Genital disorders, female; Gynecology; Infertility, female; Menstruation; Psychiatry; Reproductive system; Septicemia; Sexual dysfunction; Sexuality; Stillbirth; Women's health.

For Further Information:

Bacquet-Walsh, Caroline. "Female Genital Cutting Fact Sheet." *WomensHealth.gov*, Dec. 15, 2009.
Benedek, Wolfgang, et al., eds. *The Human Rights of Women: International Instruments and African Experiences*. London: Zed, 2002.
"Female Gential Mutilation/Cutting." *UNICEF*, May 15, 2013.
"Female Genital Mutilation." *World Health Organization*, Feb. 2013.
"Female Genital and Sexual Mutilation." *WIN News* 26, no. 2 (Spring, 2000): 51-59.
Galanti, Geri-Ann. *Caring for Patients from Different Cultures*. 4th ed. Philadelphia: University of Pennsylvania Press, 2008.
Gruenbaum, Ellen. *The Female Circumcision Controversy: An Anthropological Perspective*. Philadelphia: University of Pennsylvania Press, 2001.
James, Stanlie M., and Claire C. Robertson, eds. *Genital Cutting and Transnational Sisterhood: Disputing U.S. Polemics*. Urbana: University of Illinois Press, 2002.
Larsen, Ulla, and Sharon Yan. "Does Female Circumcision Affect Infertility and Fertility? A Study of the Central African Republic, Cote d'Ivoire, and Tanzania." *Demography* 37, no. 3 (August, 2000): 313-321.
Sarkis, Marianne. "Female Genital Cutting (FGC): An Introduction." *Female Genital Cutting Education and Networking Project*, 2003.
"Sexual Problems in Women." *MedlinePlus*, June 10, 2013.
Walker, Alice, and Pratibha Parmar. *Warrior Marks: Female Genital Mutilation and the Sexual Blinding of Women*. New York: Harcourt Brace, 1993.
Williams, Deanna Perez, William Acosta, and Herbert A. McPherson, Jr. "Female Genital Mutilation in the United States: Implications for Women's Health." *American Journal of Health Studies* 15, no. 1 (1999): 47-52.

CIRCUMCISION, MALE
Procedure

Anatomy or system affected: Genitals, reproductive system
Specialties and related fields: General surgery, pediatrics, urology
Definition: The removal of the foreskin (prepuce) covering the head of the penis.
Key terms:

chordee: the downward curvature of the penis, most apparent on erection, caused by the shortness of the skin on the downward side of the penile shaft

glans or *glans penis:* the head of the penis

necrosis: the death of one or more cells or a portion of a tissue or organ resulting from irreversible damage

phimosis: the narrowing of the opening of the skin covering the head of the penis sufficient to prevent retraction of the skin back over the glans

sepsis: an infection in the circulating blood

smegma: a pasty accumulation of shed skin cells and secretions of the sweat glands which collects in the moist areas of the foreskin-covered base of the glans

urinary tract infections: infections of the bladder, the kidneys, the urethra (which connects the bladder to the opening at the end of the penis), and the ureters (which connect the bladder to the kidneys); infection may be limited to one area of these organs or spread throughout the urinary tract

Indications and Procedures

Routine circumcision of the newborn male-in which the foreskin of the penis is stretched, clamped, and cut-is becoming an increasingly controversial procedure. Famed pediatrician Benjamin Spock once contended that circumcision is a good idea, especially if most of the boys in the neighborhood are circumcised; then a boy feels "regular." Yet, many wonder if that is justification for circumcision. Allowing routine circumcision of newborns as a religious and cultural rite still leaves the debate over medical necessity. The United States is the only country in the world that circumcises a majority of newborn males without a religious reason. In fact, circumcision has been termed a "cultural surgery."

True medical indications for the surgery are seldom present at birth. Such conditions as infections of the head and/or shaft of the penis may be indications for circumcision; an inability to retract the foreskin in the newborn (phimosis) is not an indication. Some argue that circumcision should be delayed until the foreskin has become retractable, making an imprecise surgical procedure presumably less traumatic. In 96 percent of infant boys, however, the foreskin is not fully retractable; it is normally so tight and adherent that it cannot be pulled back and the penis cleaned. By age three, that percentage decreases to 10 percent.

There are other definite contraindications to newborn circumcision. Circumcising infants with abnormalities of the penal head or shaft makes treatment more difficult because the foreskin may later be needed for use in reconstruction. Prematurity, instability, or a bleeding problem also preclude early circumcision. The foreskin is a natural protective membrane, representing 50 to 80 percent of the skin system of the penis, having 240 feet of nerve fibers, more than one thousand nerve endings, and three feet of veins, arteries, and capillaries. It keeps the sensitive head protected, facilitating intercourse, and prevents the surface of the glans from thickening and becoming desensitized. Also, within the inner surface of the foreskin are a series of tiny ridged bands that contribute significantly to stimulating the glans.

The two most persistent arguments for the operation, however, are the risks of infection and cancer in the uncircumcised. Without circumcision, smegma accumulates beneath the base of the covered head of the penis. This cheeselike material of dead skin cells and secretions of the sweat glands is thought to be a cause of cancer of the penis and prostate gland in uncircumcised men and cancer of the cervix in their female partners. Doctors who argue against circumcision, however, say that the presence of smegma in the uncircumcised is simply a sign of poor hygiene and that poor sexual hygiene, inadequate hygienic facilities, and sexually transmitted diseases cause an increased incidence of cancer in ethnic groups or populations that do not practice circumcision. Doctors who argue against circumcision also point out that complete circumcision is found as often in male partners of women without cancer of the cervix as in male partners of women who have cervical cancer. In Sweden, moreover-where newborn circumcision is not routinely practiced but where good hygiene is practiced-the rates of these cancers are essentially the same as those found in Israel, where ritualistic circumcision is practiced.

The increased incidence of urinary tract infections and sexually transmitted diseases (STDs) in uncircumcised males sufficiently argues for circumcision, say its proponents. They warn that the intact foreskin invites bacterial colonization, which leads to urethral infection ascending to the bladder that ultimately may spread upward to the kidneys and sometimes cause permanent kidney damage. On the other hand, no proof exists that uncircumcised male infants who sustain urinary tract infections will have future urologic problems. Further-

more, the operation is not a simple procedure and is not without peril. Penile amputation, life-threatening infections, and even death have been well documented.

Slightly increased rates of infection with sexually transmitted diseases in the uncircumcised argue the case for some proponents, but it is acquired immunodeficiency syndrome (AIDS) that they most fear. In Africa, where male circumcision is seldom practiced, the acquisition of AIDS by heterosexual men from infected women during vaginal intercourse is the most common mode of transmission.

Proponents say that infection with human immunodeficiency virus (HIV), the virus that leads to AIDS, depends on a break or an abrasion of the skin to gain entry. The intact foreskin provides a site for the transfer of infected cervical secretions. In Africa, doctors at the University of Nairobi noted a relationship of HIV infection to genital ulcers and lack of circumcision. Uncircumcised men had a history of genital ulcers more often than did the circumcised, and they were more often HIV-positive. They were also more frequently HIV-positive even if they did not have a history of genital ulcer disease.

Every evaluation of circumcision, pro or con, should reflect the confounding genetic and environmental variables, as well as the actual increased risks and benefits. All the pros and cons should be explained to parents before informed consent is obtained.

Uses and Complications

In 1989, the American Academy of Pediatrics" Task Force on Circumcision concluded that "newborn circumcision has potential medical benefits and advantages as well as disadvantages and risks. When circumcision is being considered, the benefits and risks should be explained to the parents and informed consent obtained." This neutral statement does not lessen the anxiety of parents who are trying to weigh the pros and cons of routine newborn circumcision, but examination of the evidence does allow parents to weigh the individual benefits and risks and see if the scale tips in either direction.

Worldwide studies of predominantly uncircumcised populations have shown a higher incidence of urinary tract infection in boys during the first few months of life, which is the reverse of what is found in older infants and children, where girls predominate. In 1986, Brooke Army Medical Center in Fort Sam Houston, Texas, took a closer look. The doctors found the incidence of urinary tract infection in circumcised infant males to be 0.11 percent but 1.12 percent in the uncircumcised. Even without proof that the uncircumcised male infants who get urinary tract infections will have future urologic problems, the proponents for the surgical procedure claim about a 1 percent advantage.

The evidence for an increase in sexually transmitted diseases (such as genital herpes, gonorrhea, and syphilis) among the uncircumcised is conflicting. Furthermore, apparent correlations between circumcision status and these diseases do not reflect confounding genetic and environmental variables. It is also difficult to factor in the risk from HIV infections.

The studies from Africa do not look at any variables in the transmission of HIV except circumcision status and previous history of genital ulcers. The nutritional and economic status of the men was not examined, even though it is known that malnourishment suppresses the immune systems. Moreover, if everyone practiced safer sex, the argument for circumcision would be moot.

Almost all the surgical complications of circumcision can be avoided if doctors performing the procedure adhere to strict asepsis, are properly trained and experienced in the procedure, remove the appropriate and correct amount of tissue, and provide adequate hemostasis. The variety of circumstances, populations, and physicians affects the incidence of complications. In the larger, teaching hospitals, often the newest physicians with the least experience or supervision perform the operation. As a result, complications may arise. Excessive bleeding is the most frequent complication. The incidence of bleeding after circumcision ranges from 0.1 percent to as high as 35 percent in some reports. Most of the episodes are minor and can be controlled by simple measures, such as compression and suturing, but some of these efforts can lead to diminished blood supply to the head and shaft of the penis with necrosis of the affected part. Chordee can result if improper technique or bad luck intervenes, and such penile deformity begets the risk of emotional distress. The urethral opening on the end of the penis can become infected or ulcerated when the glans is no longer protected by foreskin; such infection rarely occurs in the uncircumcised. Finally, any surgical procedure runs the risk of infection. These localized infections rarely spread to the blood, but death from sepsis and its sequelae has been documented.

Overall, the surgical complication rate after circumcision runs around 0.19 percent, which could be lowered with strict protocols, meticulous technique, strict asepsis, and well-trained, experienced physicians. Strict protocols, it is hoped, would ensure that absolute contraindications to the procedure-such as anomalies of the penis, prematurity, instability, or a bleeding disorder-were honored.

Another human factor must be considered. Many insurance companies do not provide payment for newborn care, since it is considered preventive medicine. In 1997, a physician's fee for performing a circumcision ranged to approximately $400, with a nationwide average of $137. Interestingly, a growing number of circumcised men are undergoing expensive foreskin restoration procedures.

In part because of an additional cost that arises with anesthesia, the vast majority of infant circumcisions are performed without pain control. The surgery is painful, yet some physicians claim that the minute that the operation ends, the circumcised baby no longer cries and frequently falls asleep. Continuing pain, therefore, is probably not present.

Another perspective to examine is the experience of adult males, who are circumcised by their own choice. Many complain of at least a week's discomfort after the operation. The most compelling argument against adult circumcision, however, comes from their answer to "Would you do it again?" In one study of several hundred men who were circumcised as adults, they were asked five years later if they would do it again. All said no.

Perspective and Prospects

Routine newborn circumcision originated in the United States in the 1860s, ostensibly as prophylaxis against disease. Some medical historians, however, believe that nonreligious circumcision was a deliberate surgical procedure to desensitize and debilitate the penis to prevent masturbation. During this era, and for nearly one hundred years afterward, most American physicians viewed masturbation as an inevitable cause of blindness, weak character, insanity, nervousness, tuberculosis, sexually transmitted disease, and even death. One physician maintained that a painful circumcision would have a salutary effect upon the newborn's mind, so that pain would be associated with masturbation. As late as 1928, the *American Medical Journal* published an editorial that justified male circumcision as an effective means of preventing the dire effects of masturbation. During World Wars I and II, soldiers were forcibly circumcised under threat of court martial, being told that the surgery was for reasons of hygiene and the prevention of epilepsy and other diseases.

Eventually, a general change in attitude occurred, notably in Great Britain and New Zealand, which virtually have abandoned routine circumcision. Rates of circumcision have also fallen dramatically in Canada, Australia, and even the United States. As recently as the mid-1970s, approximately 90 percent of US male babies were circumcised. Not until 1971 did the American Academy of Pediatrics determine that circumcision is not medically essential. In 1999, an estimated 65 percent of US male babies were circumcised; by 2010, the incidence of newborn circumcision had declined to 55 percent.

In 1971, the American Academy of Pediatrics" Committee on the Fetus and Newborn issued an advisory that said, "There are no valid medical indications for routine circumcision in the neonatal period." In 1978, when the American College of Obstetricians and Gynecologists affirmed this statement, the circumcision rate had already declined to an estimated 70 percent of newborn males, compared to previous rates of between 80 and 90 percent.

Undoubtedly, the future will bring improved surgical techniques. More emphasis will be placed on avoiding surgical complications by more rigid monitoring of the operation and who performs the procedure. It is unlikely that circumcision will disappear completely.

Organizations such as Doctors Opposing Circumcision and the National Organization to Halt the Abuse and Routine Mutilation of Males, however, are actively proposing an end to routine neonatal circumcision. Some nursing groups and concerned mothers have formed local groups to oppose circumcision in male neonates. They argue that subjecting a baby to this procedure may impair mother-infant bonding. Another question posed by some physicians and parents is the ethics involved in the unnecessary removal of a functioning body organ, particularly without the patient's consent. Others claim that the baby's rights are being violated, noting that it is the child who must live with the outcome of the decision to perform a circumcision. As a result of these efforts, the rates of circumcision will probably continue to fall.

—*Wayne R. McKinny, M.D.;*
updated by John Alan Ross, Ph.D.

See also Circumcision, female, and genital mutilation; Ethics; Genital disorders, male; Men's health; Neonatology; Pediatrics; Reproductive system; Urology, pediatric.

For Further Information:

Apuzzio, Joseph J., Anthony M. Vintzileos, and Leslie Iffy, eds. *Operative Obstetrics.* 3d ed. New York: Taylor & Francis, 2006.

Behrman, Richard E., Robert M. Kliegman, and Hal B. Jenson, eds. *Nelson Textbook of Pediatrics.* 19th ed. Philadelphia: Saunders/Elsevier, 2011.

Bigelow, Jim. *The Joy of Uncircumcising! Exploring Circumcision-History, Myths, Psychology, Restoration, Sexual Pleasure, and Human Rights.* Rev. ed. Aptos, Calif.: Hourglass, 1998.

"Circumcision." *HealthyChildren.org.* American Academy of Pediatrics, May 11, 2013.

"Circumcision." *MedlinePlus*, May 13, 2013.

Gollaher, David L. *Circumcision: A History of the World's Most Controversial Surgery.* New York: Basic Books, 2000.

Kerr, Sarah J., and Michael Woods. "Child Circumcision." *Health Library*, May 13, 2013.

King, Lowell R., ed. *Urologic Surgery in Neonates and Young Infants.* Philadelphia: W. B. Saunders, 1998.

"Male Circumcision." *Centers for Disease Control and Prevention*, Apr. 15, 2013.

Snyder, Howard M. "To Circumcise or Not." *Hospital Practice* 26 (January 15, 1991): 201-207.

Woods, Michael. "Newborn Circumcision." *Health Library*, Sept. 27, 2012.

CIRRHOSIS

Disease/Disorder

Anatomy or system affected: Liver

Specialties and related fields: Family medicine, internal medicine, psychology

Definition: The formation of scar tissue in the liver, which interferes with its normal function.

Causes and Symptoms

The liver is a large, spongy organ that lies in the upper-right abdomen. Regarded as primarily part of the digestive system because it manufactures bile, the liver has many other functions, including the synthesis of blood-clotting factors and the detoxification of such harmful substances as alcohol.

Cirrhosis describes the fibrous scar tissue (or nodules) that replaces the normally soft liver after repeated long-term injury by toxins such as alcohol or viruses. The liver may form small nodules (micronodular cirrhosis), large nodules (macronodular cirrhosis), or a combination of the two types (mixed nodular cirrhosis). Cirrhosis is a frequent cause of death among middle-aged men, and increasingly among women. While alcoholism is the most common cause, chronic hepatitis and other rarer diseases can also produce the

---

Information on Cirrhosis

Causes: Buildup of scar tissue in liver from toxins (alcohol, viruses)

Symptoms: May include jaundice, fatigue, weakness, appetite loss, easy bruising

Duration: Chronic

Treatments: None

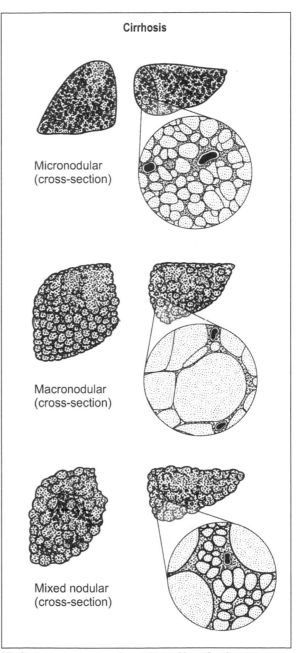

Cirrhosis

Micronodular (cross-section)

Macronodular (cross-section)

Mixed nodular (cross-section)

Cirrhosis appears in three forms, detectable under the microscope, each depending primarily on the cause of the liver damage. All are characterized by the replacement of normally soft, spongy tissue with hard, fibrous scarring. Alcohol-related cirrhosis usually produces the micronodular form.

irreversible liver damage that characterizes cirrhosis. The resulting organ is shrunken and hard, unable to perform its varied duties. Because of its altered structure, the cirrhotic liver causes serious problems for surrounding organs, as blood flow becomes difficult. The barrier to normal circulation leads to two serious complications: portal hypertension (the buildup of pressure in the internal veins) and ascites (fluid leakage from blood vessels into the abdominal cavity).

Treatment and Therapy

Diagnosis is usually made from a history of alcoholism. A physical examination may reveal jaundice; a large nodular liver or a small shrunken one, depending upon the stage; or a fluid-filled abdomen (ascites). Laboratory studies may show elevated liver enzymes released from damaged cells and low levels of products that the liver normally produces (protein, clotting factors). A definitive diagnosis can be made only by biopsy, although radiographic methods such as computed tomography (CT) scanning and magnetic resonance imaging (MRI) can be quite conclusive.

The mortality rate is very high, as the damage is irreversible. Deaths from internal vein rupture and hemorrhage (the results of portal hypertension) and from kidney failure are most common. Repeated hospitalizations attempt to control the variety of complications that arise with agents that stop bleeding, bypass tubes that relieve pressure, the removal of the ascitic fluid, and nutritional support for malnutrition. Eventually, kidney failure ensues or one of these control measures fails, and death rapidly follows. Liver transplantation is considered in some cases. Cases of mild cirrhosis, where sufficient normal tissue remains, have a clearly better course.

In 2013, a study led by Dr. W. Kim Ray, of the Mayo Clinic in Rochester, Minnesota, found a link between advanced fibrosis and higher death rates in patients with nonalcoholic fatty liver disease. The incidence of nonalcoholic fatty liver disease has risen over the last twenty-five years and it is now the most frequently occurring liver disease in the United States.

—Connie Rizzo, M.D., Ph.D.

See also Alcoholism; Endoscopic retrograde cholangiopancreatography (ERCP); Hepatitis; Jaundice; Liver; Liver cancer; Liver disorders; Liver transplantation; Nonalcoholic steatohepatitis (NASH).

For Further Information:
Dallas, Mary Elizabeth. "HealthDay: Scarring May Raise Death Risk from Fatty Liver Disease." *MedlinePlus*, Apr. 16, 2013.

Fishman, Mark, et al. *Medicine.* 5th ed. Philadelphia: Lippincott, 2004.

Goldman, Lee, and Dennis Ausiello, eds. *Cecil Textbook of Medicine.* 23d ed. Philadelphia: Saunders, 2007.

MedlinePlus. "Cirrhosis." *MedlinePlus*, Apr. 17, 2013.

Parker, James N., and Philip M. Parker, eds. *The Official Patient's Sourcebook on Primary Biliary Cirrhosis.* San Diego, Calif.: Icon Health, 2002.

Parker, James N. and Philip M. Parker. *The Official Patient's Sourcebook on Cirrhosis of the Liver: A Reference Manual for Self-Directed Patient Research.* San Diego, Calif.: Icon Health, 2004.

Wood, Debra. "Cirrhosis." *Health Library*, Oct. 11, 2012.

Zelman, Mark, et al. *Human Diseases: A Systemic Approach.* 7th ed. Upper Saddle River, N.J.: Pearson, 2010.

CLAUDICATION
Disease/Disorder
Anatomy or system affected: Blood vessels, circulatory system, legs
Specialties and related fields: Vascular medicine
Definition: Pain in the calf or thigh muscle brought on by walking and relieved by rest.

Causes and Symptoms

Claudication is pain that develops in the calf or thigh muscle during walking. The pain increases if the patient continues walking and is relieved within a few minutes after walking is terminated. The medical term for this condition is intermittent claudication. The pain is caused by a narrowing in the arteries that supply the leg with blood. This narrowing is commonly caused by atherosclerosis, in which fatty material builds up on the inside wall of the artery. At first, as the fatty material accumulates in the artery, it creates no symptoms. Only after more than 50 percent of the artery is narrowed do symptoms occur. The first symptom is mild cramping or heaviness that develops during a long walk. Over time, the narrowing increases and the distance that the individual is able to walk decreases. If not treated, the narrowing of the artery may increase further and the pain will be present all the time, signaling a more serious condition called rest pain that may lead to limb loss.

Information on Claudication

Causes: Narrowing in leg arteries from atherosclerosis; risk factors include smoking, high blood pressure, heart disease, high cholesterol, advanced age

Symptoms: Mild cramping or heaviness during long walks, progressing to leg pain at rest and sometimes amputation

Duration: Chronic, progressive without treatment

Treatments: Smoking cessation, lowering of cholesterol levels, program of long-distance walking, medications (pentoxifylline, cilostazol), surgery (angioplasty, bypass surgery, stents)

Factors that may lead to this condition include smoking, high blood pressure, heart disease, high cholesterol, and advanced age. Elderly people are more likely to develop intermittent claudication, but younger individuals with multiple risk factors for vascular disease may develop this problem at any age. Sometimes a thrombus may obstruct an artery, causing claudication symptoms to occur suddenly instead of slowly as with atherosclerosis.

The diagnosis of claudication is fairly simple. Clinically, true intermittent claudication can be differentiated from a similar but unrelated condition by noting if the symptoms happen every time that the patient walks a similar distance.

True claudication will develop every time, while pain from other conditions will occur at some times but not others.

To be more precise in diagnosing this condition, a Doppler study can be performed on an outpatient basis in a hospital or a doctor's office. The examination, called an ankle-brachial index (ABI), is simple and painless. Blood pressures are taken at the ankles and in the arms before and after exercise. If the pressure at the ankles drops with exercise and goes back to normal a few minutes later, then the diagnosis of intermittent claudication can be made. Ultrasound imaging or angiogram studies may be done to identify the exact location of the narrowing.

Treatment and Therapy

Treatment depends on the severity of the symptoms. Stopping smoking, lowering cholesterol levels, and beginning a program of long-distance walking may provide enough relief to allow some patients to return to near-normal routines. Medications such as pentoxifylline (Trental or Pentoxil) or cilostazol (Pletal) may provide limited relief from symptoms. More severe cases may require angioplasty, surgery to bypass the narrowed artery, or stenting of the diseased artery.

Perspective and Prospects

Claudication has become more common in the United States as the population ages and sedentary lifestyles become more popular. Although some treatments are effective, it is a difficult problem to manage. Education programs are available to help those at risk for this condition make necessary lifestyle changes that may lessen their chances of developing this ailment. Those changes may include getting plenty of exercise (brisk walking being the best), not smoking, lowering cholesterol, and keeping diabetes under control.

In March 2013, the US Preventive Services Task Force stated that, after reviewing available research, it did not find enough evidence to make a recommendation one way or the other about the use of ABI as a way to assess heart disease risk in patients who show no symptoms of peripheral artery disease. The task force called for more research into the matter.

—*Steven R. Talbot, R.V.T.*

See also Arteriosclerosis; Bypass surgery; Cholesterol; Circulation; Exercise physiology; Hypercholesterolemia; Lower extremities; Pain management; Plaque, arterial; Stents; Thrombosis and thrombus; Vascular medicine; Vascular system; Vasculitis.

For Further Information:

Hershey, Falls B., Robert W. Barnes, and David S. Sumner, eds. *Noninvasive Diagnosis of Vascular Disease.* Pasadena, Calif.: Appleton, 1984.
Mohler, Emile R., III. "Patient Information: Peripheral Artery Disease and Claudication (Beyond the Basics)." *UpToDate,* May 2, 2013.
Preidt, Robert. "HealthDay: Experts Question Use of Ankle Blood Pressure to Gauge Heart Risks." *MedlinePlus,* Mar. 18, 2013.
Rutherford, Robert B., ed. *Vascular Surgery.* 6th ed. Philadelphia: Saunders/Elsevier, 2005.
Zwiebel, William J., and John S. Pellerito, eds. *Introduction to Vascular Ultrasonography.* 5th ed. Philadelphia: Saunders/Elsevier, 2005.

CLEFT LIP AND PALATE
Disease/Disorder

Anatomy or system affected: Bones, musculoskeletal system

Specialties and related fields: Neonatology, otorhinolaryngology, pediatrics, plastic surgery, speech pathology

Definition: A fissure in the midline of the palate, resulting from the failure of the two sides to fuse during embryonic development; in some cases, the fissure may extend through both hard and soft palates into the nasal cavities.

Key terms:

alveolus: the bony ridge where teeth grow

ectrodactyly: a congenital anomaly characterized by the absence of part or all of one or more of the fingers or toes

hard palate: the bony portion of the roof of the mouth, contiguous with the soft palate

Logan's bow: a metal bar placed, for protection and tension removal, on the early postoperative cleft lip

obturator: a sheet of plastic shaped like a flattened dome which fits into the cleft and closes it well enough to permit nursing

soft palate: a structure of mucous membrane, muscle fibers, and mucous glands suspended from the posterior border of the hard palate

syndactyly: a congenital anomaly characterized by the fusion of the fingers or toes

uvula: the small, cone-shaped projection of tissue suspended in the mouth from the posterior of the soft palate

Causes and Symptoms

Cleft palate is a congenital defect characterized by a fissure along the midline of the palate. It occurs when the two sides fail to fuse during embryonic development. The gap may be complete, extending through the hard and soft palates into the nasal cavities, or may be partial or incomplete. It is often associated with cleft lip or "harelip." About one child in eight hundred live births is affected with some degree of clefting, and clefting is the most common of the craniofacial abnormalities.

Cleft palate is not generally a genetic disorder; rather, it is a result of defective cell migration. Embryonically, in the first month, the mouth and nose form one cavity destined to be separated by the hard and soft palates. In addition, there is no upper lip. Most of the upper jaw is lacking; only the part near the ears is present. In the next weeks, the upper lip and jaw are formed from structures growing in from the sides, fusing at

---

Information on Cleft Lip and Palate

Causes: Congenital defect

Symptoms: Craniofacial abnormalities, greater susceptibility to colds, poor muscle reactivity, dental problems

Duration: Correctable, usually between seven and twelve months of age

Treatments: Surgery

the midline with a third portion growing downward from the nasal region. The palates develop in much the same way. The fusion of all these structures begins with the lip and moves posteriorly toward, and then includes the soft palate. The two cavities are separated by the palates by the end of the third month of gestation.

If, as embryonic development occurs, the cells that should grow together to form the lips and palate fail to move in the correct direction, the job is left unfinished. Clefting of the palate generally occurs between the thirty-fifth and thirty-seventh days of gestation. Fortunately, it is an isolated defect not usually associated with other disabilities or with developmental delays.

If the interference in normal growth and fusion begins early and lasts throughout the fusion period, the cleft that results will affect one or both sides of the top lip and may continue back through the upper jaw, the upper gum ridge, and both palates. If the disturbance lasts only part of the time that development is occurring, only the lip may be cleft, and the palate may be unaffected. If the problem begins a little into the fusion process, the lip is normally formed, but the palate is cleft. The cleft may divide only the soft palate or both the soft and the hard palate. Even the uvula may be affected; it can be split, unusually short, or even absent.

About 80 percent of cases of cleft lip are unilateral; of these, 70 percent occur on the left side. Of cleft palate cases, 25 percent are bilateral. The mildest manifestations of congenital cleft are mild scarring or notching of the upper lip. Beyond this, clefting is described by degrees. The first degree is incomplete, which is a small cleft in the uvula. The second degree is also incomplete, through the soft palate and into the hard palate. Another type of "second-degree incomplete" is a horseshoe type, in which there is a bilateral cleft proceeding

almost to the front. Third-degree bilateral is a cleft through both palates but bilaterally through the gums; it results in a separate area where the teeth will erupt, and the teeth will show up in a very small segment. When the teeth appear, they may not be normally aligned. In addition to the lip, gum, and palate deviations, abnormalities of the nose may also occur.

Cleft palate may be inherited, probably as a result of the interaction of several genes. In addition, the effects of some environmental factors that affect embryonic development may be linked to this condition. They might include mechanical disturbances such as an enlarged tongue, which prevents the fusion of the palate and lip. Other disturbances may be caused by toxins introduced by the mother (drugs such as cortisone or alcohol) and defective blood. Other associated factors include deficiencies of vitamins or minerals in the mother's diet, radiation from X-rays, and infectious diseases such as German measles. No definite cause has been identified, nor does it appear that one cause alone can be implicated. It is likely that there is an interplay between genetic and chromosomal abnormalities and environmental factors.

There are at least 150 syndromes involving oral and facial clefts. Four examples of cleft syndromes that illustrate these syndromes are EEC (ectrodactyly, ectodermal dysplasia, cleft lip/palate), popliteal pterygium syndrome, van der Woude's syndrome, and trisomy 13 syndrome. EEC and trisomy 13 both result in intellectual and developmental disabilities as well as oral clefts. Popliteal pterygium has as its most common feature skin webbing (pterygium), along with clefts and skeletal abnormalities. Van der Woude's syndrome usually shows syndactyly as well as clefting and lower-lip pitting.

Problems begin at birth for the infant born with a cleft palate. The most immediate problem is feeding the baby. If the

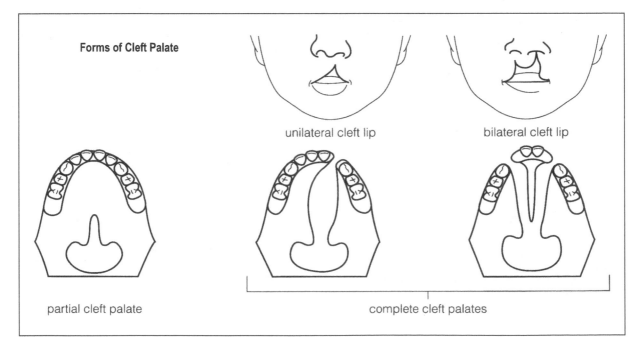

Forms of Cleft Palate

unilateral cleft lip

bilateral cleft lip

partial cleft palate

complete cleft palates

cleft is small and the lip unaffected, nursing may proceed fairly easily. If the cleft is too large, however, the baby cannot build up enough suction to nurse efficiently. To remedy this, the hole in the nipple of the bottle can be enlarged, or a plastic obturator can be fitted to the bottle.

Babies with cleft palates are more susceptible to colds than other children. Since there is an open connection between the nose and mouth, an infection that starts in either location will easily and quickly spread to the other. Frequently, the infection will spread to the middle ear via the Eustachian tube. One end of a muscle is affixed to the Eustachian tube opening, and the other end is attached to the middle of the roof of the mouth (palate). Normal contraction opens the tube so that air can travel through the tube and equalize air pressure on both sides of the eardrum. As long as the eardrum has flexibility of movement, the basics for good hearing are in place. Children with cleft palates, however, do not have good muscle contractions; therefore, air cannot travel through the tube. If the tube remains closed after swallowing, the air that is trapped is absorbed into the middle-ear tissue, resulting in a vacuum. This pulls the eardrum inward and decreases its flexibility, and hearing loss ensues. The cavity of the middle ear then fills with fluid, which can breed bacteria, causing infection. The infection may or may not be painful; if there is no pain, the infection may go unnoticed and untreated. The accumulated fluid can cause erosion of the tiny bones, which would decrease sound transmission to the auditory nerve. This conductive hearing loss is permanent. Persistent and prolonged fluid buildup can also cause accumulation of dead matter, forming a tumorlike growth called a cholesteatoma.

Other problems associated with cleft palates are those related to dentition. In some children there may be extra teeth, while in others the cleft may prevent the formation of tooth buds so that teeth are missing. Teeth that are present may be malformed; those malformations include injury during development, fusion of teeth to form one large tooth, teeth lacking enamel, and teeth that have too little calcium in the enamel. If the teeth are misaligned, orthodontia may be undertaken. Another possible problem met by patients with a cleft palate is maxillary (upper jaw) arch collapse; this condition is also remedied with orthodontic treatment.

Treatment and Therapy

One of the first questions a parent of a child with a cleft palate will pose regards surgical repair. The purpose of surgically closing the cleft is not simply to close the hole-although that goal is important. The major purpose is to achieve a functional palate. Whether this can be accomplished depends on the size and shape of the cleft, the thickness of the available tissue, and other factors.

Cleft lip surgery is performed when the healthy baby weighs at least ten pounds; it is done under a general anesthetic. If the cleft is unilateral, one operation can accomplish the closure, but a bilateral cleft lip is often repaired in two steps at least a month apart. When the lip is repaired, normal lip pressure is restored, which may help in closing the cleft in the gum ridge. It may also reduce the gap in the hard palate, if

one is present. Successive operations may be suggested when, even years after surgery, scars develop on the lip.

Surgery to close clefts of the hard and soft palate is typically done when the child is at least nine months of age, unless there is a medical reason not to do so. Different surgeons prefer different times for this surgery. The surgeon attempts to accomplish three goals in the repair procedure. The surgeon will first try to ensure that the palate is long enough to allow for function and movement (this is essential for proper speech patterns). Second, the musculature around the Eustachian tube should work properly in order to cut down the incidence of ear infections. Finally, the surgery should promote the development of the facial bones and, as much as possible, normal teeth. This goal aids in eating and appearance. All of this may be accomplished in one operation if the cleft is not too severe. For a cleft that requires more procedures, the surgeries are usually spaced at least six months apart so that complete healing can occur. This schedule decreases the potential for severe scarring.

At one time, it was thought that if surgery were performed before the child began talking, speech problems would be avoided. In reality, not only did the surgery not remedy that problem, but the early closure often resulted in a narrowing of the upper jaw and interference with facial growth as well. Thus, the trend to put off the surgery until the child was four or five years of age developed; by this age, more than 80 percent of the lateral growth of the upper jaw has occurred. However, most surgeons can perform the corrective surgery when the child is between one and two years of age without affecting facial growth.

Successful repair greatly improves speech and appearance, and the physiology of the oral and nasal cavities is also improved. Additional surgery may be necessary to improve appearance, breathing, and the function of the palate. Sometimes the palate may partially reopen, and surgery is needed to reclose it.

When the baby leaves the operating room, there are stitches in the repaired area. Sometimes a special device called a Logan's bow is taped to the baby's cheeks; this device not only protects the stitches but also relieves some of the tension on them. In addition, the baby's arms may be restrained in order to keep the baby's hands away from the affected area. (The child is fitted for elbow restraints before surgery; the elbows are encased in tubes that prevent them from bending.) A parent of a child that has just undergone cleft palate repair should not panic at the sight of bleeding from the mouth. To curb it, gauze may be packed into the repaired area and remain about five days after surgery. As mucus and other body fluids accumulate in the area, they may be suctioned out.

During the initial recovery, the child is kept in a moist, oxygen-rich environment (an oxygen tent) until respiration is normal. The patient will be observed for signs of airway obstruction or excessive bleeding. Feeding is done by syringe, eyedropper, or special nipples. Clear liquids and juices only are allowed. The child sits in a high chair to drink, when possible. After feeding, the mouth should be rinsed well with water to help keep the stitches clean. Peroxide mixed with the water may help, as well as ointment. Intake and output of fluids are measured. Hospitalization may last for about a week, or however long is dictated by speed of healing. At the end of this week, stitches are removed and the suture line covered and protected by a strip of paper tape.

An alternative to surgery is the use of an artificial palate known as an obturator. It is specially constructed by a dentist to fit into the child's mouth. The appliance, or prosthesis, is carefully constructed to fit precisely and snugly, but it must be easily removable. There must be enough space at the back so the child can breathe through the nose. While speaking, the muscles move back over this opening so that speech is relatively unaffected.

Speech problems are the most likely residual problems in the cleft palate patient. The speech of the untreated, and sometimes the treated cleft palate patient is very nasal. If the soft palate is too short, the closure of the palate may leave a space between the nose and the throat, allowing air to escape through the nose. There is little penetrating quality to the patient's voice, and it does not carry well. Some cleft palate speakers are difficult to understand because there are several faults in articulation. Certainly not all cleft lip or palate patients, however, will develop communication problems; modern surgical procedures ensure that most children will develop speech and language normally, without the help of a speech therapist.

Genetic counseling may help answer some of the family's questions about why the cleft palate occurred, whether it will happen with future children, and whether there is any way to prevent it. There are no universal answers to these questions. The answers depend on the degree and type of cleft, the presence of other problems, the family history, and the history of the pregnancy. Genetic counseling obtained at a hospital or medical clinic can determine whether the condition was heritable or a chance error and can establish the risk level for future pregnancies.

Perspective and Prospects

Oral clefts, as well as other facial clefts, have been a part of historical records for thousands of years. Perhaps the earliest recorded incidence is a Neolithic shrine with a two-headed figurine dated about 6500 BCE. The origination and causative agent of such clefts remain mysterious today.

Expectant parents are rarely alerted prior to birth that their child will be born with a cleft, so it is usually in the hospital, just after birth, that parents first learn of the birth defect. Even if it is suspected that a woman is at risk for producing a child with a cleft palate, there is no way to determine if the defect is indeed present, as neither amniocentesis nor chromosomal analysis reveals the condition. When the baby is delivered, the presence of the cleft can evoke a feeling of crisis in the delivery room.

The problems accompanying clefting may alter family morale and climate, increasing the complexity of the problem. A team of specialists usually works together to help the patient and the family cope with these problems. This team may include a pediatrician, a speech pathologist, a plastic surgeon, an orthodontist, a psychiatrist, an otologist, an audiologist, and perhaps others.

The cooperating team should monitor for the following situations: feeding problems, family and friends" reactions to the baby's appearance, how parents encourage the child to talk or how they respond to poor speech, and whether the parents are realistic about the long-term outcome for their child. The grief, guilt, and shock that the parents often feel can be positively altered by how the professional team tackles the problem and by communication with the parents. Usually the team does not begin functioning in the baby's life until he or she is older than one month. Some parents have confronted their feelings, while others are still struggling with the negative feeling that the cleft brought to bear. Therefore, the first visit that the parents have with the team is important because it establishes the foundation of a support system that should last for years.

If the cleft were only a structural defect, the solution would simply be to close the cleft. Yet, problems concerning feeding and health, facial appearance, communication, speech, dental functioning, and hearing loss, as well as the potential for psychosocial difficulties, may necessitate additional surgical, orthodontic, speech, and otolaryngological interventions. In other words, after the closure has been made, attention is focused on aesthetic, functional, and other structural deficits.

—*Iona C. Baldridge*

See also Birth defects; Cleft lip and palate repair; DiGeorge syndrome; Oral and maxillofacial surgery; Speech disorders.

For Further Information:

Berkowitz, Samuel, ed. *Cleft Lip and Palate: Diagnosis and Management*. 2d ed. New York: Springer, 2006.
"Cleft Lip and Palate" *Medline Plus*, May 4, 2012.
Clifford, Edward. *The Cleft Palate Experience*. Springfield, Ill.: Charles C. Thomas, 1987.
"Facts about Cleft Lip and Cleft Palate. *Centers for Disease Control and Prevention*, July 19, 2012.
Gruman-Trinker, Carrie T. *Your Cleft-Affected Child: The Complete Book of Information, Resources, and Hope*. Alameda, Calif.: Hunter House, 2001.
Kliegman, Robert, et al. "Cleft Lip and Palate." In *Nelson Textbook of Pediatrics*, edited by Robert Kliegman, et al. 19th ed. Philadelphia, Pa.: Elsevier, 2011.
Lorente, Christine, et al. "Tobacco and Alcohol Use During Pregnancy and Risk of Oral Clefts." *American Journal of Public Health* 90, no. 3 (March, 2000): 415-419.
Stengelhofen, Jackie, ed. *Cleft Palate*. New York: Churchill Livingstone, 1988.
Wyszynski, Diego F., ed. *Cleft Lip and Palate: From Origin to Treatment*. New York: Oxford University Press, 2002.

CLEFT LIP AND PALATE REPAIR
Procedure

Anatomy or system affected: Bones, gums, mouth, musculoskeletal system, skin

Specialties and related fields: General surgery, neonatology, otorhinolaryngology, pediatrics, plastic surgery

Definition: The surgical closure of cleft lip and cleft palate, deformities of the mouth that are often described as either the failure of tissue migration to allow fusion or the failure of tissue ingrowth (filling in).

Indications and Procedures

Cleft lip is more common in males than in females. Additionally, males tend to have more severe cleft deformities than females. Cleft lip repair is classically performed according to the rule of tens: The infant should be ten weeks old, weigh at least ten pounds, and have a white blood cell count under ten thousand (no infections) and a hemoglobin count of ten grams (not anemic). Today, many surgeons prefer to perform repairs earlier in healthy, full-term newborns ranging in age from one day to fourteen days. Cleft lip repairs typically involve making flaps around the lip area and merging the gaping sides. The muscular layer around the mouth must be sealed into a functional unit, as must the skin.

Cleft palate is more prevalent in females than males by a 2:1 ratio. A cleft palate may involve only the soft palate, or it may involve both the hard and the soft palates. Suckling can be a greater challenge with a cleft palate than with cleft lip. Moreover, middle-ear disease and infections are a greater problem for an infant with a cleft palate, because the reflux of fluids or solids into the nasal or middle-ear regions can occur. Surgical closure of a cleft palate usually is performed on infants between nine months and one year of age; delays can permanently retard speech and phonation development, while premature closure can stunt facial bone growth and contribute to dentition problems. Typically, if both the hard and the soft palates are open, they will be surgically closed at the same time. Closure of the soft palate occurs in a three-layer manner, while closure of the hard palate is done in a two-layer approach.

Cleft lip coupled with cleft palate is more common in males and tends to be left-sided more often than right-sided. Combined cleft lip and palate repair follows the same plans as described above, but there is greater concern about the well-being of an infant with the combined deformity.

—*Mary C. Fields, M.D.*

See also Birth defects; Bones and the skeleton; Cleft lip and palate; Oral and maxillofacial surgery; Pediatrics; Plastic surgery; Surgery, pediatric.

For Further Information:

Berkowitz, Samuel, ed. *Cleft Lip and Palate: Diagnosis and Management*. 2d ed. New York: Springer, 2006.

"Bonegrafting the Cleft Maxilla." *cleftline.org*, October 25, 2007.

Clifford, Edward. *The Cleft Palate Experience*. Springfield, Ill.: Charles C Thomas, 1987.

"Cleft lip and palate repair." *MedlinePlus*, June 24, 2013.

Dronamraju, Krishna R. *Cleft Lip and Palate*. Springfield, Ill.: Charles C Thomas, 1986.

Gruman-Trinker, Carrie T. *Your Cleft-Affected Child: The Complete Book of Information, Resources, and Hope*. Alameda, Calif.: Hunter House, 2001.

Watson, A. C. H. *Management of Cleft Lip and Palate*. Philadelphia: Whurr, 2001.

Wynn, Sidney K., and Alfred L. Miller. *A Practical Guide to Cleft Lip and Palate Birth Defects*. Springfield, Ill.: Charles C Thomas, 1984.

Wyszynski, Diego F. *Cleft Lip and Palate: From Origin to Treatment*. New York: Oxford University Press, 2002.

"Your child's cleft lip and palate repair." *plasticsurgery.org*, June 24, 2013.

CLINICAL TRIALS

Procedure

Anatomy or system affected: All

Specialties and related fields: All

Definition: Research studies that test new drugs or treatments on human subjects to determine whether and at what dosage they are safe, effective, and better than similar products already in use.

Key terms:

blinded or *single-blind:* a study in which the patients are not

---

The Repair of Cleft Lip

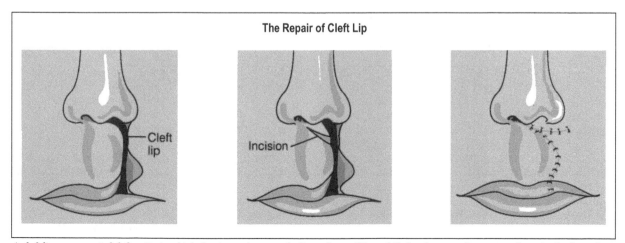

A cleft lip, a congenital deformity in which the tissues between the lip and nostril have failed to fuse, can be corrected surgically through realignment and suturing.

told whether they are in an experimental or control group

control group: a group of patients receiving either a standard treatment or a placebo, allowing comparison with the experimental treatment

double-blind: referring to a study in which neither the patients nor the research staff knows which patients are receiving which treatment

informed consent: consent for treatment by a patient who has been educated fully about the purpose, benefits, and risks of a clinical trial

Institutional Review Board (IRB): a committee that oversees informed consent, reviews the progress of clinical trials, and safeguards participants' rights

placebo: an inactive substance resembling the experimental drug that might be given to a control group, especially when no standard treatment exists

protocol: a lengthy, technical document outlining the rules for inclusion in, scientific rationale of, and procedures for a clinical trial

randomization: assigning, by chance, patients with similar characteristics to either the experimental or the control group in a clinical trial

Indications and Procedures

Clinical trials offer the most reliable process for bringing new drugs and medical treatments into public use. The process has features that can protect human participants, avoid biases, ensure that patient improvements are due to the experimental treatment and not to other factors, and allow accurate comparison of the experimental treatment with others on the market. Clinical trials are usually initiated and managed by academic institutions (often with grant funding), pharmaceutical companies, or government research agencies, such as the National Cancer Institute.

In 1998, it was estimated that the cost of developing a new drug was, on average, $500 million, and the process could take twelve to fifteen years-from discovery and laboratory testing, through clinical trials, to Food and Drug Administration (FDA) approval, and finally getting the drug to market. By the late 1990s, a new drug might go through sixty-eight clinical trials. The average number of patients enrolled in a trial was 3,800.

Clinical trials fit into one of four types. Phase I trials, which usually involve only twenty to one hundred seriously ill patients, try to determine how to administer a new drug, the maximally tolerated dose (MTD), how the human body processes the drug, and any significant side effects. Phase II trials, which are usually randomized, treat up to several hundred patients who all have measurable rates of disease. These trials study the effectiveness of the drug. Phase III trials, which are usually randomized and blinded and which treat hundreds or thousands of patients, have more relaxed criteria for inclusion and are usually multicenter (held simultaneously at more than one site). These trials try to determine whether the new drug is better than current, standard ones. Phase IV trials, conducted once a drug is on the market, are often informal. Pharmaceutical companies may simply ask physicians to

submit reports on how their patients are responding to the drug.

Uses and Complications

The 1979 Belmont Report detailed three ethical principles to guide clinical trials. They include respect for persons (abiding by their opinions and choices as autonomous agents), beneficence (doing no harm and maximizing the possible benefits while minimizing possible harm), and justice (distributing the benefits and burdens of research fairly).

Two standard features of clinical trials help ensure that ethical principles are being followed. First, all clinical trials in the United States must be approved and monitored by an Institutional Review Board (IRB), which includes both scientists and laypersons. Multicenter trials must also have a data safety and monitoring board composed of independent experts. This group monitors data from the trial regarding the treatment's effectiveness and any adverse reactions. Second, the detailed informed consent document that patients must carefully consider and sign gives a number of categories of information. Most important, anticipated physical risks and discomforts are explained, as are financial risks. Similar practices are followed in countries other than the United States as well.

Perspective and Prospects

In October, 1948, *The British Medical Journal* published an article reporting on what was probably the first study using all the methodological features of the randomized clinical trial. Since then, the randomized clinical trial has come to be regarded as perhaps the most important medical achievement of the twentieth century. It transformed biomedical research and allowed physicians to make treatment choices based on scientific evidence rather than on personal opinion and experience.

The National Cancer Institute (NCI) and other sources reported a small participation rate in clinical trials-ranging in the late 1990s from 3 to 20 percent of patients. One of many causes was that insurance companies and managed care providers frequently refused payment for experimental treatments. Their concerns were that they might be liable for adverse reactions or additional care after the trial ends and that clinical trials are more costly than conventional treatments. Because so many insurers would not cover the costs of clinical trials, researchers had trouble finding patients willing to participate, thus slowing the development of more effective drugs and treatments. Insurers gradually realized that more widespread coverage of the costs of trials might speed the development of better drugs, which could ultimately save them money. In 1998, US states began to pass laws requiring insurers to cover the routine medical costs (such as tests and office visits) of treatment in clinical trials of drugs for life-threatening diseases.

Criticism has been leveled at clinical trials for insufficient inclusion of women, children, people of color, and the aged. When these groups are underrepresented, there is no certainty that a drug will be effective or without side effects for them.

In June 2000, the FDA added a regulation that would place a clinical hold on a phase I trial of a drug or treatment for a life-threatening disease affecting both women and men if either gender was excluded because of risk to their reproductive potential. That same month, President Bill Clinton signed an executive memorandum directing Medicare to reimburse senior citizens for routine medical costs incurred in clinical trials. A major impetus for this change came from reports that only 33 percent of cancer clinical trial participants were over sixty-five, while 63 percent of all cancer patients are over sixty-five.

—*Glenn Ellen Starr Stilling, M.A., M.L.S.*

See also Animal rights vs. research; Cancer; Clinics; Death and dying; Disease; Ethics; Food and Drug Administration (FDA); Iatrogenic disorders; Invasive tests; National Cancer Institute (NCI); Noninvasive tests; Over-the-counter medications; Pharmacology; Pharmacy; Screening; Terminally ill: Extended care.

For Further Information:
Beer, Tomasz M., and Larry Axmaker. *Cancer Clinical Trials: A Commonsense Guide to Experimental Cancer Therapies and Clinical Trials.* New York: DiaMedica, 2012.
"Clinical Trials." *MedlinePlus*, May 3, 2013.
"Clinical Trials of Medical Treatments: Why Volunteer?" *US Food and Drug Administration*, Jan. 4, 2010.
Finn, Robert. *Cancer Clinical Trials: Experimental Treatments and How They Can Help You.* Sebastopol, Calif.: O'Reilly, 1999.
Green, Stephanie, Jacqueline Benedetti, and John Crowley. *Clinical Trials in Oncology.* 3d ed. Boca Raton, Fla.: Chapman & Hall, 2012.
Harrington, David P. "The Randomized Clinical Trial." *Journal of the American Statistical Association* 95, no. 449 (March, 2000): 312-315.
"Learn about Clinical Studies." *ClinicalTrials.gov*, Aug 2012.
Malay, Marilyn. *Making the Decision: A Cancer Patient's Guide to Clinical Trials.* Sudbury, Mass.: Jones and Bartlett, 2002.
"Overview of Clinical Trials." *CenterWatch Clinical Trials Listing Service*, n.d.
Quinn, Susan. *Human Trials: Scientists, Investors, and Patients in the Quest for a Cure.* Cambridge, Mass.: Perseus, 2002.

CLINICS
Health care system
Definition: Organizations that provide outpatient care to specific types of patients; they can be in-hospital or out of hospital, usually consist of a physical space with reception and examination rooms, and are staffed by doctors, nurses, and other health care professionals.

Key terms:
ambulatory surgery center: a facility providing day surgery outside a hospital setting
clinic: a site for outpatient care
hospital: an inpatient care facility that provides overnight care and in many cases intensive care, emergency care, and surgical services
inpatient care: overnight patient treatment at a hospital
outpatient care: patient treatment not requiring an overnight stay at a hospital
provider: the medical practitioner within a clinic or hospital;

providers may be physicians, nurses, dentists, or other licensed health care professionals

Organization and Functions
There are three main types of patient care facilities in North America: hospitals, ambulatory surgery centers, and clinics. Hospitals care for patients who require overnight care, emergency care, or intensive care treatment. Hospital emergency rooms are not usually considered a clinic due to the highly specialized equipment needed and the fact that many patients who are treated in the emergency room are then admitted for overnight stay at a hospital. Ambulatory surgery centers provide outpatient surgery. Clinics provide outpatient nonsurgical care. In some cases, minor procedures are performed in clinics; however, a clinic does not provide outpatient surgery.

A clinic will usually consist of at least a waiting room and patient exam rooms. The number of examination rooms and size of the clinic will depend on the number of providers and the clinic type. Clinics can range in size from a solo practice with a very small office to very large multispecialty outpatient clinics such as the Mayo Clinic or Cleveland Clinic. Specialized equipment may be part of a clinic, such as in a dental clinic. Clinics may be located within a hospital, in a private building, or in a public building. Clinics can be owned and operated by a single practitioner, a group of practitioners, a private group, a public or nonprofit group, a hospital, or a government agency.

Clinics will most often have regular business hours and are not usually open overnight. Some urgent care walk-in clinics may have extended hours. Most clinics will be closed on major holidays. Some smaller solo practitioner clinics may close for one or more weeks per year when the provider is on vacation. Some clinics will have an answering service or after-hours coverage for emergency calls.

Clinic administration will depend on the ownership of the clinic. A solo private practitioner may do administration as well as provision of care. Hospital-based clinics will generally have a clinic manager who works within the administrative system of the hospital. Some clinics may be part of a publicly held company and will have an office manager who reports to a board. Most clinics will have a clinic manager and a medical director. Larger clinics will have more administrative staff, including human resource staff and marketing staff.

Each clinic serves a specific patient population that will be determined by the primary provider or providers within the clinic. For example, a solo family practice physician will serve children and adults for treatment of common illnesses and conditions. In contrast, a pediatric clinic will see only children, and some public health clinics may provide only immunization services. There are as many clinics as there are health care specialties. Some providers will work in groups, such as a multidiscipline group that may contain internal medicine, pediatrics, and dermatology.

Clinics may accept direct fee-for-service payment, insurance, or government funding such as Medicare, Veterans Administration, or Indian Health Service. In Canada, most clinics will accept fee-for-service payment, provincial health insurance payment, or both.

A large number of combinations are possible in terms of specific services offered, number of providers, payment types accepted, clinic size, and clinic location. No matter what the combination of these features, all clinics have in common the provision of nonsurgical outpatient health care services.

Staff and Services

A health care clinic will generally be staffed by a primary provider and support staff. The primary provider will often be a medical doctor but can be another type of provider such as physical therapist, chiropractor, optometrist, dentist, or naturopath. Support staff will include nurses, physician assistants, technicians, office staff, and, in some cases, specialized paraprofessionals. Providers and other specialized staff who provide direct patient care will have licensing requirements that are specific to the state or province and that will vary depending on the field. For example, physicians and dentists will have different licensing requirements.

Depending on the clinic, patients may require referral from a physician. Other clinics such as urgent care clinics will accept walk-ins without referral. Walk-in clinics may refer patients to family practice clinics or other clinics for ongoing care of chronic disease.

Services will depend on the clinic providers. For example, a family practice clinic will provide physical examination, diagnosis, and treatment recommendations for people of all ages for general nonsurgical outpatient medical care. Diagnosis might include giving a patient requisitions to have laboratory or radiology (X-ray) or other specialized tests done at a laboratory or radiology facility. Some family practice clinics may have the capacity to do some simple laboratory tests such as a dip urinalysis or electrocardiography (ECG or EKG). Treatment may include advice, prescription for medications, or treatment of minor injuries.

Another example of a clinic would be a physical therapy clinic. This type of clinic would have one or more physical therapists as providers. These providers would provide limited physical examination, usually of the musculoskeletal system. Diagnosis would be based on the physical examination. Physical therapists would not usually order specialized testing such as X rays or magnetic resonance imaging (MRI) but might comanage a patient with a physician provider if these additional diagnostic tests were needed. Treatment within a physical therapy clinic will usually consist of specialized exercises, massage therapy, heat or cold treatment, specialized physical therapy maneuvers, and, in some cases, acupuncture.

Specialized clinics will treat only specific groups of patients. For example, an obstetrics clinic will provide care only to pregnant women. Pediatrics clinics will treat only children. Ophthalmology clinics will treat both children and adults but will care only for vision and other eye-related problems. Similarly, an orthopedic clinic will be focused on musculoskeletal disorders, and sports medicine clinics will treat sports-related injuries.

Urgent care clinics are designed to treat minor illnesses and minor injuries. More significant illness or injury would be treated in a hospital emergency room. Most urgent care clinics will operate on a walk-in basis due to the nature of the clinic focus. Some hospitals have both an urgent care clinic and an emergency room to keep the emergency room available for the more seriously ill or injured.

The Mayo Clinic and the Cleveland Clinic are examples of clinics that have grown to become very large multidisciplinary clinics that provide outpatient care. These large clinics are affiliated with hospitals that provide inpatient and surgical care.

Some clinics receive public funding to serve low-income populations. This type of clinic may operate on a sliding scale for fee payment. Often this type of clinic will be located in an urban area and may serve homeless populations as well. These clinics are sometimes staffed by volunteers, including volunteer providers.

Regardless of the clinic type, the usual practice is to have the patient check in at a desk in the reception area. Patients may have to wait in the reception area until the appropriate staff is ready and until an exam or treatment room is available. Each patient will have a paper or computerized chart that will record the examinations, diagnosis, and treatment recommendations. The patient will then be taken to the exam room, where a nurse or other specialized staff will often do some preliminary testing such as blood pressure and a preliminary history to determine what services are needed. If the chart is a paper chart, then it will be taken along with the patient to the exam room. The provider will often go from one exam room to the next to examine and treat patients. The support staff will clean each exam room as it is vacated and then room the next patient. This system allows for more efficiency for the provider. Once the provider is done with examination, diagnosis, and treatment, the patient is directed back to the reception area to book additional appointments or testing, if necessary, and is then dismissed from the clinic.

A patient who comes to a clinic with a life-threatening condition or serious injury will be directed to the nearest emergency room. In some cases, an ambulance will be called to transport a patient who is in need of inpatient care, emergency treatment, or immediate surgery.

Perspective and Prospects

The word "clinic" is derived from the Greek word for bed, *kline*. Evidence exists for the use of herbs and other natural substances for the treatment of medical conditions even in prehistoric times. The provision of health care has been historically linked with religious and spiritual beliefs. In some cases, religious leaders such as shamans or monks were the providers of health care, and illness was attributed to demons or witchcraft.

Ancient Egypt has been credited with having organized houses of medicine, and Herophilos (335-280 BCE) is considered the founder of the medical school in Alexandria, Egypt. The knowledge of human anatomy was very limited, there was no understanding of sterile technique, no understanding of germ theory, and few treatment options were available; however, these early institutions served to further medical knowledge. In the Middle Ages, medical care was provided in monasteries, which in some cases had hospitals attached.

Licensing standards vary across the world, and in some places the provision of health care is still largely unregulated. There are some areas in which the only clinics in existence are provided by volunteer organizations, and in some areas these clinics are in the form of mobile trailers.

The Mayo Clinic is one of the best known multidisciplinary clinics. It was established in the aftermath of a destructive tornado in Rochester, Minnesota, in 1883. William Mayo and his sons Charles and William joined the Sisters of St. Francis to establish a hospital and clinic to care for tornado victims. It grew to be the first and largest nonprofit multispecialty clinic serving more than one-half million patients annually at its three locations.

—*E. E. Anderson Penno, M.D., M.S., FRCSC*

See also Emergency care; Emergency rooms; Hospitals; Nursing; Physician assistants.

For Further Information:

Fauci, Anthony, et al. *Harrison's Principles of Internal Medicine.* 17th ed. New York: McGraw-Hill, 2008. Chapter 1, "The Practice of Medicine," outlines the standards for providing health care in the United States and discusses inpatient care, outpatient care, and different levels of care within hospitals.

Gonzalez-Crussi, F. *A Short History of Medicine.* New York: Modern Library, 2007. A compendium of medical care from ancient times to the early twenty-first century.

Kennedy, Michael. *A Brief History of Disease, Science, and Medicine from the Ice Age to the Genome Project.* Mission Viejo, Calif.: Asklepiad Press, 2004. History of medicine and disease.

CLONING

Procedure

Also known as: Nuclear transplantation

Anatomy or system affected: Cells

Specialties and related fields: Biotechnology, embryology, ethics, genetics

Definition: From a scientific perspective, the term "clone" signifies an exact genetic copy of a segment of deoxyribonucleic acid (DNA), cell, or organism. Cloning is a procedure conducted by teams of molecular biologists, geneticists, and embryologists to introduce the genetic information from one cell into another for the purpose of producing a clone.

Key terms:

blastocyst: the stage during early embryonic development, just prior to implantation in the uterus, in which the cells form a large hollow ball; at this point, the cells are undifferentiated

complementary DNA (cDNA): DNA that is made from messenger ribonucleic acid (mRNA) and thus represents the genes actively being expressed in a cell at a given time

eukaryotic: referring to a type of cell that contains a nucleus and membrane-bound organelles; all animal cells are

eukaryotic, as are those of plants and fungi

inner cell mass: a tight cluster of spherical cells inside the blastocyst-stage embryo of placental mammals that eventually give rise to the definitive structures of the later embryo and fetus

meiosis: a specific type of cell division that occurs in gamete-producing cells or germ cells, and results in four daughter cells each with half the number of chromosomes of the parent cell

parthenogenesis: the development of an adult from an unfertilized egg

pluripotent: a description for stem cells that have begun differentiation and are capable of forming limited cell types

stem cells: unspecialized cells capable of renewing themselves through cell division that can be induced, under certain conditions, to differentiate into particular types of cells

totipotent: an undifferentiated cell that still retains the ability to form any other cell type of the adult organism; cells of this type are commonly referred to as stem cells

transduction: the incorporation of a piece of DNA into the genome of a bacterium using a virus as a vector transformation: the incorporation into a cell of cell-free DNA from the environment

transgenic: referring to an organism that contains genetic material from two or more species

vector: a system that is used to carry a fragment of DNA for molecular cloning

Uses and Complications

Scientists use the word "cloning" to indicate an experimental process by which an exact genetic duplicate is made of a molecule, cell, or organism. It is frequently divided into three general categories. Molecular cloning involves copying genes, short segments of DNA, or cells (sometimes also called cellular cloning) for the purpose of producing multiple copies of a molecule or cell for further scientific study. The cloning of DNA is commonly called recombinant DNA technology or genetic engineering. Cell cloning isolates one particular cell from a large population of cells and places it in an environment where it can grow into a new homogeneous population of cells. Cloning at the organismal level, also called nuclear transplantation, has been used to create genetically identical organisms and has the potential to produce genetically identical tissues and organs from a donor.

The procedure for molecular cloning involves choosing a vector for the study of the target DNA. The choice of the vector depends on the size of the genetic information being studied and whether it is genomic DNA or complementary DNA (cDNA). Common vectors include plasmids (small circular pieces of bacterial DNA), viruses, and artificial chromosomes. For example, if the length of the DNA being studied is small, then the researcher may choose to insert it into a plasmid. By the process of transformation, the selected plasmid is moved into the bacteria (usually E. coli), and as the bacteria divide, cells are produced that are clones for the DNA in the plasmid vector. If the researcher is unsure what area contains the gene to be cloned, then the genome is first fragmented and the individual fragments are inserted into viruses that infect bacteria, or bacteriophages. This creates a library of genetic information. Each bacteriophage vector then infects a bacterium, and the infected bacterial cells will divide to produce a colony of bacteria that contain clones of the genetic information contained within the bacteriophage vector. These colonies may then be screened using molecular techniques to isolate a colony that contains the desired section of DNA.

If the DNA fragment is larger, as is frequently the case with studies of genomic DNA, then the researcher may decide to create an artificial chromosome. The purpose is to create a small, synthetically-derived chromosome that is replicated by the host cell prior to cell division. Bacterial artificial chromosomes (BACs) and yeast artificial chromosomes (YACs) are commonly used, but human artificial chromosomes (HACs) have also been available since 1997. In all cases, the purpose is to create cells that are genetically identical, or cloned, for a specific stretch of DNA. While this is a useful technique, molecular cloning is not able to produce an entire organism that is genetically identical to the original.

In eukaryotic organisms, sexual reproduction produces offspring that contain new combinations of the parents' genomes. While this provides variability to the species, it complicates medical research since it effectively shuffles the genome every generation. Identical, or monozygotic, twins are the closest thing to clones in humans, but between even their cells small genetic differences exist. For scientific studies of development and cell biology, large numbers of cloned cells are needed.

The process of nuclear transplantation, or cloning, as it is commonly called, has the ability to create large numbers of genetically identical multicellular organisms. In theory, cloning is not a difficult process: Simply remove the DNA from the host cell, replace it with the DNA from the donor cell, and induce the new cell to divide. Procedures such as this have been performed on amphibians since the 1950s, but nuclear transplantation in mammals is slightly more complicated, since mammalian egg cells, or oocytes, are vastly smaller than those of amphibians. Fortunately technological advances in microscopy and embryology have remedied this problem. In mammalian nuclear transplantation, the embryologist uses a microscope equipped with a micropipette. The micropipette is effectively a microscopic needle that is controlled remotely by the researcher. During the procedure, the egg is held in place by a second pipette to allow for greater control. The researcher then inserts the needle from the first pipette into the oocyte through the zona pellucida (outer covering of the oocyte) and gently removes the nucleus from the cell. At this stage, the oocyte contains only the zona pellucida, cytoplasm, and the internal organelles of the cell, such as the mitochondria. The researcher then inserts a donor cell, complete with DNA, into the area between the oocyte and the zona pellucida. At this point, there are effectively two cells alongside each other-one containing nothing but cytoplasm, the other containing the donor DNA. To form a single

cell, the plasma membranes of the two cells must be fused. This is done using a process called electrofusion, in which a small current is applied to the cells, temporarily disrupting the membranes and allowing the cytoplasm of the two cells (and the donor DNA) to mix. The end result is an egg cell than contains the DNA of a second cell.

However, this cell is not yet technically a clone. To produce an embryo that is genetically identical to the original donor cell, the oocyte must divide. In some species, the first cell divisions (cleavages) occur readily in response to electrofusion, but this is not always the case. Frequently, growth factors or other chemical signals need to be applied to make the cell divide. All the cells of the blastocyst are clones of one another and the DNA in the original donor cell. Once cell division ensues, the embryo eventually forms a hollow sphere with flat cells on the outside (trophectoderm) and a tight cluster of round cells on the inside (inner cell mass) known as a blastocyst.

Human oocytes begin as cells called "oogonia;" the progenitors of oocytes. During early fetal developing, oogonia divide and increase in numbers, but later in fetal development (18-22 weeks after conception), oogonia cease dividing, undergo one additional round of DNA synthesis and enter the first phase of meiosis, but become arrested in the first phase of meiosis, at which time it is known as a primary oocyte. Like all gametes (sex cells), oocytes undergo a special type of cell division known as meiosis in which the cell divides twice and reduces the number of chromosomes in the progeny cells by half. Primary oocytes remain arrested in the first stage of meiosis from fetal life through childhood until puberty, when a surge of luteinizing hormone from the anterior lobe of the pituitary gland stimulates the resumption of meiosis. This secondary oocyte, as it is now called, arrests at the metaphase stage of the second stage of meiosis and will not complete meiosis unless it is fertilized.

This introduction to the life of human oocytes explains why cloning human embryos has proven to be so technically difficult; the spindle chromosome apparatus that holds the chromosomes in place, poised to complete the second phase of meiosis, is a fragile structure that is easily disrupted by physical or chemical manipulation. Consequently, meiotic arrest in human oocytes is rather unstable and invasive manipulations tend to induce rapid, premature completion of meiosis, which disrupts normal reprogramming of the nucleus. To solve this problem, Shoukhrat Mitalipov and his colleagues at the Oregon Health & Science University treated human oocytes with caffeine to prevent premature exit from meiosis during the cloning procedure, which greatly increased cloning efficiency.

The development of improved technologies in nuclear transplantation has enabled scientists to create organisms that are genetically the same. In the media, the use of the term "clone" usually signifies an organism produced by this procedure. To create a cloned adult organism, the researcher must insert the blastocyst into the uterus of a surrogate mother, who will carry the embryo to term. To date cloned adult sheep, cattle, goats, mules, horses, pigs, mouflons (a wild sheep), mice, rats, dogs, cats, and rabbits have been made in the laboratory. To successfully clone adult animals (reproductive cloning), scientists have adapted the techniques of in vitro fertilization (IVF). IVF retrieves eggs from the mother and fertilizes them with sperm from the father in the laboratory. Subsequently, these embryos are grown in embryo culture, and after they grow to the blastocyst stage, the embryos are transferred into the uterus of the mother. Cloning does not require the fertilization step, since the fusion of the enucleated oocyte with the adult cell takes the place of fertilization. Theoretically, once implanted, the cloned blastocyst should develop in the same manner as an embryo made by means of a natural fertilization event.

A different use of cloning, known as therapeutic cloning, uses cloned embryos (made by means of somatic cell nuclear transfer) to generate a large number of embryonic stem cells for the purpose of treating a disease. Since embryonic stem cells are pluripotent, or have the ability to produce all adult cell types, embryonic stem cells made from a cloned embryo, which are known as "nuclear transfer embryonic stem cells (NT-ESCs) should, theoretically, have the ability to take the place of damaged or diseased cells. Embryonic stem cells (ESCs) are derived from a specific group of cells within the blastocyst called the inner cell mass (ICM). ICM cells are pluripotent cells that can be harvested and grown under laboratory conditions to form an ESC line. Under specific culture conditions, ECSs can differentiate into new tissues, such as nerves, skin, bone, fat, cartilage, or pancreas.

Stem cell scientists have used NT-ESCs to treat various diseases in laboratory animals. For example, researchers from Sloan-Kettering Institute used NT-ESCs derived from cloned mouse embryos to successfully treat animals with a rodent version of Parkinson's disease. However, the use of blood-making stem cells derived from NT-ESCs to reconstitute the immune systems of mutant mice showed that cells made from NT-ESCs can still be subject to immunological rejection under certain conditions.

Another technique to make stem cells from unfertilized eggs that have been artificially activated has been utilized. Artificial activation of eggs in the absence of fertilization can cause the egg to initiate development, and this process, by which embryonic development begins in the absence of fertilization, is known as parthenogenesis. Parthenogenesis is common in amphibians and insects, but it does not occur naturally in humans. However, if a female egg cell is chemically induced to form a blastocyst without nuclear transplantation, then the resulting stem cells derived from such blastocysts could be used to generate new organs or tissues for the female. Scientists have made several parthenogenic stem cell lines from various animals and humans, and they can be differentiated into several different cell types. However, the stability of parthenogenic stem cells has been questioned by some stem cell scientists. Parthenogenesis cannot be used in males, since sperm cells lack the cytoplasmic components found in egg cells.

Indications and Procedures

By definition, the purpose of cloning is to produce genetically identical cells or individuals for scientific studies. Yet even identical (monozygotic) twins, whose cells are derived from the same fertilized egg, are not truly identical. For example, monozygotic twins do not have the same fingerprint pattern, even though they possess the same genes for ridges on the fingers. The reason for this difference is environmental. For twins, the genes establish a general pattern, but it is the touch of the fingers on the inner wall of the uterus that establishes the final pattern of fingerprints. Environment plays a significant role in the development of the embryo, and this fact has presented a challenge for scientists who wish to produce identical genetic clones. Also, the process of DNA replication, while highly efficient, is not perfect, and DNA sequence differences between monozygotic twins and cloned individuals emerge. A study by the Seoul National University compared the genomic DNA sequence of the cloned dog (Snuppy) and the donor animal, and the genomes of two identical Korean twins. Snuppy and his donor (Tai) showed approximately the same degree of DNA sequence differences as human monozygotic twins.

Therefore, Dolly, a cloned ewe, was not an exact copy of her donor, even though she possessed the same genetic information as the donor ewe. According to Ian Wimut, the scientist whose laboratory made Dolly and other cloned sheep, the cloned sheep made in his laboratory were different sizes, and had different temperaments even though they were made from cells that came from the same donor ewe. These differences stem from the fact that Dolly and her "sisters" were raised in the uterus of a surrogate mother and thus were exposed to the minor, but important, environmental variations specific to the surrogate mother. It is known that, by a process called genomic imprinting, the mother can override certain traits in the embryo and impose her own traits, regardless of the genes present in the embryo. The mother also provides all the nutrients needed for the developing embryo, and thus any metabolic problems with the surrogate mother may inhibit proper development in the cloned embryo. Also, particular random events during embryonic and fetal development can generate unique individuals who are also genetically identical.

A potential problem with nuclear transplantation is that not all the DNA in the cell is located within the nucleus. Mitochondria, the energy factories of a cell, contain small circular pieces of DNA. The genes on this DNA are inherited along with the mother's cytoplasm, so that individuals receive all mitochondrial DNA from the maternal line. During nuclear transplantation, mitochondria are not removed from the host cell, so once transplantation is complete, the new cell contains donor DNA by both host cell and donor cell mitochondria. Because mitochondrial genetic disorders exist, it is known that the genes in the mitochondria contribute to the characteristics of the organism. In fact, in the Korean study mentioned above, the cloned animals had a significantly greater number of mitochondrial mutations.

Cells age and have a finite life span. This appears to be at least partially controlled by the length of the chromosome, specifically the ends of the chromosome called the telomeres. After each cell division, the telomeres shorten like a genetic fuse, until the cell is no longer able to divide. However, work in several species has established that the telomere length of the chromosomes is reset in the cloned embryo.

One of the greatest challenges facing the process of cloning is ethical, which involves the opinion of the general public regarding the cloning of mammals and potentially, humans. Some consider the cloning of organisms to be an unnatural event, while others question the use of cloned embryos as a source of embryonic stem cells. One of the greatest concerns among the general public regarding cloning is the moral right of people to create life by artificial processes. This objection was also applied to IVF when it was introduced in 1978. Another concern is the production of human embryos solely for the purpose of destroying them. The debate over cloning shows no signs of abating and will almost certainly continue into the foreseeable future. The majority of scientists involved in cloning research are interested in either the therapeutic benefits of cell cloning or the study of embryonic development and cell differentiation, and not the creation of a cloned human.

Perspective and Prospects

While for many people the history of cloning may appear to have begun in 1996, when Ian Wilmut of the Roslin Institute in Scotland introduced the world to Dolly the cloned ewe, the reality is that the cloning of organisms had been going on for some time. The making of cloned plants had been occurring for decades and now represents a common occurrence in agriculture. If one restricts the discussion to animals, then Dolly does not really even represent the first cloned mammal, but rather the first adult animal cloned from the cells of another adult animal.

The cloning of animals by nuclear transplantation has its roots in the late nineteenth century, when early embryologists were studying cell division in the eggs of invertebrate animals. The first experiments that transferred a nucleus from one cell to another in a vertebrate animal were conducted in the early 1950s by Robert Briggs and Thomas King. Briggs and King worked with nuclear transplantation in amphibians. These researchers were not interested in the creation of a cloned frog but rather the question of nuclear programming, or whether the cells isolated from the blastocyst had the genetic ability to form a new adult frog. These experiments examined the use of embryonic cells to produce a functionally adult organism. In later experiments, researchers, including Briggs and King, set out to determine at what age of embryonic development cells differentiate to the point where they cannot be used to produce a functioning adult. In essence, they were studying the potency of the cells and beginning to distinguish between totipotent cells and pluripotent cells. For the next several decades, scientists perfected methods of nuclear transplantation in a variety of organisms, including mammals such as mice and rabbits.

In 1996, the researchers at the Roslin Institute used tissue from the mammary gland of an adult ewe in a nuclear transplantation experiment. The result was Dolly, the first mammal to be cloned from an adult cell. Although this experiment was widely reported as producing the first cloned mammal, its real importance was the demonstration that the genes of an adult cell could be expressed in an embryo to produce a living organism. For decades, scientists had debated whether adult cells were capable of being used in cloning. Adult cells are highly specialized, and many of their developmental genes are inactivated. The experiments with Dolly demonstrated that, under the right conditions, the environment within the blastocyst allows DNA from adult cells to be used. In other words, the DNA from differentiated tissue can be used to create undifferentiated stem cells. This remains a major advance in the understanding of cellular processes.

In June 2013, Masahito Tachibana in the laboratory of Shoukhrat Mitalipov at the Oregon Health & Science University reported the derivation of human embryonic stem cells from cloned human embryos. This was the first time human NT-ESCs were produced, and it represented a remarkable technical advance.

In an earlier publication, Mitalipov's laboratory showed that replacement of an oocyte nucleus by means of somatic cell nuclear transfer, followed by fertilization, can result in a normal embryo. Several scientists suggest that this procedure might allow patients who suffer from mitochondrial genetic diseases to conceive children who do not have these destructive mutations. However, until more animal studies establish the safety of this procedure, it will remain experimental.

The question may then be asked as to why scientists pursue experiments involving the cloning of organisms. Since public opinion is against the cloning of humans and no immediate need exists to clone an individual, then research in this area would appear to be at an impasse. The reality, however, is that the process of nuclear transplantation and organism cloning gives scientists the ability to answer some important questions about cellular differentiation, especially during embryonic development, and the patterns of expression of genes within cells during development.

Furthermore, while the cloning of humans may not be morally acceptable, cloning can serve society in many other ways, such as in studies using transgenic organisms and in tissue and organ transplantation. Scientific research frequently involves the use of transgenic organisms for study. In the study of human genetics and biochemistry, mice are frequently used as a model system. The ability to study the effects of a particular gene in a transgenic organism is dependent on that organism being genetically pure (homozygous) for that trait. In animals, it can take up to fifteen generations of inbreeding to develop a pure line. For organisms with long gestation periods or a small number of offspring per generation, this becomes both cost- and time-prohibitive. The cloning of new organisms that are genetically similar to the donor can facilitate research with transgenic organisms.

Organ transplantation in humans is a difficult process. Recipients of organ transplants must be carefully matched with donors for a variety of biochemical factors to ensure that the new organ is not rejected by the recipient's immune system. Even when a match is close, the use of immunosuppressant drugs increases the chances of infection in the recipient. The process of nuclear transplantation may alleviate some of these problems. Rather than being matched with a donor, a patient would contribute genetic material for nuclear transplantation. Stem cells could then be harvested and chemically induced to form the required tissue, or someday even the entire organ. Experiments are currently under way to manufacture skin for burn victims using this type of procedure. Even though the discovery of induced pluripotent stem cells have largely marginalized NT-ESCs, many scientists still think that NT-ESCs, which are probably safer than induced pluripotent stem cells, still have an important role to play in research and regenerative medicine. The applications of nuclear transplantation are almost endless, and developments in this area of research have the potential to influence directly the lives of the majority of people alive today.

—*Michael Windelspecht, Ph.D.;*
updated by Jeffrey A. Knight, Ph.D.;
further updated by Michael A. Buratovich, Ph.D.

See also Cytology; DNA and RNA; Embryology; Ethics; Gene therapy; Genetic counseling; Genetic engineering; Genomics; Gynecology; Law and medicine; Multiple births; Obstetrics; Ovaries; Premature birth; Veterinary medicine.

For Further Information:

Buratovich, Michael A. *The Stem Cell Epistles. Letters to My Students about Bioethics, Embryos, Stem Cells, and Fertility Treatments.* Eugene, OR: Cascade Books, 2013. A readable and down-to-earth assessment of stem cells, cloning, and regenerative medicine in the form of answers to letters from his students and colleagues.

Kim, Hak-Min, et al. "Whole Genome Comparison of Donor and Cloned Dogs." *Scientific Reports* 3 (October 2013): 1-4. A comparison of the genomic sequence of Snuppy, the cloned dog, and the donor dog, Tai.

Korf, Bruce R., and Mira B. Irons. *Human Genetics and Genomics.* Hoboken, NJ: Wiley-Blackwell, 2013. A textbook of human genetics that gives a solid introduction to basic Mendelian and molecular genetics and then applies it to clinical problems and medical practice.

National Institutes of Health. Department of Health and Human Services. *Regenerative Medicine 2006.* Bethesda, MD: NIH Press, 2006. A collection of articles describing advances in stem cell and cloning technologies since this resource was first published in 2001.

Nussbaum, Martha, and Cass Sunstein, eds. *Clones and Clones: Facts and Fantasies About Human Cloning.* New York: W.W. Norton, 1999. A series of contributed essays on all aspects of human cloning, including science, ethics, and legal issues.

Trounson, Alan, and Natalie D. DeWitt. "Pluripotent Stem Cells from Cloned Human Embryos: Success at Long Last." *Cell Stem Cell* 12 (June 2013): 636-638. An excellent summary of the research that led to the first successful derivation of the first human embryonic stem cell lines from cloned human embryos.

Wilmut, Ian, and Roger Highfield. *After Dolly: The Uses and Misuses of Human Cloning.* New York: W. W. Norton, 2006. The scientist who directed the laboratory that created Dolly and other cloned sheep discusses the utility of therapeutic cloning and the dangers of reproductive cloning.

Wilmut, Ian, Keith Campbell, and Colin Tudge. *The Second Creation: Dolly and the Age of Biological Control.* New York: Farrar, Straus and Giroux, 2000. Coauthored by one of the creators of Dolly, this book examines the process of cloning and the steps that led to the cloning of the first mammal. It also provides insight into the reason why Dolly was cloned.

CLOSTRIDIUM DIFFICILE INFECTION
Disease/Disorder

Also known as: *C. difficile* disease, *C. difficile*-associated infection, *C. diff.*

Anatomy or system affected: Gastrointestinal system

Specialties and related fields: Family medicine, gastroenterology, infectious diseases

Definition: An acute, contagious gastrointestinal infection caused by the anaerobic, gram-positive, spore-forming bacillus, *Clostridium difficile.*

Causes and Symptoms

The bacteria *Clostridium difficile* that cause *C. difficile* infection are transmitted through the fecal-oral route. These bacteria are shed from feces of a colonized or infected person. When shed, they form spores as a protective mechanism when they enter the environment. They are able to survive in this form for many months on environmental surfaces. *C. difficile* infection is spread through contact with an infected or colonized patient, the environment, or the contaminated hands of a health care worker. The incubation period of *C. difficile* is unknown; however, one study suggests that it might be less than seven days.

The major risk factors for *C. difficile* infection include advanced age, hospitalization, and antibiotic use. Nearly every antibiotic has been implicated in *C. difficile* infection but clindamycin, cephalosporins, and floroquinolones are associated with a higher risk. When a patient receiving antibiotics ingests *C. difficile* spores, they germinate in the small intestine, where the normal flora has been altered. The spores multiply, flourish, and produce toxins. The toxins, toxin A and B, cause inflammation and mucosal damage leading to colitis. In severe infection, *C. difficile* can cause toxic megacolon, septic shock, and death.

When a patient becomes infected with *C. difficile*, fever, abdominal pain or tenderness, anorexia, nausea, and watery diarrhea commonly occur. In severe infection, the patient may develop pseudomembranous colitis, which may progress to toxic megacolon, a toxic dilation of the colon. If the patient develops toxic megacolon, then sepsis and death may quickly follow.

Information on *Clostridium Difficile* Infections

Causes: Bacterial infection

Symptoms: Fever, abdominal pain or tenderness, anorexia, nausea, watery diarrhea

Duration: Acute

Treatments: Antibiotics, sometimes IV fluids to prevent dehydration

Treatment and Therapy

Some cases may resolve in two to three days after discontinuing current antibiotic use. However in most cases a ten-day course of metronidazole or vancomycin orally is effective. Surgical intervention may be necessary in severe *C. difficile* infection if pseudomembranous colitis or perforation develop.

Perspective and Prospects

Before the mid 1970s, pseudomembranous colitis, an inflammatory process in the colon caused by bacterial toxins, was associated with the use of certain antibiotics; mainly lincomycin and clindamycin. It was not until 1978 that *C. difficile* was identified as the causative agent of antibiotic-associated pseudomembranous colitis. Since that time, *C. difficile* has become the leading cause of antibiotic-associated diarrhea. Between 2000 and 2007, the rate of *C. difficile*-related deaths rose 400 percent, and currently about 14,000 people in the United States die each year from such infections. Moreover, a hypervirulent strain called BI/NAP1/027 has emerged. This strain produces a type of toxin not previously seen in other strains; it is also highly resistant to the fluoroquinolone antibiotics. Many health care facilities have adopted infection prevention measures since 2010, but it is not yet clear how effective these measures have been in reducing infection rates. The American College of Gastroenterology reported in 2012 that while studies have shown that fecal microbiota transplants were effective in 91 percent of *C. diff* patients who had them, controlled trials of the treatment have not yet been performed.

—Collette Bishop Hendler, R.N., M.S., C.I.C.

See also Antibiotics; Bacterial infections; Bacteriology; Drug resistance; Emerging infectious diseases; Hospitals.

For Further Information:

Carrico, Ruth, et al. *Guide to the Elimination of* Clostridium difficile *in Healthcare Settings*. Washington, D.C.: APIC, 2008.

Centers for Disease Control and Prevention. "Healthcare-associated Infections (HAIs): *Clostridium difficile* Infection." *CDC*, Mar. 1, 2013.

Priedt, Robert. "HealthDay: Efforts to Prevent Hospital-Based Infection Falling Short, Survey Finds." *MedlinePlus*, Mar. 14, 2013.

Professional Guide to Diseases. 9th ed. Ambler, Pa.: Lippincott, 2008.

Surawicz, Christina M. "C. difficile Infection." *American College of Gastroenterology Patient Education & Resource Center*, Dec. 2012.

CLUB DRUGS

Disease/Disorder

Also known as: Designer drugs, psychedelics

Anatomy or system affected: All

Specialties and related fields: Alternative medicine, critical care, emergency medicine, pharmacology, preventive medicine, psychiatry, psychology, public health, toxicology

Definition: A slang term for a variety of substances of abuse that generally are used in social situations, have hallucinogenic properties, and may either excite or sedate the user.

Key terms:

amnesia: a diverse condition where there is complete or partial loss of memory for specific periods of time, for specific types of information, or both

blackout: memory loss, usually as a result of taking substances known to disrupt memory, in which the affected person may function as if aware of what is happening, despite having no memory of activities

psychedelic drugs: substances that cause alterations in perception and thinking, such as changes in awareness or sense of self and hallucinations

raves: social gatherings that are distinguished by long periods of music, dancing, and often a percentage of individuals using psychedelic drugs and other substances of abuse

synergistic effects: the combined effects of drugs interacting with one another, such that the effects of the drugs together have a compounded effect, greater than that of any one alone

Causes and Symptoms

Less expensive, easily accessible, intoxicating drugs can often be attractive to persons wanting a momentary high or psychedelic experience, when they are at a rave, dance party, or bar with friends. This desire, combined with a belief that club drugs seem safe, leads people to trying club drugs and sometimes using them regularly. Club drugs are often first used in dance clubs or with friends. The belief that such drugs are natural forms of prescription drugs or are not necessarily always illegal fuels a misconception of their safety. Because these drugs are psychedelic, the reactions that individual users have can vary quite significantly depending on the user's emotional state, concurrent use of other substances, underlying psychiatric conditions, personality, and past experience with the drug. Additionally, as they are street drugs, usually subject to some variability in their contents (such as being mixed with less expensive drugs), their quality may vary substantially. Finally, the individual situations where the substances are used can pose a variety of dangers of varying levels.

Club drugs go by many different names. They include substances such as gamma-hydroxybutyrate (GHB, Georgia Home Boy, Liquid X), ketamine hydrochloride (ketamine, special K), lysergic acid diethylamid (LSD, acid, blotter), methylenedioxymethamphetamine (MDMA, Adam, ecstasy, X), and rohypnol (roofies, roach, roche). They also include herbal ecstasy (herbal X, cloud nine, herbal bliss), which is a drug made from ephedrine or pseudoephedrine and caffeine. These substances vary in their effects but as a group cause a variety of positive reactions, including euphoria, feelings of well-being, emotional clarity, a decreased sense of personal boundaries, and feelings of empathy and closeness to others. They also can cause, however, significant negative reactions, including panic, impaired judgment, amnesia, impaired motor control, insomnia, paranoia, irrational behavior, flashbacks, hallucinations, rapid heartbeat, high blood pressure, chills, sweating, tremors, respiratory distress, convulsions, and violence. It is not uncommon for individuals to mix these drugs with alcohol, prescription drugs, and illegal drugs. Taken in combination, these substances can make these very dangerous reactions even worse.

Treatment and Therapy

The effects of club drugs vary somewhat by substance; as such, treatment also varies by substance. In general, though, club drugs may tend to be seen more in emergency care settings than in primary health care settings. This is due to the fact that some of the problems that they cause, as a group, are often of an emergency nature. For instance, overdose, strokes, allergic shock reactions, blackouts, loss of consciousness, and accidents related to these conditions may require emergency care. Similarly, dehydration and heat exhaustion can result from prolonged periods of dancing or other physical exertion, as can occur in rave situations, and result in a need for emergency care. Finally, because date rapes have been known to occur with these drugs, particularly rohypnol, injuries due to sexual assault also may need attention.

Certainly the long-term impact of problems like those described above may require some type of psychotherapy. In addition, problems related to the abuse of or dependence upon club drugs would be addressed in much the same manner as for other substances of abuse. General addiction treatment would be advised. A special area of treatment may also include exploration of what it is like to deal with blackouts, amnesia, and flashbacks, as these are features that are commonly reported with psychedelic drugs.

Perspective and Prospects

Club drugs emphasize that there is a continuing need for the social awareness of the dangers of substances that may otherwise seem harmless. Just because a substance is not listed as an illegal drug does not mean that it cannot be dangerous. Any drug, whether sold over the counter, by prescription, or any other place, can be misused and can be dangerous. Where drugs are used, how much is used, with whom they are used, and with what they are used can all make a difference.

Club drugs are also a reminder that in efforts to find ways of joining with each other, finding community, and discovering themselves and their relationships, people will sometimes resort to experimenting with substances. While the experimental use of psychedelic substances for psychotherapeutic work continues and may prove beneficial to certain groups of patients, such work is balanced by investigations into neurology, physiology, psychopharmacology, and psychology to ensure that the benefits do not outweigh the risks. Continued exploration of the neuronal, developmental, social, and other health effects of using club drugs is likely, as they pose a significant danger to public health, particularly that of younger populations.

—*Nancy A. Piotrowski, Ph.D.*

See also Addiction; Amnesia; Emergency medicine; Hallucinations; Herbal medicine; Intoxication; Marijuana; Panic attacks; Paranoia; Pharmacology; Seizures; Substance abuse; Tremors.

For Further Information:

Holland, Julie, comp. *Ecstasy: The Complete Guide-A Comprehensive Look at the Risks and Benefits of MDMA*. Rochester, Vt.: Inner Traditions International, 2001.

Jansen, Karl. *Ketamine: Dreams and Realities*. Ben Lomond, Calif.: Multidisciplinary Association for Psychedelic Studies, 2004.

Kuhn, Cynthia, et al. *Buzzed: The Straight Facts About the Most Used and Abused Drugs from Alcohol to Ecstasy*. 3d ed. New York: W. W. Norton, 2008.

O'Neill, John, and Pat O'Neill. *Concerned Intervention: When Your Loved One Won't Quit Alcohol or Drugs*. Oakland, Calif.: New Harbinger, 2003.

Stafford, Peter. *Psychedelics*. Berkeley, Calif.: Ronin, 2003.

CLUSTER HEADACHES

Disease/Disorder

Anatomy or system affected: Blood vessels, brain, head, nerves, nervous system

Specialties and related fields: Neurology

Definition: The most severe headache syndrome, characterized by paroxysmal onset of one side of the head, short duration, and episodic occurrence. Cluster headaches are often confused with migraine headaches, which are a similar syndrome but with different causes, patterns, and treatments.

Key terms:

alarm clock headaches: an earlier term for cluster headaches, emphasizing the characteristic awakening of sufferers during the night

circadian rhythm: the biological clockwise regularity associated with many body processes; most sufferers of cluster headaches have attacks at the same time of day during the same season of the year

cluster period: a time period, from two weeks to four months, during which cluster headaches occur; they usually disappear, or "enter remission," after the cluster period ends

paroxysmal: having a sudden, spasmlike, and painful onset

trigeminal-autonomic reflex pathway: the nerve pathway at the base of the brain activated during cluster attacks; the trigeminal nerve, the most important facial nerve for sensations such as temperature and pain, causes the "hot-poker-in-the-eye" pain typical of cluster headaches

unilateral: occurring only on one side (for example, on one side of the head or behind one eye)

Causes and Symptoms

Cluster headache is a well-defined, rare, but often misdiagnosed syndrome characterized by excruciatingly severe unilateral headaches that last from a half hour to three hours, with an average duration of forty-five minutes. Its features include paroxysmal onset of one side of the head, a short duration, and episodic occurrence. The pain often wakes sufferers one to two hours after they fall asleep. "Cluster" refers to the original perception that the headaches emerged in groups over a period of time (called the cluster period) lasting weeks to months, followed by periods that are free of pain and attacks (called remission or interim periods). The International Headache Society divides cluster headaches into episodic cluster and chronic cluster, with chronic further subclassified into primary and secondary variants. Chronic cluster headaches do not have a cessation, or interim, period but recur for years.

The precise cause of cluster headaches is unknown, although the season of the year is the most common trigger. Because they usually begin with spring or autumn, cluster headaches are often misattributed to seasonal allergies (such as hay fever) or seasonal-related stress (such as the beginning of school, final examinations, or the height of business cycles).

Positron emission tomography (PET) scanning has revealed that in cluster headaches the hypothalamus activates the trigeminal nerve, which is responsible for most of the severe pain. Located deep in the brain, the hypothalamus is also responsible for the internal biological clock that regulates the approximately twenty-four-hour sleep-wake cycle. The production and activity of the neurotransmitter serotonin, which is important in the self-regulation of these circadian rhythms, is also altered during attacks. Cluster headache is not related to the development of tumors or lesions.

Cluster headaches are rare. No more than .03 percent of the population ever experiences them. Men suffer them more than women do, although with improvements in epidemiological techniques the known ratio has been changed from 7:1 to 2:1. The age of onset is usually in the late twenties. As with migraine headaches, cluster headaches tend to run in families, with a fourteenfold increase in the chances of having them if a first-degree relative (mother, father, son, daughter, brother, or sister) suffers from the syndrome. In addition, a statistically significant incidence of migraine headaches exists in families with a cluster headache sufferer.

Cluster headache attacks, which are excruciatingly severe, debilitating, and dramatic, are almost always unilateral and occur from one to six times a day. They are most intense in, around, or behind one eye. Because the pain, commonly described as "boring" or "stabbing," often spreads into the upper teeth, jaw, neck, or temple, the headaches can be misdiagnosed as coming from dental or sinus problems. The attacks are rapid, peaking in five to ten minutes, and are occasionally, but not frequently, preceded by a visual aura. At-

tacks are much more likely to occur if tobacco and/or alcohol have been recently used, and they even more frequently will awaken sufferers during their first hour of napping or sleeping.

While migraine headache sufferers seek quiet, darkened places and try to remain still, cluster headache sufferers feel more pain if they try to lie down or recline in a chair. Typically, cluster headache sufferers are restless, pacing back and forth, or want to sit upright, holding their heads with their hands. A sufferer may even bang his or her head against a wall to obtain relief.

Treatment and Therapy

Treatments are oriented either toward abortive therapies or prophylactic therapies. Abortive approaches attempt to shorten the duration and/or intensity of an individual attack. Prophylactic approaches attempt to shorten or prevent the cluster periods themselves. While a fortunate characteristic of the attacks is their brevity, this feature also limits the range of abortive measures that can be undertaken; by the time that some agents are metabolized, the attack is over.

Although not always practical, a successful and safe abortive treatment is simply breathing 100 percent oxygen for ten to twenty minutes through a nonrebreathing mask. Also not always practical but effective are subcutaneous injections of sumatriptan (Imitrex) or intravenous, intramuscular, or subcutaneous injections of dihydroergotamine (Migranal). Other effective first-line therapies for acute intervention include zolmitriptan (Zomig) tablets, intranasal lidocane, or ergotamine (Cafergot).

Prophylactic, or preventive, treatments prevent attacks or at least lessen their intensity. All cluster headache sufferers should be on a prophylactic regimen (unless their cluster periods are less than two weeks, which is rarely the case). Verapamil (marketed as Calan, Covera, Isoptin, Tarka, and Verelan) is the most commonly prescribed medication because its mechanism as a calcium-channel blocker is well understood and it is usually effective. Occasionally, higher-than-typical doses must be employed. For those who do not respond well or receive sufficient relief on verapamil alone, a second medication such as ergotamine, lithium, methysergide (Sansert), or prednisone is often added. Sometimes, these second medications are effectively used alone, as are valproic acid and divalproex (Depakote).

In the event that pharmacology proves ineffective, several surgical or radiation techniques can block the trigeminal-autonomic reflex pathway. The benefits of these, or any, invasive treatments must be weighed against potential harm. For example, corneal anesthesia, needed to carry out these procedures, can put the eye at risk.

Perspective and Prospects

People have suffered from cluster headaches as long as people have suffered from headaches, although the rarity, seasonal occurrence, and symptoms of cluster headaches have made their recognition as a distinct syndrome difficult. Through PET scanning, neurovascular research has identified three areas of the brain particularly affected by cluster headaches. Because two of these areas are affected every time any sort of pain is felt, research is being concentrated on the third area, hypothalamic gray matter. Researchers expect that probes here will resolve their biggest debate: Is the vasodilation associated with cluster headache the primary problem or the result of activation of the trigeminal vascular system? Researchers do agree that cluster headaches, while distinct, belong to a family of related conditions, the cranial neuralgias.

—*Paul Moglia, Ph.D.*

See also Brain; Brain disorders; Head and neck disorders; Headaches; Migraine headaches; Pain; Pain management; Stress.

For Further Information:
Dalessio, Donald J. "Relief of Cluster Headache and Cranial Neuralgias." *Postgraduate Medicine* 109, no. 1 (January, 2001): 69-78.
Jasmin, Luc. "cluster Headache." *MedlinePlus*, Mar. 22, 2013
Kudrow, L. "Cluster Headache: Diagnosis and Management." *Headache* 19 (1979): 141-48.
Newman, Lawrence C., Peter Goadsby, and Richard B. Lipton. "Cluster and Related Headaches." In *Headache*, edited by Ninan T. Mathew. Philadelphia: Saunders, 2001.
Wood, Debra. "Cluster Headache." *Health Library*, Feb. 21, 2013.

COCCIDIOIDOMYCOSIS
Disease/Disorder

Also known as: San Joaquin Valley fever, valley fever
Anatomy or system affected: All
Specialties and related fields: Dermatology, family medicine, general surgery, internal medicine, microbiology, pulmonary medicine
Definition: A fungal infection acquired by inhaling the spores of particular soil-based fungi. It initially attacks the lungs and often resolves without causing symptoms, but it can cause pneumonia and disseminate throughout the body.

Key terms:
arthroconidia: asexual fungal spores that are made by the segmentation of preexisting fungal hyphae
endospores: tiny, round cells produced by spherules as they divide into smaller and smaller cells that are released upon rupture
erythema nodosum: inflammation of the fatty layer of the skin that results in red, painful bumps, usually located on the front of the legs
hyphae: the long, filamentous, often branching cells of many fungi
mycelium: a body of the fungal organism that consists of a collection of hyphae
mycetoma: a progressive and chronic fungal or bacterial infection that causes overgrowth of the infected tissue and the formation of sinuses filled with the infecting organism
pulmonary nodules: small, round growths on the lung that contain either trapped microorganisms or cancer cells
spherules: a thick-walled, spherical structure that is the tissue-specific form of *Coccidioides* species

Causes and Symptoms

Coccidioidomycosis is an infection caused by the soil-based fungi *Coccidioides immitis* (*C. immitis*) and *Coccidioides posadasii* (*C. posadasii*). These fungi are found only in the Western hemisphere, and they prefer dry, alkaline soils. *C. immitis* and *C. posadasii* are endemic to the southwestern United States (south-central California, Nevada, Arizona, New Mexico, and western Texas), those regions of Mexico that border the western United States, parts of Central America (Guatemala, Honduras, and Nicaragua), and the desert regions of South America (Argentina, Paraguay, and Venezuela).

While in the soil, *Coccidioides*, like most fungi, grows as thin, branching filaments called hyphae. A collection of hyphae is called a mycelium. When it rains, the mycelium grows quite rapidly, but once the soil dries out, it forms resting cells called arthrospores. If disturbed by wind, earthquakes, or soil excavation, these arthrospores become airborne and, if inhaled, can cause coccidioidomycosis.

Once inhaled, the arthrospore transforms into a thick-walled, spherical structure called a spherule that divides itself into hundreds of small endospores. When the spherule ruptures, it releases the endospores, which grow into spherules that form more endospores.

Information of Coccidioidomycosis

Causes: Fungal infection
Symptoms: Chest pains, chills, cough, fever, headache, spitting up blood, loss of appetite, muscle aches and stiffness, night sweats, rash, light sensitivity, excessive sweating, weight loss, wheezing
Duration: Up to three months or more
Treatments: Antifungal drugs

About 60 percent of patients show no symptoms, and the disease resolves spontaneously. Those patients who show symptoms suffer from fever, sore throat, headache, cough, fatigue, painful bumps on the skin (erythema nodosum), and chest pain approximately one to three weeks after inhaling arthrospores. About 95 percent of symptomatic patients recover without further problems after several weeks. If symptoms persist beyond three months, however, then the patient has chronic progressive coccidioidal pneumonia. Between 5 and 7 percent of patients with coccidioidal pneumonia form pulmonary nodules, which are areas of the lung where the immune system has walled-off the organism from the rest of the lung. On an X-ray, these nodules can look exactly like cancerous masses in the lung. A biopsy is often necessary to distinguish between lung cancer and coccidioidal pulmonary nodules. In 5 percent of patients with coccidioidal pulmonary nodules, the nodules enlarge to form pulmonary cavities that can become infected, rupture, and bleed, causing the release of pus between the lungs and the ribs (empyema). Small cavities (less than 2.5 centimeters) can heal after one to two years, but larger cavities can persist and cause the patient to spit up blood (hemoptysis) and allow the growth of fungi throughout the cavity (mycetoma).

A minority of patients develop disseminated coccidioidomycosis, in which the organism penetrates blood vessels, invades the bloodstream, and infects any organ in the body. Disseminated coccidioidomycosis occurs weeks or months after the primary pneumonia and can even develop in cases where there is no previous evidence of respiratory disease. Particular ethnic groups such as Filipinos and African Americans show increased risk of developing disseminated disease, as do pregnant women in the third trimester of their pregnancy, infants younger than one year old, diabetics, patients with acquired immunodeficiency syndrome (AIDS), or those taking drugs or suffering from diseases that suppress the immune system.

Treatment and Therapy

Asymptomatic or symptomatic infections are usually self-limited and require little more than supportive care. Patients with coccidioidal pneumonia require fluconazole or itraconazole treatment for at least twelve months and intravenous amphotericin B for stubborn cases. Pulmonary nodules are typically not treated, but they may require surgery. Pulmonary cavities are only treated with antifungal drugs if the patient shows symptoms. Surgical removal might also be warranted if the infection resists treatment. Disseminated coccidioidomycosis requires higher doses of fluconazole, and very sick patients may require amphotericin B or a combination of fluconazole and amphotericin B. Amphotericin B is preferred for pregnant women, since other drugs harm the developing fetus.

Perspective and Prospects

Coccidioidomycosis was first described in 1892 by Roberto Johann Wernicke and Alejandro Posadas in South America. The first case in the United States was reported in California in 1894. Two years later, Emmet Rixford and Thomas Caspar Gilchrist reported several clinical infections that were caused by an organism that, they thought, resembled the protozoan *Coccidia*. Therefore they named it *Coccidioides*, which means "*Coccidia*-like." In 1905, William Ophüls described the fungal life cycle and pathology of *C. immitis*. Charles E. Smith studied the epidemiology of coccidioidomycosis in the San Joaquin Valley of California and went on to develop the coccidioidin skin test and serological testing for the disease.

The Centers for Disease Control and Prevention released a study in 2013 that showed an increase in cases of coccidioidomycosis in the southwestern United States between 1998 and 2011. Cases in the states of Arizona, California, Nevada, New Mexico, and Utah increased from 2,265 reported in 1998 to 22,000 reported in 2011.

New treatments under investigation for coccidioidomycosis include posaconazole, voriconazole, caspofungin, and a new lipid-dispersal formulation of amphotericin B that reduces its kidney toxicity. Nikkomycin Z is another experimental agent that is very active against *Coccidioides* in culture and infected animals.

—*Michael A. Buratovich, Ph.D.*

See also Acquired immunodeficiency syndrome (AIDS); Aspergillosis; Candidiasis; Environmental diseases; Environmental health; Fungal infections; Immune system; Immunodeficiency disorders; Immunology; Immunopathology; Lungs; Microbiology; Mold and mildew; Pneumonia; Pulmonary diseases; Pulmonary medicine; Respiration.

For Further Information:

Anstead, Gregory M., and John R. Graybill. "Coccidioidomycosis." *Infectious Disease Clinics of North America* 20, no. 3 (September, 2006): 621-43.

Centers for Disease Control and Prevention. "Valley Fever Increasing in Some Southwestern States." *CDC*, Mar. 28, 2013.

Galgiani, John N. "Changing Perceptions and Creating Opportunities for Its Control." *Annals of the New York Academy of Sciences* 1111 (September, 2007): 1-18.

Kohnle, Diana. "Coccidioidomycosis." *Health Library*, Nov. 26, 2012.

Kwon-Chung, K. J., and John E. Bennett. *Medical Mycology*. Philadelphia: Lea and Febiger, 1992.

Parish, James, M., and James E. Blair. "Coccidioidomycosis." *Mayo Clinic Proceedings* 83, no. 3 (March, 2008): 343-348.

COCKAYNE DISEASE

Disease/Disorder

Also known as: Weber Cockayne syndrome, Neill-Dingwall syndrome

Anatomy or system affected: All

Specialties and related fields: Audiology, dentistry, dermatology, genetics, neurology, ophthalmology, optometry, otorhinolaryngology, pediatrics

Definition: A rare, inherited genetic disease characterized by short stature and premature aging.

Key terms:

ataxia: lack of voluntary coordination of muscle movements

contractures: the replacement of normally elastic tissues by inelastic tissues that limit flexibility and prevent normal movement

microcephaly: an abnormally small head

Causes and Symptoms

Cockayne syndrome (CS) is a rare disorder that results from mutations in the ERCC8/CSA or ERCC6/CSB genes. These genes encode proteins that repair damaged DNA.

Information on Cockayne Disease

Causes: Inherited mutations in the ERCC6 or ERCC8 genes

Symptoms: Dwarfism, mental retardation, microcephaly, growth failure, bird-like face, and photosensitivity

Duration: Cockayne syndrome I presents in childhood with death occurring by the second or third decade of life; Cockayne syndrome II presents at birth with death by age 6-7

Treatments: Protective clothing and sunscreen, dental, ophthalmologic, and neurological care; cochlear implants for hearing loss

---

Inactivating mutations in the CSA or CSB genes prevent cells from repairing their DNA, which leads to an accumulation of mutations, cell malfunction, and death. CS occurs in about 2 newborns per million live births.

There are three main types of CS, each of which differs in the age when symptoms first appear and their severity. In the case of Classical or Type I CS, symptoms usually appear after the first year of life. For the more severe, congenital Type II CS (also known as cerebro-oculo-facio-skeletal syndrome or Pena-Shokeir syndrome type II), symptoms appear at birth. Type III CS is a Cockayne Syndrome/xeroderma pigmentosum combination condition that will not be discussed further.

CS is an autosomal recessive genetic disease. Autosomal recessive diseases require that cells have two mutant copies of the gene in question in order to have the genetic disease.

CS children grow and develop at an abnormally slow rate and fail to gain weight normally (failure to thrive). In addition to microcephaly and noted mental retardation, their nervous systems deteriorate and they begin to show signs of ataxia and quick jerky movements. CS children also have skin that is highly sensitive to sun exposure (photosensitivity), thin, dry hair, hearing loss, progressive vision loss (progressive pigmentary retinopathy), and dental caries (cavities). In addition, CS children have characteristic facial features that include a pinched, narrow face with a beaked nose (bird-like face). Also, CS children who can walk have a "horse riding stance" when they stand as a result of their disproportionately long limbs, large hands and feet, and knee contractures. CS children also show accelerated aging and have an elderly look about them (progeroid appearance).

Treatment and Therapy

No cure exists for CS, but there are palliative measures that can be taken. CS patients should protect themselves from the sun at all costs; sunscreen and protective clothing are essential. Cochlear implants can minimize the effects of auditory impairment. Eye problems (optic atrophy and cataracts) require the care of an ophthalmologist. Dentists can help deal with the severe tooth decay seen in CS children. Neurological deterioration and ataxia requires consultation with a neurologist. Parents known to carry mutations in CSA or CSB should consult a geneticist for prenatal evaluation and genetic counseling.

—*Michael A. Buratovich, Ph.D.*

See also Audiology; Burns and scalds; Dentistry; Dermatology; Dermopathology; Failure to thrive; Genetic counseling; Ophthalmology; Optometry

For Further Information:

Moriwaki, Shinichi. "Hereditary Disorders with Defective Repair of UV-Induced DNA Damage." *Japanese Clinical Medicine* 4 (2013): 29-35.
Woliver, Robbie. *Alphabet Kids-From ADD to Zellweger Syndrome: A Guide to Developmental, Neurobiological and Psychological Disorders to Parents and Professionals.* London: Jessica Kingsley Publishers, 2008.

Cognitive development
Development

Anatomy or system affected: Brain, nervous system, psychic-emotional system

Specialties and related fields: Environmental health, genetics, pediatrics, psychology

Definition: The growth and age-related changes that occur over time in children's mental processes and in activities related to the faculties of attending, learning, perceiving, problem solving, thinking, and remembering.

Key terms:

adaptation: change or adjustment made to create a balance between existing thought structures and the environment

assimilation: the process of attempting to explain a new experience in terms of existing schemes

cognition: the activity of knowing and the processes through which knowledge is acquired and used

cognitive equilibrium: a term used by psychologist Jean Piaget to describe the balanced relationship between an individual's mental processes and the environment

conservation: understanding that an object's properties remain unchanged when its appearance is altered

egocentrism: seeing the world only from one's own point of view; being unable to acknowledge or recognize different perspectives

equilibration: the process of adapting or adjusting one's existing knowledge or mental structures to the new situation, thus constructing more complex and sophisticated structures

miseducation: the tendency to hurry and pressure children to perform activities and tasks for which they are not cognitively or physically ready

reflexive: referring to an automatic response to external stimuli

reversibility: the ability to negate an action by mentally reversing it or imagining its opposite

scheme: a pattern of thought constructed by the child to organize experience in a meaningful way

Physical and Psychological Factors

The mental capabilities and skills of humans develop gradually over a period of time from birth through adolescence. As a child ages, the quality of the processes by which he or she responds to and adapts thinking to particular situations and evaluates, plans, and solves problems changes over time.

In childhood, the brain develops very rapidly. At birth, the human brain already weighs about 25 percent of its adult weight. By six months of age, this figure is 50 percent. By the age of five, the child's brain has achieved 90 percent of its eventual weight. While the basic structure of the brain is genetically and biologically determined, environment and experience play a significant role in the development of cognition. Children's biological constitutions may affect the way in which they interact with and respond to their environment.

According to the Swiss psychologist Jean Piaget (1896-1980), the cognitive growth of all children follows a universal or holistic pattern of development through infancy, childhood, and adolescence. The thought processes of young children are less mature and complex than those of older children, and as children grow and experience life, their cognitive structures become more sophisticated, as well as qualitatively different from those of children in earlier or later stages of development. Cognitive structures, or "schemes" as Piaget called them, are thought patterns that children construct to explain, understand, or interpret their experiences. When children's schemes or thought processes are in harmony with their environment, they experience cognitive equilibrium. When children encounter new and puzzling events or objects, they are in a state of imbalance or disequilibrium and must achieve equilibrium via a process called equilibration. This process consists of adapting or adjusting one's existing knowledge or mental structures to the new situation, thus constructing more complex and sophisticated thought structures. Adaptation takes place through the processes of assimilation and accommodation.

Assimilation refers to the process of attempting to explain a new experience in terms of existing schemes. For example, a child who sees a pony for the first time may call it a "kitty" because a cat is the existing model of that child for four-legged animals. Noticing that there are differences between the scheme of a cat and the reality of the pony, however, the child soon attempts to modify existing mental structures to fit the new experience. This process of modification is accommodation. Through assimilation and accommodation, children organize their knowledge into schemes that better explain their observations.

Piaget's theory of cognitive development, with its emphasis on continuous and active organization and adaptation involving assimilation and accommodation, implies that children actively construct their own knowledge. This construction is based on the child's current stage of cognitive development: Piaget proposed that all children in a specific, universal cognitive stage construct similar interpretations of similar experiences.

According to Piaget, cognitive development can be divided into four major stages. The order in which these stages occur is universal, and all individuals must experience each stage. No stage can be skipped, although the rates at which children go through a stage may vary. The basis for Piaget's insistence on the unvarying sequence of cognitive stages is a concept known as epigenesis, which he used to explain the gradual development of thinking processes. Each new structure or cognitive skill is based on and develops from an earlier one. Hence, each stage, and each structure within each stage, is necessary for the development of new, more advanced structures. Piaget called this feature of development "hierarchization."

The four stages of cognitive development identified by Piaget are the sensorimotor stage (up to age two), the preoperational stage (two to seven years of age), the concrete operations stage (seven to eleven years of age), and the formal operations stage (age eleven and up).

During the sensorimotor stage, children act upon their environment and acquire knowledge of it through their senses and motor activities. In the first two years, cognition progresses from reflexive actions, such as sucking and grasping, to primitive symbolic functions or representation, such as language use and symbolic play. The sensorimotor stage can be further divided into six substages. Substage 1 lasts from birth to one month and centers on exercising basic reflexes, including eye movements, sound orientation, and vocalization, and assimilating and accommodating objects into reflexive schemes. Substage 2, from one to four months, consists of simple repetitive actions, such as thumb sucking, which are discovered by chance and acquired through repeated trials. Piaget called these actions primary circular reactions. Substage 3 appears between four and eight months of age. Piaget named this period secondary circular reactions. Infants notice stimulating events in the environment beyond their bodies-such as a noise made by squeezing a toy or a movement caused by touching an object-and attempt to re-create the events.

Between eight and twelve months of age, infants experience substage 4, or the coordination of secondary schemes. This means that infants can use two already acquired schemes to reach a simple goal. For example, they are able to remove an object to grasp a hidden toy. These early coordinations reflect intentional behavior and simple problem solving. Tertiary circular reactions are characteristic of substage 5, appearing between the ages of twelve and eighteen months. Infants display curiosity, experiment actively, and find new ways of solving problems. Their behaviors are goal-directed but are carried out through trial and error. Substage 6, from eighteen to twenty-four months, reflects inner experimentation or new mental combinations. The infant now displays symbolic functioning through language, imagery, and symbolic play. Children also begin to acquire a sense of cause and effect.

During the sensorimotor stage, children develop the ability to imitate. Piaget believed that novel actions could be imitated by infants around eight to twelve months of age and needed much practice. The ability to imitate absent models, called deferred imitation, appears between twelve and twenty-four months of age.

Another important milestone of the sensorimotor stage is the development of a sense of object permanence. Before the age of four months, objects are of interest to infants only if they can be experienced by the senses. They lose interest in objects that are hidden; such objects no longer exist for them. Between four and eight months of age, they may retain interest in partially hidden objects, and by twelve to eighteen months of age, the concept of objects is stronger. The idea that objects have permanence even when not seen appears around the age of eighteen months, when children can represent objects mentally.

The preoperational stage, the second of Piaget's stages of cognitive development, occurs between the ages of two and seven. During this stage, children increase their use of words and images to represent objects and experiences. Piaget called this stage "preoperational" because he believed that children had not yet achieved "operations," or cognitive schemes to think logically. The preoperational stage can further be divided into a preconceptual period (two to four years of age) and an intuitive period (four to seven years of age).

Characteristics of the preconceptual period include the development of symbolic representation, expressed through developing language and pretend play. Children in this stage demonstrate animism; that is, they attribute life to nonliving things. They are egocentric, seeing the world as revolving around themselves and having difficulty in understanding other points of view.

Although still egocentric during the intuitive period, children are less so than before. Piaget argued that they also display centered thinking, or the capacity to classify objects according to one feature or attribute even though several may be evident. Children in this stage find it hard to conserve, or understand that a substance or object's properties can remain unaltered even when its appearance changes. They cannot reverse actions mentally, such as realizing that water poured from a tall glass into a flat dish is the same amount of water and would look as high as before if poured back into the glass.

In the concrete operations stage, between the ages of seven and eleven, children's cognitive structures develop to include operations that help them think more competently and logically about objects and events experienced. Children are less egocentric; are able to classify, sequence, and quantify more efficiently; and display skills of conservation and reversibility. Piaget believed, however, that children are still unable to hypothesize or think about abstract concepts during this stage.

From eleven years onward, children enter the formal operations stage. They can hypothesize and reason inductively about abstract concepts such as religion, goodness, or beauty. According to Piaget, this transition from concrete to formal operations is very gradual. He also suggested that many adults reason at the formal operations level only if a problem is important or interesting to them.

Another approach to cognitive development compares individuals as information-processing systems to computers. The hardware in humans consists of physical components such as the brain, the sensory receptors, and the nervous system. The software consists of the mental processes and strategies used to store, interpret, access, and analyze information. The information-processing mechanisms of young children are elementary and immature. As children grow, as their nervous systems and brains develop, their information-processing strategies improve and become more sophisticated, like modern computers.

Humor and the appreciation of humor have also been associated with an individual's level of cognitive development. A child whose mental structures and language acquisition have developed enough to enable the child to notice incongruities or deviations from the usual and expected can perceive humor in incongruous situations. To a two-year-old, calling a bird a cat may seem hilarious or making barking sounds and pretending to be a dog may provoke much laughter. A picture of a fish in a tree will amuse a three-year-old. Seven-year-olds who can understand the double meanings inherent in language will laugh at puns and "knock-knock" jokes and can create riddles. As children's understanding of language ambiguities matures and becomes more sophisticated, they are able to appreciate more complex humor.

Sociocultural Factors

The Russian psychologist Lev Vygotsky (1896-1934) believed that cognition is sociocultural, that it is influenced by values and beliefs of cultures as well as by the specific tools that each culture uses for adaptation and problem solving. Children are born with simple mental processes such as attention, memory, perception, and sensation. These processes develop into what Vygotsky called higher mental functions, or more competent ways of using intellectual capabilities. The strategies and tools for thinking are taught to children by their culture and develop as young children interact and collaborate with capable adults or peers, who guide and model problem-solving techniques that encourage cognitive development. Vygotsky called the difference between children's level of achievement when working independently and their potential development when guided by a competent adult the zone of proximal development.

For Vygotsky, language plays an important role in cognitive growth. Adults use language to transmit the culture's ways of thinking to the child. The child uses language to plan and regulate activities and behavior and to solve problems. Language helps children organize thought and reach objectives. Younger children verbalize phrases and words aloud during this process, but older children and adults internalize speech that, although no longer uttered aloud, still organizes and guides thinking and action.

Disorders and Effects

The importance of experience on the cognitive development of children implies that when children live in intellectually impoverished environments, their cognitive development may be stunted or fail to reach its potential. Studies show the children whose parents play and interact with them in a variety of ways and provide stimulating materials to engage their interest and attention do better in school than children who lack this cognitive stimulation. Verbal interactions between parents and children, collaborative activities with competent peers, and guided activities with adults have been found to help children improve their thinking and planning abilities. Mary Ainsworth's research on mother-infant attachment showed that mothers who interacted with their infants had securely attached children who, in turn, felt confident enough to explore their environment more independently than less securely attached infants. In this way, cognitive growth was affected by social functioning. Some longitudinal studies have found that securely attached children demonstrated more cognitive competence through childhood and adolescence than children who did not have secure attachments. Parental support and responsiveness encouraged cognitive growth over time.

The effects of the curriculum within programs and schools

for children can maximize or discourage cognitive development. The Cognitively Oriented Curriculum, developed at the High/Scope Institute by David Weikart and his associates, focused on active learning. It was based on Piagetian principles and involved children in planning and other cognitively oriented activities. The games that children play can also affect their thinking and can be utilized in the curriculum. Research by Constance Kamii and Rheta DeVries has shown how the use of games and play-oriented activities can help children develop numerical thinking, language competency, and other cognitive abilities, while promoting autonomy or the ability to think independently and enhancing cooperative and social skills.

As an understanding of the negative effects of poverty and lack of enriching experiences increased during the 1950s and 1960s, initiatives such as Head Start and various other compensatory early childhood programs were established in the United States to reverse the effects of early cognitive deprivation. Initial studies on the effects of such programs were extremely encouraging, and gains in intelligence quotient (IQ) scores and cognitive performance were found to be significant. It was later discovered, however, that such gains could be lost if intellectual stimulation was not maintained. The need to continue to provide stimulating educational experiences was recognized. It was found that positive attitudes toward schooling and a sense of self-esteem also occur when compensatory education and enrichment programs are provided.

The increasing evidence of brain research concerning the importance of stimulating experiences to the developmental process during the first few years of life, as well as knowledge about the growth and weight of the brain in infancy, suggests the need to provide such experiences from a very early age. Prenatal experiences and their impact on cognitive and other areas of development are also being studied.

The concept of cognitive development as a highly active process that occurs in a series of stages has certain implications for the education and well-being of children. One implication is that children in a particular stage of development should not be hurried but should be allowed to develop and mature at their own pace. Hurrying children beyond their developmental capacity can cause mental and emotional damage. David Elkind uses the term "miseducation" to refer to the tendency to hurry and pressure children to perform activities and tasks for which they are not cognitively or physically ready. He believes that miseducation is an increasingly common problem in the United States.

Another implication of the active nature of cognitive development is that children should be given numerous opportunities to explore materials and the environment, and thus acquire knowledge for themselves. Materials, equipment, and knowledge to be discovered should be appropriate to the stage of the child and should be based on the child's existing structures and schemes.

Perspective and Prospects

The cognitive and intellectual development of children was not studied seriously or scientifically until the late nineteenth century. G. Stanley Hall was the first person to develop an instrument-the questionnaire-to study the minds of children. The twentieth century saw the emergence of developmental theories such as the psychoanalytic theory of Sigmund Freud and the psychosocial theory of Erik Erikson. Behaviorism, which viewed children's learning and development as passive and therefore controllable, dominated much of the earlier part of the century. John Watson proposed that children's minds were like blank tablets on which anything could be written. In other words, children's development was thought to be shaped solely by their environment and by the people around them. This view had been held in the seventeenth century by the philosopher John Locke. Watson's theory was extended by B. F. Skinner, who evolved a learning theory based on the use of reinforcement and external stimuli to influence and control behavior. Albert Bandura's theory of social cognition departed from the earlier passive learning theories of Watson and Skinner. He believed that individuals actively process information. Bandura also emphasized the role of observational learning, or learning by observing and mimicking others and thinking about outcomes, in the process of children's development.

During the 1950s, a cognitive revolution occurred as the theory and research of Jean Piaget became known. Piaget was interested in how children think, in their "wrong" answers as indicators of their stage of cognitive development, and in their active construction of knowledge. He observed his own children's early interactions and explorations. He also utilized the clinical method, in which he interviewed children of different ages to understand the nature of their hypotheses and problem-solving strategies. The questions in this method were flexible and depended on the responses given by the child.

Piaget's theories were later criticized and were seen to underestimate children's abilities. His assumption of the heterogeneity or universality of cognitive stages was also questioned. Critics charged that Piaget did not give enough credit to the role of cultural and social factors in cognitive development. The impact of culture and social interaction on the child's thinking and use of strategies as culturally transmitted tools of thought was studied by Lev Vygotsky. In the last decades of the twentieth century, Vygotsky's ideas aroused much interest. The difference in learning styles was also studied, and it was recognized that learning styles vary across cultures as well as from individual to individual.

Many neo-Piagetian theories attempted to integrate some Piagetian assumptions with information-processing approaches. These approaches examined cognitive processes such as memory and attention and demonstrated their influence on children's cognitive development.

The influence of the environment and various activities cannot be overemphasized in its importance to cognitive development. As technologies continue to develop for use by children, ranging from toys to educational tools, it will be crucial to consider all aspects of development carefully. One example is recent research evaluating the impact on brain development of frequent video game and computer use by children. The research suggested that activities that encourage vision and movement skills, to the exclusion of other skills important to development, may be problematic. The concern is that some capacities may become overused, while others may not receive enough stimulation to encourage adequate development. More research is certainly needed to examine the potential impact of new technologies and exposure to diverse stimuli. Important lessons can be learned from history in an effort to guard against anything that impoverishes a child's learning environment.

—*Nillofur Zobairi, Ph.D.;*
updated by Nancy A. Piotrowski, Ph.D.

See also Bonding; Developmental disorders; Developmental stages; Learning disabilities; Mental retardation; Motor skill development; Psychiatric disorders; Psychiatry, child and adolescent; Reflexes, primitive.

For Further Information:

Berk, Laura E. *Child Development*. 9th ed. Boston: Pearson/Allyn & Bacon, 2012.

Berk, Laura E., and Adam Winsler. *Scaffolding Children's Learning: Vygotsky and Early Childhood Education*. Washington, D.C.: National Association for the Education of Young Children, 1995.

Bjorklund, David F. *Children's Thinking: Developmental Function and Individual Differences*. 4th ed. Belmont, Calif.: Thomson/Wadsworth, 2005.

"Cognitive Development: One-Year-Old." *American Academy of Pediatrics*, May 11, 2013.

"Cognitive Development: Two-Year-Old." *American Academy of Pediatrics*, May 11, 2013.

Elkind, David. *Miseducation: Preschoolers at Risk*. New York: Alfred A. Knopf, 1987.

Sears, William, et al. *The Portable Pediatrician: Everything You Need to Know about Your Child's Health*. New York: Little, 2011.

Shore, Rima. *Rethinking the Brain: New Insights into Early Development*. Rev. ed. New York: Families and Work Institute, 2003.

"Zero to Three." *National Center for Infants, Toddlers, and Families*, 2012.

COGNITIVE ENHANCEMENT

Treatment

Anatomy or system affected: Brain

Specialties and related fields: Psychiatry, neurology, cognitive psychology

Definition: An increase in one or more of the cognitive processes of the brain, including learning, memory, attention, perception, problem solving, and decision making.

Key terms:

agonist: a chemical that mimics or increases the effect of a neurotransmitter

antagonist: a chemical that inhibits or decreases the effect of a neurotransmitter

mnemonic: technique used to facilitate memory by modifying the way that information is learned

neuromodulator: a brain chemical that increases or decreases the effect of a neurotransmitter

psychostimulant: any drug that increases the overall excitability of neurons in one or more neural pathways

reaction time: the amount of time required to complete a task

transcranial direct current stimulation (tDCS): a technique that uses small electrodes placed on the surface of the scalp to excite or inhibit regions deep within the brain

Perspective and Prospects

Cognitive enhancement involves the use of a specific intervention to achieve the goal of improving one or more mental processes. The processes that may be enhanced include perception, attention, working memory, long-term memory, language, problem solving, and decision making. Some cognitive enhancers are also purported to increase intelligence.

There are many ways that people attempt to enhance cognition, including nutritional supplements, over-the-counter and prescription drugs, by modifying training paradigms, with the assistance of interactive technologies, and through the direct electrical stimulation of the brain. Although many anecdotal and popular accounts of how various substances and technologies can increase cognition exist, experimental and clinical evidence suggest that there are very few, evidence-validated methods for achieving cognitive enhancement.

The ginkgo is one of the oldest surviving species of trees. The fan-shaped leaves of the Ginkgo biloba tree have been used in traditional Chinese medicine to boost memory for centuries. Though there is evidence that ginkgo leaf extract may have some memory-restoring effects for those elderly suffering from mild dementia or Alzheimer's disease, laboratory studies have failed to find any evidence for such an effect on cognition in normal, healthy individuals. Despite the lack of research support for ginkgo as a memory enhancer, it is still a popular supplement and is touted as an ingredient in so-called "energy drinks."

Energy drinks are carbonated beverages that contain high levels of caffeine and other assorted ingredients, which are purported to affect attention and learning. Along with ginkgo, the amino acid L-taurine is a common ingredient in energy drinks. Despite claims that taurine and caffeine work together to enhance cognition, researchers have failed to find any consistent positive or negative effects of adding this substance to the diet. Indeed, when positive effects on cognition were observed, they were most often attributed to the effect of caffeine on the brain.

One of the most widely used cognitive enhancers, both today and historically, is the ubiquitous alkanoid, caffeine. Caffeine is found in varying quantities in tea, coffee, soft drinks, energy drinks, and chocolate. This drug, which is classified as a psychostimulant, requires between 20-45 minutes before the effects are experienced and has a half-life of 5-6 hours. Like most stimulants, caffeine increases the level of excitation within the brain. An antagonist of the neuromodulator adenosine, caffeine indirectly increases the release of the neurotransmitters dopamine and norepinephrine by decreasing the levels of inhibition on both.

There is general agreement that moderate levels of caffeine enhance alertness, attention, and decrease reaction time, whereas high levels of caffeine have an impairing effect on attention. What is less clear is whether caffeine has any positive effect on learning and memory. The lack of consistency in experimental studies may reflect the complex way that caffeine intake, normal patterns of use (i.e., how much does one normally ingest each day), and task difficulty and demands all interact.

Nicotine is another readily available substance that may have some mild cognitive enhancing effects. This highly addictive compound, commonly found in tobacco, is an agonist of the neurotransmitter acetylcholine. The stimulating effects of nicotine on acetylcholine networks in the brain are likely responsible for the decreases in reaction time and slight increases in working memory function that have been demonstrated.

Just like nicotine and caffeine, prescription drugs that have been reported to enhance cognition are psychostimulants. Both Ritalin (methylphenidate) and Adderall (amphetamine salts) act to increase excitation within the brain by increasing the release of dopamine. Most often prescribed to ameliorate the hyperactivity associated with attention deficit hyperactivity disorder (ADHD), these drugs have been abused by non-ADHD children and adults because of their ability to increase focus and positively impact long-term memory retention. Similarly, the anti-narcolepsy drug modafinil has gained notoriety due to its purported high level of abuse by college students and professionals striving to get ahead by working long hours. Unfortunately, there are some studies that suggest that the abuse of prescription psychostimulant medications may have adverse long-term effects on the brain and other bodily systems.

Instead of taking drugs, cognition may also be enhanced by manipulating the way that information is presented and processed. As was demonstrated by Hermann Ebbinghaus in 1885, the amount of time required to learn information may be reduced drastically if the learning trials are spread out across days rather than crammed together in one day. Similarly, mnemonics can greatly enhance the amount of information that can be learned and retrieved. Techniques such as visualizing items to be remembered, anchoring new information to existing memories, and chunking large numbers of items into meaningful units, have all been shown to enhance learning and memory in both laboratory and real-life (e.g., classroom) settings.

Despite the fact that optimal results are seen when cognitive enhancing techniques are used by individuals in face-to-face settings, some mnemonic and other cognitive enhancing techniques have been integrated into computer-based "brain training" programs. Although these programs are based on neuroscientific and cognitive psychological research findings, there are few studies that have examined the effects of computer-based training on enhancing cognition directly. What studies have shown is that though there are often moderate enhancements for the specific games that are used as training (which are designed to enhance cognition in general), there is no evidence of transfer of the computer-developed skills to novel tasks, intelligence, or other areas of cognition. In the few studies that did show transfer effects outside the computer, it should be noted that the participants were required to train on the games for extended periods (i.e., hours) each day for several weeks. Thus, such prolonged and time-consuming training regimens may be prohibitive for general use.

Rather than using computers and technology to train one's brain to become more efficient and accurate, transcranial direct current stimulation (tDCS) is being used to directly stimulate portions of the brain by modifying the local electromagnetic fields in those regions. The stimulation is facilitated by placing electrodes to the scalp and applying a small electrical current. A few studies have demonstrated that tDCS enhances attention, various forms of long-term learning and memory, and working memory. Though the technique was first developed decades ago, it has only recently begun to be used in clinical and research settings. Thus, although tDCS may hold some promise for enhancing cognition, there is more that needs to be known about the safety and efficacy of this technique. For example, studies have shown that when some cognitive processes are enhanced by tDCS, others may then be impaired.

While advances in medicine and technology continue to introduce novel ways to attempt to enhance cognition, bioethicists debate whether cognitive enhancement should be pursued in the first place. Though cognitive enhancers such as nicotine and caffeine have been present for centuries, direct stimulation of the brain and abuse of prescription drugs have prompted a reexamination of the morality concerning cognitive enhancement and, even, what it means to be human.

—*Jerome L. Rekart, Ph.D.*

See also Memory loss

For Further Information:

Buchanan, Allen. *Better Than Human: The Promises and Perils of Enhancing Ourselves.* Oxford: Oxford University Press, 2011.

Hildt, Elisabeth, and Andreas G. Franke, eds. *Cognitive Enhancement: An Interdisciplinary Perspective (Trends in Augmentation of Human Performance).* New York: Springer, 2013.

Rekart, Jerome L. *The Cognitive Classroom: Using Brain and Cognitive Science to Optimize Student Success.* Lanham, PA: Rowman & Littlefield Publishers, Education Division, 2013.

Smith, Martha J., and M. Elizabeth Smith. "Are Prescription Stimulants 'Smart Pills'? The Epidemiology and Cognitive Neuroscience of Prescription Stimulant Use by Normal Health Individuals." *Psychological Bulletin* 137, no. 5 (2011): 717-741.

COLD AGGLUTININ DISEASE
Disease/Disorder

Anatomy or system affected: Blood, blood vessels, chest, circulatory system, ears, feet, hands, immune system, liver, lungs, lymphatic system, nose, respiratory system, skin, spleen, urinary system

Specialties and related fields: Bacteriology, emergency medicine, hematology, histology, immunology, oncology, pathology, pediatrics, pulmonary medicine, radiology, rheumatology, serology, urology, vascular medicine, virology

Definition: A disease characterized by the production of antibodies against red blood cells that destroy them and cause anemia.

Key terms:

anemia: a deficiency of the oxygen-carrying protein hemoglobin or the red blood cells that contain hemoglobin

antibodies: a blood protein produced by B-lymphocytes in response to the introduction of antigens into the body that binds to and neutralizes these antigens

antigens: toxins or other foreign substances introduced into the body that induce an immune response against it

complement proteins: a group of proteins in blood that initiate a biochemical cascade when an antibody is bound to a cell surface that culminates in the destruction of that cell and its clearance from the body

hemolysis: the destruction of red blood cells

plasmapheresis: a clinical procedure that removes blood from the body, separates it into liquid or plasma and cells, and then returns the cells to the body without the plasma and its components

Causes and Symptoms

Cold agglutinin disease (CAD) is one of a group of blood disorders known as autoimmune hemolytic anemias (AIHAs). The immune systems of patients who suffer from AIHAs attack their own red blood cells, which cause routine red blood cell destruction (hemolysis). Destruction of red blood cells faster than they can be replaced leads to anemia or an abnormally low number of red blood cells. Exposure to cold initiates symptoms in CAD patients, which sets it apart from other types of AIHA. Approximately 1 in 300,000 people suffer from CAD.

Everyone tends to have circulating antibodies against their own red blood cells. Because the concentration of these antibodies tends to be rather low, they usually do not cause any problems. However, in some people, the concentration of these anti-red blood cell antibodies increases. In the case of primary CAD, the increase in the concentration of these antibodies occurs for reasons that remain unclear. In the case of secondary CAD, though, certain types of bacterial and viral infections or particular kinds of white blood cell cancers boost the concentration of these red blood cell-specific antibodies.

At low body temperatures (usually between 28-31°C or 82-88°F), which usually prevail during the winter months,

the anti-red blood cell antibodies bind to the surfaces of red blood cells. The bound antibodies cause them to aggregate and activate complement proteins. Activation of the complement pathway culminates in the boring of small holes in red blood cell membranes and hemolysis. Those red blood cells that escape destruction by complement proteins are marked by them for destruction, and are filtered out by the liver and spleen and destroyed.

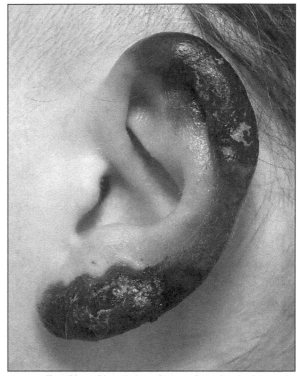

An ear affected by cold agglutinin disease. (New England Journal of Medicine)

The whole-scale destruction of red blood cells causes anemia and other symptoms as cell debris becomes lodged in small blood vessels and blocks blood flow. CAD symptoms include pain and a purplish tinge in the fingers and toes (Raynaud's phenomenon), pallor, trouble breathing (dyspnea), and fatigue. Upon physical examination, patients with CAD may show purplish discoloration of the ears, forehead, tip of the nose, and digits (acrocyanosis). Enlargement of the spleen (splenomegaly), jaundice, and fever are also seen in more severe CAD patients.

Treatment and Therapy

Most cases of secondary CAD result from diseases that are, themselves, self-limiting and only of short duration. For most cases of primary CAD, avoidance of the cold prevents the onset of symptoms. CAD patients should eat foods rich in folic acid (e.g., fresh fruits and vegetables) and iron (e.g., meat, egg yolks, beans, artichokes), which help build red blood cells.

Information on Cold Agglutinin Disease

Causes: Elevated blood levels of antibodies directed against red blood cells

Symptoms: Painful fingers; toes with a purplish tinge; passing dark urine, especially during exposure to cold; anemia; chronic fatigue; pallor; difficulty breathing

Duration: In children and young adults, acute hemolysis lasts 1-3 weeks and all evidence disappears within 6 months, but in older patients, the disease lasts as long as the patient is exposed to cold

Treatments: Avoiding cold, folic acid and iron supplementation, Rituximab, plasmapheresis, blood transfusions

For more severe cases of CAD, intravenous administration of Rituximab promptly resolves the disease. A genetically engineered antibody, Rituximab binds to the surfaces of B-lymphocytes-the cells that produce antibodies-and removes them from the body. Rituximab can provide relief for up to one year. Combination treatments with purine analogs (e.g., fludarabine, azathioprine, etc.) may achieve faster responses and longer remission times. Other immune-suppressing drugs that have been used to treat severe cases of CAD include cyclophosphamide, chlorambucil, prednisone, vincristine, and interferons, all with varying degrees of success.

For emergencies, plasmapheresis can reduce the concentration of those antibodies that bind red blood cells in the blood. Because it acts quickly, plasmapheresis provides time for drugs to act, or for the patient to undergo surgery. Blood transfusions with warmed, washed, carefully matched red blood cells are only used as a last resort.

CAD patients should strongly consider relocating to warmer climates and should wear protective clothing to prevent chilling the body.

Perspective and Prospects

Karl Landsteiner first described cold agglutinins in 1903. In 1918, M.C. Clough and I.R. Richter identi?ed the pathologic association between the presence of cold agglutinins and red blood cell destruction and its occurrence during respiratory infections. D.M. Horstmann and H. Tatlock reported the first case of secondary CAD in 1943 when they detected cold agglutinins in the serum of patients with pneumonia. In 1957, W.H. Christenson, J.H. Dacie and colleagues identified antibodies as the cold agglutinins, but H. Schubothe actually coined the phrase "cold agglutinin disease" in 1966.

Other types of drugs that have been developed to treat non-Hodgkin's lymphoma and multiple myeloma may also effectively treat CAD. For example, a drug called bortezomib prevents cells from degrading damaged or unwanted proteins and has been approved for the treatment of multiple myeloma. Bortezomib depletes B-cells and might be effective as a treatment for CAD. Other experimental drugs might also prove useful as future treatments for recalcitrant cases of CAD.

—*Michael A. Buratovich, Ph.D.*

See also Antibodies; Blood vessels; Hematology; Immunology; Immunopathology; Raynaud's phenomenon; Vascular medicine

For Further Information:

Jeskowiak, Antonia, and Tobias Goerge. "Images in Clinical Medicine: Cutaneous Necrosis Associated with Cold Agglutinins." *New England Journal of Medicine* 369 (July 2013): e1.

Rodak, Bernadette F., George A. Fritsma, and Elaine Keohane. *Hematology: Clinical Principles and Applications*. 4th ed. St. Louis: Elsevier, 2012.

Swiecicki, Paul L., Livia T. Hegerova, and Morie A. Gertz. "*Cold Agglutinin Disease*." Blood 122, no. 7 (August 2013): 1114-1121.

COLD SORES

Disease/Disorder
Also known as: Fever blisters
Anatomy or system affected: Mouth, skin
Specialties and related fields: Family medicine
Definition: An infectious disease characterized by thin-walled vesicles around the mouth.

Causes and Symptoms

Cold sores are an infectious disease caused by the herpes simplex virus. Cold sores and fever blisters are two terms used for sores that develop around the mouth. They are among the most common disorders around the mouth area, causing pain and annoyance. An estimated 45 to 80 percent of adults and children in the United States have had at least one cold sore. There are two types of herpes simplex. Type 1 usually causes oral herpes, or fever blisters, while type 2 usually causes genital herpes. About 95 percent of the cold sores located on the mouth are caused by herpes simplex type 1.

Cold sores are highly contagious, more so in the first day or two of an outbreak. Once the blister has formed a dry scab, transmission is low and the herpes simplex virus usually cannot be recovered from the site. The virus can spread to others through touch; frequently, infection spreads through kissing. The chance of infection is higher if the body's defenses are weakened by stress, illness, or injury.

Once a person is infected with oral herpes, the virus remains in the nerve located near the cold sore. It may stay dormant at this site for years. People who have had fever blisters in the past can sometimes predict when an outbreak is going to occur. The appearance of cold sores may be preceded by a few hours of a tingling, burning, or itching sensation, a phenomenon called a prodrome. Typically, the sores erupt in a small cluster, with each blister about the size of a large pimple. The blisters quickly dry to form a scab. Generally, no scarring or loss in sensation occurs. Outbreaks usually last from three to ten days.

Information on Cold Sores

Causes: Infection by herpes simplex virus
Symptoms: Sores around mouth that dry to form scabs; preceded by tingling, burning, or itching sensation
Duration: Chronic, with acute outbreaks lasting from three to ten days
Treatments: Keeping area clean and dry, avoidance of sore irritation or stress; prevention through antiviral compounds (acyclovir, valacyclovir, foscarnet)

Treatment and Therapy

Treatment includes keeping the area clean and dry to prevent bacterial infection. The patient should avoid irritating the sores, as touching them may spread the virus. For example, if a person rubs the sore and then rubs an eyelid, a new sore may appear on the eyelid in a few days. When the fever blister is contagious, kissing should be avoided. People whose cold sores appear in response to stress should try to avoid stressful situations. Some investigators have suggested that adding L-lysine to the diet or eliminating certain foods (such as nuts, chocolate, and seeds) may help, although no research studies have validated these suggestions. Even sunlight has been linked as a trigger for cold sores. The National Institute of Dental and Craniofacial Research recommends the use of sunscreen on the lips to prevent sun-induced recurrences of herpes.

Antiviral therapy of mucocutaneous herpes simplex virus infection is rarely curative, but is given for treatment of severe cases and to prevent or ameliorate recurrences. Treatment can also decrease viral shedding, making transmission to other people less likely. Available antiviral compounds include nucleoside analogues, which selectively interfere with viral deoxyribonucleic acid (DNA) replication. Oral acyclovir (Avirax or Zovirax) and valacyclovir (Valtrex), antiviral drugs that keep the virus from multiplying, can be taken to prevent recurrence. Acyclovir applied locally has also been found effective, and foscarnet (Foscavir) is useful in treating acyclovir-resistant infections. Two topical preparations, Zovirax and penciclovir (Vectavir), have been shown to influence the eruption and duration of cold sores when applied during the prodromal stage. Antibiotics may be used in treating secondary infections. An ophthalmologist should treat any eye lesions.

Some cold sore treatments that have been successful in selected people are solvents such as ether, alcohol, povidone iodine, and antiseptic mouthwash. Other patients have applied ice or toothpaste to the sores. While none of these treatments has scientific backing, eating an ice pop or applying an ice cube to the blister may relieve the discomfort.

Perspective and Prospects

Future research is aimed at determining the precise form and location of the inactive herpesvirus in nerve cells. This information might allow scientists to design antiviral drugs that can attack the virus while it lies dormant in nerves. Researchers are also trying to learn more about how sunlight, injury, and stress act as triggers so that the cycle of recurrences can be stopped.

—*Janet Mahoney, R.N., Ph.D., A.P.R.N.*

See also Blisters; Canker sores; Herpes; Lesions; Skin; Skin disorders; Stress; Stress reduction; Ulcers; Viral infections.

For Further Information:

Alan, Rick. "Cold Sores." *Health Library*, March 20, 2013.

"Cold Sore." *Mayo Clinic*, May 23, 2012.

Ignatavicius, Donna D., and M. Linda Workman, eds. *Medical-Surgical Nursing: Critical Thinking for Collaborative Care*. 7th ed. Philadelphia: Saunders/Elsevier, 2012.

Lewis, Sharon, et al., eds. *Medical-Surgical Nursing: Assessment and Management of Clinical Problems*. 8th ed. 2 vols. St. Louis, Mo.: Mosby/Elsevier, 2010.

National Institutes of Health. National Institute of Dental Research. *Fever Blisters and Canker Sores*. Rev. ed. Bethesda, Md.: Author, 1992.

Smeltzer, Suzanne C., and Brenda G. Bare, eds. *Brunner and Suddarth's Textbook of Medical-Surgical Nursing*. 12th ed.

Philadelphia: Wolters Kluwer/Lippincott Williams & Wilkins, 2010.

COLIC

Disease/Disorder

Anatomy or system affected: Gastrointestinal system, intestines, psychic-emotional system

Specialties and related fields: Gastroenterology, pediatrics

Definition: As a general term, a paroxysm of acute abdominal pain caused by spasm, obstruction, or twisting of a hollow abdominal organ. As a specific entity, infantile colic is a group of behaviors displayed by young infants including crying, facial grimacing, drawing-up of the legs over the abdomen, and clenching of the fists.

Key terms:

flatulence: the presence of excessive gas in the stomach and intestines, which is expelled from the body

irritability: a state of general overreaction to external stimuli

spasm: an involuntary muscle contraction; a painful spasm is called a cramp

Causes and Symptoms

As a general term, colic can arise from any site in the abdomen due to a spasm, obstruction, or twisting of an abdominal organ. For example, cramplike pain caused by a stone obstructing the bile ducts or a stone obstructing the urinary tract are known as biliary colic or renal colic, respectively. More specifically, the term "colic," when unmodified, generally refers to infantile colic. Infantile colic is a group of behaviours displayed by young infants including crying, facial grimacing, drawing-up of the legs over the abdomen, and clenching of the fists, which are not caused by a medical problem and typically resolve at three months of age.

The crying of colicky infants tends to be more prominent in the evening, although they cry more than other infants at other times of day. The "rule of threes" of infantile colic holds that infants with colic cry for more than three hours per day for more than three days per week for more than three weeks. The associated gestures suggest to some that the infant is experiencing abdominal pain and is responsible for the use of the term "colic" to describe the condition.

Several causes of infantile colic have been postulated, but conclusive evidence is lacking for any of them. This combination of behaviors has been interpreted as abdominal pain, leading to the idea that cramping somewhere in the intestine is the cause. Neurobehavioral explanations have been of-

---

Information on Colic

Causes: Unknown; abdominal pain suspected

Symptoms: Crying for long periods of time, facial grimacing, drawing of legs over abdomen, clenching of fists

Duration: Typically one to three months

Treatments: Switching formulas, swaddling, mimicking of in utero motion, medications

fered. The most common is that colic represents a state of agitation that may not require a noxious stimulus for agitation and crying to continue. Rarely is colic the result of organic disease, and the prevailing opinion is that it is a variant of normal infant behavior. Almost all babies display colicky symptoms to varying degrees. It appears to be unrelated to caregiving style or intensity. Other proposed mechanisms include difficult temperament, sleep disturbance, diarrhea, child abuse, and irritable bowel syndrome (IBS). Some theories ascribe colic to hypersensitivity to dietary protein-usually proteins derived from cow's milk, which can be secreted in breast milk-thus explaining the occurrence of colic in breast-fed infants. Mothers who are breastfeeding may want to remove dairy and caffeine from their diets to see if that helps their infant's colicky symptoms improve. Intestinal gas, either from air swallowed during feeding or crying or from fermentation of incompletely absorbed carbohydrates in the colon, has also been implicated. Parents of colicky infants frequently describe flatulence as an associated symptom.

Treatment and Therapy

The medical treatment of the infant with colic begins with a thorough medical history and a careful physical examination. While the likelihood of finding a cause of the infant's symptoms are slight, the thoroughness of this approach provides an effective basis for reassurance and demonstrates that the parents" complaint is taken seriously.

Infantile colic virtually always resolves spontaneously, leaving the infant healthy and thriving. The essentials of therapy are demystification, reassurance, and support for the haggard and anxious parents. Demystification is the explanation of the source of the infant's distress, which alleviates the anxiety attendant on diagnostic hypotheses that occur to or are suggested to the parents. It is important for pediatricians to deal with the anxiety aroused by the infant's symptoms with reassurance, pointing out that the baby will be fine.

Quick, superficial attempts to solve the problem with formula changes or medications, particularly when not accompanied by patient demystification and reassurance, reinforce the parents" suspicion that there is something wrong with the child, ultimately increasing parental perception of the child's vulnerability. The results of studies in the medical literature investigating the usefulness of switching formulas and using agents such as simethicone to deal with intestinal gas are mixed.

More frequent, smaller feedings may help, as may increased carrying (called "walking the floor") and rocking. One theory holds that mimicking the environment in the womb is reassuring, which can be achieved through closeness to a warm person with a detectable heartbeat (sometimes called "kangaroo care"), swaddling (wrapping the baby in a blanket to restrict movement of the extremities), and rhythmic stimulation provided by background music and car or stroller rides. One commonly used method involves placing the baby in an infant seat on top of a running washer or dryer, thus exposing the infant to constant vibration. Care must be taken to stay with the baby or to secure the infant seat to prevent injury resulting from a fall off the appliance. Caretakers should experiment to see which methods best soothe their crying infant. Most colicky infants have excessive gas, and gas pains have long been suspected as being responsible for colic. Since virtually all the gas in the intestine is swallowed air, minimizing air swallowing and maximizing burping after feedings are important measures in reducing colic. The use of cereal to ease the infant's hunger and decrease the vigor with which he or she sucks on the nipple results in less air being swallowed. Unfortunately, many parents are advised to put cereal in a bottle; this increases the negative pressure required to suck the slurry of milk and cereal and increases the amount of air swallowed. Identifying and then avoiding the dietary triggers of colic and learning how to comfort the infant during crying episodes will help to soothe the infant until the symptoms of colic subside, typically at three to four months of age.

Perspective and Prospects

One theory holds that infantile colic is related to a familial prevalence of irritable bowel syndrome, also called irritable colon or spastic colon, although the evidence for this theory is limited. Diagnosis of colic is made after carefully reviewing the familial history of the infant and performing a thorough physical examination to rule out any organic causes. Although treatment is limited, most babies outgrow the symptoms of colic by three to four months of age. In the absence of an organic disease or unexplained weight loss, colic is self-limited with no long-term adverse effects on the child's development or future health.

—*Wallace A. Gleason, Jr., M.D.*

See also Bonding; Colon; Diarrhea and dysentery; Gastroenterology, pediatric; Gastrointestinal system; Irritable bowel syndrome (IBS); Lactose intolerance; Neonatology; Pediatrics.

For Further Information:
Barr, Ronald G. "Changing Our Understanding of Infant Colic." *Archives of Pediatrics and Adolescent Medicine* 156, no. 12 (December, 2002): 1172-1175.
Ben-Joseph, Elana Pearl. "Your Colicky Baby." *Nemours Foundation*, November 2011.
Brazelton, T. Berry. *Calming Your Fussy Baby: The Brazelton Way.* Cambridge, Mass.: Perseus, 2002.
"Colic." *Mayo Clinic*, July 6, 2011.
"Colic and Crying." *Medline Plus*, August 2, 2011.
Lampe, John B. "Infantile Colic: Follow-up at Four Years of Age." *Clinical Pediatrics* 29, no. 10 (October, 2000): 620.
McCormick, David P. "The Challenge of Colic." *Clinical Pediatrics* 39, no. 7 (July, 2000): 401-402.
Thompson, June. "Infantile Colic: What Is It and Are There Effective Treatments?" *Community Practitioner* 73, no. 9 (September, 2000): 767.
Thompson, June. "Low Birth Weight and Colic Linked.'" *Community Practitioner* 73, no. 8 (August, 2000): 727.
Walling, Anne D. "Diagnosing Biliary Colic and Acute Cholecystitis." *American Family Physician* 62, no. 6 (September 15, 2000): 1386.
Waltman, Alicia Brooks. "The Crying Game." *Parenting* 14, no. 3 (April, 2000): 128-132.

White, Barbara Prudhomme, et al. "Behavioral and Physiological Responsivity, Sleep, and Patterns of Daily Cortisol Production in Infants with and Without Colic." *Child Development* 71, no. 4 (July/August, 2000): 862-877.

COLITIS
Disease/Disorder

Anatomy or system affected: Abdomen, gastrointestinal system, intestines, stomach

Specialties and related fields: Gastroenterology, internal medicine

Definition: A potentially fatal but manageable disease of the colon that inflames and ulcerates the bowel lining, occurring in both acute and chronic forms.

Key terms:

diarrhea: persistent liquid or mushy, shapeless stool

dysentery: bloody diarrhea caused by infectious agents affecting the colon

ileum: the last section of the small bowel, which passes food wastes to the colon through the ileocecal valve

inflammation: swelling caused by the accumulation of fluids and chemical agents

mucosa: the membrane of cells that lines the bowel; admits fluids and nutrients but also serves as the first-line protection against infectious agents and other materials foreign to the body

procedure: any medical treatment that entails physical manipulation or invasion of the body

stoma: an opening, formed by surgery, from the bowel to the exterior surface of the body

stool: the food wastes mixed with fluid, bacteria, mucus, and dead cells that exit the body upon defecation

ulcer: an area of the mucosa that has been abraded or dissolved by infection or chemicals, creating an open sore

Causes and Symptoms

The colon is the section of the lower bowel, or intestines, extending from the ileocecal valve to the rectum. It is wider in diameter than the small bowel, although shorter in length at about one meter. From behind the pelvis, the colon rises along the right side of the body (ascending colon), turns left to cross the upper abdominal cavity (transverse colon), and then turns down along the left side of the body (descending colon) until it joins the sigmoid (S-shaped) colon. The sigmoid colon empties into the rectum, a pouch that stores the waste products of digestion that are excreted through the anus. The colon absorbs most of the fluid passed to it from the small bowel, so that wastes solidify; meanwhile, bacteria in the colon break down undigested proteins and carbohydrates, creating hydrogen, carbon dioxide, and methane gases in the process.

A key structure in colonic activity is its mucosa. This thin sheet of cells lining the bowel wall permits passage of fluids and certain nutrients into the bloodstream but resists bacteria and toxins (poisonous chemical compounds). When the mucosa is torn or worn away, bacteria and toxins enter, infecting the bowel wall. The body responds to infection by rushing fluids and powerful chemicals to the endangered area to con-

---

Information on Colitis

Causes: Unknown; possibly bacterial or viral infection, genetic factors, exposure to antibiotics, autoimmune reaction

Symptoms: Swelling of bowel lining, ulcers, bloody diarrhea, pain, fever, severe weight loss, anemia, lack of energy, dehydration, uncontrollable urge to defecate

Duration: Chronic, with acute episodes

Treatments: Medications (anti-inflammatory agents), surgery, dietary restrictions

---

fine and kill the infecting agents. In the process, the tissues of the bowel wall swell with the fluids; this is known as "inflammation." The medical suffix denoting this response is *-itis*; when it occurs in the colon, physicians call it "colitis."

A variety of agents can cause colitis, which is divided into two major types depending on the duration of the disease: acute colitis and chronic ulcerative colitis. Acute colitis is a relatively brief, single episode of inflammation. It is often caused by bacteria or parasites. For example, *Giardia lamblia*, a bacterium in many American streams, is a common infectious agent in colitis, and the amoebas in polluted water supplies are responsible for the type of colitis known as "amebic dysentery." Some medicines, however, especially antibiotics, can also induce colitis. Acute colitis either disappears on its own or can be cured with drugs. Untreated, however, it may be fatal.

Chronic ulcerative colitis and Crohn's disease constitute a category of serious afflictions called inflammatory bowel disease (IBD), whose primary physical effects include swelling of the bowel lining, ulcers, and bloody diarrhea. Although some medical researchers think that these afflictions may be two aspects of the same disease, ulcerative colitis affects only the colon, whereas Crohn's disease can involve the small bowel as well as the colon. Moreover, colitis chiefly involves the colonic mucosa, but Crohn's disease delves into the full thickness of the bowel wall.

Chronic ulcerative colitis is a permanent disease that manifests itself either in recurring bouts of inflammation or in continuous inflammation that cannot be cleared up with drugs. It is commonly called "ulcerative colitis" because ulcers, open sores in the mucosa, spread throughout the colon and rectum, where the disease usually starts. Researchers have not yet discovered the causes of chronic ulcerative colitis although there are many theories, of which three are prominent. The first is bacterial or viral infection, and many agents have been proposed as the culprit. Because such a multitude of organisms commonly reside in or pass through the colon, researchers have enormous difficulty separating out a specific kind in order to show that it is always present during colitis attacks. Second is autoimmune reaction. Research in other diseases has shown that sometimes the body's police system, enforced by white blood cells, mistakes native, healthy tissue for a foreign agent and attacks that tissue in an attempt to destroy it. Yet no testing in chronic ulcerative colitis has yet proven the theory. Third is a combination of foreign infection and autoimmune response; it is as if the immune system overreacts to an infectious agent and continues its attack even after the agent has been neutralized. Many researchers have suspected that the disease is inherited, because certain families have higher rates of the disease than others. This genetic theory is not universally accepted, however, because it is just as likely that family members share infection rather than having passed on a genetic predisposition for the disease. Other theories propose food allergies as the cause; even toothpaste has been considered.

Regardless of the cause, there is no doubt that colitis is a painful, disabling, bewildering disease. When the bowel inflames, the tissues heat up and fever results. Cramps are common, and sufferers feel an urgent, frequently uncontrollable urge to defecate. When they reach the toilet (if they do so in time), they have soft, loose stool or diarrhea, which can seem to explode from the anus. They may have as many as ten to twenty bowel movements a day. Because ulcers often erode blood vessels, blood can appear in the stool, as well as mucus and pus from the bowel wall. Severe weight loss, anemia, lack of energy, dehydration, and anorexia often develop as the colitis persists. The symptoms may clear up on their own only to recur months or years later; attacks may come with increasing frequency thereafter. The first attack, if it worsens rapidly, is fatal in about 5 to 10 percent of patients, although the death rate can rise to 25 percent among first-time sufferers who are more than sixty years old.

Complications from colitis can be life threatening. These include perforation of the bowel wall, strictures, hemorrhaging, and toxic megacolon (hyperinflation of the colon, an emergency medical condition). If left untreated or if unresponsive to treatment, ulcerative colitis can led to bone loss or arthritis, rashes, inflammation of the eye, liver disease, or painful kidney stones. Furthermore, studies show that patients who have had ulcerative colitis for more than ten years have about a 20 percent chance of developing cancer in the colon or rectum.

Because colitis is a relapsing, embarrassing disease, patients often suffer psychological turmoil. In *Colitis* (1992), Michael P. Kelly reports the results of his study of forty-five British colitis patients. According to Kelly, they typically denied that early symptoms were the signs of serious illness, passing them off as the result of overeating or influenza. The denial continued until the continual, desperate urge to defecate made them despair of controlling their bowels without help. Often, they suffered embarrassment because they had to flee family gatherings or work in order to find a toilet or because they passed stool inadvertently in public. Many feared being beyond easy access to a toilet, shunned public places, and felt humiliated. Only then did some visit a physician, and even after chronic ulcerative colitis was diagnosed, a portion hoped they could still cope on their own. When they could not, they grew depressed, insomniac, angry at their fate, or antisocial. Even with treatment, the strain of enduring the disease can be debilitating.

Treatment and Therapy

Fortunately, medical science has several well-tested methods of controlling or curing colitis. In the case of acute colitis, patients usually resume normal bowel functions on their own and emerge as healthy as they were before the onset of symptoms. For chronic ulcerative colitis patients, however, the body is rarely the same again, and they must adjust to the effects of medication, surgery, or both-an adjustment that some authors claim is essentially a redefinition of the self.

After interviewing a patient and assessing the reported symptoms, the physician suspecting colitis orders a stool sample to check for blood, bacteria, parasites, and pus. If any of these are present, the physician directly examines the rectum and colon by inserting a fiber-optic endoscope into the rectum and up the colon. Early in the disease, the mucosa looks granular with scattered hemorrhages and tiny bleeding points. As the disease progresses, the mucosa turns spongy and has many ulcers that ooze blood and pus. An x-ray often helps determine the extent of inflammation, and tissue samples taken by endoscopic biopsy can establish if it is ulcerative colitis or infection, and not Crohn's disease, that is present.

There is no easy treatment for chronic ulcerative colitis. Dietary restrictions-especially the elimination of fibrous foods such as raw fruits and vegetables, of milk products, or of certain seasonings-may reduce the irritation to the inflamed colon, and symptoms then may improve if the disease is mild. Antidiarrheal drugs can firm the stool and reduce the patient's urgency to defecate, although such drugs must be used very cautiously to avoid dangerous dilation of the bowels.

Such nonspecific measures are seldom more than delaying tactics, and drugs are needed to counteract the colon's inflammation. The most common types are aminosalicylates, corticosteroids, oral immunosuppressants, and intravenous infliximab, an antitumor necrosis factor agent. Among the first class, sulfasalazine is a sulfa drug developed in the 1940s. It is an anti-inflammatory agent that is most effective in mild to moderate ulcerative colitis and helps prevent recurrence of inflammation. Aminosalicylates may be administered as pills, suppositories, or enemas. Corticosteroids behave like the hormones produced by the adrenal gland that suppress inflammation. Administered orally, intravenously, or rectally, these drugs work well in relieving the symptoms of moderate to moderately severe attacks. Immunosuppressants and infliximab may be prescribed for severe, unresponsive cases of ulcerative colitis. All of these types of drugs have serious side effects, so physicians must carefully tailor dosages for each patient and check repeatedly for reactions. In some patients, sulfasalazine induces nausea, vomiting, joint pain, headaches, rashes, dizziness, and hepatitis (liver inflammation). The effects of corticosteroids include sleeplessness, mood swings, acne, high blood pressure, diabetes, cataracts, thinning of the bones (especially the spine), and fluid retention and swelling of the face, hands, abdomen, and ankles. Women may grow facial hair, and adolescents may have delayed sexual maturation. In most cases, the side effects clear up when patients stop taking the drugs. Immunosuppressants and infliximab can lead to toxicity.

With medication, people who suffer mild or moderate chronic ulcerative colitis can control it for years, often for the rest of their lives. Severe colitis requires surgery, and sometimes patients with milder forms choose to have surgery rather than live with the disease's unpredictable recurrence or the ever-present side effects of drugs. In any case, surgery is the one known cure for chronic ulcerative colitis, although fewer than one-third of patients undergo surgical procedures. Several types of these surgeries have high success rates.

Because ulcerative colitis eventually spreads throughout the colon, complete removal of the large bowel and rectum is the surest way to eliminate the disease. This "total proctocolectomy" takes place in three steps. The surgeon first cuts through the wall of the abdomen, the incision extending from the mid-transverse colon to the rectum, and removes the colon. Next, the end of the ileum is pulled through a hole in the abdomen to form a stoma (a procedure called an ileostomy). Finally, the rectum is removed and the anus sutured shut. Thereafter the patient defecates through the stoma. Either of two arrangements prevents stool from simply spilling out unchecked. Most patients affix plastic bags around their stomas into which stool flows without their control; when full, the bag is either emptied and reattached or thrown away and replaced. To avoid external bags, some patients prefer a "continent ileostomy," so called because it allows them to control defecation. The surgeon constructs a pouch out of a portion of the ileum and attaches it right behind the stoma, a procedure called a "Kock pouch" after its inventor, Nils Kock of Sweden. When this pouch is full, the patient empties it with a catheter inserted through the stoma. Some patients can choose to have an ileoanal anastomosis. In this procedure, the surgeon forms the end of the ileum into a pouch, which is attached to the anus and collects wastes in place of the rectum. The patient continues to defecate through the anus rather than through a stoma.

None of these surgical procedures is free of problems, and all require extensive recovery in the hospital and rehabilitation. Moreover, both infections and mechanical failures can occur. If healthy portions of the colon are left intact, they often flare with colitis later, and more operations become necessary. Patients with stomas are vulnerable to bacterial inflammation of the small intestine, resulting in diarrhea, vomiting, and dehydration. Stomas and pouches sometimes leak or close up, and even after successful operations patients lose some capacity to absorb zinc, bile salts, and vitamin B_{12}, although food supplements can make up for these deficiencies.

Any major surgery is an emotional trial. One that leaves a basic function of the body permanently altered, as with proctocolectomy or ileostomy, is difficult to accept afterward, even when the surgery was an emergency measure to save the patient's life. Patients must live with a bag of stool on their abdomen or a pouch that they must empty with a plastic straw-bags and pouches that sometimes leak stool or gas and that, even when functioning smoothly, are not pleasant to handle. They must pay close attention to body functions that they rarely had to think about before the ulcerative colitis began. The changes can severely depress patients, who then may need psychiatric help and antidepressant drugs to recover their spirits. Patients with anastomoses, who continue to defecate through their anus, also find their bowel functions changed, although not so severely. For example, it takes many months before normal stool forms, and diarrhea plagues these patients.

After their operations, patients have access to considerable help in addition to physicians and surgeons. Special nurses train patients to care for their stomas, check regularly for infection or malfunction, and generally ease them into their new lives. Formal support groups and informal networks are common and provide the afflicted with information and reassurance.

Perspective and Prospects

Acute forms of colitis, especially amebic dysentery, have long been recognized as among the endemic diseases of polluted water, and until the development of antibiotics, they regularly killed significant portions of local populations, especially the young and elderly. Chronic ulcerative colitis was first described in 1859, but no effective treatment for it existed until the 1940s. At that time, Nana Svartz of Sweden noticed that when rheumatoid arthritis patients were given sulfasalazine, the bowel condition of those who had colitis improved as well. J. Arnold Bargen, an American physician, confirmed Svartz's observation in a formal clinical trial, and sulfasalazine soon was mass-produced for distribution in the United States and later throughout the world. Since the 1940s, medications and surgical techniques for ulcerative colitis have proliferated, although none restores a patient's original state of health.

Because the agents causing ulcerative colitis are unknown, the historical and geographical origin of the disease likewise cannot be determined. Nevertheless, three somewhat odd social facets of the disease are recognized.

Evidence suggests that ulcerative colitis is a disease of urban industrial society. Along with Crohn's disease, colitis appears to be entrenched in Scandinavia, the United States, Western Europe, Israel, and England. It rarely occurs in rural Africa, Asia, or South America, despite the poor nutrition and sanitation in some of these areas. Yet the disease does not appear to vary solely by racial type or nationality, although Jewish people tend to fall ill with it more often than any other group. For example, African Americans, whether from families long-established in the United States or recently immigrated, show an incidence of colitis as high as residents of European descent.

Furthermore, ulcerative colitis strikes the young. It most often begins between the ages of fifteen and thirty; men and women are equally likely to come down with it. This fact, taken with the high rate of inflammatory bowel disease (IBD) sufferers who have family members also with the disease (20 to 25 percent), has led some researchers to believe that a genetic factor creates a susceptibility for IBD.

Finally, IBD patients bear some social stigma or at least believe they do. Ulcerative colitis involves bowel incontinence and often ends with surgical replacement of the anus with a stoma; in such cases, bowel movements can dominate a patient's life and become obvious to family members, coworkers, and even strangers. Because the subject of stool is taboo to many and the odor offends most people, patients can feel severe embarrassment and come to see themselves as pariahs. Even though the causes of ulcerative colitis remain obscure and the treatment is often distressing, modern medicine saves people who otherwise would die.

—*Roger Smith, Ph.D.*

See also Amebiasis; Colon; Colorectal cancer; Colorectal surgery; Crohn's disease; Diarrhea and dysentery; Diverticulosis and diverticulitis; Gastroenterology; Gastrointestinal disorders; Gastrointestinal system; Giardiasis; Intestinal disorders; Intestines; Irritable bowel syndrome (IBS); Rectum; Ulcers.

For Further Information:

Beers, Mark H., et al., eds. *The Merck Manual of Diagnosis and Therapy.* 18th ed. Whitehouse Station, N.J.: Merck Research Laboratories, 2006.

Brandt, Lawrence J., and Penny Steiner-Grossman, eds. *Treating IBD: A Patient's Guide to the Medical and Surgical Management of Inflammatory Bowel Disease.* Reprint. Philadelphia: Lippincott-Raven, 1996.

Carson-DeWitt, Rosalyn, and Daus Mahnke. "Ulcerative Colitis." *Health Library*, September 10, 2012.

Crohn's and Colitis Foundation of America. http://www.ccfa.org.

Kalibjian, Cliff. *Straight from the Gut: Living with Crohn's Disease and Ulcerative Colitis.* Cambridge, Mass.: O'Reilly, 2003.

Kelly, Michael P. *Colitis.* Reprint. New York: Taylor & Francis, 2004.

Lashner, Bret A. "Ulcerative Colitis." *Center for Continuing Education, Cleveland Clinic Foundation*, March 2013.

National Digestive Diseases Information Clearinghouse. "Ulcerative Colitis." *National Institute of Diabetes and Digestive and Kidney Diseases, National Institutes of Health*, November 15, 2011.

Parker, James N., and Philip M. Parker, eds. *The Official Patient's Sourcebook on Ulcerative Colitis.* San Diego, Calif.: Icon Health, 2005.

Saibil, Fred. *Crohn's Disease and Ulcerative Colitis: Everything You Need to Know.* 3d rev. ed. Toronto, Ont.: Firefly Books, 2011.

Sklar, Jill, Manual Sklar, and Annabel Cohen. *The First Year-Crohn's Disease and Ulcerative Colitis: An Essential Guide for the Newly Diagnosed.* 2d ed. New York: Marlowe, 2007.

Steiner-Grossman, Penny, Peter A. Banks, and Daniel H. Present, eds. *The New People, Not Patients: A Source Book for Living with Inflammatory Bowel Disease.* Rev. ed. Dubuque, Iowa: Kendall/Hunt, 1997.

COLLAGEN

Biology

Anatomy or system affected: All, especially joints, ligaments, musculoskeletal system, skin, tendons

Specialties and related fields: Biochemistry, rheumatology

Definition: A fibrous protein that is the main component of most connective tissues; the most common protein in animals.

Structure and Functions

Collagen is a complex protein made up of three separate polypeptide chains that form a triple helix. These polypeptides are unusual because every third amino acid is a glycine and because prolines make up an additional 17 percent of the chains. There are at least twenty-eight types of collagen made up of forty-three distinct polypeptide chains, each coded for by a different gene. For example, type I collagen, the most common type, has two chains classified as alpha-1 and alpha-2. These peptides are initially produced on the rough endoplasmic reticulum (ER) and then processed in the ER lumen, where sequences at the ends are removed and hydroxyl groups are added to many of the chains" prolines and lysines. The triple helix then formed is called procollagen. Further processing, including preparation for secretion, takes place in the Golgi bodies. Once secreted, more end sequences are cleaved off to form collagen (also called tropocollagen). In the extracellular region, collagen molecules associate into collagen fibrils and eventually collagen fibers.

Collagen is a flexible but not stretchable protein that is an important component of most connective tissues. It is the primary component of tendons and ligaments, giving them the requisite strength to connect muscles to bones and bones to other bones or organs. Cartilage found at joints and in many other structures is mostly collagen. The connective tissues found in the dermal layer of the skin, the capsules surrounding internal organs, and blood vessels are also primarily made of collagen. Bones are initially formed from collagen, which then serves as a matrix for calcium phosphate deposition. (Collagen fragments have even been extracted from fossilized dinosaur bones.) During healing, excess collagen production can lead to scar tissue formation. Collagen can be heat-treated to produce gelatin or animal-based glues, and injected collagen is often used in cosmetic procedures to plump lips or smooth out wrinkles.

Disorders and Diseases

Collagen is associated with many disorders. Osteogenesis imperfecta (brittle bone disease) is caused by mutations in the gene for the alpha-1 protein in type I collagen. An inherited form of osteoporosis is caused by a defect in the same gene. Ehlers-Danlos syndrome, which results in hyperextensible joints and fragile, stretchable skin, is caused by defects in types III and V collagen. A form of early-onset osteoarthritis is caused by a lack of functional type VI collagen, and in all forms of osteoarthritis cartilage is lost from the ends of bones at joints. In rheumatoid arthritis, modification of type II collagen forms new antigens that are attacked by the immune system. Vitamin C deficiency decreases activity of the enzymes that add hydroxyl groups to proline, thus leading to lowered amounts of functional type I collagen, which causes scurvy.

—*Richard W. Cheney, Jr., Ph.D.*

See also Arthritis; Cartilage; Connective tissue; Joints; Ligaments; Osteoarthritis; Osteogenesis imperfecta; Rheumatoid arthritis; Rheumatology; Scurvy; Tendon disorders; Tendon repair; Wrinkles.

For Further Information:

Abreu-Velez, Ana Maria, and Michael S. Howard. "Collagen IV in

Normal Skin and in Pathological Processes." *North American Journal of Medical Sciences* 4, no. 1 (2012): 1-8.

"Collagen Vascular Disease." *Medline Plus*, February 9, 2011.

Fratzl, Peter. *Collagen: Structure and Mechanics*. New York: Springer, 2008.

Myllyharju, Joahanna, and Kari Kivirkko. "Collagen and Collagen-Related Diseases." *Annals of Medicine* 33 (2001): 7-21.

"Questions and Answers about Heritable Disorders of Connective Tissue." *National Institute of Arthritis and Musculoskeletal and Skin Diseases*, October 2011.

"Types of OI." *Osteogenesis Imperfecta Foundation*, 2012.

Whitford, David. *Proteins: Structure and Function*. Hoboken, N.J.: John Wiley & Sons, 2005.

COLLODION BABY

Disease/Disorder

Anatomy or system affected: Hair, nails, skin

Specialties and related fields: Dermatology, neonatology, pediatrics

Definition: A baby is born encased in a tight, shiny membrane.

Key terms:

desquamation: shedding of the outer layer of skin

epidermis: the outer epithelial layer of the skin

hyperkeratosis: excessive proliferation of skin cells accompanied by accelerated sloughing

Causes and Symptoms

At birth, collodion babies are encased in a tight, translucent, shiny membrane that resembles a "collodion," or a sausage skin. This membrane sloughs (desquamates) in 10-14 days to reveal the abnormal skin underneath. Ten percent of collodion babies are "self-healing" collodion babies. In this case, normal skin underlies the collodion, and peeling of the membrane leads to healing and normal skin. The incidence of collodion baby is unknown, but occurs at an estimated rate of 1 in every 100,000 births.

The two most common diseases associated with collodion babies include lamellar ichthyosis and nonbullous congenital erythroderma. Other rarer conditions associated with collodion babies include Sjögren-Larsson syndrome, Gaucher Disease type 2, Hay-Well syndrome, Trichothyodystrophy, Comel-Netherton syndrome, ectodermal dysplasia, and neutral lipid storage disease. All of these diseases result from mutations in genes that play integral roles in establishing and maintaining the outermost layer of the skin (epidermis). Dysfunctional skin cells cause accelerated turnover and thickening of the skin (hyperkeratosis).

Information on Collodion Baby

Causes: Abnormal sloughing of the skin associated with several congenital skin disorders

Symptoms: Peeling skin that scales, dries, and cracks

Duration: Extra skin sheds in 10-14 days, but duration of skin problems depends on the nature of the underlying skin condition

Treatments: High humidity, moisturizers, pain relievers, artificial tears for eyes

The sloughing of the collodion membrane reveals red, scaly skin underneath. In many cases the scaling has a plate-like appearance that resembles fish scales, but the exact nature of the scaling depends on the type of skin disease responsible for the collodion membrane. As the collodion membrane dries, it cracks. The resulting fissures compromise the barrier function of the skin, and put the baby at increased risk of infections, dehydration, and overheating or cooling. Also, the tightness of the collodion membrane physically restricts underlying tissues. These constraints can prevent the baby from properly suckling and feeding, restrict blood flow in the limbs, affect breathing, and turn the lower eyelids away from the eyeball (ectropion).

Treatment and Therapy

After birth, collodion babies are transferred to a neonatal intensive care unit and placed in a humidified incubator. During their time in the incubator, they are given intravenous fluids and fed through a feeding tube. The goal of treatment is to keep the skin soft and moist to reduce scaling. Emollients such as petrolatum are smeared on the skin to moisten it. A mild topical steroid treatment can reduce inflammation, and artificial tears can ameliorate severely dry eyes in the cases of severe ectropion.

—*Michael A. Buratovich, Ph.D.*

See also Blisters; Dehydration; Dermatology; Dermatopathology; Intensive care unit; Neonatology; Pediatrics

For Further Information:

Kinai, Miriam. *Dermatology: Ichthyosis*. Seattle: Amazon Digital Services, 2012.

Polin, Richard A., and Alan R. Spitzer. *Fetal and Neonatal Secrets*. 3rd ed. Philadelphia: Mosby, 2013.

COLON

Anatomy

Also known as: Large intestine, large bowel, large gut

Anatomy or system affected: Abdomen, gastrointestinal system, intestines, nervous system

Specialties and related fields: Alternative medicine, biochemistry, gastroenterology, general surgery, histology, internal medicine, nutrition, oncology, osteopathic medicine, pathology, pediatrics, pharmacology

Definition: The section of the gastrointestinal system where the absorption of water, sodium, and some vitamins occurs and where residual chyme is converted to semisolid feces before expulsion through the anal canal. It is connected to the small intestine through the ileo-cecal valve and is populated by commensal bacteria.

Key terms:

chyme: food in a semifluid state that reaches the large intestine after digestion in the upper gastrointestinal tract

epithelium: tissue made up of tightly adherent cells, usually lining the surfaces of the body and organs

Structure and Functions

In the average adult man, the large intestine is about 1.5 to 1.8

meters long. It is divided into the cecum; the ascending, transverse, descending, and sigmoid colon; and the rectum, ending in the anus. Its wall contains both circular and longitudinal layers of smooth muscle and innervation that controls its motility. The longitudinal musculature runs along the outside of the colon in three separate bands, called teniae coli, which converge around the sigmoid colon and the rectum. The inner layer of the large intestine consists of mucosa with sparse or no villi but with numerous invaginations (glands); it is lined with simple columnar epithelium. The glands contain goblet cells, endocrine cells, and absorptive cells. There are no digestive enzymes linked to the inner surface of the colon.

The main function of the colon is to absorb water from the chyme and to process it into feces for elimination. Most nutrients and about 90 percent of water are absorbed in the small intestine. When it reaches the large intestine, chyme still contains some electrolytes (sodium, magnesium, and chloride) and indigestible food components, such as fiber.

An abundant and varied bacterial population colonizes the human colon shortly after birth and resides in the large intestine for life. Bacteria digest fiber and produce short-chain fatty acids (acetate, propionate, and butyrate). Short-chain fatty acids promote the integrity of the colonic epithelial cells, prevent inflammation, and provide some protection against potential pathogens.

The large intestine absorbs some vitamins (mainly vitamin K) and electrolytes but mainly water-up to five liters of water per day. Water moves passively with sodium, which is mostly absorbed in the distal colon. Water absorption is in part regulated by aldosterone, a hormone that increases the absorption of sodium in response to volume depletion. Water absorption solidifies the chyme into stools.

The motility of the colon allows for mixing the contents and retaining them for prolonged periods. Periodically, the colon is swept with propulsive contractions (peristalsis) that move its contents toward the rectum. The gastrocolic reflex causes mass peristalsis after a meal. The sigmoid colon and rectum serve as a reservoir and participate in defecation.

Disorders and Diseases

A number of disorders are associated with the colon. Appendicitis is the inflammation of the vermiform appendix. It requires surgery. Constipation is the failure to empty the bowels regularly and easily. It can be linked to diet, stress, and a variety of conditions and medications. It is treated with dietary fiber and laxatives. Diarrhea involves frequent loose or liquid bowel movements. It may have many different causes and is treated mainly with loperamide or bismuth salicilate.

Diverticulitis refers to the development of outpouchings in the colon. A low-fiber diet and age are risk factors. Symptoms are linked to inflammation (diverticulosis) and are mostly treated with antibiotics. Complications may require surgical removal of the outpouchings. Hirschsprung disease (congenital aganglionic megacolon) involves the complete absence of neuronal ganglion cells (which make the intestinal muscles contract, so the stool is pushed forward) from a segment of the intestine, usually the distal colon. It requires surgery.

Inflammatory bowel disease (IBD) is a general name for diseases that cause intestinal swelling. They include ulcerative colitis (inflammation and ulcers in the top layer of the lining of the large intestine) and Crohn's disease (all layers of the intestine may be involved; healthy bowel segments alternate with affected segments). Treatment varies widely, but the condition will recur. Irritable bowel syndrome (IBS) is a functional disorder of the colon of unknown cause. Its symptoms are abdominal pain, abnormal bowel habit, bloating, and either constipation, diarrhea, or both alternating. It is worsened by stress. IBS may be linked to hypersensitivity of intestinal muscles and nerves. Its treatment varies according to symptoms.

Colorectal polyps are growths on the lining of the colon or rectum. In time, they can develop into colorectal cancer. They are removed with endoscopic microsurgery. Colorectal cancer refers to cancerous growths in the colon, rectum, and appendix, mostly thought to arise from adenomatous polyps in the colon. It requires surgery.

Perspective and Prospects

The intuition that the colon is associated with waste accumulation and release dates to antiquity. Ancient Egyptian physicians also viewed "intestinal putrefaction" as the basic cause of disease, a concept later incorporated into the humoral doctrine of disease by ancient Greeks. This concept of autointoxication lasted throughout the centuries with few adaptations. In the nineteenth century, early studies showed the presence and activity of bacteria in the colon. It was then thought that colonic bacteria generate toxic amines that shorten life span. This theory was finally abandoned by the 1920s. Later research has focused on the molecular mechanisms of water and electrolyte movements and their regulation, as well as on the pathways that modulate the secretory and absorptive functions of the colon. Recent developments in genetics and immunology have allowed a deeper understanding of inflammatory diseases of the colon. The advent of endoscopic techniques has vastly improved microsurgery and cancer prevention.

—*Donatella M. Casirola, Ph.D.*

See also Abdomen; Abdominal disorders; Anus; Appendicitis; Colitis; Colonoscopy and sigmoidoscopy; Colorectal cancer; Colorectal polyp removal; Colorectal surgery; Constipation; Crohn's disease; Diarrhea; Digestion; Diverticulitis and diverticulosis; Endoscopy; Enemas; Gastroenterology; Gastroenterology, pediatric; Gastrointestinal disorders; Gastrointestinal system; Hirschsprung's disease; Internal medicine; Intestinal disorders; Intestines; Irritable bowel syndrome (IBS); Laparoscopy; Nutrition; Obstruction; Peristalsis; Proctology; Rectum; Small intestine.

For Further Information:
Bäckhed, Fredrik, et al. "Host-Bacterial Mutualism in the Human Intestine." *Science* 307 (March 25, 2005): 1915-1920.
Barrett, Kim E. "Functional Anatomy of the GI Tract and Organs Draining into It." In *Gastrointestinal Physiology.* New York: McGraw-Hill, 2006.
"Digestive System." *MedlinePlus,* January 14, 2013.
Mahnke, Daus. "Colonoscopy." *Health Library,* February 6, 2013.
Sherwood, Lauralee. "The Digestive System." In *Human*

Physiology: From Cells to Systems. 8th ed. Belmont, Calif.: Brooks/Cole/Cengage Learning, 2013.

"Your Digestive System and How It Works." *National Digestive Diseases Information Clearinghouse (NDDIC)*, April 23, 2013.

COLON THERAPY

Treatment

Also known as: Colonic irrigation, colon hydrotherapy

Anatomy or system affected: Abdomen, anus, gastrointestinal system, intestines

Specialties and related fields: Alternative medicine

Definition: Irrigation of the colon, or large intestine, with water in order to detoxify it.

Indications and Procedures

Colon therapy involves washing out the entire approximately five-foot length of the colon with pure water in order to dislodge any impacted fecal material. Some practitioners believe that the colon may not function properly because of poor dietary habits, insufficient fluid intake, and physical or emotional stress or illness. Such malfunction can lead to a buildup of hardened, impacted fecal material, which may stagnate and decay in the colon. Bacterial decomposition of the material may create toxins that are absorbed into the bloodstream. This in turn could cause other body organs to overwork themselves as they attempt to detoxify the waste materials and could lead to a variety of illnesses, from colds to cardiovascular disease.

During this procedure, a flexible tube is inserted into the rectum and water is slowly pumped into the intestine. The pressure is regulated in order to avoid injury. Alternation of warm and cool water leads to contraction and relaxation of the intestinal walls, which helps to remove impacted pieces of dry feces from the walls. Feces, gas, mucus, and bacteria exit through the same tube. A cleaner internal surface of the colon provides more surface area for the absorption of nutrients and water. Approximately twenty gallons of water are used in the procedure, which lasts about one hour.

Uses and Complications

Irrigation of the entire colon came into prominence during the late nineteenth century in Russia. In the United States, John Harvey Kellogg espoused colonic irrigation along with other health and fitness regimes at his sanatorium in Battle Creek, Michigan, in the early twentieth century. The procedure fell into obscurity during the late 1940s, when medical research indicated no benefit to the procedure. Renewed interest in colonics in the late twentieth century led to the establishment of the International Association for Colon Hydrotherapy, which provides training and certification for practitioners. While colon therapy regained enthusiastic followers, mainstream physicians point out that waste products in the colon cannot "toxify" the body. They also believe that colonics may interfere with the natural balance of helpful bacteria that keep the intestines functioning normally.

After a procedure, some patients report feeling energized and lighter, while others report nausea, headaches, or flu-like symptoms. These symptoms generally subside within a few hours. Other side effects may include diarrhea and a loss of necessary intestinal bacteria.

—Karen E. Kalumuck, Ph.D.;
updated by LeAnna DeAngelo, Ph.D.

See also Alternative medicine; Colon; Gastrointestinal system; Hydrotherapy; Intestines; Preventive medicine.

For Further Information:

Collings, Jillie. *Principles of Colonic Irrigation: The Only Introduction You'll Ever Need.* New York: Thorsons, 1996.

Goldberg, Burton, John Anderson, and Larry Trivieri, eds. *Alternative Medicine: The Definitive Guide.* 2d ed. Berkeley, Calif.: Celestial Arts, 2002.

Jonas, Wayne, ed. *Mosby's Dictionary of Complementary and Alternative Medicine.* St. Louis, Mo.: Mosby/Elsevier, 2005.

Mayo Clinic. "Colon Cleansing: Is It Helpful or Harmful?" *Mayo Clinic*, May 19, 2012.

COLONOSCOPY AND SIGMOIDOSCOPY

Procedures

Anatomy or system affected: Gastrointestinal system, intestines

Specialties and related fields: Gastroenterology, general surgery

Definition: The insertion of a flexible tube into the rectum to look at the inside surface of the colon.

Key terms:

biopsy: removal of a piece of tissue for examination under a microscope

colitis: inflammation of the inner surface of the colon

lumen: the space inside a tubelike structure such as the colon

mucosa: the layer of tissue that lines the inside of a tubelike structure such as the colon

polyp: a small piece of tissue that extends from the surface of the colon into the lumen

Indications and Procedures

Colonoscopy and sigmoidoscopy are common procedures to evaluate the lower part of the gastrointestinal tract. Colonoscopy refers to examination of the entire large bowel, whereas sigmoidoscopy examines only the part closest to the rectum (known as the sigmoid colon). The advantage of sigmoidoscopy is that it is less time-consuming and can be performed without sedation. Since sigmoidoscopy evaluates only part of the colon, however, full colonoscopy is often preferred. The most common reason for having a colonoscopy is to screen for colon cancer. If sigmoidoscopy is used for this purpose, it must be combined with a barium enema and an x-ray to evaluate the upper part of the colon.

Prior to colonoscopy, the bowel must be cleaned of stool to enable the physician to see the underlying mucosa. Patients are often asked to go on a diet of clear liquids (such as chicken broth, gelatin, and juice) for one to three days prior to the procedure. The night before the procedure, patients ingest a purgative to clear out any residual stool. The two most common preparations are polyethylene glycol (GoLytely) and a so-

In the News:
Risks of Flat Lesions in Intestinal Lining

Approximately 0.3 percent to 0.9 percent of patients develop colon cancer a few years after having a successful colonoscopy or sigmoidoscopy. Doctors, once puzzled by this response, now attribute at least some cancer occurrence to undetected or inadequately removed flat or depressed lesions in the intestinal lining. These lesions were previously thought to be harmless. However, a study published in March, 2008, in the *Journal of the American Medical Association* cautioned that flat or depressed growths are five times more likely to be cancerous than other more easily identified lesions such as polyps.

Flat or depressed lesions are often smaller than polyps and the same color as the colon. Consequently, they innocently blend right into the surrounding healthy colon tissue. These growths also occur infrequently, comprising only 15 percent of the total lesions detected in males. They occur even less often in the female population. The danger of flat or depressed lesions makes it even more imperative that patients follow the pretest cleansing routine carefully. Remaining waste, no matter how small, may cover and hide a serious growth.

To detect flat or depressed lesions, physicians must be trained to do the test slowly, carefully look for the growths, and inject a blue dye into the colon to define the lesion. Doctors must also learn new techniques to ensure that the growths are completely removed. Physicians are encouraged to track their own success rate in detecting these difficult lesions.

Increasingly popular virtual or relatively noninvasive colonoscopies use computed tomography (CT) to detect polyps that rise from the colon wall. However, CT is not sensitive enough to detect flat or depressed lesions. Promising new techniques to readily identify these growths include narrow-band imaging, a novel illumination technology, zoom magnification, and high-definition processor technology.

—Renée Euchner, R.N.

dium phosphate mix (Fleet Phospho-Soda). Following ingestion of these solutions, patients should have clear or very light-colored liquid bowel movements. Regular medications that may cause excessive bleeding from biopsy sites, such as aspirin, warfarin, and nonsteroidal anti-inflammatory drugs (NSAIDs), are often discontinued prior to the procedure. Patients should also discontinue iron supplements, since they may create a black coating that makes it difficult for the physician to see the mucosa.

When patients enter the colonoscopy suite, they are given an intravenous (IV) catheter to administer fluids, as well as sedative and analgesic medications. Patients are asked not to eat or drink anything the day of the procedure. Sedative medications sometimes cause nausea, and any food that is present in the stomach may be vomited. Blood pressure, pulse, and oxygen saturation are monitored throughout the procedure. The patient is positioned on his or her left side, and a colonoscope is inserted through the rectum into the colon. The colonoscope is a long, flexible tube with a fiber-optic channel connected to a camera. The image of the inside of the colon is transmitted to a television screen. The colonoscope also has channels to administer air or water, as well as a suction channel. Air is introduced to expand the walls of the colon, enabling better viewing. Water is used to remove residual stool that may obstruct the view of the colon. The colonoscope is advanced to the cecum (the first part of the large bowel) or even the terminal ileum (the last part of the small bowel). The instrument is then slowly withdrawn while any abnormalities in the mucosa are noted. Following the procedure, patients are often observed for a period of time to make sure that no complications occur. If sedative medications were used, patients should not drive or operate machinery for the rest of the day.

Uses and Complications

In addition to screening for colon cancer, colonoscopy and sigmoidoscopy can be used to evaluate blood in the stool, chronic diarrhea or other changes in bowel habits, and unexplained abdominal pain. Common findings include polyps, which may be biopsied. It is common practice to remove a polyp completely, in case it turns out to be the precancerous type (known as an adenomatous polyp). Other findings include diverticula, small outpouchings of the colon which have very thin walls and are prone to spontaneous bleeding. They may also become infected, resulting in a condition known as diverticulitis. Other findings during colonoscopy may be useful in establishing the presence of a particular disease. Yellowish pseudo-membranes line the gut in colitis associated with the bacterium *Clostridium difficile*. A dusky hue is often seen in cases of ischemic colitis caused by diminished blood supply to the colon. Characteristic findings are also seen in inflammatory bowel disease.

Colonoscopy is a very safe procedure. One common aftereffect is abdominal discomfort as a result of the air used to distend the colon. This condition usually resolves over a few hours as the air is passed. The most serious complications of colonoscopy are perforation and bleeding. Perforation refers to a hole in the colon. It is an extremely rare occurrence, but it can be deadly. Patients with perforations often have severe abdominal pain and a rigid abdomen. If it is large and results in free air in the abdomen, a perforation requires emergency surgery. Rarely, very small perforations can be treated with observation and antibiotics. Bleeding is a risk if a biopsy is taken during the procedure. Most of the time, the bleeding stops by itself, but in some cases a repeat colonoscopy may be required to control the bleeding. Rarely, bleeding may occur a few hours to several days after colonoscopy, so patients should report these symptoms to their physician. Whenever sedation is used, there is a risk of too much being given, which can lead to respiratory or cardiac arrest. Other possible complications include pain and inflammation at the site of the catheter and allergic reactions to sedative or analgesic medications.

—Ahmad Kamal, M.D.

See also Colon; Colorectal cancer; Colorectal polyp removal; Colorectal surgery; Diverticulitis and diverticulosis; Endoscopy; Enemas; Gastroenterology; Gastrointestinal system; Intestines; Invasive tests; Oncology; Proctology; Screening; Tumor removal; Tumors.

For Further Information:

Church, James M. *Endoscopy of the Colon, Rectum, and Anus*. New York: Igaku-Shoin, 1995.

Drossman, Douglas A., et al., eds. *Handbook of Gastroenterologic Procedures*. 4th ed. Philadelphia: Lippincott Williams & Wilkins, 2005.

HealthDay. "Prepping for a Colonoscopy: Why It's a Necessary Evil." *MedlinePlus*, May 30, 2013.

Health Library. "Colonoscopy." *Health Library*, February 6, 2013.

Health Library. "Flexible Sigmoidoscopy." *Health Library*, September 10, 2012.

Longstreth, George F. "Sigmoidoscopy." *MedlinePlus*, October 8, 2012.

MedlinePlus. "Colonoscopy." *MedlinePlus*, June 7, 2013.

Waye, Jerome D., Douglas K. Rex, and Christopher B. Williams, eds. *Colonoscopy: Principles and Practice*. 2d ed. Malden, Mass.: Blackwell, 2009.

COLOR BLINDNESS
Disease/Disorder

Anatomy or system affected: Eyes

Specialties and related fields: Brain, optometry

Definition: An inability to distinguish certain colors resulting from an inherited defect in the light receptor cells in the retina of the eye.

Causes and Symptoms

The retina of the eye is a thin, fragile membrane that contains millions of photoreceptor cells. They convert light energy into an electrical signal, which is transmitted to the brain via the optic nerve. On a microscopic scale, the structure of the retina is like a carpet with its many fibers sticking upward. There are two types of photoreceptor cells, called rods and cones because of their distinctive shapes. Only the cones are important for color vision. There are three varieties of cones with peak sensitivities for red, green, and blue, respectively. The shades and tints of all other colors are mixtures of these three.

Color blindness involves a deficiency in these photoreceptor cells. A deficiency of green photoreceptor cells is much more common than a deficiency of red photoreceptors. Some people are totally color-blind, which means that they are completely unable to distinguish among red, orange, yellow, and green. Color blindness is quite rare in females (less than 1 percent of the population) but is more prevalent in males (about 8 percent).

Diagnostic tests are available to determine the extent of color blindness. The Ishihara color test, named after a Japanese ophthalmologist, consists of a mosaic of colored dots

---

Information on Color Blindness

Causes: Genetic defect resulting in photoreceptor deficiency

Symptoms: Inability to distinguish between certain colors (red, orange, yellow, green)

Duration: Lifelong

Treatments: None

---

containing a letter of the alphabet made up of dots of a different color-for example, yellow dots in a background of green ones. Color-blind individuals would be unable to distinguish the letter because yellow and green look the same to them.

A more precise diagnostic test makes use of the Nagel anomaloscope, which has two colored light sources whose brightness can be adjusted. The patient tries to match a given color by superimposing the two light beams while varying their intensities. For normal eyes, red and green lights of similar intensities can be superimposed to create yellow. However, a patient who requires a considerably larger green component to create yellow evidently has a deficiency of green photoreceptor cells.

Treatment and Therapy

Color blindness is a genetic defect from birth, not a disease. No procedure is known by which it can be corrected. Color-blind people must find ways to counter the effects of their condition. For example, they can obtain driver's licenses because they learn that stoplights are always red on top, yellow in the middle, and green on the bottom. Color-blind individuals may need help, however, with tasks such as clothing selection. Good color discrimination is required for some occupations, such as interior decorating, graphic design, advertising, or airplane piloting. Fortunately, color blindness is not a deterrent for most jobs.

—*Hans G. Graetzer, Ph.D.*

See also Eye infections and disorders; Eyes; Genetic diseases; Vision; Vision disorders.

For Further Information:

Cameron, John R., James G. Skofronick, and Roderick M. Grant. *Medical Physics: Physics of the Body*. Madison, Wis.: Medical Physics, 1992.

"Color Blindness." *MedlinePlus*, June 1, 2011.

Kasper, Dennis L., et al., eds. *Harrison's Principles of Internal Medicine*. 18th ed. New York: McGraw-Hill, 2012.

Stresing, Diane. "Color Blindness." *Health Library*, March 15, 2013.

"Vision." In *Encyclopaedia Brittanica*. 15th ed. Chicago: Encyclopaedia Britannica, 2002.

COLORECTAL CANCER
Disease/Disorder

Also known as: Large bowel cancer

Anatomy or system affected: Abdomen, anus, gastrointestinal system, intestines, lymphatic system

Specialties and related fields: Gastroenterology, genetics, immunology, oncology, proctology

Definition: Cancer occurring in the large intestine, which is the second deadliest type of this disease.

Causes and Symptoms

With an estimated 51,000 deaths per year in the United States, cancer of the colon and rectum is the second most deadly cancer, ranking only behind lung cancer. About 90 percent of colorectal cancers arise from the glandular epithelium lining the inner surface of the large bowel and are termed adenocarcinomas. The cells of this layer are constantly being replaced by new cells. This fairly rapid cell division, along with the relatively hostile environment within the bowel, promotes internal cellular errors that lead to the formation of aberrant cells. These cells can become disordered and produce abnormal growths or tumors. Often, colorectal tumors protrude into the lumen (the spaces within the bowel), forming growths called polyps. Some polyps are benign and do not spread to other parts of the body, but they may still disturb normal bowel functions. Other polyps become malignant by forming more aggressive cell types, which allows them to grow larger and spread to other organs. The cancer can grow through the layers of the colon wall and extend into the body cavity and nearby organs such as the urinary bladder. Cancer cells can also break away from the main tumor and spread (metastasize) through the blood or lymphatic vessels to other organs, such as the lungs or liver. If not controlled, the spreading cancer eventually causes death by impairment of organ and system functions.

The tendency to develop colorectal polyps and cancer can be inherited; this genetic predisposition may be responsible for about 5 to 7 percent of all colorectal cancers. One example is an inherited disorder called familial adenomatous

> ### Information on Colorectal Cancer
>
> **Causes:** Hereditary and/or environmental factors, dietary habits, colon polyps, long-standing ulcerative colitis
> **Symptoms:** Fatigue, weakness, shortness of breath, change in bowel habits, narrow stools, diarrhea or constipation, red or dark blood in stool, weight loss, abdominal pain, cramps, bloating
> **Duration:** Chronic
> **Treatments:** Surgery, chemotherapy, radiation

polyposis (FAP), in which multiple polyps develop in the colon; it often leads to colorectal cancer. Some of the defective genes that cause this and other types of colorectal cancers have been identified and are being studied to determine their role. Irritable bowel syndrome (IBS) and exposure to certain occupational carcinogens are also known to increase the risk.

Treatment and Therapy

The chances for survival are greatly increased when colorectal cancer is detected and treated at an early stage. Early detection in the general population is possible with the

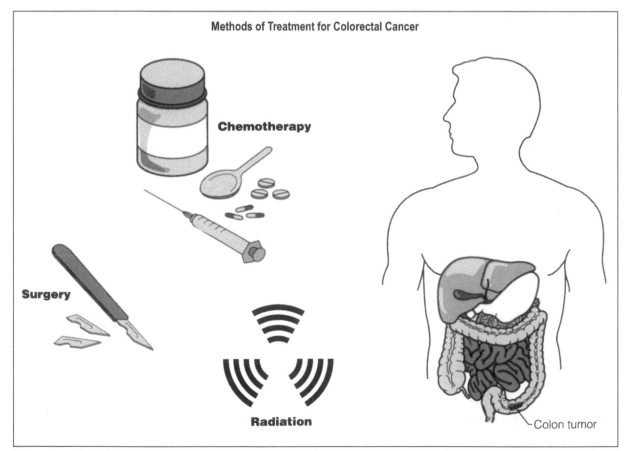

Methods of Treatment for Colorectal Cancer

Chemotherapy

Surgery

Radiation

Colon tumor

The presence of a malignant tumor in the colon requires some form of treatment or a combination of treatments, usually beginning with its surgical removal and followed by radiation therapy and/or chemotherapy (the use of anticancer drugs).

use of a number of available medical tests: digital rectal examination, in which the physician checks the inner surface of the rectal wall with a gloved finger for abnormal growths; fecal occult blood test, in which a stool sample is tested for hidden blood that may have emanated from a cancerous growth; sigmoidoscopy, in which the physician examines the rectal and lower-colon inner lining with a narrow tubular optical instrument inserted through the anus; colonoscopy, in which an optical instrument, inserted through the anus, assesses more of the colon and can remove tissue for pathological examination; virtual colonoscopy, which is a noninvasive test to assess the colon through use of X-rays; and double contrast barium enema, in which X-rays are taken after a liquid containing barium is put into the rectum. Newer screening tests, called fecal DNA testing, continue to be under study. These tests look for early genetic changes in the colon cells that are sloughed off into the stool.

Once cancer is suspected, further tests will be done to arrive at a diagnosis. These tests may include a computed tomography (CT) scan, double-contrast barium enema X-ray series, and colonoscopy. The CT scan and contrast X-rays reveal abnormal growths, and colonoscopy is similar to sigmoidoscopy but uses a longer, flexible tube in order to inspect the entire colon. During sigmoidoscopy and colonoscopy, the physician can remove polyps and obtain tissue samples for biopsy. Microscopic examination of the tissue samples by a pathologist can determine the stage or extent of growth of the cancer. This is important because it helps determine the type of treatment needed. In one type of staging, the following criteria are used: stage 0 (cancer confined to epithelium lining of the bowel), stage 1 (cancer confined to the bowel wall), stage 2 (cancer penetrating through all layers of the bowel wall and possibly invading adjacent tissues), stage 3 (cancer invading lymph nodes and/or adjacent tissues), and stage 4 (cancer spreading to distant sites, forming metastases).

Surgery is the primary treatment for colorectal cancer. Very small tumors in stage 0 can be removed surgically with the colonoscope. Tumors in more advanced stages require abdominal surgery in which the tumor is removed along with a portion of the bowel and possibly some lymph nodes. For cases in which the bowel cannot be reconnected, an opening is created through the abdominal wall (colostomy). This is usually a temporary procedure, and the hole will be closed when the bowel can be rejoined. Some advanced cancers cannot be cured by surgery alone. Adjuvant therapies-chemotherapy, radiation therapy, and biological therapy-may be used in combination with surgery. Chemotherapy drugs kill spreading cancer cells. The most common is 5-fluorouracil (5-FU), a chemical that interferes with the production of deoxyribonucleic acid (DNA) in dividing cells. 5-FU is more effective when given together with leucovorin (a compound similar to folic acid) and levamisole (an immune system stimulant).

In 2004, the Food and Drug Administration (FDA) approved the use of the Eloxatin injection in combination with 5-FU and leucovorin for the treatment of patients whose cancer has recurred or become worse following initial drug ther-

apy. This approach was shown to shrink tumors in some patients and delay resumed tumor growth. Levamisole and other treatments that reinforce the immune system are forms of biological therapy. Radiation therapy, given either before or after surgery, is helpful in killing undetected cancer cells near the site of the tumor.

Perspective and Prospects

More than 608,000 people worldwide die of colorectal cancer each year, or roughly 8 percent of all cancer deaths. The incidence of colorectal cancer is lower among women than men and rises dramatically after the age of fifty. Colorectal cancer is more common in developed countries and in densely populated, industrialized regions. Populations moving from low-risk parts of the world for developing colorectal cancer, such as Asia or Africa, to high-risk areas, such as the United States or Europe, take on the higher risk within a generation or two, and vice versa.

Research is ongoing to determine the risk factors of colorectal cancers. Recent epidemiological evidence has supported the use of nonsteroidal anti-inflammatory drugs (NSAIDs) as a means of reducing the risk of cancers of the colon and rectum, as well as the risk of intestinal cancers resulting from exposure to carcinogens. The studies focused only on the daily use of aspirin, but similar results have been reported following long-term use of sulindac and indomethacin. Sulindac has shown an ability to induce regression of colon polyps in patients with familial adenomatous polyposis. Researchers are still working on finding the right balance in dose and frequency since sulindac has potentially severe side effects and aspirin may induce bleeding if high doses are maintained on a daily basis. Regular cardiovascular exercise and a healthy diet have also been shown to reduce the risk of developing colorectal cancer.

—*Rodney C. Mowbray, Ph.D.;*
updated by Connie Rizzo, M.D., Ph.D.

See also Biopsy; Cancer; Chemotherapy; Colon; Colon therapy; Colonoscopy and sigmoidoscopy; Colorectal polyp removal; Colorectal surgery; Ileostomy and colostomy; Intestinal disorders; Intestines; Malignancy and metastasis; National Cancer Institute (NCI); Oncology; Radiation therapy; Rectum; Stomach, intestinal, and pancreatic cancers; Tumor removal; Tumors.

For Further Information:
Adrouny, Richard. *Understanding Colon Cancer*. Jackson: University Press of Mississippi, 2002.
Bub, David S., et al. *One Hundred Questions and Answers About Colorectal Cancer*. 2d ed. Sudbury, Mass.: Jones and Bartlett, 2008.
De Vita, Vincent T., Jr., Samuel Hellman, and Steven A. Rosenberg, eds. *Cancer: Principles and Practice of Oncology*. 9th ed. Philadelphia: Lippincott Williams & Wilkins, 2011.
Dollinger, Malin, et al. *Everyone's Guide to Cancer Therapy*. 5th ed. Kansas City, Mo.: Andrews McMeel, 2008.
Eyre, Harmon J., Dianne Partie Lange, and Lois B. Morris. *Informed Decisions: The Complete Book of Cancer Diagnosis, Treatment, and Recovery*. 2d ed. Atlanta: American Cancer Society, 2002.
Goldman, Lee, and Dennis Ausiello, eds. *Cecil Textbook of Medicine*. 23d ed. Philadelphia: Saunders/Elsevier, 2007.
LaRusso, Laurie. "Colon Cancer." *Health Library*, February 28,

2013.

Levin, Bernard, et al., eds. *American Cancer Society's Complete Guide to Colorectal Cancer*. Atlanta: American Cancer Society, 2006.

Miskovitz, Paul, and Marian Betancourt. *What to Do If You Get Colon Cancer: A Specialist Helps You Take Charge and Make Informed Choices*. New York: Wiley, 1997.

Parker, James N., and Philip M. Parker, eds. *The Official Patient's Sourcebook on Colon Cancer*. San Diego, Calif.: Icon Health, 2002.

"What Is Colorectal Cancer?" *American Cancer Society*, January 17, 2013.

COLORECTAL POLYP REMOVAL
Procedure

Anatomy or system affected: Abdomen, anus, gastrointestinal system, intestines

Specialties and related fields: Gastroenterology, general surgery, proctology

Definition: The surgical removal of overgrowths of the tissue lining the rectum and colon.

Indications and Procedures

Rectal and colon polyps are growths of tissue that occur in the mucous membranes lining the colon and rectum. They are usually not malignant. Common types of colorectal polyps are juvenile polyps, Peutz-Jeghers polyps (hamartomas), hyperplasias, adenomas, and mixed hyperplastic-adenomatous polyps. Adenomas are both the most dangerous and the most common type of colon polyp.

Rectal or colon polyps are removed when they are found, even if they cause no symptoms, because identifying the kind of polyp helps doctors determine whether cancer is likely to develop. The type of polyp is determined in the laboratory after surgical removal, using microscopic techniques.

The presence of polyps does not mean that a patient has cancer, although larger polyps (greater than one centimeter) indicate a higher risk for cancer than do smaller ones. Certain types of polyps also are more likely than others to develop into cancer. Hyperplasias are polyps with no potential to develop into cancer. Juvenile polyps and Peutz-Jeghers polyps are associated with inherited disorders that indicate an increased risk for colon cancer, but they do not always develop into malignant tumors. Colorectal adenomas are particularly dangerous when they occur in conjunction with a genetic condition known as familial adenomatous polyposis (FAP). In patients with FAP, untreated colorectal adenomas develop into colon cancer virtually 100 percent of the time. Mixed hyperplastic-adenomatous polyps, although not as risky as pure adenomas, can develop into colon cancer, and patients with a diagnosis of this type of polyp should be closely monitored.

Colon polyps often cause no symptoms. They are usually detected by routine screening for colorectal cancers. The most common symptoms, when they occur, are bleeding from the anus (visible on underwear or toilet paper), constipation or diarrhea lasting more than a week, and blood in the stool, which can appear as red streaks or an overall darkening of fe-

cal matter. The fecal occult blood test will detect blood that is not visible.

When polyps are suspected, the physician will perform a rectal examination or special tests such as barium enema x-rays, flexible sigmoidoscopy, or colonoscopy. In a rectal examination, the doctor feels the rectal tissue with his or her fingers, looking for abnormalities. Barium makes healthy intestinal tissue look white on an x-ray, and polyps appear dark against the white background. The sigmoidoscope is a flexible fiber-optic tube that can be inserted through the anus. The tube has a small video camera and a light so that the doctor can visualize the lower third of the large intestine. Colonoscopy is similar to sigmoidoscopy, but the colonoscope allows the physician to visualize the entire intestine.

Removal is most commonly accomplished using colonoscopy to visualize the polyps and specialized forceps to detach and remove the growths. Snare forceps can be used to surround a polyp and cut it from the lining of the colon or rectum. Other methods of removal include a laser beam, burning, or ultrasound, depending on the size of the polyp. Bleeding during the procedure can be controlled with electrocautery forceps, which use heat to sever the polyp from the surrounding healthy tissue and seal off blood vessels, or by pressing epinephrine-soaked gauze against the removal site.

Special precautions must be taken during surgery to remove gas from the colon so that the combustion of hydrogen or methane gas does not occur. These gases are normally produced by bacteria that inhabit the colon.

A polyp in the lower portion of the colon may be removed using similar procedures during the sigmoidoscopy. In some cases, the patient may undergo surgery to remove the polyp through the abdomen.

Uses and Complications

Since colonoscopy is somewhat uncomfortable for the patient, sedatives are usually given, but general anesthesia is usually not necessary. Rectal and colon polyp removal is typically done as an outpatient procedure.

Because of the gas that enters the intestine during the procedure, patients may experience bloating, pressure, and intestinal cramps in the twenty-four hours following removal. This discomfort subsides as the gas passes out of the intestine.

Repeat colonoscopy should be performed so that recurrent polyps can be removed and examined for malignancy. Colorectal cancer is the second leading cause of cancer deaths in the United States, and the majority of these cancers arise from colorectal polyps.

—Matthew Berria, Ph.D.,
and Douglas Reinhart, M.D.;
updated by Caroline M. Small

See also Biopsy; Cancer; Colon; Colonoscopy and sigmoidoscopy; Colorectal cancer; Colorectal surgery; Electrocauterization; Endoscopy; Enemas; Gastroenterology; Gastrointestinal system; Hemorrhoid banding and removal; Hemorrhoids; Intestinal disorders; Intestines; Oncology; Polyps; Proctology; Rectum; Screening.

For Further Information:

Ades, Terri, Katie Couric, and Bernard Levin. *American Cancer Society's Complete Guide to Colorectal Cancer*. Chicago: American Cancer Society, 2012.

Burke, Carol, and James Church, eds. *Hereditary Colorectal Cancer Syndromes*. New York: Blackwell, 2007.

Corman, Marvin L. *Colon and Rectal Surgery*. 5th ed. Philadelphia: Lippincott Williams & Wilkins, 2005.

Greenberger, Norton J., R. S. Blumberg, and Robert Burakoff. *Current Diagnosis & Treatment: Gastroenterology, Hepatology, & Endoscopy*. 2d ed. New York: McGraw-Hill Medical, 2012.

Health Library. "Colorectal Polyps." *Health Library*, February 8, 2013.

Longo, Walter E., and John M. A. Northover, eds. *Reoperative Colon and Rectal Surgery*. New York: Martin Dunitz, 2003.

Longstreth, George F. "Colorectal Polyps." *MedlinePlus*, October 8, 2012.

National Institutes of Health and National Cancer Institute. *Cancer of the Colon and Rectum*. Rev. ed. Bethesda, Md.: Author, 1991.

National Institutes of Health and National Cancer Institute. *What You Need to Know About Cancer of the Colon and Rectum*. Rev. ed. Bethesda, Md.: Author, 2006.

Zollinger, Robert M., Jr., Robert M. Zollinger, Sr., et al. *Zollinger's Atlas of Surgical Operations*. 9th ed. New York: McGraw-Hill, 2011.

COLORECTAL SURGERY

Procedure

Anatomy or system affected: Abdomen, anus, gastrointestinal system, intestines

Specialties and related fields: Gastroenterology, general surgery, proctology

Definition: Surgery that is required to correct pathologies of the colon, rectum, and anus.

Key terms:

abscess: a pocket of infection or inflammation

acute: referring to a short, immediate disease state

chronic: referring to an enduring disease state

ulcer: a lesion that destroys tissue

Indications and Procedures

The large intestine, or colon, is shaped like an inverted *U*. It starts at the lower right side of the pelvis, where the small intestine empties into the cecum. The colon rises from the cecum to the center of the abdomen, crosses to the left, and descends to the S-shaped sigmoid colon, the rectum, and the anus. Common disorders of the colon, rectum, and anus that require surgery are hemorrhoids, Crohn's disease, ulcerative colitis, cancer, diverticulosis, and diverticulitis.

Hemorrhoids are swollen veins in the lower part of the rectum and the anus. They protrude as nodes or lumps that can cause severe pain, itching, and inflammation. Hemorrhoids can be tied off with tiny rubber bands. After a few days, they fall off painlessly. Medications can shrink internal hemorrhoids, or hemorrhoidal tissue can be removed by photocoagulation, a process that uses electromagnetic energy to eradicate affected tissues. Sometimes, a hemorrhoidectomy is required. This procedure involves the extensive excision of hemorrhoidal tissue and can be quite painful.

Crohn's disease and ulcerative colitis are chronic inflammatory bowel diseases (IBDs) that can affect the colon.

Crohn's disease usually occurs in the small intestine, although it may be limited to the colon. When Crohn's disease is severe and restricted to the colon, the surgeon may perform a colectomy and ileostomy. This procedure involves removing the entire lower intestine, rectum, and anus. The anal opening is closed, and a new opening, or stoma, is made in the abdominal wall. The ileum, the lower end of the small intestine, is then attached to the opening. A removable pouch is sealed to the opening to collect fecal matter, which must be emptied manually.

Ulcerative colitis may exist with no symptoms other than an occasional flare-up, or it can be a chronic, serious, or life-threatening disease. It is characterized by a series of ulcers on the inner wall of the colon. Bloody diarrhea, abdominal pain, and painful bowel movements are symptoms. In severe cases, there is danger of perforation of the colon wall or of swelling (toxic megacolon), either of which can be life-threatening. Ulcerative colitis may also be a precursor of colon cancer. In severe cases of ulcerative colitis, surgery is required. Colectomy and ileostomy are the surgical procedures usually performed, but recently developed is a procedure called ileoanal anastomosis. As in ileostomy, the surgeon removes the entire colon and rectum but leaves the anal sphincter muscles. The ileum is then attached to the anus. This procedure allows the patient to have natural bowel movements and avoids the necessity of the ileostomy pouch.

Cancers of the colon or rectum, called colorectal cancers, are major causes of morbidity and mortality. The possibility of colon cancer is often signaled by the presence of polyps on the lower intestinal wall. Symptoms such as mucus or blood in the stool may alert the physician to look for polyps and determine whether they are likely to become cancerous. Benign polyps are usually removed surgically.

When polyps are likely to become cancerous, and in the presence of actual colorectal cancer, surgery is usually performed to remove diseased tissue. This often requires excising part or all of the colon. Sometimes a colectomy and colostomy are performed, an operation similar to an ileostomy. In this procedure, the diseased sections of the colon, the rectum, and the anus are removed. The anal opening is sealed, and the remaining colon is brought to an opening in the abdominal wall. This opening, or stoma, is fitted with a removable colostomy bag or pouch to collect fecal matter.

Diverticula are small, sac-like pouches that develop in the colon wall, most often in the sigmoid colon. Their presence is known as diverticulosis. These sacs can collect stagnant fecal matter and become inflamed, resulting in diverticulitis. Abscesses and infection may develop. As inflammation progresses or recurs, the wall of the colon thickens, reducing the width of the passage and increasing the possibility of obstruction and distension of the colon. Perforations in the colon wall may develop and cause peritonitis (infection of the membrane that covers the abdomen).

In severe cases, it may be necessary to perform a temporary colostomy. The diseased section of colon is removed, and the rectum and anus are closed. A stoma is made in the abdominal wall and attached to the remaining colon and covered by a pouch to collect fecal matter. After the bowel has healed, the rectum and anus can be reopened and attached to the colon.

Uses and Complications

Patients with permanent ileostomies and colostomies have a hole in their abdomens that is often five or more centimeters (two or more inches) in diameter. Patients are required to wear removable pouches sealed to their stomas to collect fecal matter so that it can be eliminated. The apparatus is cumbersome, and the entire process can be unpleasant enough to cause serious depression in the patient. Patients" spouses and other family members are often involved in changing and emptying the bags, particularly with older, infirm persons. Ileoanal anastomosis solves some of these problems because it allows natural bowel movements, but it is useful only in certain conditions.

Perspective and Prospects

Current surgical procedures are often effective in serious colorectal conditions. The success rate of these surgeries for the treatment of cancer is quite high if the cancer is caught before it spreads to other parts of the body. Nevertheless, patients may have to endure the inconvenience of ostomy bags and paraphernalia for the rest of their lives. Ostomy equipment has been improved: Better sealing adhesives are now in use so that the bags do not slip or leak as they once did. The configuration of belts, bags, and other appliances has been altered to make them more convenient and easier to live with. New surgical procedures that could maintain normal bowel function for more patients, however, would be a major advancement.

—*C. Richard Falcon*

See also Abdomen; Abdominal disorders; Biopsy; Cancer; Colitis; Colon; Colonoscopy and sigmoidoscopy; Colorectal cancer; Colorectal polyp removal; Crohn's disease; Diverticulitis and diverticulosis; Electrocauterization; Endoscopy; Enemas; Fistula repair; Gastroenterology; Gastrointestinal system; Hemorrhoid banding and removal; Hemorrhoids; Hernia repair; Hernias; Ileostomy and colostomy; Intestinal disorders; Intestines; Oncology; Proctology; Rectum; Tumor removal; Tumors.

For Further Information:

Feldman, Mark, Lawrence S. Friedman, and Lawrence J. Brandt, eds. *Sleisenger and Fordtran's Gastrointestinal and Liver Disease: Pathophysiology, Diagnosis, Management.* 9th ed. 2 vols. Philadelphia: Saunders/Elsevier, 2010.

Kapadia, Cyrus R., James M. Crawford, and Caroline Taylor. *An Atlas of Gastroenterology: A Guide to Diagnosis and Differential Diagnosis.* Boca Raton, Fla.: Pantheon, 2003.

Litin, Scott C., ed. *Mayo Clinic Family Health Book.* 4th ed. New York: HarperResource, 2009.

Phillips, Robert H. *Coping with an Ostomy: A Guide to Living with an Ostomy for You and Your Family.* Wayne, N.J.: Avery, 1986.

Zollinger, Robert M., Jr., Robert M. Zollinger, Sr., et al. *Zollinger's Atlas of Surgical Operations.* 9th ed. New York: McGraw-Hill, 2011.

COMA. *See* MINIMALLY CONSCIOUS STATE.

COMMON COLD
Disease/Disorder

Anatomy or system affected: Chest, lungs, nose, respiratory system

Specialties and related fields: Family medicine, internal medicine, otorhinolaryngology, public health, virology

Definition: A class of viral respiratory infections that form the world's most prevalent illnesses.

Key terms:

acute: referring to a disease process of sudden onset and short duration

chronic: referring to a disease process of long duration and frequent recurrence

coronavirus: a microorganism causing respiratory illness; one of the most prevalent causes of the common cold

pathogen: any disease-causing microorganism

rhinovirus: a microorganism causing respiratory illness; one of the most prevalent causes of the common cold

virus: an extremely small pathogen that can replicate only within a living cell

Causes and Symptoms

One of the reasons that no cure has ever been found for the common cold is that it is caused by literally hundreds of different viruses. More than two hundred distinct strains from eight genera have been identified, and no doubt more will be discovered. Infection by one of these viruses may confer immunity to it, but there will still be scores of others to which that individual is not immune. The common cold is usually restricted to the nose and surrounding areas-hence its medical name, rhinitis (*rhin* meaning "nose" and *itis* meaning "inflammation").

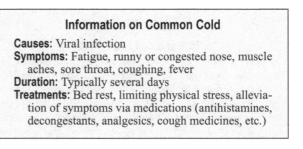

Information on Common Cold

Causes: Viral infection
Symptoms: Fatigue, runny or congested nose, muscle aches, sore throat, coughing, fever
Duration: Typically several days
Treatments: Bed rest, limiting physical stress, alleviation of symptoms via medications (antihistamines, decongestants, analgesics, cough medicines, etc.)

Children get the most colds, averaging six to eight per year until they are six years old. From that age, the number diminishes until, for adults, the rate is three to five colds per year. Colds and related respiratory diseases are the largest single cause of missed workdays and school days. Colds and related respiratory diseases are probably the world's most expensive illnesses. In the United States alone, about a million person-years are lost from work each year; this figure accounts for one-half of all absences. Worldwide, the costs of lost workdays, medications, physician's visits, and complications that may require extensive medical care are incalculable.

Among the virus types that cause the common cold are rhinovirus, coronavirus, influenza virus, parainfluenza virus, enterovirus, adenovirus, respiratory syncytial virus, and coxsackie virus. They are not all equally responsible for cold infections. Rhinoviruses and coronaviruses between them are thought to cause 25 to 60 percent of all colds. Rhinoviruses appear to be responsible for colds that occur in the peak cold seasons of late spring and early fall. Coronaviruses appear to be responsible for colds that occur when rhinovirus is less active, such as in the late fall, winter, and early spring. Enteroviruses are the most common cause of the "summer cold." During the summer months up to 20 percent of children may be shedding one of these viruses and thus are infective.

A respiratory syncytial virus can cause the common cold in adults; in children it causes much more severe diseases, including pneumonia and bronchiolitis (inflammation of the bronchioles, small air passages in the lungs). Similarly, influenza and parainfluenza viruses, adenoviruses, and enteroviruses can be responsible for rhinitis and sore throat, but they are also capable of causing more serious illnesses such as pneumonia and meningitis.

Viruses are the smallest of the invading microorganisms that cause disease, so small that they are not visible using ordinary microscopes. They can be seen, however, with an electron microscope, and their presence in the body can be detected through various laboratory tests.

Viruses vary enormously in their size and structure. Some consist of three or four proteins with a core of either deoxyribonucleic acid (DNA) or ribonucleic acid (RNA); some have more than fifty proteins and other substances. Viruses can replicate only within living cells. They invade the body and produce disease conditions in different ways. Some travel through the body to find their target host cells. A good example is the measles virus, which enters through the mucous membranes of the nose, throat, and mouth and then finds its way to target tissues throughout the body. Some, such as the viruses that cause the common cold, enter the body through the nasal passages and settle directly into nearby cells.

Rhinoviruses are members of the Picornaviridae family (*pico*- from "piccolo," meaning "very small"; *rna* from RNA, the genetic material that it contains; and *viridae* denoting a virus family). Coronaviruses are members of the Coronaviridae family, and they also contain RNA. Most viruses that are pathogenic to humans can thrive only at the temperature inside the human body, 37 degrees Celsius (98.6 degrees Fahrenheit). Rhinoviruses prefer the cooler temperatures found in the nasal passages, 33 to 34 degrees Celsius (91.4 to 93.2 degrees Fahrenheit). More than one hundred different rhinovirus types have been identified.

Exactly how a patient contracts a cold is better understood than it once was. Exposure to a cold environment-for example, getting a chill in winter weather-does not cause a cold unless the individual is exposed to the infecting virus at the same time. Fatigue or lack of sleep does not increase susceptibility to the cold virus, and even the direct exposure of nasal tissue to cold viruses does not guarantee infection.

A group in England, the Medical Research Council's Common Cold Unit, studied the disease from 1945 to 1990 and made many fundamental discoveries-even though the researchers never found a cure, or, for that matter, any effective methods to prevent the spread of the disease. As part of their research, they put drops containing cold virus into the noses of volunteers. Only about one-third of the subjects thus inoculated developed cold symptoms, showing that direct exposure to the infecting agent does not necessarily bring on a cold.

What appears to be essential in the spread of the disease is bodily contact, particularly handshaking or touching. The infected individual wipes his or her nose or coughs into his or her hand, getting nasal secretions on the fingers. These infected secretions are then transferred to the hand of another person who, if susceptible, can become infected by bringing the hand up to the mouth or nose. Sneezing and coughing also spread the disease. Many viral and bacterial diseases are transmissible through nasopharyngeal (nose and throat) secretions; these include measles, mumps, rubella, pneumonia, influenza, and any number of other infections.

One or more individuals in a group become infected and bring the disease to a central place, such as a classroom, office, military base, or day care center. In the case of the common cold, transferring infected particles by touch exposes another person to the infection. In other respiratory diseases, breathing, sneezing, or coughing virus-laden particles into the air will spread the disease. The infected individual then becomes the means by which the disease is brought into the home. By far, the largest number of colds are brought into the family by children who have contracted the infection in classrooms or day care centers.

The pathogenesis of the common cold-that is, what happens when an individual is exposed to the cold virus-is not fully understood. It is believed that the virus enters the nasal passages

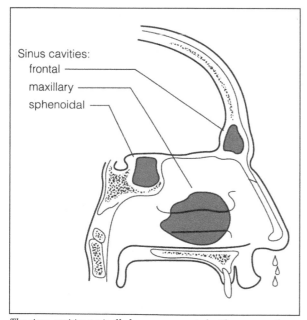

Sinus cavities:
frontal
maxillary
sphenoidal

The sinus cavities typically become congested with mucus as the body fights the virus that has caused the cold.

and attaches itself to receptors on a cell of the nasal mucous membrane and then invades the cell. Viruses traveling freely in the blood or lymphatic system are subject to attack by white blood cells called phagocytes in what is part of the body's nonspecific defense system against invading pathogens.

Once inside the host cell, the virus replicates itself by stealing elements of the protoplasm of the cell and using them to build new viruses under the direction of the RNA component. These new viruses are released by the host cell to infect other cells. This process can injure or kill the host cell, activating the body's specific immune response system and starting the chain of events that will destroy the invading virus and create immunity to further infection from it.

In response to cell death or injury, certain chemicals are released that induce inflammation in the nasal passages. Blood vessels in the nasal area enlarge, increasing blood flow to the tissues and causing swelling. The openings in capillary walls enlarge and deliver lymphocytes, white blood cells that produce antibodies to fight the virus, as well as other specialized white blood cells.

Nasal mucosa swell and secretions increase, a condition medically known as rhinorrhea (-rrhea meaning "flowing," denoting the runny nose of the common cold). During the first few days of infection, these secretions are thin and watery. As the disease progresses and white blood cells are drawn to the area, the secretions become thicker and more purulent, that is, filled with pus. A sore throat is common, as is laryngitis, or inflammation of the larynx or voice box. Fever is not a usual symptom of the common cold, but a cough will often develop as excess mucus or phlegm builds up in the lungs and windpipe.

As mucus accumulates and clogs nasal passages, the body attempts to expel it by sneezing. In this process, impulses from the nose travel to the brain's "sneeze reflex center," where sneezing is triggered to help clear nasal passages. Similarly, as phlegm accumulates in the windpipe and bronchial tree of the lungs, a message is sent to the "cough reflex center" of the brain, where coughing is initiated to expel the phlegm.

The common cold is self-limiting and usually resolves within five to ten days, but there can be complications in some cases. Patients who have asthma or chronic bronchitis frequently develop bronchoconstriction (narrowing of the air passages in the lungs) as a result of a common cold. If severe purulent tracheitis and bronchitis develop, there may be a con-comitant bacterial infection. In some patients, the infection may spread to other organs, such as the ears, where an infection called otitis media can develop. Sinusitis, infection of the cavities in the bone of the skull surrounding the nose, is common. If the invading organism spreads to the lungs, bronchitis or pneumonia may develop.

Other possible complications of the common cold depend on the individual virus. Rhinoviruses, usually limited to colds, may infrequently cause pneumonia in children. Coronaviruses, also usually limited to colds, infrequently cause pneumonia and bronchiolitis. A respiratory syncytial virus causes pneumonia and bronchiolitis in children, the common cold in adults, and pneumonia in the elderly. Parainfluenza virus, which causes croup and other respiratory diseases in children, can cause sore throat and the common cold in adults and, rarely, may cause tracheobronchitis in these patients. Influenza B virus, an occasional cause of the common cold, also causes influenza and, infrequently, pneumonia.

Another condition that can closely resemble the common cold, but which is not caused by a virus, is allergic rhinitis. The major form of allergic rhinitis is hay fever. It has many of the same symptoms as the common cold: sneezing, runny

---

In the News:
Gene Studies May Help Find a Treatment for the Common Cold

Genomic mapping has been completed for the human rhinovirus (HRV). In a collaborative effort among four research institutions, all ninety-nine strains of the common cold virus, the human rhinovirus (HRV), have been genetically sequenced. This data set provides an important baseline framework for future analysis of new HRVs that may be identified, according to the study authors Ann C. Palmenberg from the University of Wisconsin, and her colleagues at University of Maryland School of Medicine and the J. Craig Venter Institute in Rockville, Maryland. The database will help inform future research in the development of antiviral agents and vaccines.

Rhinoviruses can alter human genes. A University of Calgary study published in the *American Journal of Respiratory and Critical Care* in 2008 found that rhinoviruses causes cold symptoms not by triggering an immune response in the host, but by altering the host cellular genes that control inflammation and antiviral responses. The randomized study involved nasal scrapings from thirty-five healthy volunteers, half of whom were inoculated with rhinovirus. Changes in gene expression were analyzed for nasal scraping taken at eight and forty-eight hours after inoculation. While eight-hour samples found no differences in cellular genes between groups, the forty-eight-hour sample found more than 6,500 genes altered in the inoculation group when compared with the control group. Two affected groups of genes were genes involved in the inflammatory process and antiviral genes, according to study authors David Proud and colleagues. A faulty visperin gene, known to play a role in other viral infections such as influenza, hepatitis, and cytomegalovirus was identified. The identification of altered human genes associated with rhinovirus infection provides potential new direction for therapeutic research.

Poor sleep habits can reduce resistance to common cold. A study published in January, 2009, in the *Archives of Internal Medicine* by Sheldon Cohen and colleagues suggests there is a simple way to reduce the risk of acquiring the common cold. A study of 153 healthy men and women found that participants who got less than seven hours of sleep a night for fourteen consecutive nights were almost three times as likely to get a cold after receiving nasal drops containing rhinovirus. The researchers concluded that poor sleep habits reduce resistance to viruses such as the common cold virus.

—*Sandra Ripley Distelhorst*

nose, nasal congestion, and, sometimes, sore throat. In addition, the hay fever victim may suffer from itching in the eyes, nose, mouth, and throat. Hay fever is an allergic reaction to certain pollens. Because the pollens that cause hay fever are abundant at certain times of the year, it may be prevalent at the same times as some colds. Spring is a peak season for the common cold and also for hay fever, because of the many tree pollens that are carried in the air. In the fall, weed pollens, such as those of ragweed, affect hay-fever sufferers during another peak period for colds. Colds occur less frequently in summer, but summer is another peak season for hay fever.

Treatment and Therapy

The nose is the first barrier of defense against the bacteria and viruses that cause upper respiratory infections. The nasal cavity is lined with a thin coating of mucus, a thick liquid that is constantly replenished by the mucous glands. Inner nasal surfaces are filled with tiny hairs, or cilia. Dust, bacteria, and other foreign matter are trapped by the mucus and moved by the cilia toward the nasopharynx to be expectorated or swallowed.

The blood vessels in the nasopharyngeal bed respond automatically to stimulation from the brain. Certain stimuli cause the vessels to constrict, widening air passages and at the same time reducing the flow of mucus. Other stimuli, such as those that are sent in response to a viral infection, allergen, or other irritant, cause blood vessels to dilate and increase the flow of mucus. Nasal passages become swollen, and airways are blocked.

The mucus-covered lining of the nasal passages contains various substances that help ward off infection and irritation by allergens. Lysozyme (*lyso* meaning "dissolution" and *zyme* from "enzyme," a catalyst that promotes an activity) attacks the cell walls of certain bacteria, killing them. It also attacks pollen granules. Mucus also contains glycoproteins that temporarily inhibit the activity of viruses. Mucus has small amounts of the antibodies immunoglobulin IgA and IgC that also may inhibit the activity of invading viruses.

Bed rest is usually the first element of treatment for a common cold. Limiting physical stress may help keep the cold from worsening and may avoid secondary infections. The medications used to treat the common cold are directed at relieving individual symptoms; there is no available medication that will kill the viruses that cause it. Most cases of the common cold are treated at home with over-the-counter cold preparations. Children's colds and the complications that may arise from colds, such as bacterial and viral superinfection, may require the services of a physician.

Many medications for the common cold contain antihistamines. Histamine is a naturally occurring chemical in the body that is released in response to an allergen or an infection. It is a significant cause of the inflammation, swelling, and runny nose of hay fever. When these symptoms are seen with the common cold, however, they are probably caused by the body's inflammatory defense system rather than by histamine.

When antihistamines were first discovered, it was thought that they could inhibit the inflammatory defense against a cold. Patients were advised to take antihistamines at the first sign of a cold, in the hope of avoiding a full infection. Current thinking is that antihistamines have little value in the treatment of the common cold. They may have a minor effect on a runny nose, but there are better agents for this purpose. Antihistamines are usually highly sedative-most over-the-counter sleeping pills are antihistamines-so they may cause drowsiness. Patients taking many antihistamines are cautioned to avoid driving or operating machinery that could be dangerous.

The mainstays of therapy for the common cold are the decongestants that are applied topically (that is, directly to the mucous membranes in the nose) or taken orally. They are also called sympathomimetic agents because they mimic the effects of certain natural body chemicals that regulate many body processes. A group of these, called adrenergic stimulants, regulate vasoconstriction and vasodilation-in other words, they can narrow or widen blood vessels, respectively. Their vasoconstrictive capability is useful in managing the common cold, because it reduces the size of the blood vessels in the nose, reduces swelling and congestion, and inhibits excess secretion.

Topical decongestants are available as nasal sprays or drops. The sprays are squirted up into each nostril. The patient is usually advised to wait three to five minutes and then blow his or her nose to remove the mucus. If there is still congestion, the patient is advised to take another dose, allowing the medication to reach farther into the nasal cavity. Nose drops are taken by tilting the head back and squeezing the medication into the nostrils through the nose-dropper supplied with the medication. Clearance of nasal congestion is prompt, and the patient can breathe more easily. Nasal irritation is reduced, so there is less sneezing. Some nasal sprays and drops last longer than others, but none works around-the-clock, so applications must be repeated throughout the day.

Patients who use nasal sprays and drops are advised to follow the manufacturer's directions exactly. Applied too often or in too great a quantity, these preparations can cause unwanted problems, such as rhinitis medicamentosa, or nasal inflammation caused by a medication (also called rebound congestion). As the vasoconstrictive effect of the drugs wears down, the blood vessels dilate, the area becomes swollen, and secretions increase. This reaction may be attributable to the fact that the drug's vasoconstrictive effect has deprived the area of blood, and thus excited an increased inflammatory state, or it may simply be attributable to irritation by the drug. Use of sprays or drops should be limited to three or four days.

Oral decongestants are also effective in reducing swelling and relieving a runny nose, although they do not have as great a vasoconstrictive effect concentrated in the nasal area as sprays or drops. Because they circulate throughout the body, their vasoconstrictive effects may be seen in other vascular beds. Patients with high blood pressure; diabetes; heart disease; or who are taking certain drugs such as monoamine oxidase inhibitors (MAOIs), guanethidine, bethanidine, or debrisoquin sulfate are advised not to use oral decongestants unless they are under the care of a physician.

Three kinds of coughs may accompany colds: coughs that produce phlegm or mucus; hyperactive nagging coughs, which result from overstimulation of the cough reflex; and dry, unproductive coughs. If the phlegm or mucus collecting in the lungs is easily removed by occasional coughing, a soothing syrup, cough drop, or lozenge may be all that the patient requires. If the cough reflex center of the brain is overstimulated, there may be hyperactive or uncontrollable coughing, and a cough suppressant, such as dextromethorphan, may be needed. Dextromethorphan works in the brain to raise the level of stimulus that is required to trigger the cough reflex. Some antihistamines, such as diphenhydramine hydrochloride, are effective cough suppressants. If coughing is unproductive-that is, if the mucus has thickened and dried and is not easily removed-an expectorant should be taken. Currently, the only expectorant used in over-the-counter drugs is guaifenesin. It helps soften and liquefy mucus deposits, so that coughs become productive. When the cough of a cold is serious enough for a physician to be consulted, prescription drugs may need to be used, such as codeine to stop hyperactive coughing and potassium iodide for unproductive coughs.

For allergic rhinitis or hay fever, avoidance of allergens is recommended but is not always possible. For hay-fever outbreaks, antihistamines are the mainstays of therapy, with other agents added to relieve specific symptoms. For example, topical and oral decongestants may be required to relieve a runny nose.

Perspective and Prospects

Viruses are among the most intriguing and baffling challenges to medical science. Great progress has been made in preventing some virus diseases, such as by immunization against smallpox and hepatitis B. There has been only limited success, however, in finding agents to cure viral diseases, and so far nothing has been found to prevent or cure the common cold. Vaccines have been developed against certain rhinoviruses, and no doubt many more will be developed. Yet because the common cold is caused by so many different types of virus-more than two hundred-and vaccines against one virus are not necessarily effective against others, it is questionable whether such vaccines would ever be useful. A helpful vaccine would be one that could immunize against an entire family of viruses such as rhinoviruses or coronaviruses, the two leading causes of the common cold.

The search goes on for agents to cure the common cold. Substances, such as interferons, have been found that are effective against a wide range of viruses. One of the interferons was used by the British Medical Research Council's Common Cold Unit. Those researchers reported that interferon applied as an intranasal spray was effective in protecting subjects from cold infection. After some years, however, experimentation with interferon in the common cold was abandoned because the agent had significant side effects, nasal congestion among them.

The science of virology only began in the 1930s, so it is not surprising that viruses continue to baffle scientists. Nevertheless, many fundamental discoveries have been made and one can predict increasing success. As scientists unravel the intricacies of viral infections, they find clues that help them devise ways of interfering with virus life processes. In some cases, effective drugs have been developed, such as the interferons, acyclovir for herpes simplex, and amantadine for the influenza virus. It is likely that the cure for the common cold will continue to be elusive, unless a broad-spectrum antiviral agent could be developed that works against multiple viral infections in the way that broad-spectrum antibiotics work against multiple bacterial infections.

—*C. Richard Falcon*

See also Allergies; Antihistamines; Bronchitis; Coughing; Decongestants; Fever; Influenza; Nasopharyngeal disorders; Nausea and vomiting; Noroviruses; Otorhinolarnygology; Pneumonia; Rhinitis; Rhinoviruses; Sinusitis; Sore throat; Viral infections.

For Further Information:

Biddle, Wayne. *A Field Guide to Germs*. 2d ed. New York: Anchor Books, 2002.

Carson-DeWitt, Rosalyn. "Common Cold." *Health Library*, January 9, 2013.

"Common Cold." *National Institute of Allergy and Infectious Diseases*, February 11, 2011.

Gallo, Robert. *Virus Hunting*. New York: Basic Books, 1991.

Kimball, Chad T. *Colds, Flu, and Other Common Ailments Sourcebook*. Detroit, Mich.: Omnigraphics, 2001.

Krinsky, Daniel L., et al. *Handbook of Nonprescription Drugs*. 17th ed. Washington, D.C.:American Pharmaceutical Association, 2011.

Litin, Scott C., ed. *Mayo Clinic Family Health Book*. 4th ed. New York: HarperResource, 2009.

Woolf, Alan D., et al., eds. *The Children's Hospital Guide to Your Child's Health and Development*. Cambridge, Mass.: Perseus, 2002.

Young, Stuart H., Bruce Dobozin, and Margaret Miner. *Allergies*. Rev. ed. New York: Plume, 1999.

COMPUTED TOMOGRAPHY (CT) SCANNING
Procedure

Also known as: Computed axial tomography, CAT scan

Anatomy or system affected: Circulatory system, endocrine system, gastrointestinal system, musculoskeletal system, nervous system, reproductive system, respiratory system

Specialties and related fields: Biotechnology, cardiology, emergency medicine, endocrinology, gastroenterology, internal medicine, oncology, preventive medicine, psychiatry, radiology, vascular medicine

Definition: The use of X rays and a computer to produce detailed cross-sectional images of most body regions to aid in diagnosis.

Key terms:

cathode: an electrode that produces electrons

cathode-ray tube (CRT): a vacuum tube whose cathode emits electrons accelerated through a high voltage anode, focused on a fluorescent image screen

slice: a CT cross section of a body part

soft tissue: tissue other than bone

tomogram: the three-dimensional image of a CT slice

X ray: high-energy electromagnetic radiation

Indications and Procedures

Computed tomography (CT) scanning collects X-ray data and uses a computer to produce three-dimensional images, called tomograms, of body cross sections, or slices. The noninvasiveness of CT scanning yields easy and safe body part analysis based on varying tissue opacity to X-rays. Bone absorbs X-rays well and appears white. Air absorbs them poorly, so the lungs are dark. Fat, blood, and muscle absorb X-rays to varying extents, yielding different shades of gray. Tumors and blood clots, for example, appear as areas of abnormal shades in normal tissue.

CT scanning is used to analyze disorders of the brain (brain CT) and most body parts (body CT), yielding tomograms that are hundreds of times more definitive than conventional X-rays. For example, conventional abdominal X-rays show bones and faintly outline the liver, kidneys, and stomach. Tomograms clearly depict all abdominal organs and large blood vessels.

Physicians call CT scanning the most valuable diagnostic method because, without it, the symptoms that patients describe may not be identified clearly as minor, serious, or life-threatening. For example, a subjective description of repeated headache does not reveal whether the cause is tension, stroke, or brain cancer. Before CT scanning, an accurate diagnosis often required complex or dangerous identification methods.

A CT patient changes into a hospital gown, removes any metal possessions, and lays on a table that can be raised, lowered, or tilted. During a scan, the patient enters a doughnut-shaped scanner that holds an X-ray source, detectors, and computer hookups. In brain CT, the patient's head is in the scanner. Some CT patients have experienced claustrophobia, which can be prevented with faster scanner speeds and less-enclosed scanners. A patient who must stay still for an extended time may be given a sedative. If small anomalies are

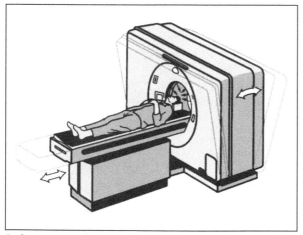

In the imaging technique called computed tomography (CT) scanning (formerly known as a CAT scan), multiple X-ray pictures are taken as the scanner tilts and rotates around the patient. These images are then assembled by a computer to create a three-dimensional view of a body part, such as the head.

foreseen, then contrast materials are given before or during the procedure. These materials include barium salts and iodine, X-ray blockers that allow better visualization of specific tissues. Subjects may take the materials orally, by enema, or intravenously.

The CT scanner generates a continuous, narrow X-ray beam while moving in a circle around the patient's head or body. The beam is monitored by X-ray detectors sited around the aperture through which the patient passes. Slices are produced as the scanner circles the head or body. Between slices, the table moves through the scanner. Slices become tomograms seen on a cathode-ray tube (CRT) and are stored in a computer. The procedure used to take twenty to forty minutes in a standard scanner. However, in the newer spiral CT, which is now standard in most hospitals, a patient is scanned rapidly as the X-ray tube rotates in a spiral. There are no gaps, as with slices, and tissue-volume tomograms are produced. A simple spiral scan is completed while the patient holds his or her breath, aiding the detection of small lesions and decreasing scan artifacts. Spiral CT, twenty times faster than standard CT, is useful in all patients, from restless children to the critically ill.

Uses and Complications

CT scanning detects organ abnormalities, and a major use is in diagnosing and treating brain disease. Even the earliest scanners could distinguish tumors from clots, aiding in the diagnosis of cancer, stroke, and certain birth defects. Furthermore, brain CT saves lives as physicians avoid risky methods requiring opening of the brain for pretreatment diagnosis. In addition, postsurgical scans can find recurrences or metastases.

Body CT allows for better damage appraisal of broken bones than does conventional X-ray analysis. Another use of body spiral CT is in the diagnosis of pulmonary embolism; it is safer than using pulmonary angiography, which maneuvers a catheter from the heart to the pulmonary artery. CT scans can also guide surgery, biopsy, and abscess drainage and can help fine-tune radiation therapy. Speed and excellent soft tissue elucidation make CT scanning invaluable for trauma detection in emergency rooms.

There are few side effects to CT scanning. Preparation for a scan may be mildly uncomfortable, but it is rarely dangerous. Before body CT, subjects often fast, take enemas to clear the bowels, and receive contrast materials through enemas or IVs. If contrast materials are used, then physicians must be told of allergies, especially to iodine. Contrast materials-enhancers of specific tissue CT-may cause hot flashes. Barium enemas for lower gastrointestinal tract scans cause full feelings and urges to defecate.

Perspective and Prospects

British engineer Godfrey Hounsfield and American physicist Allan Cormack won the 1979 Nobel Prize in Physiology or Medicine for the theory and development of computed tomography. CT scanning was first used in 1972, after Hounsfeld made a brain scanner holding an X-ray generator,

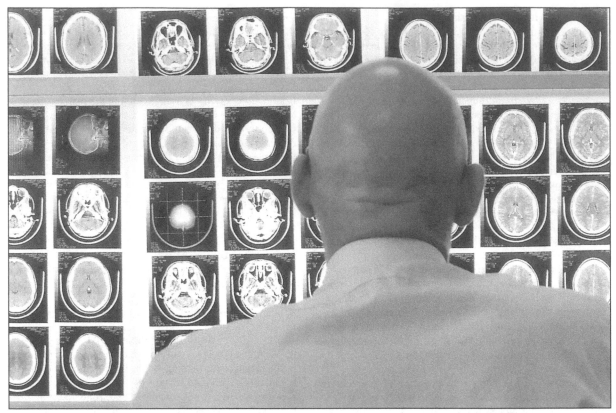

A doctor can use CT scans to detect abnormalities in brain tissue, such as tumors. (Digital Stock)

a scanner rotated around a circular chamber, a computer, and a CRT. The patient laid on a gurney, head in the scanner, and emitter detectors rotated 1 degree at a time for 180 degrees. At each position, 160 readings entered the computer, so 28,800 readings were processed.

CT scanning is essential to radiology, which began in 1885 after Wilhelm Conrad Röntgen discovered X-rays. The rays soon became medical aids, and for years broad X-ray beams were sent through body parts to exit onto film, yielding conventional X-ray images. Bones absorb X-rays well, appearing white, and conventional images can show bone fractures and give some soft tissue data. However, soft tissue evaluation is poor, the tissues superimpose, and estimating their condition is difficult. CT scans allow convenient, noninvasive analysis.

CT scans and stereotaxic neurosurgery, later joined, have improved diagnosis and treatment. For example, the implantation of electrodes in a brain can be monitored using CT, enhancing accuracy. Similar techniques are used in breast biopsy. Current progress in CT scans includes thinner slices, spiral scans, and fast-operating standard scanners. Because complex scans expose patients to more radiation than do conventional X-rays, fast scans are preferred to minimize patient risk.

—Sanford S. Singer, Ph.D.

See also Brain; Brain disorders; Headaches; Imaging and radiology; Magnetic resonance imaging (MRI); Neuroimaging; Noninvasive tests; Nuclear medicine; Positron emission tomography (PET) scanning; Single photon emission computed tomography (SPECT); Strokes; Tumors; Ultrasonography.

For Further Information:

"CT Scans." *MedlinePlus*, June 12, 2013.

Durham, Deborah L. *Rad Tech's Guide to CT: Imaging Procedures, Patient Care, and Safety.* Malden, Mass.: Blackwell Scientific, 2002.

Hsieh, Jiang. *Computed Tomography: Principles, Design, Artifacts, and Recent Advances.* 2d ed. Bellingham, Wash.: SPIE Press, 2009.

Kalender, Willi A. *Computed Tomography: Fundamentals, System Technology, Image Quality, Applications.* 3rd ed. Weinheim, Germany: Wiley VCH, 2009.

McCoy, Krisha, and Brian Randall. "CT Scan (General)." *Health Library*, Nov. 26, 2012.

"Radiation-Emitting Products: Full-Body CT Scans " What You Need to Know." *US Food and Drug Administration*, Apr. 6, 2010.

Slone, Richard M., et al., eds. *Body CT: A Practical Approach.* New York: McGraw-Hill, 2000.

CONCEPTION

Biology

Anatomy or system affected: Cells, reproductive system, uterus

Specialties and related fields: Embryology, gynecology, obstetrics

Definition: The process of creating new life, encompassing all the events from deposition of sperm into the female to the first cell divisions of the fertilized ovum.

Key terms:

cervix: the lowest part of the uterus in contact with the vagina; contains an opening filled with mucus through which sperm can pass

ejaculation: the reflex activated by sexual stimulation that results in sperm mixed with fluid being expelled from the male's body

fertilization: the union of the sperm and the ovum, which usually occurs in the female's oviduct

menstruation: the process of shedding the lining of the uterus that occurs about once a month

oviduct: the thin tube that leads from near the ovary to the upper part of the uterus; also called the Fallopian tube

ovulation: the process by which the mature ovum is expelled from the ovary

ovum: the round cell produced by the female that carries her genetic material; also called the egg

sperm: the motile cells produced within the male that carry his genetic material

uterus: the organ above the vagina through which the sperm must pass on their way to the ovum; also called the womb

vagina: the stretchy, tube-shaped structure into which the male's penis is inserted during intercourse; the site of sperm deposition

Process and Effects

The process of conception begins with the act of intercourse. When the male's penis is inserted into the female's vagina, the stimulation of the penis by movement within the vagina triggers a reflex resulting in the ejaculation of sperm. During ejaculation, involuntary muscles in many of the male reproductive organs contract, causing semen, a mixture of sperm and fluid, to move from its sites of storage out through the urethra within the penis.

The average volume of semen in a typical human ejaculation is only 3.5 milliliters, but this small volume normally contains two hundred million to four hundred million sperm. Other constituents of semen include prostaglandins, which cause contractions of involuntary muscles in both the male and the female; the sugar fructose, which provides energy to the sperm; chemicals that adjust the activity of the semen; and a number of enzymes and other chemicals.

In a typical act of intercourse, the semen is deposited high up in the woman's vagina. Within a minute after ejaculation, the semen begins to coagulate, or form a clot, because of the activation of chemicals within the semen. Sperm are not able to leave the vagina until the semen becomes liquid again, which occurs spontaneously fifteen to twenty minutes after ejaculation.

Once the semen liquefies, sperm begin moving through the female system. The path to the ovum (if one is present) lies through the cervix, then through the hollow cavity of the uterus, and up through the oviduct, where fertilization nor-

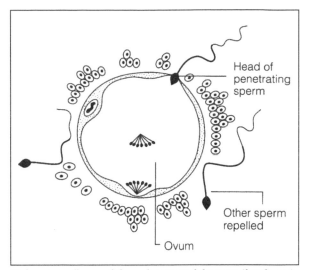

Male sperm cells propel themselves toward the ovum (female egg) by the swimming movements of their tails; fertilization occurs when a sperm cell penetrates the layers surrounding the ovum and fuses its membrane with the membrane of the ovum.

mally occurs. The sperm are propelled through the fluid within these organs by the swimming movements of their tails called flagella, as well as by female organ contractions that are stimulated by the act of intercourse and by prostaglandins contained in the semen. The contractions allow sperm to reach the oviduct within five minutes after leaving the vagina, a rate of movement that far exceeds their own swimming abilities.

Although some sperm can reach the oviduct quite rapidly, others never enter the oviduct at all. Of the two hundred million to four hundred million sperm deposited in the vagina, it is estimated that only one hundred to one thousand enter the oviducts. Some of the other millions of sperm may be defective, lacking the proper swimming ability. Other apparently normal sperm may become lost within the female's organs, possibly trapped in clefts between cells in the organ linings. The damaged and lost sperm will eventually be destroyed by white blood cells produced by the female.

Sperm movement through the female system is enhanced around the time of ovulation. For example, at the time of ovulation, the hormones associated with ovulation cause changes in the cervical mucus that aid sperm transport. The mucus at that time is extremely liquid and contains fibers that align themselves into channels, which are thought to be used by the sperm to ease their passage through the cervix. The hormones present at the time of ovulation also increase the contractions produced by the uterus and oviduct, and thus sperm transport through the structures is enhanced as well.

During transport through the female system, sperm undergo a number of important chemical changes, collectively called capacitation, that enable them to fertilize the ovum successfully. Freshly ejaculated sperm are not capable of penetrating the layers surrounding the ovum, a fact that was uncovered when scientists first began to experiment with in vitro fertilization (the joining of sperm and ovum outside the body). Capacitation apparently occurs during transport of the sperm through the uterus and possibly the oviduct, and it is presumably triggered by some secretion of the female reproductive system. With in vitro fertilization, capacitation is achieved by adding female blood serum to the dish that contains the sperm and ovum. Capacitation is not instantaneous; it has been estimated that this process requires an hour or more in humans. Even though the first sperm may arrive in the vicinity of the ovum within twenty minutes after ejaculation, fertilization cannot take place until capacitation is completed. In 2003, scientists discovered that sperm has a type of chemical sensor that causes the sperm to swim vigorously toward concentrations of a chemical attractant. While researchers long have known that chemical signals are an important component of conception, the 2003 findings were the first to demonstrate that sperm will respond in a predictable and controllable way, a fact promising for future contraception and fertility research.

The site where ovum and sperm typically come together is within the oviduct. At the time of ovulation, an ovum is released from the surface of the ovary and drawn into the upper end of the oviduct. Once within the oviduct, the ovum is propelled by contractions of the oviduct and possibly by wavelike motions of cilia, hairlike projections that line the inner surface of the oviduct. It takes about three days for the ovum to travel the entire length of the oviduct to the uterus, and since the ovum only remains fertilizable for twelve to twenty-four hours, successful fertilization must occur in the oviduct.

Upon reaching the ovum, the sperm must first penetrate two layers surrounding it. The outermost layer, called the corona radiata, consists of cells that break away from the ovary with the ovum during ovulation; the innermost layer, the zona pellucida, is a clear, jellylike substance that lies just outside the ovum cell membrane. Penetration of these two layers is accomplished by the release of enzymes carried by the sperm. Once through the zona pellucida, the sperm are ready to fertilize the ovum.

Fertilization occurs when a sperm fuses its membrane with the membrane of the ovum. This act triggers a protective change in the zona pellucida that prevents any additional sperm from reaching the ovum and providing it with extra chromosomes. Following fusion of the fertilizing sperm and ovum, the chromosomes of each become mingled and pair up; the resulting one-celled zygote contains a complete set of chromosomes, half contributed by the mother and half by the father.

It is at the moment of fertilization that the sex of the new child is decided. Genetic sex is determined by a pair of chromosomes denoted X and Y. Female body cells contain two Xs, and each ovum produced contains only one X. Male body cells contain an X and a Y chromosome, but each sperm contains either an X or a Y chromosome. Men usually produce equal numbers of X- and Y-type sperm. The sex of the new individual is determined by which type of sperm fertilizes the ovum: If it is a Y-bearing sperm, the new individual will be male, and if it is an X-bearing sperm, the new individual will be female. Since entry of more than one sperm is prohibited, the first sperm to reach the ovum is the one that will fertilize it.

Following fertilization, the zygote or early embryo begins a series of cell divisions while it travels down the oviduct. When it arrives at the uterus about three days after ovulation, the zygote will be in the form of a hollow ball of cells called a blastocyte. Initially, this ball of cells floats in the fluid-filled cavity of the uterus, but two or three days after its arrival in the uterus (five to six days after ovulation), it will attach to the uterine lining. In 2003, researchers made an exciting discovery when they identified how embryos stop and burrow into the lining of a woman's uterus. A protein, called L-selectin, on the surface of the embryo acts like a puzzle piece when it touches and quickly locks into carbohydrate molecules found on the uterine surface. This implantation process must occur in exact synchrony during a very short time in a woman's cycle. (If it occurs outside the uterus, usually in one of the Fallopian tubes, then the result is an ectopic pregnancy, which is often a medical emergency.) In the weeks following conception, the cells of the zygote will form the fetus and the placenta, which surrounds and provides nutrients to the fetus. Over the next nine months, the fetus will increasingly take on a human form, developing muscle tissue, bone, organs, and skin. Pregnancy typically lasts for forty weeks from conception until childbirth. .

Complications and Disorders

Three factors limit the time frame in which conception is possible: the fertilizable lifetime of the ovulated ovum, estimated to be between twelve and twenty-four hours; the fertilizable lifetime of ejaculated sperm in the female tract, usually assumed to be about forty-eight hours; and the time required for sperm capacitation, which is one hour or more. The combination of these factors determines the length of the fertile period, the time during which intercourse must occur if conception is to be achieved. Taking the three factors into account, the fertile period is said to extend from forty-eight hours prior to ovulation until perhaps twenty-four hours after ovulation. For example, if intercourse occurs forty-eight hours before ovulation, the sperm will be capacitated in the first few hours and will still be within their fertilizable lifetime when ovulation occurs. On the other hand, if intercourse occurs twenty-four hours after ovulation, the sperm will still require time for capacitation, but the ovum will be near the end of its viable period. Thus the later limit of the fertile period is equal to the fertilizable lifetime of the ovum, minus the time required for capacitation.

Obviously, a critical factor in conception is the timing of ovulation. In a typical twenty-eight-day menstrual cycle, ovulation occurs about halfway through the cycle, or fourteen days after the first day of menstrual bleeding. In actuality, cycle length varies widely from month to month. It appears that generally the first half of the cycle is more variable in length, with the second half more stable. Thus, no matter how long the entire menstrual cycle is, ovulation usually occurs fourteen days prior to the first day of the next episode of menstrual bleeding. Therefore, it is relatively easy to determine when ovulation occurred by counting backward, but difficult to predict the time of ovulation in advance.

Assessment of ovulation time in women is notoriously difficult. There is no easily observable outward sign of ovulation. Some women do detect slight abdominal pain about the time of ovulation; this is referred to as *Mittelschmerz*, which means, literally, pain in the middle of the cycle. This slight pain may be localized on either side of the abdomen and is thought to be caused by irritation of the abdominal organs by fluid released from the ovary during ovulation. Other signs of ovulation are an increased volume of the cervical mucus and flexibility of the cervix and a characteristic fernlike pattern of the mucus when it is dried on a glass slide. There is also a slight rise in body temperature after ovulation, which again makes it easier to determine the time of ovulation after the fact rather than in advance. It is also possible to measure the amount of lutcinizing hormonc (LH) in urine or blood; this hormone shows a marked increase about sixteen hours prior to ovulation. Home test kits to detect LH levels are available for urine samples. There are additional signs of the time of ovulation, such as a slight opening of the cervix and a change in the cells lining the vagina, that can be used by physicians to determine the timing and occurrence of ovulation.

Since ovulation time is so difficult to detect in most women on an ongoing basis, most physicians would counsel that, to achieve a pregnancy, couples should plan on having intercourse every two days. This frequency will ensure that sperm capable of fertilization are always present, so that the exact time of ovulation becomes unimportant. A greater frequency of intercourse is not advised, since sperm numbers are reduced when ejaculation occurs often. Approximately 85 to 90 percent of couples will achieve pregnancy within a year when intercourse occurs about three times a week.

Couples often wonder if it is possible to predetermine the sex of their child by some action taken in conjunction with intercourse. Scientists have found no consistent effect of diet, position assumed during intercourse, timing of intercourse within the menstrual cycle, or liquids that are introduced into the vagina to kill one type of sperm selectively. In the laboratory, it is possible to achieve partial separation of sperm in a semen sample by subjecting the semen to an electric current or other procedure due to the physical difference of X- and Y-containing sperm. The separated sperm can then be used for artificial insemination (the introduction of semen through a tube into the uterus). This method is not 100 percent successful in producing offspring of the desired sex and so is available only on an experimental basis.

Some couples have difficulty in conceiving a child, in a few cases as a result of some problem associated with intercourse. For example, the male may have difficulty in achieving erection or ejaculation. The vast majority of these cases are caused by psychological factors such as stress and tension rather than any physiological problem. Fortunately, therapists can teach couples how to overcome these psychological problems.

About 10 to 15 percent of couples suffer from some type of biological infertility-that is, infertility that persists for more than one year when intercourse occurs successfully. In about 10 to 20 percent of the cases of infertility, doctors are unable to establish a cause. About one-third of infertility cases are caused by the female partner's problems, while another one-third of infertility cases are caused by the male partner's problems. The remaining cases of infertility are caused by both male and female problems or are unexplained..

In men, the most commonly diagnosed cause of infertility is low sperm count. Sometimes low sperm count is caused by a treatable imbalance of hormones. If not treatable, this problem can sometimes be circumvented by the use of pooled semen samples in artificial insemination or through in vitro fertilization. In vitro fertilization may also be a solution for men who produce normal numbers of sperm but whose sperm lack swimming ability. Another cause of male infertility is blockage of the tubes that carry the semen from the body, which may bc caused by a previous infection. Surgery is sometimes successful in removing such a blockage. Another problem, called varicocele, occurs when the veins on the testicle are too large or do not properly circulate blood. This causes the testicles to overheat, which may affect the number or the viability of the sperm. Varicocelectomy, the surgical correction of this problem, may be performed on an outpatient basis.

In women, a common cause of infertility is a hormonal problem that interferes with ovulation. Polycystic ovarian syndrome (PCOS) is a hormone imbalance that affects normal ovulation and is the most common cause of female infertility. Women with PCOS typically have high levels of androgens and many ovarian cysts. Treatment with one of a number of so-called fertility drugs may be successful in promoting ovulation. Clomiphene, a selective estrogen receptor modulator (SERM), is the most commonly prescribed fertility medication. Fertility drugs, however, have some disadvantages: They have a tendency to cause ovulation of more than one ovum, thus raising the possibility of multiple pregnancy, which is considered risky; and they may alter the environment of the uterus, making implantation of a resulting embryo less likely. Therefore, other causes of infertility, both male and female, should be ruled out before fertility drugs are used.

Another common cause of female infertility is blockage of the oviducts or the fallopian tubes resulting from scar tissue formation in the aftermath of some type of infection or prior surgery. Because surgery is not always successful, this condition may require the use of in vitro fertilization or the new technique of surgically introducing ova and sperm directly into the oviduct at a point below the blockage. Another cause of female infertility is an abnormally shaped uterus, which may interfere with the fertilized egg's ability to attach to the uterine wall. Uterine fibroids, noncancerous growths in the uterus, are very common among women and most often cause no symptoms; however, in certain cases, uterine fibroids can make it difficult for the fertilized egg to attach to the uterine wall. Surgery may be performed to shrink or remove the fibroids.

Finally, some cases of infertility result from biological incompatibility between the man and the woman. It may be that the sperm are unable to penetrate the cervical mucus, or perhaps that the woman's immune system treats the sperm cells as foreign, destroying them before they can reach the ovum. Techniques such as artificial insemination and in vitro fertilization offer hope for couples experiencing these problems.

Perspective and Prospects

For most of history, the events surrounding conception were poorly understood. For example, microscopic identification of sperm did not occur until 1677, and the ovum was not identified until 1827 (although the follicle in which the ovum develops was recognized in the seventeenth century). Prior to these discoveries, people held the belief espoused by early writers such as Aristotle and Galen that conception resulted from the mixing of male and female fluids during intercourse.

There was also confusion about the timing of the fertile period. Some early doctors thought that menstrual blood was involved in conception and therefore believed that the fertile period coincided with menstruation. Others recognized that menstrual bleeding was a sign that pregnancy had not occurred; they assumed that the most likely time for conception to result was immediately after the menstrual flow ceased. It was not until the 1930s that the first scientific studies on the timing of ovulation were completed.

Since there was little scientific understanding of the processes involved in conception, medical practice for most of human history was little different from magic, revolving around the use of rituals and herbal treatments to aid or prevent conception. Gradually, people rejected these practices, often because of religious teachings. By the twentieth century, conception had been established as an area of intense privacy, thought by physicians and the general public to be unsuitable for medical intervention.

In the early part of the twentieth century, the role of physicians in aiding conception was mostly limited to educating and advising couples finding difficulty in conceiving. There were few techniques, other than artificial insemination and fertility drug treatment, available to assist in conception at that time.

The situation changed with the first successful in vitro fertilization in 1978. This event ushered in an era of intense medical and public interest in assisting conception. Other methods to aid conception were soon introduced, including embryo transfer, frozen storage of embryos, and surgical placement of ova and sperm directly into the oviduct.

Paralleling the development of these techniques has been demand on the part of society for medicine to apply them. In most developed countries, infertility rates have been gradually increasing. One reason for increased infertility has been the increasing age at which couples decide to start a family, since the fertility of women appears to undergo a decline past the age of thirty-five. Another factor affecting fertility rates of both men and women has been an increased incidence of various sexually transmitted diseases, which can result in chronic inflammation of the reproductive organs and infertility caused by scar tissue formation.

People's attitudes toward medical intervention in conception have also changed. The earlier taboos against interference in conception have been somewhat relaxed, although some individuals still do not approve of certain methods of fertility management. Although there remain ethical issues to be resolved, the general public seems to have accepted the idea that medicine should provide assistance to those who wish to, but cannot, conceive children.

—Marcia Watson-Whitmyre, Ph.D.;
updated by Alexander Sandra, M.D.

See also Assisted reproductive technologies; Childbirth; Cloning; Contraception; Gamete intrafallopian transfer (GIFT); Gynecology; In vitro fertilization; Infertility, female; Infertility, male; Menstruation; Multiple births; Obstetrics; Pregnancy and gestation; Reproductive system; Sperm banks; Uterus.

For Further Information:

Doherty, C. Maud, and Melanie M. Clark. *Fertility Handbook: A Guide to Getting Pregnant.* Omaha, Nebr.: Addicus Books, 2002.
Harkness, Carla. *The Infertility Book: A Comprehensive Medical and Emotional Guide.* Rev 2d ed. Berkeley, Calif.: Celestial Arts, 1992.
"Infertility." *Medline Plus*, February 26, 2012.
"Infertility Fact Sheet." *US Department of Health and Human Services-Office on Women's Health*, July 16, 2012.
"In Vitro Fertilization (IVF)." *Medline Plus*, February 26, 2012.
Jones, Richard E., and Kristin H. Lopez. *Human Reproductive Biology.* 4th ed. Burlington, Mass.: Academic Press/Elsevier, 2013.
Kearney, Brian. *High-Tech Conception: A Comprehensive Handbook for Consumers.* New York: Bantam Books, 1998.
"Pregnancy: Condition Information." *Eunice Kennedy Shriver National Institute of Child Health and Human Development*, April 3, 2013.
Weschler, Toni. *Taking Charge of Your Fertility.* Rev. ed. New York: Collins, 2006.
Wisot, Arthur L., and David R. Meldrum. *Conceptions and Misconceptions: The Informed Consumer's Guide Through the Maze of In Vitro Fertilization and Other Assisted Reproduction Techniques.* 2d ed. Point Roberts, Wash.: Hartley & Marks, 2004.

Concussion

Disease/Disorder

Anatomy or system affected: Brain, head, nerves, nervous system

Specialties and related fields: Critical care, emergency medicine, neurology, sports medicine

Definition: Mild brain injury that briefly impairs neurological functions.

Key terms:

amnesia: memory loss

disorientation: lack of comprehension of reality

unconsciousness: lack of awareness of one's surroundings

Causes and Symptoms

Concussions can be caused by a variety of traumatic events: motor vehicle accidents, penetrating injuries, sports injuries, and falls. Recent studies indicate that the number of concussions from motor vehicle accidents and falls have decreased, while penetrating injuries (gunshot wounds) and sports-related injuries are on the increase. Concussion is a common athletic injury experienced by approximately 300,000 youths each

---

Information on Concussion

Causes: Brain trauma from car accidents, falls, sports injuries, etc.

Symptoms: Unconsciousness, memory loss, headache, dizziness, nausea, disorientation, double vision, hearing problems, lack of coordination, sensitivity to light and noises, sensory changes in smell and taste

Duration: Ranges from several seconds to minutes immediately after impact

Treatments: Dependent on severity; none (mild), rest and alleviation of symptoms (moderate), neck immobilization and hospitalization (severe)

---

year. Recent information suggests that children heal more slowly than adults following head trauma. Although concussions are the mildest traumatic brain injuries, they can result in irreversible damage or death if a person suffers another head trauma prior to recovering fully from the initial injury.

People who have experienced head trauma that disrupts brain activity and sometimes causes brief unconsciousness, ranging from several seconds to minutes immediately after an impact, are considered to have sustained a concussion. Direct, sudden, powerful blows to the head or an impact to the body that jars the head cause the brain to bounce inside the skull and suffer tissue bruising. Nerve fibers tear, and chemical reactions are altered.

Concussions are described as mild, moderate, or severe, though there is a lack of standardized definitions for each type of concussion. A mild concussion may or may not involve a brief period of unconsciousness; the brain generally recovers quickly and without long-term damage. However, approximately 15 percent of those injured will continue to experience symptoms one year after the initial injury. These symptoms may range from headaches to emotional or behavioral problems. The US Centers for Disease Control and Prevention (CDC) and the National Center for Injury Prevention and Control have developed recommendations for standardized terminology, treatment, and prevention of mild traumatic brain injuries. A severe concussion is considered an emergency and requires an extended period of time for recovery.

Headache, dizziness, nausea, and disorientation immediately following the injury are considered risk factors for long-term complications from the head injury. Each person's brain and injury are unique. Therefore, a wide variety of symptoms may occur. Patients may experience double vision and suffer hearing problems. People with concussions also report becoming uncoordinated and sensitive to light and noises, and they may experience sensory changes in smell and taste. Patients may become moody, cognitively impaired, unable to concentrate, or fatigued.

Researchers have determined that the major neuropsychological complications of concussion may occur in the brain's memory, learning, and planning functions.

Some concussion patients taking tests, such as the Wechsler Abbreviated Scale of Intelligence, have revealed decreased concentration, reaction, and processing skills in performing intellectual tasks. Their strategies to solve problems are impaired when compared to people who have not suffered concussions.

Medical professionals assess patients with a head injury by physical examination, radiological tests, and a standardized scale that measures level of consciousness called the Glasgow Coma Scale. Computed tomography (CT) and magnetic resonance imaging (MRI) scans may also be used. The American Academy of Neurology emphasizes the duration of loss of consciousness to determine the severity of concussions. Evaluations also consider orientation and posttraumatic amnesia. Medical professionals assess patients" responses to stimuli and memory of incidents before their injury, defining the concussion according to the level of confusion, amnesia, and duration of loss of consciousness. Physicians ask patients questions about who and where they are and about the time and date. The duration of amnesia after the brain trauma helps medical professionals to determine the extent of the injury and treatments that would be most effective to heal the brain. The Colorado Medical Society developed a popular system, assigning Grades 1 (mild), 2 (moderate), and 3 (severe) to aoncussions, to guide athletic personnel in examining players who suffer concussions during games and deciding how long they must refrain from participation in order to prevent additional damage.

Brain damage and death can result from serial concussions. Postconcussion complications may include second impact syndrome: If a patient suffers another concussion before healing is complete following the first injury, then the second concussion can be the catalyst for rapid cerebral swelling that causes increased pressure within the structure of the brain. This pressure can cause the brain to press on the brain stem and result in respiratory failure and death. This condition is usually fatal.

More common is postconcussive syndrome (PCS), which consists of such cognitive and physical symptoms as headache, anxiety, vertigo, nausea, and hallucinations. An estimated 30 percent of professional football players suffer from PCS. Researchers have determined that people who experience several concussions, such as athletes and soldiers, are more vulnerable to becoming clinically depressed.

Treatment and Therapy

Research has found that patients who rest for one week following a concussion, with a slow return to previous activities to allow the brain to heal, have fewer long-term complications than do patients who resume activities more quickly. Although most patients recover, some experience long-term concussion-related conditions, such as memory loss and neurological impairment.

Severe concussions with increased brain pressure require hospitalization, often in a neurological intensive care unit. The patient's head is maintained in a neutral position. The patient is at risk for stopped breathing due to increased brain pressure. This risk is decreased by placing the patient on a mechanical ventilator. The patient may have suffered internal bleeding in the brain because of the injury, and blood clots can form there. Surgery may be required to remove these clots. Patients with preexisting conditions such as epilepsy and diabetes may develop complications related to those diseases and require longer recovery times.

Physicians recommend wearing helmets to absorb shocks sustained during athletic activities involving the risk of head injury in order to prevent or minimize concussions. The American Academy of Neurology has demanded a ban on boxing because the sport involves knocking out opponents by inflicting concussions. Boxers often suffer permanent brain damage and are at a heightened risk for neurological diseases.

Perspective and Prospects

Concussions were first described in medical literature by Muslim physician Rhazes (850-923). He differentiated between a head injury that caused neurological symptoms from those injuries that resulted in lesions and structural damage. In the nineteenth century, medical researchers developed hypotheses, often controversial, regarding the physical and emotional influences of concussion symptoms. Second impact syndrome was first defined in 1984.

The development of sports medicine increased the interest in studying concussions. The understanding of the internal brain damage involved in concussions did not significantly advance, however, until neuroimaging technologies such as CT scanning and magnetic resonance imaging (MRI) were developed in the late twentieth century. In the twenty-first century, medical professionals utilize those techniques to view brain tissues and to observe the physiological reactions to concussion-causing trauma. Positive emission tomography (PET) has been developed to measure chemical changes in the brain. In the case of concussion, the PET scan can be used to evaluate changes that signal areas of injury in the brain. These technologies will likely yield more accurate diagnostic exams for concussions.

—Elizabeth D. Schafer, Ph.D.;
updated by Amy Webb Bull, D.S.N., A.P.N.

See also Amnesia; Bleeding; Brain; Brain damage; Brain disorders; Coma; Dizziness and fainting; First aid; Head and neck disorders; Nausea and vomiting; Nervous system; Neuroimaging; Neurology; Sports medicine; Subdural hematomas; Unconsciousness.

For Further Information:

Arbogast, Kristy B., et al. "Cognitive Rest and School-Based Recommendations Following Pediatric Concussion: The Need for Primary Care Support Tools." *Clinical Pediatrics* 52, no. 5 (April, 2013): 397-402.

Evans, Randolph W., ed. *Neurology and Trauma*. 2d ed. New York: Oxford University Press, 2006.

Kennedy, Jan, Robin Lumpkin, and Joyce Grissom. "A Survey of Mild Traumatic Brain Injury Treatment in the Emergency Room and Primary Care Medical Clinics." *Military Medicine* 171, no. 6 (June, 2006): 516-521.

Kerr, Mary, and Elizabeth Crago. "Acute Intracranial Problems." In *Medical-Surgical Nursing*. Edited by Sharon Lewis, Margaret Heitkemper, and Shannon Dirksen. 6th ed. St. Louis, Mo.: Mosby, 2004.

Metzl, Jordan. "Concussion in the Young Athlete." *Pediatrics* 117, no. 5. (May, 2006): 1813.

National Center for Injury Prevention and Control. *Report to Congress on Mild Traumatic Brain Injury in the United States: Steps to Prevent a Serious Public Health Problem*. Atlanta: Centers for Disease Control and Prevention, 2003.

Shannon, Joyce Brennfleck, ed. *Sports Injuries Sourcebook*. 4th ed. Detroit, Mich.: Omnigraphics, 2012.

Smoots, Elizabeth. "Concussion." *Health Library*, September 30, 2012.

Wrightson, Philip, and Dorothy Gronwall. *Mild Head Injury: A Guide to Management*. New York: Oxford University Press, 1999.

CONGENITAL ADRENAL HYPERPLASIA
Disease/Disorder

Also known as: Adrenogenital syndrome, 21-hydroxylase deficiency

Anatomy or system affected: Endocrine system, genitals, reproductive system

Specialties and related fields: Endocrinology, genetics, urology

Definition: A family of genetic conditions that affect hormone production by the adrenal glands.

Key terms:

adrenal glands: endocrine glands located above the kidneys that produce glucocorticoid, mineralocorticoid, and androgenic hormones

aldosterone: a mineralocorticoid that controls sodium retention

androgens: hormones that regulate sexual differentiation, development, and maintenance of male sex characteristics

cortisol: a glucocorticoid that raises blood sugar levels; elevated in response to physical or psychological stress

glucocorticoids: drugs or hormones that regulate carbohydrate metabolism

hydrocortisone: a pharmaceutical term for cortisol

mineralocorticoids: hormones that regulate the balance of water and electrolytes

salt-wasting: a condition in which there is an inappropriately large excretion of salt; symptoms include poor feeding, weight loss, vomiting, dehydration, and hypotension and can progress to adrenal crisis and death

virilization: the development of masculine sex characteristics in a female

---

Information on Congenital Adrenal Hyperplasia

Causes: Genetic defect in hormone production

Symptoms: Ambiguous genitalia in girls, enlarged penis, salt-wasting, very early puberty, irregular menstrual cycles, infertility

Duration: Lifelong; can be fatal during infancy if untreated

Treatments: Hormone therapy, genital reconstructive surgery

Causes and Symptoms

Congenital adrenal hyperplasia (CAH) is a family of autosomal recessive conditions that affect the production of hormones by the adrenal glands. It is caused by an inherited deficiency in one of the enzymes that is necessary to convert cholesterol to cortisol. About 95 percent of cases of CAH are caused by a deficiency in the enzyme 21-hydroxylase, but deficiencies in 3-beta hydroxysteroid dehydrogenase, 11-beta-hydroxylase, 17-alpha-hydroxylase, or cholesterol desmolase can also cause the condition.

If an individual has a mutation in one copy of the gene that codes for one of these enzymes, then he or she will not have any clinical symptoms but is considered a carrier of CAH. If both parents are carriers, then there is a 25 percent chance that their child will inherit both of these mutations. Individuals with two mutated copies of a gene will have a deficiency of the corresponding enzyme and will be clinically affected with CAH.

Individuals with CAH have reduced levels of cortisol production. They may also have decreased aldosterone production and increased production of androgens, such as testosterone.

Girls who are born with classic CAH often have virilized or ambiguous external genitalia, while boys may have enlarged penises. Affected infants may also experience weight loss, dehydration, vomiting, and salt-wasting crises. If left untreated, affected individuals may experience very early puberty, irregular menstrual cycles, infertility, and short stature in adulthood. There is also a nonclassic form of CAH that is less severe and develops in late childhood or early adulthood.

A diagnosis of CAH is usually made based on biochemical testing. Affected individuals typically have decreased serum levels of cortisol, aldosterone, sodium, chloride, and total carbon dioxide. They also have elevated levels of the steroid hormone 17-hydroxyprogesterone (17-OHP) and serum DHEA sulfate (an androgen). Genetic testing for CAH is also available. Newborn screening for CAH is routine and is done by measuring the concentration of 17-OHP on a filter paper blood spot sample.

Treatment and Therapy

The principal treatment for CAH is lifelong hormone replacement therapy. The aim of this therapy is to replace deficient glucocorticoid, reduce the production of androgens, prevent the development of secondary male sex characteristics in females, optimize growth, and promote fertility.

In children, oral hydrocortisone is usually given in two to three daily doses. Individuals with the salt-wasting form of CAH may also need supplemental sodium chloride and mineralocorticoids. Serum concentrations of 17-OHP and other hormones must be checked regularly to assess hormonal control. Overtreatment with glucocorticosteroids can result in elevated cortisol levels and can lead to Cushing's syndrome. Signs of Cushing's syndrome include an accumulation of fat between the shoulders; a full, rounded face; muscle weakness; stretch marks on the skin of the abdomen, thighs, and breasts; high blood pressure; and bone loss.

Girls with virilization or genital ambiguity may need corrective surgery to ensure proper urinary, sexual, and reproductive functioning. Males are at risk for testicular adrenal rest tumors and require periodic imaging of the testes with ultrasound or magnetic resonance imaging (MRI).

If a couple is known to be at risk for having a pregnancy affected with CAH, then oral dexamethasone can be given to the mother during pregnancy to prevent virilization of a female fetus. To be effective, however, treatment must be started early in the pregnancy, before testing can be done to determine the sex of the fetus or if the fetus is affected with CAH. This often results in unnecessary treatment of a male or unaffected fetus. However, universal screening of all newborn infants improves early detection of the often fatal salt-wasting form of CAH in both girls and boys.

Perspective and Prospects

Luigi De Crecchio, an Italian anatomist, is credited with the earliest known description of a case of probable CAH. In 1865 he wrote an account of Joseph Marzo, a man who had passed away following an episode of vomiting and diarrhea. Although Marzo had a male appearance, he had ambiguous external genitalia and internal female reproductive organs.

J. Phillips helped to identify CAH as a genetic condition when he reported in 1887 the case of a family with four children who had been born hermaphrodites and passed away in early infancy with wasting disease. Then, in 1905, J. Fibiger noted that some infants with prolonged vomiting and dehydration had enlarged adrenal glands.

Lawson Wilkins, a researcher at Johns Hopkins Medical School, concluded that the impaired ability to produce cortisol led to adrenal hyperplasia and overproduction of adrenal androgens in individuals with CAH. In 1950, he reported that adrenal cortical extracts could be used to treat children with CAH. By the late 1950s, hydrocortisone, fludrocortisone, and prednisone were available and could be used for treatment. By 1990, many of the causative genes and enzymes had been identified.

Research continues on improving the hormone replacement regimen for individuals with CAH. Excess adrenal androgen secretions need to be suppressed while still allowing for normal growth and development. There is also continuing research on the psychological effects of CAH. The degree to which prenatal androgen exposure may affect psychosexual development in females with CAH is an ongoing subject of research.

—Laura Garasimowicz, M.S.

See also Corticosteroids; Cushing's syndrome; Endocrine disorders; Endocrinology; Endocrinology, pediatric; Genetic diseases; Hormones; Hyperplasia.

For Further Information:

"Congenital Adrenal Hyperplasia (CAH)." *Eunice Kennedy Shriver National Institute of Child Health and Human Development*, April 3, 2013.

Hsu, C. Y., and Scott A. Rivkees. *Congenital Adrenal Hyperplasia: A Parents" Guide.* Bloomington, Ind.: AuthorHouse, 2005.

Kliegman R. M., et al. "Congenital Adrenal Hyperplasia and Related Disorders." In *Nelson Textbook of Pediatrics* . 19th ed.

Philadelphia: Saunders/Elsevier, 2011.

Mayo Clinic. "Congenital Adrenal Hyperplasia." *Mayo Clinic*, March 4, 2011.

Parker, Philip M. *Congenital Adrenal Hyperplasia: A Medical Dictionary, Bibliography, and Annotated Research Guide to Internet References.* San Diego, Calif.: ICON Group, 2004.

Stresing, Diane. "Congenital Adrenal Hyperplasia." *Health Library*, November 26, 2012.

Congenital disorders

Disease/Disorder

Anatomy or system affected: All

Specialties and related fields: Genetic counseling, genetics, neonatology, obstetrics, pediatrics

Definition: An abnormality present at birth, which may be due to a genetic defect, exposure to a toxic or infectious agent in utero, or a deficiency or lack of a substance necessary for fetal development.

Key terms:

amniocentesis: withdrawal of fluid from the amniotic sac for genetic analysis

aneuploidy: an abnormal number of chromosomes

chorionic villus sampling (CVS): removal of a small portion of chorionic villi (placental tissue) for genetic analysis

chromosomes: paired structures that contain genetic material (DNA)

Down syndrome: a highly studied genetic defect caused by an extra twenty-first chromosome

genetics: the study of the hereditary transmission of characteristics

triple test: a blood test that screens for genetic defects

trisomy: the presence of an extra chromosome; for example, Down syndrome is trisomy 21

Causes and Symptoms

Congenital disorders can be the result of genetic factors, environmental exposure, infection during pregnancy, or a deficiency or lack of a substance required for proper fetal development.

Genetic defects include defective genes, extra chromosomal material, and missing chromosomal material. Examples of defects from a single gene include Huntington's disease, cystic fibrosis, and Tay-Sachs disease. Huntington's disease is caused by an autosomal dominant gene (inheritance of the gene from one parent will produce the disease). Cystic fibrosis and Tay-Sachs disease are autosomal recessives (inheritance of the gene from both parents is necessary for expression of the disease). Huntington's disease is a progressive and fatal deterioration of the central nervous system with an onset in middle age. Patients with cystic fibrosis produce excessive mucus in the lungs, pancreas, and other secretory organs. The secretions in the lungs clog respiratory passages, causing pulmonary damage, and subject the patient to life-threatening infection. Secretions in the pancreas prevent the flow of enzymes into the intestines and damage the pancreatic islet cells, resulting in diabetes. Tay-Sachs disease is a fatal disorder in which a fatty substance known as

---

Information on Congenital Disorders

Causes: Vary; genetic abnormality, exposure to toxic or infectious agent in utero, deficiency or lack of substance necessary for fetal development

Symptoms: Vary from mild to profound, can affect one or more organ systems

Duration: Often lifelong; some defects correctable through surgery or medication

Treatments: Vary by specific disorder

---

ganglioside G_{M2} builds up in tissues and nerve cells in the brain. Even with meticulous medical care, death usually occurs by age four.

In some types of defects caused by recessive genes, the possession of one abnormal gene can be detrimental. One example is sickle cell disease and sickle cell trait, which is an abnormality of the red blood cells. Individuals with two defective genes are much more severely affected than those with one. Some defective genes reside on the sex chromosomes. Females have two X chromosomes, and males have one X and one Y chromosome. The Y chromosome is shorter than the X chromosome and has less genetic material. A defective gene on an X chromosome in the area with no corresponding material on the Y chromosome will always express itself; therefore, these diseases affect males much more frequently than females. An example of an X-linked disease is red-green color blindness, in which individuals cannot distinguish between red and green.

Ethnicity is also a factor in the inheritance of genetic disorders. For example, Tay-Sachs disease is most common among Eastern European Jews (Ashkenazi), sickle cell disease is most common among individuals of African descent, and thalassemia (a blood disease) is most common among people of Mediterranean descent.

A number of congenital disorders are the result of aneuploidy, which is the presence of extra or missing chromosomes. The normal human complement is twenty-two pairs of autosomes and one pair of sex chromosomes (X and Y). A number of defects due to extra chromosomal material are trisomies. Two examples of trisomies are Down syndrome (trisomy 21) and Edwards syndrome (trisomy 18). Down syndrome is characterized by delayed mental development and physical deformities such as an enlarged tongue, poor muscle tone, and cardiac abnormalities. Trisomy 18 is characterized by profound physical deformities and developmental disabilities; about 95 percent of affected individuals die before birth or within the first year of life, and those who live rarely survive beyond childhood. Turner syndrome is an example of aneuploidy caused by a missing chromosome. Affected individuals have only one X chromosome and no Y chromosome. They are typically sterile and may have physical characteristics such as short stature and a webbed neck.

Toxic substances ingested by a woman during pregnancy can affect a developing fetus, often to a much greater extent than the mother. Toxins that can cause congenital disorders include alcohol, cocaine, and nicotine. Fetal alcohol syndrome is characterized by delayed mental development, low birth weight, and facial deformities. The syndrome has occurred in infants whose mothers reportedly consumed as little as two drinks per day (one drink is defined as 1.25 ounces of 80 proof liquor, twelve ounces of beer, or six ounces of wine). Infants born of mothers who use cocaine may have low birth weight and disproportionately small heads. They may have learning difficulties; some research suggests that a variety of congenital disorders are prevalent in these children. Mothers who smoke cigarettes during pregnancy are more likely to deliver infants with low birth weights or respiratory problems. Although most congenital disorders resulting from toxins are related to maternal exposure, paternal exposure is a factor in some cases. For example, cocaine use by the father at the time of conception has been reported to affect the fetus. This is thought to be the result of the lodging of the cocaine molecule on the spermatozoa head; these molecules are passed to the ovum during fertilization. In general, use of a toxic substance increases the risk of fetal loss and premature birth.

Infectious agents that cause congenital disorders include rubella, human immunodeficiency virus (HIV), and syphilis. A pregnant woman who becomes infected with the rubella virus, particularly during the first trimester (three months), may give birth to an infant with the rubella syndrome. The syndrome is characterized by auditory, cerebral, cardiac, and ophthalmic defects. Symptoms range from mild to severe. If a woman with HIV does not undergo treatment during pregnancy, transmission of the virus to the fetus is likely. Infants born with congenital syphilis may appear healthy at birth; however, they can subsequently develop central nervous system, bone, teeth, and eye disorders.

Poor nutrition during pregnancy can likewise result in congenital disorders. Folic acid deficiency has been implicated in the development of neural tube defects such as spina bifida, anencephaly, and encephalocele. Spina bifida is caused by failure of the spinal column to close during fetal development. The severity of symptoms depends on the location and size of the defect. Affected infants may have varying degrees of paralysis of the lower extremities as well as problems with bowel and bladder control. Anencephaly is caused by the lack of the formation of a cranium (skull cap); as a result, the brain does not form at all or in major part. This disorder is always fatal. An encephalocele is a skull defect that exposes a portion of the brain. This disorder may be fatal or result in varying degrees of developmental disability.

Treatment and Therapy

As is the case with all disorders, prevention is preferable to treatment. Avoidance of harmful substances (mind-altering drugs, alcohol, and tobacco) during pregnancy is essential, and adequate nutrition, including vitamin supplements, is extremely important. Exposure to infectious agents (rubella, HIV, syphilis) should be avoided. Certain medications can increase the risk of congenital disorders, including isotretinoin and etretinate, used for the treatment of acne, and phenytoin and carbamazepine, used to treat epilepsy. Any woman who is pregnant or contemplating pregnancy should consult a health care professional in regard to any medication, prescription or nonprescription.

Screening tests such as the triple test are blood tests that can screen for genetic abnormalities. Chorionic villus sampling (CVS) and amniocentesis can definitively diagnose genetic abnormalities that cause disorders such as Down syndrome and trisomy 18. Single-gene defects can also be diagnosed with CVS or amniocentesis, particularly when a family history of the defect is present. Prenatal diagnosis allows parents the ability to choose whether to continue with a pregnancy. If they opt to continue with the pregnancy, it gives them time to seek counseling and join support groups to help them cope with caring for a child with a congenital disorder.

Treatment for congenital disorders ranges from nonexistent to complete. For example, anencephaly has no known treatment. Phenylketonuria (PKU), a metabolic defect that leads to developmental disabilities, is caused by an inability to metabolize the amino acid phenylalanine. As such, a special low-phenylalanine diet can markedly reduce progression of the disease. Surgery can correct some congenital disorders, such as cardiac defects related to Down syndrome and spinal defects associated with spina bifida.

Advances in medical science and supportive therapy have greatly improved the longevity of patients with genetic disorders. For example, for centuries, many children with cystic fibrosis died in childhood. However, according to the Cystic Fibrosis Foundation, by the early twenty-first century, many individuals with access to medical treatment were able to live well into adulthood.

Perspective and Prospects

Genetic disorders have been recognized for centuries; however, the genetic basis was not understood until the latter half of the twentieth century. Down syndrome and cystic fibrosis are two typical examples. English physician John Down noted that Down syndrome was a specific type of mental disability with distinct physical features. For centuries, the foreheads of children with cystic fibrosis were licked; if a salty taste was noted, the child was deemed to be bewitched and expected to die soon. It was not until the 1990s that the mutated gene that causes the disease was identified.

In addition to Down syndrome and cystic fibrosis, rapid progress has been made in the past decades in regard to genetic abnormalities. The locations of defective genes have been mapped, and alleles (different forms of a gene) have been identified. Research into the treatment of congenital disorders caused by genetic abnormalities is ongoing. Currently, treatment is mainly limited to surgical correction of defects (correction of a cardiac abnormality in an individual with Down syndrome), medical therapy (enzyme therapy for an individual with cystic fibrosis), and supportive care (pulmonary therapy to loosen secretions in an individual with cystic fibrosis). The most promising treatment for specific gene defects rests in the field of stem cell research. Single-gene defects may be curable via gene therapy in the near future. To date, most of the studies have been animal or in vitro (laboratory) studies.

The outlook is much poorer for trisomies, which involve a significant amount of extra chromosomal material. The outlook is extremely poor for severe disorders such as trisomy 18 and virtually hopeless for disorders such as anencephaly. In the case of anencephaly, the best option at present is early diagnosis via CVS or amniocentesis and pregnancy termination.

There now exists an increased public awareness of the impact of exposure to toxins and infections on pregnancy. This increased awareness has the potential to reduce the incidence of these preventable disorders. For example, awareness of the benefits of folic acid can reduce the incidence of neural tube defects. Aggressive therapy for children with a disorder caused by exposure to a toxin can sometimes reverse the damage. For example, speech therapy and other behavioral support can reverse central nervous disorders resulting from congenital cocaine exposure. The therapy must be initiated promptly when symptoms are recognized, while the developing brain is in its formative phase. Therapy is most effective before the age of five.

—*Robin L. Wulffson, M.D.*

See also Amniocentesis; Batten's disease; Birth defects; Breast cancer; Cardiology, pediatric; Cerebral palsy; Childbirth; Childbirth complications; Chorionic villus sampling; Cleft lip and palate; Cleft lip and palate repair; Colon cancer; Color blindness; Congenital heart disease; Congenital hypothyroidism; Cornelia de Lange syndrome; Cystic fibrosis; Diabetes mellitus; DiGeorge syndrome; DNA and RNA; Down syndrome; Dwarfism; Embryology; Endocrinology, pediatric; Environmental diseases; Enzymes; Fetal alcohol syndrome; Fetal surgery; Fragile X syndrome; Fructosemia; Gaucher's disease; Gene therapy; Genetic counseling; Genetic diseases; Genetic engineering; Genetics and inheritance; Genomics; Gigantism; Glycogen storage diseases; Hemochromatosis; Hemophilia; Huntington's disease; Hydrocephalus; Immunodeficiency disorders; Klinefelter syndrome; Klippel-Trenaunay syndrome; Laboratory tests; Leukodystrophy; Maple syrup urine disease (MSUD); Marfan syndrome; Mental retardation; Metabolic disorders; Mucopolysaccharidosis (MPS); Multiple sclerosis; Muscular dystrophy; Mutation; Neonatology; Neurofibromatosis; Niemann-Pick disease; Obstetrics; Oncology; Pediatrics; Phenylketonuria (PKU); Polycystic kidney disease; Porphyria; Prader-Willi syndrome; Pregnancy and gestation; Premature birth; Progeria; Proteomics; Rubinstein-Taybi syndrome; Screening; Severe combined immunodeficiency syndrome (SCID); Sickle cell disease; Spina bifida; Tay-Sachs disease; Teratogens; Thalassemia; Thalidomide; Thrombocytopenia; Turner syndrome; Von Willebrand's disease; Wilson's disease; Wiskott-Aldrich syndrome.

For Further Information:
A.D.A.M. Medical Encyclopedia. "Genetic Counseling." *MedlinePlus*, May 31 2012.
American Pregnancy Assn. http://www.americanpregnancy.org.
Amniocentesis Report. http://www.amniocentesis.org.
Cummings, Michael. *Human Heredity: Principles and Issues*. 8th ed. Belmont, Calif.: Brooks/Cole, 2008.
Cystic Fibrosis Foundation. http://www.cff.org.
Lewis, Ricki. *Human Genetics*. 8th ed. New York: McGraw-Hill, 2007.
March of Dimes. http://www.marchofdimes.com.
National Center for Birth Defects and Developmental Disabilities.

"Pediatric Genetics." *Centers for Disease Control and Prevention*, March 12, 2012.
Rapp, Rayna. *Testing Women, Testing the Fetus: The Social Impact of Amniocentesis in America*. New York: Routledge, 2000.
Scriver, Charles. *The Metabolic and Molecular Bases of Inherited Disease*. 8th ed. 4 vols. New York: McGraw-Hill, 2007.
World Health Organization. "Congenital Anomalies." *World Health Organization*, October 2012.

CONGENITAL HEART DISEASE

Disease/Disorder

Anatomy or system affected: Chest, circulatory system, heart

Specialties and related fields: Cardiology, neonatology, pediatrics, vascular medicine

Definition: Conditions resulting from malformations of the heart that occur during embryonic and fetal development, accounting for about 25 percent of all congenital defects.

Key terms:

atria: heart chambers that receive blood, the left from the lungs and the right from the body

great arteries and veins: large vessels channeling blood into and out of the heart, including the aorta (to the body), the pulmonary artery (to the lungs), the vena cava (from the body), and the pulmonary veins (from the lungs)

heart failure: the inability of the heart to pump adequate amounts of blood to maintain the organs and tissues of the body; often results in tissue fluid retention and congestion

murmur: a sound made by the heart other than the normal two-step beat; murmurs are caused by the turbulent movement of blood and may indicate a heart defect

septum: a membrane that serves as a wall of separation; in the heart, the interatrial septum divides the two atria and the interventricular septum divides the two ventricles

ventricles: heart chambers that pump blood out of the heart, the left to the body and the right to the lungs

Causes and Symptoms

Congenital heart disease includes various structural and functional defects of the heart and blood vessels resulting from errors that occur during embryonic development. The defects may cause heart murmurs, high or low blood pressure, congestive heart failure, cyanosis (blue skin), abnormal heart rhythms and rates, and incidences of low oxygen (hypoxia). Congenital heart disease is detected in about 0.7 percent of live births and more than 10 percent of stillbirths. Some babies born with congenital heart disease have difficulty during

---

Information on Congenital Heart Disease

Causes: Genetic and environmental factors

Symptoms: Shortness of breath, fatigue, sweating while eating, inability to gain weight, lung congestion, altered blood pressure, hypoxia, congestive heart failure

Duration: Ranges from short-term to lifelong

Treatments: Surgery, medications, insertion of balloon catheter

the first few weeks of life. Some problems, however, are not easily detected at the time of birth and are discovered at various stages of life. Heart defects may be inherited from parents, induced by environmental agents such as drugs, or caused by an interaction of genetic and environmental factors. Defects are more common in children with genetic disorders such as Down syndrome. With intensive treatment, including surgery, many forms of congenital heart disease can be corrected, allowing those affected to lead normal lives.

Tetralogy of Fallot

A relatively common congenital heart defect, tetralogy of Fallot comprises four defects: an overriding or displaced aorta, pulmonary stenosis (a narrowed pulmonary valve), a ventricular septal defect (a hole in the ventricular septum), and a thickened, or enlarged, right ventricle. These together result in cyanosis: poor blood oxygenation.

Knowledge of normal heart development will help in understanding how congenital heart disease occurs and will provide a means for categorizing these defects. Near the end of the third week of embryonic development, the heart begins to form from two cords of tissue that hollow out and fuse to form a primitive heart tube. This tube undergoes some constrictions and dilations to form the early divisions of the heart, including a receiving chamber, the atrium, and a pumping chamber, the ventricle, which exits into a muscular tube called the truncus arteriosus. At about twenty-two days, the heart begins to contract and pump blood. A day later, it bends or loops upon itself to form an S shape, with the atrium on one side, the truncus arteriosus on the other side, and the ventricle in the middle. If it bends to the left instead of to the right, a rare heart defect called dextrocardia results. The heart will be displaced to the right side of the body and may have some accompanying abnormalities.

During the fourth and fifth week of development, the heart begins to divide into four chambers by first forming a septum (dividing membrane) in the canal between the atrium and the ventricle. This septum is formed by heart tissue called the endocardial cushions. Failure of this septum to form properly causes atrioventricular canal defects. These are often associated with Down syndrome. During the fifth week of development, a spiral septum forms in the truncus arteriosus that divides it into two vessels: the pulmonary artery, which connects to the right ventricle, and the aorta, which connects to the left ventricle. The formation of this septum and the ventricular connections are subject to error and may result in a group of anomalies called conotruncal defects.

As these large arteries are forming, a shunt (bypass) develops between them called the ductus arteriosus. This short vessel allows the blood to be diverted away from the nonfunctional fetal lungs into the aorta and on to the placenta, where it will receive oxygen and nutrients. Persistence of this shunt after birth is responsible for a defect called patent ductus. A septum dividing the atrium into right and left halves also forms during the fourth and fifth weeks of development; however, blood is allowed to pass from the right atrium to the left

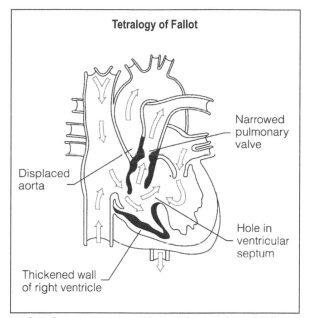

Tetralogy of Fallot

Narrowed pulmonary valve

Displaced aorta

Hole in ventricular septum

Thickened wall of right ventricle

A relatively common congenital heart defect, tetralogy of Fallot comprises four defects: an overriding or displaced aorta, pulmonary stenosis (a narrowed pulmonary valve), a ventricular septal defect (a hole in the ventricular septum), and a thickened, or enlarged, right ventricle. These together result in cyanosis: poor blood oxygenation.

atrium through a small hole in this septum called the foramen ovale. This hole normally closes after birth but is necessary during fetal life to shunt blood away from the fetal lungs and toward the placenta in a manner similar to that of the ductus arteriosus. At about the same time, a septum forms from the floor of the ventricle and divides it into right and left halves. Failure of the atrial and ventricular septa to form properly and to close at the time of birth results in septal defects.

After the appearance of the four chambers, two pairs of valves form in the heart to prevent the backflow of blood and to ensure greater efficiency in pumping. The semilunar valves (also called the pulmonary and aortic valves) form between the ventricles and their respective outlet arteries (pulmonary artery and aorta), and the atrioventricular valves (bicuspid or mitral on the left and tricuspid on the right) form between the atria and the ventricles. Improperly formed valves can lead to flow defects. During development, the heart also makes connections with veins returning from the general circulation and the lungs. Errors in these connections and other structural errors cause several other less common congenital heart defects.

The most common congenital heart defects are the septal defects and patent ductus, which together account for about 37 percent of all heart defects. After birth, because the pressure becomes higher in the left side of the heart, blood moves from left to right through the openings in the heart that come with such defects, causing too much to flow to the lungs and a mixing of systemic and pulmonary blood. The child's lungs will be congested, causing difficulty in breathing and eventually heart failure.

About 29 percent of congenital heart defects are categorized as right-heart and left-heart flow defects. These defects impede the flow of blood from either the right or the left side of the heart to its normal destination. Right-heart flow defects include bicuspid pulmonary valve (a valve with two cusps instead of three), pulmonary valve stenosis (a narrowing of the valve), dysplastic pulmonary valve (a malformed valve), peripheral pulmonary stenosis (a narrowing of the walls of the pulmonary artery), infundibular pulmonary stenosis (a narrowing below the valve), and hypoplastic right ventricle (incomplete formation of the valve). These defects impede blood flow to the lungs, which results in poor oxygenation of the blood (cyanosis). Left-heart flow defects include bicuspid aortic valve, aortic valve stenosis, coarctation of the aorta (narrowing), aortic atresia (a blocked aorta), and hypoplastic left ventricle. These defects impede blood flow to the body and often result in altered blood pressure, hypoxia of body tissues, and congestive heart failure.

The principal conotruncal defects, which account for about 17 percent of heart defects, are tetralogy of Fallot and transposition of the great arteries. Tetralogy of Fallot includes four defects that result in cyanosis: pulmonary stenosis, a ventricular septal defect, an overriding or displaced aorta, and hypertrophy or enlargement of the right ventricle. With transposition of the great arteries, the aorta connects to the right ventricle and the pulmonary artery to the left ventricle, the opposite of the normal formation. The blood is not properly oxygenated, and survival is not possible without medical intervention or a natural shunt such as patent ductus. Other rare conotruncal defects include double outlet right ventricle (the aorta and the pulmonary artery attached to right ventricle), truncus arteriosus (failure of the truncus to separate into the aorta and the pulmonary artery), and aortopulmonary window (an opening between the aorta and the pulmonary artery).

Defects resulting from improper fusion of the endocardial cushions and surrounding tissues cause atrioventricular defects, which affect about 9 percent of congenital heart disease cases. Complete atrioventricular canal defect occurs in about 20 percent of Down syndrome cases, but it is rare outside this group. The defect produces a large open space in the center of the heart, allowing blood to intermix freely between the right and left sides of the heart. The defect is sometimes accompanied by hypoplastic ventricle. If the condition is not treated, the heart will fail. Patent foramen primum or ostium primum is a milder form of atrioventricular canal defect in which the atrial septum fails to fuse with the endocardial cushions, resulting in a problem similar to atrial septal defect. In addition, the mitral valve is usually deformed.

Other less common defects include looping defects such as dextrocardia, in which the apex of the heart points to the right instead of to the left. This change in symmetry normally does not affect heart function, but some looping defects are associated with other problems such as transposition of the great arteries. Another less common defect is anomalous venous return, in which the veins returning blood to the heart from the lungs attach to the right atrium or return to the right atrium by attaching to other large veins rather than to the left atrium. Errors in the coronary artery connections may also occur, causing poor circulation of blood to the heart muscles. Very rarely, the heart may protrude through the chest wall at birth, causing a difficult-to-treat problem called ectopia cordis.

Treatment and Therapy

Congenital heart disease can often be diagnosed shortly after birth, especially if the baby experiences certain symptoms such as cyanosis, shortness of breath, fatigue and sweating while eating, and inability to gain weight. A physical examination by a physician will include checking the heart and breathing rates for abnormalities and listening to the heart for possible murmurs. Heart murmurs are whooshing sounds caused by turbulent movement of blood that may indicate faulty valves, patent ductus, and other heart defects. A cardiologist will make the definitive diagnosis by administering such tests as the electrocardiogram, the Doppler-echocardiogram, and the cardiac catheterization. The electrocardiogram measures the rhythmic electrical signal that passes through the heart with each beat. An abnormal signal will often indicate problems with a particular region of the heart and is especially useful in identifying rhythm disorders. The echocardiogram produces visual images of the heart by sending out ultrasound waves that bounce off and return to a receiving device. Most structural heart defects can be detected with this technique, and many are discovered prenatally with routine fetal ultrasound monitoring. At the same time, a second receiving device (the Doppler) analyzes ultrasound signals from blood moving through the heart and is able to provide information about the speed and direction of blood flow within the heart. This helps detect abnormal functions such as reverse blood flow. The Doppler-echocardiogram has revolutionized congenital heart disease diagnosis and, in most cases, provides enough information to define the patient's problem accurately.

If the cardiologist believes it to be necessary, then further tests can be done. A chest X-ray may be taken to determine if there is any lung involvement in the disorder. Cardiac catheterization can add information about the internal heart blood pressures and blood oxygen levels and can help visualize some defects better with the administration of contrast dyes in combination with X-ray analysis. Special monitors can be used to record the electrocardiogram for one or two days to check for intermittent rhythm irregularities, and older children can be monitored while exercising to see how the heart performs under stress. These and other tests allow physicians to assess the seriousness of the problem and to recommend timely and appropriate treatment.

Serious heart malformations need to be treated immediately upon diagnosis. Often these include defects that cause cyanosis, including transposition of the great arteries, left-heart flow defects such as coarctation of the aorta, and defects that cause heart failure, such as truncus arteriosus. Immediate emergency surgery may be needed to save the life of the newborn infant. Additional follow-up surgeries may also be required to correct the defect completely. For example, one way of correcting transposition of the great arteries is by performing an atrial switch operation in which systemic blood returning from the body is diverted to the left side of the heart (so it can be pumped to the lungs) and pulmonary blood from the lungs is diverted to the right side of the heart (so it can be pumped to the body). This is accomplished by first enlarging the foramen ovale with a balloon catheter, a procedure called Rashkind balloon atrial septostomy. A second operation several months later enlarges the opening between the two atria further and installs a flap to enhance the cross flow of blood. This is known as a Mustard or Senning atrial switch operation. A more recently developed procedure for correcting this defect requires only one operation. The misplaced aorta and pulmonary artery are both cut and then reattached to the correct heart chamber; this is called a Jatene arterial switch operation. At the same time, the coronary arteries are moved to the new aorta.

Some defects require no surgery but can be treated with drugs and other less traumatic procedures, such as the balloon catheter. Drugs are also used to help improve heart performance before and after surgery. When fluid accumulates in the lungs or other body tissues, the heart has problems pumping all the blood that returns to it because of the congestion. The overworked heart suffers under this stress, and thus the condition is called congestive heart failure. Diuretics such as Lasix (furosemide) improve the kidneys" ability to remove the excess fluid and relieve the congestion. Another drug, digitalis, can be helpful in treating congestive heart failure by slowing the heart rate and causing the heart to beat more forcefully. An open ductus is beneficial to children born with cyanotic heart defects because it allows a more even distribution of oxygenated blood. Treatment with prostaglandin E1 helps to keep the ductus open until corrective surgery can be performed. Indomethacin has the opposite effect and is often used to promote closing of a patent ductus in premature babies. As in adults, drugs such as digitalis, beta-blockers, and calcium channel blockers can be used to treat abnormal heart rhythms (arrhythmia) in children with congenital heart disease. The balloon catheter is used to enlarge narrow vessels and passages and has been used successfully to treat pulmonary and aortic valve stenosis in a technique called balloon valvuloplasty.

Types of surgery done later in infancy or childhood include closed-heart operations such as repair of a patent ductus and partial treatment of some types of cyanosis with a Blalock-Taussig shunt (connecting the subclavian artery to the pulmonary artery to bring more blood to the lungs). Open-heart surgery is used to repair defects inside the heart such as septal defects. A heart-lung machine is used to bypass the heart and lungs while the operation is under way, and the body is cooled so that the brain and other tissues require less oxygen. Children with very serious heart defects such as hypoplastic right or left ventricles may require a series of corrective surgical operations, and for some the only hope is a heart transplant. For example, children with hypoplastic right ventricle are given a Blalock-Taussig shunt shortly after birth to improve blood flow to their lungs and then are later given

the Fontan operation, which involves closing off the Blalock-Taussig shunt and connecting the pulmonary artery to the right atrium so that blood returning from the body will flow directly to the lungs, completely bypassing the defective right ventricle.

Some heart defects require no treatment. For example, most small septal defects close on their own during the first one or two years of life. Also, mild disorders such as benign valve defects usually require no treatment, and many children with heart murmurs have no detectable problems.

Perspective and Prospects

In the late nineteenth and early twentieth centuries, physicians were beginning to understand that certain congenital heart defects such as patent ductus could be diagnosed by listening to the heart. Treatment, however, was not possible at that time. The *Atlas of Congenital Cardiac Disease* was published in 1936 by Maude Abbot of McGill University. This manual greatly assisted physicians in recognizing and diagnosing congenital heart disease. In 1939, Robert Gross of Boston repaired a patent ductus, and in 1944, Alfred Blalock and Helen Taussig developed and performed their shunt operation in order to treat children with tetralogy of Fallot. Open-heart surgery was not performed until the mid-1950s, when the heart-lung machine was perfected. Even then, open-heart surgery could be performed only on older children. These operations were pioneered by Walton Lillehei of the University of Minnesota and John Kirlin of the Mayo Clinic. Open-heart surgery on newborn infants was developed in the 1970s by Brian Barratt-Boyes of New Zealand.

During the period while heart surgery was being developed, cardiac catheterization was also advancing. It was used primarily for diagnosis, but in 1966, William Rashkind of Philadelphia began to use the balloon catheter to enlarge openings in the atrial septum in order to treat transposition of the great arteries. Microsurgical catheters are currently being developed to repair patent ductus and other heart defects without the need for major surgery. The echocardiogram was pioneered by Inge Edler in the 1950s, and the Doppler-echocardiogram came into widespread use as a diagnostic tool in the 1980s. This instrument has greatly reduced the need for other diagnostic tests that were used in the past.

The modern strategy for treatment of congenital heart defects is to perform the corrective surgery as early in infancy as possible. This eliminates the need for numerous hospitalizations and diagnostic tests and reduces the need for extensive drug treatment. Children with multiple defects may still need more than one surgery. Modern treatment also emphasizes the roles of the child, the family, and health care personnel in fostering an understanding of the condition, treatment, and outcome. Even children who have been successfully treated will sometimes have physical limitations. These children need to be encouraged and supported by their families and allowed to pursue their goals to the fullest extent possible. Overcoming congenital heart disease is now possible for the vast majority of those who are afflicted.

—Rodney C. Mowbray, Ph.D.

See also Arrhythmias; Birth defects; Blue baby syndrome; Bypass surgery; Cardiology; Cardiology, pediatric; Congenital disorders; Cyanosis; DiGeorge syndrome; Echocardiography; Genetic diseases; Heart; Heart disease; Heart failure; Heart transplantation; Mitral valve prolapse; Neonatology; Shunts.

For Further Information:

"Congenital Heart Disease." *Medline Plus*, December 5, 2011.

Gersh, Bernard J., ed. *The Mayo Clinic Heart Book*. 2d ed. New York: William Morrow, 2000.

Koenig, Peter, Ziyad M. Hijazi, and Frank Zimmerman, eds. *Essential Pediatric Cardiology*. New York: McGraw-Hill, 2004.

Kramer, Gerri Freid, and Shari Mauer. *Parent's Guide to Children's Congenital Heart Defects: What They Are, How to Treat Them, How to Cope with Them*. New York: Three Rivers Press, 2001.

Moore, Keith L., T. V. N. Persaud, and Mark G. Torchia. *The Developing Human: Clinically Oriented Embryology*. 9th ed. Philadelphia: Saunders/Elsevier, 2011.

Neill, Catherine A., Edward B. Clark, and Carleen Clark. *The Heart of a Child: What Families Need to Know About Heart Disorders in Children*. 2d ed. Baltimore: Johns Hopkins University Press, 2001.

Park, Myung K. *The Pediatric Cardiology Handbook*. 4th ed. St. Louis, Mo.: Mosby/Elsevier, 2010.

Porter, Robert S., et al., eds. *The Merck Manual of Diagnosis and Therapy*. 19th ed. Whitehouse Station, N.J.: Merck, 2011.

Sherwood, Lauralee. *Human Physiology: From Cells to Systems*. 8th ed. Pacific Grove, Calif.: Brooks/Cole, 2012.

CONGENITAL HYPOTHYROIDISM

Disease/Disorder

Also known as: Infantile hypothyroidism, cretinism

Anatomy or system affected: Endocrine system, musculoskeletal system, neck, nervous system

Specialties and related fields: Endocrinology, internal medicine, perinatology, preventive medicine

Definition: Retardation of mental and physical growth arising from prenatal or neonatal hypothyroidism.

Key terms:

goiter: the sometimes gross enlargement of the thyroid gland in an effort to produce hormones when insufficient iodine is available

L-thyroxine (T₄): a less potent thyroid hormone than the T_3 form that can be converted in the cells to T_3

L-triiodothyronine (T₃): the most potent of the thyroid hormones

thyroid gland: the endocrine gland in humans that produces the hormones that control metabolism

Causes and Symptoms

In humans, the thyroid gland consists of two connected lobes in the front of the neck, on either side of the thyroid cartilage or Adam's apple. It produces the thyroid hormones, the most important of which are L-triiodothyronine (T_3) and L-tetraiodothyroxine or L-thyroxine (T_4). These compounds circulate in the blood serum to the body's cells and regulate virtually all metabolism: the production and consumption of proteins, carbohydrates, fats, and vitamins and the generation of energy that makes body heat. In these activities, the T_3 molecule (which can be derived in the cells from T_4) has two

---

Information on Congenital Hypothyroidism

Causes: Thyroid disorder

Symptoms: Mental retardation, low body temperature, poor appetite, decreased activity, flabbiness, low pulse rate, delayed union of skull bones, feeding difficulties, off-color skin

Duration: Lifelong

Treatments: Thyroid replacement therapy from birth

---

to four times the effectiveness of T_4. Because of the high iodine content of both T_3 and T_4, sufficient dietary iodine must be supplied to maintain normal thyroid function.

Abnormal levels of T_3 and T_4 have a profound effect on all bodily functions. In adults, the low production of T_3 and T_4, known as hypothyroidism, leads to reduced mental and physical activity, weight gain, general weakness, and other symptoms. Elevated thyroid activity, or hyperthyroidism, produces restlessness and irritability, weight loss, and symptoms generally the opposite of those seen with hypothyroidism. When either of these conditions develops in adults, surgery or drug regimens, or both, are available to control them and to produce normal metabolism in the patient. When these conditions occur in utero, however, there is almost no way to counteract their effects.

A child born with congenital hypothyroidism (CH) has developmental disabilities with little or no chance of improvement and, unless immediately treated with thyroid hormones, may also be physically disabled or dwarfed, with the bone ends not growing or maturing normally. The typical infant with CH can show a variety of symptoms: low body temperature, poor appetite, decreased activity, flabbiness, low pulse rate, delayed union of bones of the skull, feeding difficulties even to the point of choking and cyanosis (turning blue from lack of oxygen), and thickened, off-color skin.

Treatment and Therapy

For the child born with CH, no treatment is available for the brain damage that has taken place. Thyroid replacement therapy from birth, using either natural or synthetic hormones, will avert most physical effects, but the intellectual disability is irreversible.

The most effective way to avoid this problem is to ensure that a pregnant woman consumes enough iodine to be made into the T_3 and T_4 molecules by her fetus. The thyroid hormones do not transfer readily from the placental blood supply to that of the fetus, but the iodide ion does. This alone is enough, when made available before the end of the second trimester of pregnancy, to allow the fetal thyroid gland to develop normally, and the unborn fetus to have proper neurological and musculoskeletal function. Iodide ions are most easily supplied in iodized salt, but they can also be given as an injection of iodized oil or by the oral administration of a number of iodine-containing medicines, such as Lugol's iodine solution.

When hypothyroidism develops in the older child or adolescent-often appearing as a goiter, in addition to the other symptoms described above-iodine therapy is sometimes sufficient to return thyroid function to normal levels. Oddly, such therapy can also be counterproductive. The complex mechanisms that maintain proper hormone levels in blood serum can be misled by artificially high iodine concentrations and may close down hormone production because it appears high. For this condition, only thyroid hormone administration is effective.

Perspective and Prospects

Hypothyroidism, goiter, and CH are worldwide health problems because of the body's dependence on dietary iodine. Many places in the world have low soil levels of iodine, leading to low iodine levels in crops and thus inadequate iodine intake from food. Such areas include high mountain country, such as the Himalayas, where glacial meltwater leaches iodine from the soil with no replacement from higher geologic formations, and the Ganges River basin, where the sheer volume of water removes iodine from crop lands. Some mountainous areas of the United States-such as the hill country of West Virginia, Kentucky, and Tennessee-have been, historically, centers of endemic goiter formation. Supplying iodine to inhabitants of these areas is a medical necessity but, like so many such problems, is complicated by logistic and political considerations.

—*Robert M. Hawthorne, Jr., Ph.D.*

See also Birth defects; Congenital disorders; Dwarfism; Endocrine system; Endocrinology, pediatric; Growth; Hashimoto's thyroiditis; Malnutrition; Mental retardation; Nutrition; Thyroid disorders; Thyroid gland; Vitamins and minerals.

For Further Information:

"Another Reason for Iodine Prophylaxis." *The Lancet* 335, no. 8703 (June 16, 1990): 1433-1434.

Buyukgebiz, Atilla. "Newborn Screening for Congenital Hypothyroidism." *Journal of Clinical Research in Pediatric Endocrinology* 5 (March, 2013): 8-12.

Cao, Xue-Yi, et al. "Timing of Vulnerability of the Brain to Iodine Deficiency in Endemic Cretinism." *New England Journal of Medicine* 331, no. 26 (December 29, 1994).

"Key Findings: Congenital Hypothyroidism." *Centers for Disease Control and Prevention*, September 7, 2011.

Gomez, Joan. *Thyroid Problems in Women and Children*. Alameda, Calif.: Hunter House, 2003.

Hetzel, Basil S. "Iodine and Neuropsychological Development." *Journal of Nutrition* 130, no. 2S (1999): 493S-495S.

Kronenberg, Henry M., et al., eds. *Williams Textbook of Endocrinology*. 11th ed. Philadelphia: Saunders/Elsevier, 2008.

Maberly, Glen F. "Iodine Deficiency Disorders: Contemporary Scientific Issues." *Journal of Nutrition* 124, no. 8 (August, 1994): 1473-1478S.

"Neonatal Hypothyroidism." *Medline Plus*, June 28, 2011.

Rosenthal, M. Sara. *The Thyroid Sourcebook*. 5th ed. New York: McGraw-Hill, 2009.

Woeber, K. A. "Iodine and Thyroid Disease." *Medical Clinics of North America: Thyroid Diseases* 75, no. 1 (January, 1991): 169-178.

CONGESTIVE HEART FAILURE. *See* **HEART FAILURE.**

CONJUNCTIVITIS

Disease/Disorder
Also known as: Pinkeye
Anatomy or system affected: Eyes, immune system
Specialties and related fields: Bacteriology, family medicine, microbiology, ophthalmology, optometry, virology
Definition: An acute inflammatory disease of the eye caused by infection or irritation.

Causes and Symptoms

Conjunctivitis, or pinkeye, is one of the most common eye disorders. The conjunctiva is a thin translucent membrane that overlies the white part of the eye and the inner surface of the eyelids. It protects the eye from foreign objects and infection.

The conjunctiva may become inflamed through infection with a virus or bacterium, allergic reactions, and exposure to certain chemicals. Inflammation of the conjunctiva brings increased blood flow to the eye, producing a red or bloodshot appearance. Conjunctivitis causes a feeling of irritation, burning, or mild pain. A discharge often occurs, which may form a crust on the eyelids when it dries. Conjunctivitis does not cause visual loss, fever, or severe pain. It is typically mild and short-lived, lasting from a few days to a few weeks.

Most conjunctivitis is caused by infection and is highly contagious, spreading quickly from one eye to the other and from person to person by touch. Viral conjunctivitis will resolve without treatment, although symptoms may persist as long as a few weeks. Upper-respiratory symptoms may occur simultaneously because similar viruses cause the common cold. These viruses may live on surfaces for several hours and can be transmitted in poorly chlorinated swimming pools. Bacterial conjunctivitis causes a thicker discharge and more severe crusting. It is caused by various bacteria, and all respond well to topical antibiotics.

Allergic conjunctivitis may be stimulated by a reaction to dust, mold, animal dander, or pollen. It causes burning or itching in both eyes and occurs in a seasonal pattern. Chemicals, wind, dust, smoke, and chronic dry eyes can also cause direct irritation of the conjunctiva.

Treatment and Therapy

For viral conjunctivitis, no therapy is required, but the patient may be contagious for as long as two weeks. Common bacterial conjunctivitis resolves quickly with antibiotic eyedrops or ointment. A person remains contagious with bacterial conjunctivitis until after twenty-four hours of antibiotic

---

Information on Conjunctivitis

Causes: Viral or bacterial infection, allergic reactions, exposure to chemicals or irritants
Symptoms: Red or bloodshot eye, burning sensation, mild pain, discharge forming crust on eyelids
Duration: Ranges from a few days to a few weeks
Treatments: None or topical antibiotics

treatment. The spread of infection can be prevented by washing one's hands frequently, using separate towels, and isolating an infected child from interaction with other children for the first twenty-four hours of treatment. For allergic conjunctivitis, avoiding the offending allergen and using topical antihistamines or artificial tears are effective treatments.

Perspective and Prospects

Conjunctivitis is generally benign and rarely causes permanent injury. However, in many developing countries, conjunctivitis is a leading cause of blindness. In areas of extreme poverty, repeated infections with trachoma, a bacterial infection spread by flies, can lead to permanent scarring of the eyes. Newborns may also contract severe bacterial conjunctivitis from the mother's cervix during birth. For this reason, most developed nations require that all newborns receive antibiotic eyedrops at birth.

—*Christopher D. Sharp, M.D.*

See also Allergies; Bacterial infections; Blindness; Childhood infectious diseases; Eye infections and disorders; Eyes; Keratitis; Trachoma; Viral infections; Vision; Vision disorders.

For Further Information:

Badash, Michelle. "Conjunctivitis (Pink Eye)." *Health Library*, November 26, 2012.

"Conjunctivitis (Pink Eye). *Centers for Disease Control and Prevention*, June 4, 2010.

Johnson, Gordon J., et al., eds. *The Epidemiology of Eye Disease*. 3rd ed. London: World Scientific, 2012.

Longo, Dan, et al., eds. *Harrison's Principles of Internal Medicine*. 18th ed. New York: McGraw-Hill, 2011.

Parker, James N., and Philip M. Parker, eds. *The Official Patient's Sourcebook on Conjunctivitis*. San Diego, Calif.: Icon Health, 2002.

Stoffman, Phyllis. *The Family Guide to Preventing and Treating One Hundred Infectious Illnesses*. New York: John Wiley & Sons, 1995.

CONNECTIVE TISSUE
Anatomy

Anatomy or system affected: Blood, bones, ligaments, musculoskeletal system, tendons

Specialties and related fields: Biochemistry, hematology, orthopedics, rheumatology

Definition: A category of tissue composed of adipose (fat), blood, bone, cartilage, ligaments, and tendons; the function of connective tissue is to connect, support, bind, protect, and store materials.

Structure and Function

Cells, the structural and functional units of life, are organized into tissue, a group of different types of cells and their nonliving intracellular matrix, or glue, that performs a specialized function. The four groups of tissues are epithelial (covering and lining tissue; also glands); connective (adipose, blood, bone, cartilage, ligament, and tendon); muscle (skeletal, cardiac, and smooth); and nervous (brain and spinal cord).

Connective tissue typically has cells widely scattered throughout a large amount of intracellular matrix (that is, a substance in which the cells are embedded), unlike epithelial tissue that typically has cells arranged in an orderly manner and has a limited amount of intracellular matrix.

Connective tissues are categorized as loose (areolar), dense, and specialized. Some connective tissues are difficult to classify, with the distinction between "loose" and "dense" not clearly defined. Also, dense connective tissue may be called fibrous connective tissue because of the large amount of collagen or elastin fibers contained.

Because a tissue is defined as a collection of different cells, several types of cells may be found in various types of connective tissue: fibroblasts, which secrete collagen and other elements of the extracellular matrix, thereby creating and maintaining the matrix; adipocytes, which store excess caloric energy in the form of fat; and mast cells, macrophages, leukocytes, and plasma cells, which have immune functions and, therefore, an active role in inflammation. The components of the matrix are different in the various types of connective tissue and may include fibers, amorphous ground substances (glycoproteins, proteins, and proteoglycans), and tissue fluid. Each type of connective tissue has a characteristic pattern of cells and a distinctive amount and type of matrix. For example, bone matrix includes minerals, while blood has plasma for a matrix.

Loose connective tissue is the most common type of connective tissue; it holds organs in place and attaches epithelial tissue to underlying tissues. Loose connective tissue can be further categorized based on the type of fibers and how the fibers are arranged: collagenous fibers, which are composed of collagen and are arranged as coils; elastic fibers, which are composed of elastin and are able to stretch; and reticular fibers, which join connective tissue to other tissues. Loose connective tissue has a relatively large amount of cells, matrix, or both, and a relatively small amount of fibers. Loose connective tissue is found in the hypodermis and fascia (the connective tissue that loosely binds structures to one another).

Dense connective tissue is identified by the high density of fibers in the tissue and a low density of cells and matrix. The type of fiber that predominates determines the type of dense connective tissue. Dense collagenous connective tissue, for example, contains an abundance of collagen fibers and is found in structures where tensile strength is needed, such as the sclera (white) of the eye, tendons, and ligaments. Dense elastic connective tissue contains an abundance of elastin fibers and is found in structures where elasticity is needed (for example, the aorta).

Specialized connective tissues include adipose tissue, cartilage, bone, and blood. Adipose tissue is a form of loose connective tissue that stores fat. It is found in the fatty layer around the abdomen, in bone marrow, and around the kidneys. Cartilage is a form of fibrous connective tissue. It is composed of closely packed collagenous fibers embedded in a gelatinous intracellular matrix called chondrin. While the skeleton of human embryos are composed of cartilage, cartilage does not become bone but rather is replaced by bone. The replacement is not universal; cartilage provides flexible support for ears (external pinnae), nose, and trachea. Bone is a type of mineralized connective tissue, and it contains collagen and calcium phosphate. Cells found in bone include osteoblasts, which form new bone for growth, repair, or remodeling, and osteoclasts, which break down bone for growth and remodeling. The living cells are found in spaces in the calcified matrix. These spaces are called lacunae and are interconnected by small channels called canaliculi that eventually join up with blood vessels in the bone organ. Thus, even in a solidified matrix, living cells are able to obtain nutrients and expel wastes.>

Blood too is a type of specialized connective tissue. Blood may seem to be an unlikely connective tissue, but it fits the definition: different cells widely dispersed in intracellular matrix, working together to perform a specific function. Unlike other connective tissues, blood has no fibers. Blood does have several types of cells: red blood cells or erythrocytes, white blood cells or leukocytes (with subdivisions of monocytes, macrophages, eosinophils, lymphocytes, neutrophils, and basophils), and platelets or thrombocytes. The matrix is liquid and contains enzymes, hormones, proteins, carbohydrates, and fats.

Disorders and Diseases

Connective tissue, like any other tissue, is subject to disorders and diseases. Some disorders are inherited (passed from one generation to the next by means of DNA in chromosomes), while other disorders are related to environmental factors (such as a lack of specific nutrients).

Some inherited connective tissue disorders are Marfan syndrome and osteogenesis imperfecta. In Marfan syndrome, connective tissue grows outside the cell, having deleterious effects on the lungs, heart valves, aorta, eyes, central nervous system, and skeletal system. People with Marfan syndrome are often unusually tall with long, slender arms, legs, and fingers. In osteogenesis imperfecta, or brittle bone disease, the quantity and quality of collagen is insufficient to produce healthy bones. People with this disorder have multiple spontaneous bone breaks. Other connective tissue diseases are environmental, such as scurvy, which is caused by a lack of vitamin C required for the production and maintenance of collagen. Without sufficient vitamin C in the diet, and subsequent lack of collagen, the patient will develop spots on the skin, particularly the legs and thighs; will be tired and depressed; and may lose teeth. Osteoporosis has many factors, but lack of vitamin D and calcium in the diet will lead to a thinning of the bone, subjecting the patient to fractures, primarily of the hip, spine, and wrist.

Connective tissue diseases may also be classified as systemic autoimmune disease and may have both genetic and environmental causes. In these situations, the immune system is spontaneously overactivated and extra antibodies are produced. Examples of systemic autoimmune diseases include systemic lupus erythematosus and rheumatoid arthritis. Systemic lupus erythematosus can damage the heart, joints, skin, lungs, blood vessels, liver, kidneys, and nervous system. More woman than men are diagnosed with lupus, and more

black women than other groups. Rheumatoid arthritis is caused when immune cells attack the membrane around joints and destroys the cartilage of the joint; it can also affect the heart and lungs and interfere with vision.

—*M. A. Foote, Ph.D.*

See also Blood and blood disorders; Bones and the skeleton; Cartilage; Ligaments; Tendon disorders.

For Further Information:
Gordon, Caroline, and Wolfgang Gross. *Connective Tissue Diseases: An Atlas of Investigation and Management.* Oxford: Clinical Publishing, 2011.
Lundon, Katie. *Orthopedic Rehabilitation Science: Principles for Clinical Management of Nonmineralized Connective Tissue.* Boston: Butterworth-Heinemann, 2003.
"Mixed Connective Tissue Disease." *Mayo Clinic*, May 30, 2012.
Price, Sylvia Anderson, and Lorraine McCarty Wilson, eds. *Pathophysiology: Clinical Concepts of Disease Processes.* St. Louis: Mosby, 2003.
"Questions and Answers about Heritable Disorders of Connective Tissue." *National Institute of Arthritis and Musculoskeletal and Skin Diseases*, October 2011.
Royce, Peter M., and Beat Steinmann, eds. *Connective Tissue and Its Heritable Disorders: Molecular, Genetic, and Medical Aspects.* New York: Wiley-Liss, 2002.

CONSTIPATION
Disease/Disorder

Anatomy or system affected: Abdomen, gastrointestinal system, intestines
Specialties and related fields: Family medicine, gastroenterology, internal medicine
Definition: The slow passage of feces through the bowels or the presence of hard feces.

Causes and Symptoms

People of every age group, from infants to the elderly, can experience the unpleasant symptoms of constipation, which is characterized primarily by discomfort. Certain disease states such as diabetes mellitus, paralysis of the legs, colon cancer, and hypothyroidism predispose a person to constipation. Possible causes of constipation are medications, iron supplements, toilet training procedures, pregnancy, lack of adequate fluids, a low-fiber diet, and lack of physical activity.

Treatment and Therapy

Most cases of constipation can be treated by the patient at home. Drinking adequate fluids makes it easier for fecal

---

Information on Constipation

Causes: Lack of fiber or adequate fluids in diet, certain medications, iron supplements, pregnancy, lack of physical activity, aging
Symptoms: Uncomfortable passage of stools, bloating, abdominal discomfort
Duration: Ranges from short-term to chronic
Treatments: Adequate hydration, high-fiber diet, exercise, laxatives

material to pass through the large intestine. Without adequate hydration, a person may experience small, pelletlike stools. Eight to ten glasses of liquids per day are recommended, including water, milk, fruit juice, herbal tea, and soup. Once adequate hydration is achieved, a high-fiber diet can gradually be started. Without enough fluids, a high-fiber diet can worsen the problems of constipation. A high-fiber diet adds bulk to the bowel movement (increasing stool volume, decreasing pressure within the colon, and decreasing the intestinal transit time of foods) and thus can lead to more regular bowel habits and partial relief of the symptoms. One can increase fiber in the diet by eating high-fiber breakfast cereals, beans or legumes, raw fruits and vegetables, prunes, and whole-grain breads. To minimize gastrointestinal discomforts such as increased flatulence (gas), it is recommended to increase one's fiber consumption gradually.

In addition to adequate liquids and a high-fiber diet, exercise is important in treating constipation. Any sort of physical activity, such as walking, running, or swimming, can help to stimulate the activity of the large intestine.

Laxatives and enemas should not be used until after a discussion with a physician. Mineral oil should also not be used because many essential fat-soluble vitamins (such as vitamins A, D, E, and K) may be excreted as well. Persistent constipation should be evaluated by a physician.

—*Martha M. Henze, M.S., R.D.*

See also Colon; Diarrhea and dysentery; Enemas; Fiber; Gastroenterology; Gastroenterology, pediatric; Gastrointestinal disorders; Gastrointestinal system; Hemorrhoid banding and removal; Hemorrhoids; Indigestion; Intestinal disorders; Intestines; Obstruction; Over-the-counter medications; Rectum.

For Further Information:

Berkson, D. Lindsey. *Healthy Digestion the Natural Way.* New York: Wiley, 2000.

Capasso, Francesco. *Laxatives: A Practical Guide.* New York: Springer, 1997.

"Chart of High-Fiber Foods." *Mayo Clinic*, November 17, 2012.

"Constipation." *National Digestive Diseases Information Clearinghouse*, February 21, 2012.

"Constipation. in Children." *National Digestive Diseases Information Clearinghouse*, February 21, 2012.

Gitnick, Gary, and Karen Cooksey. *Freedom from Digestive Distress.* New York: Crown, 2000.

Parker, James N., and Philip M. Parker, eds. *The Official Patient's Sourcebook on Constipation.* San Diego, Calif.: Icon Health, 2002.

Peikin, Steven R. *Gastrointestinal Health.* 3d ed. New York: Quill, 2005.

Wexner, Steven D., and Graeme S. Duthie, eds. *Constipation: Etiology, Evaluation, and Management.* 2d ed. London: Springer, 2006.

Whorton, James C. *Inner Hygiene: Constipation and the Pursuit of Health in Modern Society.* New York: Oxford University Press, 2000.

CONTRACEPTION

Procedure

Anatomy or system affected: Genitals, reproductive system, uterus

Specialties and related fields: Gynecology, obstetrics, urology

Definition: The use of techniques to prevent pregnancy, which may interfere with ovulation, sperm transport, or implantation of an embryo.

Key terms:

barrier method: a contraceptive that physically prevents sperm from meeting an egg

cervix: the entrance to the uterus from the vagina

ejaculation: the release of semen from the male's body during sexual activity

hormone: a chemical signal carried in the blood that allows distant body parts to coordinate their actions

implantation: the process in which the embryo attaches to the uterine lining

ovulation: the monthly release of a mature egg from the ovary

spermicide: a chemical that kills sperm after they are ejaculated

toxic shock syndrome: an infection normally caused by staphylococci that can develop rapidly into severe untreatable shock, which can be fatal

uterus: the organ that supports the embryo during its development

vagina: the tube-shaped cavity of the female into which the male's penis is inserted during intercourse

vas deferens: the tubes in the male reproductive system that carry sperm

Methods and Effectiveness

Contraception is defined as the avoidance of conception by either natural means (abstinence) or artificial means (physical barriers, chemicals, hormones). Pregnancy can be prevented by interfering with the process of conception at any number of sites in the male or female anatomy.

Barrier methods. A male condom, or prophylactic, is a thin sheath made to fit an erect penis. It can be made of latex (a type of rubber), polyurethane (a type of plastic), or natural products such as lamb's intestines. A condom prevents semen, which contains sperm, from entering a woman's vagina during intercourse. The latex or polyurethane condom is one of the few forms of contraception that can also protect against sexually transmitted diseases (STDs). Men who are not allergic to latex should use latex condoms, as they are the best at preventing pregnancy and STDs. Polyurethane condoms break more easily, and natural condoms are not as effective at preventing STDs.

Male condoms should be used any time a man has intercourse with his partner and desires to prevent STDs or pregnancy. If the condom does not have space at the end called a sperm repository, then 0.25 inches of the condom should be left at the tip of the penis to collect semen. To increase the protective birth control value, spermicidal foam or jelly can be used in addition to the condom. According to the American College of Obstetricians and Gynecologists, this combination is 99 percent effective. Vaseline or other types of petroleum jelly, lotion, or oils should not be used as lubricants with condoms because they weaken the latex rubber. Non-oil-based lubricants or even water can be used with latex condoms. Condoms come in a variety of sizes and can be purchased over the counter at drugstores and pharmacies and in coin machines in many public restrooms. There is no age restriction on buying condoms.

The female condom is a lubricated, thin polyurethane or nitrile tube that has a flexible ring that facilitates insertion and an outside ring that helps keep the condom in place around the vulva. The closed end of the tube is inserted into the vagina, and the other end remains outside the vagina, slightly covering the labia and providing some enhanced protection against skin-borne infections. With proper use, the female condom is similar to the male condom in effectiveness, and it may be more accepted by male partners who do not wish to wear a condom. Female condoms, however, are more expensive and harder to find. Recent introduction of a new nitrile female condom, FC2, has lowered the price, and many public health and reproductive health advocates are working to make the method more accepted and widely available. Like the male condom, the female condom should be used only once per intercourse, and female and male condoms should not be used together.

A diaphragm is a dome-shaped rubber disk with a flexible rim, which covers the cervix so that sperm are unable to enter the uterus. A diaphragm, which must be prescribed and sized by a health care professional, is designed to be used with a spermicide that is applied inside the dome and around the rim. The diaphragm provides birth control protection up to six hours after insertion. A new application of spermicide should be inserted into the vagina with an applicator and with the diaphragm in place for repeated intercourse. To be effective, the diaphragm must remain in the vagina six hours after the last intercourse, but never longer than twenty-four hours because of the risk of toxic shock syndrome. The diaphragm is approximately 83 percent effective as a birth control method.

The cervical cap is a soft rubber or plastic cup with a round rim, which fits snugly over the cervix. As with a diaphragm, it must be fitted by a health care professional. The cervical cap should be used in combination with a spermicidal cream or jelly for optimal effectiveness. It can provide birth control protection for up to forty-eight hours. The cervical cap should be removed after forty-eight hours because of a low risk of toxic shock syndrome. It does not provide any protection against STDs.

Vaginal spermicides include creams, jellies, films, foams, suppositories, and tablets. They contain sperm-killing chemicals and act somewhat as a barrier to sperm entering the uterus. Spermicides used by themselves are up to 79 percent effective for birth control, but when used properly with condoms, they are up to 99 percent effective. They are available without a prescription. For spermicides to be effective, they should be inserted into the woman's vagina up to twenty minutes before intercourse and stay in the vagina at least eight hours. A new application of spermicide should be applied for repeated intercourse. Spermicides do not protect against STDs unless they are used in combination with condoms.

Hormonal methods. Oral contraceptives or birth control pills, often simply called "the pill," are the most popular form

of reversible birth control in the United States. They contain synthetic hormones that interact with a woman's natural hormones to prevent pregnancy. There are two types of birth control pills: combination estrogen-progestin and progestin alone.

Combination birth control pills stop the ovaries from releasing eggs. Available only by prescription, combination pills come in packages of twenty-one or twenty-eight pills per month, although there are new pills designed for continuous or extended cycling that come in packages with more than a month's supply. There are twenty-one active pills in the twenty-one-day pack. The twenty-eight-day pack contains twenty-one active pills and seven placebo or sugar pills, with the exception of some newer formulations that extend the active pill cycle to more than twenty-one pills, reducing the number of inactive or placebo pills. Menstruation occurs during the week with no pills or inactive pills, although extended or continuous cycling involves a longer or continuous regimen of active pills and delays menstruation until a pill-free interval.

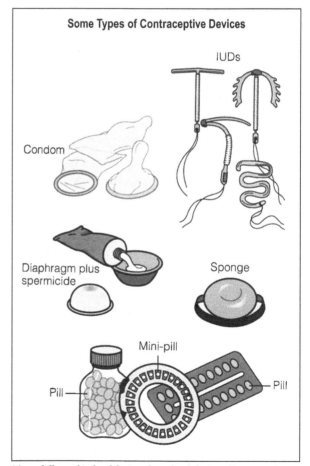

Some Types of Contraceptive Devices

Many different kinds of devices have been designed to prevent pregnancy, from barrier methods such as condoms and diaphragms to hormonal methods such as birth control pills. Each method has its own advantages, disadvantages, and failure rates.

Some other form of contraception should be used for the first month in addition to the birth control pill. By the second month, the pill should provide the needed birth control. Pills should be taken at the same time of the day each day. Oral contraceptives are 98 to 99 percent effective in providing birth control, but they provide no protection against STDs. Oral contraceptives can be taken safely by most women, but they are not recommended for women over thirty-five who smoke. A benefit of oral contraceptives is that they can make a woman's menstrual cycle regular and lighter, and they are protective against pelvic inflammatory disease (PID), ovarian cancer, and endometrial cancer.

The second form of oral contraception is the mini-pill. It contains only one hormone, progestin, and works by thickening the cervical mucus so that sperm is unable to reach the egg. Progestin also changes the lining of the uterus so that implantation cannot occur. Mini-pills are 95 percent effective in preventing pregnancy, but their effectiveness diminishes if they are not taken on time. The pill taken more than two hours from the set time for a daily dose constitutes a missed pill and significantly raises the chance of unintended pregnancy.

Ortho Evra is a thin patch that releases a combination of estrogen and progestin. It is worn on the upper outer arm, upper torso (excluding the breast), buttocks, or abdomen. Once attached, it delivers hormones through the skin and into the bloodstream. The patch will remain in place during exercise or bathing and in humid conditions. It is worn for three weeks, then removed for one week before a new patch is worn. The patch offers approximately 99 percent birth control protection, but no protection from STDs. It has been found to be significantly less effective in women weighing more than 198 pounds.

NuvaRing is a transparent flexible ring that is inserted into the vagina, and normally stays around the cervix. The ring releases estrogen and progestin into the vagina to stop ovulation, to thicken cervical mucus, and to prevent implantation if fertilization occurs. The ring is worn for three weeks, followed by a week off, during which menstruation occurs. Vaginal rings must be replaced each month. If the ring slips out of the vagina, the patient can wash the ring with cold to lukewarm water (avoiding hot water) and reinsert it. The chance of pregnancy is increased if the ring is outside the vagina for more than three hours; if this occurs, the woman should use a backup method for another seven days to obtain maximum protection against pregnancy. Both NuvaRing and Ortho Evra share the same contraindications and benefits as combined oral contraceptives.

Depo-Provera (depo-medroxyprogesterone acetate, or DMPA) contains only the hormone progestin and is given by a health care provider as an injection every twelve weeks. DMPA comes in two formulations and can be given by intramuscular or subcutaneous injection. Patients need to be aware that irregular bleeding (which may include brownish spotting) and probable lack of normal menses is an expected side effect of DMPA, not a sign of a serious adverse affect. For some women who discontinue using DMPA, delayed fertility can last up to one year beyond the end of the injections. DMPA works in the same way as the mini-pill.

Those who use DMPA should be cautious, as both adolescents and adults have experienced a significant loss of bone density. This bone loss is thought to correct itself when the injections are discontinued, with the exception of women in perimenopause, who may not have enough time to reclaim bone mass before menopause. Furthermore, DMPA leads to weight gain in some women, through increased appetite. Women should be cautioned against overeating once beginning DMPA as their birth control method.

Emergency contraceptive pills can be used after a sexual assault, after intercourse without contraception, after finding that a condom broke during or after sex, or after the failure of some other method. Emergency contraception can be performed through a progestin-only formulation that involves taking two pills as soon as possible after unprotected sex, but within seventy-two hours (based on strong evidence, some clinical practices recommend emergency contraception as effective for up to five days after unprotected intercourse). A woman should have her menstrual cycle within ten to twenty-one days of taking emergency contraception pills, and thereafter her cycle should return to normal. These pills prevent conception, rather than causing a miscarriage, by thickening the cervical mucus, thus preventing sperm from fertilizing the egg. In 2003, a Food and Drug Administration (FDA) panel recommended that these morning-after pills, as they came to be known, be made available over the counter. They initially became available over the counter to girls and women seventeen years of age and older. Girls under the age of seventeen needed a prescription from a health care provider to obtain emergency contraception. In 2011, the FDA was ready to lift this age restriction but was blocked by Secretary of Health and Human Services Kathleen Sebelius. When a federal judge ordered the FDA to certify the drug for nonprescription use in 2013, the Obama administration initially tried to block the order before deciding to drop its appeal. On June 20, 2013, the FDA approved Plan B One-Step (levonorgestrel) as an over-the-counter emergency

---

In the News:
New Contraception Option Implanon

Implanon, an etonogestrel-releasing implant effective for up to three years, was approved in July, 2006. Implanon has advantages over Norplant, a contraceptive implant no longer available in the United States. It requires implantation of one rod into the upper arm instead of Norplant's six, making insertion and removal easier. Additionally, blood levels appear to vary less with Implanon. Fertility is regained within a few days following removal. Implanon is highly associated with irregular bleeding. Other side effects are similar to those from oral contraceptives. Because the product is progestin-only, it may be appropriate for some women who cannot use estrogens. Trial data suggest that Implanon in combination with injectable testosterone may be effective as a male contraceptive. Further study is needed for this indication.

—*Karen M. Nagel, R.Ph., Ph.D.*

contraceptive without age or point-of-sale restrictions.

Additional but less widely used methods of emergency contraception include the Yuzpe method, involving high doses of combined oral contraceptives, and insertion of an IUD following unprotected intercourse.

Intrauterine devices (IUDs). The IUD is a small device that is inserted into a woman's uterus by a health care provider in a simple office procedure. Two IUDs are currently available in the United States. Both are shaped like a capital *T*, and both have a silky or plastic thread that extends out into the cervix, allowing for easy removal. The ParaGard T 380A contains copper, but no hormones, and can be kept in the uterus for ten years. Mirena is an IUD that contains a progestin that releases slowly throughout the time that the device is in place. It can be kept in the uterus for five years. While ParaGard may result in some increased bleeding, a woman will have regular menses. Mirena greatly decreases menstrual flow but can result in irregular spotting, especially in the first three months of insertion, and some women stop having menses altogether. An IUD is thought to prevent pregnancy because it is a foreign object whose presence causes the woman's uterus to function improperly. The IUD interferes with sperm reaching the egg and prevents the egg from implanting in the uterus. IUDs that contain copper are thought to work by releasing of copper ions into the uterus. The copper in the uterine cavity stops sperm from moving through the vagina and into the uterus. IUDs are 97 to 99 percent effective in preventing pregnancy but provide no protection from STDs.

Sterilization. Essure is a sterilization device shaped much like a spring. The device is threaded through a thin tube through the vagina and into the Fallopian tubes. Two Essure devices are inserted, one in each Fallopian tube. Once they are in place, a meshlike substance inside the devices irritates the Fallopian tubes, causing scarring of the Fallopian tubes over time. The scarring finally causes permanent closing of the tube. Since this process of blockage in the tubes takes time, women are advised to use another form of birth control for the first three months after the insertion of Essure. The device then provides more than 99 percent effectiveness as birth control. It provides no protection from STDs.

Female sterilization through tubal ligation is one of the most common forms of contraception in the United States. An estimated 700,000 women undergo tubal ligation each year. The procedure involves surgically sealing the Fallopian tubes in order to prevent eggs from being released into the uterus. This surgery also prevents a male's sperm from entering the Fallopian tube, where fertilization normally occurs. The procedure is performed in a hospital or an outpatient surgical clinic under general anesthesia. One or two small incisions are made in a woman's abdomen, and a laparoscope is inserted. Instruments are also inserted and used to burn or seal the passages into the Fallopian tubes. Patients are usually able to return home a few hours after surgery. This procedure is more than 99 percent effective as birth control but provides no protection from STDs.

Male sterilization through vasectomy can be performed in a doctor's office. Local anesthesia is applied and a small incision is made in the upper part of the scrotum. The vas deferens is cut and sealed. This simple operation prevents sperm from traveling out of the testes. There is also a nonsurgical technique in which the doctor locates the vas deferens and holds it in place with a small clamp. A tiny puncture is made in the skin, and the opening is stretched so that the vas deferens can be cut and tied. This procedure requires no stitches because the punctures heal quickly on their own. With either of these methods, a man is able to return home immediately after the procedure and usually needs only a day of rest before resuming his normal activities. It is recommended that another form of birth control be used during the first nine or ten ejaculations to ensure that the seminal fluid no longer contains sperm. This method is 99 to 100 percent effective in preventing pregnancy; however, it provides no protection against STDs.

Perspective and Prospects

Even though highly effective contraceptive techniques are available both over the counter and through health care providers, almost 60 percent of pregnancies in the United States are not planned, and many are unwanted. The contraception and reproductive branch of the National Institute of Child Health and Human Development (NICHD), which has as one of its goals the prevention of acquired immunodeficiency syndrome (AIDS) and other STDs, is looking into the development of new microcides with spermicidal activity that can provide birth control as well as simultaneous protection against major STDs. One of the top objectives is to link contraceptive technology to HIV/AIDS prevention.

—*Clair Kaplan, A.P.R.N./M.S.N.;*
additional material by Toby R. Stewart, Ph.D.

See also Abortion; Conception; Ethics; Gynecology; Hormones; Hysterectomy; Men's health; Menstruation; Over-the-counter medications; Pregnancy and gestation; Reproductive system; Semen; Sterilization; Tubal ligation; Uterus; Vasectomy; Women's health.

For Further Information:
Centers for Disease Control and Prevention. "Reproductive Health: Contraception." *CDC*, April 26, 2013.
Connell, Elizabeth B. *The Contraception Sourcebook.* Chicago: Contemporary Books, 2002.
Global Campaign for Microbicides. *Global Campaign for Microbicides*, n. d.
Keyzer, Amy Marcaccio. *Family Planning Sourcebook.* Detroit, Mich.: Omnigraphics, 2001.
MedlinePlus. "Birth Control." *MedlinePlus*, June 24, 2013.
National Institutes of Health. "Contraception and Birth Control: Condition Information." *NIH Eunice Kennedy Shriver National Institute of Child Health and Human Development*, November 30, 2012.
Porter, Robert S., et al., eds. *The Merck Manual Home Health Handbook.* Whitehouse Station, N.J.: Merck Research Laboratories, 2009.
Thornton, Yvonne S. *Woman to Woman: A Leading Gynecologist Tells You All You Need to Know About Your Body and Your Health.* New York: E. P. Dutton, 1998.
US Food and Drug Administration. "FDA Approves Plan B One-Step Emergency Contraceptive for Use without a Prescription for All Women of Childbearing Potential." *FDA*, June 20, 2013.

CORNEAL TRANSPLANTATION

Procedure

Anatomy or system affected: Eyes

Specialties and related fields: General surgery, ophthalmology

Definition: A delicate surgical operation involving the removal and replacement of the cornea, the transparent outer covering of the eye.

Key terms:

endothelium: the inner surface of the cornea, which is separated from the rest of the eye by an essential layer of transparent fluid

keratoplasty: surgery on the cornea

lamellar keratoplasty: the partial removal or transplantation of a portion of the cornea; usually possible in younger patients or those with less advanced disorders

penetrating keratoplasty: the surgical transplantation of the entire thickness of the cornea, which is made up of four distinct layers of tissue

trephine: a specialized surgical instrument that is used to cut a perfectly vertical incision to remove corneas from both the donor and the recipient

Indications and Procedures

The cornea, which has four distinct layers, is the transparent outer coating of the eye. It serves both to protect the eye and to provide the main refracting surface as light reaches the eye and is transmitted to the lens and retina. Its total thickness is approximately 0.52 millimeter. The layers of specialized tissue are the epithelium, the stroma, Descemet's membrane, and the endothelium, or inner surface of the cornea.

Several types of corneal disorders may lead to a decision to perform partial or total keratoplasty. Most of these fall under the general term "corneal dystrophy." The most common, or classical, cases of corneal dystrophy involve the deposit of abnormal material in the cornea, resulting in irritation and eventually damage. Frequently, such disorders stem from genetic factors, making it possible to diagnose the dystrophy during the patient's childhood and perform a lamellar keratoplasty. Other dystrophies include granular dystrophy and macular dystrophy. The former involves lesions in the center of the cornea, which may multiply and coalesce. At that stage, they may extend into the deeper layers of the stroma, the second layer of the cornea. Macular dystrophy actually begins in the stroma, causing all layers to become opaque.

Entirely different types of disorders that may call for corneal transplantation are interstitial keratitis (a type of inflammation) and trachoma. The latter condition can reach near epidemic levels in underdeveloped areas of the world, where low levels of hygiene allow the implantation and rapid multiplication of bacteria in the cornea. The effect is a breakdown of tissue accompanied by the discharge of mucus.

Whether the cornea has been affected by disease or injury, the goal of corneal transplantation is to eliminate any opacity that can hamper vision. The graft operation itself may be de-

scribed in only a few stages, each marked by the need for a high degree of technical skill to increase the likelihood of success. First, the surgeon must calculate the exact size of the graft in question. This is done through the use of a special tool called a trephine, which will make the cuts to remove both the donor and the host eye corneas. Some trephines are equipped with transparent lenses to give the surgeon maximum levels of accuracy. When the two vital incisions are made, great care is taken to obtain a perfectly vertical cut.

Beginning with this initial stage, the surgeon may add a bubble of air through the incision to protect the endothelium and reduce the likelihood of an immune system reaction once the donor cornea has been transplanted. As the transfer occurs, another air bubble is introduced. After suturing, this bubble will be replaced by a balanced salt solution called acetylcholine.

This suturing, which must be very precise, almost always begins with four sutures at the cardinal points to ensure even tension. The last stage of the operation involves checking the wound for leakage of acetylcholine. This step is necessary not only to avoid infection but also to guard against rejection of the cornea by the host organ.

Uses and Complications

Significant differences in the healing process following corneal transplantation occur according to the method of suturing. A choice is made between a continuing or an interrupted series of sutures around the circumference of the cornea. Interrupted sutures may be preferred if there is a chance of uneven healing of the wound, something the physician may judge following examination of the degree of vascularization in particular corneal graft beds. In some cases, surgeons may opt for double suturing.

The chief complication that can follow corneal transplantation is rejection by the immune system. Surgeons try to obviate this risk by close study of the factors that can affect the receptivity of the eye to a new cornea. Earlier literature on corneal transplantation tended to assume that there was a lack of antigenicity-the production of disease-fighting antigens, or antibodies, as a defense system against viruses, bacteria, or foreign tissues-in the cornea. As ophthalmologists developed a fuller understanding of the immunological role of blood vessels and the lymphatic system, however, the need to give considerable attention to the degree of vascularization of the graft bed zone became more obvious. One method that surgeons can use to reduce antigen activity and enhance host acceptance is part of the transplantation operation itself: constant maintenance of a liquid layer between the host tissue and the new cornea tissue being transplanted. In the late 1990s, researchers at the University of Texas Southwestern Medical Center at Dallas announced the creation of an oral vaccine that may prevent rejection. Processed corneal cells in liquid form fed to laboratory mice produced a marked reduction in rejection rates. Current studies focus on the success of the vaccine with humans.

Although the period for healing and suture removal varies from patient to patient, the surgeon looks for the normal development of a gray-tinged scar tissue in the incision area as a sign of success. Failure, if discovered in time, may lead to a second transplantation attempt.

Perspective and Prospects

The first attempts to perform corneal transplantation-all unsuccessful-date from the nineteenth century. In the 1820s, German doctor F. Reisinger experimented with corneal grafts using rabbits and chickens. In the 1830s, Samuel Bigger of Ireland and R. S. Kissam of the United States tried to pioneer surgical grafts on humans, but both made the error of trying to replace human corneas with animal corneas. Success with living tissue (as opposed to the application of a glass product) finally came in 1905 when Moravian doctor Edward Zirm transplanted a child donor's cornea to the eye of a chemical burn victim. Zirm's success was based on cumulative medical knowledge of antiseptics, anesthesia, and technical aids such as the ophthalmoscope and the trephine. After a long period without major changes, in 1935 a Russian scientist named Filatov experimented with two innovations that were copied in other countries: the use of egg membrane to enhance a firm fix and the insertion of a delicate spatula between the cornea and lens to protect the intraocular tissues.

The greatest advances were made soon after antibiotics and steroids were introduced in the 1940s. By the 1950s, the use of extremely delicate surgical needles helped reduce postsurgical rejection rates. Major contributions to the development of delicate surgical instruments were made by the Spanish ophthalmologist Ramón Castroviejo, who performed many operations in the United States. By the 1980s, Castroviejo was urging others to follow the example of Townley Paton, who founded New York's first eye bank some two decades earlier.

By the turn of the twenty-first century, forty thousand people in the United States had received corneal transplants using cells taken from the eyes of donors who had died. However, many patients with severe corneal damage cannot be helped by conventional cornea transplants. Two research teams, one in Taiwan, at the University of Taoyuan, and one at the University of California at Davis School of Medicine, used stem cells to continually produce new corneal cells within the eye. In Taiwan, stem cells were placed on amniotic membrane, taken from placentas, to grow the tissue. In California, cells were first grown in laboratory dishes and then placed on the amniotic membrane to produce the tissue, which was transplanted to the damaged corneas. The use of this kind of tissue showed improved or restored vision for patients with corneal damage. While these procedures hold great potential for worldwide application, they have been called "investigational" and by no means eliminate the need for cornea donors.

The prospects for increasingly higher success rates in the field of corneal transplantation are linked to technical progress in donor organ conservation and the level of precision that can be achieved in carrying out transplantation operations.

—*Byron D. Cannon, Ph.D.*

See also Eye infections and disorders; Eye surgery; Eyes; Grafts and grafting; Keratitis; Ophthalmology; Trachoma; Transplantation; Vision; Vision disorders.

For Further Information:

Brightbill, Frederick S., ed. *Corneal Surgery: Theory, Technique and Tissue*. 4th ed. St. Louis, Mo.: Mosby, 2009.

De la Rocha, Kelly. "Corneal Transplant." *Health Library*, February 28, 2012.

Foster, C. Stephen, Dimitri T. Azar, and Claes H. Dohlman, eds. *Smolin and Thoft's The Cornea: Scientific Foundations and Clinical Practice*. 4th ed. Philadelphia: Lippincott Williams & Wilkins, 2005.

Parker, James N., and Philip M. Parker, eds. *The Official Patient's Sourcebook on Corneal Transplant Surgery*. San Diego, Calif.: Icon Health, 2002.

Spaeth, George L., ed. *Ophthalmic Surgery: Principles and Practice*. 4th ed. Philadelphia: W. B. Saunders, 2012.

Sutton, Amy L., ed. *Eye Care Sourcebook: Basic Consumer Health Information About Eye Care and Eye Disorders*. 3d ed. Detroit, Mich.: Omnigraphics, 2008.

Vorvick, Linda J. "Corneal Transplant." *MedlinePlus*, September 3, 2012.

CORNELIA DE LANGE SYNDROME
Disease/Disorder

Also known as: Amsterdam dwarfism, Brachmann-de Lange syndrome

Anatomy or system affected: Arms, brain, ears, eyes, feet, hair, hands, head, heart, immune system, legs, mouth, nose, teeth

Specialties and related fields: Genetics, neurology, pediatrics, physical therapy

Definition: A disorder with distinctive physical abnormalities and mental retardation usually apparent at birth.

Causes and Symptoms

Cornelia de Lange syndrome occurs at an estimated rate of 1 per 10,000 to 30,000 live births. Sometimes siblings have this syndrome, reinforcing the hypothesis that it is hereditary. Although the precise causation is unknown, researchers are investigating the possibility that mutations in the NIPBL, SMC1A, and SMC3 genes cause Cornelia de Lange syndrome.

Patients with this syndrome are smaller in size and weight than average infants, and their growth and motor develop-

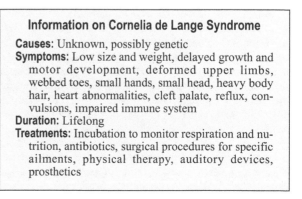

Information on Cornelia de Lange Syndrome

Causes: Unknown, possibly genetic

Symptoms: Low size and weight, delayed growth and motor development, deformed upper limbs, webbed toes, small hands, small head, heavy body hair, heart abnormalities, cleft palate, reflux, convulsions, impaired immune system

Duration: Lifelong

Treatments: Incubation to monitor respiration and nutrition, antibiotics, surgical procedures for specific ailments, physical therapy, auditory devices, prosthetics

ment are usually delayed. Upper limbs are often deformed, with missing tissues. Although legs attain average size and development appropriate to patients" age, sometimes toes are webbed. Hands tend to be small. Patients share similar facial characteristics. Heads are abnormally small with upturned nostrils and thin lips and eyebrows. Heavy body hair often grows.

Intellectual development is impeded, particularly affecting vocalization. Hearing and vision sometimes are affected. Patients often suffer heart abnormalities, cleft palate, reflux, and convulsions. They are vulnerable to infections because of impaired immune systems.

Prenatal ultrasounds can reveal if fetuses have physical deficiencies that might be associated with Cornelia de Lange syndrome. Physicians identify the syndrome by observing characteristics evident in infants and toddlers. Genetic professionals confirm diagnoses, especially in patients whose symptoms are less obvious.

Treatment and Therapy

Many newborns with Cornelia de Lange syndrome require incubation to monitor respiration and nutrition. Antibiotics and other medications, as well as surgical procedures, are administered to treat specific ailments affecting these individuals. Physical therapy, auditory devices, and prosthetics can aid children. Some patients have shortened life spans and are unable to live autonomously. Heart conditions cause most of the deaths associated with this syndrome.

Although no known cure or prevention exists, medical awareness and treatment of this syndrome can extend the life span and enhance the quality of life for many patients. Some patients with milder conditions survive to average life expectancies. Adults with this syndrome attain a height from four to five feet and undergo puberty at normal ages. Various therapies can assist patients who exhibit aggressive and self-destructive behaviors and improve communication and social skills.

Perspective and Prospects

In 1916, Winfried R. Brachmann became the first physician to document this syndrome's characteristics in an infant. Dutch pediatrician Cornelia C. de Lange clinically described two patients in 1933 and discussed her work at neurological conferences. By the early twenty-first century, researchers had established a Cornelia de Lange syndrome database to coordinate information. Geneticists, particularly Ian Krantz and his colleagues at the University of Pennsylvania's Department of Genetics, conducted molecular investigations to determine the genetic causation of this syndrome. A mutation in a gene known as NIPBL is now known to be one cause of this relatively rare disorder. This gene provides directions for the making of a protein, delangin, which is very important in developmental regulation of a number of body parts in the fetus.

—Elizabeth D. Schafer, Ph.D.;
updated by Lenela Glass-Godwin, M.W.S.

See also Birth defects; Congenital disorders; Dwarfism; Genetic diseases; Genetics and inheritance; Mental retardation.

For Further Information:
"About CdLS." *Cornelia de Lange Syndrome Foundation*, 2010.
Benson, M. "Cornelia de Lange Syndrome: A Case Study." *Neonatal Network* 21, no. 3 (April, 2002): 7-13.
Berg, J. M., et al. *The De Lange Syndrome*. New York: Pergamon Press, 1970.
Braunholz, Diana, et al. "Isolated NIBPL Missense Mutations That Cause Cornelia de Lange Syndrome Alter MAU2 Interaction." European Journal of Human Genetics 20, no. 3 (March, 2012): 271-276.
"Cornelia de Lange Syndrome." *Genetics Home Reference*, July 2012.
Gardner, R. J. M. "Another Explanation for Familial Cornelia de Lange Syndrome." *American Journal of Medical Genetics* 118A, no. 2 (April 15, 2003): 198.
Gilbert, Patricia. *Dictionary of Syndromes and Inherited Disorders*. 3d ed. Chicago: Fitzroy Dearborn, 2000.

CORNS AND CALLUSES
Disease/Disorder
Anatomy or system affected: Feet, hands, skin
Specialties and related fields: Dermatology, podiatry
Definition: Areas of thickened skin that form as a result of constant pressure or friction over a bony prominence.

Causes and Symptoms

Both corns (clavi) and calluses (tylomas or tyloses) occur when chronic pressure or friction causes hypertrophy of the dermal skin layer and a proliferation of keratin as a protective response. Both corns and calluses usually occur on the feet. Corns develop from pressure on normally thin skin. Calluses develop over areas where the skin is normally thicker. They commonly develop on the plantar (sole) surface of the foot and on the palmar (palm) surface of the hand. Corns are frequently painful, whereas calluses usually are not painful. Corns are small, flat, or slightly elevated lesions with a smooth, hard surface. Calluses cover a larger area than corns and are less well demarcated.

There are two classifications of corns: hard and soft. Hard corns have a conical structure composed of keratin, with the point of the cone directed inward, causing pain when pressed into the soft, underlying tissue. Hard corns have a circumscribed border that demarcates the lesions from the surrounding soft tissue. Hard corns usually develop on the top or sides of the toes, where shoes press on the interphalangeal joints of the toes, or the plantar surface of the foot, where pressure is exerted against bony prominences.

Soft corns develop in areas where a bony prominence causes constant pressure against soft tissue, resulting in a

---

Information on Corns and Calluses

Causes: Constant pressure or friction over bony prominence, often from improperly fitting shoes
Symptoms: Pain, inflammation, rough skin
Duration: Typically short-term, occasionally chronic
Treatments: Better-fitting footwear, over-the-counter medications, occasionally surgery

blanched thickening of the skin. Because soft corns commonly develop on interdigital surfaces, such as between the fourth and fifth toe, they are characteristically moist and macerated and can become inflamed.

Calluses develop as a protection against continual pressure. They do not have the central core of keratin and as a result are not sensitive to pressure. Normal skin markings are present over callused areas. Calluses usually develop on weight-bearing areas of the foot under the metatarsal heads and the heel. Calluses on the palm are frequently the result of manual occupations.

Treatment and Therapy

Treatment of corns and calluses depends on symptoms. Since corns and calluses are caused by chronic pressure, preventive measures include removing the source of friction or pressure. Well-fitting shoes that do not crowd the toes relieve pressure on interdigital areas. Soft, sufficiently wide or open-toed shoes are good choices. Soft insoles and properly fitting socks or stockings also reduce pressure. Wrapping lamb's wool or other padding over pressure points can increase air circulation and reduce pressure and discomfort. Corns and calluses can be treated with over-the-counter keratolytic agents. Salicylic acid plasters are used to soften the tissue, which can then be removed with a pumice stone. When corns, or occasionally calluses, become inflamed or painful, they can be removed by paring or trimming. This should be done by a health care provider, especially in patients with compromised circulation to the feet. In rare circumstances, surgery may be required if a corn or callus becomes infected or if the chronic pressure on particular areas is caused by a structural abnormality of the foot, such as a hammertoe, an abnormal bend in the toe joint.

—*Roberta Tierney, M.S.N., J.D., A.P.N.*

See also Bedsores; Bunions; Dermatology; Feet; Foot disorders; Hammertoe correction; Hammertoes; Hypertrophy; Podiatry; Skin; Skin disorders.

For Further Information:

Copeland, Glenn, and Stan Solomon. *The Foot Doctor: Lifetime Relief for Your Aching Feet*. Rev. ed. Toronto, Ont.: Macmillan Canada, 1996.
"Corns and Calluses." *American Orthopaedic Foot and Ankle Society*, 2012.
"Corns and Calluses." *Mayo Clinic*, April 5, 2011.
"Do You Abuse Your Feet?" *Harvard Medical School*, March 19, 2009.
Lippert, Frederick G., and Sigvard T. Hansen. *Foot and Ankle Disorders: Tricks of the Trade*. New York: Thieme, 2003.
Lorimer, Donald L., et al., eds. *Neale's Disorders of the Foot*. 7th ed. New York: Churchill Livingstone/Elsevier, 2006.
Mackie, Rona M. *Clinical Dermatology*. 5th ed. New York: Oxford University Press, 2003.

CORONARY ARTERY BYPASS GRAFT
Procedure

Anatomy or system affected: Circulatory system, heart
Specialties and related fields: Cardiac surgery, cardiology

Definition: A surgical procedure in which a healthy blood vessel is taken from another part of the body and grafted into a segment of a coronary artery in order to bypass a blockage.

Key terms:

angina: pain in the chest caused by insufficient blood flow to the heart muscle

angioplasty: surgical procedure to reduce blockages in a coronary artery that uses a catheter

atherosclerosis: a process in which plaque builds up on the walls of blood vessels

catheter: a flexible tube inserted into a small opening or incision in the body

heart-lung bypass machine: equipment that pumps and oxygenates the blood during heart surgery

ischemia: insufficient blood flow to a part of the body

plaque: fat deposits on the blood vessel walls

saphenous vein: a vein from the upper leg often used to bypass a blocked coronary artery

Indications and Procedures

Atherosclerosis is a disease in which fat deposits called plaque accumulate on the walls of arteries and restrict blood flow. Although plaque can form in any arteries in the body, the effect is most noticeable in the coronary arteries, which supply blood to the heart muscle. Since the heart must pump continuously, it needs a steady supply of oxygenated blood. When the plaque in a coronary artery gets too thick, an area of the heart muscle will not receive enough blood, resulting in a condition called ischemia. The result is often chest pain called angina. Patients with angina are high risk for having a heart attack.

To alleviate angina and restore sufficient blood flow to the heart muscle, coronary artery bypass graft surgery may be performed. The patient is given general anesthesia for the procedure. The breastbone or sternum is sawed in two, and the chest is opened to expose the heart. At the same time, an assistant removes a healthy vein from an arm or leg. Most commonly, the saphenous vein from the upper leg is used. The heart is stopped and the patient is put on a heart-lung bypass machine that pumps the blood during the surgery. While the heart is stopped, the surgeon cuts the coronary artery above the blockage, and the healthy vessel which was removed from another part of the body is attached. Then the coronary artery is cut below the blockage and the other end of the healthy vessel is attached. This procedure effectively reroutes the blood flow through the grafted vessel and around the blockage, thereby giving it the name bypass graft. Because the normal blood flow is restored, the angina is alleviated and the risk of heart attack is decreased. Another approach is to use the internal mammary artery, which is already attached to the aorta, for a blood source. Only one incision below the blockage needs to be made to establish good blood flow. After the bypass is completed, the heart is restarted and the machine is removed. The sternum is wired together and the incision is sutured.

Uses and Complications

Coronary artery bypass surgery is used to restore sufficient blood flow through a coronary artery that is narrowed or blocked with plaque. In patients with coronary artery disease it is common to have more than one artery narrowed or blocked. In this case, multiple bypasses may be completed in one surgery. Double, triple, and quadruple bypass surgeries are common. In these cases, the grafting procedure is repeated as many times as necessary to bypass all narrowed or blocked arteries.

One major problem for postoperative cardiac patients who have had bypass surgery is the threat of additional blockages developing. Sometimes patients need to have additional bypass surgeries several years later to bypass new blockages that have developed. Therefore, after surgery most patients will be referred to a cardiac rehabilitation program, or cardiac rehab. In cardiac rehab, patients learn to exercise safely, eat right, and manage stress better. By making lifestyle changes patients can delay or prevent the development of additional plaque obstructions.

Perspective and Prospects

Bypass graft surgery is one way to restore blood flow through a blocked coronary artery. It has been widely used since the 1970s and has been safe and effective. However, it is a major surgical procedure that causes great discomfort to the patient. With advances in technology that are less invasive, such as cardiac catheters, other options are now available.

A procedure that competes with coronary artery bypass surgery is angioplasty. Instead of a major incision through the chest, angioplasty uses a catheter inserted through a small incision in an arm or the groin. The catheter is run through the blood vessels and into the heart. When the catheter reaches the narrowed area, the surgeon inflates a small balloon that compresses the plaque against the wall of the artery. Like bypass surgery, this procedure also improves blood flow to the heart muscle. Unfortunately, not all patients are good candidates for angioplasty and the more invasive bypass surgery must be used. As technology continues to improve, however, more patients will be able to have angioplasty.

—*Bradley R. A. Wilson, Ph.D.*

See also Angina; Angioplasty; Arteriosclerosis; Bypass surgery; Cardiac surgery; Cardiology; Cardiology, pediatric; Circulation; Heart; Heart disease; Heart valve replacement; Vascular medicine; Vascular system.

For Further Information:

Chizner, Michael A. *Clinical Cardiology Made Ridiculously Simple.* 4th ed. Miami: MedMaster, 2012.

Health Library. "Coronary Artery Bypass Grafting." *Health Library,* September 26, 2012.

MedlinePlus. "Coronary Artery Bypass Surgery." *MedlinePlus,* June 10, 2013.

NIH National Heart, Lung, and Blood Institute. "What Is Coronary Artery Bypass Grafting?" *NIH National Heart, Lung, and Blood Institute,* February 23, 2012.

Rippe, James. *Heart Disease for Dummies.* Hoboken, N.J.: Wiley, 2004.

Sheridan, Brett C., et al. *So You're Having Heart Bypass Surgery.* Hoboken, N.J.: John Wiley & Sons, 2003.

CORONAVIRUSES

Disease/Disorder

Anatomy or system affected: Immune system, lungs, lymphatic system, respiratory system

Specialties and related fields: Environmental health, epidemiology, immunology, public health, pulmonary medicine, virology

Definition: Viruses frequently infecting the upper respiratory system and capable of producing either the common cold or severe acute respiratory syndrome (SARS).

Key terms:

common cold: an acute respiratory tract infection including stuffy or running nose, sore throat, sneezing, fever, wheezing, and nasal pressure headache

epidemiology: the study of epidemic disease; that which determines the onset, distribution, and course of disease within populations

rhinoviruses: spherical, non-enveloped, positive single-strand RNA viruses with a diameter of about thirty nanometers and the most common viral agent infecting humans; infection results in upper respiratory distress

severe acute respiratory syndrome (SARS): a deadly, novel coronavirus disease originating in China in 2002 that became a global epidemic in 2003

virion: a single virus particle

Causes and Symptoms

Coronaviruses are spherical, enveloped virion particles sixty to two hundred nanometers in diameter with twenty-nanometer-long surface projections resembling ball-topped points of a crown. They are positive-strand ribonucleic acid (RNA) viruses with nonsegmented genomes containing roughly thirty thousand nucleotides. Coronaviruses are widespread in the environment and exist in a large range of hosts, including humans, dogs, cats, mice, cattle, swine, turkeys, and chickens, and may also be present in rats and rabbits.

The dominant mode of coronavirus transmission is uncertain. Coronaviruses are usually transmitted through contact with infected carrier animals who act as vectors for the virus without becoming ill themselves or contact with surfaces or body fluids contaminated with the virus. Depending on environmental conditions, the virus can survive minutes to hours on exposed surfaces or within discharged fluids.

Information on Coronaviruses

Causes: Usually contact with infected carrier animals or with surfaces or body fluids

Symptoms: High fever, headache, nasal discharge, cough, sore throat, general lethargy, diarrhea, breathing difficulties; in severe cases, collapsed lungs, massively reduced white blood cell count, depleted platelet reserves, blood cells leaking into glands and major organs, dead tissue in glands and major organs

Duration: Two to eighteen days

Treatments: Fever-reducing drugs, extra oxygen, ventilator support (if needed), some antiviral drugs

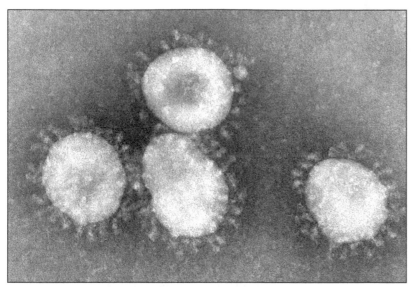

Coronavirus virions seen with an electron microscope. (CDC/Dr. Fred Murphy)

Human coronaviruses were first identified in 1965, and continuing epidemiological research suggests coronaviruses are prime agents of respiratory illness in humans, though the viruses can infect nerve cells and immune system cells as well. Coronaviruses are second only to rhinoviruses as causes of upper respiratory illnesses collectively known as the common cold; coronaviruses are likely responsible for 10 to 15 percent of such infections in adults. Most people have endured at least one bout of coronavirus infection before reaching adulthood. Coronaviruses may also result in severe secondary infections of the lower respiratory system if the patient has an existing health condition such as asthma.

The first identified case of SARS can be traced back to November 16, 2002, in Foshan, China. The patient was diagnosed with pneumonia and sent home to recover. Soon a large number of people in the area became ill with the same symptoms of respiratory distress. Chinese authorities took no action to contain the disease. By February 2003, the disease had spread to Hong Kong, and guests at the Metropole Hotel began to fall ill. Many international guests of the hotel, showing no symptoms, boarded planes and traveled home only to become symptomatic after arriving at their destinations. As more and more people in Hong Kong, and then in distant locations, became severely ill, an intense effort was mounted to find the cause: a coronavirus.

The coronavirus responsible for SARS was traced back to specific locations in China where wild mammals were being sold in meat markets as exotic food. While the carrier animals were immune to the virus, a mutation in the virus's genes allowed it to infect humans and then spread from person to person. The global spread of SARS was precipitated by air travel from China, initiating outbreaks in a number of countries in a matter of days. Once the source of the outbreak was identified and scientists discovered the infection was caused by a coronavirus, efforts to stop the spread of SARS were initiated worldwide. The World Health Organization (WHO) and the US Centers for Disease Control and Prevention issued global alerts. Airports and rail stations in many countries set up infrared scanners to detect travelers with fevers and quarantine them until they were screened for the virus. In some cities with identified cases of SARS, entire blocks, districts, and buildings were quarantined; sporting events, school attendance, international conferences, and religious services were canceled. Within four months of its outbreak, SARS had spread to twenty-four nations on four continents.

Eventually, the SARS epidemic was suppressed by breaking the chain of human transmission with quarantines. Globally, more than eight thousand individuals were diagnosed with

In humans, two to ten days after exposure, symptoms appear, including fever with high temperature, headache, nasal discharge, cough and sore throat, general lethargy, diarrhea, and breathing difficulties. In severe cases, patients may experience collapsed lungs, massively reduced white blood cell count, depleted platelet reserves, blood cells leaking into glands and major organs, and dead tissue in glands and major organs. In animals, symptoms of coronavirus infection include stresses to digestive, respiratory, reproductive, renal, and central nervous systems.

Treatment and Therapy

It is not possible to distinguish coronavirus infections from rhinovirus infections based on symptoms alone. Diagnosis of a coronavirus infection requires laboratory tests, which may include organ or cell cultures, electron microscopy, immunofluorescence, nucleic acid hybridization, reverse transcription-polymerase chain reaction, and serology, the most effective method being an enzyme-linked immunoassay. Though there is presently no direct line of evidence linking back to respiratory infection, coronaviruses are tenuously implicated in a number of nonrespiratory diseases, including highly infectious mononucleosis, pancreatitis, thyroiditis, nephropathy, pericarditis, and multiple sclerosis.

Besides the common cold, the most notable coronavirus infection is associated with highly contagious severe acute respiratory syndrome (SARS), which produces an atypical pneumonia and a resulting high death rate.

Coronaviruses have an incubation period of two days to two weeks. There are two to eighteen days of active infection, and reinfections are common.

Treatment consists of fever-reducing drugs, extra oxygen, ventilator support if needed, and some antiviral drugs.

SARS, and there were more than seven hundred deaths. There is no effective treatment for SARS beyond supporting the patient toward recovery. Although the international medical community was able to contain the disease in the human population, it is unknown whether the virus remains active in animals.

In 2012, researchers identified a new coronavirus capable of causing severe respiratory illness in those infected. By May 2013, the WHO had confirmed about forty cases of the virus, more than half in Saudi Arabia.

—*Randall L. Milstein, Ph.D.*

See also Common cold; Environmental diseases; Environmental health; Epidemiology; Microbiology; Pneumonia; Pulmonary diseases; Pulmonary medicine; Severe acute respiratory syndrome (SARS); Viral infections; Zoonoses.

For Further Information:

Global Alert and Response. "Coronavirus Infections." *World Health Organization*, May 14, 2013.

Kleinman, A., and J. Watson, eds. *SARS in China: Prelude to Pandemic?* Stanford, Calif.: Stanford University Press, 2006.

National Center for Immunization and Respiratory Diseases, Division of Viral Diseases. "Coronavirus." *Centers for Disease Control and Prevention*, March 12, 2013.

National Center for Immunization and Respiratory Diseases, Division of Viral Diseases. "Novel Coronavirus." *Centers for Disease Control and Prevention*, May 14, 2013.

National Institute of Allergy and Infectious Diseases. "Common Cold." *National Institutes of Health*, May 20, 2011.

Peiris, M., et al., eds. *Severe Acute Respiratory Syndrome*. Malden, Mass.: Blackwell, 2005.

Schmidt, A., M. H. Wolff, and O. Weber, eds. *Coronaviruses with Special Emphasis on First Insights Concerning SARS*. Boston: Birkhäuser, 2005.

Siddell, Stuart G., ed. *The Coronaviridae*. New York: Plenum Press, 1995.

CORTICOSTEROIDS

Biology

Also known as: Glucocorticoids, mineralocorticoids

Anatomy or system affected: Endocrine system, immune system

Specialties and related fields: Biochemistry, endocrinology, family medicine, immunology

Definition: Steroid hormones such as cortisol and aldosterone synthesized and secreted by the adrenal cortex, or their synthetic equivalents.

Key terms:

Addison's disease: a disease characterized by hypoadrenalism caused by cortisol deficiency

cortisol: a steroid hormone of the adrenal cortex that has many physiological actions

Cushing's syndrome: a disease characterized by hyperadrenalism caused by an excess secretion or exogenous administration of cortisol

glucocorticoid: a steroid hormone such as cortisol from the adrenal cortex that has many physiological actions, including the regulation of glucose metabolism

mineralocorticoid: a steroid hormone from the adrenal cortex that regulates salt and water balance

Structure and Functions

Corticosteroids are steroid hormones produced by the cortex of the adrenal glands. They have several physiological actions, including regulation of glucose, lipid and protein metabolism, regulation of inflammation and the immune response, maintenance of homeostasis during stress, and control of water and electrolyte balance and blood pressure.

Corticosteroids that have their primary effects on glucose metabolism are glucocorticoids, whereas those that have the control of electrolyte and water balance as their main functions are mineralocorticoids. Cortisol is the primary glucocorticoid, although significant amounts of corticosterone and cortisone are secreted. Aldosterone is the primary mineralocorticoid.

Glucocorticoids promote an increase in blood glucose by stimulating the synthesis of glucose (gluconeogenesis). They also stimulate the catabolism of lipids and proteins. Thus, glucocorticoids increase blood glucose and are antagonistic to insulin.

The synthesis of corticosteroids is controlled by adrenocorticotropic hormone (ACTH) produced by the pituitary gland. Corticotropin-releasing hormone (CRH) produced by the hypothalamus controls the secretion of ACTH. A feedback loop exists so that when cortisol levels are high, the release of CRH and ACTH is inhibited, and when cortisol levels are low, CRH and ACTH are released.

Aldosterone is primarily responsible for the control of salt and water balance by promoting the excretion of potassium and the retention of sodium and water. Through its effect on salt and water balance, aldosterone can increase blood pressure. Plasma levels of aldosterone are controlled by a variety of mechanisms, including plasma volume and potassium ion concentration.

Disorders and Diseases

Addison's disease results from adrenal insufficiency (hypocortisolism). Although most cases are caused by a disorder of the adrenal glands (primary adrenal insufficiency), some cases are caused by a disorder of the pituitary gland (secondary adrenal insufficiency). An autoimmune disorder that destroys the adrenal cortex is the major cause of primary adrenal insufficiency. Secondary adrenal insufficiency is usually caused by a lack of ACTH. Pituitary tumors, surgical removal of the pituitary, and loss of blood flow to the pituitary are the major causes of secondary adrenal insufficiency. Major symptoms of adrenal insufficiency include loss of appetite, weight loss, fatigue, muscle weakness, and hypotension. Addison's disease can be diagnosed by administering ACTH and monitoring the adrenal gland's response by measuring serum and urine cortisol levels. Adrenal insufficiency is treated by oral administration of hydrocortisone, a synthetic form of cortisol. If aldosterone is also deficient, then fludrocortisone is administered.

Adrenal insufficiency is often caused by a mutation in one of the enzymes synthesizing cortisol. These cases are referred to as congenital adrenal hyperplasia (CAH). Since serum cortisol is low or absent, the pituitary gland stimulates the adrenal gland to produce more cortisol. The precursor steroids and their metabolic products that accumulate can cause varying degrees of virilization of female fetuses and infants. Replacement therapy is the treatment of choice. Surgery to reconstruct the genital organs may be necessary in severe cases.

Hypercortisolism can lead to Cushing's syndrome. Major symptoms include obesity, osteoporosis, fatigue, hypertension, hyperglycemia, and amenorrhea (absence of menstruation). Cushing's syndrome may be caused by prolonged use of glucocorticoids or by an overproduction of glucocorticoids by the adrenal glands. The major causes of an overproduction of glucocorticoids are pituitary and adrenal tumors. Diagnosis of Cushing's syndrome is most commonly made by determining the amount of cortisol in the urine. Cushing's syndrome can be treated by reducing administered glucocorticoids or by treatment of the tumor causing the disease through surgical removal, radiation, and/or chemotherapy.

Hypoaldosteronism is a condition in which the adrenal cortex does not produce an adequate amount of aldosterone, which results in an inability to control and regulate blood volume and blood pressure. Blood pressure can fall to dangerously low levels.

Synthetic corticosteroids such as prednisone, prednisolone, methylprednisolone, hydrocortisone, and dexamethasone have an immunosuppressive effect and are used to treat a variety of chronic autoimmune and inflammatory diseases. They can reduce the pain, swelling, itching, inflammation, and redness associated with arthritis, bursitis, asthma, dermatitis, eczema and psoriasis, lupus erythematosus, Crohn's disease, and various ear, eye, and skin infections and allergic reactions.

Prolonged use of corticosteroids can lead to medically induced Cushing's syndrome, suppression of the immune system, hypertension, hypokalemia (low serum potassium), and hypernatremia (high serum sodium).

Perspective and Prospects

In 1855, Thomas Addison became the first physician to describe the clinical symptoms of adrenal insufficiency. In the early 1930s, Frank Hartman, Wilbur Swingle, and Joseph Pfiffner were the first to prepare active adrenal extracts capable of treating the symptoms of adrenal insufficiency. By the mid-1930s, Pfiffner, Edward Calvin Kendall, Oskar Wintersteiner, and Tadeus Reichstein had isolated and crystallized some of the adrenal hormones. In 1944, Lewis Sarett became the first to synthesize cortisone. In the late 1940s, Philip Showalter Hench discovered that the administration of cortisone could alleviate the symptoms of arthritis.

In recent years, it has been shown that corticosteroids express their effect by modulating the expression of a variety of genes involved in many physiological functions, including metabolism and the immune or inflammatory response.

—*Charles L. Vigue, Ph.D.*

See also Addison's disease; Adrenal glands; Adrenalectomy; Cushing's syndrome; Endocrine disorders; Endocrine glands; Endocrinology; Endocrinology, pediatric; Glands; Hormones; Kidneys; Osteonecrosis; Steroids.

For Further Information:

"Corticosteroids." *NHS*, April 18, 2013.

Griffin, James E., and Sergio R. Ojeda, eds. *Textbook of Endocrine Physiology*. 5th ed. New York: Oxford University Press, 2004.

Lüdecke, Dieter K., George P. Chrousos, and George Tolis, eds. *ACTH, Cushing's Syndrome, and Other Hypercortisolemic States*. New York: Raven Press, 1990.

Riedemann, Therese, Alexandre Patchev, Kwangook Cho, and Osborne F. X. Almeida. "Corticosteroids." *Molecular Brain* 3 (2010): 2-21.

Vaughan, Darracott E., and Robert M. Carey. *Adrenal Disorders*. New York: Thieme Medical, 1989.

Vinson, Gavin P., Barbara Whitehouse, and Joy Hinson. *The Adrenal Cortex*. Englewood Cliffs, N.J.: Prentice Hall, 1992.

"What Are Corticosteroids?" *healthychildren.org*, May 11, 2013.

COSMETIC SURGERY. *See* PLASTIC SURGERY.

COUGHING
Disease/Disorder

Anatomy or system affected: Chest, immune system, lungs, respiratory system

Specialties and related fields: Family medicine, internal medicine, pulmonary medicine

Definition: A physiological act in which air is forcibly expelled from the lungs.

Causes and Symptoms

The energy that is consumed during the breathing process is used to stretch the chest cavity and allow air to flow into the lungs. This amounts to about 1 percent of the basic energy requirements of the body but increases considerably during periods of exercise or respiratory system illness.

When the respiratory tract is invaded by irritants (such as smoke, perfume, and pollen) or there is an excessive accumulation of secretions in the lungs, coughing takes place. It arises via a reflex mechanism that starts with the stimulation of the nerves that supply the larynx, trachea (windpipe), and bronchial tubes. The pressure within the chest cavity is increased by the action of chest muscles and the diaphragm. The glottis, the opening of the windpipe at the back of the mouth, remains closed in order to allow the pressure to rise. Within a few seconds, the glottis opens again and a rapid, noisy release of air is allowed through the bronchial tubes and the windpipe. Any foreign substance is expelled through the mouth.

Treatment and Therapy

Coughing is an important symptom of diseases that affect any

Information on Coughing

Causes: Various diseases, allergens, lung infection, environmental factors

Symptoms: Breathlessness, chest and lung pain

Duration: Ranges from short-term to chronic

Treatments: Antibiotics, anti-inflammatory drugs

part of the respiratory system, such as the nasal cavities, the pharynx (throat), the larynx, the trachea, the bronchi, and lung tissue. By coughing, foreign matter called sputum, which is chiefly composed of mucus, that has accumulated in the respiratory system is expectorated. Sputum formation during coughing is an important evidence of a disease, such as bronchitis. In this case, the lining of the bronchi enlarges dramatically and sputum production may increase to 60 milliliters per day. An irritative cough without sputum may be due to the extension of the disease to the bronchial tube and eventually to nearby organs. The use of antibiotics and anti-inflammatory agents to reduce the discomfort is part of the standard treatment.

The presence of blood in the sputum (called hemoptysis) is important and should alert patients or their caregivers to call a doctor. This symptom often arises from an existing infection, inflammation, or tumor. It is also a sign of tuberculosis. In this case, extensive and reliable tests will identify the real cause of the bleeding.

Polluted air increases the possibility of chronic bronchitis. Common air pollutants include vehicle exhaust, chemical fumes, smoke, smog, molds, and pollen. They are all responsible for a decrease in arterial oxygen and an increase in carbon dioxide tension in the lungs. The use of air-conditioning, air filters, and inhalers and an increased-oxygen environment can provide relief for people with respiratory problems.

—*Soraya Ghayourmanesh, Ph.D.*

See also Allergies; Asbestos exposure; Aspergillosis; Avian influenza; Bronchi; Bronchitis; Choking; Common cold; Croup; Cystic fibrosis; Diphtheria; Immune system; Influenza; Laryngitis; Lung cancer; Lungs; Otorhinolaryngology; Over-the-counter medications; Pneumonia; Pulmonary diseases; Pulmonary medicine; Pulmonary medicine, pediatric; Respiration; Sore throat; Tuberculosis; Wheezing; Whooping cough.

For Further Information:

Adelman, Daniel C., et al., eds. *Manual of Allergy and Immunology.* 5th ed. Philadelphia: Lippincott Williams & Wilkins, 2012.

Braga, Pier Carlo, and Luigi Allegra, eds. *Cough.* New York: Raven Press, 1989.

Chung, Kian Fan, John G. Widdicombe, and Homer A. Boushey, eds. *Cough: Causes, Mechanisms, and Therapy.* Malden, Mass.: Blackwell, 2008.

"Cough." *Mayo Clinic*, May 24, 2013.

Glenn, Jim. *Colds and Coughs.* Springhouse, Pa.: Springhouse, 1986.

"How Is Cough Treated?" *National Heart, Lung, and Blood Institute*, October 1, 2010.

Kimball, Chad T. *Colds, Flu, and Other Common Ailments Sourcebook.* Detroit, Mich.: Omnigraphics, 2001.

Korpás, Juraj, and Z. Tomori. *Cough and Other Respiratory Reflexes.* New York: S. Karger, 1979.

"What Is Cough?" *National Heart, Lung, and Blood Institute*, October 1, 2010.

Woolf, Alan D., et al., eds. *The Children's Hospital Guide to Your Child's Health and Development.* Cambridge, Mass.: Perseus, 2002.

CRANIOSYNOSTOSIS
Disease/Disorder
Anatomy or system affected: Bones, head
Specialties and related fields: Orthopedics, plastic surgery
Definition: The premature closing of the open areas between the bones in an infant's skull.

Causes and Symptoms

Craniosynostosis is a craniofacial abnormality that occurs in a variety of forms. The skull of a newborn infant contains several open areas between the bones that make up the skull. These areas, called fontanelles, allow the skull to expand as the child's brain grows. Craniosynostosis is the premature closure of one or more of these open areas, resulting in the abnormal shaping of the head and face. Craniosynostosis may occur alone or in association with other defects.

Treatment and Therapy

During the 1960s the French surgeon Paul Tessier developed improved techniques for treating craniosynostosis. Treatment of craniosynostosis is often done with a surgical procedure known as fronto-orbital advancement. This technique involves cutting the skull in such a way that the frontal bone (the portion of the skull behind the forehead) and the supraorbital rim (the portion of the skull above and to the sides of the eyes) can be moved forward. These portions of the skull are then attached to the rest of the skull in their new positions with surgical wire. For some types of craniosynostosis, it may also be necessary to cut the frontal bone and the supraorbital rim down the middle to allow them to be reshaped. Fronto-orbital advancement usually takes place after the patient is three months old.

Correction of craniosynostosis is a complicated procedure, requiring the patient to be monitored in a special hospital bed for at least four or five days after surgery. After the surgery, the patient will experience severe swelling of the eyelids and scalp. Most patients will be unable to open their eyes until several days after surgery, and the swelling may not completely disappear for a few months. Care must be taken to keep the incision clean.

Information on Craniosynostosis

Causes: Birth defect
Symptoms: Abnormal head and face shape
Duration: Typically correctable, with side effects of surgery lasting several months
Treatments: Fronto-orbital advancement

In some cases, craniosynostosis can be treated through a less invasive surgery in which a surgeon uses very small tools to remove bone from the skull through small incisions in the child's scalp. This surgery is usually performed on patients younger than six months. The recovery period is typically shorter than that of the more invasive surgery, although the patient must usually wear protective headgear for a time.

—*Rose Secrest*

See also Birth defects; Bone disorders; Bones and the skeleton; Growth; Surgery, pediatric.

For Further Information:
A.D.A.M. Medical Encyclopedia. "Craniosynostosis." *MedlinePlus*, November 7, 2011.

A.D.A.M. Medical Encyclopedia. "Craniosynostosis Repair." *MedlinePlus*, November 2, 2012.

Cohen, M. Michael, Jr., and Ruth E. MacLean, eds. *Craniosynostosis: Diagnosis, Evaluation, and Management.* 2d ed. New York: Oxford University Press, 2000.

Galli, Guido, ed. *Craniosynostosis.* Boca Raton, Fla.: CRC Press, 1984.

Hayward, Richard, et al., eds. *The Clinical Management of Craniosynostosis.* New York: Cambridge University Press, 2004.

Mayo Foundation for Medical Education and Research. "Craniosynostosis." *Mayo Clinic*, September 29, 2011.

McCarthy, Joseph G., ed. *Distraction of the Craniofacial Skeleton.* New York: Springer, 1999.

Moore, Keith L., and T. V. N. Persaud. *The Developing Human.* 8th ed. Philadelphia: Saunders/Elsevier, 2008.

Sadler, T. W. *Langman's Medical Embryology.* 11th ed. Philadelphia: Lippincott Williams & Wilkins, 2009.

Turvey, Timothy A., Raymond J. Fonseca, and Katherine W. Vig, eds. *Facial Clefts and Craniosynostosis: Principles and Management.* Philadelphia: W. B. Saunders, 1996.

CRANIOTOMY
Procedure

Anatomy or system affected: Brain, head

Specialties and related fields: Critical care, neurology

Definition: A means of exposing or gaining access to the brain and cranial nerves so that intracranial disease can be treated surgically.

Indications and Procedures

Problems requiring craniotomy include tumors, abscesses, hematomas, and vascular lesions. The cranium may also be opened to excise an area of cortex or to disrupt various nerves and fiber tracts for the relief of pain, seizures, tremors, or spasms that do not respond to pharmacologic therapy. Skull fractures and other traumatic head wounds may be repaired by opening the cranium. Bony defects, dural tearing, bleeding, and removal of penetrating objects are also treated with this procedure. In case of a neoplasm (tumor), the goal of surgery is to remove the pathology completely while preserving the normal neural and vascular structures.

In craniotomy, the skin is cut to the skull bone. Small bleeding arteries are sealed with electric current, and the skin is pulled back. Three burr holes are drilled into the skull, and a fine-wire Gigli's saw is used to connect the holes. The skull piece is hinged open, and the dura mater, a tough membrane covering the brain, is dissected away. After the required procedure on the brain is completed, the dura mater is stitched together, the bone flap is replaced and secured with soft wire, and the scalp incision is closed.

An intracranial operation can be considered a planned head injury, and the complications are similar. Postoperatively, the degree of impairment depends on the extent of damage to neural tissue caused both by the neurological disorder and by surgical manipulation. Damage may be transient or permanent.

Uses and Complications

With craniotomy, complications include cerebral edema (swelling), which is a normal reaction to the manipulation

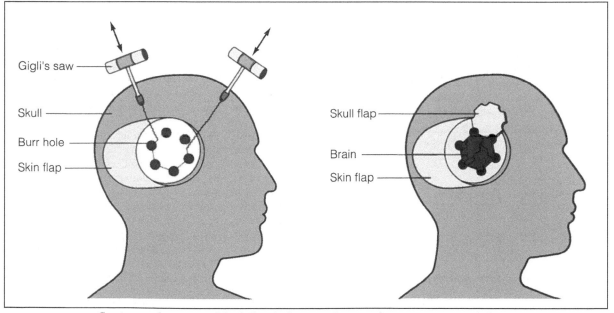

Craniotomy, the opening of the skull, is the first step taken to perform neurosurgery on the brain.

and retraction of brain tissue. Periorbital edema and ecchymosis (bleeding under the skin) usually follow frontal and temporal surgery. Focal motor deficits result from cerebral edema and are transitory. Permanent focal motor deficits may occur and are a direct and predictable consequence of the surgical procedure or the result of a complication such as stroke. Hematomas are the most devastating and dreaded complication. The clots may be extradural, intradural, or both and usually are caused by a single bleeding vessel rather than a generalized bleed.

Pain and discomfort are expected following cranial surgery, with headache being most common. Pain control may be accomplished with mild analgesics. Fever may occur following operations in the region of the upper brain stem and hypothalamus, and it requires vigorous treatment. Infection may occur, with the risk being greater following open head trauma and if a cerebrospinal fluid leak is present. Postoperative seizure risk is related to the underlying pathological condition and the degree of damage caused by surgery. Diabetes insipidus and the syndrome of inappropriate antidiuretic hormone (SIADH) secretion are also possible complications of craniotomy. These endocrine disorders may be transient or permanent. If unchecked, either may be life-threatening because of the severity of the fluid and electrolyte imbalance precipitated.

A cerebrospinal fluid leak may occur immediately following surgery but usually appears later in the postoperative course. Fluid seeps from the wound edges. Discharge from the nose (rhinorrhea) or ears (otorrhea) of cerebrospinal fluid is frequent with basal skull fractures, but these conditions may also occur following surgery in the frontal sinus or mastoid cavity. Anosmia (loss of sense of smell) frequently occurs following head injury or frontal craniotomy. Visual loss may be caused by damage to the optic nerve, resulting in blindness and lack of response to direct light. Hydrocephalus may develop as a result of postoperative adhesions secondary to blood sealing the subarachnoid space. Postoperative meningitis, abscess formation, and osteomyelitis of the bone flap occur as complications of a break in sterility or the introduction of organisms as a result of a contaminated open wound.

—*Jane C. Norman, Ph.D., R.N., C.N.E.*

See also Bones and the skeleton; Brain; Brain disorders; Hydrocephalus; Neuroimaging; Neurology; Neurology, pediatric; Neurosurgery.

For Further Information:

Aminoff, Michael J., David A. Greenberg, and Roger P. Simon. *Clinical Neurology*. 8th ed. New York: McGraw-Hill Medical, 2012.

Bakay, Louis. *An Early History of Craniotomy: From Antiquity to the Napoleonic Era*. Springfield, Ill.: Charles C Thomas, 1985.

Jasmin, Luc. "Brain Surgery." *MedlinePlus*, February 9, 2011.

Kellicker, Patricia Griffin. "Craniotomy." *Health Library*, February 6, 2013.

Rowland, Lewis P., ed. *Merritt's Textbook of Neurology*. 12th ed. Philadelphia: Lippincott Williams & Wilkins, 2010.

Samuels, Martin A., ed. *Manual of Neurologic Therapeutics*. 7th ed. New York: Lippincott Williams & Wilkins, 2004.

CRETINISM. *See* CONGENITAL HYPOTHYROIDISM.

CREUTZFELDT-JAKOB DISEASE (CJD)
Disease/Disorder

Anatomy or system affected: Brain, nervous system

Specialties and related fields: Environmental health, epidemiology, microbiology, neurology, public health, virology

Definition: Creutzfeldt-Jakob disease (CJD) is a human central nervous system disorder that is characterized by distinctive lesions in the brain, progressive dementia, lack of coordination, and eventual death. Although uncommon, it is the most prevalent of the human spongiform encephalopathies, inherited or transmissible illnesses of uncertain etiology associated with proteinaceous molecules called prions. Mad cow disease is a spongiform encephalopathy that affects cattle but may be transmissible to humans, leading to a new variant of CJD. It is important to note, however, that the new form variant of CJD is different from classic CJD.

Key terms:

dementia: an organic mental disorder characterized by personality disintegration, confusion, disorientation, stupor, deterioration of intellectual function, and impairment of memory and judgment

encephalopathy: any abnormality in the structure or function of the brain

knockout mouse: a mouse in which a specific gene has been inactivated or "knocked out"

myoclonus: involuntary twitching or spasm of muscle

spongiform: shaped like or resembling a sponge

Causes and Symptoms

Spongiform encephalopathies are inherited or transmissible neurological diseases that are associated with abnormalities in proteinaceous molecules called prions, which can aggregate, leading to spongelike lesions in the brain and causing disruptions in brain function. Prions are found in all species from yeast to humans, but their normal role is not known. Their evolutionary persistence in so many species implies an important purpose, although knockout mice lacking prions do not appear to be deleteriously affected.

Inherited spongiform encephalopathies are primarily attributed to mutations in the prion gene, producing abnormal prions that adopt an unusual conformation and clump together over time to cause the brain pathology and neurological symptoms characteristic of this type of disease. The diseases can be transmitted to a susceptible animal by inserting a fragment or extract from diseased tissue into the brain or blood or, much less efficiently, by oral ingestion. The infectious agent seems to be the abnormal prion itself, which apparently recruits normal prions in the brain to adopt the abnormal conformation, leading to their aggregation and the disruption of brain function. This is an unorthodox etiology, in that the infectious agent appears to be devoid of nucleic acid (RNA or DNA); its mode of action is not fully understood, nor is this etiology universally accepted.

> **Information on Creutzfeldt-Jakob Disease (CJD)**
>
> **Causes:** Prion disease; can be acquired through ingestion of infected cow tissue
> **Symptoms:** Dementia, lack of coordination, personality change
> **Duration:** Weeks to months; death typically occurs within one year
> **Treatments:** None

Creutzfeldt-Jakob disease (CJD), known since the 1920s, is the major spongiform encephalopathy in humans, although it occurs in only one per million persons worldwide. It has different forms, namely sporadic, inherited, infectious, and, recently, new variant.

The sporadic form has no known basis, accounts for 85 percent of the cases, and usually affects individuals aged fifty-five to seventy years of age. The pathologic findings are limited to the central nervous system, although the transmissible agent can be detected in many organs. Researchers noted in 2002 that psychiatric and neurological symptoms are often present within four months of the disease's onset. Common symptoms include withdrawal, anxiety, irritability, insomnia, and a loss of interest. Within a few weeks or months, a relentlessly progressive dementia becomes evident, and myoclonus is often present at some point. Deterioration is usually rapid, with 90 percent of victims dying within one year. CJD patients do not have fevers, and their blood and cerebrospinal fluid are normal.

The inherited or familial form has been noted in some one hundred extended families, accounting for 15 percent of the cases of CJD. At least seven different point mutations and one insertion mutation in the prion gene have been identified. Some prion mutations result in slightly different symptoms and are classified as different diseases. Other mutations may lead to the sporadic, infectious, or new variant forms.

The infectious form is rare and generally has been associated with medical procedures, such as organ transplants, inadvertent infection from contaminated surgical instruments, or treatment with products derived from human brains. Because the infectious agent is highly resistant to denaturation, thorough decontamination of surgical instruments has proven essential in minimizing transmission. A number of cases occurred in individuals receiving growth hormone extracts derived from human pituitary glands, a practice discontinued in the United States in 1985. The infectious form also appears to be the basis for kuru, a disease previously endemic among the Fore people of the eastern highlands of Papua New Guinea. Typically, it was characterized by cerebellar dysfunction, dementia, and progression to death within two years. Evidence indicates that the kuru agent was transmitted through the ritual handling and consumption of affected tissues, especially brains, from deceased relatives. With discontinuation of these cultural practices, kuru has virtually disappeared.

A new variant CJD (nvCJD) was first reported in Britain in 1996. It differed from sporadic CJD in affecting younger persons (aged sixteen to thirty-nine) and in its behavioral symptoms, pathology, and longer course. This variant followed the British epidemic of bovine spongiform encephalopathy (BSE), known as mad-cow disease. Contaminated beef consumption was suspected as the source of nvCJD, which has subsequently been shown to have a molecular signature similar, if not identical, to that for BSE. Furthermore, nvCJD has been observed only in countries with BSE.

BSE first appeared in Britain in 1986 and has subsequently been diagnosed in twelve other countries. It occurs in adult cattle between two and eight years of age and is fatal. In the course of the disease, the animals lose coordination and show extreme sensitivity to sound, light, and touch. While it may be transmitted from mother to calf, the major cause of the BSE epidemic in Britain is attributed to feed containing contaminated ruminant-derived protein. Following a ban on incorporating such protein into cattle feed, the incidence has decreased. Since the beginning of the epidemic, a total of 200,000 cattle have been diagnosed with the disease; fewer than 1,000 new cases are currently reported per year. In the United States, a surveillance program is in effect, importation of beef from affected countries is prohibited, and incorporating ruminant-derived protein into cattle feed has been banned. Nevertheless, an infected cow was discovered in 2003 on a farm in Washington State. It had been imported from Canada.

When the British BSE outbreak occurred, concern arose for its human health implications, despite the fact that scrapie, the comparable condition in sheep, was long known not to be a risk to human consumers. A surveillance unit was established in 1990, and ten cases of the new variant form of CJD were reported in 1996. In 2000, twenty-eight cases were recorded in Britain. The numbers began to slow soon afterward, but fears of another epidemic remained.

Treatment and Therapy

Research on experimental animals has been crucial to understanding the unusual etiology of these diseases. Brain tissue from patients dying of kuru was inoculated into the brains of chimpanzees that, after a prolonged incubation period, developed a similar disease. CJD, BSE, and scrapie have been similarly transmitted to a wide variety of laboratory animals. Mouse models have been particularly useful. Knockout mice lacking their normal prion gene are not susceptible to transmissible disease, indicating the importance of endogenous brain prions in the etiology. Transgenic mice, whose own prions have been replaced with those from other species or with specific mutations, exhibit different susceptibilities to various infectious particles.

Because none of the spongiform encephalopathies stimulates a specific immune response, diagnosis of these diseases in living persons or animals is difficult. Postmortem identification of brain lesions is necessary to verify the diagnosis. The use of antibodies to prions is permitting rapid confirmation of the diagnosis from specimens obtained by brain biopsy or postmortem examination. As of 2013, no effective treatment was available for these diseases, which are uniformly fatal. Treatment focuses on alleviating pain and other symptoms. Although these diseases can be transmitted to health care workers and others having contact with CJD patients, the risk is no higher than for the general population. Isolation of patients is not suggested, but reasonable care should be exercised. No organs, tissues, or tissue products from these patients or others with an ill-defined neurologic disease should be used for transplantation, replacement therapy, or pharmaceutical manufacturing.

Perspective and Prospects

Clinically, Creutzfeldt-Jakob disease can be mistaken for other disorders that cause dementia in the elderly, especially Alzheimer's disease. CJD, however, usually has a shorter clinical course and includes myoclonus. While nvCJD has a longer clinical course, it generally affects younger persons.

Continued monitoring of CJD and especially nvCJD in the United Kingdom is warranted. In addition, surveillance of the food supply in the United States and other countries should persist to prevent meat from BSE cattle from reaching consumers. Above all, further research into the etiology of these pathologies is needed. Research into prion biology and disease epidemiology, including studies of nvCJD clusters, must be pursued until the progression of these diseases is fully understood. Early detection and effective treatment await this understanding.

—James L. Robinson, Ph.D.

See also Brain; Brain disorders; Dementias; Food poisoning; Prion diseases; Viral infections; Zoonoses.

For Further Information:

Badash, Michelle. "Creutzfeldt-Jakob Disease." *Health Library*, March 15, 2013.
Balter, Michael. "Tracking the Human Fallout from Mad Cow Disease." *Science* 289 (September, 2000): 1452-1453.
Bloom, Floyd E., M. Flint Beal, and David J. Kupfer, eds. *The Dana Guide to Brain Health*. New York: Dana Press, 2006.
"Creutzfeldt-Jakob Disease." *Mayo Clinic*, October 23, 2012.
"Creutzfeldt-Jakob Disease." *National Institute of Neurological Disorders and Stroke*, May 1, 2013.
Marieb, Elaine N., and Katja Hoehn. *Human Anatomy and Physiology*. 9th ed. San Francisco: Pearson/Benjamin Cummings, 2010.
Nolte, John. *Human Brain: An Introduction to Its Functional Anatomy*. 6th ed. Philadelphia: Mosby/Elsevier, 2009.
Prusiner, Stanley B. "The Prion Diseases." *Scientific American* 272, no. 1 (January, 1995): 48-57.
Prusiner, Stanley B. *Prion Biology and Diseases*. 2d ed. Cold Spring Harbor, N.Y.: Cold Spring Harbor Laboratory Press, 2004.
Schwartz, Maxime. *How the Cows Turned Mad*. Translated by Edward Schneider. Berkeley: University of California Press, 2003.
Spencer, Charlotte A. *Mad Cows and Cannibals: A Guide to the Transmissible Spongiform Encephalopathies*. Upper Saddle River, N.J.: Prentice Hall, 2004.
Transmissible Spongiform Encephalopathies in the United States. Ames, Iowa: Council for Agricultural Science and Technology, 2000.

CRITICAL CARE

Specialty

Anatomy or system affected: All

Specialties and related fields: Anesthesiology, cardiology, emergency medicine, gastroenterology, geriatrics and gerontology, neurology, nursing, obstetrics, pharmacology, pulmonary medicine, radiology, sports medicine, toxicology

Definition: The care of patients who are experiencing severe health crises-short-lived or prolonged, accidental or anticipated-that require continuous monitoring.

Key terms:

asphyxia: an impaired exchange of oxygen and carbon dioxide in the lungs; if prolonged, this condition leads to death

aspirate: to suck fluid or a foreign body into an airway of the lungs, which frequently leads to aspiration pneumonia

debridement: the excision of bruised, injured, or otherwise devitalized tissue from a wound site

electrocardiogram (EKG or ECG): a graphic record of the electrical activity of the heart, obtained with an electrocardiograph and displayed on a computer screen or paper strip

emphysema: an increase in the size of air spaces at the terminal ends of bronchioles in the lungs; this damage reduces the ability of the lungs to exchange oxygen and carbon dioxide

esophagus: the portion of the digestive system connecting the mouth and stomach; it is muscular, propelling food during the act of swallowing

hypothermia: a subnormal body temperature; clinically, it is a sustained cooling of the body to lower-than-normal temperatures

resuscitation: the restoration to life after apparent death; the methods used to restore normal organ functioning, primarily referring to the heart

sternum: the breastbone; found in the midline of the chest cavity and lying over the heart

trauma: an injury caused by rough contact with a physical object; it can be accidental or induced

Science and Profession

Critical care is the branch of medicine that provides immediate services, usually on an emergency basis. It also encompasses some forms of ongoing care provided in a hospital setting for patients who are so sick that they are medically unstable and must be monitored constantly. Such patients are at an ongoing high risk for disastrous complications.

Critical care personnel must be specially trained, and standards for training and evaluation in this field have been prepared for physicians, nurses, and other hospital personnel. Approximately 90 percent of hospitals in the United States with fewer than two hundred beds have a single critical care unit, usually called an intensive care unit (ICU). Only 9 percent of these hospitals have a second intensive care facility, typically dedicated solely to the care of heart attack victims. In total, 7 to 8 percent of all hospital beds in the United States are used for intensive care. Because ICU facilities are at a premium and are expensive to operate, patients are transferred to a regular hospital bed as quickly as possible, given the severity of their specific medical condition. Of the physicians who are certified in critical care, most are anesthesiologists, followed by internists.

Critical care facilities are available in several varieties, providing specialized care to particular patients. The most common type of ICU is for individuals who require care for medical crises. These patients frequently have a short-term condition or disease that can be treated successfully. Others are admitted to a medical ICU for multiple organ system failure. These people are often very sick with conditions that overwhelm even the best available care and equipment. Heart attack victims are often admitted to a coronary ICU, which has specialized equipment for support and resuscitation if needed. Once medically stable, coronary ICU patients are transferred to a regular hospital bed.

Larger hospitals may have an ICU for surgical patients. Typically, these individuals are admitted to the surgical ICU from the operating room after a procedure. In the ICU, they are stabilized while the effects of anesthesia wear off. They, too, are transferred to a normal hospital room as soon as is medically safe. Neonatal ICUs exist in some larger hospitals to provide care for premature and very sick infants. Such infants may stay in neonatal ICUs for extended periods of time (weeks to months) depending on their specific condition. There may also be a pediatric ICU specially designed for very sick children.

Diagnostic and Treatment Techniques

Critical care is synonymous with immediate care: Swift action is required on an emergency basis to sustain or save a life. The most immediate of critical care needs are to establish and maintain a patent airway for ventilation and to maintain sufficient cardiac functioning to provide minimal perfusion or blood supply to critical organs of the body.

Resuscitation is the support of life by external means when the body is unable to maintain itself. Basic life support is for emergency situations and consists of delivering oxygen to the lungs, maintaining an airway, inflating the lungs if necessary, and assisting with circulation. These methods are collectively known as cardiopulmonary resuscitation (CPR). Oxygen can be transferred from one mouth to another by forceful breathing or by the means of pumps and pure oxygen from a container. The airway is commonly maintained by positioning the head and neck so as to extend the chin and open the trachea. It is also possible to make an incision in the trachea, insert a tube, and provide oxygen through the tube. The lungs may be inflated by using the force of exhaled air from one person breathing into another's mouth or by utilizing a machine that inflates the lungs to a precise level and delivers oxygen in accurate, predetermined amounts. When a victim's heart is not working, the circulation of blood is provided by external compression of the chest. This action squeezes the heart between the sternum and the spine, forcing blood into the circulatory system.

Advanced life support includes attempts to restart a nonfunctioning heart. This goal is commonly accomplished by electrical means (defibrillation). The heart is given a brief shock that is sufficient to start it beating on its own. Drugs can also be used to restore spontaneous circulation in cardiac arrest. Epinephrine (adrenaline) is the most commonly used drug, although sodium bicarbonate is used for some conditions. A heart can be restarted by manual compression. This technique requires direct access to the heart and is limited to situations in which the heart stops beating during a surgical procedure involving the thorax, when the heart is directly accessible.

Prolonged life support is administered after the heart has been restarted and is concerned chiefly with the brain and other organs such as the kidneys that are sensitive to oxygen levels in the blood. Drugs and mechanical ventilation are used to supply oxygen to the lungs. Prolonged life support uses sophisticated technology to deliver oxygenated blood to the organs continuously. The body can be maintained in this manner for long periods of time. Once begun,

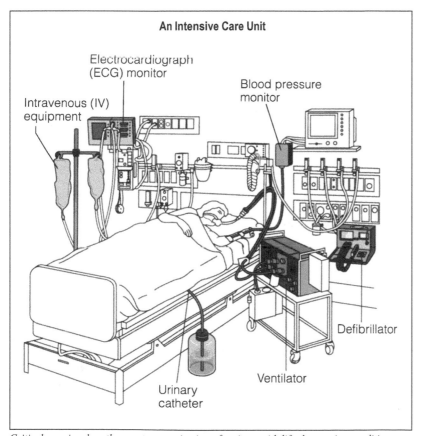

An Intensive Care Unit

Electrocardiograph (ECG) monitor

Intravenous (IV) equipment

Blood pressure monitor

Defibrillator

Ventilator

Urinary catheter

Critical care involves the constant monitoring of patients with life-threatening conditions. This care is usually provided in an intensive care unit (ICU).

prolonged life support is continued until the patient regains consciousness or until brain death has been certified by a physician. A patient's state of underlying disease may be determined to be so severe that continuing prolonged life support becomes senseless. The factors entering into a decision to terminate life support are complex and involve a patient's family, the physician, and other professionals.

Individuals who are critically ill must be closely monitored. Many of the advancements in the care of these patients have been attributable to improvements in monitoring. While physiologic measurements cannot replace the clinical impressions of trained professionals, monitoring data often provide objective information that reinforces clinical opinions. More people die from the failure of vital organs than from the direct effects of injury or disease. The most commonly monitored events are vital signs: heart rate, blood pressure, breathing rate, and temperature. These are frequently augmented by electrocardiograms (ECGs or EKGs). Other, more sophisticated electronic methods are available for individuals in intensive care units.

Vital signs are still frequently assessed manually, although machinery is available to accomplish the task. Modern intensive care units are able to store large amounts of data that can be analyzed by computer programs. Data can be transmitted to distant consoles, thus enabling a small number of individuals to monitor several patients simultaneously. Monitoring data can also be displayed on computer screens, allowing more rapid evaluation. Automatic alarms can be used to indicate when bodily functions fall outside predetermined parameters, thus rapidly alerting staff to critical or emergency situations.

Breathing-or, more correctly, ventilation-can be monitored extensively. The volume of inspired air can be adjusted to accommodate different conditions. The amount of oxygen can be changed to compensate for emphysema or other loss of oxygen exchange capacity. The rate of breathing can also be regulated to work in concert with the heart in order to provide maximum benefit to the patient. The effectiveness of pulmonary monitoring is itself monitored by measuring the amount of oxygen in arterial blood. This, too, can be accomplished automatically, with adjustments made by instruments.

Common situations that require critical care are choking, drowning, poisoning, physical trauma, psychological trauma, and environmental disasters.

Choking. Difficulty in either breathing or swallowing is termed choking. The source of the obstruction may be either internal or external. Internal obstructions can result from a foreign body becoming stuck in the mouth (pharynx), throat (esophagus or trachea), or lungs (bronchi). The blockage may be partial or total. A foreign body that is caught in the esophagus will create difficulty in swallowing; one that is caught in the trachea will obstruct breathing. Any foreign body may become lodged and create a blockage. Objects that commonly cause obstructions include teeth (both natural and false), food (especially meat and fish bones), and liquids such as water and blood.

Obstructions can occur externally. Examples of external causes of choking include compression of the larynx or trachea as a result of blunt trauma (a physical blow or other injury sustained in an accident), a penetrating projectile such as a bullet or stick, and toys or small items of food that are swallowed accidentally. An object that becomes stuck in the lungs frequently does not cause an acute shortage of breath, but this situation can lead to aspiration pneumonia, which is extremely difficult to treat.

The symptoms of choking are well known: gagging, coughing, and difficulty in breathing. Pain may or may not be present. Frequently, there is a short episode of difficulty in breathing followed by a period when no symptoms are experienced. The foreign body may be moved aside or pushed deeper into the body by the victim's initial frantic movements. A foreign body lodged in the esophagus will not interfere with breathing but may cause food or liquids to spill into the trachea and become aspirated; as with an object in the lungs, this usually leads to pneumonia or other serious respiratory conditions.

Drowning. Drowning is defined as the outcome (usually death) of unanticipated immersion into a liquid (usually water). Consciousness is an important determinant of how an individual reacts to immersion in water. A person who is conscious will attempt to escape from the fluid environment, which involves attempts to regain orientation and not to aspirate additional liquids. An unconscious person has none of these defenses and usually dies when the lungs fill rapidly with water. Normal persons can hold their breath for thirty seconds or more. Frequently, this is sufficient time for a victim to escape from immersion in a fluid environment. When a victim exhales just prior to entering water, this time period is not available; indeed, panic frequently develops, and the victim aspirates water.

Most but not all victims of drowning die from aspirating water. Approximately 10 percent of drowning victims die from asphyxia while underwater, possibly because they hold their breath or because the larynx goes into spasms. The brain of the average person can survive without oxygen for about four minutes. After that time, irreversible damage starts to occur; death follows in a matter of minutes. After four minutes, survival is possible but unlikely to be without the permanent impairment of mental functions.

The physical condition of the victim exerts a profound influence on the outcome of a drowning situation. Physically fit persons have a far greater chance of escaping from a drowning environment. Individuals who are in poor condition, who are very weak, or who have disabilities must overcome these conditions when attempting to escape from a drowning situation; frequently, they are unable to remove themselves and die in the process.

Another physical condition such as exhaustion or a heart attack may also be present. An exhausted person is weak and may not have the physical strength or endurance to escape. A person who experiences a heart attack at the moment of immersion is at a severe disadvantage. If the heart is unable to deliver blood and nutrients to muscles, even a physically fit person is weakened and may be less likely to escape a drowning situation.

The temperature of the water is critical. Immersing the face in cold water (below 20 degrees Celsius or 56 degrees Fahrenheit) initiates a reflex that slows the person's heart rate and shunts blood to the heart and brain, thus delaying irreversible cerebral damage. Immersion in water even colder leads to hypothermia (subnormal body temperature). In the short term, hypothermia reduces the body's consumption of oxygen and allows submersion in water for slightly longer periods of time. There have been reports of survival after immersion of ten minutes in warm water and forty minutes in extremely cold water. Age is also a factor: Younger persons are more likely to tolerate such conditions than older persons.

Poisoning. Whether intentional or accidental, poisoning demands immediate medical care. Intoxication can also initiate a crisis that requires critical care. Alcohol is the most common intoxicant, but a wide range of other substances are accidentally ingested. When an individual is poisoned, the toxic substance must be removed from the body. This removal may be accomplished in a variety of ways and is usually done in a hospital. Supportive care may be needed during the period of acute crisis. The brain, liver, and kidneys are usually at great risk during a toxic crisis; steps must be taken to protect these organs.

Physical trauma. Trauma is the leading cause of death in persons under the age of forty. Motor vehicle accidents alone account for nearly 2 percent of all deaths worldwide. Globally, nearly six million people die each year from accidental or violence-related injury, accounting for nearly 9 percent of total global mortality. The three leading causes of trauma-related deaths are motor vehicle accidents, suicide, and homicide.. Trauma is commonly characterized as either blunt or penetrating.

Blunt trauma occurs when an external force is applied to tissue, causing compression or crushing injuries as well as fractures. This force can be applied directly from being hit with an object or indirectly through the forces generated by sudden deceleration. In the latter event, relatively mobile organs or structures continue moving until stopped by adjacent, relatively fixed organs or structures. Any of these injuries can result in extensive internal bleeding. Damage may also cause fluids to be lost from tissues and lead to shock, circulatory collapse, and ultimately death.

The most frequent sources for penetrating wounds are knives and firearms. A knife blade produces a smaller wound; fewer organs are likely to be involved, and adjacent structures are less likely to sustain damage. In contrast, gunshot wounds are more likely to involve multiple tissues and to damage adjacent structures. More energy is released by a bullet than by a knife. This energy is sufficient to fracture a bone and usually leads to a greater amount of tissue damage.

The wound must be repaired, typically through surgical exploration and suturing. Extensively damaged tissue is removed in a process called debridement. Any visible sources of secondary contamination must also be removed. With both knife and firearm wounds often comes contamination by dirt, clothing, and other debris; this contamination presents a seri-ous threat of infection to the victim and is also a problem for critical care workers. The wound is then covered appropriately, and the victim is given antibiotics to counteract bacteria that may have been introduced with the primary injury.

Psychological trauma. Critical care is often required in situations that lead to psychological stress. Individuals taking drug overdoses require critical supportive care until the drug has been metabolized by or removed from the body. Respiratory support is needed when the drug depresses the portion of the brain that controls breathing. Some drugs cause extreme agitation, which must be controlled by sedation.

Severe trauma to a loved one can initiate a psychological crisis. Psychological support must be provided to the victim; frequently, this is done in a hospital setting. An entire family may require critical care support for brief periods of time in the aftermath of a catastrophe. Severe trauma, disease, or the death of a child may require support by outsiders. Most hospitals have professionals who are trained to provide such support. In addition, people with psychiatric problems sometimes fail to take the medications that control mental illness. Critical care support in a hospital is often needed until these people are restabilized on their medications.

Environmental disasters. The need for psychological support, as well as urgent medical care, is magnified with natural or environmental disasters such as earthquakes, hurricanes, floods, or tornadoes. Environmental disasters seriously disrupt lives and normal services; they can arise with little or no warning. The key to providing critical care in a disaster situation is adequate prior planning.

Responses to disasters occur at three levels: institutional (hospital), local (police, fire, and rescue), and regional (county and state). The plan must be simple and evolve from normal operations; individuals respond best when they are asked to perform tasks with which they are familiar and for which they are trained. The response must integrate all existing sources of emergency medical and supportive services. Those who assume responsibilities for overall management must be well trained and able to adapt to different and rapidly changing conditions that may be encountered. Because no two disasters are ever alike, such flexibility is essential. Summaries of individual duties and responsibilities should be available for all involved individuals. Finally, the disaster plan should be practiced and rehearsed using specific scenarios. Experience is the single best method to ensure competency when a disaster strikes.

Environmental disasters such as earthquakes, hurricanes, floods, or tornadoes cause loss of life and extensive property damage. Essential services such as water, gas, electricity, and telephone communication are often lost. Victims must be provided food, shelter, and medical care on an immediate basis. Critical care is usually required at the time of the disaster, and the need for support may continue long after the immediate effects of the disaster have been resolved.

Perspective and Prospects

One of the most important issues with regard to critical care is sometimes controversial: when to discontinue life support.

Life-support equipment is usually withdrawn as soon as patients are able to function independent of the machinery. These patients continue to recover, are discharged from the hospital, and complete their recovery at home. For some, however, the outcome is not as positive. Machines may be used to assist breathing. For a patient who does not improve, or who deteriorates, there comes a point in time when a decision to stop life support must be made. This is not an easy decision, nor should it be made by a single individual.

The patient's own wishes must be paramount. These wishes, however, must have been clearly communicated while the individual was in good health and had unimpaired thought processes. A patient's family is entitled to provide input in the decision to terminate care, but others are also entitled to provide input: the patient's physician, representatives of the hospital or institution, a representative of the patient's religious faith, and the state.

Medical science has developed criteria for death. The application of these criteria, however, is not uniform. The final decision to terminate life support is frequently a consensus of all the parties mentioned above. When there is a dispute, the courts are often asked to intervene. Extensive disagreements exist concerning the ethics of terminating critical care. It is beyond the scope of this discussion to provide definitive guidelines. This logical extension of critical care may not have a uniform resolution; the values and beliefs of each individual determine the outcome of each situation.

—*L. Fleming Fallon, Jr., M.D., Ph.D., M.P.H.*

See also Accidents; Aging: Extended care; Choking; Coma; Critical care, pediatric; Death and dying; Disease; Drowning; Electrocardiography (ECG or EKG); Electroencephalography (EEG); Emergency medicine; Ethics; Euthanasia; Hospice; Hospitals; Hyperbaric oxygen therapy; Intensive care unit (ICU); Living will; Nursing; Palliative medicine; Paramedics; Poisoning; Psychiatric disorders; Respiration; Resuscitation; Surgery, general; Terminally ill: Extended care; Tracheostomy; Unconsciousness; Wounds.

For Further Information:

"A Primer on Critical Care for Patients and Their Families." *American Thoracic Society*, December 11, 1999.

Bongard, Frederick, and Darryl Y. Sue, eds. *Current Critical Care Diagnosis and Treatment.* 3d ed. New York: McGraw-Hill Medical, 2008.

"Critical Care Statistics." *Society of Critical Care Medicine*, January 4, 2012.

Hogan, David E., and Jonathan L. Burstein. *Disaster Medicine.* 2d ed. Philadelphia: Lippincott Williams & Wilkins, 2007.

Legome, Eric, and Lee W. Shockley. *Trauma: A Comprehensive Emergency Medicine Approach.* Cambridge: Cambridge University Press, 2011.

Limmer, Daniel, et al. *Emergency Care.* 12th ed. Boston: Prentice Hall, 2011.

Markovchick, Vincent J., Peter T. Pons, and Katherine A. Bakes. *Emergency Medicine Secrets.* 5th ed. Philadelphia: Mosby/Elsevier, 2010.

Safar, Peter, and Nicholas G. Bircher. *Cardiopulmonary Cerebral Resuscitation: Basic and Advanced Cardiac and Trauma Life Support-An Introduction to Resuscitation Medicine.* 3d ed. Philadelphia: W. B. Saunders, 1988.

Vincent, Jean-Louis, et al., eds. *Textbook of Critical Care.* 6th ed. Philadelphia: Elsevier Saunders, 2011.

"Worldwide Injuries and Violence." *Centers for Disease Control and Prevention*, June 10, 2011.

CROHN'S DISEASE
Disease/Disorder

Also known as: Regional enteritis

Anatomy or system affected: Gastrointestinal system, intestines

Specialties and related fields: Gastroenterology, immunology, nutrition, pediatrics

Definition: A chronic disease process in which the bowel becomes inflamed, leading to scarring and narrowing of the intestines.

Key terms:

abscess: a localized collection of pus (dead cells and a mixture of live and dead bacteria)

antigen: a foreign substance in the body causing an immunological response that produces antibodies

fissure: a break in the surface tissue of the anal canal or the wall of the gastrointestinal tract

fistula: an abnormal connection between two hollow structures or between a hollow structure and the skin surface

Causes and Symptoms

Crohn's disease is a chronic disease of the digestive system. It is one of two diseases labeled as inflammatory bowel disease (IBD); the other is ulcerative colitis. With both diseases, patients suffer from diarrhea, abdominal pain, bleeding from the rectum, and fever. The cell lining of the bowel (usually the small intestine) becomes inflamed, leading to erosion of tissues and bleeding.

Crohn's disease may affect areas of the gastrointestinal system from the mouth to the anus. The inflammatory process may spread to include the joints, skin, eyes, mouth, and sometimes liver. In children, IBD involves a substantial risk of slow or interrupted growth.

The most common early sign is abdominal pain, often felt over the navel or on the right side. Diarrhea and subsequent weight loss often follow. Other early signs of Crohn's disease include sores in the anal area (skin tabs), hemorrhoids, fissures (cracks), fistulas (abnormal openings from the intestines to the skin surface or other organs), abscesses (uncommon in children), and nausea and vomiting, especially in young children. Children as young as ten may develop this disease; however, in the majority of cases the onset is between the ages of thirteen and twenty-five. Some sources re-

---

Information on Crohn's Disease

Causes: Infection

Symptoms: Diarrhea, abdominal pain, rectal bleeding, fever, weight loss, anal sores, hemorrhoids, fissures, fistulas, abscesses, nausea, vomiting

Duration: Chronic

Treatments: Medications for symptom alleviation

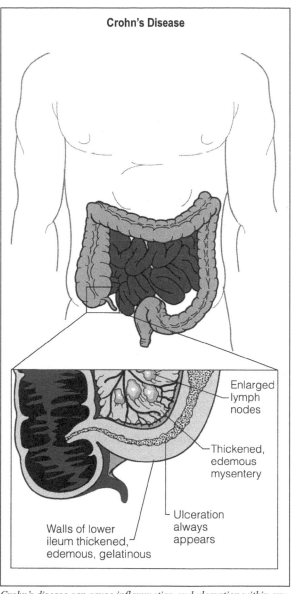

Crohn's Disease

Enlarged
lymph
nodes

Thickened,
edemous
mysentery

Ulceration
always
appears

Walls of lower
ileum thickened,
edemous, gelatinous

Crohn's disease can cause inflammation and ulceration within any region of the digestive tract, but most often in the ileum.

(disruptions in the intestinal lining). In Crohn's disease, these ulcerations involve the full thickness of the intestinal lining.

When the inflamed intestine heals, it may become scarred around the areas previously inflamed. This may lead to a narrowing of the bowel, or stricture, which can lead to partial or total blockage of the intestinal flow (bowel obstruction).

Treatment and Therapy

Crohn's disease is a baffling, unpredictable disease for which a truly successful treatment has not been found. Some of the medications used in treatment are corticosteroids, such as prednisone and adrenocorticotropic hormone (ACTH), and sulfasalazine-type drugs, such as Azulfidine. Both have limited benefits and some side effects. Prednisone-type drugs reduce tissue inflammation and thereby relieve symptoms such as rectal bleeding, abdominal pain, and fever. They may cause side effects, including rounding of the face, increased facial hair, fluid retention, bone loss (osteoporosis), high blood pressure, and high blood sugar levels. These drugs also may cause mood swings. They are prescribed conservatively by most doctors. Sulfasalazine contains two active ingredients, a sulfa preparation(sulfapyridine) and an aspirin-like drug (5-aminosalicylic acid, or 5-ASA), which are bonded together. The 5-ASA medication is thought to act on the surface of the lining of the intestine, suppressing tissue inflammation.

The drug 6-mercaptopurine, or 6-MP, is an immunosuppressive, a substance that alters the body's normal immune response to a disease or antigen. Immunosuppressive drugs have been used to treat autoimmune diseases, conditions in which the immune system attacks healthy tissues, among them Crohn's disease. It is believed that these drugs can stop the mechanism that causes the body to attack itself.

Drugs can offer relief of symptoms, but no drug has yet been found to alter the long-term progression or natural course of Crohn's disease. Following a special diet may help to alleviate some of the symptoms of Crohn's disease, as certain foods, such as alcohol or high-fiber foods, may irritate the lining the bowel further. Surgical removal of the diseased intestine is usually reserved for cases in which medical treatment has failed. The recurrence rates of Crohn's disease following surgery are high.

Perspective and Prospects

Unlike ulcerative colitis, which affects only the inner lining of the intestines, Crohn's disease affects the full thickness of the bowel wall. Both types of IBD occur in predominantly Western or developed countries, especially Scandinavia, the United Kingdom, Western Europe, Israel, and the United States. In recent years, IBD has been reported in Japan. IBD is seen rarely in Africa, most of Asia, and parts of South America. IBD seems to cluster in families, suggesting a genetic factor. Up to 20 percent of people with IBD have one or more blood relatives with the disease.

American gastroenterologist Burrill B. Crohn first identified Crohn's disease in 1932. The prognosis for sufferers was poor, and their quality of life was limited. Prednisone was the

port that Crohn's disease is slightly more common in women. The incidence is greater in persons of Jewish ethnic origin.

Diagnosis often is made after a series of abdominal X-rays, an upper gastrointestinal series, or a colonoscopy (visual inspection of the intestines with a camera). The gastrointestinal (GI) tract is best pictured as a continuous tube that begins at the mouth and ends at the anus. The mucosal layer of intestine that absorbs nutrients contains immune cells that act as defenders of the body (antibodies). Sometimes, this mucosal layer breaks down, and harmful bacteria enter the deep layers of the intestine. The resulting inflammatory process can entail swelling (edema), increased blood flow, and ulcerations

first of the above-mentioned medications to be used to treat Crohn's disease. Investigation into the causes and treatment of IBD continues in many areas, including genetic studies. Current research offers reason for optimism that the causes of IBD will be found and that a cure will follow.

—*Lisa Levin Sobczak, R.N.C.*

See also Colitis; Colon; Diarrhea and dysentery; Gastroenterology; Gastroenterology, pediatric; Gastrointestinal system; Immune system; Intestinal disorders; Intestines; Irritable bowel syndrome (IBS); Nausea and vomiting.

For Further Information:

Baumgart, Daniel C., and William J. Sandborn. "Crohn's Disease." *Lancet* 380, no. 9853 (November, 2012): 1590-1605.

Brandt, Lawrence J., and Penny Steiner-Grossman, eds. *Treating IBD: A Patient's Guide to the Medical and Surgical Management of Inflammatory Bowel Disease.* Reprint. Philadelphia: Lippincott-Raven, 1996.

Carson-DeWitt, Rosalyn. "Crohn's Disease." *Health Library*, February 7, 2013.

"Crohn's Disease." *Medline Plus*, October 29, 2012.

Kalibjian, Cliff. *Straight from the Gut: Living with Crohn's Disease and Ulcerative Colitis.* Cambridge, Mass.: O'Reilly, 2003.

Murray, Michael T. *Stomach Ailments and Digestive Disturbances: How You Can Benefit from Diet, Vitamins, Minerals, Herbs, Exercise, and Other Natural Methods.* Rocklin, Calif.: Prima, 1997.

Saibil, Fred. *Crohn's Disease and Ulcerative Colitis: Everything You Need to Know.* Rev. ed. Toronto, Ont.: Firefly Books, 2009.

Sklar, Jill, Manuel Sklar, and Annabel Cohen. *The First Year-Crohn's Disease and Ulcerative Colitis: An Essential Guide for the Newly Diagnosed.* 2d ed. New York: Marlowe, 2007.

Steiner-Grossman, Penny, Peter A. Banks, and Daniel H. Present, eds. *The New People, Not Patients: A Source Book for Living with Inflammatory Bowel Disease.* Rev. ed. Dubuque, Iowa: Kendall/ Hunt, 1997.

Zonderman, Jon, and Ronald S. Vender. *Understanding Crohn Disease and Ulcerative Colitis.* Jackson: University Press of Mississippi, 2000.

CROSSED EYES. *See* **STRABISMUS.**

CROUP

Disease/Disorder

Also known as: Viral croup, spasmodic croup, laryngotracheobronchitis

Anatomy or system affected: Lungs, respiratory system, throat

Specialties and related fields: Emergency medicine, otorhinolaryngology, pediatrics, preventive medicine, virology

Definition: An inflammation of the larynx, throat, and upper bronchial tubes causing hoarseness, cough, and difficult breathing.

Key terms:

cortisone: a steroid hormone used to reduce inflammation

epiglottis: a small piece of cartilage that covers the entry to the windpipe during swallowing

epiglottitis: a serious condition caused by a bacterial infection sometimes confused with croup

larynx: the voice box

stridor: the characteristic noisy, labored breathing present with croup

trachea: the windpipe

Causes and Symptoms

Croup is an inflammation of the larynx, trachea, and upper bronchial tubes of the lungs affecting children between the ages of six months and five years. Two-year-olds seem to be the most commonly affected. The inflammation of the trachea causes a narrowing of the child's already small airways, making breathing difficult. Technically, croup is a syndrome, or collection of symptoms associated with several different kinds of infections. These symptoms include hoarseness, a distinctive cough most often described as "barky" and noisy, and labored breathing known as stridor.

Croup occurs in three different forms. The first, viral croup, usually begins with a cold and is most commonly caused by parainfluenza viruses. Indeed, studies indicate that the parainfluenza viruses are responsible for about 70 to 75 percent of croup cases. Viral croup is often accompanied by a low-grade fever. A second type of croup is called spasmodic croup. This condition tends to occur with changes of the weather or the seasons, and the child does not usually run a fever. Allergies are often thought to be responsible for this kind of croup. A third, but rare, form is a bacterial infection caused by mycoplasma. This form can be very serious and is often identified by the extreme difficulty that the child experiences with breathing.

Studies indicate that attacks of croup most commonly occur in October through March and generally strike at night. In general, boys are somewhat more likely to be affected by croup than are girls.

Information on Croup

Causes: Viral or bacterial infection, allergens, change in environment (seasonal change)

Symptoms: Hoarseness, "barking" cough, difficulty breathing

Duration: Acute

Treatments: Medications (cortisone, antibiotics), humidifier; if severe, emergency care and oxygen tent

---

A serious, but rare, condition known as epiglottitis can sometimes be mistaken for croup. In this condition, the epiglottis, the flap that covers the windpipe during swallowing, becomes inflamed and swollen, potentially cutting off the child's air supply. The symptoms of epiglottitis are similar to those of croup, but the child's difficulty in breathing is much more severe, and the child will often run a high fever, drool, and be unable to make voiced sounds. Epiglottitis develops quickly; a child's life can be in jeopardy in only a few hours. Consequently, this condition must be treated as an emergency, requiring hospital care.

Treatment and Therapy

A number of treatments are generally used to bring relief to the child suffering from viral or spasmodic croup. The use of a cool mist humidifier can ward off an attack in the child who exhibits a tendency toward developing croup. A mild attack can also be alleviated through use of the humidifier. If the attack of croup is well under way or if it is severe, however, a cool mist humidifier may not be adequate. Many doctors recommend that after an attack of croup, a cool mist humidifier should be run in the child's room for the next three or four evenings. Another commonly used treatment is to take the child, properly dressed, outside at night. Usually the cold, damp air will soothe the child's inflamed airways.

Still another technique reported to relieve the symptoms of croup is to fill the bathroom with steam by running a hot shower. Setting the child in the steam-filled room for fifteen to twenty minutes often eases the child's breathing. The most successful use of this treatment requires that the child be held, not placed on the floor, because steam rises.

Neither cough syrups nor antibiotics are appropriate treatments for croup. Cough syrups prevent the expulsion of phlegm, while antibiotics have no effect on viral infections. Croup caused by mycoplasma, however, is treated with an antibiotic, generally erythromycin.

Pediatricians recommend that the child's doctor be called in the event of a croup attack. Serious attacks are generally treated in a hospital emergency room. There, the child may be given cortisone by injection or by mouth. In addition, hospitals can administer breathing treatments.

Bacterial croup is also treated at a hospital with antibiotics and an oxygen tent as needed. Indeed, immediate emergency room treatment is called for if there is a whistling sound in the breathing that seems to grow louder, if the child does not have enough breath to speak, or if the child is struggling to breathe.

Perspective and Prospects

Accounts of croup can be found in medical literature dating back to the eighteenth century. Membranous croup, also known as diphtheria, was a great killer of children and adults alike in the past. Immunization made this kind of croup extremely rare, however, by the mid-twentieth century.

During the last quarter of the twentieth century, doctors continued to research the uses of corticosteroids in the treatment of croup, as well as the most effective way to deliver these drugs.

—*Diane Andrews Henningfeld, Ph.D.*

See also Bacterial infections; Bronchi; Bronchitis; Childhood infectious diseases; Coughing; Diphtheria; Epiglottitis; Laryngitis; Lungs; Respiration; Sore throat; Trachea; Viral infections; Wheezing.

For Further Information:

American Medical Association. *American Medical Association Family Medical Guide.* 4th rev. ed. Hoboken, N.J.: John Wiley & Sons, 2004.
"Croup." *Medline Plus*, March 22, 2013.
Kliegman, Robert M., et al. *Nelson Textbook of Pediatrics*. 19th ed. Philadelphia, Pa.: Elsevier, 2011.
Nathanson, Laura Walter. "Coping with Croup." *Parents* 70, no. 9 (September, 1995): 29-31.
Niederman, Michael S., George A. Sarosi, and Jeffrey Glassroth. *Respiratory Infections*. 2d ed. Philadelphia: Lippincott Williams & Wilkins, 2001.
Shelov, Steven P., et al. *Caring for Your Baby and Young Child: Birth to Age Five*. 5th ed. New York: Bantam Books, 2009.
Spock, Benjamin, and Robert Needlman. *Dr. Spock's Baby and Child Care*. 9th ed. New York: Gallery Books, 2011.
West, John B. *Pulmonary Pathophysiology: The Essentials*. 7th ed. Philadelphia: Wolters Kluwer/Lippincott Williams & Wilkins, 2008.
Wood, Debra. "Croup (Laryngotracheobronchitis)." *Health Library*, September 10, 2012.
Woolf, Alan D., et al., eds. *The Children's Hospital Guide to Your Child's Health and Development*. Cambridge, Mass.: Perseus, 2002.

CROWNS AND BRIDGES
Treatment

Also known as: Restorative dentistry, indirect restorations
Anatomy or system affected: Mouth, teeth
Specialties and related fields: Dentistry
Definition: Structures that restore the function of the mouth after teeth have been broken or lost. A crown covers and protects a single tooth, while a bridge is a false tooth suspended between two crowns to replace a missing tooth.

Key terms:

abutment: a tooth protected by a crown that serves to anchor one end of a bridge

indirect restoration: a restoration that is fabricated outside the mouth, such as a crown or bridge

restoration: an item or material that is used to restore the structure and function of a compromised tooth

root canal: treatment in which the nerve and pulp of a damaged or infected tooth are removed

Indications and Procedures

A crown may be needed to protect a tooth from cracking or breaking, especially one that already has a large filling. It may also be used to cover a tooth that has already broken, become infected, and required endodontic treatment (commonly called a "root canal"). A crown provides a whole new chewing surface, so it must be able to withstand tremendous jaw pressure. Crowns are indirect restorations that may be made of tooth-colored porcelain, ceramic, or resin; metal, preferably gold; or a combination of porcelain and metal. In this combination, the porcelain is fused to gold, palladium, or platinum. In all-metal crowns, gold is preferable because it can be cast accurately for a tight fit and it will not corrode. In some cases, all that is needed is a partial crown, or onlay, which preserves more of the natural tooth beneath.

The first step in the preparation of a crown is to modify the tooth to receive a crown. Then, an impression of the tooth is made, and from this, a mold is made in which to cast the crown. Once produced, the crown is polished and contoured to approximate a natural tooth. Any porcelain is colored and glazed to match the shade of the patient's natural teeth. Once the crown is finished, the dentist adjusts its fit in the patient's mouth and secures the crown in place with a photosensitive resin. This process has traditionally been accomplished in two visits; the patient is given a temporary crown, usually acrylic, to wear while the permanent one is being made.

A bridge is indicated when one or several teeth in a row are missing and there are stable teeth on either side of the gap to serve as abutments. It is important to fill the gap to maintain optimal function for chewing and speaking by preventing the remaining teeth from shifting and losing their proper alignment.

Models of the patient's mouth are made that indicate the shapes and positions of the abutting teeth that will receive crowns to support the bridge and the gap to be filled by the artificial tooth or teeth. The components of the bridge may be made of metal, porcelain, or a combination of the two. The dentist will indicate to the bridge fabricator what shade from a standard color system to make the porcelain to best match the patient's natural teeth. Once the bridge is made, the dentist adjusts the fit in the patient's mouth and cements the bridge in place. The entire process may require several visits; the patient is given a temporary acrylic bridge to protect the area while the permanent one is being made.

Uses and Complications

Because the preparation of crowns and bridges involves drilling on teeth, the dentist provides local anesthetic to numb the area. This numbness may last a while, and the patient must be careful not to bite the lips or tongue.

While the permanent restoration is being fabricated, the patient wears a temporary piece that is held in place with a light adhesive so it may be easily removed later. However, it may become dislodged before the next dental appointment. It is important that the temporary crown or bridge be replaced as soon as possible to keep the prepared teeth protected and stable. Should their shape or position change, the finished restoration would no longer fit properly.

Fabricating and fitting indirect restorations requires skill and patience. Any excess space inadvertently left between the tooth and the crown or bridge increases the risk of decay or infection because food may become trapped. This is especially problematic for teeth that have not had root canal treatment because a painful abscess may form under the crown. Excess space in bridgework creates the possibility of teeth shifting, which the bridge was originally designed to avoid.

When the crown or bridge is delivered, it might feel high and contact the teeth on the opposite jaw sooner than expected. The dentist will make adjustments at the time of delivery, but a return visit may be necessary if further discomfort is felt.

The teeth involved may be somewhat sensitive to cold following delivery of the restoration. This sensitivity may last for weeks, but it typically resolves on its own.

Perspective and Prospects

Indirect restorations were initially unattractive but functional metal structures. Later, fabrication with porcelain allowed for a less obvious appearance. Advances in materials science have led to the development of stronger, more fracture-resistant ceramics. These contribute to longer lasting, more aesthetically pleasing restorations.

Technology is partnering with dentistry to generate computer-aided design and computer-aided manufacturing (CAD/CAM) for use in crown and bridge fabrication. Dentists and dental laboratory technicians are using CAD/CAM technology to increase the precision of individual restorations by capturing each tooth's exact size, shape, and position. Digital impressions are more comfortable for the patient and less technique-dependent than customary alginate impressions. The resulting three-dimensional image appears on a computer screen, and the dentist can electronically draw the restoration design on the image instead of sculpting wax on a stone model. The details can then be transmitted digitally without distortion to the dental lab technician, who uses a CAD/CAM machine to mill a ceramic material into a detailed replica of the drawing. By looking at the same electronic image before manufacturing, the dentist and the dental laboratory technician can clearly communicate their needs and expectations for an accurate preparation that will result in a quality custom restoration. Digital impressions are also now making same-day crowns feasible.

—Bethany Thivierge, M.P.H., E.L.S.

See also Aging; Bone disorders; Cavities; Dental diseases; Dentistry; Dentures; Teeth.

For Further Information:
Christensen, Gordon J. "Salvaging Crowns and Fixed Prostheses: When and How to Do It." *Journal of the American Dental Association* 139 (December, 2008): 1679-1682.
"Dental Bridges." *Cleveland Clinic Foundation*, October 11, 2012.
"Dental Crowns." *Cleveland Clinic Foundation*, December 10, 2011.
Jacobsen, Peter. *Restorative Dentistry: An Integrated Approach.* Malden, Mass.: Blackwell, 2008.
"Porcelain Fixed Bridges." *American Academy of Cosmetic Dentistry*, 2011.
Stahl, Rebecca J., and Marcin Chwistek. "Dental Crown (Dental Cap)." *Health Library*, March 15, 2013.
Walmsley, A. Damien, et al. *Restorative Dentistry.* 2d ed. New York: Churchill Livingstone/Elsevier, 2007.
"What Are Crowns?" *Academy of General Dentistry*, January, 2012.

CRYOSURGERY

Procedure

Also known as: Cryotherapy

Anatomy or system affected: All

Specialties and related fields: Dermatology, family medicine, general surgery, gynecology, neurology, oncology, otorhinolaryngology, plastic surgery, urology

Definition: The destruction of undesired or abnormal body tissues by exposure to extreme cold.

Key terms:

cryogenic agent: a substance (such as liquid nitrogen) that produces low temperatures

cryoprobe: a liquid nitrogen-cooled, probelike tool used in cryosurgery

lesion: abnormal or diseased tissue

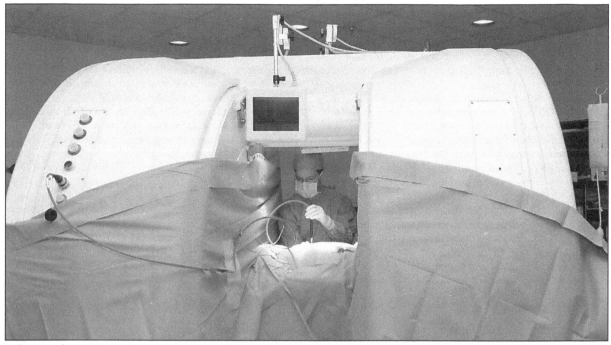

A doctor performs MRI renal cryosurgery, a procedure in which a surgical tube with a freezing tip at the end is used to destroy cancerous kidney tumors while the patient is monitored with MRI. (AP/Wide World Photos)

Indications and Procedures

Cryosurgery, the therapeutic use of extreme cold, is used to remove minor skin lesions such as freckles and warts as well as cancers of the skin and other tissues. Skin heals well after cold injury, and skin pathologies were among the first lesions treated cryosurgically. Although cryosurgery is not the first treatment choice for all skin problems, it is a popular one because of the availability of liquid nitrogen, the main cryogenic agent. In addition, cryosurgery is inexpensive, compared to other procedures, and can be performed without surgical facilities. For example, family physicians and dermatologists use it to treat minor skin lesions at their offices.

Cryosurgery kills tissue via extracellular and intracellular ice. When cells freeze, extracellular ice squeezes them together and changes their extracellular/intracellular volumes. Thawing causes similar, opposite changes that break cell membranes. The rapid temperature drops used in cryosurgery produce intracellular ice, another major source of cell destruction. The result is altered solute concentrations in tissue fluid, electrolyte loss from cells, disrupted membranes, and protein inactivation and transmigration. Reversed temperature gradients cause more destruction during thawing.

Cryosurgery results in tissue hyperemia, discoloration, and ice buildup. On thawing, edema (swelling) develops, yielding necrosis (cell death) in four days. Dead tissue sloughs off in three more days. Within a month, it is replaced by granulation tissue, which yields normal tissue.

Cryosurgery uses between one and five freeze-thaw cycles (FTCs). The freeze speed is 300 degrees Celsius per minute with a drop from 37 degrees Celsius to -196 degrees Celsius followed by crash (about ten-second), short (one-minute), medium (about three-minute), or long (ten-minute) thaws, depending on the type of lesion treated.

For external tissue treatment, liquid nitrogen (at -196 degrees Celsius) may be applied by swab or in a spray. More often, liquid nitrogen-cooled cryoprobes are pressed on lesions. Cryoprobes are cylindrical, with flat contact surfaces. The duration of cryoprobe use depends on the lesion size and type. For example, genital warts of the cervix are treated by quick freeze, a several-minute thaw, and refreezing.

Treating cancer is more complex. In treating internal cancer, liquid nitrogen is circulated through a cryoprobe touching the lesion. Its position and cell freezing are monitored by ultrasound, which also minimizes the destruction of healthy tissue and identifies the extent of cancer death. The size of the cryoprobe depends on the size of the lesion. If a lesion is not destroyed entirely, then the number of FTCs and the treatment time can be lengthened at follow-up visits.

Uses and Complications

The complexity of cryosurgery varies. Cervical warts require one FTC and a cryoprobe, without any anesthetic. Because of the possibility of postoperative fainting, patients are observed for twenty minutes and should arrange for a ride home. Mild abdominal cramps or vaginal discharge may occur. The surgeon should be contacted about prolonged bleeding, infection, or cramps lasting more than twenty-four hours.

Most skin cancers, most often basal and squamous cell carcinomas, can be treated cryosurgically. Often, three or four

FTCs are used. Ear, eyelid, and nose cartilage sites are good targets because scarring and necrosis of surrounding tissue are rare. Superficial basal cell carcinoma exhibits a near 100 percent cure rate, as do nose and ear lesions, because these cancers rarely enter cartilage. Squamous cell carcinoma often does, however, and is harder to treat without creating scars. Cryosurgery is the treatment of choice for facial Bowen's squamous cell carcinoma, with a cure rate near 100 percent, and for cancers of the cervix or penis; removing these cancers does not leave scars. Treating lesions on the eyelids, however, may cause them to swell shut.

Cryosurgery can also be used for localized prostate cancer. Warm saline is passed through a urethral catheter to prevent freezing. Cryoprobe placement is achieved through incisions between the anus and scrotum, guided by ultrasound. As with conventional surgery, anesthesia is needed for pain. The appearance of prostate tissue changes during cryosurgery, and damage to healthy tissue can be minimized through the observation of ultrasound images. The prostate gland swells postoperatively, and a catheter in the bladder is used to prevent urination stoppage. This complication and bruises from probe insertion sites can result in hospital stays. However, cryosurgery causes less bleeding, shorter hospitalization and recovery periods, and less pain than does surgical removal of the prostate. Assurance of complete cancer destruction requires follow-up with radiation or chemotherapy.

Cryosurgery is also used to treat liver, pancreas, and breast cancers, and the applicability of cryosurgery to bone, brain, and spinal cancers is under study. In these cases, cryosurgery is part of a mixed treatment, including conventional surgery and radiation or chemotherapy. Initial reports are encouraging, but the long-term effectiveness here is unknown. When standard treatments fail or are unusable in primary or secondary liver cancer, cryosurgery may be used alone. If the surgical removal of cancer from other internal organs is impossible, then cryosurgery may be used to increase symptom-free survival time.

With all cryosurgeries, the discoloration of treated areas and minor scarring may occur. The skin can lose pigment, sweat glands, and hair follicles. Therefore, cryosurgery is less desirable for dark skin and is not suggested for lesions at sites where alopecia (hair loss) would be a problem.

Perspective and Prospects

The first use of cryosurgery was in the early twentieth century through liquid air freezing for skin cancer treatment and cosmetic surgery. In the mid-1950s, improved cryotools began the expansion of cryosurgery to its modern state. This progress was enhanced by the availability of liquid nitrogen, which enabled clinicians to work at temperatures of -196 degrees Celsius.

Cryosurgery is a standard method used in cosmetic surgery and the treatment of skin cancers and is accepted for use with other cancers, including prostate, liver, pancreatic, uterine, lung, and brain cancers. Cryosurgery is employed alone and with other treatments (such as traditional surgery), or when other methods fail. After cryosurgery, many patients re-

gain a high quality of life and are pain-free. Moreover, they are often outpatients, spend little time in surgery, have short hospitalizations, and recuperate rapidly. Scarring is minimal, and cure rates are high.

Cryosurgery has side effects, though they are less severe than those of traditional surgery. In treatment of the liver, cryosurgery may damage bile ducts or blood vessels, causing hemorrhage or infection. In the treatment of prostate cancer, it may cause incontinence and impotence. The main disadvantage, unclear long-term value in internal cancer surgery, is sure to be addressed.

—*Sanford S. Singer, Ph.D.*

See also Cancer; Cervical procedures; Dermatology; Electrocauterization; Lesions; Melanoma; Moles; Prostate cancer; Skin; Skin cancer; Skin disorders; Skin lesion removal; Tumor removal; Tumors; Warts.

For Further Information:
"Cryosurgery in Cancer Treatment: Questions and Answers." *National Cancer Institute*, Sept. 10, 2003.
"Cryotherapy." *RadiologyInfo.org*. Radiological Society of North America, Aug. 10, 2012.
Dehn, Richard W., and David P. Asprey, eds. *Clinical Procedures for Physician Assistants*. Philadelphia: W. B. Saunders, 2002.
Jackson, Arthur, Graham Colver, and Rodney Dawber. *Cutaneous Cryosurgery: Principles and Clinical Practice*. 3d ed. New York: Taylor & Francis, 2006.
Korpan, Nikolai N., ed. *Basics of Cryosurgery*. New York: Springer, 2001.
Lask, Gary P., and Ronald L. Moy, eds. *Principles and Techniques of Cutaneous Surgery*. New York: McGraw-Hill, 1996.
Peterson, Elizabeth A., Michael J. Fucci. "Cardiac Catheter Cryoablation." *Health Library*, Nov. 26, 2012.
Vorvick, Linda J., and David Zieve. "Cryotherapy." *MedlinePlus*, Aug. 14, 2012.
Xu, Kecheng, Nikolai N. Korpan, and Lizhi Niu. *Modern Cryosurgery for Cancer*. Singapore: World Scientific, 2012.

CT SCANNING. *See* **COMPUTED TOMOGRAPHY (CT) SCANNING.**

CULDOCENTESIS
Procedure
Anatomy or system affected: Abdomen, reproductive system
Specialties and related fields: General surgery, gynecology
Definition: A diagnostic procedure in which fluid in the cul-de-sac of Douglas, the space behind the uterus and in front of the rectum, is removed using a needle inserted through the vagina.

Indications and Procedures

Culdocentesis is indicated in cases where a woman is suspected of having fluid in the abdomen or pelvis with an unclear cause. The patient may have an acutely painful and tender abdomen. Culdocentesis can identify the presence of fluid in the pelvis as well as distinguish whether the fluid is the result of active bleeding, infection, a perforated organ, or other causes.

For culdocentesis, the patient lies on her back with her legs in stirrups, as for a pelvic examination. A speculum is inserted into the vagina to visualize the cervix, and the cervix is gently lifted with a grasping instrument. A long, thin needle is inserted through the vagina, behind the cervix, and into the cul-de-sac of Douglas. Any fluid in this cul-de-sac is aspirated, and analysis of the fluid is subsequently performed.

Uses and Complications

Culdocentesis is not common, as noninvasive imaging modalities such as pelvic ultrasound with vaginal transducer have replaced this procedure to evaluate fluid collections in the abdomen and pelvis. Nevertheless, culdocentesis can yield useful information regarding the nature of abdominal or pelvic fluid, and hence it can assist in diagnosis and treatment decisions. For instance, nonclotted bloody fluid can be consistent with active bleeding, such as from a ruptured ectopic pregnancy or hemorrhagic ovarian cyst. Either of these conditions may require immediate surgery to stop the bleeding. The fluid aspirated from the cul-de-sac may be bile or bowel contents, indicating perforation of the gastrointestinal tract and possible need for urgent surgery. Infected fluid suggests pelvic inflammatory disease (PID) or abscess, for which surgery may not be the first line of treatment. Nonbloody, noninfected fluid may be caused by the rupture of a benign ovarian cyst, which would not require intervention.

Complications associated with culdocentesis are very rare. They include perforation of internal organs, such as the bowel or uterus, with the needle. In almost all cases, no serious aftereffects occur from these perforations, as the needle used is thin, but there are case reports of bleeding from organ perforations that require surgical intervention. Other examples of risks involved with culdocentesis are infection and bleeding from the puncture site.

—*Anne Lynn S. Chang, M.D.*

See also Abdomen; Abscess drainage; Abscesses; Cyst removal; Cysts; Ectopic pregnancy; Gynecology; Invasive tests; Pelvic inflammatory disease (PID); Rectum; Reproductive system; Uterus; Women's health.

For Further Information:

Doherty, Gerard M., and Lawrence W. Way, eds. *Current Surgical Diagnosis and Treatment.* 13th ed. New York: Lange Medical Books/McGraw-Hill, 2010.
Roberts, James R., et al. *Clinical Procedures in Emergency Medicine.* 5th ed. Philadelphia: Saunders/Elsevier, 2010.
Rock, John A., et al., eds. *Te Linde's Operative Gynecology.* 10th ed. Philadelphia: Lippincott Williams & Wilkins, 2011.
Stenchever, Morton A., et al. *Comprehensive Gynecology.* 5th ed. St. Louis, Mo.: Mosby, 2007.
Vorvick, Linda J. "Culdocentesis." *MedlinePlus*, February 26, 2012.

CUSHING'S SYNDROME
Disease/Disorder

Anatomy or system affected: Abdomen, back, blood, bones, endocrine system, glands, hair, muscles, skin
Specialties and related fields: Endocrinology, family medicine, immunology, internal medicine, nutrition, radiology, urology

Definition: A hormonal disorder caused primarily by chronic exposure of body tissues to excessive levels of cortisol.

Causes and Symptoms

Cushing's syndrome is a group of abnormalities that result from either excessive levels of hormones produced by the outer layer of the adrenal glands or the taking of steroid hormones. The primary source of the disorder is the hormone cortisol. This condition is typically triggered by an excess production of adrenocorticotropic hormone (ACTH) from the pituitary gland. ACTH in turn stimulates the adrenal glands to produce hormones, particularly cortisol. Excessive production of ACTH may result from a pituitary gland tumor or a tumor associated with other organs or as a side effect from taking steroid hormones used to treat asthma, rheumatoid arthritis, and other serious diseases. Adrenal gland tumors also produce excess amounts of cortisol. Though extremely rare, an inherited tendency to develop endocrine gland tumors is another cause of Cushing's syndrome.

Since the hormones produced by the adrenal glands regulate processes throughout the body, excess production can cause widespread disorders. Some of the more common symptoms of Cushing's syndrome are a rounded face, an obese trunk with thin arms and legs, fat pads over the neck and shoulders, purple stretch marks on the skin, easy bruising, muscle weakness, poor wound healing, fractures in weakened bones, high blood pressure, diabetes mellitus, emotional instability, and severe fatigue. Men can experience diminished desire for sex, while women may experience increased hairiness, acne, and decreased or absent menstrual periods. Children are usually obese, and their growth rate is slow.

Treatment and Therapy

Cushing's syndrome is treated by restoring the hormonal balance within the body, which may take several months. If Cushing's syndrome is left untreated, it can lead to death. The disease is diagnosed through blood and urine tests to determine excess amounts of cortisol. Pituitary tumors and tumors at other locations in the body that have been diagnosed as producing ACTH are surgically removed, when possible, or are treated with radiation or chemotherapy. Cortisol replacement therapy is provided after surgery until cortisol production resumes. Lifelong cortisol replacement therapy may be

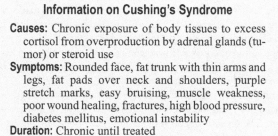

Information on Cushing's Syndrome

Causes: Chronic exposure of body tissues to excess cortisol from overproduction by adrenal glands (tumor) or steroid use
Symptoms: Rounded face, fat trunk with thin arms and legs, fat pads over neck and shoulders, purple stretch marks, easy bruising, muscle weakness, poor wound healing, fractures, high blood pressure, diabetes mellitus, emotional instability
Duration: Chronic until treated
Treatments: Restoration of hormonal balance, surgical removal of tumor, discontinuance of steroid use

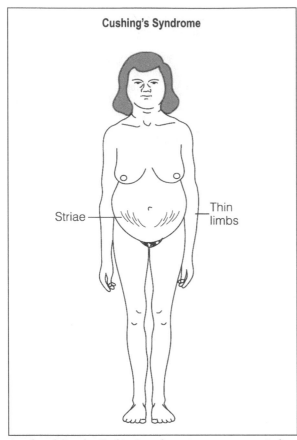

Cushing's Syndrome

Striae

Thin limbs

An adrenal disorder, Cushing's syndrome causes symptomatic fatty deposits, striae, and thin limbs and may be associated with a variety of mild to serious conditions.

necessary. If steroids are not being used to control a life-threatening illness, then their use should be discontinued.

Adrenal and pituitary tumors are always surgically removed. The remaining adrenal gland, which has usually diminished in size as a result of inactivity, will return to its normal size and function. As it is doing so, steroid hormones are administered to supply the needed cortisol and then tapered off over time. Some tumors may recur after surgical excision.

Perspective and Prospects

The first diagnosis of Cushing's syndrome was made by Harvey Cushing in 1912. In 1932, he linked the syndrome to an abnormality in the pituitary gland that stimulated an overproduction of cortisol from the adrenal glands; this condition is known as Cushing's disease. Pituitary tumors cause approximately 70 percent of cases of Cushing's syndrome. The syndrome is more common in women than in men, with most cases occurring between the ages of twenty-five and forty-five. The disease can be very serious, possibly even fatal, unless diagnosed and treated early.

—*Alvin K. Benson, Ph.D.; updated by*
Sharon W. Stark, R.N., A.P.R.N., D.N.Sc.

See also Addison's disease; Adrenal glands; Corticosteroids; Endocrine disorders; Endocrine glands; Endocrinology; Endocrinology, pediatric; Hormones; Tumors.

For Further Information:
A.D.A.M. Medical Encyclopedia. "Cushing Syndrome." *MedlinePlus*, December 11, 2011.
Badash, Michelle. "Cushing's Syndrome." *HealthLibrary*, May 1, 2013.
Fox, Stuart Ira. *Human Physiology*. 11th ed. Boston: McGraw-Hill, 2010.
Kronenberg, Henry M., et al., eds. *Williams Textbook of Endocrinology*. 11th ed. Philadelphia: Saunders/Elsevier, 2008.
National Endocrine and Metabolic Diseases Information Service. "Cushing's Syndrome." *National Institutes of Health*, April 6, 2012.

CUTIS MARMORATA TELANGIECTATICA CONGENITA
Disease/Disorder
Also known as: Van Lohuizen syndrome, congenital generalized phlebectasia, nevus vascularis reticularis, congenital phlebectasia, livedo telangiectatica, congenital livedo reticularis

Anatomy or system affected: Arms, blood vessels, brain, circulatory system, eyes, legs, nervous system, skin

Specialties and related fields: Dermatology, neonatology, neurology, ophthalmology, orthopedics, pediatrics, vascular medicine

Definition: Congenital abnormalities of the small blood vessels in the skin that are also usually associated with other congenital abnormalities.

Key terms:
capillaries: smallest of the body's blood vessels

hemangiomas: small, benign skin tumors that result from overgrowth of the endothelial cells that line the inside of blood vessels

nevus flammeus: a congenital malformation of that causes a pink, red or purplish spot on the skin; also known as a birthmark, port wine stain, or stork bite

phlebectasia: dilation of veins

telangiectasia: small, widened blood vessels in the skin

Information on
Cutis Marmorata Telangiectatica Congenita

Causes: Unknown

Symptoms: Skin mottling, atrophy, and ulcerations, blood vessels abnormalities, birthmarks and small skin growths, glaucoma, asymmetric limbs, neurologic abnormalities

Duration: Highly variable, but skin lesions usually fade in the first 3-5 years of life although more serious abnormalities may remain for a lifetime

Treatments: Orthopedic surgery for skeletal abnormalities, ophthalmologic surgery for eye problems, neurological consultation for neurological problems, but often no treatment is required

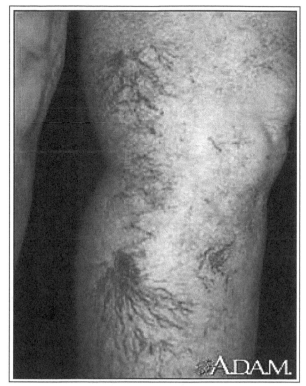

Essential telangiectasia often appears over the lower extremities, beginning in adolescence, and continuing throughout adult life. (Penn Medicine)

Causes and Symptoms

Cutis Marmorata Telangiectatica Congenita (CMTC) is a congenital, sporadic malformation of blood vessels characterized by red to purple net-like patches on the trunk, extremities, or face. Generally, these patches are present at birth or appear soon thereafter. These net-like patches do not disappear with warming, which distinguishes CMTC from cutis marmorata, in which the patches appear in a cold environment and disappear with warming. The cause and incidence of CMTC remain unknown.

Babies with CMTC also tend to have other abnormalities: 25-43 percent CMTC babies show body asymmetry in which one limb or one side of the face is larger than the other, while 15-37 percent has red to purple skin splotches that result from abnormal collections of capillaries (nevus flammeus) or small tumor-like outgrowths of blood vessels (hemangiomas). Other CMTC babies show dilated, varicose veins (phlebectasia), and almost 20 percent have red, flat marks that result from widened small blood vessels in the skin (telangiectasia). Approximately 6 percent have atrophy of the skin, particularly in the lower extremities, which results in skin ulcers or missing patches of skin (aplasia cutis). Other rarer conditions associated with CMTM include glaucoma and retinal detachment, fusion of the digits (syndactyly), cleft palate, hip malformation, clubfoot, underdevelopment of the kidneys (renal hypoplasia), and neurological abnormalities.

Treatment and Therapy

Usually treatment of CMTC is unnecessary, since the skin lesions tend to improve with time. The net-like patches and skin ulcers tend to disappear within the first 3-5 years of life.

More permanent abnormalities require treatment. Glaucoma and retinal detachment require ophthalmological intervention. Pulse-dye laser treatment effectively treats retinal detachments. Medicines that reduce intraocular pressure and eye surgeries that increase drainage in the eye (trabeculectomy) and subsequently reduce intraocular pressure can mitigate glaucoma. Skeletal abnormalities sometimes self-correct with time, but the more severe and persistent problems may require orthopedic surgeries for correction. Neurological abnormalities may require neurology consultations.

—*Michael A. Buratovich, Ph.D.*

See also Blood vessels; Dermatology; Dermopathology; Epidermal nevus syndromes; Neonatology; Neurology; Orthopedics; Pediatrics

For Further Information:
Calonje, J. Eduardo, Thomas Brenn, Alexander J. Lazar, and Phillip H. McKee. *McKee's Pathology of the Skin.* 4th ed. Philadelphia: Saunders, 2011.
Hook, Kristen P. "Cutaneous Vascular Anomalies in the Neonatal Period." *Seminars in Perinatology* 37, no. 1 (2013): 40-48.
Levy, Rebecca, and Joseph M. Lam. "Cutis Marmorata Telangiectatica Congenita: A Mimicker of a Common Disorder." *Canadian Medical Association Journal* 183, no. 4 (March 2011): E249-E251.

CYANOSIS
Disease/Disorder

Anatomy or system affected: Blood, skin
Specialties and related fields: Hematology, internal medicine, pulmonary medicine, toxicology
Definition: Dark blue discoloration of the skin and nail beds resulting from decreases in the oxygenation of hemoglobin in the red blood cells in the arteries.
Key terms:
arterial blood: blood from an artery receiving blood from the left ventricle; usually bright red
hemoglobin: the protein in red cells that combines reversibly with oxygen to form oxyhemoglobin; also referred to as reduced hemoglobin or deoxyhemoglobin
hemoglobin saturation: the portion of total hemoglobin that is combined with oxygen, usually expressed as a percentage
methemoglobin: oxidized hemoglobin, which is present

Information on Cyanosis

Causes: Inadequate oxygenation of hemoglobin in arterial blood from various injuries, illnesses, and disorders
Symptoms: Dark blue discoloration of skin and nails
Duration: Chronic until treated
Treatments: Oxygen administration, treatment of underlying disorder

normally as up to 1 percent of total hemoglobin; it does not combine reversibly rapidly with oxygen and cannot serve in oxygen transport

oxyhemoglobin: a reversibly oxygenated form of hemoglobin

sulfhemoglobin: the reaction product of hemoglobin with certain toxic agents (oxidants)

venous blood: blood from a vein conducting blood to the right ventricle, before passage through the lungs

Causes and Symptoms

Cyanosis, a dark blue discoloration of the skin and nail beds, is a sign of a disorder, not a disease in itself, and it may have several causes. It is also not a symptom sensed by a patient but a physical finding. To appear, cyanosis requires a concentration in arterial blood of 4 to 5 grams per deciliter of reduced hemoglobin. Anemic patients may not show cyanosis even though their hemoglobin saturations are low. Its presence indicates one or more of the following: inadequate oxygenation of arterial blood (a decrease of oxygen saturation to 85 percent or less), the presence of a normal constituent (methemoglobin) in increased concentration, or the presence of an abnormal constituent (sulfhemoglobin).

Inadequate oxygenation of normally circulating blood. The obstruction of large airways (the tracheobronchial system) can occur from external compression or the aspiration of solid or semisolid materials (foodstuffs, particularly ground meat). Laryngospasm may be a factor. The aspiration of aqueous fluids, as in drowning in freshwater, can fill the alveoli and decrease or prevent the contact of inspired air with the blood in the pulmonary capillaries. Freshwater can pass rapidly into the blood and eventually free the alveoli for gas exchanges. Drowning in seawater is usually accompanied by marked laryngospasm. If the hypertonic seawater reaches the alveoli, then water will cross from the blood into the alveoli and produce even more fluid and froth in the lungs (pulmonary edema).

The inhalation of certain toxic agents, available industrially or used in warfare, can damage the alveoli and the pulmonary capillaries and produce pulmonary edema. Typical agents are chlorine and phosgene. Smoke inhalation is another possible cause of lung damage. Pulmonary edema from cardiac failure can occur as a result of increased pressure in the alveolar capillaries. Respiratory distress syndrome, or noncardiogenic pulmonary edema, occurs probably as the end result of a variety of initiators (shock, sepsis) culminating in the production of damaging free radicals.

Pharmacologically active agents such as heroin and morphine injected intravenously, as by drug abusers, can produce fulminating pulmonary edema extremely rapidly, possibly as the result of alpha-adrenergic discharge. Substances such as ethchlorvynol can also produce this condition if injected intravenously, although they may be innocuous if taken orally.

Pulmonary infections such as pneumococcal pneumonia can cause edema through the perfusion of alveoli that are filled with fluid, that is, nonventilated. This condition is essentially venous admixture, and it can occur when three or more lobes of the lungs are involved. Chronic obstructive pulmonary disease (COPD) can produce cyanosis because of destruction of lung tissue (emphysema) and because of obstruction to air movement. Oxygenation is incomplete, and cyanosis is a common feature of advanced disease.

Low oxygen concentration in ambient atmosphere occurs with ascent to high altitudes. In certain caves, oxygen may be displaced by carbon dioxide. Incorrect gas mixtures may be administered to patients under anesthesia or on artificial respiration. The oxygen of the ambient atmosphere may be decreased in closed environments such as submarines. Polycythemia (increased numbers of red blood cells per unit volume of blood) may occur as a result of chronic exposure to high altitudes or as a spontaneous problem (polycythemia vera). The oxygen content of the blood may be normal or high, but the unoxygenated portion may be increased so that a ruddy cyanosis may be present.

Admixture of venous and arterial blood flows. Patent ductus arteriosus is a heart defect that produces blue baby syndrome. It offers a classic example of the direct entry of venous blood into the arterial system, as the lungs are partially bypassed. Other cardiopulmonary abnormalities, such as right-to-left shunts, can also produce cyanosis.

Localized circulatory problems. Frostbite and Raynaud's phenomenon are examples of localized occurrence of cyanosis. In these conditions, vascular changes limit blood flow, leading to congestion and unsaturation.

Increased concentrations of methemoglobin or sulfhemoglobin. Naturally occurring methemoglobin is present at about the 1 percent level in blood. From 0.5 to 3 percent of the total hemoglobin is oxidized each day and returned to deoxyhemoglobin through enzymatic reductase activity. In congenital forms of methemoglobinemia, cyanosis appears when the concentration of methemoglobin approaches 10 percent of the total (about 1.4 grams per deciliter).

Acquired increased concentration can be caused by a variety of agents (such as sodium perchlorate, Paraquat, nitroglycerine, and inhaled butyl and isobutyl nitrites) by oxidizing hemoglobin to methemoglobin through the formation of free radicals. Nitrates, absorbed by mouth, are transformed into nitrites in the gut and also produce methemoglobin. Sulfhemoglobin can also be formed and produces cyanosis at concentrations of 0.5 gram per deciliter.

Treatment and Therapy

Treatment is directed not to the cyanosis itself but to the underlying problem. Oxygen administration is crucial in many but not all cases.

For airway obstruction, the Heimlich maneuver may be lifesaving, as may an emergency tracheostomy. Drowning requires artificial respiration, positioning of the body so that drainage of fluid from the lungs is facilitated, and administration of oxygen, if available. Full cardiopulmonary resuscitation (CPR) may be needed. Pulmonary edema from cardiac failure or respiratory distress syndrome calls into use a variety of approaches, but oxygen is almost always provided. Artificial respiration and oxygen are usually required in heroin, morphine, and ethchlorvynol pulmonary edema. COPD and emphysema are chronic, progressive disorders in which oxygen, bronchodilators, antibiotics, steroids, and surgical interventions (lung volume reduction) may be used. In methemoglobinemia, the congenital forms may not require any treatment. If the cyanosis is the result of exposure to nitrites and other potential oxidants, then methylene blue is usually effective.

Perspective and Prospects

Cyanosis has been recognized for centuries as a sign or indicator of an underlying problem. The focus of investigations has been on identifying these problems. The properties of the hemoglobins have been investigated by physiologists and hematologists, leading to an understanding of their structures and functions. Surgical correction of the vascular abnormalities of so-called blue babies by Alfred Blalock and Helen Taussig led to the development of the field of cardiovascular surgery. Molecular biology has provided knowledge of the enzymatic and genetic factors involved in the development of methemoglobinemia.

—Francis P. Chinard, M.D.

See also Accidents; Altitude sickness; Asphyxiation; Blood and blood disorders; Blue baby syndrome; Cardiac surgery; Cardiology; Cardiology, pediatric; Choking; Chronic obstructive pulmonary disease (COPD); Circulation; Congenital heart disease; Edema; Emphysema; Frostbite; Heart; Heart failure; Heimlich maneuver; Hyperbaric oxygen therapy; Lungs; Poisoning; Pneumonia; Pulmonary diseases; Pulmonary medicine; Pulmonary medicine, pediatric; Respiration; Respiratory distress syndrome; Toxicology; Vascular system.

For Further Information:

A.D.A.M. Medical Encyclopedia. "Cyanotic Heart Disease." *MedlinePlus*, November 21, 2011.

A.D.A.M. Medical Encyclopedia. "Skin Discoloration-Bluish." *MedlinePlus*, May 25, 2011.

Dickerson, Richard E., and Irving Geis. *Hemoglobin: Structure, Function, Evolution, and Pathology.* Menlo Park, Calif.: Benjamin/Cummings, 1983.

Heart Information Center. "Cyanosis." *Texas Heart Institute*, August 2012.

Icon Health. *Cyanosis: A Medical Dictionary, Bibliography, and Annotated Research Guide to Internet References.* San Diego, Calif.: Author, 2004.

Nagel, Ronald L., ed. *Hemoglobin Disorders: Molecular Methods and Protocols.* Totowa, N.J.: Humana Press, 2003.

Weibel, Ewald R. *The Pathway for Oxygen: Structure and Function in the Mammalian Respiratory System.* Cambridge, Mass.: Harvard University Press, 1984.

CYST REMOVAL

Procedure

Anatomy or system affected: Breasts, genitals, glands, joints, reproductive system, skin

Specialties and related fields: Dermatology, general surgery, gynecology, plastic surgery

Definition: A surgical procedure to remove a fluid-filled nodule, performed in a physician's office or a hospital depending on the type and location of the cyst.

Key terms:

aspirate: to remove a substance using suction; a cyst can be aspirated using a needle and syringe to withdraw its contents

cyst: a sac containing a fluid or semifluid substance

incision: a cut made with a scalpel during a surgical procedure

laparoscope: a small surgical tube which can be inserted through a small incision into the abdominal cavity to view and perform surgery on abdominal organs

Indications and Procedures

Many types of cysts can develop in the body. The vast majority of them are noncancerous, although in rare cases small areas of cancerous tissue may be found within a cyst. The indications and procedures for removing cysts depend on the type of cyst, its location, and whether it is causing symptoms. Examples of common types of cysts are Baker's, Bartholin's, ovarian, sebaceous, thyroglossal, and breast cysts.

Baker's cysts are small lumps that form behind the knee. Fluid-filled sacs found around joints, known as "bursas," normally protect the moving joint from causing damage to overlying skin, tendons, and muscles. When the bursas behind the knee accumulate excess fluid, they can expand and form a Baker's cyst. This fluid accumulation often occurs if the knee is arthritic. Physicians usually apply pressure bandages to reduce the bursal swelling. If this does not work, then the cyst must be excised surgically.

Bartholin's gland cysts are formed when the Bartholin's glands found in the external female genitalia (specifically the vulva) become occluded and swollen with fluid. Infections can occur in the ducts of these glands, causing pain and scarring. Bartholin's cysts are treated with conservative measures such as warm water soaks, antibiotics, and placement of a catheter, which continuously drains the cyst. If these methods fail, then the cyst may be incised in the operating room and then marsupialized, a procedure that sutures the inner cyst wall to the vulval skin and keeps the cyst open and draining.

Ovarian cysts do not usually need to be removed, and many of them are physiologic and come and go with the menstrual cycle. When an ovarian cyst becomes large (greater than 6 centimeters in diameter), it may cause the ovary to twist, a condition called "ovarian torsion." A twisted ovary is at risk for necrosis, since its blood supply is cut off. In this case, the ovarian cyst needs to be removed. Other reasons for removing an ovarian cyst include a cyst that is persistent and growing with time and a cyst with characteristics upon ultrasound examination that suggest malignancy.

If an ovarian cyst is thought to be noncancerous, then it can usually be removed through the abdomen using a laparoscope. The laparoscope enables visualization of the cyst, while manipulation of the ovary and cyst is accomplished through incisions and tools placed on the sides of the abdomen. The cyst is usually shelled out from the remainder of the ovary using blunt dissection, and the remaining ovary is inspected for areas of bleeding, which may be cauterized. Many patients do not need to be hospitalized if the surgery is straightforward. If there is a concern about cancer within an ovarian cyst, then an open abdominal surgery is indicated. In this case, the abdomen is opened surgically and the cyst is removed, along with any other abnormal-appearing tissue surrounding the cyst.

A sebaceous cyst may develop when a duct from a sebaceous gland in the skin becomes blocked and the oily fluid is unable to escape. These glands, which are associated with hair follicles, secrete sebum to lubricate the hair and skin. If the sebaceous cyst is very large or infected with bacteria, then surgical removal is usually indicated. This operation can be done in a physician's office under local anesthesia. A small incision is made in the skin, and the entire cyst is removed or drained. The complete wall of the cyst is removed in order to prevent recurrence. A few sutures are usually placed to close the wound.

Thyroglossal cysts usually arise because of a congenital defect in which the duct that connects the base of the tongue to the thyroid gland fails to disappear. If a cyst develops in this area, a noticeable swelling will occur above the thyroid cartilage (Adam's apple). This cyst nearly always becomes infected and thus should be removed surgically. This procedure involves an incision just above the thyroid cartilage and gland. The surgeon then separates surrounding tissue up to the base of the tongue to gain access to the cyst. The cyst can then be removed and the skin sutured.

Breast cysts are common and can come and go with the menstrual cycle. They are usually detected as a breast lump on physical examination. If they are persistent, then they can be visualized on ultrasound (or mammogram) to confirm that they are fluid filled (rather than solid, which could be indicative of cancer). Breast cysts can be drained using a needle and the fluid sent for pathological analysis. If the fluid is benign, then no further procedures are indicated.

Uses and Complications

The uses of cyst removal in general are to relieve pain and discomfort, minimize the chance of infection, and preserve the normal anatomy and function of surrounding organs. In addition, the cyst can be sent for pathological analysis after it is removed, in order to determine if any portions suggest cancer.

Complications common to all cyst removal procedures include bleeding at the site where the cyst has been removed, damage to organ structures surrounding the cyst during the excision process, and risk of infection from the excision procedure itself, as foreign instruments are introduced into the field. Another complication is that the cysts may recur, necessitating further intervention. In addition, each type of cyst removal has its own specific risks. For instance, thyroglossal cyst removal surgery may inadvertently remove thyroid tissue, which can lead to thyroid hormone deficiency and the need for thyroid medication for hormone replacement.

—*Matthew Berria, Ph.D.,*
and Douglas Reinhart, M.D.;
updated by Anne Lynn S. Chang, M.D.

See also Abscess drainage; Abscesses; Biopsy; Breast biopsy; Breast disorders; Breasts, female; Colorectal polyp removal; Colorectal sur-gery; Cysts; Dermatology; Fibrocystic breast condition; Ganglion removal; Genital disorders, female; Glands; Gynecology; Hydroceles; Laparoscopy; Myomectomy; Nasal polyp removal; Ovarian cysts; Ovaries; Polyps; Reproductive system; Skin; Skin disorders; Skin lesion removal.

For Further Information:

A.D.A.M. Medical Encyclopedia. "Cyst." *MedlinePlus*, November 20, 2012.
Doherty, Gerard M., and Lawrence W. Way, eds. *Current Surgical Diagnosis and Treatment*. 12th ed. New York: Lange Medical Books/McGraw-Hill, 2006.
Icon Health. *Ovarian Cysts: A Medical Dictionary, Bibliography, and Annotated Research Guide to Internet References*. San Diego, Calif.: Icon Health, 2004.
Kasper, Dennis L., et al., eds. *Harrison's Principles of Internal Medicine*. 18th ed. 2 vols. New York: McGraw-Hill, 2011.
Moynihan, Timothy J. "Tumor vs. Cyst: What's the Difference?." *Mayo Foundation for Medical Education and Research*, January 11, 2011.
Tierney, Lawrence M., Stephen J. McPhee, and Maxine A. Papadakis, eds. *Current Medical Diagnosis and Treatment 2013*. New York: McGraw-Hill Medical, 2013.

CYSTIC FIBROSIS

Disease/Disorder

Anatomy or system affected: Chest, lungs, respiratory system, most bodily systems

Specialties and related fields: Genetics, neonatology, pediatrics, pulmonary medicine

Definition: A disease that affects the exocrine glands and, secondarily, most physical systems, resulting in death usually between the ages of sixteen and thirty.

Key terms:

chloride transport: the movement of one of the ions found in ordinary salt across a membrane from the inside of a cell to the outside; this transport is common in human cells and is critical for many important metabolic functions

cystic fibrosis transmembrane-conductance regulator (CFTR): the protein product of the cystic fibrosis gene and a chloride transport channel

meconium ileus: the puttylike plug found in the intestines of some cystic fibrosis babies when they are born

mutation: an alteration in the deoxyribonucleic acid (DNA) sequence of a gene, which usually leads to the production of a nonfunctional enzyme or protein and thus a lack of a normal metabolic function

recessive genetic disease: a disease caused by mutated genes that must be inherited from both parents for that individual to show its symptoms

secretory epithelium: tissues or groups of cells that have the ability to move substances, such as chloride ions, from the inside of cells to a duct or tube

Causes and Symptoms

Genetic diseases are inherited rather than caused by any specific injury or infectious agent. Thus, unlike many other types of diseases, genetic diseases range throughout a person's lifetime and often begin to exert their debilitating effects prior to

Information on Cystic Fibrosis

Causes: Genetic defect
Symptoms: Severe malnutrition, production of bulky stools, chronic respiratory infections, constant coughing, compromised fertility
Duration: Chronic and progressive
Treatments: Alleviation of symptoms with dietary supplements, balanced diet, backslapping to break up mucus, antibiotics

birth. Since in many cases the primary defect or underlying cause of the disease is unknown, treatment is difficult or impossible and is usually restricted to treating the symptoms of the disease. Genetic diseases include sickle cell disease, thalassemia, Tay-Sachs disease, and cystic fibrosis (also known as CF).

In each disease, a specific normal function is missing because of a mutation in the individual's genes. Genes are sequences of deoxyribonucleic acid (DNA) contained on the chromosomes of an individual that are passed to the next generation via ova and sperm. Usually, the primary defect in a genetic disease is the inability to produce a normal enzyme, the class of proteins used to speed up, or catalyze, the chemical reactions that are necessary for cells to function. A mutation in a gene may not allow the production of a necessary enzyme; therefore, some element of metabolism is missing from an individual with such a mutation. This lack of function leads to the symptoms associated with a genetic disease, such as the lack of insulin production in juvenile diabetes or the inability of the blood to clot in hemophilia. In the 1940s and 1950s, when the understanding of basic cellular metabolism made clear the relationship between mutant genes and lack of enzyme function, the modern definition of genetic disease came into routine medical use.

Cystic fibrosis, one such genetic disease, has several major effects on an individual. These effects begin before birth, extend into early childhood, and become progressively more serious as the affected individual ages. The primary diagnosis for the disease is a very simple test that looks for excessive saltiness in perspiration. Although the higher level of salt in the perspiration is not life threatening, the associated symptoms are. Because these other symptoms may vary from one individual to the next, the perspiration test is a very useful early diagnostic tool.

Major symptoms of cystic fibrosis include the blockage of several important internal ducts. This blockage occurs because the cystic fibrosis mutation has a critical effect on the ability of certain internal tissues called secretory epithelia to transport normal amounts of salt and water across their surfaces. These epithelia are often found in the ducts that contribute to the digestive and reproductive systems.

The blockage of ducts resulting from the production and export of overly viscous secretions reduces the delivery of digestive enzymes from the pancreas to the intestine; thus, proteins in the intestine are only partly digested. Fat-emulsifying compounds, called bile salts, are often blocked as well on their route from the pancreas to the intestine, so the digestion of fats is often incomplete. These two conditions often occur prior to birth. Approximately 10 to 20 percent of newborns with cystic fibrosis have a puttylike plug of undigested material in their intestines called the meconium ileus. This plug prevents the normal movement of foods through the digestive system and can be very serious.

Because of their overall inefficiency of digestion, young children with cystic fibrosis can seem to be eating quite normally yet remain severely undernourished. They often produce bulky, foul-smelling stools as a result of the high propor-

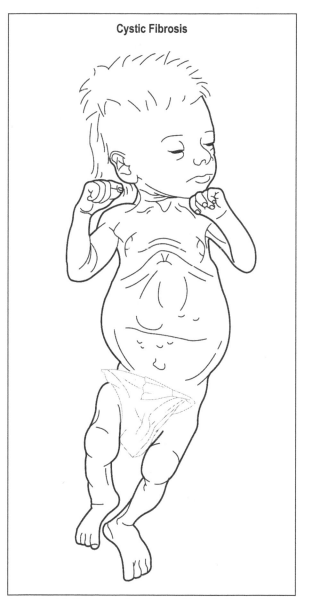

Cystic Fibrosis

Approximately 10 percent of newborns with cystic fibrosis have a puttylike plug of undigested material in their intestines called the meconium ileus, which results in emaciation with a distended abdomen.

tion of undigested material. This symptom serves as an indicator of the progress of the disease, as such digestive problems often increase as the affected child ages.

As individuals with cystic fibrosis grow older, their respiratory problems increase because of the secretion of a thick mucus on the inner lining of the lungs. This viscous material traps white blood cells that release their contents when they rupture, which makes the mucus all the more thick and viscous. The affected individuals constantly cough in an attempt to remove this material. Of greater importance is that the mucus forms an ideal breeding ground for many types of pathogenic bacteria, and the affected individual suffers from continual respiratory infections. Male patients are almost always infertile as a result of the blockage of the ducts of the reproductive system, while female fertility is sometimes reduced as well.

Traditional treatments for cystic fibrosis have improved an individual's chance of survival and have dramatically affected the quality of life. In the 1950s, a child with cystic fibrosis usually lived only a year or two. Thus, cystic fibrosis was originally described as a children's disease and was intensively studied only by pediatricians. Today, aggressive medical intervention has increased survival rates dramatically. Affected individuals are treated with a package of therapies designed to alleviate the most severe symptoms of the disease, and taken together, these therapies have allowed many patients with cystic fibrosis to live well into adulthood. It is difficult to calculate an average life expectancy for individuals with cystic fibrosis, as data from some regions is largely unavailable. In addition, life expectancy varies greatly depending on the age at which a patient was diagnosed, the extent of medical care available, and various environmental factors. Individuals with access to the necessary treatments may live into middle age.

The available treatments, however, do not constitute a cure for the disease. The major roadblock to developing a cure was that the primary genetic defect remained unknown. All that was clear until the mid-1980s was that many of the secretory epithelia had a problem transporting salt and water. By the late 1980s, the defect was further restricted to a problem in the transport of chloride ions, one of the two constituents of ordinary salt and a critical chemical in many important cellular processes. Because individuals who had severe forms of cystic fibrosis could still live, however, this function was deemed important but not absolutely essential for survival. Furthermore, only certain tissues and organs in the body seemed to show abnormal functions in a cystic fibrosis patient, while other organs-the heart, brain, and nerves-seemed to function normally. Thus, the defect was not uniform.

The pattern of inheritance of cystic fibrosis was relatively easy to determine. The disease acts as a recessive trait. Humans, like most animals, have two copies of each gene: one that is inherited on a chromosome from the egg, and the other on a similar chromosome from the sperm. There is a gene in all humans that controls some normal cellular function related to the transport of chloride from the inside of a cell to the outside. If this function is missing or impaired, the individual

shows the symptoms of cystic fibrosis.

A recessive trait is one that must be inherited from both the mother and the father in order to take effect. Inheriting only a single copy of the mutation from one parent does not have a deleterious effect on an individual, who would not demonstrate any of the disease symptoms. Such a person, however, is a carrier of the disease and can still pass that mutation on to his or her own children. Thus, genetic diseases caused by recessive mutations, such as cystic fibrosis, can remain hidden in a family for many generations. When two carriers of the disease procreate, their children may be born with the disease. The rules of genetics, as first described by Gregor Mendel in the nineteenth century, predict that in such a union, approximately one in four children will have cystic fibrosis. Another one-fourth will not have the mutated gene, and the remaining half will be carriers of the disease like their parents. Because the production of eggs and sperm involves a random shuffling of genes and chromosomes, however, the occurrence of unaffected individuals, carriers, and affected individuals cannot be predicted; only average probabilities can be discussed.

Treatment and Therapy

The treatment of cystic fibrosis typically focuses on preventing or delaying lung damage and optimizing growth and nutrition. Traditional treatments usually include dietary supplements that contain the digestive enzymes and bile salts that cannot pass through the blocked ducts; these must be taken daily. Individuals with cystic fibrosis are also placed on balanced diets to ensure proper nutrition despite their difficulties in digesting fats and proteins. One characteristic of cystic fibrosis treatment is the long daily ritual of backslapping, which is designed to help break up the thick mucus in the lungs; individuals with cystic fibrosis may also use high-frequency chest wall oscillation vests for the same purpose. Aggressive antibiotic therapy can keep infections of the lungs from forming or spreading. In the 1990s, an additional therapy was begun using a special enzyme that can break down DNA in the lung mucus when inhaled. Many white blood cells rupture while trapped in the thick mucus lining of the lungs, and the release of their DNA adds to the high viscosity of the mucus. Genetically engineered deoxyribonuclease (DNase), an enzyme produced from bacteria, has been found to be helpful in degrading this extra DNA, thus making it easier to break up and cough out the mucus found in the lungs of affected patients.

Another treatment approach for cystic fibrosis focused on determining the nature of the primary genetic defect. The ultimate goal was to determine which of the thousands of human genes was the one that, when defective, led to cystic fibrosis. Once accomplished, the next step would be to determine the normal function of this gene so that therapies designed to replace this function could be developed.

The classic approach to studying any genetic phenomenon involves mapping the gene. First, it must be determined which of a human's twenty-three chromosomes contains the DNA that makes up the gene. By studying the inheritance of the disease, along with other human traits, researchers located the gene on chromosome number 7. To localize the gene more precisely, however, modern molecular techniques had to be applied. Success came when two independent groups announced that they had identified the location of the gene in 1989. The groups were led by Lap-Chee Tsui of the Hospital for Sick Children in Toronto, Canada, and Francis Collins of the University of Michigan in Ann Arbor. The groups not only located the exact chromosomal location of the gene but also purified the gene from the vast amount of DNA in a human cell so that it could be studied in isolation. Then the structure of the normal form of the gene was compared to the DNA structure found in individuals with the disease.

DNA from more than thirty thousand individuals with cystic fibrosis was analyzed, and to the surprise of most, more than 230 differences between the mutated genes and normal genes were found. Although about 70 percent of the affected individuals did have a single type of DNA difference or mutation, the other 30 percent had a tremendous variety of differences. Thus, unlike sickle cell disease, which seems to be attributable to the same defect in every affected individual, cystic fibrosis is based on a widely varying group of differences, which accounts for the range in severity of its symptoms. More important, this enormous diversity of defects makes developing a single, simple DNA-based screening procedure difficult. The only thing that all these individuals had in common was that, in each case, the same gene and gene product were affected.

Tsui's and Collins's groups, as well as several others, tried to determine the normal function of the protein that was coded by the cystic fibrosis gene. This protein was called cystic fibrosis transmembrane-conductance regulator (CFTR) because it was soon shown to create a channel or passage by which cells move chloride ions across their membranes. In an individual with cystic fibrosis, this channel does not work properly; both the salt and the water balance of the affected cell, and ultimately of the whole tissue, is disturbed. The thick mucus buildup in the lungs is a direct consequence of this disturbance, as is the high salt concentration in the patient's perspiration.

Remarkably, CFTR is an enormous protein that is embedded in the membrane of cells found in the lungs, pancreas, and reproductive tracts. CFTR contains 1,480 amino acids linked end to end. The CFTR found in 70 percent of individuals with cystic fibrosis contains the same amino acids as normal genes, with one exception: the 508th amino acid found in a normal individual is missing. Thus, the extensive debilitating symptoms of this disease result from the mere omission of one amino acid from a long chain containing 1,479 identical ones. The other mutations affect different parts of this protein and, in all cases, reduce the ability of the CFTR protein to carry out its normal function.

In the cases of several other genetic diseases, screening programs have been developed to help patients make informed choices about having children. For Tay-Sachs disease, a fatal neurological disease found in 1 in 3,600 Ashke-nazi Jews, a screening program coupled with a strong educational program combined to reduce the incidence of the disease from approximately one hundred births a year in the 1970s to an average of thirteen by the early 1980s. Similar screening programs have been developed for a rare genetic disease called phenylketonuria (PKU). A screening program for cystic fibrosis, however, would be much more difficult for several reasons.

First, the population at risk for cystic fibrosis is much larger; hence, the costs and scope of the program would be enormous. Second, since there are many different mutations that can affect the gene responsible for causing cystic fibrosis, it may not be easy to develop a simple test that could detect this enormous variation accurately without missing affected individuals or falsely concluding that some normal individuals are affected. Finally, the symptoms shown by individuals affected with cystic fibrosis range from quite severe to very mild, thus making it even more difficult to provide definitive genetic counseling. For such counseling to be truly effective, large numbers of individuals from groups known to be at risk for the disease would have to undergo screening and counseling. Furthermore, a prenatal diagnostic test would need to be available to allow couples at risk to ascertain with some degree of certainty whether any particular child is going to be born with the disease. Developing these tests and coupling them with widely available, low-cost counseling remain major challenges to the medical community.

Therapies for cystic fibrosis, like those for any genetic disease, once consisted solely of ways to treat the symptoms. Since every cell in the affected individual lacked a particular metabolic function as a result of the disease, there was no easy way to replace these functions. For cystic fibrosis, this problem was exacerbated by the lack of understanding of the primary defect. The work of Tsui's and Collins's teams allowed a more direct assault on the actual defect. Gene therapy involves either replacing a defective gene with a normal one in affected cells or adding an additional copy or copies of the normal gene to affected cells, in an attempt to restore the same functional enzymes and thus reestablish a normal metabolic process. In the case of cystic fibrosis, animal studies have shown that it is possible to produce normal lung function when either genes or genetically engineered viruses containing normal genes are sprayed into the lungs of affected animals. Yet since there is no similar direct route for getting engineered viruses or purified genes to the pancreas or reproductive system, because of their location deep within the body, other procedures will need to be developed. In the case of the lung cells, only those cells that actually receive the purified gene change, becoming normal. Since the cells lining the lung are continuously being replenished, lung gene therapy would need to be an ongoing process.

Perspective and Prospects

Patients with the symptoms of cystic fibrosis were first described in medical records dating back to the eighteenth century. The disease was initially called mucoviscidosis and later cystic fibrosis of the pancreas. It was not clear that these symptoms were related to a single specific disease, however, until the work of Dorothy Anderson of Columbia University in the late 1930s. Anderson studied a large number of cases of persons who died with similar lung and pancreas problems. She noticed that siblings were sometimes affected and thus suspected that the disease had a genetic cause. Anderson was responsible for naming the disease on the basis of the fibrous cysts on the pancreas that she often saw in autopsies performed on affected individuals.

Because treatment of cystic fibrosis is largely confined to managing the disease's symptoms, a premium has been placed on the development of inexpensive and accurate diagnostic procedures, which along with good genetic counseling could greatly reduce the incidence of cystic fibrosis in the population. Yet, since carriers experience no symptoms and often do not realize that they are indeed carrying the gene, conventional genetic counseling cannot easily reduce the incidence of the mutation in human populations at risk. Only the widespread use of a DNA-based diagnostic procedure could serve to identify the large population of carriers, but even then, since three-fourths of the children of two carriers would not have the disease, counseling would be fraught with severe ethical problems. Why such a deleterious gene exists in such high frequencies in the population remains a mystery.

—*Joseph G. Pelliccia, Ph.D.*

See also Birth defects; Congenital disorders; Coughing; Genetic counseling; Genetic diseases; Lungs; Respiration; Wheezing.

For Further Information:

A.D.A.M. Medical Encyclopedia. "Cystic Fibrosis." *MedlinePlus*, May 16, 2012.

A.D.A.M. Medical Encyclopedia. "Neonatal Cystic Fibrosis Screening." *MedlinePlus*, May 16, 2012.

Carson-DeWitt, Rosalyn. "Cystic Fibrosis (CF)." *HealthLibrary*, November 26, 2012.

Cystic Fibrosis Foundation (CFF). http://www.cff.org.

Harris, Ann, and Anne H. Thompson. *Cystic Fibrosis: The Facts*. 4th ed. New York: Oxford University Press, 2008.

Kepron, Wayne. *Cystic Fibrosis: Everything You Need to Know*. Buffalo, N.Y.: Firefly Books, 2004.

Orenstein, David. *Cystic Fibrosis: A Guide for Patient and Family*. 3d ed. Philadelphia: Lippincott Williams & Wilkins, 2004.

Parker, James N., and Philip M. Parker, eds. *The Official Patient's Sourcebook on Cystic Fibrosis*. Rev. ed. San Diego, Calif.: Icon Health, 2002.

Pierce, Benjamin A. *The Family Genetic Sourcebook*. New York: John Wiley & Sons, 1990.

Tsui, Lap-Chee. "Cystic Fibrosis, Molecular Genetics." In *The Encyclopedia of Human Biology*, edited by Renato Dulbecco. 2d ed. Vol. 2. New York: Academic Press, 1997.

US Congress. Office of Technology Assessment. *Cystic Fibrosis and DNA Tests: Implications of Carrier Screening*. Washington, D.C.: Government Printing Office, 1992.

US Congress. Office of Technology Assessment. *Genetic Counseling and Cystic Fibrosis Carrier Screening: Results of a Survey-Background Paper*. Washington, D.C.: Government Printing Office, 1992.

Yankaskas, James R., and Michael R. Knowles, eds. *Cystic Fibrosis in Adults*. Philadelphia: Lippincott-Raven, 1999.

Cystitis

Disease/Disorder

Anatomy or system affected: Bladder, urinary system

Specialties and related fields: Bacteriology, gynecology, urology

Definition: An inflammation of the bladder, primarily caused by bacteria and resulting in pain, a sense of urgency to urinate, and sometimes hematuria (blood in the urine).

Key terms:

cytoscopy: a minor operation performed so that the urologist can examine the bladder

dysuria: painful urination, usually as a result of infection or an obstruction; the patient complains of a burning sensation when voiding

Escherichia coli: bacteria found in the intestines that may cause disease elsewhere

hematuria: the abnormal presence of blood in the urine

perineum: the short bridge of flesh between the anus and vagina in women and the anus and base of the penis in men

ureters: the two tubes that carry urine from the kidneys to the bladder

urethra: the tube carrying urine from the bladder to outside the body

Causes and Symptoms

The term "cystitis" is a combination of two Greek words: *kistis*, meaning hollow pouch, sac, or bladder, and *itis*, meaning inflammation. Cystitis is often used generically to refer to any nonspecific inflammation of the lower urinary tract. Specifically, however, it should be used to refer to inflammation and infection of the bladder. Three true symptoms denote cystitis: dysuria, frequent urination, and hematuria.

The symptoms of cystitis may appear abruptly and, often, painfully. One of the trademark symptoms signaling an onset is dysuria (burning or stinging during urination). It may precede or coincide with an overwhelming urge to urinate, although the amount passed may be extremely small. In addition, some sufferers may experience nocturia (sleep disturbance because of a need to urinate). In many cases there may be pus in the urine. Origination of hematuria (blood in the urine), which often occurs with cystitis, may be within the bladder wall, in the urethra, or even in the upper urinary tract. These painful symptoms should be enough to spur one to seek medical attention; if left untreated, the bacteria may progress up the ureters to the kidneys, where a much more serious infection, pyelonephritis, may develop. Pyelonephritis can cause scarring of the kidney tissue and even life-threatening kidney failure. Usually kidney infections are accompanied by chills, high fever, nausea or vomiting, and back pain that may radiate downward.

Acute cystitis can be divided into two groups. One is when infection occurs with irregularity and with no recent history of antibiotic treatments. This type is commonly caused by the bacteria *Escherichia coli*. Types of bacteria other than *E. coli* that can cause cystitis are *Proteus*, *Klebsiella*, *Pseudomonas*, *Streptococcus*, *Enterobacter*, and, rarely, *Staphylococcus*.

Information on Cystitis

Causes: Bacterial infection
Symptoms: Pain and burning upon urination, sense of urgency to urinate, sometimes blood in urine
Duration: Acute
Treatments: Antibiotics

The second group of sufferers have undergone antibiotic treatment; those bacteria not affected by the antibiotics can cause infection. Most urinary tract infections are precipitated by the patient's own rectal flora. Once bacteria enter the bladder, whether they will cause infection depends on how many bacteria are present, how well the bacteria can adhere to the bladder wall, and how strongly the bladder can defend itself. The bladder's inherent defense system is the most important of the factors.

One of the natural defense mechanisms employed by the bladder is the flushing provided by regular urination at frequent intervals. If fluid intake is sufficient-most urologists consider this amount to be sixty-four ounces daily-there will be regular and efficient emptying of the bladder, which can wash away the bacteria that have entered. This large volume of fluid also helps dilute the urine, thereby decreasing bacterial concentration. Another defense mechanism is the low pH of the bladder, which also helps control bacterial multiplication. It may be, too, that the bladder lining employs some means to repel bacteria and to inhibit their adherence to the wall. Some researchers theorize that genetic, hormonal, and immune factors may help determine the defensive capability of the bladder.

Cystitis occurs most frequently in women, in large part because of the length and positioning of the urethra. Many women experience their first episode of cystitis as they become sexually active. So-called honeymoon cystitis, that related to sexual activity, comes about when intercourse (penetrative or nonpenetrative) forces bacteria upward through the urethra. From the urethra, the bacteria travel to the bladder. Unless they are voided through urination upon conclusion of intercourse, they may multiply, causing inflammation and infection. Bathing after intercourse is too late to prevent the *E. coli* from being pushed into the urethral opening. Some instances of cystitis may be reduced if there is adequate vaginal lubrication prior to intercourse and vaginal sprays and douches are avoided.

Women who use a diaphragm as birth control are more likely to develop urinary tract infections than other sexually active women. The reason for this increased likelihood may be linked to the more alkaline vaginal environment in diaphragm users, or perhaps to the spring in the rim of the diaphragm that exerts pressure on the tissue around the urethra. Urine flow may be restricted, and the stagnant urine is a good harbor for bacterial growth.

When urine remains in the bladder for an extended period of time, its stagnation may allow for the rapid growth of bacteria, thereby leading to cystitis. Urine flow may be restricted by an enlarged prostate or pregnancy. Diabetes mellitus may also lead to cystitis, as the body's resistance to infection is lowered. Infrequent urination for whatever reason is associated with a greater likelihood of cystitis.

Less frequently, cases have been linked to vaginitis as a result of *Monilia* or *Trichomonas*. Yeasts such as these change the pH of the vaginal fluid, which will allow and even encourage bacterial growth in the perineal region. Sometimes, it is an endless cycle: A patient takes antibiotics for cystitis, which kills her protective bacteria and allows the overgrowth of yeasts. The yeasts cause vaginitis, which may promote another case of cystitis, and the cycle continues. In fact, recurrent cystitis may be a result of an inappropriate course of antibiotic treatment; the antibiotic is not specific to the bacteria. More rarely, recurrent cases may be a result of constant seeding by the kidneys or a bowel fistula. The most common cause of recurrent cystitis, however, is new organisms from the rectal area that invade the perineal area. This new pool may be inadvertently changed by antibiotic treatment.

A less common but often more severe kind of cystitis is interstitial cystitis, an inflammation of the bladder caused by nonbacterial causes, such as an autoimmune or allergic response. With this type of cystitis, there may be inflammation or ulceration of the bladder, which may result in scarring. These problems usually cause frequent and painful urination and possible hematuria. What separates interstitial cystitis from acute cystitis is that it primarily strikes women in their early to mid-forties and that, while urine output is normal, soon after urination, the urge to void again is overwhelming. Delaying urination may cause a pink tinge to appear in the urine. This minimal bleeding is most often a result of an overly small bladder being stretched so that minute tears in

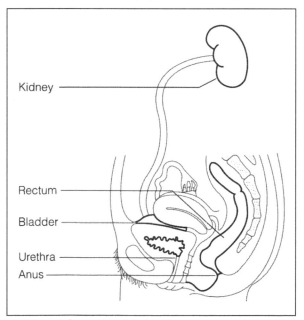

Cystitis, an inflammation of the bladder, may progress to the kidneys if left untreated.

the bladder wall bleed into the urine. This form is often hard to diagnose, as the symptoms may be mild or severe and may appear and disappear or be constant.

Treatment and Therapy

Medical students are typically underprepared to deal with the numerous cases of cystitis. The student is told to test urine for the presence of bacteria, prescribe a ten-day course of antibiotics, sometimes take a kidney x-ray or perform a cytoscopy, and then perhaps prescribe more antibiotics. If the patient continues to complain, perhaps a painful dilation of the urethra or cauterizing (burning away) of the inflamed skin is performed. None of these procedures guarantees a cure.

Diagnosis of cystitis should be relatively easy; however, in a number of cases it is misdiagnosed because the doctor has failed to identify the type of bacteria, the patient's history of past cases, and possible links between cystitis and life factors (sexual activity, contraceptive method, and diet, for example). A more appropriate antibiotic given at this point might lower the risks of frequent recurrences. Diagnosis of urinary tract infection takes into account the medical history, a physical examination of the patient, and performance of special tests. The history begins with the immediate complaints of the patient and is completed with a look back at the same type of infections that the patient has had from childhood to the present. The physician should conduct urinalysis but be cognizant that if the urine is not examined at the right time, the bacteria may not have survived and thus a false-negative reading may occur.

One special test, a cytoscopy, is used to diagnose some of the special characteristics of cystitis. These include redness of the bladder cells, enlarged capillaries with numerous small hemorrhages, and in cases of severe cystitis, swelling of bladder tissues. Swelling may be so pronounced that it partially blocks the urethral opening, making incomplete emptying of the bladder likely to occur. Pus pockets may be visible.

In the case of women who first experience cystitis when they become sexually active, doctors usually instruct the patients to be alert to several details. They should wash or shower before intercourse and be warned that certain contraceptive methods and positions during intercourse may increase their chances of becoming infected. To decrease the chance of introducing the contamination of bowel flora to the urethra, wiping from front to back after urination and defecation is advised.

Children are not immune to attacks of cystitis; in fact, education at an early age may aid children in lowering their chances of developing cystitis. Some of the following may be culprits in causing cystitis and maintaining a hospitable environment for bacteria to grow: soap or detergent that is too strong, too much fruit juice, overuse of creams and ointments, any noncotton underwear, shampoo in the bath water, bubble bath, chlorine from swimming pools, and too little fluid intake. Once children reach the teenage years, many of the above remain causes. Added to them are failure to change underwear daily, irregular periods, use of tampons, and the use of toiletries and deodorants. Careful monitoring of these conditions can greatly reduce the risk of recurrent infections.

The symptoms of cystitis are often urgent and painful enough to alert a sufferer to visit a physician as quickly as possible. Such a visit not only makes the patient feel better but also decreases the chances that the bacteria will travel toward and even into the kidney, causing pyelonephritis. Antibiotic therapy is the typical mode of treating acute or bacterial cystitis. The antibiotics chosen should reach a high concentration in the urine, should not cause the proliferation of drug-resistant bacteria, and should not kill helpful bacteria. Some antibiotics used to treat first-time sufferers of cystitis with a high success rate (80 to 100 percent) are TMP-SMX, sulfisoxazole, amoxicillin, and ampicillin. Typically, a three-day course of therapy not only will see the patient through the few days of symptoms but also will not change bowel flora significantly. When *E. coli* cause acute cystitis, there is a significant chance that one dose of an antibiotic such as penicillin will effectively end the bout, and again, the bowel flora will not be upset. Such antibiotics, when chosen carefully by the physician to match the bacteria, are useful in treating cystitis because they act very quickly to kill the bacteria. Sometimes, enough bacteria can be killed in one hour that the symptoms begin to abate immediately.

Yet antibiotics are not without their drawbacks: they may cause nausea, loss of appetite, dizziness, diarrhea, and fatigue and may increase the likelihood of yeast infections. The most common problem is the one posed by antibiotics that destroy all bacteria of the body. When the body's normal bacteria are gone, yeasts may proliferate in the body's warm, moist places. In one of the areas, the vagina, vaginitis causes a discharge that can seep into the urethra, causing the symptoms of cystitis to begin all over again.

For those suffering from recurrent cystitis, the treatment usually is a seven- to ten-day course of antibiotic treatment that will clear the urine of pus, indicating that the condition should be cured. If another bout recurs fairly soon, it is probably an indication that treatment was ended too quickly, as the infective bacteria were still present. To ensure that treatment has been effective, the urine must be checked and declared sterile.

Because cystitis is so common, and because many are frustrated by the inadequacies of treatment, self-treatment has become very popular. Self-treatment does not cure the infection but certainly makes the patient more comfortable while the doctor cultures a urine specimen, determines the type of bacteria causing the infection, and prescribes the appropriate antibiotic. Monitoring the first signs that a cystitis attack is imminent can save a victim from days of intense pain.

Those advocating home treatment do not all agree, however, on the means and methods that reduce suffering. All agree that once those first sensations are felt, the sufferer should start to drink water or water-based liquids; there is some disagreement on whether this intake should include fruit juice, especially cranberry juice. Some believe that the high acidic content of the juice may act to kill some of the bacteria, while others believe that the acid will only decrease the pH of the urine, causing a more intense burning sensation as the acidic urine passes through the inflamed urethra. An increased fluid intake produces more copious amounts of urine and, by diluting the urine, decreases its normal acidity. The excess urine acts to leach the bacteria from the bladder. More dilute urine will relieve much of the burning discomfort during voiding. If a small amount of sodium bicarbonate is added to the water, it will aid in alkalinizing the urine. The best self-treatment is to drink one cup of water every twenty minutes for three hours; after this period, the amount can be decreased. A teaspoonful of bicarbonate every hour for three or four hours is safe, unless the person suffers from blood pressure problems or a heart condition. Additionally, the patient may wish to take a painkiller such as acetaminophen. If lifestyle permits, resting will enhance the cure, especially if a heating pad is used to soothe the back or stomach. After the frequent visits to the toilet, cleaning the perineal area carefully can reduce continued contamination.

Diagnosis of interstitial cystitis can be made only using a cytoscope. Since the cause is not bacterial, antibiotics are not effective in treating this type of cystitis. To enhance the healing process of an inflamed or ulcerated bladder as a result of interstitial cystitis, the bladder may be distended and the ulcers cauterized; both procedures are done under anesthesia. Corticosteroids may be prescribed to help control the inflammation.

Perspective and Prospects

Infection in males is far less frequent than in females, although it does occur. Unfortunately, most urologists are better versed in male problems. Female specialists, gynecologists, treat the reproductive system but may not have studied female urinary dysfunction. If a man suffers from urinary dysfunction, he should seek the services of a urologist. A woman who has interstitial cystitis should also see a urologist, specifically one who knows about this form of cystitis. If a woman is experiencing recurrent cystitis, she is probably already seeing a gynecologist or an internist; however, if she is not getting relief, she should avail herself of a urologist, especially one specializing in female urology, if possible.

A strong social stigma is associated with bladder dysfunction, which may create an obstacle when treatment is necessary. From the time of infancy, some children are taught that anything to do with bladder or bowel function is shameful or dirty. Therefore, when dysfunction occurs, self-esteem may be decreased. As a result, the sufferer may fail to ask for help. Such a reaction must be overcome if there is to be significant progress in treating and conquering cystitis.

—*Iona C. Baldridge*

See also Antibiotics; Bacterial infections; Hematuria; Kidneys; Urethritis; Urinalysis; Urinary disorders; Urinary system; Urology; Urology, pediatric; Women's health.

For Further Information:

A.D.A.M. Medical Encyclopedia. "Cystitis-Acute." *MedlinePlus*, September 17, 2010.
A.D.A.M. Medical Encyclopedia. "Cystitis-Noninfectious." *MedlinePlus*, April 16 2012.
Chalker, Rebecca, and Kristene E. Whitmore. *Overcoming Bladder Disorders*. New York: HarperCollins, 1990.
Cohen, Barbara J. *Memmler's The Human Body in Health and Disease*. 11th ed. Philadelphia: Wolters Kluwer Health/Lippincott Williams & Wilkins, 2009.
Gillespie, Larrian, with Sandra Blakeslee. *You Don't Have to Live with Cystitis*. Rev. ed. New York: Quill, 2002.
Parker, James N., and Philip M. Parker, eds. *The Official Patient's Sourcebook on Urinary Tract Infection*. San Diego, Calif.: Icon Health, 2002.
Riley, Julie. "Acute Cystitis." *HealthLibrary*, April 12, 2013.
Schrier, Robert W., ed. *Diseases of the Kidney and Urinary Tract*. 8th ed. Philadelphia: Wolters Kluwer Health/Lippincott Williams & Wilkins, 2007.

CYSTOSCOPY

Procedure

Anatomy or system affected: Bladder, reproductive system, urinary system

Specialties and related fields: Gynecology, oncology, urology

Definition: An endoscopic procedure that utilizes a water or carbon dioxide distension system to visualize the urethra and bladder.

Indications and Procedures

Cystoscopy is indicated in patients for whom visual inspection of the urethra, bladder mucosa, and ureteral orifices is likely to yield a diagnosis. This includes patients who have hematuria (blood in the urine), incontinence, and irritative bladder symptoms for whom all obvious causes have been ruled out. In addition, patients who have undergone difficult abdominal or pelvic surgery may receive cystoscopy to verify that the bladder and the ureters, the tubes that carry urine from the kidneys to the bladder, are intact.

Cystoscopy is performed with the patient in a supine position with legs in stirrups. The cystoscope consists of a small metal tube, through which distension medium is passed. The light source, which enables visualization, also passes through this tube. The cystoscope can be attached to a video screen, or the clinician can visualize the urethral and bladder mucosas directly through the cystoscope. The cystoscope may be angled at 0 degrees, 30 degrees, or 70 degrees to facilitate visualization of different parts of the bladder. The procedure involves passing the cystoscope into the urethra and then the bladder under direct visualization. Cystoscopy is performed in a systematic fashion to ensure complete coverage of the urethral and bladder mucosas. Abnormal areas can be biopsied. The ureteral orifices can be visualized using the cystoscope, and the presence of urine flow from the orifices confirms patency (lack of obstruction) of the ureters.

Uses and Complications

Cystoscopy can be used to diagnose a variety of benign and malignant conditions of the lower urinary tract. Among the benign conditions commonly found through cystoscopy are endometriosis of the bladder, interstitial cystitis, foreign bodies, and anatomic abnormalities such as fistulas (communicating tracts between the bladder and another organ such as the bowels) or diverticula (small outpouchings of the bladder or urethra). By filling the bladder with distension fluid during cystoscopy, it is also possible to perform limited bladder function tests. Malignant conditions that may be found on cystoscopy include bladder cancers and cancers of adjacent pelvic organs, such as the cervix, which may invade the bladder.

Cystoscopy is an extremely safe procedure. Theoretical risks include the possibility of bladder injury or perforation from the cystoscope.

—*Anne Lynn S. Chang, M.D.*

See also Bladder cancer; Bladder removal; Cervical, ovarian, and uterine cancers; Cystitis; Diverticulitis and diverticulosis; Endometriosis; Endoscopy; Fistula repair; Hematuria; Incontinence; Invasive tests; Urethritis; Urinalysis; Urinary disorders; Urinary system; Urology; Urology, pediatric.

For Further Information:

Doherty, Gerard M., and Lawrence W. Way, eds. *Current Surgical Diagnosis and Treatment*. 13th ed. New York: Lange Medical Books/McGraw-Hill, 2010.

Miller, Brigitte E. *An Atlas of Sigmoidoscopy and Cystoscopy*. Boca Raton, Fla.: Parthenon, 2002.

Randall, Brian. "Cystoscopy." *Health Library*, April 17, 2013.

Rock, John A., and Howard W. Jones III, eds. *Te Linde's Operative Gynecology*. 10th ed. Philadelphia: Lippincott Williams & Wilkins, 2011.

Stenchever, Morton A., et al. *Comprehensive Gynecology*. 5th ed. St. Louis, Mo.: Mosby/Elsevier, 2007.

Vorvick, Linda J. "Cystoscopy." *MedlinePlus*, June 18, 2012.

CYSTS
Disease/Disorder
Anatomy or system affected: All
Specialties and related fields: All
Definition: A walled-off sac that is not normally found in the tissue where it occurs. To be a true cyst, a lump must have a capsule around it. Cysts usually contain a liquid or semisolid core (center) and vary in size from microscopic to very large. They may occur in any tissue of the body in a person of any age.

Key terms:
asymptomatic: not causing any symptoms

benign: not malignant; noncancerous

capsule: the wall that encloses a cyst

computed tomography (CT) scan: a technique that generates detailed pictures from a series of X rays

genetic: inherited

magnetic resonance imaging (MRI): a radiologic technique that uses radio signals and magnets and a computer to produce highly detailed images of tissues

malignant: cancerous; able to spread into and destroy nearby tissues and to spread to distant areas

renal: pertaining to the kidney

sebaceous: pertaining to glands in the skin that secrete an oily substance called sebum

ultrasonography: the use of sound waves to create an image of the soft tissues of the body

---

Information on Cysts

Causes: Unknown; likely arise when hair follicles becomes blocked

Symptoms: Lumps in skin or areas such as the breast, brain, or bone; may put pressure on surrounding organs, causing pain

Duration: Varies

Treatments: Surgical drainage, sometimes antibiotics to prevent infection

---

Causes and Symptoms

Cysts can be caused by a many different processes, including infections, defects in the development of an embryo during pregnancy, various obstructions to the flow of body fluids, tumors, a number of different inflammatory conditions, and genetic diseases.

Cysts may have no symptoms at all, or they may be quite noticeable, depending on their size and location. For example, a person with a cyst in the skin or breast will most likely be able to feel the lump. On the other hand, a cyst on an internal organ may not produce any symptoms unless it becomes so large that it keeps the organ from functioning properly or presses on another organ. Many times, internal cysts are discovered by chance on an X ray, computed tomography (CT) scan, magnetic resonance imaging (MRI) scan, or ultrasound for an unrelated condition.

It is impossible to list all the different types of cysts that might form in the body, but they are usually benign. Only very rarely are cysts associated with cancer or with serious infection. One common type of cyst is a sebaceous cyst, found in the oil-secreting glands of the skin. Sebacious cysts may become quite large and contain a foul-smelling, cheesy substance within the capsule. Breast cysts are filled with fluid and may enlarge and recede with the changing hormones of the menstrual cycle. Just before menses, breast cysts may be quite tender. Ganglion cysts occur over joints and on the tendons of the body. A chalazion, or cyst in the eyelid, is usually not painful but can be quite irritating.

Some cyst development is part of a particular disease or disorder. For example, cysts form on the ovaries in a disorder called polycystic ovary syndrome. There are also a number of different renal diseases that involve the development of cysts on the kidney.

Treatment and Therapy

The treatment for cysts depends on their size and location and whether they are causing symptoms. A small, asymptomatic cyst is often simply monitored.

When surgery is performed to remove a cyst, it is usually "shelled out" so that the entire capsule and its contents are removed. (If the capsule is left intact, then it might simply fill up again.) Depending on the location of the cyst, this may be performed in an office using local anesthesia or in the operating room of a hospital. When cancer is a possibility, the cell wall and any fluids are evaluated microscopically to determine whether any malignant cells are present.

Aspiration is another technique for treating cysts. A needle is inserted into the middle of the cyst, and any fluid is removed (aspirated) through the needle. If the cyst is deep within the body, then the aspiration may be guided by ultrasound or another radiologic technique. Aspiration may make the cyst disappear, or it may fill up again.

Some cysts are treated by incision and drainage. An opening is made in the cyst, and all the material in the core is removed. The cyst is then packed with gauze to ensure that the surgical incision does not close and allow the cyst to fill up again. The gauze is replaced periodically until healing takes place.

Ganglion cysts on tendons or joints may be successfully treated by injection with a steroid. If the cyst is part of another medical condition such as polycystic ovary syndrome, then any treatment is usually aimed at the medical condition rather than the cyst itself.

—*Rebecca Lovell Scott, Ph.D., PA-C*

See also Abscess removal; Abscesses; Acne; Bone disorders; Bones and the skeleton; Breast disorders; Breasts, female; Cyst removal; Fibrocystic breast condition; Ganglion removal; Hydroceles; Kidney disorders; Kidneys; Ovarian cysts; Ovaries; Plastic surgery; Reproductive system; Skin; Skin disorders; Tendon disorders.

For Further Information:

American Medical Association. *American Medical Association Family Medical Guide*. 4th rev. ed. Hoboken, N.J.: John Wiley & Sons, 2004.

Berman, Kevin. "Cyst." *MedlinePlus*, November 20, 2012.

Komaroff, Anthony, ed. *Harvard Medical School Family Health Guide*. New York: Free Press, 2005.

Stoppard, Miriam. *Family Health Guide*. London: DK, 2006.

CYTOLOGY

Specialty

Anatomy or system affected: Cells, immune system

Specialties and related fields: Bacteriology, hematology, histology, immunology, oncology, pathology, serology

Definition: The study of the appearance of cells, usually with the aid of a microscope, to diagnose diseases.

Key terms:

cell: a tiny baglike structure within which the basic functions of the body are carried out

chromosomes: rodlike cell parts made up of the genes that are the blueprints for every feature of the body; located in the nucleus of almost all cells

electron: a tiny particle with an electronic charge; a component of an atom

enzyme: a protein that is able to speed up a particular chemical reaction in the body

membranes: sheetlike structures that enclose each cell and separate the various organelles from one another

nucleus: the "control center" of plant and animal cells; a large spherical mass occupying up to one-third of the volume of a typical cell

organelles: specialized parts of cells

pathologist: a physician who is specially trained to use cytology and related methods to diagnose disease

protein: an abundant kind of molecule found in cells; proteins have many functions, from acting as enzymes to forming mechanical structures such as tendons and hair

Science and Profession

Cytology is the study of the appearance of cells, the fundamental units that make up all living organisms. Cells are complex structures constructed from many different subcomponents that work together in a precisely regulated fashion. Each cell must also cooperate with neighboring cells within the organism. A cell is like a complex automobile: Many separate components must be synchronized, and the cell (or car) must follow a strict order of function to coordinate successfully with its neighbors. Because illness results from the malfunction of cells, physicians must be able to measure key cell functions accurately. The normal and abnormal function of cells can be evaluated in many different ways; cytology is the study of cells using microscopes. A sophisticated collection of cytological techniques is available to pathologists; with these a precise diagnosis of cellular malfunction is possible.

All cells share several basic features. They are surrounded by a membrane, a flexible, sheetlike structure which encloses the fluid contents of the cell but allows required materials to move into the cell and waste products to move out of it. The complex salty fluid contained by the membrane is the cytoplasm; the other subcomponents of the cell, called organelles, are suspended in this substance. Each cell contains a set of genes, located on chromosomes, which function as blueprints for all other structures of the cell; the genes are inherited from an individual's parents. In plant and animal cells, the chromosomes are contained in a prominent organelle called the nucleus, which is surrounded by its own membrane inside the cell. Cells must also have a collection of enzymes used to convert food into energy to power the cell. In the cells of animals and plants, these enzymes are packaged into organelles called mitochondria. Membranes, the nucleus, and the mitochondria are the most prominent parts of a cell that are visible with a microscope, but cells also contain a variety of other specialized parts that are required for them to function properly. In addition, cells can also export (secrete) a variety of materials. For example, secreted materials make up bone, cartilage, tendons, mucus, sweat, and saliva.

Despite these basic features, the different types of cells have very distinct appearances. The cells of bacteria, plants, and animals are easily distinguishable from one another using a microscope. Bacterial cells are simplified, lacking organized nuclei and mitochondria. Different kinds of bacteria can be precisely distinguished; for example, strep throat is caused by spherical bacteria that form chains, like beads of a necklace. Some dangerous bacteria can be colored with dyes that do not stain harmless bacteria. Because so many human diseases are caused by bacteria, highly accurate procedures have been developed for their identification.

The adult human body is made up of approximately sixty to ninety trillion individual cells. Although much larger than bacteria, all of these are far too small to be seen with the naked eye (typically about 20 microns in diameter). Each organ of the body-the brain, liver, kidney, skin, and so on-is made up of several kinds of cells, specialized for particular functions. They must cooperate closely: Mistakes in the activities of any of these many cells can cause disease. A pathologist is able to recognize small changes in the appearance of each of many different cell types.

A few of the characteristic cell types in the human body include nerve, muscle, secretory, and epithelial cells. Nerve cells are designed to pass information throughout the nervous system. The nerve cells function much like electrical wires, so they have slender wirelike extensions that can be several feet long. Defects in the wiring circuits-for example, in patients with Alzheimer's disease-can be readily detected. Muscle cells are easily identified because they are elongated

cylinders packed with special fibers that cause muscular contraction. Secretory cells produce and release such substances as digestive enzymes. Such cells are often filled with membrane-bound packets of their specialized product, ready to be released from the cell. The skin and the surfaces of various internal organs are encased in a cell type called epithelium. Epithelial cells are tilelike and are often fastened tightly to neighboring epithelial cells by special kinds of connectors. Numerous other specialized cell types are found in the body as well, but these four types represent the most common cell designs.

Cells are sophisticated and delicate structures that carry out specific functions efficiently. The structure and function of normal cells are stable and predictable. If significant numbers of cells are somehow damaged, disease is the result. Such defective cells change in their appearance in character-

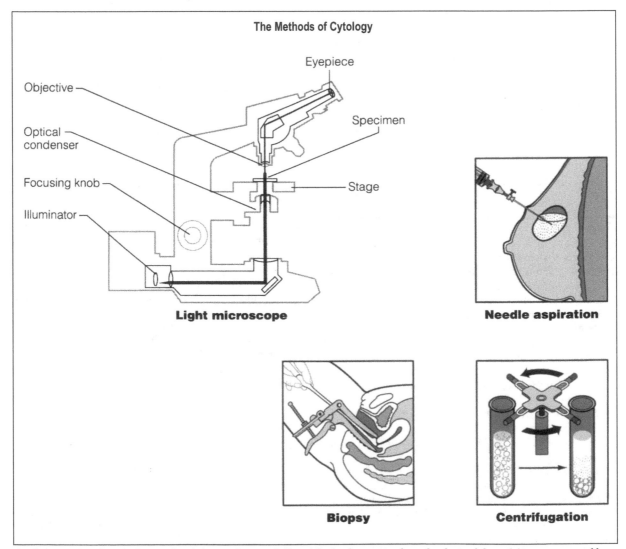

Cytologists study cells in both normal and abnormal states. Cells and fluid to be examined may be obtained through biopsy, separated by centrifugation, and studied under a light microscope.

istic ways. Therefore, cytology is an important element in the diagnosis of many diseases and for monitoring the cellular response to therapy.

Many different types of stress can cause cell damage. One of the most common stresses is oxygen deprivation, known as hypoxia. Even a brief interruption of oxygen can cause irreversible damage to cells because it is needed for energy production. Since oxygen is transported in the blood, the most common cause of hypoxia is loss of blood supply, which can occur with trauma, blockage by blood clots or narrowed blood vessels, and several kinds of lung or heart problems. Carbon monoxide poisoning results from interference with the blood's ability to absorb and carry oxygen, while the poison cyanide interferes with a cell's ability to make use of oxygen.

Poisons such as cyanide can damage cells in many other ways, as can drugs and alcohol. Prolonged use of barbiturates or alcohol can damage liver cells. These cells are also sensitive to common chemicals such as carbon tetrachloride, once used widely as a household cleaning agent. The liver is where foreign chemicals are changed to harmless forms, which explains why the liver cells are often damaged. Even useful chemicals, however, can cause harm to cells in some circumstances. Constant high levels of glucose, a sugar used by all cells, may overwork certain cells of the pancreas to the point where they become defective. Some foods (especially fats) and certain food additives, if they are eaten in excess, can interfere with cell function.

Physical damage to cells-caused, for example, by blows to the body-can dislocate parts of cells, preventing their proper coordination. Extreme cold can interfere with the blood supply, causing hypoxia; extreme heat can cause cells to speed up their rate of metabolism, again exceeding the oxygen-carrying capacity of the circulatory system. The "bends," the affliction suffered by surfacing deep-sea divers, results from tiny bubbles of nitrogen that block capillaries. Various kinds of radiant energy, such as radioactivity or ultraviolet light, can damage specific chemicals of cells, causing them to malfunction. Electrical energy generates extreme local heat within the body, which can damage cells directly.

Many small living organisms can interfere with cellular function as well. Viruses are effective parasites of cells, using cells for their own survival. This relationship can result in cell death, as in poliomyelitis; in depressed cell function, as in viral hepatitis; or in abnormal cell growth, as in cancers. (Cancer occurs when the genetic material of a cell becomes damaged, causing mutations that lead to uncontrolled cell growth and division. Several viruses are known to cause cancer, including the human papillomavirus, or HPV.) Bacteria can also live as parasites, releasing toxins that interfere with cellular function in a variety of ways. Malaria is caused by a single-celled animal that damages blood cells, athlete's foot is caused by a fungus, and tiny worms called nematodes can invade cells and cause them to work improperly.

All cell types are not equally sensitive to damage by each agent. Liver cells are particularly sensitive to damage by toxic chemicals. Nerve and muscle cells are the first to be injured by hypoxia. Kidney cells are also easily damaged by loss of blood supply. Lung cells are affected by anything that is inhaled.

Diagnostic and Treatment Techniques

Before cells can be successfully observed, they must be prepared through several steps. First, it is necessary to select a relatively small sample of a particular organ for closer scrutiny. Such a sample is called a biopsy when it is collected by a physician who wishes to test for a disease. The biopsy must then be preserved, or fixed, so that its parts will not deteriorate. Next, the specimen must be encased within a solid substance so that it can be handled without damage. Most often, the fixed specimen is soaked in melted paraffin, which then is allowed to solidify in a mold. For some kinds of microscopes, harder plastic materials are used. Next, the specimen must be thinly sliced so that the internal details can be seen. The delicate slices are mounted on a support, typically a thin glass slide for light microscopy. Finally, the parts of the cell must be colored, or stained. Without this coloring, the cell parts would be transparent and thus unobservable.

The basic tool of the cytologist is the light microscope. It can magnify up to about one thousand times. Numerous sophisticated methods are used with light microscopy. Specific stains have been developed for distinguishing the different molecules that make up cells. For example, Alcian blue is a dye that stains a type of complex sugar that accumulates outside certain abnormal cells, making it easier to identify these cells. Also, specially prepared antibodies can recognize particular proteins within cells. Disease-causing proteins, including the proteins of dangerous viruses and bacteria, can be precisely identified in this way.

A major advance in cytology is the electron microscope. It forms images in essentially the same way as a light microscope does, but using electrons rather than visible light. Because of the properties of electrons, this type of microscope can magnify up to one million times beyond life size. A wide range of new cell features has been revealed with the electron microscope. The details of how genes work, how materials enter and leave cells, how energy is produced, and how molecules are synthesized have been made clearer. The steps for preparing specimens for electron microscopy are delicate, time-consuming, and demanding. Furthermore, the electron microscope itself is complex and expensive. Considerable skill is required to use it effectively. For these reasons, electron microscopy is not commonly used for routine medical diagnoses.

Cell injury causes predictable changes in cells that can be interpreted by a pathologist to suggest the underlying cause of the damage and how best to treat it. Almost all forms of reversible injury cause changes in the size and shape of cells. Cellular swelling is an obvious symptom that almost always reflects a serious underlying problem. Such cells also have a characteristic cloudy appearance. Swelling and cloudiness indicate loss of energy reserves and abnormal uptake of water into the cell through improperly functioning cell-surface membranes. An indication of serious damage is the accumulation within the cell of vacuoles-small, fluid-filled sacs that have a characteristic clear appearance when viewed through a microscope. More severe injury can cause the formation of vacuoles that contain fat, giving the cells a foamy appearance. Such damage is most often seen in cells of the heart, kidneys, and lungs. These changes appear to reflect both membrane abnormalities and the defective metabolism of fats.

Cells that are damaged beyond the point of repair will die, a process called necrosis. The two key processes in necrosis are the breakdown and mopping up of cellular contents, and large changes in structure of cellular proteins in ways that can be identified using a microscope. The most conspicuous and reliable indicators of necrosis are changes in the appearance of the nucleus, which can shrink or even break into pieces and which eventually disappears completely. Ultimately, the entire cell disappears.

Cancer provides a good illustration of how cytology is employed in the diagnosis of a specific disease. A skilled cytologist can detect cells at an early stage of cancer development and, with accuracy, can gauge how dangerous a cancer cell is or is likely to become. Cancer is a disease of abnormal growth. Cancer cells may have few abnormal features other than their improper growth; tumors made up of such cells are generally not dangerous and so are labeled benign. Malignant tumor cells, on the other hand, are highly abnormal. They can damage and invade other parts of the body, making these cells much more dangerous.

The cells of benign tumors may have nearly the same appearance as the cells of the normal tissue from which they arose. Benign cancers of skin, bone, muscle, and nerve maintain the obvious structures that allow these highly specialized cell types to carry out their normal functions. Ironically, however, continued normal function can itself become a problem, because there are too many cells producing specialized products. For example, tumors in tissues that produce hormones can result in massive excesses of such hormones, causing severe imbalances in the function of the body's organs. Malignant tumor cells, on the other hand, have lost some or all of the functional and cytological features of their parent normal cells. They have a simpler and more primitive appearance, termed anaplasia by pathologists. The degree of anaplasia is one of the most reliable hallmarks of how malignant a cell has become.

Almost any part of the cell can become anaplastic. A common change is in the chromosomes of a cancer cell. The number, size, and shape of chromosomes change, and detailed analysis of these changes is often important in diagnosis, as in leukemia. Many malignant tumor cells secrete enzymes that attack surrounding connective tissue, changing its appearance in characteristic ways. Membrane systems of anaplastic cells are also abnormal, with serious consequences. The movement of materials in and out of cells becomes defective, and energy production mechanisms are upset, causing the characteristic changes in appearance described above. A general feature of tumors made up of anaplastic cells is the variability among individual cells. Some cells can appear virtu-

ally normal, while other tumor cells nearby can appear highly abnormal in several ways.

The cells of benign tumors remain where they arose. The cells of malignant tumors, however, have the ability to spread through the body (metastasize), penetrating and damaging other organs in the process. These abilities, to invade and metastasize, have serious effects on the rest of the body. Invading cells often can be identified easily with a microscope. Extensions of the tumor cells may reach into surrounding normal organ parts. Tumor cells can be observed penetrating into blood and lymph vessels and other body cavities, such as the abdominal cavity and air pockets in the lung. Small clusters of tumor cells can be found in blood and identified in distant organs. These cells can begin the process of invasion all over again, producing so-called secondary tumors in other organs. How malignant cancer cells can cause so much harm becomes clear.

Perspective and Prospects

Of the diagnostic procedures that are available to physicians, cytologic techniques are among the most effective. Because the cells being examined are so tiny, the microscopes used must be able to magnify the cells enough to allow observation of their characteristics. Historically, the use of cytology in medical practice has closely paralleled the development of adequate microscopes and methods for preparing specimens.

Magnifying lenses by themselves lack the power required for observing cells. A microscope of adequate power must use several such lenses stacked together. The first crude microscopes with this design appeared late in the sixteenth century. During the next several hundred years, microscopes were mostly used to observe cells of plant material because the woody parts of plants can be thinly sliced and then observed directly, without the need for further preparation. The word "cell" was first employed by Robert Hooke (1635-1703) in a paper published in 1665. He observed small chambers in pieces of cork, which were where cells had been located in the living cork tree. These chambers reminded Hooke of monks" cells in a monastery, hence the name.

The great anatomist Marcello Malpighi (1628-1694) may have been the first to observe mammalian cells, within capillaries. The real giant of this era, however, was the Dutch microscopist Antoni van Leeuwenhoek (1632-1723), who greatly improved the quality of microscopes and then used them to observe single-celled animals, bacteria, sperm, and the nuclei within certain blood cells. Although most progress continued to be made with plants, numerous observations accumulated during the seventeenth and eighteenth centuries which suggested that animals are made up of tiny saclike units, and Hooke's word "cell" was applied to describe them. This concept was clearly stated in 1839 by Theodor Schwann (1810-1882); his idea that all animals are composed of cells and cellular products quickly gained acceptance. At this time, however, there was essentially no comprehension of how cells work. Without an understanding of normal cell function, cytology was still of little use in identifying and understanding disease.

During the late nineteenth and early twentieth centuries, the appearance of different cell types was carefully described. The main organelles of cells were identified, and such fundamental processes as cell division were observed and understood. At last it was possible to utilize cytology for medical purposes. The principles of medical cytology were established by the great pathologist Rudolf Virchow (1821-1902), who suggested for the first time that diseases originate from changes in specific cells of the body.

Rapid progress in cytology was made in the 1940s and 1950s, for two reasons. First, improved microscopes were developed, allowing greater accuracy in observing cell structure. The second reason-rapid progress in genetics and biochemistry-greatly increased the knowledge of how cells function and of the significance of specific changes in their appearance. Because cells are the basic units of life, scientists will continue to study them in detail, and the medical world will benefit directly from further, improved understanding in this field.

—*Howard L. Hosick, Ph.D.*

See also Bacterial infections; Bacteriology; Biopsy; Blood and blood disorders; Blood testing; Cancer; Cells; Cytopathology; Diagnosis; Gram staining; Hematology; Hematology, pediatric; Histology; Karyotyping; Laboratory tests; Malignancy and metastasis; Microbiology; Microscopy; Oncology; Pathology; Prognosis; Serology; Urinalysis; Viral infections.

For Further Information:
Cibas, Edmund S., and Barbara S. Ducatman. *Cytology: Diagnostic Principles and Clinical Correlates.* 3d ed. Philadelphia: Saunders Elsevier, 2009.
"Cytologic Evaluation." *Medline Plus*, August 16, 2011.
Gray, Winnifred, and Gabrijela Kocjan. *Diagnostic Cytopathology.* 3d ed. Philadelphia: Churchill Livingston, 2010.
Kumar, Vinay, et al., eds. *Robbins Basic Pathology.* 9th ed. Philadelphia: Saunders/Elsevier, 2012.
Taylor, Ron. *Through the Microscope.* Vol. 22 in *The World of Science.* New York: Facts On File, 1986.
Wolfe, Stephen L. *Cell Ultrastructure.* Belmont, Calif.: Wadsworth, 1985.

CYTOMEGALOVIRUS (CMV)
Disease/Disorder

Anatomy or system affected: Blood, brain, cells, ears, eyes, gastrointestinal system, immune system, liver, lungs

Specialties and related fields: Family medicine, gastroenterology, hematology, immunology, obstetrics, pediatrics, virology

Definition: A viral disease normally producing mild symptoms in healthy individuals but severe infections in the immunocompromised. Congenital infection may lead to malformations or fetal death.

Key terms:
hepatitis: inflammation of the liver; usually caused by viral infections, toxic substances, or immunological disturbances
hepatosplenomegaly: enlargement of the liver and spleen such that they may be felt below the rib margins
heterophil antibodies: antibodies that are detected using antigens other than the antigens that induced them
jaundice: yellow staining of the skin, eyes, and other tissues and excretions with excess bile pigments in the blood
latency: following an acute infection by a virus, a period of dormancy from which the virus may be reactivated during times of stress or immunocompromise
microcephaly: a congenital condition involving an abnormally small head associated with an incompletely developed brain

Causes and Symptoms

Cytomegalovirus (CMV) is a member of the herpesvirus group that includes such viruses as the Epstein-Barr virus, which causes infectious mononucleosis, and the varicella-zoster virus, which causes chickenpox. CMV is a ubiquitous virus that is transmitted in a number of different ways. A newly infected woman may transmit the virus across the placenta to her unborn child. Infection may also occur in the birth canal or via mother's milk. Young children commonly transmit CMV by means of saliva. Sexual transmission is common in adults. Blood transfusions and organ transplants may also transmit cytomegalovirus to recipients. As many as 80 percent of adults worldwide have antibodies indicating exposure to cytomegalovirus.

Congenital cytomegaloviral infection is universally common and especially prevalent in developing nations. According to the Centers for Disease Control and Prevention, about 0.7 percent of children are born infected. Most congenitally infected infants exhibit no symptoms. Normal development may follow, but some infants experience problems such as hearing loss, visual impairment, and developmental disabilities. Approximately 10 to 20 percent exhibit clinically obvious evidence of cytomegalic inclusion disease: hepatosplenomegaly, jaundice, microcephaly, deafness, seizures, cerebral palsy, and blood disorders such as thrombocytopenia (a decrease in platelets) and hemolytic anemia (in which red blood cells are destroyed). Giant cells having nuclei containing large inclusions are found in affected organs. Cytomegalovirus is a leading cause of developmental disabilities and has also been linked to microcephaly.

In immunocompetent adults and older children, cytomegalovirus can cause heterophil-negative mononucleosis, an infectious mononucleosis in which no heterophil antibodies are formed. Such antibodies are found in infectious

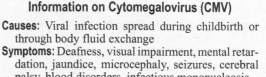

Information on Cytomegalovirus (CMV)

Causes: Viral infection spread during childbirth or through body fluid exchange
Symptoms: Deafness, visual impairment, mental retardation, jaundice, microcephaly, seizures, cerebral palsy, blood disorders, infectious mononucleosis
Duration: Varies
Treatments: Antiviral drugs (ganciclovir, foscarnet)

mononucleosis caused by the Epstein-Barr virus. Heterophil-negative mononucleosis is characterized by fever, hepatitis, lethargy, and abnormal lymphocytes in blood.

Severe systemic cytomegalovirus infections are frequently seen in the immunocompromised. Transplant patients are intentionally immunosuppressed to reduce the likelihood of graft rejection, making them vulnerable to infection by cytomegalovirus either by reactivation or by acquisition of the virus from the donor organ. Resulting systemic infections are manifested in diseases such as pneumonia, hepatitis, and retinitis. In addition to these CMV diseases, acquired immunodeficiency syndrome (AIDS) patients may experience infections of the central nervous system and gastrointestinal tract. Their blood cells may also be affected, resulting in disorders such as thrombocytopenia. AIDS patients frequently have intestinal CMV infections leading to chronic diarrhea. Cytomegalovirus retinitis in AIDS patients is particularly serious and may lead to retinal detachment and blindness. This is the most common sight-damaging opportunistic eye infection found in AIDS patients.

Treatment and Therapy

Ganciclovir, valganciclovir, foscarnet, and cidofovir are all antiviral agents that have been found useful in treating CMV infections in immunocompromised patients. Toxic properties, however, can limit their long-term administration. Ganciclovir exhibits hematopoietic toxicity; that is, it has an adverse affect on blood cells that may result in neutropenia, a decrease in the number of neutrophils in the blood. Foscarnet has more side effects than ganciclovir. It is a nephrotoxic substance, which means that it may damage the kidneys and thus cannot be used in patients with renal failure.

Valganciclovir, the oral form of ganciclovir, has been used effectively to prevent CMV infection in transplant recipients. It is administered to CMV-seronegative transplant patients receiving organs from CMV-seropositive donors as well as in CMV-seropositive recipients who will be undergoing immunosuppression to prevent rejection of transplanted organs. Another material employed as a prophylaxis for bone marrow and renal transplant recipients is intravenous cytomegalovirus immune globulin.

Therapy for CMV retinitis involves intravenous treatment with either ganciclovir, foscarnet, or cidofovir plus oral probenecid or oral valganciclovir. Alternatively, an intraocular ganciclovir implant may be used along with one of the systemic treatments mentioned above. Therapy of retinitis as well as other types of CMV infection in AIDS patients should be accompanied by highly effective antiretroviral therapy (HAART) to treat the human immunodeficiency virus and improve the immune function in the the patient. Successful HAART may allow the CMV antiviral therapy to be discontinued, but the patient must be carefully monitored for relapse of the CMV infection.

Retinal detachment is another complication arising from cytomegalovirus retinitis. It may occur even in those undergoing successful antiviral treatment. Surgical intervention is required to restore functional vision in these cases.

Perspective and Prospects

The term *cytomegalia* was first used in 1921 to describe the condition of an infant with intranuclear inclusions in the lungs, kidney, and liver. This condition in an adult was first attributed to a virus of the herpes group in 1925. Twenty-five cases of apparent cytomegalic inclusion disease had been described by 1932. Cytomegalovirus was pursued and isolated in the mid-1950s by researcher Margaret Smith. Around the same time, independently and serendipitously, groups in Boston, Massachusetts, and Bethesda, Maryland, also isolated the virus.

Development of new antiviral drugs and measures to reduce the immunocompromised state should continue to progress and improve the outcomes for patients infected with CMV.

—*Nancy Handshaw Clark, Ph.D.;*
updated by H. Bradford Hawley, M.D.

See also Acquired immunodeficiency syndrome (AIDS); Birth defects; Epstein-Barr virus; Eye surgery; Eyes; Hepatitis; Herpes; Immune system; Immunodeficiency disorders; Immunology; Mental retardation; Mononucleosis; Pregnancy and gestation; Stillbirth; Transplantation; Viral infections; Vision disorders.

For Further Information:

A.D.A.M. Medical Encyclopedia. "Cytomegalovirus Infections." *MedlinePlus*, May 2, 2013.

A.D.A.M. Medical Encyclopedia. "Cytomegalovirus Retinitis." *MedlinePlus*, December 6, 2011.

Bellenir, Karen, and Peter D. Dresser, eds. *Contagious and Noncontagious Infectious Diseases Sourcebook*. Detroit, Mich.: Omnigraphics, 1996.

National Center for Immunization and Respiratory Diseases, Division of Viral Diseases. "Cytomegalovirus (CMV) and Congenital CMV Infection." *Centers for Disease Control and Prevention*, December 6, 2010.

Roizman, Bernard, ed. *Infectious Diseases in an Age of Change: The Impact of Human Ecology and Behavior on Disease Transmission*. Washington, D.C.: National Academy Press, 1995.

Roizman, Bernard, Richard J. Whitley, and Carlos Lopez, eds. *The Human Herpesviruses*. New York: Raven Press, 1993.

Scheld, W. Michael, Richard J. Whitley, and Christina M. Marra, eds. *Infections of the Central Nervous System*. 3d ed. Philadelphia: Lippincott Williams & Wilkins, 2004.

Wagner, Edward K., and Martinez J. Hewlett. *Basic Virology*. 3d ed. Malden, Mass.: Blackwell Science, 2008.

CYTOPATHOLOGY

Specialty

Anatomy or system affected: Cells, immune system

Specialties and related fields: Bacteriology, cytology, forensic pathology, hematology, histology, oncology, pathology, serology

Definition: The medical field that deals with changes in cell structure or physiology as a result of injuries, infectious agents, or toxic substances.

Science and Profession

The profession of cytopathology deals with the search for lesions or abnormalities within individual cells or groups of cells. Generally speaking, a pathologist is a physician trained in pathology, the study of the nature of diseases. Observations of tissue or cell lesions are utilized in the diagnosis of disease or other agents associated with damage to cells.

Cell damage may result from endogenous phenomena, including the aging process, or from exogenous agents such as biological organisms (viruses or bacteria), chemical agents (bacterial toxins or other poisons), and physical agents (heat, cold, radiation, or electricity). For example, particular biological agents produce recognizable lesions that may be useful in the diagnosis of disease, such as the crystalline structures characteristic of certain viral infections.

The type of necrosis, or cell death, encountered is useful in diagnosing the problem. For example, certain types of enzymatic dissolution of cells, which result in areas of liquefaction, are the result of bacterial infection. Gangrenous necrosis often follows the restriction of the blood supply, because of either infection or a blood clot.

Pathologic changes within the cell can also help pinpoint the time of death. Organelles degenerate at a rate dependent on their use of oxygen. For example, mitochondria, which utilize significant amounts of oxygen, are among the first organelles to degenerate.

Diagnostic and Treatment Techniques

The diagnosis and treatment of cancer are prime examples of the use of cytopathology. The extent of pleomorphism in cell size and shape, irregularity of the nucleus, and presence (or absence) of organelles all provide the basis for the choice of treatment and help determine the ultimate prognosis. Specific organelles are stained with characteristic histochemicals, followed by microscopic observation. A preponderance of large, irregularly shaped cells provides for a poorer prognosis than if cells appear more normally differentiated. The nuclei in highly malignant tumors show a greater variation in size and chromatin pattern, as compared with those of cells from benign growths. Such differences lead directly to decisions on the choice of treatment: surgical removal, chemotherapy, or radiation.

—*Richard Adler, Ph.D.*

See also Bacteriology; Biopsy; Blood and blood disorders; Blood testing; Cancer; Cells; Cytology; Diagnosis; Gram staining; Hematology; Hematology, pediatric; Histology; Laboratory tests; Malignancy and metastasis; Microbiology; Microscopy; Oncology; Pathology; Prognosis; Serology; Toxicology; Tumors; Urinalysis.

For Further Information:

"About Cytopathology." *American Society of Cytopathology*, 2013.

Geisinger, Kim R., et al. *Modern Cytopathology*. Philadelphia: Churchill Livingstone/Elsevier, 2004.

Kumar, Vinay, et al., eds. *Robbins Basic Pathology*. 9th ed. Philadelphia: Saunders/Elsevier, 2012.

Lewin, Benjamin, et al., eds. *Cells*. 2d ed. Sudbury, Mass.: Jones and Bartlett, 2010.

MacDemay, Richard. *The Art and Science of Cytopathology*. 2d ed. Chicago: American Society for Clinical Pathology, 2011.

Majno, Guido, and Isabelle Joris. *Cells, Tissues, and Disease: Principles of General Pathology*. 2d ed. New York: Oxford University Press, 2004.

Silverberg, Steven G., ed. *Silverberg's Principles and Practice of Surgical Pathology and Cytopathology*. 4th ed. New York: Churchill Livingstone/Elsevier, 2006.

DEAFNESS

Disease/Disorder

Also known as: Hearing loss, hearing impairment, presbycusis

Anatomy or system affected: Ears, nervous system

Specialties and related fields: Audiology, geriatrics and gerontology, speech pathology

Definition: Deafness is either partial or complete loss of hearing. Hearing loss occurs most often in older adults, but people may be born deaf or become deaf at young ages.

Key terms:

acquired: not present at birth; developing after birth

auditory: pertaining to hearing

cerumen: earwax produced by specialized glands to protect and lubricate the ear canal

cochlea: the organ of hearing in the inner ear that takes the vibrations from the middle ear organs and converts them into nerve impulses for the brain to interpret

congenital: present at birth

eighth cranial nerve: also known as the auditory nerve or the vestibulocochlear nerve; the nerve running between the ear and the brain, involved with hearing and balance

genetic: inherited

ossicles: the chain of tiny bones in the middle ear which carry the vibrations of the tympanic membrane to the cochlea

ototoxic: toxic or harmful to the ears

tympanic membrane: also called the eardrum; a thin membrane that separates the external or outer ear from the middle ear

Causes and Symptoms

To understand deafness, it is first necessary to understand how sound is heard. The sound waves produced by any noise travel through the air and are funneled down the ear canal by the external ear, which is specially shaped for this function. The sound waves then cause the tympanic membrane to vibrate, which in turn causes the chain of tiny ossicles to vibrate. This mechanical energy of vibration is then transformed by the cochlea into nerve impulses that travel along the eighth cranial nerve to the spinal cord. These impulses are transmitted to the auditory cortex (center) of the brain, where they are interpreted. The ability to hear depends on all these elements working properly.

Deafness can occur when any particular part of this hearing pathway is not functioning as it should. If the ear canal is blocked with cerumen (earwax), a foreign body, fluid, or the products of infection or inflammation, then the sound waves are unable to travel to the eardrum. If the eardrum has ruptured or become stiff (sclerosed), then it cannot vibrate. If the ossicles have been damaged in any way, then they cannot vibrate. If the middle ear is filled with fluid from inflammation or infection, then the eardrum and ossicles cannot work properly. If the cochlea, auditory nerve, or both have been damaged through trauma, disease, or use of an ototoxic drug, then they cannot do their job of converting vibration into nerve impulses and transmitting them to the brain. If the auditory center of the brain is damaged, then it cannot interpret the nerve

impulses correctly.

Hearing loss is classified by the cause: conductive, sensory, or neural. Conductive losses are those that affect the conduction of sound waves; they involve problems with the external ear, ear canal, tympanic membrane, and ossicles. The sensory and neural causes are usually classified together as "sensorineural"—these losses affect the cochlea, auditory nerve, or auditory cortex of the brain.

The most common cause of hearing loss in children is otitis media, or middle-ear infection, which causes fluid to build up behind the tympanic membrane. It is usually reversible with time and treatment. This is a type of conductive loss, as is hearing loss attributable to cerumen impaction (excessive buildup of earwax), which can occur in both children and adults. Sensorineural losses are caused by such things as excessive noise exposure, ototoxic drugs, exposure to toxins in the environment, and diseases such as rubella (German measles). The type of sensorineural loss that many people experience as they get older is called presbycusis, which means "a condition of elder hearing." Many people with sensorineural losses have a genetic predisposition for hearing loss.

Congenital deafness is deafness that is present at the time a baby is born. Before the widespread availability of immunization against rubella, mothers who contracted the disease during pregnancy were at great risk of having a baby with congenital deafness. Congenital deafness may also be genetic. For example, if a child inherits a defective copy of the *GJB2* gene from each parent, then that child will be deaf even if both parents can hear.

Likewise, deafness that occurs after birth may be either acquired or genetic. Deafness associated with exposure to loud noises is acquired, for example, while many forms of deafness that occur in older age are genetic. About one-third of people over the age of sixty-five have hearing loss.

Treatment and Therapy

According to the World Health Organization, as of early 2013, about half of all cases of hearing loss worldwide were preventable. Indeed, the best treatment for deafness is prevention. Immunization against rubella, protection of ears from excessive noise, and avoidance of too much aspirin are all examples of preventative measures.

Information on Deafness

Causes: Aging; ear canal blockage (earwax, foreign body, fluid); ruptured or stiff eardrum; middle-ear infection; cochlea or auditory nerve damage (excessive noise exposure, ototoxic drugs, environmental toxins); genetic defect or predisposition

Symptoms: Hearing loss ranging from moderate to total

Duration: Acute, permanent, or progressive

Treatments: Depends on cause; for permanent loss, hearing aids, cochlear implants, other assistive devices

---

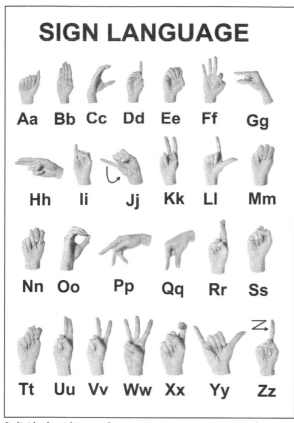

Individuals with severe hearing impairment may use sign language to communicate. (© Stephen Coburn/Dreamstime.com)

Once hearing impairment has occurred, determination of the cause is essential. The primary care provider, an otorhinolaryngologist (ear, nose, and throat doctor), an audiologist (hearing specialist), and a neurologist may be involved in this assessment. Reversible causes of deafness or hearing loss can be addressed medically or surgically, as in the removal of earwax. For nonreversible causes, hearing aids and other assistive hearing devices may be helpful. These devices have become increasingly sophisticated. Some allow the wearer to adjust the hearing aid to specific circumstances, while older versions amplified all sounds equally.

Cochlear implants are electronic devices that give profoundly deaf persons a sense of sound that helps them understand speech and other noises. A microphone picks up sounds, which are processed, converted to electric impulses, and sent to different areas of the auditory nerve.

In addition to these products, many assistive devices are available to help persons with severe hearing impairment function independently. For example, special telephones, alarm clocks, and doorbells that flash a light or shake the bed in addition to ringing are readily available.

—Rebecca Lovell Scott, Ph.D., PA-C

See also Aging; Audiology; Ear infections and disorders; Ear surgery; Ears; Hearing; Hearing aids; Hearing loss; Hearing tests; Neu-

ralgia, neuritis, and neuropathy; Otorhinolaryngology; Sense organs; Speech disorders.

For Further Information:
A.D.A.M. Medical Encyclopedia. "Hearing Loss." *MedlinePlus*, May 22, 2012.

American Medical Association. *American Medical Association Family Medical Guide*. 4th rev. ed. Hoboken, N.J.: John Wiley & Sons, 2004.

Carmen, Richard, ed. *The Consumer Handbook on Hearing Loss and Hearing Aids: A Bridge to Healing*. 3d rev. ed. Sedona, Ariz.: Auricle Ink, 2009.

Dillon, Harvey. *Hearing Aids*. New York: Thieme, 2001.

Komaroff, Anthony, ed. *Harvard Medical School Family Health Guide*. New York: Free Press, 2005.

National Center on Birth Defects and Developmental Disabilities. "Hearing Loss in Children." *Centers for Disease Control and Prevention*, March 22, 2013.

National Institute on Deafness and Other Communication Disorders. "Hearing, Ear Infections, and Deafness." *National Institutes of Health*, September 8, 2011.

Romoff, Arlene. *Hear Again: Back to Life with a Cochlear Implant*. New York: League for the Hard of Hearing, 1999.

Stoppard, Miriam. *Family Health Guide*. London: DK, 2006.

World Health Organization. "Millions Have Hearing Loss That Can Be Improved or Prevented." *World Health Organization*, February 27, 2013.

DEATH AND DYING

Disease/Disorder

Anatomy or system affected: Psychic-emotional system, all bodily systems

Specialties and related fields: Family medicine, geriatrics and gerontology, psychology

Key terms:

anticipatory depression: a depressive reaction to the awaited death of either oneself or a significant other; also called anticipatory grieving, preparatory grieving, or preparatory depression

bereavement: the general, overall process of mourning and grieving; considered to have progressive stages which include anticipation, grieving, mourning, postmourning, depression, loneliness, and reentry into society

depression: a general term covering mild states (sadness, inhibition, unhappiness, discouragement) to severe states (hopelessness, despair); typically part of normal, healthy grieving; considered the fourth stage of death and dying, between bargaining and acceptance

grief: the emotional and psychological response to loss; always painful, grieving is a type of psychological work and requires some significant duration of time

mourning: the acute phase of grief; characterized by distress, hopelessness, fear, acute loss, crying, insomnia, loss of appetite, anxiety, guilt, and restlessness

reactive depression: depression occurring as a result of overt events that have already taken place; it universally occurs in the bereaved

thanatology: the study and investigation of life-threatening actions, terminal illness, suicide, homicide, death, dying, grief, and bereavement

uncomplicated bereavement: a technical psychiatric label describing normal, average, and expectant grieving; despite an experience of great psychological pain, grieving is considered normal and healthy unless it continues much beyond one year

Causes and Symptoms

Medicine determines that death has occurred by assessing bodily functions in either of two areas. Persons with irreversible cessation of respiration and circulation are dead; persons with irreversible cessation of ascertainable brain functions are also dead. There are standard procedures used to diagnose death, including simple observation, brain-stem reflex studies, and the use of confirmatory testing such as electrocardiography (ECG or EKG), electroencephalography (EEG), and arterial blood gas analysis (ABG). The particular circumstances—anticipated or unanticipated, observed or unobserved, the patient's age, drug or metabolic intoxication, or suspicion of hypothermia—will favor some procedures over others, but in all cases both cessation of functions and their irreversibility are required before death can be declared.

Between 60 and 75 percent of all people die from chronic terminal conditions. Therefore, except in sudden death (as in a fatal accident) or when there is no evidence of consciousness (as in a head injury which destroys cerebral functions while leaving brain-stem reflexive functions intact), dying is both a physical and a psychological process. In most cases, dying takes time, and the time allows patients to react to the reality of their own passing. Often, they react by becoming vigilant about bodily symptoms and any changes in them. They also anticipate changes that have yet to occur. For example, long before the terminal stages of illness become manifest, dying patients commonly fear physical pain, shortness of breath, invasive procedures, loneliness, becoming a burden to loved ones, losing decision-making authority, and facing the unknown of death itself.

As physical deterioration proceeds, all people cope by resorting to what has worked for them before: the unique means and mechanisms which have helped maintain a sense of self and personal stability. People seem to go through the process of dying much as they have gone through the process of living—with the more salient features of their personalities, whether good or bad, becoming sharper and more prominent. People seem to face death much as they have faced life.

Medicine has come to acknowledge that physicians should understand what it means to die. Indeed, while all persons should understand what their own deaths will mean, physicians must additionally understand how their dying patients find this meaning.

In 1969, psychiatrist Elisabeth Kübler-Ross published the landmark *On Death and Dying,* based on her work with two hundred terminally ill patients. Though the work of Kübler-Ross has been criticized for the nature of the stages described and whether or not every person experiences every stage, her model has retained enormous utility to those who work in the area of death and dying. Technologically driven, Western medicine had come to define its role as primarily dealing with

extending life and thwarting death by defeating specific diseases. Too few physicians saw a role for themselves once the prognosis turned grave. In the decades that followed the publication of *On Death and Dying,* the profession has reaccepted that death and dying are part of life and that, while treating the dying may not mean extending the length of life, it can and should mean improving its quality.

Kübler-Ross provided a framework to explain how people cope with and adapt to the profound and terrible news that their illness is terminal. Although other physicians, psychologists, and thanatologists have shortened, expanded, and adapted her five stages of the dying process, neither the actual number of stages nor what they are specifically called is as important as the information and insight that any stage theory of dying yields. As with any human process, dying is complex, multifaceted, multidimensional, and polymorphic.

Well-intentioned, but misguided, professionals and family members may try to help move dying patients through each of the stages only to encounter active resentment or passive withdrawal. Patients, even dying patients, cannot be psychologically moved to where they are not ready to be. Rather than making the terminally ill die the "right" way, it is more respectful and helpful to understand any stage as a description of normal reactions to serious loss, and that these reactions normally vary among different individuals and also within the same individual over time. The reactions appear, disappear, and reappear in any order and in any combination. What the living must do is respect the unfolding of an adaptational schema which is the dying person's own. No one should presume to know how someone else should prepare for death.

Complications and Disorders

Kübler-Ross defined five stages of grief. Denial is the first stage defined by Kübler-Ross, but it is also linked to shock and isolation. Whether the news is told outright or gradual self-realization occurs, most people react to the knowledge of their impending death with existential shock: Their whole selves recoil at the idea, and they say, in some fashion, "This cannot be happening to me." Broadly considered, denial is a complex cognitive-emotional capacity that enables temporary postponement of active, acute, but in some way detrimental, recognition of reality. In the dying process, this putting off of the truth prevents a person from being overwhelmed while promoting psychological survival. Denial plays an important stabilizing role, holding back more than could be otherwise managed while allowing the individual to marshal psychological resources and reserves. It enables patients to consider the possibility, even the inevitability, of death and then to put the consideration away so that they can pursue life in the ways that are still available. In this way, denial is truly a mechanism of defense.

Many other researchers, along with Kübler-Ross, report anger as the second stage of dying. The stage is also linked to rage, fury, envy, resentment, and loathing. When "This cannot be happening to me" becomes, "This is happening to me. There was no mistake," patients are beginning to replace denial with attempts to understand what is happening to and inside them. When they do, they often ask, "Why me?" Though it is an unanswerable question, the logic of the question is clear. People, to remain human, must try to make intelligible their experiences and reality. The asking of this question is an important feature of the way in which all dying persons adapt to and cope with the reality of death.

People react with anger when they lose something of value; they react with greater anger when something of value is taken away from them by someone or something. Rage and fury, in fact, are often more accurate descriptions of people's reactions to the loss of their own life than is anger. Anger is a difficult stage for professionals and loved ones, more so when the anger and rage are displaced and projected randomly into any corner of the patient's world. An unfortunate result is that caregivers often experience the anger as personal, and the caregivers" own feelings of guilt, shame, grief, and rejection can contribute to lessening contact with the dying person, which increases his or her sense of isolation.

Bargaining is Kübler-Ross's third stage, but it is also the one about which she wrote the least and the one that other thanatologists are most likely to leave unrepresented in their own models and stages of how people cope with dying. Nevertheless, it is a common phenomenon wherein dying people fall back on their faith, belief systems, or sense of the transcendent and the spiritual and try to make a deal—with god, life, fate, a higher power, or the universe. They ask for more time to help family members reconcile or to achieve something of importance. They may ask if they can simply attend their child's wedding or graduation or if they can see their first grandchild born. Then they will be ready to die; they will go willingly. Often, they mean that they will die without fighting death, if death can only be delayed or will delay itself.

At some point, when terminally ill individuals are faced with decisions about more procedures, tests, surgeries, or medications or when their thinness, weakness, or deterioration becomes impossible to ignore, the anger, rage, numbness, stoicism, and even humor will likely give way to depression, Kübler-Ross's fourth stage and the one reaction that all thanatologists include in their models of how people cope with dying.

The depression can take many forms, for indeed there are always many losses, and each loss individually or several losses collectively might need to be experienced and worked through. For example, dying parents might ask themselves who will take care of the children, get them through school, walk them down the aisle, or guide them through life. Children, even adult children who are parents themselves, may ask whether they can cope without their own parents. They wonder who will support and anchor them in times of distress, who will (or could) love, nurture, and nourish them the way that their parents did. Depression accompanies the realization that each role, each function, will never be performed again. Both the dying and those who love them mourn.

Much of the depression takes the form of anticipatory grieving, which often occurs both in the dying and in those who will be affected by their death. It is a part of the dying process experienced by the living, both terminal and nonterminal. Patients, family, and friends can psychologically anticipate what it will be like when the death does occur and what life will, and will not, be like afterward. The grieving begins while there is still life left to live.

Bereavement specialists generally agree that anticipatory grieving, when it occurs, seems to help people cope with what is a terrible and frightening loss. It is an adaptive psychological mechanism wherein emotional, mental, and existential stability are painfully maintained. When depression develops, not only in reaction to death but also in preparation for it, it seems to be a necessary part of how those who are left behind cope to survive the loss themselves. Those who advocate or advise cheering up or looking on the bright side are either unrealistic or unable to tolerate the sadness in themselves or others. The dying are in the process of losing everything and everyone they love. Cheering up does not help them; the advice to "be strong" only helps the "helpers" deny the truth of the dying experience.

Both preparatory and reactive depression are frequently accompanied by unrealistic self-recrimination, shame, and guilt in the dying person. Those who are dying may judge themselves harshly and criticize themselves for the wrongs that they committed and for the good that they did not accomplish. They may judge themselves to be unattractive, unappealing, and repulsive because of how the illness and its treatment have affected them. These feelings and states of minds, which have nothing to do with the reality of the situation, are often amenable to the interventions of understanding and caring people. Financial and other obligations can be restructured and reassigned. Being forgiven and forgiving can help finish what was left undone.

Kübler-Ross's fifth stage, acceptance, is an intellectual and emotional coming to terms with death's reality, permanence, and inevitability. Ironically, it is manifested by diminished emotionality and interests and increased fatigue and inner (many would say spiritual) self-focus. It is a time without depression or anger. Envy of the healthy, the fear of losing all, and bargaining for another day or week are also absent. This final stage is often misunderstood. Some see it either as resignation and giving up or as achieving a happy serenity. Some think that acceptance is the goal of dying well and that all people are supposed to go through this stage. None of these viewpoints is accurate. Acceptance, when it does occur, comes from within the dying person. It is marked more by an emotional void and psychological detachment from people and things once held important and necessary and by an interest in some transcendental value (for the atheist) or god (for the theist). It has little to do with what others believe is important or "should" be done. It is when dying people become more intimate with themselves and appreciate their separateness from others more than at any other time.

Perspective and Prospects

Every person will eventually die, and the fact of death in each life is one that varies by culture in terms of its meaning. For some cultures, dying is seen as the ultimate difficulty for dying people and their loved ones. For other cultures, it is seen as not difficult at all, but more so like passing on to another realm of existence. In Western cultures, however, dying has very much become a medical process, and it is often a process filled with challenging questions. Patients ask questions that cannot be answered; families in despair and anger seek to find cause and sometimes to lay blame. It takes courage to be with individuals as they face their deaths, struggling to find meaning in the time that they have left. Given this, in Western medicine, a profession that prides itself on how well it intervenes to avoid outcomes like death, it takes courage to witness the process and struggle involved in death. Working with death also reminds professionals of their own inevitable death. Facing that fact inwardly, spiritually, and existentially also requires courage.

Cure and treatment become care and management in the dying. They should live relatively pain-free, be supported in accomplishing their goals, be respected, be involved in decision making as appropriate, be encouraged to function as fully as their illness allows, and be provided with others to whom control can comfortably and confidently be passed. The lack of a cure and the certainty of the end can intimidate health care providers, family members, and close friends. They may dread genuine encounters with those whose days are knowingly numbered. Yet the dying have the same rights to be helped as any of the living, and how a society assists them bears directly on the meaning that its members are willing to attach to their own lives.

Today, largely in response to what dying patients have told researchers, medicine recognizes its role to assist these patients in working toward an appropriate death. Caretakers must determine the optimum treatments, interventions, and conditions which will enable such a death to occur. For each terminally ill person, these should be unique and specific. Caretakers should respond to the patient's needs and priorities, at the patient's own pace and as much as possible following the patient's lead. For some dying patients, the goal is to remain as pain-free as is feasible and to feel as well as possible. For others, finishing whatever unfinished business remains becomes the priority. Making amends, forgiving and being forgiven, resolving old conflicts, and reconciling with one's self and others may be the most therapeutic and healing of interventions. Those who are to be bereaved fear the death of those they love. The dying fear the separation from all they know and love, but they fear as well the loss of autonomy, letting family and friends down, the pain and invasion of further treatment, disfigurement, dementia, loneliness, the unknown, becoming a burden, and the loss of dignity.

The English writer C. S. Lewis said that bereavement is the universal and integral part of the experience of loss. It requires effort, authenticity, mental and emotional work, a willingness to be afraid, and an openness to what is happening and what is going to happen. It requires an attitude that accepts, tolerates suffering, takes respite from the reality, reinvests in whatever life remains, and moves on. The only way to cope with dying or witnessing the dying of loved ones is by grieving through the pain, fear, loneliness, and loss of meaning. This process, which researcher Stephen Levine has likened to opening the heart in hell, is a viscous morass for most, and all people need to learn their own way through it and to have that learning respected. Healing begins with the first halting, unsteady, and frightening steps of genuine grief, which sometimes occur years before the "time of death" can be recorded.

—Paul Moglia, Ph.D.

See also Acquired immunodeficiency syndrome (AIDS); Aging; Depression; Ethics; Euthanasia; Grief and guilt; Hospice; Living will; Midlife crisis; Palliative medicine; Phobias; Psychiatry; Psychiatry, child and adolescent; Psychiatry, geriatric; Stress; Sudden infant death syndrome (SIDS); Suicide; Terminally ill: Extended care.

For Further Information:

Becker, Ernest. *The Denial of Death*. New York: Free Press, 1997. Written by an anthropologist and philosopher, this is an erudite and insightful analysis and synthesis of the role that the fear of death plays in motivating human activity, society, and individual actions. A profound work.

Cook, Alicia Skinner, and Daniel S. Dworkin. *Helping the Bereaved: Therapeutic Interventions for Children, Adolescents, and Adults*. New York: Basic Books, 1992. Although not a self-help book, this work is useful to professionals and nonprofessionals alike as a review of the state of the art in grief therapy. Practical and readable. Of special interest for those becoming involved in grief counseling.

Corr, Charles A., Clyde M. Nabe, and Donna M. Corr. *Death and Dying, Life and Living*. 6th ed. Belmont, Calif.: Wadsworth/Cengage Learning, 2009. This book provides perspective on common issues associated with death and dying for family members and others affected by life-threatening circumstances.

Forman, Walter B., et al., eds. *Hospice and Palliative Care: Concepts and Practice*. 2d ed. Sudbury, Mass.: Jones and Bartlett, 2003. A text that examines the theoretical perspectives and practical information about hospice care. Other topics include community medical care, geriatric care, nursing care, pain management, research, counseling, and hospice management.

Kübler-Ross, Elisabeth, ed. *Death: The Final Stage of Growth*. Reprint. New York: Simon & Schuster, 1997. A psychiatrist by training, Kübler-Ross brings together other researchers' views of how death provides the key to how human beings make meaning in their own personal worlds. Addresses practical concerns over how people express grief and accept the death of those close to them, and how they might prepare for their own inevitable ends.

Kushner, Harold. *When Bad Things Happen to Good People*. 20th anniversary ed. New York: Schocken Books, 2001. The first of Rabbi Kushner's works on finding meaning in one's life, it was originally his personal response to make intelligible the death of his own child. It has become a highly regarded reference for those who struggle with the meaning of pain, suffering, and death in their lives.

McFarlane, Rodger, and Philip Bashe. *The Complete Bedside Companion: No-Nonsense Advice on Caring for the Seriously Ill*. New York: Simon & Schuster, 1998. A comprehensive and practical guide to caregiving for patients with serious illnesses. The first section deals with the general needs of caring for the sick, while the second section covers specific illnesses in depth. Includes bibliographies and lists of support organizations.

DECONGESTANTS

Treatment

Anatomy or system affected: Circulatory system, ears, nose, respiratory system, throat

Specialties and related fields: Family medicine, otorhinolaryngology

Definition: Oral and topical medications that are used to relieve nasal and sinus congestion and to promote the opening of collapsed Eustachian tubes.

Key terms:

adjunctive: referring to the treatment of symptoms associated with a condition, not the condition itself

contraindication: a condition that makes a particular treatment not advisable; contraindications may be absolute (should never be used) or relative (should be used only with caution when the benefits outweigh the potential problems)

evidence-based medicine: a method of basing clinical medical practice decisions on systematic reviews of published medical studies

systemic: affecting the entire body; systemic treatments may be administered orally, directly into a vein, into the muscle, or through mucous membranes

topical: referring to treatments applied directly to the skin or mucous membranes that affect primarily the area in which they are applied

upper respiratory tract: the nose, sinuses, throat, ears, Eustachian tubes, and trachea

Indications and Procedures

Decongestants are used to shrink inflamed mucous membranes, promote drainage, or open collapsed Eustachian tubes. They are often used for the temporary relief of congestion caused by an upper respiratory tract infection (a cold), a sinus infection, or hay fever and other nasal allergies by promoting both nasal and sinus drainage. They are also often used as adjunctive therapy in the treatment of middle-ear infection (otitis media) to decrease congestion around the openings of the Eustachian tubes, and they may relieve the ear pressure, blockage, and pain experienced by some people during air travel. Careful scientific evaluation of the effectiveness of decongestants, however, has shown somewhat contradictory results.

The action of decongestants is accomplished primarily through stimulation of specific receptors in the smooth muscle of the upper respiratory tract, which in turn leads to constriction of the blood vessels and shrinkage of the mucous membranes. This improves air flow through the upper respiratory tract and relieves the sensation of stuffiness.

Uses and Complications

Decongestants may be applied topically, as sprays or drops, or taken by mouth. Commonly used decongestants include ephedrine, epinephrine, naphazoline, oxymetazoline, phenylephrine, pseudoephedrine, tetrahydrozoline, and xylometazoline. Some of these drugs are available over the counter and some by prescription only.

Oral preparations must be used with caution in elderly persons, children, and people with high blood pressure or other cardiac problems. If used as directed, decongestants do not usually cause excessive increases in blood pressure, overstimulate the heart, or change the distribution of blood in the circulatory system. The topical preparations are somewhat safer, because they are less likely to cause side effects, but they must also be used with caution.

The major advantage of oral decongestants is their long duration of action. Topical decongestants work more quickly but last a shorter period of time and are more likely to cause irritation of the tissues to which they are applied. If used too often or for too long a period of time (more than three to five days), nasal preparations may lead to a condition called rhinitis medicamentosa or rebound congestion, in which the congestion may be worse than before the person started using the medication.

People who take a certain type of antidepressant medication called a monoamine oxidase inhibitor (MAOI) and those with severe high blood pressure or heart disease should not take decongestants at all. People with thyroid disease, diabetes mellitus, glaucoma, or an enlarged prostate gland should take these drugs only after consulting a health care professional. Specific decongestants are contraindicated in infants and children.

People who take excessive doses of decongestants or who take them with other drugs that stimulate the central nervous system may experience insomnia, restlessness, dizziness, tremors, or nervousness. Overdose or long-term use of high doses may lead to hallucinations, convulsions, cardiovascular collapse, or even death.

Perspective and Prospects

Although decongestants have been widely used for decades, evidence-based medicine reveals few good studies indicating that decongestants do, in fact, treat illnesses. Systematic and careful reviews of the scientific studies available in the medical literature suggest that a single dose of a decongestant may relieve the stuffiness associated with the common cold in adults, but that no evidence exists for the usefulness of repeated doses. In people with a cough, a combination decongestant-antihistamine provides some relief in adults but not in children. In children with otitis media, there is a small statistical benefit from use of a combination decongestant-antihistamine, but it is not clear that the children benefit clinically. An evidence-based medicine review suggests that they not be used in children, especially given the increased risk of side effects from these medications in this age group.

—*Rebecca Lovell Scott, Ph.D., PA-C*

See also Allergies; Antihistamines; Anti-inflammatory drugs; Blood vessels; Common cold; Ear infections and disorders; Hay fever; Host-defense mechanisms; Immune system; Immunology; Inflammation; Multiple chemical sensitivity syndrome; Nasopharyngeal disorders; Otorhinolaryngology; Over-the-counter medications; Pharmacology; Pharmacy; Sinusitis; Smell.

For Further Information:

American Academy of Otolaryngology—Head and Neck Surgery. "Antihistamines, Decongestants, and Cold Remedies." *American Academy of Otolaryngology—Head and Neck Surgery*, December, 2010.

FamilyDoctor.org. "Decongestants: OTC Relief for Congestion." *FamilyDoctor.org*, February, 2012.

Flynn, C. A., G. Griffin, and F. Tudiver. "Decongestants and Antihistamines for Acute Otitis Media in Children." In *The Cochrane Library, Issue 4*. New York: John Wiley & Sons, 2003.

Komaroff, Anthony, ed. *Harvard Medical School Family Health Guide*. New York: Free Press, 2005.

Lacy, Charles F. *The Drug Information Handbook*. 20th ed. Hudson, Ohio: Lexi-Comp, 2011.

Schiff, Donald, and Steven Shelov, eds. *American Academy of Pediatrics Guide to Your Child's Symptoms: The Official, Complete Home Reference, Birth Through Adolescence*. New York: Villard, 1999.

Schroeder, K., and T. Fahey. "Over-the-Counter Medications for Acute Cough in Children and Adults in Ambulatory Settings." In *The Cochrane Library, Issue 4*. New York: John Wiley & Sons, 2003.

Taverner, D., L. Bickford, and M. Draper. "Nasal Decongestants for the Common Cold." In *The Cochrane Library, Issue 4*. New York: John Wiley & Sons, 2003.

DEEP VEIN THROMBOSIS
Disease/Disorder

Also known as: Blood clots, hypercoagulation

Anatomy or system affected: Blood, blood vessels, circulatory system, legs

Specialties and related fields: Family medicine, hematology

Definition: The formation of a blood clot (thrombus) in a deep vein that prevents blood circulation.

Key terms:

anticoagulant: a substance that hinders the clotting of blood

enzyme: a complex protein produced by living cells that catalyzes certain biochemical reactions at body temperature

fibrin: a fibrous insoluble protein formed from fibrinogen by the action of thrombin, especially in the clotting of blood

fibrinogen: a protein produced in the liver that is present in blood plasma and is converted to fibrin during the clotting of blood

platelet: a minute disk of vertebrate blood that assists in blood clotting

thrombin: an enzyme that facilitates the clotting of blood by catalyzing a conversion of fibrinogen to fibrin

Causes and Symptoms

Deep vein or venous thrombosis (DVT) is a blood clot (thrombus) in a deep vein. In vessels that transport blood toward the heart, various disorders including skin infections or phlebitis (inflammation of the vein) can occur; however, specific tests are required to diagnose the existence of DVT. While phlebitis afflicts superficial veins, DVT occurs in deep veins, usually in the legs.

Because of the possibility of its breaking loose, lodging in the lungs, and creating a potentially fatal pulmonary embolism (blockage of blood to the lungs), a clot in the leg is highly dangerous. Clots in veins in the legs generally form following

---

Information on Deep Vein Thrombosis

Causes: Prolonged inactivity, surgery, cancer, pregnancy, oral contraceptive use

Symptoms: Pain, redness, warmth; often none

Duration: Three to six months, possibly longer

Treatments: Anticoagulation drugs (heparin, coumadin)

---

long periods of inactivity or lengthy bed rest, pregnancy, obesity, smoking, estrogen therapy, oral contraceptive medication, or surgery.

With DVT, the afflicted leg begins to swell, turn red, become warm, and throb. Occasionally, the area is tender to touch or movement. However, about one-half of the instances of DVT produce no symptoms, and it is frequently referred to as a silent killer.

Treatment and Therapy

Treatment for deep vein thrombosis begins with anticoagulants (blood thinners), specifically heparin, administered intravenously in the hospital, or through self-injections given at home. The anticoagulant warfarin (Coumadin), given as pills, are then prescribed daily to prevent clots from becoming larger. Frequent check-ups with a physician are mandatory to maintain a certain level of medication effectiveness; depending upon the risk of further clotting, Coumadin can be required anywhere from three months to the remainder of the patient's life. Patients may also be advised to elevate the afflicted leg or apply a heating pad to the area. Walking is sometimes recommended, as is wearing tight-fitting stockings or compression stockings to reduce pain and swelling. In the event that Coumadin is unable to prevent blood clots, a filter may be surgically placed into the vena cava, the large vein carrying blood from the lower body to the heart, to prevent clots from entering the lungs. Also, a large clot may be removed through surgery or may be treated with powerful clot-destroying drugs.

Perspective and Prospects

Inquiries into the mysteries of blood coagulation have existed since 400 BCE, when Hippocrates observed that blood appeared to congeal as it cooled. By the nineteenth century, Pierre Andral, the founder of hematology (the branch of biology that deals with the blood and the blood-forming organs) and one of the first physicians to study the chemistry of the blood, formulated the classical hypothesis of blood coagulation. He found that the process of blood coagulation follows two pathways: the intrinsic, wherein, within seconds, platelets form a hemostatic plug at the site of the injury (primary hemostasis, or stoppage of bleeding); and the extrinsic, wherein fibrin molecules react in a complex cascade or network (secondary hemostasis) that ultimately moves into a third stage, wherein protein factors combine with the enzyme thrombin and contribute to the clotting of blood. Twentieth-century research determined, however, that the tissue pathway (formerly known as the extrinsic) is a series of enzymes generated to participate with thrombin and catalyze fibrinogen into fibrin, which is essential to blood clotting. These factors are responsible for any abnormalities in the clotting of blood.

While the most commonly known blood clotting disorder is hemophilia, or uncontrolled bleeding, its opposite condition, hypercoagulation, specifically the formation of abnormal clots in veins, can also be life-threatening. In 1994, the clotting disorder factor V Leiden (named for the Dutch city in which it was discovered) was identified as a hereditary resistance to activated protein C. An estimated 30 percent of those individuals who suffer from hypercoagulation are afflicted by this enzyme mutation that encourages the overproduction of thrombin and, consequently, causes excessive clotting. Most of these persons are unaware of their condition or its dangers. Treatment and control of this disorder depends largely on antiplatelet medication, such as aspirin or clopidogrel (Plavix), that is designed to prevent platelets from sticking together. Maintaining a heart-healthy lifestyle by getting regular caradiovascular exercise, maintaining a healthy weight, avoiding smoking, and controlling blood pressure and cholesterol levels can significantly reduce an individual's risk of developing lethal blood clots.

Continued research into the complexities of coagulation account for new developments in medications, including thrombin inhibitors or molecular products that target enzymes controlling specific coagulation factors.

—Mary Hurd

See also Bleeding; Blood and blood disorders; Blood vessels; Circulation; Disseminated intravascular coagulation (DIC); Embolism; Hematology; Hematology, pediatric; Hemophilia; Lower extremities; Thrombus; Varicose vein removal; Vascular medicine; Vascular system.

For Further Information:

American Medical Association. *Family Medical Guide.* 4th ed. New York: John Wiley, 2004.
"Are You at Risk for Deep Vein Thrombosis?" *Centers for Disease Control and Prevention*, March 7, 2011.
"Fact Sheet: Deep Vein Thrombosis and Pulmonary Embolism." *SurgeonGeneral.gov*, n.d.
Johnston, Bernard, ed. *Collier's Encyclopedia.* 24 vols. New York: Collier's, 1997.
Owen, Charles A. *History of Blood Coagulation.* Edited by William L. Nichols and E. J. Walter Bowie. Rochester, Minn.: Mayo Foundation for Medical Education and Research, 2001.
"What Is Deep Vein Thrombosis?" *National Heart, Lung, and Blood Institute*, October 28, 2011.
Wood, Debra. "Deep Vein Thrombosis." *Health Library*, May 7, 2013.

DEFIBRILLATION

Procedure

Also known as: Cardioversion, defib, shock

Anatomy or system affected: Blood, blood vessels, brain, cells, chest, circulatory system, heart, nervous system, respiratory system

Specialties and related fields: Anesthesiology, biotechnology, cardiology, critical care, emergency medicine, ethics, exercise physiology, family medicine, forensic medicine, general surgery, internal medicine, nursing, occupational health, pulmonary medicine, sports medicine, toxicology, vascular medicine

Definition: A procedure that shocks the heart with therapeutic volts of electricity. Applied correctly and in the right circumstances, these shocks can change a life-threatening heart rhythm to a normal cardiac rhythm.

Key terms:

automated external defibrillators (AEDs): portable and automated devices that deliver life-saving shocks

cardiac: referring to the heart

normal sinus rhythm: the heart's normal electrical activity

pulseless ventricular tachycardia (VT), ventricular fibrillation (VF): abnormal heart rhythms needing immediate defibrillation

Indications and Procedures

Heart tissue beats in a rhythmic manner as a result of electrical signals generated by the heart tissue. Sometimes, the normal heart rhythm, known as "normal sinus rhythm," goes awry. Many different abnormal heart rhythms can develop from a variety of causes. These abnormal heart rhythms, known as "arrhythmias," can be deadly since the heart cannot effectively pump blood when the heart is not in normal sinus rhythm. "Cardioversion" refers to any procedure that seeks to correct an arrhythmia and return the heart to normal sinus rhythm. Defibrillation, or electrical cardioversion, delivers short bursts of direct electrical current across the chest to the heart.

Although cardioversion is used for a variety of abnormal and dangerous heart rhythms, defibrillation treats two very deadly arrhythmias, known as "ventricular fibrillation (VF)" and "pulseless ventricular tachycardia (VT)." The heart has four chambers: two atria and two ventricles. The ventricles pump blood to the lungs and body. In VF, the heart's electrical activity is chaotic and disorganized. This electrical chaos results in the ventricles fibrillating (quivering like a bag of wiggling worms) and unable to pump blood. If blood is not pumped, the body will die in a manner of minutes. Therefore, defibrillation is of urgent and lifesaving importance.

In VT, the ventricles are beating very fast. If the patient is unconscious and has no pulse (this can happen if the ventricles are beating too fast to fill up with enough blood to circulate), then VT treatment includes defibrillation.

A person with VF is unconscious because that person will have no cardiac output and no pulse. If the patient is placed on a cardiac monitor, a distinctive abnormal electrical pattern is displayed. The patient will shortly die if the fibrillation is not resolved quickly. The electrical current delivered during defibrillation shocks the heart tissue. This electrical shock stops all electrical heart activity, a process called "depolarization," and resets the heart's electrical activity. Once the heart resets with defibrillation, normal sinus rhythm can take over.

Electrical cardioversion is also used as an elective, nonemergency procedure for rhythm control in patients with atrial fibrillation (an arrhythmia originating in the atrium) and in cases of VT with a pulse.

Uses and Complications

Advanced cardiac life-support ambulance units and hospitals use devices equipped with electrical paddles and heart rhythm monitors for defibrillation. An unconscious patient with no pulse, showing the characteristic pattern of VF or VT on the cardiac monitor, will be urgently shocked with specified doses of electricity. The paddles are placed firmly on the patient's chest wall. Firm pressure, along with electrode paste, gel, or saline pads, helps ensure good electrical contact between the paddles and the chest wall.

Before discharging the electricity through the paddles, health care providers check the area surrounding the patient to ensure that no one is in physical contact with the patient or anything touching the patient. The electricity will shock anyone in direct contact with the patient or any metal touching the patient. This shock can change normal sinus rhythm into an abnormal rhythm. The health care provider delivering the shock must quickly look around the area and shout "clear" and must avoid touching metal objects (such as the stretcher frame) with any body part. Hands in the paddles are safely insulated from the delivered electricity.

Defibrillation protocols specify the sequencing and amount of electricity delivered during defibrillation. These protocols are quite detailed, involving cardiopulmonary resuscitation (CPR) and various medications.

Complications of defibrillation include damage to the heart muscle, which is rare unless repeated high energy shocks are used; blood clots dislodging from the heart and traveling to the body and lungs, causing problems when the clots block off blood supply; other abnormal heart rates emerging after defibrillation; fluid and blood backing up into the lungs, resulting in pulmonary edema (swelling); and low blood pressure that usually resolves in three to four hours.

Perspective and Prospects

Automated external defibrillators (AEDs) are lifesaving devices that have gained in prominence and availability since the late twentieth century. AEDs are portable machines often found in public areas, such as airports, sports arenas, shopping malls, or office buildings. They differ from the larger cart-based defibrillators found in health care facilities in several ways, so that they are easier and simpler to use. AED electrodes are attached to the patient with adhesive pads, rather than pressed down by hands and paddles, allowing hands-free operation. AEDs have microprocessors built into the system that detect ventricular fibrillation or ventricular tachycardia. If the device senses VF or VT, then the device advises the operator to deliver a shock.

The portable and automated nature of AEDs saves lives. Defibrillation is needed to reset the heart's electrical activity within minutes of the patient losing consciousness as the result of VF or VT. When defibrillation is indicated, earlier treatment is better. The increasing availability of AEDs, along with the ability of people trained to use the automated device in the right circumstances, promises to save even more lives in future.

An automatic implantable cardioverter defibrillator (ICD) has been developed for those with unpredictable fibrillation. An ICD incorporates a pacemaker component and, much like an external defibrillator, can deliver large electrical jolts directly to the heart to restore normal rhythm.

—*Richard P. Capriccioso, M.D.*

See also Arrhythmias; Cardiac arrest; Cardiology; Cardiology, pediatric; Cardiopulmonary resuscitation (CPR); Emergency medicine; Emergency medicine, pediatric; Heart; Heart attack; Pacemaker implantation; Paramedics; Resuscitation.

For Further Information:

A.D.A.M. Medical Encyclopedia. "Cardioversion." *MedlinePlus*, June 22, 2012.

A.D.A.M. Medical Encyclopedia. "Implantable Cardioverter-Defibrillator." *MedlinePlus*, November 8, 2010.

Calvagna, Mary, and Michael J. Fucci. "Automatic Cardioverter Defibrillator Implantation." *Health Library*, November 26, 2012.

"Cardioversion." *Health Library*, November 26, 2012.

Chan, Paul S., et al. "Delayed Time to Defibrillation After In-Hospital Cardiac Arrest." *New England Journal of Medicine* 358, no. 1 (January 3, 2008): 9–17.

Picard, André. "School Defibrillators Could Be Lifesavers." *Globe and Mail*, March 31, 2009.

Rull, Gurvinder. "Defibrillation and Cardioversion." *Patient.co.uk*, January 22, 2010.

"2005 American Heart Association Guidelines for Cardiopulmonary Resuscitation and Emergency Cardiovascular Care." *Circulation* 112, no. 24 supp. (December 13, 2005): IV-1–IV-5.

DEHYDRATION

Disease/Disorder

Anatomy or system affected: Brain, cells, circulatory system

Specialties and related fields: Exercise physiology, family medicine, sports medicine, vascular medicine

Definition: Excessive loss of body water, which is often accompanied by disturbances in electrolyte balance.

Key terms:

electrolytes: elements dissolved within body fluids that help regulate metabolism

plasma: the fluid portion of the blood

relative humidity: the percent moisture saturation of ambient air

Causes and Symptoms

The average adult's total body weight is approximately 60 percent water. Daily water requirements vary based on age, gender, level of physical activity, and climate. Dehydration, loss of 3 to 5 percent or more of body weight, is often accompanied by the loss of essential electrolytes such as sodium, potassium, and chloride. Conditions that deplete body water faster than it is absorbed include fever-induced sweating, diarrhea, vomiting, acidosis, anorexia nervosa, bulimia, diabetes mellitus and insipidus, poor nutrition, obesity, and lack of acclimatization to heat stress. People exercising in hot, humid environments provide an excellent example of how dehydration develops and progresses. Symptoms of dehydration may include dry mouth, lips, and skin; decreased salivation; dizziness; dark-colored urine; weakness; constipation; and confusion.

Information on Dehydration

Causes: Fever-induced sweating, diarrhea, vomiting, acidosis, diabetes mellitus and insipidus, anorexia nervosa, bulimia, malnutrition, obesity, sedentary lifestyle, lack of acclimatization to heat stress

Symptoms: Flushed skin, dark yellow urine, cramps, and heat exhaustion or stroke, causing cool and clammy skin, low blood pressure, rapid but weak heart rate, faintness, dizziness, headaches

Duration: Acute

Treatments: Rapid restoration of fluid volume and electrolyte balance

Heat gain is higher and evaporative heat loss is lower during physical exertion for children than adults, predisposing children to more rapid and severe dehydration. Both child and adult bodies attempt to reduce the buildup of metabolic heat through blood flow adjustments and sweat gland secretion. Flushed, red skin indicates that peripheral blood vessels have dilated, carrying blood and internal heat to the body surface for cooling. Once the heat is carried to the periphery by the bloodstream, dissipation occurs mainly by sweat evaporation. Large quantities of sweat may roll off the skin in a high humidity environment, but cooling only occurs when the sweat evaporates. Children exhibit a higher number of sweat glands per unit of body surface area than do adults, with each immature sweat gland producing about 40 percent as much sweat as an adult sweat gland. Children also gain heat from the environment faster than do adults because of their larger body surface area to body weight ratio; they dehydrate quicker as a result of lower overall fluid storage capacity. A large portion of the fluid released as sweat comes from the circulating blood plasma, making fluid consumption to rebuild blood plasma volume and to replenish lost water weight very important. Children acclimatize to a heat stress environment such as a sauna more slowly than do adults. They generally need at least six exposures before adjusting, whereas adults need only about three acclimation bouts.

The effects of dehydration are of particular concern in infants and young children, since their electrolyte balance can become precarious.

Treatment and Therapy

Rapid restoration of fluid volume and electrolyte balance are primary treatment goals that may require intravenous infusion if sufficient fluid cannot be ingested orally.

"Prehydrating" the body by consuming liberal amounts of fluid before anticipated heat stress and "trickle hydrating" while losing body fluid are critical. Cool fluids of about 40 degrees Fahrenheit (about 5 degrees Celsius) empty from the gastrointestinal tract and supply the dehydrated cells more quickly than warmer or colder temperature fluid. Studies of fluid absorption indicate that excessive sugar in electrolyte drinks slows water movement into the bloodstream. Children have been shown voluntarily to drink nearly twice as much when flavored fluids, as compared to plain water, are allowed.

Monitoring body weight before and after dehydration episodes and drinking enough water to regain lost weight is important. Nearly all body weight lost during exercise is attributable to water loss, not fat loss. Consuming 1 pint (473 milliliters) of fluid will replenish 1 pound (9.45 kilograms) of water weight loss. People should drink back all lost water weight even though they may not feel thirsty, as the human thirst mechanism is not a good indicator of actual need. Checking the urine is also recommended, as dark yellow urine indicates that more water consumption is needed and clear, nearly colorless urine indicates that adequate rehydration has been achieved. Wearing light-colored, loose-fitting clothing in the heat is recommended, as rubberized or tight-weave clothing interferes with sweat evaporation and body cooling.

Other suggestions for countering dehydration include getting into good physical condition and acclimatizing to the heat. Conditioning increases the body's metabolic efficiency, so that fewer of the calories burned accumulate as heat; enhances blood plasma volume to enable a larger sweat reserve; and reduces fat weight that insulates the body and retards heat dissipation. Eating a carbohydrate-enriched diet will retain water in muscle cells at a rate of nearly 3 grams of water per 1 gram of stored glycogen, whereas stored fat retains minimal water.

Perspective and Prospects

Many episodes of dehydration can be prevented from developing into heat cramps, heat exhaustion, and heatstroke during sporting events by adhering to the aforementioned guidelines. Heat cramps, especially muscle spasms in the calves and stomach, may occur during intense sweating, with the accompanying loss of electrolytes. Mineral loss, however, is always of secondary importance to fluid loss because water provides the medium in which all cellular processes occur.

Heat exhaustion occurs when increased sweating and peripheral blood flow reduce venous return of blood to the heart, resulting in cool and clammy skin, lower-than-normal blood pressure, and a rapid but weak heart rate. Less blood is pumped to the brain, causing weakness, faintness, dizziness, headaches, and a grayish look to the face. Treatment includes lying down in a shaded, breezy place, drinking cool fluids, removing excess clothing, and replenishing electrolytes. Heatstroke occurs when the brain can no longer maintain thermal balance, as evidenced by the cessation of sweating, hot (sometimes white to gray) skin, rapid and full pulse, and a rise in body temperature over 104 degrees Fahrenheit leading to disorientation and unconsciousness. Heatstroke is rare but requires immediate medical attention to reduce body temperature. The body temperature should be lowered quickly by placing cool cloths or ice packs to the groin, neck, and under the arms. Cool sheets may be placed over and under the patient. The patient should not be allowed to shiver, which increases the body temperature. Caretakers should be alert for seizures and the possible need to perform cardiopulmonary resuscitation (CPR). The most effective treatment is prevention through proper hydration.

—Daniel G. Graetzer, Ph.D.;
updated by Amy Webb Bull, D.S.N., A.P.N.

See also Anorexia nervosa; Appetite loss; Bulimia; Cardiovascular system; Constipation; Diabetes mellitus; Diarrhea and dysentery; Dizziness and fainting; Emergency medicine; Emergency medicine, pediatric; Enterocolitis; Exercise physiology; Fever; Headaches; Heat exhaustion and heatstroke; Malnutrition; Motion sickness; Nausea and vomiting; Nutrition; Obesity; Pyloric stenosis; Seizures; Sweating; Well-baby examinations.

For Further Information:

Brody, Jane E. "For Lifelong Gains, Just Add Water. Repeat." *The New York Times*, July 11, 2000, p. F8.

"Dehydration and Oral Rehydration." *JAMA Pediatrics*, August 2010.

"Dehydration." *Nemours Foundation*, July 2013.

"How Do I Know If I'm Dehydrated?" *Harvard Medical School*, February 22, 2011.

Martini, Frederic H., and Edwin F. Bartholomew. *Essentials of Anatomy and Physiology*. 6th ed. Boston: Pearson, 2012.

McArdle, William, Frank I. Katch, and Victor L. Katch. *Exercise Physiology: Energy, Nutrition, and Human Performance*. 7th ed. Boston: Lippincott Williams & Wilkins, 2010.

Sawka, Michael N., Samuel N. Cheuvront, and Robert Carter. "Human Water Needs." *Nutrition Reviews* 63, no. 6 (June, 2005): S30–S39.

Sawka, Michael N., and Scott J. Montain. "Fluid and Electrolyte Supplementation for Exercise Heat Stress." *American Journal of Clinical Nutrition* 72, no. 2S (August, 2000): S564–S572.

Sturt, Patty Ann. "Environmental Conditions." In *Mosby's Emergency Nursing Reference*, edited by Julia Fulz and Sturt. 3d ed. St. Louis, Mo.: Mosby/Elsevier, 2005.

Delirium

Disease/Disorder

Anatomy or system affected: Central nervous system

Specialties and related fields: Neurology, gerontology, internal medicine

Definition: A neurocognitive disorder characterized by a change in attention and awareness (i.e., reduced ability to direct, focus, sustain, and shift attention).

Key terms:

cognition: mental processes including memory, attention, language, judgment and problem-solving

dementia: a syndrome wherein the person loses cognitive ability over time

inattention: the inability to focus, stay on subject or easily follow a conversation

polypharmacy: the use of more than one medication together

Causes and Symptoms

Usually by treating the cause of the delirium, the delirious state will resolve. The most common causes of delirium are substance intoxication, substance withdrawal, medication-induced or delirium due to a medical condition. In addition, a person's baseline frailty contributes to his or her vulnerability to delirium. Elderly persons and those with underlying brain diseases such as dementia, Parkinson's, and stroke are more likely to suffer delirious states.

Substance intoxication can be of any illicit or legal substance that could potentially change a person's mental status. Examples include illicit drugs such as marijuana or psychotropic drugs such as Lysergic acid diethylamide (LSD). Legal substances like alcohol can also cause delirious states. Withdrawal from these same types of drugs may also cause delirium including anti-anxiety medication, antidepressants and pain medication.

Medication-induced delirium is delirium caused by the side effect of a medication. Medications that commonly cause delirium are anti-anxiety medications, opioid painkillers such as morphine, sedative medications for sleep, and stimulant-type medications such as those taken for attention-deficit disorder. More commonly, delirium can be caused by polypharmacy, which is the use of more than one medication together. In this case, the interactions between those drugs may either enhance one drug over another, or the combination of drugs may cause a synergistic effect.

Delirium can also be due to a medical condition. Dehydration, malnutrition, cancer, and infection are common causes of medical conditions that may precipitate into delirium. Furthermore, delirium is commonly seen in postoperative patients. Though this phenomenon is not linked to the use of anesthesia or sedation, underlying medical conditions (including preexisting neurocognitive disorders), overall health status and pain controls are correlated to delirium.

Change in awareness or attention. People who are delirious have a difficult time focusing their attention and have a change in their level of awareness. This may present as drowsiness or fatigue in a person, and can easily be missed. Inattention presents as their inability to focus (i.e., easily distractible), stay on subject or easily follow a conversation. It is easy to see why early signs of delirium are easily missed, as these attributes could be attributable to any variety of factors.

Change in cognition. Cognition is the ability for one to think, understand, learn, or remember. During delirious states, a person will have a change in cognition. This may be as abrupt as the loss of speech or incoherent speech, or it may be as subtle as being slightly confused. Memory may be impaired, and the person may not be able to recall names, dates, or places. These impairments can be confusing or frightening to people, and may cause them to be agitated and anxious.

Fluctuation over time. The last hallmark of delirium is the time course of the condition. Delirium comes on over hours to days and can last days to months. The relative quick onset of delirium distinguishes it from dementia, which is characterized by its slow and insidious presentation. Even within the day, a person's mental status can change. Often, the affected person may seem perfectly lucid in the morning and may become progressively more confused during the day and into the night.

Treatment and Therapy

The best treatment for delirium is prevention, especially as this relates to medication-induced or medically related delirium. Medications should be reviewed for their side effects, and special care should be taken for frail patients with underlying neurocognitive disorders or those on many medications. Prevention of intoxication, dehydration, and malnutrition are almost always modifiable and can make a person less vulnerable to delirium. Identifying and treating infections early would also help in preventing delirium.

Most delirium occurs in hospital settings. When this occurs, the medical team will try to find the cause of the delirium. Usually, this has to do with identifying likely medication(s) or an underlying medical reason that caused the delirium. If known, it is possible to give an antidote for a particular medication; sometimes this is not possible, and withdrawing from the medication and awaiting the outcome is the only option. When the underlying condition is thought to be medical, the team will treat the medical condition. For example, if uncontrolled pain is the likely source of the delirium, pain control will be offered and monitored; or if a bacterial infection caused the delirium, antibiotics will be used to treat the infection.

In the meanwhile, supportive therapies will contribute to the well-being of the person who is delirious. Adequate nutrition and hydration are mainstays of therapy. Because the person may be bedbound during his or her delirium, keeping the person as active as possible without risking injury is also important. Family members and caretakers can help orient the person to time and place, talk about memories they have shared together, and bring in familiar items to make them feel safe.

Oftentimes, because confusion leads to frustration and anger for the person suffering from delirium, medications such as lorazepam or haloperidol may be given in low doses to help control disruptive, agitated, or combative behaviors.

—*Maki Matsumura*

See also Dehydration; Dementia; Fluid-electrolyte imbalance; Malnutrition; Parkinson's disease; Surgery

For Further Information:
Diagnostic and Statistical Manual of Mental Disorders, 5th Edition: DSM-5. Arlington, VA: American Psychiatric Publishing, 2013.
Francis, J., and G.B. Young. "Diagnosis of Delirium and Confusional States." *UpToDate,* edited by M.J. Aminoff, K.E. Schmader, and J.L. Wilterdink. Retrieved from http://www.uptodate.com/contents/diagnosis-of-delirium-and-confusional-states?detectedLanguage=en&source=search_result&search=delirium&selected Title=1~150&provider=noProvider.

DEMENTIAS
Disease/Disorder
Anatomy or system affected: Brain, nervous system, psychic-emotional system
Specialties and related fields: Geriatrics and gerontology, neurology, psychiatry
Definition: A group of disorders involving pervasive, progressive, and irreversible decline in cognitive functioning resulting from a variety of causes; differs from mental retardation, in which the affected person never reaches an expected level of mental growth.
Key terms:
basal ganglia: a collection of nerve cells deep inside the brain, below the cortex, that controls muscle tone and automatic actions such as walking
cortical dementia: dementia resulting from damage to the brain cortex, the outer layer of the brain that contains the bodies of the nerve cells
delirium: an acute condition characterized by confusion, a fluctuating level of consciousness, and visual, auditory, and even tactile hallucinations; often caused by acute disease, such as infection or intoxication
hydrocephalus: a condition resulting from the accumulation of fluid inside the brain in cavities known as ventricles; as fluid accumulates, it exerts pressure on the neighboring brain cells, which may be destroyed
subcortical dementia: dementia resulting from damage to the area of the brain below the cortex; this area contains nerve fibers that connect various parts of the brain with one another and with the basal ganglia
vascular dementia: dementia caused by repeated strokes, resulting in interference with the blood supply to parts of the brain

Causes and Symptoms
Dementia affects an estimated 35.6 million people worldwide, according to the World Health Organization, and is a major cause of disability in individuals over sixty. Its prevalence increases with age. Dementia is characterized by a permanent memory deficit affecting recent memory in particular and of sufficient severity to interfere with the patient's ability to take part in professional and social activities. Dementia is not part of the normal aging process. It also is not synonymous with benign senescent forgetfulness, which is more common and affects recent memory. Although the latter is a source of frustration, it does not significantly interfere with the individual's professional and social activities because it tends to affect only trivial matters (or what the individual considers trivial). Furthermore, patients with benign forgetfulness usually can remember what was forgotten by using a number of strategies, such as writing lists or notes to themselves and leaving them in conspicuous places. Individuals with benign forgetfulness also are acutely aware of their memory deficit, while those with dementia, except in the early stages of the disease or for specific types of dementia, generally have no insight into their memory deficit and often blame others for their problems.

In addition to the memory deficit, patients with dementia often show evidence of impaired abstract thinking, impaired judgment, or other disturbances of higher cortical functions such as aphasia (the inability to use or comprehend language), apraxia (the inability to execute complex, coordinated movements), or agnosia (the inability to recognize familiar objects).

Dementia may result from damage to the cerebral cortex (the outer layer of the brain), as in Alzheimer's disease, or from damage to the subcortical structures (the structures below the cortex), such as white matter, the thalamus, or the basal ganglia. Although memory is impaired in both cortical and subcortical dementias, the associated features are different. In cortical dementias, for example, cognitive functions

Information on Dementias

Causes: Aging, diseases (Alzheimer's, Pick's, Parkinson's), stroke, chronic infections, head trauma

Symptoms: Impaired abstract thinking, impaired judgment, inability to use or comprehend language, inability to recognize familiar objects, inability to execute complex movements

Duration: Chronic

Treatments: None; alleviation of symptoms

such as the ability to understand speech and to talk and the ability to perform mathematical calculations are severely impaired. In subcortical dementias, on the other hand, there is evidence of disturbances of arousal, motivation, and mood in addition to a significant slowing of cognition and of information processing.

Alzheimer's disease, the most common cause of presenile dementia, is characterized by progressive disorientation, memory loss, speech disturbances, and personality disorders. Pick's disease is another cortical dementia, but unlike Alzheimer's disease, it is rare, tends to affect younger patients, and is more common in women. In the early stages of Pick's disease, changes in personality, absence of inhibition, inappropriate social and sexual conduct, and lack of foresight may be evident—features that are not common in Alzheimer's disease. Patients also may become euphoric or apathetic. Poverty of speech is often present and gradually progresses to mutism, although speech comprehension is usually spared. Pick's disease is characterized by cortical atrophy localized to the frontal and temporal lobes.

Vascular dementia is another common cause of dementia in patients over the age of sixty-five and is responsible for an estimated 20 to 30 percent of all dementia cases. It is caused by interference with the blood flow to the brain. Although the overall prevalence of vascular dementia is decreasing, there are some geographical variations, with the prevalence being higher in countries with a high incidence of cardiovascular and cerebrovascular diseases, such as Finland and Japan. Some patients with dementia have both Alzheimer's disease and vascular dementia. Several types of vascular dementia have been identified.

Multiple infarct dementia (MID) is the most common type of vascular dementia. As its name implies, it is the result of multiple, discrete cerebral infarcts (strokes) that have destroyed enough brain tissue to interfere with the patient's higher mental functions. The onset of MID is usually sudden and is associated with neurological deficit, such as the paralysis or weakness of an arm or leg or the inability to speak. The disease characteristically progresses in steps: With each stroke experienced, the patient's condition suddenly deteriorates and then stabilizes or even improves slightly until another stroke occurs. In some cases, however, the disease displays an insidious onset and causes gradual deterioration. Most patients also show evidence of arteriosclerosis and other factors predisposing them to the development of strokes, such as hypertension, cigarette smoking, high blood cholesterol, diabetes mellitus, narrowing of one or both carotid arteries, or cardiac disorders, especially atrial fibrillation (an irregular heartbeat). Somatic complaints, mood changes, depression, and nocturnal confusion tend to be more common in vascular dementias, although there is relative preservation of the patient's personality. In such cases, magnetic resonance imaging (MRI) or a computed tomography (CT) scan of the brain often shows evidence of multiple strokes.

Strokes are not always associated with clinical evidence of neurological deficits, since the stroke may affect a "silent" area of the brain or may be so small that its immediate impact is not noticeable. Nevertheless, when several of these small strokes have occurred, the resulting loss of brain tissue may interfere with the patient's cognitive functions. This is, in fact, the basis of the lacunar dementias. The infarcted tissue is absorbed into the rest of the brain, leaving a small cavity or lacuna. Brain-imaging techniques and especially MRI are useful in detecting these lacunae.

A number of neurological disorders are associated with dementia. The combination of dementia, urinary incontinence, and muscle rigidity causing difficulties in walking should raise the suspicion of hydrocephalus. In this condition, fluid accumulates inside the ventricles (cavities within the brain) and results in increased pressure on the brain cells. A CT scan demonstrates enlargement of the ventricles. Although some patients may respond well to surgical shunting of the cerebrospinal fluid, it is often difficult to identify those who will benefit from surgery. Postoperative complications are significant and include strokes and subdural hematomas.

Dementia has been linked to Parkinson's disease, a chronic, progressive neurological disorder that usually manifests itself in middle or late life. It has an insidious onset and a very slow progression rate. Although intellectual deterioration is not one of the classical features of Parkinson's disease, dementia is being recognized as a late manifestation of the disease, with as many as 50 to 80 percent of patients eventually being afflicted. The dementing process also has an insidious onset and slow progression rate. Some of the medication used to treat Parkinson's disease also may induce confusion, particularly in older patients.

Subdural hematomas (collections of blood inside the brain) may lead to mental impairment and are usually precipitated by trauma to the head. Usually, the trauma is slight and the patient neither loses consciousness nor experiences any immediate significant effects. A few days or even weeks later, however, the patient may develop evidence of mental impairment. By that time, the patient and caregivers may have forgotten about the slight trauma that the patient had experienced. A subdural hematoma should be suspected in the presence of a fairly sudden onset and progressing course. Headaches are common. A CT scan can reveal the presence of a hematoma. The surgical removal of the hematoma is usually associated with a good prognosis if the surgery is done in a timely manner, before irreversible brain damage occurs.

Brain tumors may lead to dementia, particularly if they are slow growing. Most tumors of this type can be diagnosed by

CT scanning or MRI. Occasionally, cancer may induce dementia through an inflammation of the brain.

Many chronic infections affecting the brain can lead to dementia; they include conditions that, when treated, may reverse or prevent the progression of dementia, such as syphilis, tuberculosis, slow viruses, and some fungal and protozoal infections. Human immunodeficiency virus (HIV) infection is also a cause of dementia, and it may be suspected if the rate of progress is rapid and the patient has risk factors for the development of HIV infection. Although dementia is part of the acquired immunodeficiency syndrome (AIDS) complex, it may occasionally be the first manifestation of the disease.

It is often difficult to differentiate depression from dementia. Nevertheless, sudden onset—especially if preceded by an emotional event, the presence of sleep disturbances, and a history of previous psychiatric illness—is suggestive of depression. The level of mental functioning of patients with depression is often inconsistent. They may, for example, be able to give clear accounts of topics that are of personal interest to them but be very vague about, and at times not even attempt to answer, questions on topics that are of no interest to them. Variability in performance during testing is suggestive of depression, especially if it improves with positive reinforcement.

Treatment and Therapy

It is estimated that dementia affects about 1 percent of the population aged sixty to sixty-four years. By age eighty-five and higher, however, it affects anywhere from 25 to 50 percent of individuals. While different surveys may yield different results, depending on the criteria used to define dementia, it is clear that this is a significant problem.

For physicians, an important aspect of diagnosing patients with dementia is detecting potentially reversible causes that may be responsible for the impaired mental functions. A detailed history followed by a meticulous and thorough clinical examination and a few selected laboratory tests are usually sufficient to reach a diagnosis. Various investigators have estimated that reversible causes of dementia can be identified in 10 percent to 20 percent of patients. Recommended investigations include brain imaging (CT scanning or MRI), a complete blood count, and tests of erythrocyte sedimentation rate, blood glucose, serum electrolytes, serum calcium, liver function, thyroid function, and serum B_{12} and folate. Some investigators also recommend routine testing for syphilis. Other tests, such as those for the detection of HIV infection, cerebrospinal fluid examination, neuropsychological testing, drug and toxin screening, serum copper and ceruloplasmin analysis, carotid and cerebral angiography, and electroencephalography, are performed when appropriate.

It is of paramount importance for health care providers to adopt a positive attitude when managing patients with dementia. Although at present little can be done to treat and reverse dementia, it is important to identify its cause. In some cases, it may be possible to prevent the disease from progressing. For example, if the dementia is the result of hypertension, adequate control of this condition may prevent further brain damage. Moreover, the prevalence of vascular dementia is decreasing in countries where efforts to reduce cardiovascular and cerebrovascular diseases have been successful. Similarly, if the dementia is the result of repeated emboli (blood clots reaching the brain) complicating atrial fibrillation, then anticoagulants or aspirin may be recommended.

Even after a diagnosis of dementia is made, it is important for the physician to detect the presence of other conditions that may worsen the patient's mental functions, such as the inadvertent intake of medications that may induce confusion and mental impairment. Medications with this potential are numerous and include not only those that act on the brain, such as sedatives and hypnotics, but also hypotensive agents (especially if given in large doses), diuretics, and antibiotics. Whenever the condition of a patient with dementia deteriorates, the physician meticulously reviews all the medications that the patient is taking, both medical prescriptions and medications that may have been purchased over the counter. Even if innocuous, some over-the-counter preparations may interact with other medications that the patient is taking and lead to a worsening of mental functions. Inquiries are also made into the patient's alcohol intake. The brain of an older person is much more sensitive to the effects of alcohol than that of a younger person, and some medications may interact with the alcohol to impair the patient's cognitive functions further.

Many other disease states also may worsen the patient's mental functions. For example, patients with diabetes mellitus are susceptible to developing a variety of metabolic abnormalities including a low or high blood glucose level, both of which may be associated with confusional states. Similarly, dehydration and acid-base or electrolyte disorders, which may result from prolonged vomiting or diarrhea, may also precipitate confusional states. Infections, particularly respiratory and urinary tract infections, often worsen the patient's cognitive deficit. Finally, patients with dementia may experience myocardial infarctions (heart attacks) that are not associated with any chest pain but that may manifest themselves with confusion.

The casual observer of the dementing process is often overwhelmed with concern for the patient, but the process is often more difficult for the patient's family. Dementia patients themselves experience no physical pain or distress, and except in the very early stages of the disease, they are oblivious to their plight as a result of their loss of insight. Health care professionals therefore are alert to the stress imposed on the caregivers by dealing with loved ones with dementia. Adequate support from agencies available in the community is essential.

When a diagnosis of dementia is made, the physician discusses a number of ethical, financial, and legal issues with the family, and also the patient if it is believed that he or she can understand the implications of this discussion. Families are encouraged to make a list of all the patient's assets, including insurance policies, and to discuss this information with an attorney to protect the patient's and the family's assets. If the patient is still competent, it is recommended that he or she select a trusted person to have durable power of attorney. Unlike the regular power of attorney, the former does not become invalidated when the patient becomes mentally incompetent and remains in effect regardless of the degree of mental impairment of the person who executed it. Because durable power of attorney cannot be easily reversed once the person is incompetent, great care should be taken when selecting a person, and the specific powers granted should be clearly specified. It is also important for the patient to make his or her desires known concerning advance directives and the use of life-support systems.

Courts may appoint a guardian or conservator to have charge and custody of the patient's property (including real estate and money) when no responsible family members or friends are willing or available to serve as guardian. Courts supervise the actions of the guardian, who is expected to report all the patient's income and expenditures to the court once a year. The court may also charge the guardian to ensure that the patient is adequately housed, fed, and clothed and receiving appropriate medical care.

Perspective and Prospects

Dementia is a very serious and common condition, especially among the older population. Dementia permanently robs patients of their minds and prevents them from functioning adequately in their environment by impairing memory and interfering with the ability to make rational decisions. It therefore deprives patients of their dignity and independence.

Because dementia is mostly irreversible, cannot be adequately treated at present, and is associated with a fairly long survival period, it has a significant impact not only on the patient's life but also on the patient's family and caregivers and on society in general. The expense of long-term care for patients with dementia, whether at home or in institutions, is staggering. Every effort, therefore, is made to reach an accurate diagnosis and especially to detect any other condition that may worsen the patient's underlying dementia. Finally, health care professionals do not treat the patient in isolation but also concern themselves with the impact of the illness on the patient's caregivers and family.

Much progress has been made in defining dementia and determining its cause. Terms such as *senile dementia* are no longer in use, and even the use of the term *dementia* to diagnose a patient's condition is frowned upon because there are so many types of dementia. The recognition of the type of dementia affecting a particular patient is important because of its practical implications, both for the patient and for research into the prevention, management, and treatment of dementia.

There is little that can be done to cure dementia and no effective means to regenerate nerve cells. Researchers, however, are feverishly trying to identify factors that control the growth and regeneration of nerve cells. Although no single medication is expected to be of benefit to all types of dementia, it is hoped that effective therapy for many dementias will be developed. In 2012, the World Health Organization announced that the number of people living with dementia would likely double by 2030 and triple by 2050, further rein-forcing the need to develop improved treatments and methods for diagnosing dementia's many causes.

—*Ronald C. Hamdy, M.D.,*
Louis A. Cancellaro, M.D.,
and Larry Hudgins, M.D.;
updated by Nancy A. Piotrowski, Ph.D.

See also Aging; Aging: Extended care; Alzheimer's disease; Amnesia; Brain; Brain disorders; Delusions; Frontotemporal dementia (FTD); Hallucinations; Hospice; Memory loss; Parkinson's disease; Pick's disease; Psychiatric disorders; Psychiatry; Psychiatry, geriatric; Strokes; Terminally ill: Extended care.

For Further Information:
A.D.A.M. Medical Encyclopedia. "Dementia." *MedlinePlus*, September 26, 2011.
Alzheimer's Association. "What Is Dementia?" *Alzheimer's Association*, 2013.
Ballard, Clive, et al. *Dementia: Management of Behavioural and Psychological Symptoms*. New York: Oxford University Press, 2001.
Carson-DeWitt, Rosalyn. "Dementia." *HealthLibrary*, September 27, 2012.
Coons, Dorothy H., ed. *Specialized Dementia Care Units*. Baltimore: Johns Hopkins University Press, 1991.
Dana.org. http://www.dana.org.
Hamdy, Ronald C., J. M. Turnbull, and M. M. Lancaster, eds. *Alzheimer's Disease: A Handbook for Caregivers*. 3d ed. St. Louis, Mo.: Mosby Year Book, 1998.
Howe, M. L., M. J. Stones, and C. J. Brainerd, eds. *Cognitive and Behavioral Performance Factors in Atypical Aging*. New York: Springer, 1990.
Kovach, Christine, ed. *Late-Stage Dementia Care: A Basic Guide*. Washington, D.C.: Taylor & Francis, 1997.
Mace, Nancy L., and Peter V. Rabins. *The Thirty-Six-Hour Day: A Family Guide to Caring for People with Alzheimer Disease, Other Dementias, and Memory Loss in Later Life*. 4th ed. Baltimore: Johns Hopkins University Press, 2006.
National Center for Chronic Disease Prevention and Health Promotion. "Dementia/Alzheimer's Disease." *Centers for Disease Control and Prevention*, December 16, 2011.
O'Brien, John, et al., eds. *Dementia*. 3d ed. New York: Oxford University Press, 2006.
US Congress. Office of Technology Assessment. *Confused Minds, Burdened Families: Finding Help for People with Alzheimer's and Other Dementias*. Washington, D.C.: Government Printing Office, 1990.
World Health Organization. "Dementia Cases Set to Triple by 2050 but Still Largely Ignored." *World Health Organization*, April 11, 2012.

Dengue fever
Disease/Disorder

Also known as: Break-bone fever

Anatomy or system affected: Bones, eyes, glands, gums, head, mouth, musculoskeletal system, nose, skin

Specialties and related fields: Family medicine, internal medicine, microbiology, public health, virology

Definition: A flulike viral illness, contracted by humans through the bite of an infected *Aedes* mosquito.

Key terms:

endemic: something commonly found in a specific geographic area or population

Flaviviridae: a family of single-strand RNA viruses that spread via mosquitoes and ticks

Causes and Symptoms

Although dengue fever is primarily confined to the tropics, each year it causes nearly four hundred million infections worldwide. Dengue is caused by the dengue virus (DENV) that belongs to the Flaviviridae family. This viral family includes several other members, such as the yellow fever virus and the West Nile encephalitis virus, all of which have emerged as serious public health concerns over the years. All four serotypes of dengue virus (DENV-1 through DENV-4) are capable of causing the full spectrum of clinical manifestations, from asymptomatic presentation to dengue fever to the more severe dengue hemorrhagic fever or dengue shock syndrome. These forms are primarily found in hyperendemic areas that have all four serotypes of dengue virus.

Dengue virus enters the human host via the bite of an infected *Aedes* mosquito, primarily *A. aegypti* and occasionally *A. albopictus*. These vector populations are difficult to control because they are highly invasive and over time have accumulated adaptations that make them extremely resilient. Once inside the *Aedes* mosquito, having entered it via a blood meal, the dengue virus needs to incubate for about eight to twelve days in the mosquito before it can initiate another round of infection in a healthy host. An *Aedes* mosquito that has acquired the dengue virus will forever act as a vector.

After being bitten by the infected *Aedes* mosquito, a human host will typically start showing symptoms anywhere between four to seven days; symptoms last for as long as three to ten days. Once inside the human body, the dengue virus first replicates inside the dendritic cells. The replicated virus then infects macrophages and lymphocytes before entering the patient's bloodstream. Dengue fever patients can show a variety of symptoms, from mild feverishness to high fever of abrupt onset along with severe headache, pain behind the eyes (retro-orbital pain), flushing of the face, malaise, generalized joint and muscle pains, nausea, vomiting, and rash.

In dengue hemorrhagic fever and dengue shock syndrome, the more severe forms of dengue, clinical manifestations include fever, hemorrhage (diagnosed with a tourniquet test), low platelet count (thrombocytopenia), and increased vascular permeability. Some signs of hemorrhage seen in dengue hemorrhagic fever patients include pinpoint-sized red dots (petechiae), fragile capillaries that could lead to passage of blood from the ruptured blood vessels into subcutaneous tissue (purpura), and blood stains in vomit and stool (melena). The severity of dengue hemorrhagic fever depends on the extent of plasma leakage (detected by a rise in hematocrit level) from the capillaries that results in hypovolemia. As plasma continues to leak into the interstitial spaces, the patient can go into hypovolemic shock, a situation that can be fatal. These symptoms are typically accompanied by liver failure and increase in liver size (hepatomegaly). Concomitantly, as one would expect, viremia titers (indicating the presence of virus in the bloodstream) are much more pronounced in cases of dengue hemorrhagic fever and dengue shock syndrome as compared to dengue fever.

Information on Dengue Fever

Causes: Viral infection transmitted by mosquitoes
Symptoms: High fever, rash, joint and muscle pain, vomiting
Duration: Subacute
Treatments: Symptomatic treatment

Clinical diagnosis of dengue virus infection is based on signs of leukopenia (low white blood cell count), thrombocytopenia, and high serum transaminase levels in blood tests. Since rash is a common component of dengue fever, often the extent, nature, and location of the rash is used in the diagnostic process—for example, dengue rash is usually seen on the trunk and inner surfaces of the thighs and arms. With an increase in number of dengue cases, some unusual neurological complications, such as convulsions, spasticity, and encephalopathy (resulting from water intoxication), have also been reported. To date, the exact molecular mechanism that underlies the pathogenesis seen in dengue hemorrhagic fever and dengue shock syndrome is not very well understood and is still under investigation.

Treatment and Therapy

Patients who have been diagnosed with dengue virus infection are required to maintain adequate hydration levels. Often, the key to successful management of a patient with dengue hemorrhagic fever or dengue shock syndrome involves a careful monitoring of the patient's fluid level and replenishing any deficits with isotonic solution administered intravenously. Antipyretics such as acetaminophen are used for pain and fever management; patients are advised to avoid using aspirin and nonsteroidal anti-inflammatory drugs (NSAIDs), since they may accentuate the bleeding problem associated with certain types of dengue infection. Blood transfusions and oxygen therapy may also be used to treat dengue hemorrhagic fever.

The adaptive immune response of the patient plays an important role in clearing of the infection as well as providing immunity against reinfection. Infection with a DENV serotype (1–4) protects the individual only against reinfection by the same serotype. Since there are four serotypes of dengue virus, in theory, a person can get dengue as many as four times during his or her lifetime. Efforts are underway to design a vaccine; the ideal vaccine would provide lifelong protection against all four DENV serotypes. Dengue vaccine candidates that are currently being investigated include live attenuated vaccines, inactivated virus vaccines, recombinant subunit vaccines, and deoxyribonucleic acid (DNA) vaccines.

Perspective and Prospects

Dengue is considered an emerging infectious disease. As with the Ebola virus, the four serotypes are believed to have originated in monkeys in Africa or Southeast Asia and then mutated to move on to the human host several hundred years ago. Until the mid-twentieth century, dengue was largely a localized infection, primarily affecting populations in Southeast Asia. It is believed that the spread of the *Aedes* mosquito vector, and thus the dengue virus pathogen, via cargo ships to different parts of the world contributed to the global threat that the world is currently experiencing. Approximately 2.5 billion people now live in areas where dengue virus is endemic.

—Sibani Sengupta, Ph.D.

See also Bleeding; Ebola virus; Encephalitis; Epidemiology; Fever; Hemorrhage; Marburg virus; Tropical medicine; Viral hemorrhagic fevers; Viral infections; West Nile virus; Yellow fever; Zoonoses.

For Further Information:

A.D.A.M. Medical Encyclopedia. "Dengue Fever." *MedlinePlus*, January 11, 2013.

A.D.A.M. Medical Encyclopedia. "Dengue Hemorrhagic Fever." *MedlinePlus*, November 10, 2012.

DeWitt, Rosalyn. "Dengue Fever." *Health Library*, December 30, 2011.

Halstead, S. B. "More Dengue, More Questions." *Emerging Infectious Diseases* 11, no. 5 (May, 2005): 740–741.

Hirshler, Ben. "Experts Triple Estimate of World Dengue Fever Infections." *Reuters Health Information*, April 7, 2013.

National Center for Emerging and Zoonotic Infectious Diseases, Division of Vector-Borne Diseases. "Dengue." *Centers for Disease Control and Prevention*, February 6, 2013.

Whitehead, S. S., et al. "Prospects for a Dengue Virus Vaccine." *Nature Reviews Microbiology* 5 (July, 2007): 518–528.

DENTAL DISEASES

Disease/Disorder

Anatomy or system affected: Gums, mouth, teeth
Specialties and related fields: Dentistry
Definition: Diseases that affect the teeth, such as dental caries, and the gums, such as gingivitis, pyorrhea, or cancer.

Key terms:

dental caries: tooth decay

dentin: a hard, bonelike tissue lying beneath the tooth enamel

enamel: the hard surface covering of teeth

gingivae: the soft tissue surrounding the teeth; the gums

gingivitis: an inflammation of the gums

periodontal diseases: diseases characterized by inflammation of the gingivae

pyorrhea: the second stage of gingivitis

tooth pulp: the tissue at the center of teeth, surrounded by dentin

Vincent's infection: a bacterial infection of the gingivae, also known as trench mouth

Causes and Symptoms

Dental diseases fall into four major categories: dental caries, or tooth decay; periodontal disease, including gingivitis and pyorrhea; Vincent's infection, or trench mouth; and oral cancer. The first of these diseases was the largest contributor to tooth loss among people under thirty-five in the United States before the widespread fluoridation of drinking water was begun; it remains a major cause of tooth loss in much of the world. Periodontal disease in its two stages, gingivitis and pyorrhea, is the most widespread dental problem for people over thirty-five. Most people who suffer the loss of all of their teeth do so because of this condition. Vincent's infection, which shares many characteristics with gingivitis, is bacterial. The infection flares up, is treated, and disappears, whereas gingivitis is more often a continuing condition that requires both persistent home treatment and specialized treatment. The most serious but least frequently occurring dental disease is oral cancer. It is the only dental disease commonly considered life threatening, and there is a risk that it may spread to other parts of the body.

Dental caries occur because the food that one eats becomes trapped in the irregularities of the teeth, creating lactic acids that penetrate the enamel through holes (often microscopic) in it. Once lodged between the teeth or below the gum line, carbohydrates and starches combine with saliva to form acids that, over time, can penetrate a tooth's enamel, enter the dentin directly below it, and progressively destroy the dentin while spreading toward the tooth's center, the pulp.

This process often is not confined to a single tooth. As decay spreads, adjoining teeth may be affected. Some people have much harder tooth enamel than others. Therefore, some individuals may experience little or no decay, whereas others who follow similar diets and practice similar methods of dental hygiene may develop substantial decay.

Toothache occurs when decay eats through the dentin and enters the nerve-filled dental pulp, causing inflammation, infection, and pain. A dull, continuous ache, either mild or severe and often pulsating, may indicate that the infection has entered the jawbone beneath the tooth. An aching or sensitivity in the back teeth during chewing is sometimes a side effect of sinusitis.

One of dentistry's nagging problems is periodontal disease, which results from a buildup of calculus, or tartar, formed by hardened plaque. Plaque is formed when food, particularly carbohydrates and starches, interacts with the saliva that coats the teeth, creating a yellowish film. If this film is not removed, it inevitably lodges between the gums and the teeth, where, within twenty-four hours, it hardens into calculus. Dental hygienists can remove most of this calculus mechanically. If it is allowed to build up over extended periods,

---

Information on Dental Diseases

Causes: Tooth decay, periodontal disease (gingivitis, pyorrhea), Vincent's infection (trench mouth), oral cancer

Symptoms: Vary; may include dull, continuous ache; gum soreness, swelling, and bleeding; receding gums forming pockets for infections; bone destruction and tooth loss; fever; persistent mouth sores

Duration: Short-term to chronic

Treatments: Dependent on condition; may include medications (dextrose, antibiotics), tooth implantation, gum surgery, laser treatment, radiation, chemotherapy, surgery

however, the calculus will irritate the gums, causing the soreness, swelling, and bleeding that signal gum infection. Eventually, this infection becomes entrenched and difficult to treat.

Periodontists can control but not cure most periodontal disease. In its early manifestations, periodontal disease results in gingivitis, marked by inflammation and bleeding. Untreated, it progresses to pyorrhea, which is characterized by gums that recede from the teeth and form pockets in which infections flourish. As pyorrhea advances, the bone that underlies the teeth and holds them in place is compromised and ultimately destroyed, causing looseness and eventual tooth loss.

Vincent's infection (trench mouth) is communicable through kissing or sharing eating utensils. Although it is sometimes mistaken for gingivitis, Vincent's infection has one distinguishing characteristic that gingivitis does not have: it is accompanied by a fever stemming from sustained bacterial infection, which also causes extremely foul breath. Vincent's infection is curable through proper treatment. It is unlikely to recur unless one is again exposed to the infection.

Oral cancer is the most serious of oral diseases. It often spreads quickly, destroying the tissues of the mouth during its ravaging advance. It not only threatens its original site but also can spread to other areas of the body and to vital organs. Fortunately, oral cancer is uncommon. Nevertheless, dentists look vigilantly for signs of it when they perform mouth examinations because early detection is vital to successful treatment, containment, and cure. People who have persistent mouth sores that do not heal may be experiencing the early manifestations of oral cancer and should see their dentists or physicians immediately.

Two other dental conditions afflict many people: malocclusion and toothache. Malocclusion occurs when, for a variety of reasons, the teeth are out of alignment. People with malocclusion are prime candidates for dental caries and periodontal disease, largely because their teeth are difficult to reach and hard to clean. Malocclusion may also cause one or more teeth to strike the teeth above or below them, causing injury to teeth and possibly fracturing them.

Treatment and Therapy

Modern dentistry has succeeded in controlling most dental diseases. In the United States, dental caries have been almost eliminated in the young by the addition of fluoride to most water systems. Used over time, fluoride strengthens the teeth by increasing the hardness of the enamel, making it resistant to the acids that form in the mouth and cause decay. Countries such as the United Kingdom, Canada, Singapore, and Israel have likewise implemented fluoridation programs in an attempt to prevent tooth decay. Fluoride has also been added to toothpaste and mouthwash, which offer considerable protection from dental caries.

Researchers discovered in the mid-1960s that a substance found in the mouth's streptococcal bacteria creates dextran. Dextran enables bacteria to cling to the surface of the teeth and invade them with the lactic acid that they generate. Re-

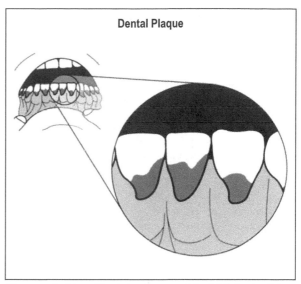

Dental Plaque

Plaque—a buildup of bacteria, mucus, and food debris—leads to dental caries (tooth decay) if not regularly removed by brushing, flossing, and professional tooth cleaning.

searchers ultimately discovered dextranase, an enzyme effective in dissolving dextran. Strides are being made to use dextranase in toothpaste or mouthwash to reduce or eliminate the effects of dextran.

Some people's teeth seem to be impervious to tooth decay. It has been determined that such people have a common substance in their blood that protects their teeth from dental caries. Attempts are being made to identify and isolate this substance and to make it generally available to the public and to dentists in an applicable form. Some dentists coat the teeth with a durable plastic substance to make them resistant to penetration by the acids that cause dental decay, creating a hard protective coating above the enamel and making it difficult for food to lodge between the teeth or in irregularities in the teeth.

Because malocclusion, or poor spacing, can lead to tooth decay, dentists have become increasingly aware of the need to replace lost teeth so that the alignment of the remaining teeth will not be disturbed. Tooth implantation, a process by which a tooth, either artificial or natural, is anchored directly and permanently in the gum, solves many dental problems that in the past were addressed by attaching artificial teeth to existing ones beside them. In situations where malocclusion is caused by malformations, the use of orthodontic braces results in a more regular alignment.

Nutrition has come to the forefront of recent research in dental health. A lack of calciferol, a form of vitamin D_2, may result in dental abnormalities, including malocclusion. Among substantial numbers of hospital patients who suffer from nutritional problems, the earliest symptoms occur in the soft tissue of the mouth.

Brushing the teeth after meals and before bed controls plaque, as does regular flossing. Such daily attention must be supplemented by twice-yearly cleaning, performed by a dentist or dental hygienist, and by annual or biennial whole-mouth x-rays to reveal incipient decay. Various mouthwashes also contain substances that control decay.

People who cannot brush after every meal should use a mouthwash or rinse the mouth out with water after eating, then brush as soon as they can. Special attention must be given to the back surfaces of the lower front teeth because the salivary glands are located there. This area is a breeding ground for the bacteria that cause the formation of lactic acid. Routine home care of this kind, particularly daily flossing, will help prevent both tooth decay and periodontal disease and can also reverse some of the inroads that periodontal disease has made. When gingivitis advances to pyorrhea, however, dental surgery may be necessary.

The major villain in both gingivitis and pyorrhea is tartar, or calculus, which is produced when plaque hardens. When tartar accumulates beneath the gums, it causes an irritation that can lead to infection. Sometimes, this infection moves to other parts of the body, causing joint problems and other difficulties.

People can control plaque by practicing daily dental hygiene at home. They must also have accumulated tartar regularly scraped away or removed by ultrasound in the dentist's office. Malocclusions and defects in the production of saliva can be corrected by dentists and can greatly reduce the progress of periodontal disease.

When gum surgery is advised for the removal of the deep gum pockets that occur with pyorrhea, further surgery can usually be avoided with regular home care. Meanwhile, researchers are trying to develop a vaccine to immunize its recipients against the bacteria that cause tooth decay. Other decay-inhibiting agents are being studied closely with the expectation that they may in time be added to common foods and beverages.

Vincent's infection is successfully treated with antibiotics, accompanied by a prescribed course of dental hygiene that is begun in the dentist's office and continues at home on a daily basis. Some patients have found a peroxide mouthwash helpful in treating this disease.

When dentists find evidence of oral cancer, they usually refer patients to their primary physicians, who coordinate referrals to oncologists. An oncologist will determine if the patient has cancer and will determine the best ways to treat it. Laser treatment and radiation are used in controlling oral cancer, as are chemotherapy and surgery. The most important element in cancer treatment is time. It is essential, therefore, that specialized treatment be initiated as soon as oral cancer is discovered or suspected. In cases of oral cancer, a delay of even days can affect outcomes negatively.

The most immediate treatments for toothache range from the application of cold compresses to the taking of aspirin or another analgesic every few hours. If the decayed part of the tooth is visible and reachable, sometimes applying a mixture of oil of cloves and benzocaine to the decayed area with a small swab soothes the pain. These treatments, however, offer only temporary relief.

Dentists resist treating toothache by removing the tooth, although removal offers an immediate solution to the problem. In some cases, dentists can drill out the decay and fill the tooth with silver amalgam, gold, or plastic. Quite often, by the time a tooth begins to ache, the pulp and dentin have been ravaged by decay. The best solution is endodontistry, or root canal, which will preserve the tooth but may necessitate the attachment of a crown.

Perspective and Prospects

Great strides have been made in preventing and treating dental disease, as researchers have reached deeper understandings of the root causes of such disease. Dentistry has become increasingly less painful through the use of anesthetics and high-speed, water-cooled drills. The public at large has grown aware of the close relationship between dental health and general health. People are unwilling to accept tooth loss as a natural consequence of aging. They have also begun to realize that orthodontistry is more than a cosmetic procedure. Rather, it is a necessary procedure for correcting misalignments of the teeth that can result in difficulty if uncorrected.

Advances in preventing and treating dental disease are constantly being made. Through genetic engineering, it is almost inevitable that substances will soon be available to increase an individual's resistance to tooth decay. Nevertheless, controlling the buildup of calculus, the major factor in periodontal disease, will probably remain the responsibility of individuals through daily home care and twice-yearly visits to their dentists.

—*R. Baird Shuman, Ph.D.*

See also Canker sores; Cavities; Crowns and bridges; Dentistry; Dentistry, pediatric; Dentures; Endodontic disease; Fluoride treatments; Fracture repair; Gingivitis; Gum disease; Jaw wiring; Oral and maxillofacial surgery; Orthodontics; Periodontal surgery; Periodontitis; Plaque, dental; Root canal treatment; Teeth; Teething; Tooth extraction; Toothache; Wisdom teeth.

For Further Information:
Anderson, Pauline C., and Alice E. Pendleton. *The Dental Assistant.* 7th ed. Albany, N.Y.: Delmar, 2001.
Diamond, Richard. *Dental First Aid for Families.* Ravensdale, Wash.: Idyll Arbor, 2000.
Fairpo, Jenifer E. H., and C. Gavin Fairpo. *Heinemann Dental Dictionary.* 4th ed. Boston: Butterworth-Heinemann, 1997.
Foster, Malcolm S. *Protecting Our Children's Teeth: A Guide to Quality Dental Care from Infancy Through Age Twelve.* New York: Insight Books, 1992.
Gluck, George M., and William M. Morganstein. *Jong's Community Dental Health.* 5th ed. St. Louis, Mo.: Mosby, 2003.
Langlais, Robert P., and Craig S. Miller. *Color Atlas of Common Oral Diseases.* 4th ed. Philadelphia: Lippincott Williams & Wilkins, 2009.
MedlinePlus. "Gum Disease." *MedlinePlus*, April 25, 2013.
MedlinePlus. "Tooth Decay." *MedlinePlus*, April 24, 2013.
National Center for Chronic Disease Prevention and Health Promotion, Division of Oral Health. "Oral Health Resources." *Centers for Disease Control and Prevention*, April 11 2013.
Newman, Michael G., Henry H. Takei, and Perry R. Klokkevold, eds. *Carranza's Clinical Periodontology.* 10th ed. St. Louis, Mo.: Saunders/Elsevier, 2006.
Ring, Malvin E. *Dentistry: An Illustrated History.* New York:

Abradale, 1992.

Woodall, Irene R., ed. *Comprehensive Dental Hygiene Care*. 4th ed. St. Louis, Mo.: Mosby, 1993.

Your Dental Health: A Guide for Patients and Families. Farmington: Connecticut Consumer Health Information Network, University of Connecticut Health Center, 2008.

DENTISTRY

Specialty

Anatomy or system affected: Gums, mouth, teeth

Specialties and related fields: Anesthesiology, orthodontics

Definition: The field of health involving the diagnosis and treatment of diseases of the teeth and related tissues in the oral cavity.

Key terms:

dental caries: the scientific term for tooth decay

dentist: a doctor with specialized training to diagnose and treat diseases of the teeth and oral tissues

endodontics: the dental specialty that treats diseases of infected pulp tissue

oral surgery: the dental specialty that surgically removes diseased teeth and oral tissues and treats fractures of the jawbone

orthodontics: the dental specialty that treats malocclusions or improperly aligned teeth by straightening the teeth in the jaws

pedodontics: the dental specialty that treats children

periodontics: the dental specialty that treats the diseases of the supporting tissues of the teeth

prosthodontics: the dental specialty that restores missing teeth with fixed or removable dentures

Science and Profession

The practice of dentistry is a specialized area of medicine that treats the diseases of the teeth and their surrounding tissues in the oral cavity. Dental education normally takes four years to complete, with predental training preceding it. Prior to entering a dental school, students are usually required to have a bachelor's degree. This degree should have major emphasis in biology or chemistry. Predental courses are concentrated in both inorganic and organic chemistry. The biology courses can cover such subjects as comparative anatomy, histology, physiology, and microbiology. Other courses that can help students to prepare for both dental school and the future practice of dentistry are English, speech skills, physics, and computer technology. Upon entering dental school, students are faced with two distinct parts of their education: didactics and techniques.

Some Conditions Treated in Dentistry

Care of the teeth and supporting structures may involve the treatment of such dental diseases as gingivitis (infection of the gums), the removal of dental plaque (hard deposits on the teeth), the surgical excision of impacted molars (teeth trapped beneath the gums), and the fitting of a crown (an artificial covering for a tooth) following root canal treatment.

The didactic courses offered in dental schools are required to achieve knowledge of the human body, most particularly the head and neck. Some of the courses required are human anatomy, physiology, biochemistry, microbiology, general and oral histology and pathology, dental anatomy, pharmacology, anesthesiology, and radiology. One course specific to dental school is occlusion, which emphasizes the structure of the temporomandibular joint and its accompanying neurology and musculature.

In addition, students must know the properties of the materials used in the practice of dentistry. The physical properties of metals, acrylic plastics, gypsum plasters, impression materials, porcelains, glass ionomers, dental composites, sealant resins, and other substances must be thoroughly understood to determine the proper restorations for diseased tissues in the mouth. Knowledge of resistance to wear by chewing forces, thermal conductivity, and corrosion and staining by mouth fluids and foods is important. Information concerning the materials used in dental treatment in terms of resistance to recurrent decay, possible toxicity, or irritation to the hard and soft tissues of the oral cavity is also necessary.

The technical phase of dental education addresses the practical use of this didactic knowledge in treating diseases of the mouth. Students are trained to operate on diseased teeth and to prepare the teeth to receive restorations that will function as biomechanical prostheses in, or adjacent to, living tissue. An understanding of anatomy, physiology, and pathology is necessary for successful restoration of the teeth. During this course of study, students are required to construct fillings, cast-gold crowns and inlays, fixed and removable dentures, porcelain crowns and inlays, and other restorations on mannequins, plastic models, or extracted teeth. These activities are undertaken prior to working on patients. Through practice and repetition of these techniques, dental students soon become aware of the importance of mastering this phase of the education prior to their application in a clinical environment.

The clinical phase of dental education integrates the didactic and technical instruction that has taken place throughout the first years of professional study. Students learn to treat patients under the close supervision of their instructors. The treatment of patients in all the specialties of dentistry is required of students before they receive the degree for general dentistry. Some students may opt for extra training in one of several specialties. To become a specialist, postgraduate education is required. This education commonly encompasses two years of study but is sometimes longer.

Upon graduation, students receive their professional degrees. Before they can legally practice dentistry in the United States, however, they must successfully pass an examination offered by the board of dental examiners in their chosen state. National exams in didactics are offered during dental school, and most states accept them as part of their state examination. The technical portion of the exam may only be taken after the student has received a doctorate from an accredited college or university. The emphasis regarding techniques may vary from state to state. Many states allow reciprocity, which means that a student who has passed the examination in one state may become licensed to practice in another. In states that do not accept reciprocity, the student must pass the practical examination of that state prior to obtaining a license. There have been attempts to make reciprocity universal among all states, but several states insist on governing the quality of their dental health care.

Dental education can be quite expensive. After a dentist receives a license to practice, the cost of equipping an office must also be borne. A dental office must have dental chairs, office and reception room furniture, a dental laboratory, a sterilizing room, x-ray units, instruments, and various supplies. Because of these expenses, new dentists often initially practice as an associate or partner of an established dentist, as an employee of a dental clinic, in the military or Public Health Service, or in state institutions. Some dentists enjoy the academic atmosphere of dental schools and return to become part-time or full-time educators.

Diagnostic and Treatment Techniques

The practice of dentistry is quite different in modern times compared to the past. While some techniques and materials are still in use, there have been improvements in materials and instruments because of expanded knowledge in many scientific fields. This knowledge has increased to such an extent that dentistry has divided into several specialties. While the general dentist uses all disciplines of dentistry to treat patients, complex problems often require referral and the expertise of a specialist.

The general dentist is involved primarily in the treatment of caries or tooth decay and the replacement of missing teeth. Bacterial acids that dissolve the enamel and dentin of teeth cause caries. A diseased or damaged tooth must be prepared mechanically by the removal of the decayed material using a dental drill and tough, sharp bits called burs. The amount of damage and the position of the tooth in the mouth determine the type of restoration. In the posterior or back teeth, initial cavities may be restored with bonded composite resins. In addition to removing the decayed tooth structure, the dentist must take into consideration the closeness of the dental pulp, the chewing forces of the opposing teeth, and the aesthetics of the finished restoration. In the anterior or front teeth, aesthetic restorative materials are used to fill small cavities. In this case also, the size and position of the defect determine the choice of restorative material.

When the amount of tooth destruction caused by decay becomes too large for conservative filling materials, the remaining tooth structure must be reinforced by the use of cast metal or porcelain restorations. The tooth is prepared for the specific restoration, and accurate impressions are taken of the prepared teeth. The crown or inlay is fabricated on hard plaster models reproduced from the impressions and then cemented into place on the tooth. This process is also used for fixed partial dentures, or bridges, which are used to replace one or more missing teeth. Two or more teeth are prepared on either end of the space of missing teeth to support the span. The bridge is constructed with metal and porcelain as a single unit. It is then cemented on the prepared abutment teeth.

The health of the supporting tissues of the teeth, the periodontium, is necessary for the long-term retention of any mechanical restoration. When teeth become loose in the jaws because of periodontal disease, or pyorrhea, the restoration of these teeth often depends on the treatment by a periodontist, the specialist in this field. Periodontists treat the diseased tissues by scraping off harmful deposits on the roots of the teeth and by removing the diseased soft tissue and bone through curettage, surgery, or both techniques. At present, there is no means to regenerate or regrow bone lost by periodontal disease. Some newer techniques of grafting the patient's bone with sterile freeze-dried bone, implanting stainless steel pins, or using other artificial materials show great promise.

If the tooth decay reaches the dental pulp and infects it, there are two choices of treatment: removal of the tooth or endodontic therapy, commonly known as root canal treatment. If the tooth is well supported by a healthy periodontium, it is better to save the tooth by endodontics. The basic procedure of a root canal is to enter the tooth through the chewing surface on teeth toward the rear of the mouth or the inside surface or lingual aspect of teeth in the front of the mouth. Files, reamers, and broaches to the tip of the root remove diseased or decaying (necrotic) material of the dental pulp. The now-empty canal is filled by cementing a point that fits into it. Although the tooth is now nonvital, meaning that it has lost its blood supply and nerve, it can remain in the mouth for many years and provide good service.

The maintenance of the health of the primary dentition, or baby teeth, is very important. These deciduous teeth, although lost during childhood and adolescence, are important not only to the dental health of the child but to the permanent teeth as well. The deciduous teeth act as guides and spacers for the correct placement of adult teeth when they erupt. A pediodontist, who specializes in the practice of dentistry for children, must have a good knowledge of the specific mechanics of children's mouths in treating primary teeth. This specialist must also have a thorough foundation in the treatment of congenital diseases. The pediodontist prepares the way for dental treatment by an adult dentist and often assists an orthodontist by doing some preliminary straightening of teeth.

An orthodontist treats malocclusions, or ill-fitting teeth (so-called bad bites) with mechanical appliances that reposition the teeth into an occlusion that is closer to ideal. These appliances, known commonly as braces, move the teeth through the bone of the jaws until the opposing teeth occlude in a balanced bite. The side benefit of this treatment is that the teeth become properly positioned for an attractive smile and easier cleaning.

Sometimes the teeth or their supporting tissues become so diseased that there is no alternative but to remove them. A general dentist often does routine extractions of these diseased teeth. If the patient has complications beyond the training of a general dentist or is medically compromised by systemic illness, an oral surgeon, with specialized training, is typically consulted. This specialist not only removes teeth under difficult conditions but also is trained to remove tumors of the oral cavity, treat fractures of the jaws, and perform the surgical placement of dental implants.

Although the total loss of teeth is becoming rarer, there are still many patients who are without teeth. Often, they have been wearing complete, removable dentures that, over a period of time, have caused the loss or resorption of underlying bone. Prosthodontists are specialists trained to construct fixed and removable dentures for difficult cases. The increased success of titanium implants in the jaws and the appliances connected to them have aided prosthodontists in treating the complex cases. They also construct appliances to replace tissues and structures lost from cancer surgery of the oral cavity and congenital deformities such as cleft palate.

Perspective and Prospects

In the past, dentistry only treated pain caused by a diseased tooth; the usual mode of treatment was extraction. Today, the prevention of disease, the retention of teeth, and the

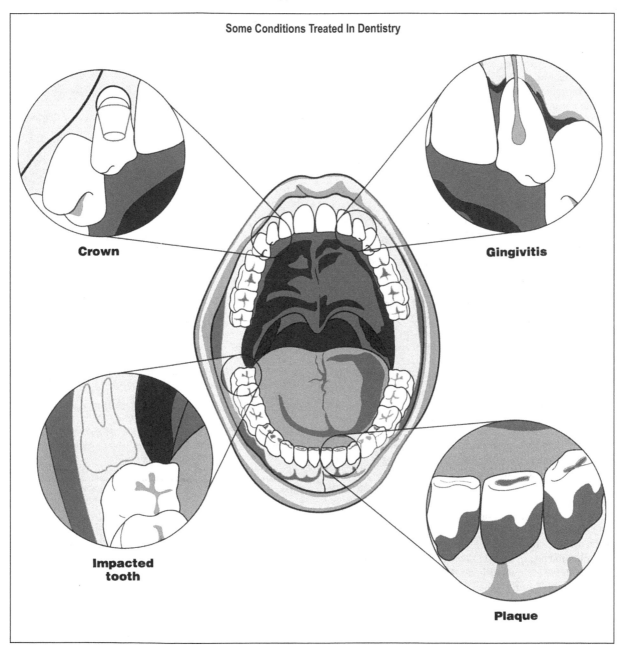

Some Conditions Treated In Dentistry

Crown

Gingivitis

Impacted tooth

Plaque

Care of the teeth and supporting structures may involve the treatment of such dental diseases as gingivitis (infection of the gums), the removal of dental plaque (hard deposits on the teeth), the surgical excision of impacted molars (teeth trapped beneath the gums), and the fitting of a crown (an artificial covering for a tooth) following root canal treatment.

restoration of the dentition are the treatment goals of dentists.

The development of composite resins has successfully addressed many aesthetic problems associated with restorations. Although metal fillings of silver amalgam (actually a mixture of silver, lead, and mercury) and cast-gold restorations were often the treatments of choice in the past, composite fillings have become the treatment of choice. Plastic composite materials that are chemically bonded to the enamel and dentin of teeth are more aesthetically pleasing than metals. They have also shown great promise for longevity. There is still some concern about the resistance of these materials to chewing forces and leakage of the bonding to the tooth, but the techniques and materials are improving.

Dental porcelains improved greatly in the last half of the twentieth century. Although porcelain fused to metal crowns is often the material of choice, in certain cases crowns, inlays, and fixed bridges of a newer type of porcelain are being used. Thin veneers of porcelain are also used to restore front teeth that are congenitally or chemically stained. The result is cosmetically more appealing. Through a similar bonding process of composites, these veneers on the front surfaces of the teeth offer maximum aesthetics with minimum destruction of tooth structure.

While implantation of metals into the jawbones to support dentures and other prosthetic appliances is not new, the recent use of titanium implants and precision techniques promises long-term retention. Special drills are used to prepare the implant site, and titanium cylinders are either threaded into the bone or pushed into the jaw. The implant is covered by the gum tissue and allowed to heal for six to eight months, so that the process of osseointegration (joining of bone and metal) can occur. The bone will actually fuse to the pure metal, anchoring the implant for an eventual prosthetic appliance.

Laser technology is an exciting field has yielded some important applications in dentistry. Lasers have been used in gum surgery. Some theorists believe that if the enamel surface of the teeth were to be fused, it would be highly resistant to decay. The heat generated by lasers is a concern, but steps are being taken to control this problem. One of the most promising uses of lasers is in the specialty of endodontics. A thin laser fiber-optic probe advanced down the root canal, preparing and sterilizing the canal prior to filling, vaporizes diseased or degenerating pulp.

Computer science is also being integrated into the treatment phase of dentistry. For example, after scanning a patient's mouth, projected results of treatment can be displayed on a computer screen. In addition, restorations can be developed using the concept of computer-aided design/computer-aided manufacturing (CAD/CAM). A computer scans a prepared tooth for a crown or inlay. The restoration is then designed for a three-dimensional model on the screen. After the model restoration has been chosen, the computer transfers the data to a computer-activated milling machine in the dental laboratory, and a restoration is reproduced in a ceramic or composite resin material in the designed image. The restoration is then cemented into the prepared tooth.

Such improvements in techniques and materials have advanced dentistry into a new era in providing treatment for patients. The basic fundamentals of treatment of the teeth and their surrounding tissues must be maintained, however, in view of the peculiar anatomy and physiology of the teeth.

—William D. Stark, D.D.S.; updated by
L. Fleming Fallon, Jr., M.D., Ph.D., M.P.H.

See also Anesthesia; Anesthesiology; Braces, orthodontic; Canker sores; Cavities; Crowns and bridges; Dental diseases; Dentistry, pediatric; Dentures; Endodontic disease; Fluoride treatments; Fracture repair; Gastrointestinal system; Gingivitis; Gum disease; Halitosis; Head and neck disorders; Jaw wiring; Oral and maxillofacial surgery; Orthodontics; Periodontal surgery; Periodontitis; Plaque, dental; Root canal treatment; Teeth; Teething; Temporomandibular joint (TMJ) syndrome; Tooth extraction; Toothache; Wisdom teeth.

For Further Information:

Bird, Doni L., and Debbie S. Robinson. Modern Dental Assisting. 10th ed. St. Louis, Mo.: Elsevier Saunders, 2011.

Darby, Michelle L. Mosby's Comprehensive Review of Dental Hygiene. 7th ed. St. Louis, Mo.: Mosby, 2011.

Foster, Malcolm S. *Protecting Our Children's Teeth: A Guide to Quality Dental Care from Infancy Through Age Twelve.* New York: Insight Books, 1992.

Gluck, George M., and William M. Morganstein. *Jong's Community Dental Health.* 5th ed. St. Louis, Mo.: Mosby, 2003.

Heymann, Harald O., Edward J. Swift Jr., and Andre V. Ritter. *Sturdevant's Art and Science of Operative Dentistry.* 6th ed. St. Louis, Mo.: Elsevier, 2012.

Kendall, Bonnie L. *Opportunities in Dental Care Careers.* Edited by Blythe Camenson. New York: McGraw-Hill, 2006.

Moss, Stephen J. *Growing Up Cavity Free: A Parent's Guide to Prevention.* New York: Edition Q, 1994.

Parker, James N., and Philip M. Parker, eds. *The Official Patient's Sourcebook on Gingivitis.* San Diego, Calif.: Icon Health, 2002.

Parker, James N., and Philip M. Parker, eds. *The Official Patient's Sourcebook on Periodontitis.* San Diego, Calif.: Icon Health, 2002.

Ring, Malvin E. *Dentistry: An Illustrated History.* New York: Abrams, 1985.

Smith, Rebecca W. *The Columbia University School of Dental and Oral Surgery's Guide to Family Dental Care.* New York: W. W. Norton, 1997.

"What Is Laser Dentistry?" *Academy of General Dentistry,* January 2012.

Your Dental Health: A Guide for Patients and Families. Farmington: Connecticut Consumer Health Information Network, University of Connecticut Health Center, 2008.

DENTURES

Treatment

Anatomy or system affected: Gums, mouth, teeth

Specialties and related fields: Dentistry

Definition: Removable artificial teeth worn to replace missing or diseased teeth, thus restoring both facial appearance and the ability to speak clearly and chew food by maintaining the shape of the jaw.

Indications and Procedures

With the aging process, disease of the teeth and surrounding tissues often increases, leading to the eventual loss of some or all the teeth. When teeth are missing, the remaining teeth can change position, drifting into the surrounding space. Teeth that are out of position can damage tissues in the mouth. It is also more difficult to clean thoroughly between crooked teeth, resulting in an increased risk of tooth decay, gum disease, and additional loss of teeth. The solution is to replace the missing teeth with a denture. In 1999, more than thirty-two million Americans were wearing some type of denture, and the majority were over fifty-five years of age.

When a large number of teeth are missing, and a sufficient number of adjacent teeth are not present to support a bridge, or fixed partial denture, a removable partial denture is the solution. It consists of replacement teeth attached to pink or gum-colored plastic bases, which are connected by a metal framework. This prosthetic device is usually secured by clasping it to several of the remaining teeth. The clasps are typically made out of gold or a cobalt-steel alloy. Although more costly, precision attachments are nearly invisible and generally more aesthetically pleasing than metal clasps. Crowns on the adjacent natural teeth may improve the fit of a removable partial denture, and they are usually required with precision attachments.

When all the teeth need replacement, a full denture is constructed. It is usually made of acrylic, occasionally reinforced with metal. Full dentures replace all the teeth in either jaw and are generally held in place by suction created between saliva and the soft tissues of the mouth. A temporary soft liner can be placed in a new or old denture to help improve the health of the gum tissues by absorbing some of the pressures of mastication and providing maximum retention by fitting around undercuts in the bone and gums.

Uses and Complications

A common misconception is that when all the teeth are extracted and replaced by full dentures, all teeth problems cease. In fact, properly fitted full dentures at best are only about 25 to 35 percent as efficient as natural teeth. Many elderly have little trouble adjusting, but some find it difficult to adapt to and learn to use dentures properly. Furthermore, the tissues of the mouth undergo constant changes, which may result in loose or bad-fitting dentures, which may cause damage to the mouth tissues. Consequently, a person who wears dentures should continue to see a dentist for regular annual checkups.

Full and partial dentures are removable and must be taken out frequently and cleansed. In addition, the supporting soft tissues of the mouth need thorough cleansing with a soft mouth brush two to three times daily. It typically takes a few weeks to get used to inserting, wearing, eating with, removing, and maintaining dentures. Careful attention to all the instructions given by the dentist is vital.

—Alvin K. Benson, Ph.D.

See also Aging; Bone disorders; Cavities; Crowns and bridges; Dental diseases; Dentistry; Otorhinolaryngology; Periodontitis; Teeth; Tooth extraction.

For Further Information:

American Academy of Cosmetic Dentistry. "Dentures." *AACD*, 2011.

Devlin, Hugh. *Complete Dentures: A Clinical Manual for the General Dental Practitioner.* New York: Springer, 2002.

MedlinePlus. "Dentures." *MedlinePlus*, May 16, 2013.

Schillingburg, Warren, et al. *Fundamentals of Fixed Prosthodontics.* 4th ed. Hanover Park, Ill.: Quintessence Pub., 2012.

Smith, Rebecca W. *The Columbia University School of Dental and Oral Surgery's Guide to Family Dental Care.* New York: W. W. Norton, 1997.

Woodforde, John. *The Strange Story of False Teeth.* New York: Universe Books, 1983.

DEPARTMENT OF HEALTH AND HUMAN SERVICES

Organization

Definition: A division of the executive branch of the U.S. government, with representation in the cabinet of the president, that is responsible for public health.

Key terms:

Head Start: local preschool programs that help prepare children of economically disadvantaged or recent immigrant families for entry into regular primary school grades; encouraged by the Department of Health and Human Services through selective funding

Medicaid: a health care program, made available by the Department of Health and Human Services in conjunction with most states, to those with low-level income or those who are disabled and unable to pay health insurance premiums

Medicare: a governmental health insurance system for persons sixty-five years of age and older, supported by obligatory payroll withholding

History and Mission

Although several efforts were made in earlier decades to create a federal authority responsible for public health, it was not until Dwight D. Eisenhower's administration in the 1950s that a formal agency became part of the executive branch of government. Presidents Franklin D. Roosevelt and Harry S. Truman in particular had hoped, but failed, to create a federally administered health program as an added component of the Social Security Act put in place by Roosevelt in 1935. The Department of Health, Education, and Welfare (HEW)—restructured in 1979 as the Department of Health and Human Services (HHS)—began operations in April 1953. For a number of years, until 1995, the Social Security Administration remained under the HHS. A number of legislative reorganization acts expanded and diversified responsibilities assigned to the HHS. Among these was the major milestone when, as part of the Social Security Act of 1965 (a piece of President Johnson's Great Society legislation), two government-funded health care programs—Medicare and Medicaid—were placed under the administration of the secretary of HEW.

The shift in party control of the executive branch of government that came with Republican Richard M. Nixon's election in 1968 raised some question that there might be declining support for HHS activities. This would not occur, however, mainly because public perceptions of the need for government responsibilities for health and social welfare had become a political given. In fact, there would be an expanding pattern of activities of, as well as budgetary allowances for, HHS in the latter decades of the twentieth and first part of the twenty-first centuries.

The Department of Education Organization Act of 1979 provided for the creation of a separate Department of Education, while the HHS retained responsibilities for operations relating to public health and welfare. In part, the evolving scope of HHS operations reflected changing perceptions of the social definition of public health, as well as the impact on US agencies of global health concerns, particularly those relating to HIV/AIDS and the avian and H1N1 influenza pandemics.

Since its inception as HEW and following restructuring as DHHS in 1980, as of 2009 there had been twenty-one secretaries appointed to head this executive branch of the U.S. government.

Overview

Overall responsibility for the activities of the HSS rests with the secretary of Health and Human Services, assisted by the Office of Inspector General, whose task it is to report to the secretary and to Congress detailing both the budgetary soundness and managerial effectiveness of the activities assigned to more than ten subagencies of the department.

In general terms, work carried on by the HHS falls into three categories: provision of direct services to specific groups within the overall population; gathering and disseminating technical information vital to the maintenance of optimal public health and safety standards within the United States; and support for scientific research that can contribute to the same health-related goals.

Closer examination of activities sponsored by several key HHS subagencies suggests that many of their activities can be complementary. A first grouping, for example, consists of agencies providing direct assistance: Centers for Medicare and Medicaid (CMM), the Administration for Children and Families (ACF), the Administration on Aging, the Indian Health Service, and the Substance Abuse and Mental Health Services Administration (SAMHSA). In particular, SAMHSA is an example of complementary functions bridging several agencies.

Medicare and Medicaid clearly occupy the most public and politically sensitive position among all of HHS's agencies. Unlike Medicare, which is fully funded by the federal government through withholding taxes on individual incomes, Medicaid programs involve budgetary and organizational cooperation between HHS and each state. This fact of decentralization means that HHS has the responsibility of monitoring a wide variety of state-run programs that set up eligibility standards (for example, low-income resources, disabilities, pregnancy) before providing free health care to Medicaid applicants. Some states include as much as half the cost of Medicaid services in their budgets, but others depend on HHS for well over half of their expenditures. Nearly fifty million persons received Medicaid services across the country in 2008 at an estimated federal (HHS) cost of more than $200 billion. Because many state programs have faced budgetary cuts that could decrease their ability to maintain Medicare services, measures were put in place at the end of 2008 to allow participating states to introduce minimal premiums and higher copayments for Medicaid recipients. The Patient Protection and Affordable Care Act of 2010 laid plans for expanding Medicaid eligibility in 2014.

The ACF, organized with ten regional offices across the country, provides financial assistance to needy families, enforces child support obligations, and assists children held back by various economic or developmental disadvantages. Head Start is ACF's widely recognized program to help prepare children of qualifying economically disadvantaged families for entry into the regular school system. Grants are made available to local public and private nonprofit institutions to develop methods—ideally methods involving parent participation with their children—to develop necessary social and cognitive skills that may be lacking as a result of disadvantaged social and economic environments. Enrollments in Head Start since its inception in 1965 increased (although not steadily) from about 500,000 to more than 900,000 participants in 2010. Budgetary support also rose steadily, passing the billion dollar mark in 1985. By 2011, appropriations were close to $8.1 billion.

The activities of other important agencies of HHS involve support for scientific research and dissemination of research findings to the general public. The National Institutes of Health (NIH) is the best known such agency focusing on "pure" scientific research. For its part, the Agency for Health Care Policy and Research, created in 1989 and reauthorized in 1999 as the Agency for Healthcare Research and Quality (AHRQ), supports research that gauges the effectiveness of existing or proposed health care programs around the country. These programs are studied, for example, in terms of costs, accessibility, and reduction of safety risks for patients. One should also note the social relevance of a number of AHRQ research projects, including studies of ethnic and racial disparities in access to health care. AHRQ also makes vital practical health care information available to the public. This is clear in the activities of one program in particular: the Office of Consumer Assessment of Healthcare Providers and Systems.

In the broader domain of informational services relating to public health, two agencies—the Food and Drug Administration (FDA) and Centers for Disease Control and Prevention (CDC)—stand out. The FDA is responsible for testing and approving (or rejecting) a broad spectrum of products proposed by manufacturers for the consumer market. These range from the obvious—vaccines and new pharmaceutical products or generic equivalents of brand-name drugs—through many categories of food additives and dietary supplements to cosmetics and tobacco products. FDA recommendations reach the public through a variety of media, most notably regular publications outlining the characteristics of individual drugs or providing advice on buying medicines online (including warnings on counterfeit products). Potentially the most direct protective impact of the FDA is the power to recall drugs or food items that, although they succeed in reaching the consumer market, later reveal dangerous health or safety risks. A number of FDA activities extend beyond US borders, both with the aim of sharing vital research information and encouraging cooperation when international public health safety questions (most notably in combating pandemic diseases) are involved. In these areas, the FDA coordinates its functions with the CDC, which has a program providing relevant disease risk information to travelers going abroad.

The CDC not only deals with common widespread infectious diseases such as influenza, hepatitis, and HIV/AIDS (as well as major debilitating chronic diseases such as diabetes and cancer) but also maintains specialized branches responsible for health and safety in the workplace as well as emergency preparedness in the event of bioterrorism, chemical and radiation disasters, and health hazards that stem from natural disasters.

SAMHSA has a wide range of programs that are either preventive or, when drug or alcohol abuse or mental health issues require treatment, provide referrals to appropriate public health institutions. It also maintains an online database, the National Registry of Evidence-Based Programs and Practices, which reviews modes of preventing or treating, or both, the most common mental disorders and cases of substance abuse. SAMHSA also provides funding to support qualified community programs involved in either substance abuse prevention or treatment. Grants in 2009, for example, included almost $2.5 million awarded to local juvenile court systems to help develop their ability to provide substance abuse treatment and some $15 million for the same need in geographically concentrated areas of particular need (mainly, but not solely, in large urban zones). A major sum (grants totaling $60 million) was earmarked in 2009 for local groups with existing or planned drug-free-community programs. Grants

Other agencies of HHS carry on programs whose importance to public health can be said to be visible in the very names they bear. For example, the Agency for Toxic Substances and Disease Registry (ATSDR) is responsible not only for monitoring dangerous substances that are easily recognizable by the general public (asbestos, lead, DDT, and mercury, for example), but for conducting research that can reveal new dangers in unsuspected places. Another responsibility of ATSDR is to monitor both public and specialized toxic waste sites across the country. The Indian Health Service and the Administration on Aging are two other agencies whose work within important subsectors of the US population is easily recognized as a vital public service.

Perspective and Prospects

Because the budget for HHS must be reviewed by Congress, a certain degree of uncertainty may surround the ongoing work of its several agencies. Some programs, like Medicare and Medicaid, are subject to close scrutiny not only because of their critical place within the total US budget but also because of their importance as part of the health care reform debate,

which came to center stage following the election of President Barack Obama in 2008 and continued to be debated after the Patient Protection and Affordable Care Act, commonly called Obamacare, was signed into law in 2010. Other HHS agencies, without being as politically "supercharged" as Medicare and Medicaid, are clearly identified in the public's mind because they represent easily visible dilemmas affecting everyday life. Within the brief period of two decades, questions of substance abuse and dysfunctional families, for example, have become the focus of major media attention. Because budgetary and political debates over the relative importance of the multidimensional activities of the HHS can arise at any time, its administrators must be prepared for possible calls for prioritization.

—*Byron D. Cannon, Ph.D.*

See also Centers for Disease Control and Prevention (CDC); Environmental health; Epidemiology; Health care reform; Medicare; National Institutes of Health (NIH); Occupational health; Preventive medicine; World Health Organization.

For Further Information:

Centers for Disease Control and Prevention. US Department of Health and Human Services, 2013.
Daschle, Thomas, Scott Greenberger, and Jeanne Lambrew. *Critical: What We Can Do About the Health-Care Crisis*. New York: Thomas Dunne Books, 2008.
HHS.gov. US Department of Health and Human Services, 2013.
Institute of Medicine. *An Assessment of the CDC Anthrax Vaccine Safety and Efficacy Research Program*. Washington, DC: National Academy Press, 2003.
McCormick, Joseph B., Susan Fisher-Hoch, and Leslie Alan Horvitz. *Level 4: Virus Hunters of the CDC*. Atlanta: Turner, 1996.
Medicaid.gov. Centers for Medicare and Medicaid Services. US Department of Health and Human Services, 2013.
Medicare.gov. Centers for Medicare and Medicaid Services. US Department of Health and Human Services, 2013.
Moon, Marilyn, and Janemarie Mulvey. *Entitlements and the Elderly*. Washington, DC: Urban Institute Press, 1996.
National Institutes of Health. US Department of Health and Human Services, 2013.
National Research Council, Committee on the Organizational Structure of the National Institutes of Health. *Enhancing the Vitality of the National Institutes of Health*. Washington, DC: National Academy Press, 2003.
Office of Head Start. Administration for Children and Families. US Department of Health and Human Services, 2013.
SAMHSA. Substance Abuse and Mental Health Services Administration. US Department of Health and Human Services, 2013.
FDA: US Food and Drug Administration. US Department of Health and Human Services, 2013.

DEPRESSION
Disease/Disorder

Anatomy or system affected: Brain, heart, musculoskeletal system, psychic-emotional system

Specialties and related fields: Family medicine, geriatrics and gerontology, psychiatry, psychology

Definition: One of the most common psychiatric disorders to occur in most lifetimes, caused by biological, psychological, social, and/or environmental factors.

Key terms:

bipolar disorders: mood disorders characterized by symptoms of mania and symptoms of depression

cyclothymia: a mood disorder characterized by fewer and less intense symptoms of elevated mood and depressed mood than bipolar disorders

dysthymia: a mood disorder characterized by symptoms similar to depression that are fewer in number but last for a much longer period of time

electroconvulsive therapy (ECT): the use of electric shocks to induce seizure in depressed patients as a form of treatment

major depressive disorder: a pattern of major depressive episodes that form an identified psychiatric disorder

major depressive episode: a syndrome of symptoms characterized by depressed mood; required for the diagnosis of some mood disorders

manic episode: a syndrome of symptoms characterized by elevated, expansive, or irritable mood; required for the diagnosis of some mood disorders

psychopharmacology: the drug treatment of psychiatric disorders

psychosurgery: the surgical removal or destruction of part of the brain of depressed patients as a form of treatment

psychotherapy: the "talk" therapies that target the emotional, social, and other contributors to and consequences of depression

seasonal affective disorder (SAD): a mood disorder associated with the winter season, when the amount of daylight hours is reduced

---

Information on Depression

Causes: Genetic factors, psychosocial stressors, neurochemical dysfunction, certain medications

Symptoms: Irritable mood, diminished interest in previously pleasurable activities, significant weight loss or gain, insomnia or hypersomnia, physical excitation or slowness, loss of energy, feelings of worthlessness or guilt, indecisiveness, recurrent thoughts of death

Duration: Ranges from short-term to chronic

Treatments: Drug therapy, individual and group psychotherapy, light therapy, electroconvulsive therapy

---

Causes and Symptoms

The word "depression" is used to describe many different things. For some, it defines a fleeting mood, for others an outward physical appearance of sadness, and for others a diagnosable clinical disorder. In any year, millions of adults suffer from a clinically diagnosed depression, a mood disorder that often affects personal, vocational, social, and health functioning. The *Diagnostic and Statistical Manual of Mental Disorders: DSM-5* (5th ed., 2013) of the American Psychiatric Association delineates a number of mood disorders that include clinical depression, known as major depression.

A major depressive episode is a syndrome of symptoms, present during a two-week period and representing a change from previous functioning. The symptoms include at least five of the following: depressed or irritable mood, diminished interest in previously pleasurable activities, significant weight loss or weight gain, insomnia or hypersomnia, physical excitation or slowness, loss of energy, feelings of worthlessness or guilt, indecisiveness or a diminished ability to concentrate, and recurrent thoughts of death. The clinical depression cannot be initiated or maintained by another illness or condition, and it cannot be a normal reaction to the death of a loved one (some symptoms of depression are a normal part of the grief reaction).

In major depressive disorder, the patient experiences a major depressive episode and does not have a history of mania or hypomania. Major depressive disorder is often first recognized in the patient's late twenties, while a major depressive episode can occur at any age, including infancy. Women are twice as likely to suffer from the disorder than are men.

There are several potential causes of major depressive disorder. Genetic studies suggest a familial link with higher rates of clinical depression in first-degree relatives. There also appears to be a relationship between clinical depression and levels of the brain's neurochemicals, specifically dopamine, norepinephrine, and serotonin, as well as hormones. It is important to keep in mind, however, that anywhere from 15 to 40 percent of adults will experience depression in their lifetimes. Furthermore, not everyone has a biological cause for this depression. Common causes of clinical depression also include psychosocial stressors such as the death of a loved one, financial stress, loss of a job, interpersonal problems, or world events. It is unclear, however, why some people respond to a specific psychosocial stressor with a clinical depression and others do not. Finally, certain prescription medications have been noted to cause or be related to clinical depression. These drugs include muscle relaxants, heart medications, hypertensive medications, ulcer medications, oral contraceptives, painkillers, narcotics, and steroids. Thus there are many causes of clinical depression, and no single cause is sufficient to explain all clinical depressions.

Another category of depressive disorder is bipolar disorders. Bipolar disorders occur in about 1 percent of the population as a whole. In persons over the age of eighteen, about two to three persons out of one hundred are diagnosed. Bipolar I disorder is characterized by one or more manic episodes along with persisting symptoms of depression. A manic episode is defined as a distinct period of abnormally and persistently elevated, expansive, or irritable mood. Three of the following symptoms must occur during the period of mood disturbance: inflated self-esteem, decreased need for sleep, unusual talkativeness or pressure to keep talking, racing thoughts, distractibility, excessive goal-oriented activities (especially in work, school, or social areas), and reckless activities with a high potential for negative consequences (such as buying sprees or risky business ventures). For a diagnosis of bipolar disorder, the symptoms must be sufficiently severe to cause impairment in functioning and/or concern regarding the person's danger to himself/herself or to others, must not be superimposed on another psychotic disorder, and must not be initiated or maintained by another illness or condition. Bipolar II disorder is characterized by symptoms of a history of a major depressive episode and symptoms of hypomania.

Cyclothymia is another cyclic mood disorder related to depression. Considered a mild form of bipolar disorder, it involves symptoms of both depression and mania. However, the manic symptoms are without marked social or occupational impairment and are known as hypomanic episodes. Similarly, the symptoms of major depressive episodes do not meet the clinical criteria (less than five of the nine symptoms described above), but the symptoms must be present for at least two years. Cyclothymia cannot be superimposed on another psychotic disorder and cannot be initiated or maintained by another illness or condition. This mood disorder is a particularly persistent and chronic disorder with an identified familial pattern.

Dysthymia is another chronic mood disorder affecting approximately 6 percent of the population in a lifetime. Dysthymia is characterized by at least a two-year history of depressed mood and at least two of the following symptoms: poor appetite, insomnia or hypersomnia, low energy or fatigue, low self-esteem, poor concentration or decision making, or feelings of hopelessness. There cannot be evidence of a major depressive episode during the first two years of the dysthymia or a history of manic episodes or hypomanic episodes. The individual cannot be without the symptoms for more than two months at a time, the disorder cannot be superimposed on another psychotic disorder, and it cannot be initiated or maintained by another illness or condition. Dysthymia is more common in adult females, equally common in both sexes of children, and with a greater prevalence in families. The causes of dysthymia are believed to be similar to those listed for major depressive disorder, but the disorder is less well understood than is depression.

A final variant of clinical depression is known as seasonal affective disorder. Patients with this illness demonstrate a pattern of clinical depression during the winter, when there is a reduction in the amount of daylight hours. For these patients, the reduction in available light is thought to be the cause of the depression.

Treatment and Therapy

Crucial to the choice of treatment for clinical depression is determining the variant of depression being experienced. Each of the diagnostic categories has associated treatment approaches that are more effective for a particular diagnosis. Multiple assessment techniques are available to the health care professional to determine the type of clinical depression. The most valid and reliable is the clinical interview. The health care provider may conduct either an informal interview or a structured, formal clinical interview assessing the symptoms that would confirm the diagnosis of clinical depression. If the patient meets the criteria set forth in the DSM-5, then the patient is considered for depression treatments. Patients who meet many but not all diagnostic criteria are sometimes diagnosed with a "subclinical" depression. These

patients might also be considered appropriate for the treatment of depression, at the discretion of their health care providers.

Another assessment technique is the "paper-and-pencil" measure, or depression questionnaire. A variety of questionnaires have proven useful in confirming the diagnosis of clinical depression. Questionnaires such as the Beck Depression Inventory, Hamilton Depression Rating Scale, Zung Self-Rating Depression Scale, and the Center for Epidemiologic Studies Depression Scale are used to identify persons with clinical depression and to document changes with treatment. This technique is often used as an adjunct to the clinical interview and rarely stands alone as the definitive assessment approach to diagnosing clinical depression.

Laboratory tests, most notably the dexamethasone suppression test, have also been used in the diagnosis of depression. The dexamethasone suppression test involves injecting a steroid (dexamethasone) into the patient and measuring the production levels of another steroid (cortisol) in response. Studies have demonstrated, however, that certain severely depressed patients do not reveal the suppression of cortisol production that would be expected following the administration of dexamethasone. The test has also failed to identify some patients who were depressed and has mistakenly identified others as depressed. Research continues to determine the efficacy of other measures of brain activity, including computed tomography (CT) scanning, positron emission tomography (PET) scanning, and magnetic resonance imaging (MRI). However, laboratory and imaging tests are not a reliable diagnostic strategy for depression.

Once a clinical depression (or a subclinical depression) is identified, several types of treatment options are available. These options are dependent on the subtype and severity of the depression. They include psychopharmacology (drug therapy), individual and group psychotherapy, light therapy, family therapy, electroconvulsive therapy (ECT), and other less traditional treatments. These treatment options can be provided to the patient as part of an outpatient program or, in certain severe cases of clinical depression in which the person is a danger to himself/herself or others, as part of a hospitalization.

Clinical depression often affects the patient physically, emotionally, and socially. Therefore, prior to beginning any treatment with a clinically depressed individual, the health care provider will attempt to develop an open and communicative relationship with the patient. This relationship will allow the health care provider to provide patient education on the illness and to solicit the collaboration of the patient in treatment. Supportiveness, understanding, and collaboration are all necessary components of any treatment approach.

Three primary types of medications are used in the treatment of clinical depression: cyclic antidepressants, monoamine oxidase inhibitors (MAOIs), and lithium salts. These medications are considered equally effective in decreasing the symptoms of depression, which begin to resolve in several weeks after initiating treatment. The health care professional will select an antidepressant based on side effects, dosing convenience (once daily versus three times a day), and cost.

The cyclic antidepressants are the largest class of antidepressant medications. As the name implies, the chemical makeup of the medication contains chemical rings, or "cycles." There are unicyclic (buproprion and fluoxetine, or Prozac), bicyclic (sertraline and trazodone), tricyclic (amitriptyline, desipramine, and nortriptyline), and tetracyclic (maprotiline) antidepressants. These antidepressants function to either block the reuptake of neurotransmitters by the neurons, allowing more of the neurotransmitter to be available at a receptor site, or increase the amount of neurotransmitter produced. The side effects associated with the cyclic antidepressants—dry mouth, blurred vision, constipation, urinary difficulties, palpitations, and sleep disturbance—vary and can be quite problematic. Some of these antidepressants have deadly toxic effects at high levels, so they are not prescribed to patients who are at risk of suicide. The newer drugs are more specific in terms of the drug action. For instance, fluoxetine is a selective serotonin reuptake inhibitor (SSRI) and works specifically on the neurotransmitter serotonin. Similarly, buproprion is a norepinephrine and dopamine reuptake inhibitor (NDRI) and works specifically on the neurotransmitters norepinephrine and dopamine. More specific drugs generally create fewer side effects. Fewer side effects can be associated with greater medication compliance, potentially making these drugs a more effective treatment.

Monoamine oxidase inhibitors (isocarboxazid, phenelzine, and tranylcypromine) are the second class of antidepressants. They function by slowing the production of the enzyme monoamine oxidase. This enzyme is responsible for breaking down the neurotransmitters norepinephrine and serotonin, which are believed to be responsible for depression. By slowing the decomposition of these transmitters, more of them are available to the receptors for a longer period of time. Restlessness, dizziness, weight gain, insomnia, and sexual dysfunction are common side effects of the MAOIs. MAOIs are most notable because of the dangerous adverse reaction (severely high blood pressure) that can occur if the patient consumes large quantities of foods high in tyramine (such as aged cheeses, fermented sausages, red wine, foods with a heavy yeast content, and pickled fish). Because of this potentially dangerous reaction, MAOIs are not usually the first choice of medication and are more commonly reserved for depressed patients who do not respond to the cyclic antidepressants.

A third class of medication used in the treatment of mood disorders are mood stabilizers, the most notable being lithium carbonate, which is used primarily for bipolar disorder. Lithium is a chemical salt that is believed to affect mood stabilization by influencing the production, storage, release, and reuptake of certain neurotransmitters. It is particularly useful in stabilizing and preventing manic episodes and preventing depressive episodes in patients with bipolar disorder.

Psychotherapy refers to a number of different treatment techniques used to deal with the psychosocial contributors and consequences of clinical depression. Psychotherapy is a common supplement to drug therapy. In psychotherapy, the patients develop knowledge and insight into the causes and treatment for their clinical depression. In cognitive psychotherapy, symptom relief comes from assisting patients in modifying maladaptive, irrational, or automatic beliefs that can lead to clinical depression. In behavioral psychotherapy, patients modify their environment such that social or personal rewards are more forthcoming. This process might involve being more assertive, reducing isolation by becoming more socially active, increasing physical activities or exercise, or learning relaxation techniques. Research on the effectiveness of these and other psychotherapy techniques indicates that psychotherapy is as effective as certain antidepressants for many patients and, in combination with certain medications, is more effective than either treatment alone.

Electroconvulsive (or "shock") therapy is the single most effective treatment for severe and persistent depression. If the clinically depressed patient fails to respond to medications or psychotherapy and the depression is life-threatening, electroconvulsive therapy is considered. It is also considered if the patient cannot physically tolerate antidepressants, as with elders who have other medical conditions. This therapy involves inducing a seizure in the patient by administering an electrical current to specific parts of the brain. The therapy has become quite sophisticated and much safer than it was in the mid-twentieth century, and it involves fewer risks to the patient. Patients undergo several treatments over a period of time, such as a week, and show marked treatment benefit. Some temporary memory impairment is a common side effect of this treatment. In the past, however, more memory impairment, of lasting duration for some, was more common.

A special treatment used for individuals with seasonal affective disorder is light therapy, or phototherapy. Light therapy involves exposing patients to bright light for a period of time each day during seasons of the year when there is decreased light. This may be done as a preventive measure and also during depressive episodes. The manner in which this treatment approach modifies the depression is unclear and awaits further research, but some believe it affects the internal clock of the body, or circadian rhythm. Studies of the effectiveness of light therapy have been mixed, but interest in this promising treatment is strong, as it may prove useful for working with nonseasonal mood disorders as well. It should be noted, however, that light therapy does have some risks associated with it. Caution must be used to protect the eyes and use the light as directed. Additionally, the intensity of light must be correct so as to achieve therapeutic effects and not cause other problems. Finally, some individuals can experience manic episodes if they are exposed to too much light, so caution must be exercised in terms of the length of time for light exposure treatment sessions.

Psychosurgery, the final treatment option, is quite rare. It refers to surgical removal or destruction of certain portions of the brain believed to be responsible for causing severe depression. Psychosurgery is used only after all treatment options have failed and the clinical depression is life-threatening. Approximately 50 percent of patients who undergo psychosurgery benefit from the procedure.

Perspective and Prospects

Depression, or the more historical term "melancholy," has had a history predating modern medicine. Writings from the time of the ancient Greek physician Hippocrates refer to patients with a symptom complex similar to the present-day definition of clinical depression.

The rates of clinical depression have increased since the early twentieth century, while the age of onset of clinical depression has decreased. Women appear to be at least twice as likely as men to suffer from clinical depression, and people who are happily married have a lower risk for clinical depression than those who are separated, divorced, or dissatisfied in their marital relationship. This data, along with recurrence rates of 50 to 70 percent, indicate the importance of this psychiatric disorder.

While most psychiatric disorders are nonfatal, clinical depression can lead to death. About 60 percent of individuals who commit suicide have a mood disorder such as depression at the time. In a lifetime, however, only about 7 percent of men and 1 percent of women with lifetime histories of depression will commit suicide. Though these numbers are very high, what this means is that not everyone who is depressed will commit suicide. In fact, many receive help and recover from this illness. There are, however, other costs of clinical depression. Billions of dollars are spent on clinical depression, divided among the following areas: treatment, suicide, and absenteeism (the largest). Clinical depression obviously has a significant economic impact on a society.

The future of clinical depression lies in early identification and treatment. Identification will involve two areas. The first is improving the social awareness of mental health issues to include clinical depression. By eliminating the negative social stigma associated with mental illness and mental health treatment, there will be an increased level of the reporting of depression symptoms and thereby an improved opportunity for early intervention, preventing the progression of the disorder to the point of suicide. The second approach to identification involves the development of reliable assessment strategies for clinical depression. Data suggests that the majority of those who commit suicide see a physician within thirty days of the suicide. The field will continue to strive to identify biological markers and other methods to predict and/or identify clinical depression more accurately. Treatment advances will focus on further development of pharmacological strategies and drugs with more specific actions and fewer side effects. Adjuncts to traditional drug therapies need continued development and refinement to maximize the success of integrated treatments.

—Oliver Oyama, Ph.D.;
updated by Nancy A. Piotrowski, Ph.D.

See also Antianxiety drugs; Antidepressants; Anxiety; Bipolar disorders; Brain; Death and dying; Dementias; Eating disorders; Emotions, biochemical causes and effects of; Geriatrics and gerontology; Grief and guilt; Hypochondriasis; Light therapy; Midlife crisis; Neurology; Neurology, pediatric; Neurosis; Neurosurgery; Obsessive-compulsive disorder; Palliative medicine; Panic attacks; Paranoia; Pharmacology; Phobias; Postpartum depression; Post-traumatic stress disorder; Psychiatric disorders; Psychiatry; Psychiatry, child and adolescent; Psychiatry, geriatric; Psychoanalysis; Psychosomatic disorders; Seasonal affective disorder; Shock therapy; Stress; Suicide; Terminally ill: Extended care.

For Further Information:

"About Mood Disorders." *Depression and Bipolar Support Alliance*, 2013.
American Psychiatric Association. *Diagnostic and Statistical Manual of Mental Disorders: DSM-5*. 5th ed. Washington, DC: Author, 2013.
"Bipolar Disorder." *MedlinePlus*, 30 July 2013.
DePaulo, J. Raymond, Jr., and Leslie Ann Horvitz. *Understanding Depression: What We Know and What You Can Do About It*. New York: Wiley, 2003.
"Depression." *MedlinePlus*, 29 July 2013.
"Depression." *National Institute of Mental Health*, 2013.
Jones, Steven. *Coping with Bipolar Disorder: A Guide to Living with Manic Depression*. Oxford, England: Oneworld, 2002.
Koplewicz, Harold S. *More than Moody: Recognizing and Treating Adolescent Depression*. New York: Penguin, 2003.
"Mood Disorders." *MedlinePlus*, 4 July 2013.

DERMATITIS

Disease/Disorder
Also known as: Eczema
Anatomy or system affected: Hair, skin
Specialties and related fields: Dermatology
Definition: A wide range of skin disorders, some the result of allergy, some caused by contact with a skin irritant, and some attributable to other causes.

Key terms:

allergen: a substance that excites an immunologic response; also called an antigen
crusting: the appearance of slightly elevated skin lesions made up of dried serum, blood, or pus; they can be brown, red, black, tan, or yellowish
immunoglobulin E (IgE): ordinarily, a relatively rare antibody; in patients with atopic dermatitis, levels can be significantly higher than in the general population
lesion: any pathologic change in tissue
scaling: a buildup of hard, horny skin cells
secondary infection: a bacterial, viral, or other infection that results from or follows another disease
wheal: a small swelling in the skin

Causes and Symptoms

The term *dermatitis* refers not to a single skin disease but to a wide range of disorders. *Dermatitis* is often used interchangeably with *eczema*. The two most common dermatitides are atopic (allergic) dermatitis, in which the individual appears to inherit a predilection for the disease, and contact dermatitis, in which the individual's skin reacts immediately on contact with a substance or develops sensitivity to it.

Atopic dermatitis often occurs in individuals with a personal or family history of allergy, such as hay fever or asthma.

Between 50 and 70 percent of children with severe atopic dermatitis develop asthma, a rate that is more than five times higher than for the general population. These people often have high serum levels of a certain antibody, immunoglobulin E (IgE), which may be associated with their skin's tendency to break out, although a specific antigen-antibody reaction has not been demonstrated.

There are many distinct characteristics of atopic dermatitis, some of which depend on the age of the patient. The disease usually starts early in childhood. It is often first discovered in infants in the first months of life when redness and weeping, crusted lesions appear mostly on the face, although the scalp, arms, and legs may also be affected. There is intense itching. Papules (pimples), vesicles (small, blisterlike lesions filled with fluid), edema (swelling), serous exudation (discharge of fluid), and scaly crusts may be seen. At one year of age, oval, scaly lesions appear on the arms, legs, face, and torso. In older children and adults, the lesions are usually localized in the crook of the elbow and the back of the knees, and the face and neck may be involved. The course of the disease is variable. It usually subsides by the third or fourth year of life, but periodic outbreaks may occur throughout childhood, adolescence, and adulthood. Cases persisting past the patient's middle twenties, or beginning then, are the most difficult to treat.

Dryness and itching are always present in atopic dermatitis. People with atopic dermatitis seem to lose skin moisture more readily than average people: Rather than soft, pliable skin, they develop dry, rough, sensitive skin that is particularly prone to chapping and splitting. The skin becomes itchy, and the individual's tendency to scratch significantly aggravates the condition in what is called the "itch-scratch-itch" cycle or the "scratch-rash-itch" cycle: the individual scratches to relieve the itching, which causes a rash, which in turn causes increased itching, which invites increased scratching and increased irritation. After years of itching and scratching, the skin of older children and adults with atopic dermatitis develops red, lichenified (rough, thickened) patches in the crook of the arm and behind the knees as well as on the eyelids, neck, and wrists.

Constant chafing of the affected area invites bacterial infection and lymphadenitis (inflammation of lymph nodes). Furthermore, patients with atopic dermatitis seem to have altered immune systems. They appear to be more susceptible than others to skin infections, warts, and contagious skin diseases. *Staphylococcus aureus* and certain streptococci are common infecting bacteria in these patients. Pyoderma is often seen as a result of bacterial infection in atopic dermatitis. This condition features redness, oozing, scaling, and crusting as well as the formation of small pustules (pus-filled pimples).

Patients with atopic dermatitis are also particularly sensitive to herpes simplex and vaccinia viruses. Exposure to either could cause a severe skin disease called Kaposi's varicelliform eruption. Vaccinia virus (the agent that causes cowpox) is used in the preparation of smallpox vaccine. Therefore, patients with atopic dermatitis must not be vacci-

---

Information on Dermatitis

Causes: Allergies, infection, contact irritation, altered immune system
Symptoms: Dry and itchy skin, rashes, inflammation, pain
Duration: Short-term to chronic
Treatments: Topical corticosteroids or antihistamines, antibiotics, dietary changes, and specialized lotions, soaps, or shampoos

---

nated against smallpox. Furthermore, they must be isolated from patients with active herpes simplex and those recently vaccinated against smallpox.

Patients with atopic dermatitis may also develop contact dermatitis, which can greatly exacerbate their condition. They are also sensitive to a wide range of allergens, which can bring on outbreaks, as well as to low humidity (such as in centrally heated houses in winter), which can contribute to dry skin. They may not be able to tolerate woolen clothing.

A condition called keratosis pilaris often develops in the presence of atopic dermatitis. It is not seen in young infants, but it does appear in childhood. Hair follicles on the torso, buttocks, arms, and legs become plugged with horny matter and protrude above the skin, giving the appearance of goose bumps or "chicken skin." The palms of the hands of patients with atopic dermatitis have significantly more fine lines than those of average people. In many patients, there is a tiny "pleat" under the eyes. They are often prone to cold hands and may have pallor, seen as a blanching of the skin around the nose, mouth, and ears.

When ordinary skin is lightly rubbed with a pointed object, almost immediately there is a red line, followed by a red flare, and finally, a wheal or slight elevation of the skin along the line. In patients with atopic dermatitis, however, there is a completely different reaction: The red line appears, but almost instantly it becomes white. The flare and the wheal do not appear.

About 4 to 12 percent of patients with atopic dermatitis develop cataracts at an early age (some estimates range as high as nearly 40 percent). Normally, cataracts do not appear until the fifties and sixties; those with atopic dermatitis may develop them in their twenties. These cataracts usually affect both eyes simultaneously and develop quickly.

Psychologically, children with atopic dermatitis often show distinct personality characteristics. They are reported to be bright, aggressive, energetic, and prone to fits of anger. Children with severe, unmanageable cases of atopic dermatitis may become selfish and domineering, and some go on to develop significant personality disorders.

It is not known exactly what happens to cause the itching and dry skin that are the fundamental signs of atopic dermatitis and the root of many of its complications. Theories suggest various origins. It is by definition an allergic disorder, but the allergens that are specifically involved and how they produce the signs of atopic dermatitis are unknown. One of the most interesting theories involves the antibody IgE. Theoretically, the union of IgE with an antigen causes certain cells to release pharmacologic mediators, such as histamine, bradykinin, and slow-reacting substance (SRS-A), that cause itching and thus begin the cycle of scratching and irritation characteristic of atopic dermatitis. The fact that patients with atopic dermatitis have higher than normal levels of IgE, and that there is a relationship between IgE levels and the severity of atopic dermatitis, seems to lend support to this theory.

Contact dermatitis resembles atopic dermatitis at certain stages, but the dry skin of atopic dermatitis may not be seen. Contact dermatitis is usually characterized by a rash consisting of small bumps, itchiness, blisters, and general swelling. It occurs when the skin has been exposed to a substance to which the body is sensitive or allergic. If the contact dermatitis is caused by direct irritation by a caustic substance, it is called irritant contact dermatitis. The causative agents are primary irritants that cause inflammation at first contact. Some obvious irritants are acids, alkalis, and other harsh chemicals or substances. An example is fiberglass dermatitis, in which fine glass particles from fiberglass fabrics or insulation enter the skin and cause redness and inflammation.

If the dermatitis is caused by allergic sensitivity to a substance, it is called allergic contact dermatitis. In this case, it may take hours, days, weeks, or years for the patient to develop sensitivity to the point where exposure to these substances causes allergic contact dermatitis. Agents that may cause allergic contact dermatitis include soaps, acetone, skin creams, cosmetics, poison ivy, and poison sumac.

Allergic contact dermatitis comprises the largest variety of contact dermatitides, many of them named for the allergens that cause them. Hence, there is pollen dermatitis; plant and flower dermatitis, such as poison ivy or poison oak; clothing dermatitis; shoe, and even sandal strap, dermatitis; metal and metal salt dermatitis; cosmetic dermatitis; and adhesive tape dermatitis, among others. They all have one thing in common: the skin is exposed to an allergen from any of these sources and becomes so sensitive to it that further exposure causes a rash, itching, and blistering.

The development of sensitivity to an allergen is an immunological response to exposure to that substance. With many allergens, the first contact elicits no immediate immunological reaction. Sensitivity develops after the allergen has been presented to the T lymphocytes that mediate the immune response.

Because it often takes a long time to develop sensitivity, patients are surprised to discover that they have become allergic to substances that they have been using for years. For example, a patient who has been applying a topical medication to treat a skin condition may one day find that the medication causes an outbreak of dermatitis. Ironically, some of the ingredients in medications commonly used to treat skin conditions are among the major allergens that cause allergic contact dermatitis. These include antibiotics, antihistamines, topical anesthetics, and antiseptics as well as the inactive ingredients used in formulating the medications, such as stabilizers.

Other substances to which the patient may develop sensi-

tivity include the chemicals used in making fabric for clothing, tanning chemicals used in making leather, dyes, and ingredients in cosmetics. Many patients develop sensitivity to allergens found in the workplace. The list of potential allergens in the industrial setting is virtually endless and includes solvents, petroleum products, chemicals commonly used in manufacturing processes, and coal tar derivatives.

In some cases, the allergen requires sunlight or other forms of light to precipitate an outbreak of contact dermatitis. This is called photoallergic contact dermatitis, and it may be caused by such agents as aftershave lotions, sunscreens, topical sulfonamides, and other preparations applied to the skin. Another light reaction, termed phototoxic contact dermatitis, can be caused by exposure to sunlight after exposure to perfumes, coal tar, certain medications, and various chemicals.

A different form of dermatitis involves the sebaceous glands, which secrete sebum, a fatty substance that lubricates the skin and helps retain moisture. Sebaceous dermatitis is usually seen in areas of the body with high concentrations of sebaceous glands, such as on the scalp or face, behind the ears, on the chest, and in areas where skin rubs against skin, such as the buttocks and the groin. It is seen most often in infants and adolescents, although it may persist into adulthood or start at that time.

In infants, sebaceous dermatitis can begin within the first month of life and appears as a thick, yellow, crusted lesion on the scalp called cradle cap. There can be yellow scaling behind the ears and red pimples on the face. Diaper rash may be persistent in these infants. In older children, the lesion may appear as thick, yellow plaques in the scalp. When sebaceous dermatitis begins in adulthood, it starts slowly, and usually its only manifestation is scaling on the scalp (dandruff). In severe cases, yellowish-red scaling pimples develop along the hairline and on the face and chest. Its cause is unknown, but a yeast commonly found in the hair follicles, *Pityrosporum ovale*, may be involved.

There are many other kinds of dermatitis. Diaper dermatitis, or diaper rash, is a complex skin disorder that involves irritation of the skin by urine and feces, irritation by constant rubbing, and secondary infection by *Candida albicans*. Nummular dermatitis is characterized by crusting, scaly, disc-shaped papules and vesicles filled with fluid and often pus. Pityriasis alba is a common dermatitis with pale, scaly patches. In lichen simplex chronicus, there is intense itching, with lesions caused and perpetuated by scratching and rubbing. Stasis dermatitis occurs at the ankles; brown discoloration, swelling, scaling, and varicose veins are common. Hyperimmunoglobulin E (Hyper IgE) syndrome is characterized by extremely high IgE levels, ten to one hundred times higher than normal, and a family history of allergy; the patient has frequent skin infections, suppurative (pus-forming) lymphadenitis, pustules, plaques, and abscesses. Pompholyx occurs on the hands and soles of the feet; there is excessive sweating, with eruptions of deep vesicles accompanied by burning or itching.

Friction can also cause dermatitis. In intertrigo, the friction of skin rubbing against skin causes inflammation that can become infected. In frictional lichenoid dermatitis, or sandbox dermatitis, it is thought that the abrasive action of sand or other gritty material on the skin causes the characteristic lesions. Winter eczema seems to be caused by the skin-drying effects of low humidity as well as by harsh soaps and overfrequent bathing; dry skin and itching are common. The acrodermatitis diseases may be limited to the hands and feet, or, like acrodermatitis enteropathica, may erupt in other parts of the body, such as around the mouth and on the buttocks. In fixed-drug eruption, lesions appear in direct response to the administration of a drug; the lesions are generally in the same parts of the body, but they may spread. Swimmer's itch is a parasitic infection from an organism that lives in freshwater lakes and ponds, while seabather's eruption seems to be caused by a similar saltwater organism.

Treatment and Therapy

Many dermatitides resemble one another, and it is important for a physician to identify the patient's complaint precisely to treat it effectively. Therefore, the physician will confirm the identity of the condition through a process known as differential diagnosis. This method allows him or her to rule out all similar conditions, pinpoint the exact nature of the patient's problem, and develop a therapeutic regimen to treat it.

In treating atopic dermatitis, one of the first goals is to relieve dryness and itching. The patient is cautioned not to bathe excessively, as this dries the skin. Lotions are used to lubricate the skin and retain moisture. The patient is advised not to scratch, because this could break the skin and invite infection. The patient is also advised to avoid any known offending agents and cautioned not to apply any medication to the skin without the doctor's knowledge.

Wet compresses can bring relief to patients with atopic dermatitis. Topical corticosteroids are used to help resolve acute flare-ups, but only for short-term therapy, because their prolonged use might produce undesirable side effects. Oral antihistamines are often given to relieve itching and to help the patient sleep. Diet may play a role in atopic dermatitis in infants; some pediatric dermatologists and other physicians recommend elimination of milk, eggs, tomatoes, citrus fruits, wheat products, chocolate, spices, fish, and nuts from the diets of these patients. Soft cotton clothing is recommended, as is the avoidance of pets or fuzzy toys that might be allergenic. For secondary infections that arise from atopic dermatitis, the physician prescribes appropriate antibiotic therapy.

In primary irritant contact dermatitis, the offending agent is eliminated or avoided. In allergic contact dermatitis, one of the main goals is to discover the offending agent so that the patient can avoid contact with it. Sometimes this information can be elicited from the patient interview, and sometimes it is necessary to conduct a series of patch tests. In this procedure, known allergens are applied to the skin of the patient to find those that cause irritation. Avoidance of the offending agent can cause the patient some difficulty if the agent happens to be something that is found everywhere. An example is the metal nickel, which is in coins, jewelry, and hundreds of other objects. Patients who insist on wearing jewelry containing nickel are advised to paint it with clear nail polish periodically to avoid contact of the metal with the skin. Similarly, many other allergens are in common use. Patients are advised to read cosmetics labels and food and medical ingredients lists to avoid contact with agents to which they are sensitive.

Because there is such a wide range of allergic contact dermatitides, treatments vary considerably. Topical and oral steroids are used, as well as antihistamines. Sometimes the physician finds it necessary to drain large blisters and apply drying agents to weeping lesions. Sometimes the condition calls for wet compresses to relieve itching and soothe the patient. Specialized lotions, soaps, and shampoos are also used, some to treat dryness and others, as in the case of sebaceous dermatitis, to remove scales and to relieve oiliness.

Other treatments depend on the type of dermatitis from which the patient suffers. Patients with photoallergic or phototoxic dermatitis are advised to avoid light. Acrodermatitis enteropathica is caused by a zinc deficiency; in addition to palliative therapy to relieve the symptoms, these patients are given zinc sulfate, which results in complete remission of the disease. As with atopic dermatitis, bacterial infections occurring as a result of a flare-up of allergic contact dermatitis are treated with appropriate antibiotic therapy.

Perspective and Prospects

The skin is the largest organ of the human body, and it is subject to an extraordinary range and number of diseases, with atopic dermatitis and contact dermatitis among the most common. They may afflict patients of all ages, but they are particularly prevalent in children. Many of the dermatitides start in the first weeks of life and continue through childhood. In many cases, the disease is resolved by the time that the child reaches adolescence, but in some it continues into adulthood.

In spite of the fact that disorders of the skin are readily apparent, understanding of them has been imperfect throughout history. For example, the allergic nature of many of the dermatitides was not explained until the twentieth century. In addition, because their symptoms are similar to one another and to diseases that are not properly classified as dermatitides, there has been much confusion in identifying them. It has been suggested that many of the biblical lepers were in fact suffering only from a form of dermatitis. With prolonged exposure, however, they probably contracted leprosy in time.

The dermatitides are often highly complex diseases involving genetic, allergic, metabolic, and immune and infective factors, among many others. They are not usually life threatening, but they take an enormous toll in pain, discomfort, and disfigurement, with an equal toll in psychological distress that can be suffered by patients.

Understanding of these disorders improves constantly, and with understanding comes new methods of treating them. Nevertheless, progress will probably be limited. There is the possibility that patients can be desensitized to allow them to tolerate the allergens that bring about their eruptions, as many hay fever sufferers have been desensitized against the pollens and dusts that trigger their allergies. It is unlikely, however, that there will ever be vaccines to immunize against this group of diseases, nor can many of them be cured, except in the sense that the discomfort that they bring can be treated and the agents that cause them can be avoided.

—*C. Richard Falcon*

See also Acne; Allergies; Blisters; Dermatology; Dermatology, pediatric; Dermatopathology; Diaper rash; Eczema; Hives; Itching; Multiple chemical sensitivity syndrome; Poisonous plants; Psoriasis; Rashes; Rosacea; Scabies; Skin; Skin disorders.

For Further Information:

A.D.A.M. Medical Encyclopedia. "Atopic Dermatitis." *MedlinePlus*, November 20, 2012.

A.D.A.M. Medical Encyclopedia. "Contact Dermatitis." *MedlinePlus*, November 21, 2012.

Adelman, Daniel C., et al., eds. *Manual of Allergy and Immunology.* 4th ed. Philadelphia: Lippincott Williams & Wilkins, 2002.

American Academy of Dermatology. http://www.aad.org.

Bair, Brooke, et al. "Cataracts in Atopic Dermatitis: A Case Presentation and Review of the Literature." *Archives of Dermatology* 147, no. 5 (May, 2011): 585–88.

Hellwig, Jennifer. "Contact Dermatitis." *HealthLibrary*, October 11, 2012.

Litin, Scott C., ed. *Mayo Clinic Family Health Book.* 4th ed. New York: HarperResource, 2009.

Middlemiss, Prisca. *What's That Rash? How to Identify and Treat Childhood Rashes.* London: Hamlyn, 2002.

National Institute of Arthritis and Musculoskeletal and Skin Diseases. "Handout on Health: Atopic Dermatitis." *National Institutes of Health*, August 2011.

Parker, James N., and Philip M. Parker, eds. *The Official Patient's Sourcebook on Atopic Dermatitis.* San Diego, Calif.: Icon Health, 2002.

Rietschel, Robert L., and Joseph F. Fowler, eds. *Fisher's Contact Dermatitis.* 6th ed. Lewiston, N.Y.: Marcel Decker, 2008.

Titman, Penny. *Understanding Childhood Eczema.* New York: Wiley, 2003.

Weston, William L., et al. *Color Textbook of Pediatric Dermatology.* 4th ed. St. Louis, Mo.: Mosby/Elsevier, 2007.

Williams, Hywel C., ed. *Atopic Dermatitis: The Epidemiology, Causes, and Prevention of Atopic Eczema.* New York: Cambridge University Press, 2000.

DERMATOLOGY

Specialty

Anatomy or system affected: Hair, immune system, nails, skin

Specialties and related fields: Cytology, histology, immunology, oncology, public health

Definition: The study of a variety of irritations or lesions affecting one of several layers of the skin.

Key terms:

allergens: foreign substances in the surrounding environment that may cause an allergic response, such as a skin reaction

dermatitis: a general term for nonspecific skin irritations that may be caused by bacteria, viruses, or fungi

keratin: a fibrous molecule essential to the tissue structure of hair, nails, or the skin

melanin: a polymer made up of several compounds (including the amino acid tyrosine) that causes pigmentation in the skin, hair, and eyes

Science and Profession

Dermatology is the subfield of medicine that deals with diseases of the skin. Some disorders affecting the hair and fingernails may also fall under this category.

Dermatological study requires attention to three distinct layers of the skin, each of which can be affected differently by different disorders. The deepest layer is the subcutaneous tissue, where fat is formed and stored. It is also here that the deeper hair follicles and sweat glands originate. Blood vessels and nerves pass from this layer to the dermis. The dermis is mainly connective tissue that contains the oil-producing, or sebaceous, glands and shorter hair follicles. On the surface of the skin is the epidermis, which is itself multilayered. The innermost basal layer is made up of specialized keratin- and melanin-forming cells, whereas the outermost, horny cell layer consists of keratinized dead cells.

The diagnosis of apparent skin disease requires dermatologists to determine whether symptomatic sores, or lesions, are primary (the original symptoms of suspected disease) or secondary (such as infection or irritation caused by scratching, which may overshadow the original disorder). Dermatologists are trained to recognize categories of lesions and to determine whether they represent actual diseases or relatively common disorders characteristic of age, or even genetic predispositions. The most common categories of lesions include vesicles, bullae, and crusts; scaling; keratosis; lichenification; pustules; atrophy; and tumors.

Vesicles and bullae are bubblelike eruptions filled with clear serous fluid. As primary lesions, they are often the symptoms of diseases such as chickenpox and herpes zoster. Crusts are formed by tissue fluid that remains in a dried form after the rupture of microscopic vesicles.

Scaling is noticeably different from crusting. These flakes on the surface of the skin may represent a subsiding stage of earlier inflammation. Scaling may be a secondary lesion associated with psoriasis. Keratoses are rough lesions that show strongly adherent (not loose) flaking. Lichenification involves a thickening of the epidermis, with a more pronounced visibility of lined patterns on the skin surface. Pustules are lesions filled with pus, which serves as a growth medium for microorganisms. Atrophy involves shrinkage of skin tissues, creating in some cases visible depressions in the area of the lesion. The last category of primary lesions, tumors, may be found either on the surface of or underneath the skin. Tumorous growths can signal a condition as benign as seborrheic keratosis (the appearance of thick scales in isolated spots, particularly as age advances) or as serious as one of several forms of skin cancer.

Secondary lesions appear as the primary, or causal, skin disorder progresses, creating different symptoms in the secondary stage. Examples of secondary lesions include scales (dandruff and psoriasis), crusts (impetigo), ulcers (advanced syphilis), and scarring, the growth of connective tissue that actually replaces damaged tissues following burns or other traumatic injuries.

In addition to these general categories of lesions associated with dermatological diseases, a number of localized problems in blood flow—called vascular nevoid lesions, or birthmarks—may be visible at or soon after birth. Dermatologists assume that some of these lesions may be caused by genetic factors. The most common vascular nevi categories are nevus flammeus (port-wine stain), a purple discoloring of the skin resulting from dilated dermal vessels, and capillary hemangioma (strawberry mark), which begins as a bruiselike lesion but soon grows into a protruding mass. Unlike port-wine stains, which remain throughout the individual's lifetime unless they are removed through laser surgery, strawberry marks will usually subside and disappear on their own, leaving at most visible puckering of the skin. Unless there are complications (such as ulceration), treatment is usually simple, consisting of the application of elastic bandages to maintain constant pressure, thus reducing the distortion caused by the rapid expansion of skin tissue in a localized area.

Probably the most commonly recognized dermatological disorder, acne, usually occurs among adolescents and young adults. Although this problem is likely to occur as part of the normal process of maturation, lack of proper care of acne may cause complications and lifelong scarring. Acne, as with equally common cases of seborrheic dermatitis (which causes dandruff), afflicts those areas of the body where oil gland secretions are plentiful and where many forms of bacteria are present on the skin (mainly the face, neck, and upper trunk). The points of lesion for acne are always specific: the hair follicles that are so numerous in these areas of the body. Two phenomena, so-called blackheads and the pimples associated with acne, occur when the normal draining of follicle secretions is blocked in a sac called a comedo. Blackheads occur when the residue trapped in the comedo—keratin, sebum, and various microorganisms—becomes chemically oxidized. When conditions associated with acne appear, an increase in bacterial growth within the comedones produces characteristic pimples which, if traumatized by scratching or picking, may burst, leading to the possibility of further infection. There is no way to prevent acne from appearing, but dermatological therapy to soothe the effects of advanced cases may be recommended.

Another relatively benign but persistently insoluble dermatological problem, the appearance of warts, occurs most often among the middle-aged or older segment of the adult population. Modern dermatological research dating from the 1960s has determined that warts are associated with particular viral strains (papillomaviruses). At least four subtypes have been associated with the appearance of warts on the human body. Warts may vary greatly in appearance—from plantar warts, which grow well below the skin surface and exhibit a drier consistency; to plane warts, which are even with the skin surface; to a very visible brownish and moist lump, which is often found on the face or hands. All warts are localized viral infections that destroy the normal skin tissue in the area of infection. Despite their common occurrence—dermatologists experience a high rate of patient demand for their removal—warts have always carried a certain social stigma. As viruses, they may be transferred to others through contact, particularly if the lesion is an open one.

The term "seborrheic dermatitis" can refer to the recurrent and common problem of dandruff (redness and scaling mainly in skin areas where body hair is present). Like acne, seborrheic dermatitis is more a condition resulting from secretion imbalances and chemical reactions affecting the skin than an actual disease. Dermatological complications arise when excessive scratching of sensitive areas causes secondary lesions to form.

Beyond these categories of common skin disorders are far more serious diseases that require professional dermatological treatment. For example, psoriasis, although varying in possible locations all over the body (including the hands and feet), seems to share symptoms with seborrheic dermatitis, specifically the flaking away of dry skin. What begins as limited patches of flaking, usually on elbows or in the armpits, however, may spread rapidly and have traumatic effects. Dermatologists usually associate psoriasis with stress and anxiety. When irritations are limited in scope, treatment through topical medications—including corticosteroids, salicylic acid, and coal tar—may be successful. Advanced cases may demand systemic treatment with more sophisticated drugs. Phototherapy (light therapy) may also be used for treatment.

Herpes simplex is another common viral infection that leads directly to surface lesions that may be communicable, in this case cold sores. As with warts, folk knowledge has it that improper hygienic practices lead to the much more virulent eruptions associated with herpes simplex. Medical observations have shown, however, that various factors may unleash a dermatological reaction from latent viral sources in an individual. A herpes simplex reaction to increased levels of exposure to sunlight is a good example. On the other hand, many cases of herpes simplex occur in both the male and female genital areas. Although these eruptions are not necessarily connected with much more serious sexually transmitted diseases, their communicability is clearly associated with levels of hygiene in intimate sexual contact. Whatever the cause of herpes simplex, its highly contagious nature may demand dermatological attention to avoid more serious complications. Any occurrence of herpes simplex inflammation near a vital organ, for example, must be treated immediately to prevent the spread of viral infection, particularly in the area surrounding the eyes.

Herpes zoster, commonly referred to as shingles, is thought to be a recurrence in the adult years of a common viral infection that most people experience at an earlier age: chickenpox. The persistence of the symptoms of shingles among adults, however, is not comparable to the mild effect of the virus during childhood. The appearance of painful lesions, usually but not always in the trunk area, may come after a short period of tingling. Although inflammation may pass, many elderly patients, especially those suffering from systemic diseases such as diabetes mellitus, are plagued by continuous long-term discomfort. In addition to discomfort, there may be (as in herpes simplex) a danger of complications if the area of inflammation is close to vulnerable tissues or key organs, such as the eyes or ears. In cases where lesions may affect the eyes, dermatologists must go beyond topical treatment to enhance the healing process. Additional emergency therapy may include corticosteroid treatments.

Diagnostic and Treatment Techniques

The diagnosis of specific dermatoses, or potentially serious skin diseases, may or may not require cutaneous biopsies; because their symptoms are not shared by other diseases, a diagnosis can often be made by observation alone. Less easily recognized problems include lichen planus, an uncommon chronic pruritic disease; such potentially dangerous bullous diseases as pemphigus vulgaris, which is characterized by flat-topped papules on the wrists and legs that resemble poison ivy reactions; and skin cancer. Such conditions usually require biopsy to ensure that a mistaken diagnosis does not lead to the wrong treatment. Several methods of biopsy are employed, according to the nature of the lesion under examination. For example, the cutaneous punch technique, which utilizes a special surgical tool that penetrates to about four millimeters, may not be appropriate if the lesion is close to the surface. In this case, either curettage (scraping) or shave biopsy (cutting a layer corresponding to the thickness of the lesion) may be used in combination with the cutaneous punch method.

The total number of dermatoses that can be diagnosed is far too great for review here. The conditions that are most commonly treated, however, range from mildly serious but clearly irritating lesions such as acne or warts to much more serious phenomena such as psoriasis and lupus erythematosus. Several early and potentially dangerous conditions, such as basal cell carcinoma, may deteriorate into fatal skin cancers.

Dermatologists classify serious skin diseases under several key divisions. Pruritic dermatoses are characterized by itching. Vascular dermatoses, including several categories of urticaria, are all characterized by sudden outbreaks of papules—some temporary in their irritation and therefore merely disorders, as with hives as a reaction to poison ivy or medicines such as penicillin; and others more serious, such as swelling of the glottis, which may accompany angioneurotic edema. Papulosquamous dermatoses include psoriasis and lichen planus, both localized irritations that involve redness and flaking. In addition to these categories of dermatoses, a wide variety of common dermatologic viruses demand special medical attention because they are socially communicable. These include herpes simplex and herpes zoster. Other serious viruses affecting the skin, such as smallpox and measles, have been controlled by preventive vaccinations. Impetigo, once common during childhood in certain environments, is a bacterial infection, not a viral one. One formerly lethal sexually transmitted disease is syphilis, a form of spirochetal infection. Although far from eradicated, syphilis has been treatable through the use of benzathine penicillin since the mid-twentieth century.

The most serious challenge to dermatologists is the early diagnosis and treatment of skin cancer. The most common forms of skin cancer are basal cell epithelioma, which origi-

nates in the epidermis, often as a result of excessive exposure to the sun, and squamous cell carcinoma, which may affect the epidermis or mucosal surfaces (the inside of the mouth or throat). Early diagnosis of both types is essential to prevent metastasis (spreading). The most dangerous skin cancer is malignant melanoma, which may reveal itself through changes in size or color of a body mark such as a mole. This cancer can metastasize very rapidly and endanger the life of the patient.

Possible treatments for different types of skin disease vary considerably. Surgical operations, although certainly not unknown, tend to be associated with more extreme disorders, most notably skin cancer. In such cases, it is usually not the dermatologist but a specialized surgeon who performs the procedure.

The most common treatments used by dermatologists involve the application of various pharmaceutical preparations directly to the surface of the skin. For the treatment of common skin disorders, dermatologists may choose between a variety of medications.

The effect of antipruritic agents (menthol, phenol, camphor, or coal tar solutions) is to reduce itching. Keratoplastic agents (salicylic acid) and keratolytic agents (stronger doses of salicylic acid, resorcinol, or sulfur) affect the relative thickness or softness of the horny layer of the skin. They are associated with the treatment of diseases or disorders characterized by flaking.

Antieczematous agents, including coal tar solutions and hydrocortisone, halt oozing from vesicular lesions. By far the most commonly used drugs in dermatology are antiseptics which, according to their classification, control or kill bacteria, fungi, and viruses. Ointments to combat viral infections are much less common on the pharmaceutical market; however, some are available, mainly for the treatment of infection by herpes labialis (cold sores), herpes zoster (shingles), or varicella zoster (chickenpox).

These and many other topical applications may be only the first steps, however, in soothing the irritating side effects of more serious or chronically persistent dermatological diseases. Doctors may turn to more active therapies to treat specific ailments, beginning with the general category of electrosurgery, of which there are five specialized subtreatments: electrodesiccation, or the drying of tissues; electrocoagulation, which involves more intense heat; electrocautery, the actual burning of tissues; electrolysis, which produces the cauterization of lesions by chemical reaction; and electrosection, or the removal of tissues by cutting, achieved by the focus of electrical currents produced by various forms of vacuum tubes. By the 1990s, rapid progress in laser beam technology—particularly the carbon dioxide laser, which is a beam of infrared electromagnetic energy with an almost infinitesimal wavelength of 10,600 nanometers—began to replace some of these time-tested methods in cases in which electrosurgery had been commonplace for almost half a century.

Other modes of treatment that penetrate the subsurface layers of the skin include radiation therapy and cryosurgery, which is the immediate freezing of tissues by application of agents such as solid carbon dioxide (below -78.5 degrees Celsius) or liquid nitrogen (below -195.8 degrees Celsius). Another treatment option is phototherapy, or light therapy, in which skin is exposed to ultraviolet light for a set amount of time. These methods are used to treat conditions ranging from psoriasis and pruritic dermatoses to skin cancer.

Perspective and Prospects

One common feature—visible body surface symptoms— means that the medical identification and attempted treatment of human skin diseases can be traced to almost all cultures in all historical periods. An outstanding example of ancient peoples" concerns for eruptions on the skin can be found in the Old Testament or Talmud in Leviticus. In this text, however, as well as in many medieval texts, one sees that a variety of skin diseases tended to be classified as leprosy. The physical location of skin lesions often determined the results of very general attempts at diagnosis.

It was not until the last quarter of the eighteenth century that Viennese physicians ushered in what could be called the first phase of scientific study of the skin and its disorders, or dermatology. This early Viennese school insisted on the study of the morphological nature of the lesions. Until this time, physicians had grouped skin diseases according to their appearance in different places on the body. By the mid-nineteenth century another Austrian, Ferdinand von Hebra, made considerable progress in classifying skin diseases.

Because so many lesions of the skin could potentially lead to diagnoses of sexually transmitted diseases, early generations of dermatologists concentrated most of their emphasis in this area. Discovery of a treatment for syphilis in the early twentieth century freed researchers to diversify their physiological investigations, opening the field to broader applications of biochemistry for treatment of different skin conditions, a field developed by the American doctor Stephen Rothman in the 1930s. Some categories, such as fungal diseases, were brought under control by treatments that were developed fairly quickly. By the second half of the century, dermatologists could alleviate most of the complications caused by psoriasis. Then, during the last quarter of the twentieth century, impressive advances in the discovery and patenting of sophisticated drugs brought most of the major dermatological diseases, including those caused in large part by nervous stress, under general control.

Although the treatment of life-threatening diseases, particularly skin cancers, continues to fall short of guaranteed cures, early recognition of their symptoms has steadily increased patients" chances for survival.

—*Byron D. Cannon, Ph.D.*

See also Abscess drainage; Abscesses; Acne; Age spots; Albinos; Athlete's foot; Bedsores; Biopsy; Birthmarks; Blisters; Boils; Bruises; Burns and scalds; Cancer; Carcinoma; Chickenpox; Collagen; Cryosurgery; Cyst removal; Cysts; Dermatitis; Dermatology, pediatric; Dermatopathology; Diaper rash; Eczema; Electrocauterization; Fifth disease; Fungal infections; Glands; Grafts and grafting; Hair; Hair loss and baldness; Hair transplanta- tion; Hand-foot-and-mouth disease; Healing; Histology; Hives; Human papillomavirus (HPV); Itching; Impetigo; Lesions; Lice, mites, and ticks; Melanoma; Moles; Multiple chemical sensitivity syndrome; Nail removal; Necrotizing fasciitis; Neurofibromatosis; Pigmentation; Plastic surgery; Poisonous plants; Psoriasis; Rashes; Ringworm; Rosacea; Scabies; Sense organs; Skin; Skin cancer; Skin disorders; Skin lesion removal; Styes; Sunburn; Systemic lupus erythematosus (SLE); Tattoo removal; Tattoos and body piercing; Touch; Warts; Wrinkles.

For Further Information:

Braverman, Irwin M. *Skin Signs of Systemic Disease.* 3d ed. Philadelphia: W. B. Saunders, 1998.

Ceaser, Jennifer. *Everything You Need to Know About Acne.* Rev. ed. New York: Rosen, 2003.

Hall, John C., and Gordon C. Sauer. *Sauer's Manual of Skin Diseases.* 10th ed. Philadelphia: Lippincott Williams & Wilkins, 2010.

"Health Information Index." *National Institute of Arthritis and Musculoskeletal and Skin Diseases,* 2013.

Jacknin, Jeanette. *Smart Medicine for Your Skin.* New York: Putnam, 2001.

Monk, B. E., R. A. C. Graham-Brown, and I. Sarkany, eds. *Skin Disorders in the Elderly.* Boston: Blackwell Scientific, 1992.

"Skin Cancer Information." *Skin Cancer Foundation,* 2013.

"Skin Conditions." *MedlinePlus,* 10 July 2013.

Turkington, Carol, and Jeffrey S. Dover. *The Encyclopedia of Skin and Skin Disorders.* 3d ed. New York: Facts On File, 2007.

Weedon, David. *Skin Pathology.* 3d ed. New York: Churchill Livingstone/Elsevier, 2010.

DERMATOPATHOLOGY

Specialty

Anatomy or system affected: Immune system, skin

Specialties and related fields: Cytology, dermatology, forensic medicine, histology, immunology, oncology, pathology

Definition: The study of the causes and characteristics of diseases or changes involving the skin.

Key terms:

basal cells: cells at the base of the epidermis that migrate upward and become the principal source of epidermal tissue

dermatoses: disorders of the skin

dermis: the layer of skin just below the surface, in which is found blood and lymphatic vessels, sebaceous (oil) glands, and nerves; also called the corium

epidermis: the outer layer of the skin, consisting of a dead superficial layer and an underlying cellular section

Science and Profession

Dermatopathology is the medical specialty that utilizes external clinical features of the body's surface, as well as histological changes that are observed microscopically, to define diseases of the skin. The dermatopathologist is a physician who has specialized in pathology, the clinical study of disease, and/or in histology, the microscopic study of cells and tissues. Although the specific clinical field of this specialty involves the skin, the practitioner has also received broader training in pathology.

The skin is the tough, cutaneous layer that covers the entire surface of the body. In addition to the epidermal tissue of the surface, the skin contains an extensive network of underlying structures, including lymphatic vessels, nerves and nerve endings, and hair follicles. The dead cells on the surface of the epidermis continually slough off, to be replaced by dividing cells from the underlying basal layers. As these cells proceed to the surface, they mature and die, forming the outer layer of the skin.

When a disease or condition of the skin is being diagnosed, the initial observations are often carried out by a general practitioner or dermatologist. This person will make a gross observation; if warranted, biopsies or samples of the lesion may then be provided to the dermatopathologist for examination. The most common forms of skin lesions are those associated with allergies, such as contact dermatitis associated with exposure to plant oils (such as poison ivy) or chemicals (such as antibiotics). More serious dermatologic diseases may also require diagnosis. Specific types of disease are often represented by specific kinds of lesions; these may include a variety of forms of skin cancers, lesions associated with bacterial or viral infections (such as impetigo or herpes simplex), and autoimmune disorders (such as lupus). The dermatopathologist may also be concerned with diseases of underlying tissue, such as lymphoid cancers or lesions penetrating into mucous membranes.

The dermatopathologist is involved in the diagnosis of the problem but generally is not involved with specific forms of treatment. Nevertheless, his or her recommendations may certainly influence any decisions. The major role of the dermatopathologist is observation; this may then be followed by an interpretation of results, including a possible prognosis or outcome.

Diagnostic and Treatment Techniques

The clinical examination of skin lesions initially falls within the realm of the dermatologist. If the gross observations are insufficient to warrant diagnosis, however, a sample of the lesion can be sent to the dermatopathologist for further examination. In addition to the tissue sample, information on the age, sex, and skin color of the patient should be included, along with any history of the suspected condition.

If the lesion is superficial, as in dermatoses such as warts or even certain types of cancer, a superficial shave biopsy is sufficient for examination. If the lesion involves an infiltrating tumor, inflammation, or possible metabolic problems, a deeper section of tissue is necessary. The specimen is immediately placed in a fixative solution, such as formalin, to prevent deterioration.

The dermatopathologist initially embeds the sample in paraffin, which can be sectioned into thin slices after hardening. The tissue is stained, most commonly with hematoxylin and eosin (H & E), and observed microscopically.

Anything about the cells that is out of the ordinary may be helpful in the diagnosis of the problem. For example, in the case of basal cell carcinoma, the cells may be abnormally shaped, with enlarged nuclei. They may also be observed infiltrating other layers of tissue. With contact dermatitis, the lesion is characterized by infiltration of large numbers of white blood cells, particularly lymphocytes, with their easily observed large nuclei. Edema, the abnormal accumulation of fluid, is also common with these types of lesions.

The presence of bacteria, as with boils or impetigo, warrants the use of antibiotics, unlike other inflammatory lesions. In this matter, the dermatopathology of the sample can determine the appropriate form of treatment.

While dermatopathology is primarily observational, recommendations regarding treatment may be made by its practitioners. For example, the study of a sample for the type and extent of cancer may lead to a recommendation concerning how extensive the surgical removal of the tumor should be.

Perspective and Prospects

The use of the physical appearance of the skin as a means of diagnosis represents one of the earliest attempts to understand disease. With the microscopic examination of tissue, first performed during the nineteenth century, it became possible to match the presence of histological lesions to specific diseases and to differentiate these diseases from one another.

The field of dermatopathology was greatly refined during the twentieth century. The development of differential and immunological staining methods allowed for a greater understanding of the roles played by the wide variety of cells in the body. For example, the dendritic cells of the skin were found to have a critical function in the immune responses that begin at that level.

In many Western countries, there was a significant shift during the twentieth century in the types of skin disease most commonly seen, mostly reflecting changes in lifestyle. The prevalence of malignant melanomas and basal cell carcinomas became much higher as a result of increased exposure to sun during leisure hours. The recognition of such problems has become an important aspect of the training of clinicians less specialized than dermatopathologists, such as family physicians.

—*Richard Adler, Ph.D.*

See also Autoimmune disorders; Bacterial infections; Biopsy; Cancer; Carcinoma; Cytopathology; Dermatitis; Dermatology; Diagnosis; Edema; Electrocauterization; Grafts and grafting; Herpes; Histology; Human papillomavirus (HPV); Lesions; Melanoma; Microscopy; Oncology; Pathology; Pigmentation; Plastic surgery; Skin; Skin cancer; Skin disorders; Skin lesion removal; Systemic lupus erythematosus (SLE); Viral infections; Warts.

For Further Information:

Busam, Klaus J., ed. *Dermatopathology*. Philadelphia: Saunders/Elsevier, 2010.

Caputo, Ruggero, and Carlo Gemetti. *Pediatric Dermatology and Dermatopathology: A Concise Atlas*. Washington, DC: Taylor & Francis, 2002.

"Health Information Index." *National Institute of Arthritis and Musculoskeletal and Skin Diseases*, 2013.

McKee, Phillip. *A Concise Atlas of Dermatopathology*. New York: Gower Medical, 1993.

Mehregan, Amir H., et al. *Pinkus" Guide to Dermatohistopathology*. 6th ed. Norwalk, Conn.: Appleton & Lange, 1995.

"Skin Conditions." *MedlinePlus*, 10 July 2013.

Tierney, Lawrence M., Stephen J. McPhee, and Maxine A. Papadakis, eds. *Current Medical Diagnosis and Treatment*. New York: McGraw-Hill Medical, 2010.

Weedon, David. *Skin Pathology*. 3d ed. New York: Churchill Livingstone/Elsevier, 2010.

"What Is a Dermatopathologist?" *American Academy of Dermatology*, 2013.

DEVELOPMENTAL DISORDERS
Disease/Disorder

Also known as: Pervasive developmental disorders

Anatomy or system affected: Nervous system, psychic-emotional system

Specialties and related fields: Psychiatry, psychology

Definition: A group of conditions that indicate significant delays in or a lack of social skill development with deficiencies in adaptive behaviors, poor language skills, and a limited capacity to communicate effectively.

Key terms:

antipsychotic medication: a category of drugs helpful in the treatment of psychosis

Asperger's disorder: severe and sustained impairment in social interactions, often involving limited interests

disintegrative disorder: deterioration in functioning following a period of normal development

encephalopathy: disorder of the brain

infantile autism: the first term coined in 1943 for a diagnosis of autistic disorder

microcephaly: abnormal smallness of the head

regression: reverting to a pattern of behavior seen at an earlier age of development

Causes and Symptoms

According to the revised fourth edition of the *Diagnostic and Statistical Manual of Mental Disorders* (known as the DSM-IV-TR), published in 2000 by the American Psychiatric Association, the developmental disorders may be categorized into five distinct disorders that all share the central feature of childhood development that is outside the norm in some manner. These disorders are included under the heading of pervasive developmental disorders in the DSM-IV-TR. The term *pervasive* is used to indicate the extensive developmental deficits found among these disorders. The five pervasive developmental disorders in the DSM-IV-TR are autistic disorder, Rett syndrome, childhood disintegrative disorder, Asperger syndrome, and pervasive developmental disorder not otherwise specified (PDD-NOS).

Autistic disorder is probably the best known of the disorders in the developmental disorders group. The disorder has an onset before age three but may not be formally diagnosed until some years later. Children with autistic disorder do not commonly show any unusual physical characteristics, but they demonstrate a number of behavioral, social, and affective symptoms. There are usually major deficiencies in the capacity to show social relatedness to others, including parents. The social smile is absent during infancy, and autistic children continue to show deficits in play activities and social attachments throughout their lives. There is an inability to understand or infer the feelings and mental state of other people around them. Language development is usually limited, with difficulties in communicating ideas even when the vocabulary is present. Delayed mental development occurs in a high percentage of children with autism, with greatest deficits in abstract reasoning and social understanding. Children from an early age do not show interactive play activity but rather engage in repetitive actions such as rocking and other unusual mannerisms. Children with autism usually form attachments to inanimate objects rather than to people. Their mood is usually marked with sudden changes and potentially aggressive outbursts. Although the exact cause in unknown, autistic disorder is considered to have a biological cause with a high genetic vulnerability. Research has indicated that two regions on chromosomes 2 and 7 contain genes involved with autistic disorder. Studies suggest that abnormal levels of serotonin and other neurotransmitters in the brain are found because there is a disruption of normal brain development early in fetal development caused by defects in the genes. The temporal lobe area of the brain has been implicated in the development of autism since this area is strongly associated with social development.

Rett syndrome features a period of normal development for approximately six months after birth that is followed by deterioration of functioning. Symptoms such as encephalopathy, seizures, breathing difficulties, loss of purposeful hand movements, loss of social engagement with others, poor coordination, and severely impaired language development then develop. The growth of the head circumference slows and produces microcephaly. The child begins to show repetitive movements such as hand-wringing and problems walking. The condition is progressive, and the skill level remains at the level of the first year of life. Children may live for ten years or more but must use a wheelchair as a result of muscle wasting. The cause of Rett syndrome has been identified as related to a genetic mutation. The gene is located at the Xq28 site on the X chromosome. Only one of the two X chromosomes need have the mutation in order for it to cause the disorder. This means that it is an X-linked dominant disorder. Rett syndrome is a rare condition usually found in females.

Childhood disintegrative disorder is diagnosed when there is marked regression or deterioration in a number of areas of functioning after age two. Children with this disorder begin to lose language and social skills previously developed in the first two years of life. Both bowel and bladder control as well as manual skills can be lost. It is common for these children to exhibit high levels of anxiety as the deterioration progresses. Children with this disorder also typically develop seizures. The cause of childhood disintegrative disorder is unknown, but it is considered to be related to some central nervous system pathology.

Asperger syndrome is marked with symptoms of severe and sustained impairments in social interactions. Repetitive patterns of behavior are commonly seen. In contrast to autism, children with Asperger syndrome do not exhibit signifi-

---

Information on Developmental Disorders

Causes: Genetic and biological causes
Symptoms: Impairment in language, cognitive abilities, social skills, communication
Duration: Chronic
Treatments: Structured educational and behavioral interventions

---

cant delays in language or cognitive development. Common characteristics of Asperger syndrome include a lack of empathy toward the feelings of others, minimal social interactions, limited ability to form friendships, pedantic and monotonic speech, and intense fascination with trivial topics learned in rote fashion. The cause of Asperger syndrome is unknown but is believed to have a genetic base. Current research suggests that a tendency toward the condition may run in families. Children with Asperger syndrome are also at risk for other psychiatric problems, including depression, attention-deficit disorder, schizophrenia, and obsessive-compulsive disorder. Persons with Asperger syndrome have a variable prognosis depending upon their cognitive abilities and language skills, but all continue into adulthood showing an awkward manner toward other adults and lack of comfort in social settings. Asperger syndrome is usually first diagnosed in children between the ages of two and six.

PDD-NOS is the fifth developmental disorder described in the DSM-IV-TR. It is viewed as a severe impairment in communication skills with deficiencies in social behavior. It differs from autistic disorder in terms of the severity of symptoms, and persons diagnosed with this disorder experience better functioning into adulthood than those with autistic disorder.

Treatment and Therapy

The goal for treatment of autistic disorder is to increase socially acceptable behaviors and decrease or extinguish unusual actions such as rocking and self-injurious behaviors. Therapy attempts to improve verbal and nonverbal communication skills to enhance interactions with other people. Therapy usually involves both educational and behavioral interventions with structured classroom training using behavioral techniques that employ rewards or positive reinforcements. Treatments for children with autistic disorder require a great deal of structure and repetition. Family members often participate in counseling sessions to help with the stressors of raising a child with autistic disorder. Medications are used as an adjunct to educational and behavioral treatments to diminish temper tantrums, self-injurious behaviors such as head banging, and hyperactivity. Antipsychotic medications such as risperidone and haloperidol are the most commonly used adjunctive treatments.

Rett syndrome has limited treatment options. The focus is on providing symptomatic relief whenever possible and structured behavioral techniques of positive rewards to concentrate on positive behaviors. Anticonvulsive medications are used to control seizures that can develop in this disorder and also diminish self-injurious behaviors. Physical therapy can assist with the distress associated with muscle deterioration.

Childhood disintegrative disorder is treated with similar methods as used in autistic disorder. Highly structured educational and behavioral programs are used to maintain the limited language and cognitive skills that had developed prior to the onset of the disorder.

Asperger syndrome treatments depend upon the level of functioning present among those with this disorder. Emphasis is usually placed upon improving social skills and adaptive functioning in social situations.

Treatment for PDD-NOS is largely the same as used with autistic disorder. Children with this disorder have a higher functioning of language skills than found with autistic disorder; consequently, the educational and behavioral treatments are supplemented with individual psychotherapy.

Perspective and Prospects

Autistic disorder was initially identified in 1867 by psychiatrist Henry Maudsley, but it was not until 1943 that Leo Kanner coined the term *infantile autism* and carefully described the associated signs and symptoms of the condition. Even with this description, many children with autism received the diagnosis of childhood schizophrenia. This tendency toward misdiagnosis continued into the 1980s. When considering the causes for the development of infantile autism, Kanner initially hypothesized that infantile autism was caused by emotionally unresponsive or "refrigerator" mothers who were unable to provide nurturance and emotional warmth to their newborn infants. Some children reacted to this emotional coldness by turning inward as a defense mechanism. Because of this defense, the child with autism focused on his or her inner world and did not develop communication skills. The child with autism usually focuses on inanimate objects rather than people and exhibits repetitive or self-stimulating behaviors such as rocking to gain personal satisfaction. Additions to this theoretical idea focused on the unresponsiveness of both parents toward the child and feelings of rage directed toward the child. Theories focusing on parental factors have since been discarded in favor of the current emphasis on identifying biological and genetic factors in the development of autism.

Rett syndrome was first identified by pediatrician Andreas Rett in 1966. Practicing in Austria, Rett based his descriptions on a pool of twenty-two girls who had developed normally until they were around six months of age. Rett published his findings in several German medical journals, but the information was largely ignored in the rest of the world. Awareness about the disorder increased when Rett published a description of the disease in English in 1977, but it was a 1983 article that appeared in the mainstream English-language journal *Annals of Neurology* that finally raised the recognition of this disorder.

Childhood disintegrative disorder was first described in 1908 by Viennese remedial teacher Theodor Heller. He described six children who had unexpectedly developed a severe mental deterioration between their third and fourth years of life, after previously normal development. Heller termed the condition dementia infantilis, and it was subsequently called Heller's syndrome. The disorder is more often diagnosed in males than in females. Although the DSM-IV-TR uses two years of age as the standard for its diagnosis, most cases emerge when a child is between three and four years of age.

Asperger syndrome was first described in 1944 by Austrian pediatrician Hans Asperger, who called the condition autistic psychopathy. Asperger described a number of children, and his descriptions were close to Kanner's idea of infantile autism. Asperger's portrayals differed from Kanner's, however, in that speech was less commonly delayed and the onset appeared to be somewhat later. The children that Asperger described were seen to have social behavior that was labeled as odd or unusual. Asperger called the children with this condition "little professors" because of their formal manner when talking about their favorite topics using great detail. Asperger also suggested that similar problems could be observed in the children's family members, particularly their fathers. Most of the scientific literature concerning Asperger's discovery initially appeared in European professional journals until Asperger syndrome was made official in 1994, when the diagnosis was added to the DSM-IV.

In 2013, the American Psychiatric Association published the fifth edition of the *Diagnostic and Statistical Manual of Mental Disorders*, known as DSM-5. This edition made significant changes to a number of classification systems, perhaps most notably the classification of pervasive developmental disorders. Autistic disorder, Asperger syndrome, childhood disintegrative disorder, Rett syndrome, and PDD-NOS were subsumed under the category autism spectrum disorder. This change was met with criticism from some members of the medical community; however, others argued that the new system would aid medical professionals in making diagnoses.

—*Frank J. Prerost, Ph.D.*

See also Antianxiety drugs; Anxiety; Asperger's syndrome; Autism; Bonding; Cognitive development; Developmental stages; Learning disabilities; Mental retardation; Neuroimaging; Psychiatric disorders; Psychiatry; Psychiatry, child and adolescent; Speech disorders.

For Further Information:

Aman, M., et al. "Medication and Parent Training in Children with Pervasive Developmental Disorders and Serious Behavior Problems: Results from a Randomized Clinical Trial." *Journal of the American Academy of Child and Adolescent Psychiatry* 23 (October, 2009): 1025–38.

American Psychiatric Association. *Diagnostic and Statistical Manual of Mental Disorders*. 5th ed. Washington, D.C.: American Psychiatric Publishing, 2013.

Bopp, K., et al. "Behavior Predictors of Language Development over Two Years in Children with Autism Spectrum Disorders." *Journal of Speech, Language, and Hearing Research* 52 (October, 2009): 1106–20.

Elder, J., et al. "Supporting Families of Children with Autism Spectrum Disorders: Questions Parents Ask and What Nurses Need to Know." *Pediatric Nursing* 35 (July/August, 2009): 240–45.

National Institute of Mental Health. "Autism Spectrum Disorders (Pervasive Developmental Disorders." *National Institutes of Health*, May 23, 2013.

National Institute of Neurological Disorders and Strokes. "NINDS Pervasive Developmental Disorders." *National Institutes of Health*, May 7, 2013.

Noterdaeme, M., et al. "Asperger's Syndrome and High-Functioning Autism: Language, Motor, and Cognitive Profiles." *European Child and Adolescent Psychiatry* 8 (October, 2009): 875–925.

DEVELOPMENTAL STAGES

Development

Anatomy or system affected: Brain, nervous system, psychic-emotional system

Specialties and related fields: Neurology, psychiatry, psychology

Definition: The growth and changes that occur over time in children's mental and physical processes as they develop from birth to adulthood.

Key terms:

attachment: special relationship of mutual closeness established between an infant and a caregiver; based on consistent caring, it confers an anticipation of security in relationships

concrete operations stage: Jean Piaget's cognitive stage in which concrete, easily visualized objects can be grouped together, combined, and transformed in equivalent ways; "concrete" contrasts with "formal" operations, which involve abstract and hypothetical transformations

initiative versus guilt: Erik Erikson's characterization for the young child's imaginative exploration of wishes and impulses in fantasy and dramatic play, restrained by emerging pangs of conscience

mental operations: comprehension of the reversibility of such events as regrouping objects into different categories or transferring a fixed quantity of a substance into containers of different shapes

preoperational stage: Piaget's transitional stage of young childhood in which absent objects can be remembered from mental representations but cannot be grouped or logically manipulated

sensorimotor stage: Piaget's stage in infancy in which objects can be recognized by appropriate habitual reactions to them

stage: a period in a progressive, invariant sequence of events when specified cognitive and motivational events are programmed to occur

Physical and Psychological Factors

The development of the human being from infant to child to adolescent to adult is a story of increasing physical, cognitive, social, and emotional adequacy in coping with environmental demands. Major observers of human development have added a key corollary concerning the nature and pace of this development: It occurs in stages.

Development in stages implies several features about the process. The first implication is that developmental changes are not simply quantitative but also qualitative, changes not only in degree but also in kind. With advancement to another stage, perceptions, thoughts, motives, and social interactions are fundamentally altered. A second implication is that development is uneven in its pace—sometimes flowing and sometimes ebbing, sometimes fast and sometimes slow and steady in apparent equilibrium. A third implication is that the order of the stages is invariant: one always moves from lower to higher stages. No individual skips stages; each subsequent stage is a necessary antecedent to the more mature or advanced stages to come. The invariant sequence is preordained by the biological maturation of neurological systems and by the necessary requirements of human societies.

Descriptions of development in terms of stages are found in the writings of many psychologists, especially cognitive psychologists, who are interested in age-related changes in thinking styles, and psychoanalytic psychologists, influenced by Sigmund Freud, who concern themselves with changes in the growing child's emotional involvements. The most significant, influential, and comprehensive of stage descriptions of development are those of two seminal scientists, Jean Piaget (1896–1980) and Erik Erikson (1902–94).

Piaget, a cognitive developmental psychologist, outlined a series of shifts in children's cognition, their ways of thinking about and interpreting the world. They include the sensorimotor stage in infancy, the preoperational stage beginning in toddlerhood, the intuitive preoperational substage of the preschool child, the concrete operations stage of the school-age child, and the formal operations stage beginning in adolescence.

Erikson, who updated psychoanalytic theory, outlined a series of age-related shifts in motives and ways of relating to others, each one related to a psychosocial crisis. These psychosocial stages include an infancy stage of trust versus mistrust, a toddlerhood stage of autonomy versus shame and doubt, a preschool childhood stage of initiative versus guilt, a school-age stage of competence versus inferiority, and an adolescent stage of identity versus role diffusion.

The approaches of Piaget and Erikson originated independently, each emphasizing different aspects of development. The stages that they describe, however, should be viewed as complementary. Since the social changes result in large part from shifts in the child's thinking, the psychosocial stages of Erikson closely parallel the cognitive stages outlined by Piaget.

In infancy, a period lasting from birth to about eighteen months, sensorimotor cognitive development is initiated by rapid brain development. During the first six months of life, the nerve cells in the forebrain that control coordinated movements, refined sensory discriminations, speech, and intellect increase greatly in number and size and develop a rich network of connections. This neural growth makes possible dramatic progress in the child's ability to discriminate relevant objects and to coordinate precise movements of arms, legs, and fingers in relating to these objects. The infant who was capable of only a few reflexes at birth by six months can grasp a dangling object. The infant who was born with very poor vi-

sual acuity by six months can recognize detailed patterns in toys and faces. The infant shows recognition and knowledge of an object by relating to it repeatedly with the same pattern of movements. During the first few months of life, the infant has very limited ability to recall objects when they are not directly seen or heard and, in fact, will fail to look for a toy when it is not in view. Sensorimotor integrations, therefore, form the infant's principal method of representing reality. Only gradually does attention span increase and does the infant acquire the capacity to think about missing objects. The capacity to keep out-of-sight objects in mind, the gradual appreciation of object permanence, is a key achievement of the sensorimotor stage.

The corresponding psychosocial stage of infancy is built around the establishment of trust, some sort of sustaining faith in the stability of the world and the security of human relationships. Crucial to the establishing of this trust is the stability of the infant's relationship with a primary caregiver, most commonly a mother. Babies begin to pay special attention to the caregiver on a schedule determined by their cognitive development. The primary caregiving adult is among the first significant objects identified by the infant. Indeed, it appears that infants are wired to be especially responsive to a human caregiver. Infants of only two or three months of age find the human face the most interesting object and will focus on faces and facelike designs in preference to almost any other stimulus object. By the age of six months, infants clearly recognize the caregiver as special but for some time cannot appreciate that the caregiver continues to exist during absences. Thus, conspicuous anxiety sometimes occurs when the caregiver leaves.

It is little wonder that an infant perceives the caregiver as special. The human caregiver is wonderfully reinforcing to the infant. Relief from all kinds of pain, smiling responses to infantile smiles, vocal responses to infant babbling, soft and warm cuddling contact, and games all offer to the infant what is most craved. By six to nine months of age, the baby seems dependent on the caregiver for a basic feeling of security. Until the age of two or three, most infants seem more secure when their mother or primary caregiver is physically present. The relationship between the quality and warmth of infant-mother interactions and the infant's feelings of security has been supported by voluminous research on mother-infant attachment.

By about age two, neural and physical developments make possible the advance to more adaptive styles of cognitive interpretations. Piaget characterized the cognitive stage of toddlerhood as preoperational. Brain centers important for language and movement continue to develop rapidly. Now the child can deal cognitively with reality in a new way, by representing out-of-sight and distant objects and events by words, images, and symbols. The child can also imitate the actions of people not present. Thinking during this stage remains limited. The child cannot yet hold several thoughts simultaneously in mind and manipulate them—that is, perform mental operations. This stage is, therefore, "preoperational."

Erikson described the psychosocial crisis of toddlerhood

as autonomy versus shame and doubt. This crisis results in part from the child's cognitive growth. The preoperational child has acquired an increasing ability to appreciate the temporary nature of a caregiver's absence and to move about independently. The toddler can now assert autonomy and often does so emphatically. Resistance to parental demands is possible, and the toddler seems to delight in such resistance. "No" becomes a favorite word. Since this period corresponds to the time when children are toilet trained, parent-child tugs-of-war often involve issues of bowel control and cleanliness. The beginning of shame, the humiliation that comes from overextending freedom foolishly and making mistakes, begins to serve as a self-imposed check on this autonomy.

Piaget characterized the thinking of three-, four-, and five-year-olds as "intuitive." This thinking is still preoperational. Children can represent to themselves all sorts of objects but cannot keep these objects in the focus of attention long enough to classify them or consider how these objects could be regrouped or transformed. If six tin soldiers are stretched into three groups of two, the preschool child assumes that there are now more than before. Thinking is egocentric because children lack the ability to put themselves in the perspective of others while keeping their own perspective. Yet preschool children make all sorts of intuitive attempts to fit remembered events and scenes into underlying plots or themes. Fanciful attempts to understand events often result in misconstruing the nature of things. Children at this stage are easily misled by appearances. A man in a tiger suit could become a tiger; a boy who wears a dress could become a girl and grow up to be a mother. Appearance becomes reality.

Erikson characterized the corresponding psychosocial stage of the preschool child as involving the crisis of initiative versus guilt. The child's new initiative is expressed in playful exploration of fanciful possibilities. Children can pretend and transform themselves in play as never before and never again. From dramatic play, the child's conceptions of the many possibilities of the world of bigger people are enacted. The earlier psychoanalyst, Freud, focused particularly on how children experience their first sexual urges at this time of life and sometimes weave into their ruminations fantastic themes of possession of the opposite-sex parent and jealous triumph over the same-sex parent. To Erikson, such themes are merely examples of the many playful fantasies essential to later, more realistic involvements.

Piaget characterized the cognitive stage of the school-age child as the concrete operations stage. The child is capable of mental operations. The school-age child can focus on several incidents, objects, or events simultaneously. Now it is obvious that six tin soldiers sorted into three pairs of two could easily be transformed back into a single group of six. Regardless of grouping, the total quantity is the same. The formerly egocentric child becomes cognitively capable of empathetic role taking, of assuming the perspective of another person while keeping the perspective of the self in mind. In making ethical choices, the child can now appreciate the impact of alternative possibilities on particular people in particular situations. The harshness of absolute dictates is softened by empathetic understanding of others.

Erikson characterized the psychosocial crisis of the school-age child as one of competence versus inferiority. Now is the time for children to acquire the many verbal, computational, and social skills that are required for adequate adulthood. Learning experiences are structured and planned, and performances are evaluated. Newly empathetic children are only too aware of how their skill levels are perceived by others. Adequacy is being assessed. The schoolchild must not only be good but also be good at something.

The cognitive stage of the adolescent was described by Piaget as formal operational. The dramatic physical changes that signal sexual maturity are accompanied by less obvious neural changes, especially a fine tuning of the frontal lobes of the brain, the brain's organizing, sequencing, executive center. Cognitively, the adolescent becomes capable of dealing with formal operations. Unlike concrete operations, which can be visualized, formal operations include abstract possibilities that are purely hypothetical, abstract strategies useful in ordering a sequence of investigations, and "as if" or "let us suppose" propositions.

Erikson's corresponding psychosocial crisis of adolescence was that of identity versus role diffusion. The many physical and mental changes and the impending necessity of finding occupational, social, marital, religious, and political roles in the adult world impel a concern with the question, "Who am I?" To interact as an adult, one must know what one likes and loathes, what one values and despises, and what one can do well, poorly, and not at all. Most adolescents succeed in finding themselves—some by adopting the identity of family and parents, some after a soul-searching struggle.

Disorders and Effects

Stage theories define success as advancement through the series of stages to maturity. Psychosocially, each successful advance yields a virtue that makes life endurable: hope, will, purpose, competence, and finally fidelity to one's own true self. As a final reward for normal developmental success, one can enjoy the benefits of adulthood: intimacy, or the sharing of one's identity with another, and generativity, or the contribution of one's own gifts to the benefit of the next generation and to the collective progress of humankind. Cognitively, maturity means the capacity for formal operational thought. Hypothetical thinking of this type is basic to most fields of higher learning, to the sciences, to philosophy, and even to the comprehension of such abstract moral principles as justice.

Advancement to each subsequent stage of cognitive development is dependent on both neurological maturation and a culture that presents appropriate problems. Adults who fail to attain concrete operational thought are considered intellectually disabled. A failure in neurological maturation is a frequent cause. Failures to attain formal operational thought, on the other hand, are not unusual among normal adults. Cultural experience must nourish advancement to formal operational thinking within a domain of inquiry by the provision of moderately novel and challenging but not overwhelming tasks. When people are not confronted with such complex problems within some domain, then abstract, formal operational thought fails to occur. Abstract ethical reasoning is a case in point. Cross-cultural studies suggest that concepts of justice that involve the application of abstract rules are rare in cultures where people seldom confront questions of ethical complexity.

Psychosocial pathology is evidenced by development arrested in one of the immature stages of psychosocial development. It results from a social environment that fails to foster growth or exaggerates the particular apprehensions that are most acute in one of the developmental stages.

The development of trust in infancy requires a loving, available, and sensitive caretaker. If the infant's caretaker is unavailable, missing, neglectful, or abusive, the pathology of mistrust develops. The world is perceived as unstable. Close personal relationships are viewed as unreliable, fickle, and possibly malicious. Later, closeness in relationships may be rejected. Confident exploration of the possibilities of life may never be attempted.

Similarly, the apprehensions of each subsequent psychosocial stage can be exaggerated to the point of pathology. The toddler, shamed out of troublesome expressions of autonomy, may compensate for doubts with the rigidly excessive controls of the compulsive lifestyle. The preschool child can become so overwhelmed with guilt over playful fantasies, particularly sexual and aggressively tinged fantasies, that adult possibilities become severely restricted. The school-age child can become so wounded by humiliations in a harshly competitive school environment that the child becomes beaten down into enduring feelings of inferiority. An adolescent may so fear the risks of exploring the possibilities of life that future adulthood becomes a shallow diffusion of roles, a yielding to social pressures and whims unguided by any knowledge of who one really is.

The successful confrontation of the tasks of adulthood—finding a partner to share intimacy and caring for the next generation—are most easily attainable for adults who have overcome each of these earlier developmental hurdles.

Perspective and Prospects

Stage theories of development are found as early as 1900 in the work of American psychologist James Mark Baldwin and in Freud's psychoanalysis. Baldwin, much influenced by Charles Darwin's theory of evolution by natural selection, hypothesized that the infant emerges from a sensorimotor stage of infancy to a symbolic mode of thinking, an advancement yielding enormous evolutionary advantages. Freud, the Viennese psychoanalyst, based his conception of emotional development on what he called psychosexual stages. Progression occurs from an oral period of infancy, when sensory pleasure is concentrated on the mouth region, to an anal stage of toddlerhood, when anal pleasures and the control of such pleasures become of concern. When sexual pleasure shifts to the genital region in the three-year-old, the love of the opposite-sex parent becomes sexually tinged, and the child becomes jealous of the same-sex parent. Working through these so-called Oedipal fantasies was, to Freud, crucial to the formation of personality.

Neither Baldwin nor Freud and his followers were the sort of rigorous scientists most respected by scientific psychology in the mid-twentieth century. Far more influential in American psychology between 1920 to about 1960 were behavioral conceptions of the developmental process as steady, incremental growth. To behaviorists such as B. F. Skinner, becoming an adult was conceived as a process of continuously being reinforced for learning progressively more adequate responses.

The stage approaches of Piaget and Erikson were introduced to most American psychologists in 1950, the year that both Piaget's *Psychology of Intelligence* and Erikson's *Childhood and Society* were published in English. Piaget's description of cognitive stages was much more complete than Baldwin's earlier account and was much better supported by clever behavioral observations. Erikson's thesis of psychosocial stages incorporated most of Freud's observations about stages. Erikson treated the social environmental pressures intrinsic to each stage as events of primary importance and shifts in the locus of bodily pleasures as secondary.

By the 1970s, Piaget's and Erikson's accounts of stages were awarded an important place in most developmental texts. This influence occurred for several reasons. First, researchable hypotheses were derived, and most of this research was supportive. Cross-cultural comparisons suggested that these stages could be found in a similar sequence in differing cultures. Second, the theses of Piaget and Erikson were mutually supportive. The stage-related cognitive changes, in fact, would seem to explain the corresponding psychosocial concerns. Finally, these approaches generated productive spinoffs in related theory and research. In 1969, basing his work on the cognitive changes outlined by Piaget, Lawrence Kohlberg elaborated a stage sequence of progressively more adequate methods of moral reasoning. In 1978, basing her work on Erikson's hypotheses about trust, Mary Ainsworth began a productive research program on the antecedents and consequents of stable and unstable mother-infant attachment styles.

The most recent challenges to cognitive and psychosocial stage theory arise from the alternative perspectives of biopsychology and information-processing theory. Some psychologists argue that biologically rooted temperament, rather than the social environment, affects both styles of attachment and identity formation. Not only do babies respond to caregivers, but caregivers respond to babies as well. A baby who begins with a shy, passive temperament may be more susceptible to an avoidant attachment style and more likely to elicit detached, unresponsive caregiver behavior. Temperament, it is maintained, is more important than psychosocial environment.

Information processing theorists have challenged the discontinuity implied by stage concepts. They suggest that the appearance of global transformations in the structure of thought may be an illusion. Development is a continuous growth of efficiency in processing and problem solving. The growing child combines an expanding number of ideas, increases the level and speed of processing by increments, and learns more effective problem-solving strategies. To select particular points in this continuous development and call them "stages," they argue, is purely arbitrary.

The final research to settle the question of the ultimate nature of stages has not been performed. A psychosocial stage theorist can acknowledge the role of temperament but still maintain that loving, trust-creating environments are also significant in encouraging the child to apply temperamental potential in positive social directions rather than in angry antagonism or frightened withdrawal. At the very least, Piagetian and Eriksonian stage concepts have the practical usefulness of highlighting significant developmental events and interpersonal reactions to these events. The warmth of caregivers for infants, the later tolerance of children's struggles to become themselves, and environments that present challenging problems appropriate to the child's developmental level are vital to emotional and intellectual growth.

For some purposes, it may be instructive to break the achievement of cognitive and emotional growth into increments that can be seen as if under a microscope. For other purposes, it is instructive to go up for an aerial view to gain perspective on the nature and direction of such achievements. The aerial view is the contribution of stage theories of development.

—*Thomas E. DeWolfe, Ph.D.*

See also Bed-wetting; Bonding; Cognitive development; Developmental disorders; Motor skill development; Puberty and adolescence; Reflexes, primitive; Separation anxiety; Soiling; Speech disorders; Teething; Thumb sucking; Toilet training; Weaning.

For Further Information:

Berk, Laura E. *Child Development*. 9th ed. Boston: Pearson/Allyn & Bacon, 2013.

Bukatko, Danuta, and Marvin W. Daehler. *Child Development: A Thematic Approach*. 6th ed. Belmont, Calif.: Wadsworth/Cengage, 2012.

Charlesworth, Rosalind. *Understanding Child Development*. 8th ed. Belmont, Calif.: Wadsworth/Cengage, 2011.

Feldman, Robert S. *Development Across the Life Span*. 6th ed. Upper Saddle River, N.J.: Pearson/Prentice Hall, 2011.

Ginsburg, Herbert, and Sylvia Opper. *Piaget's Theory of Intellectual Development*. 3d ed. Englewood Cliffs, N.J.: Prentice Hall, 1988.

Hall, Calvin S., Gardner Lindzey, and John B. Campbell. *Theories of Personality*. 4th ed. New York: John Wiley & Sons, 1998.

Karen, Robert. "Becoming Attached." *Atlantic Monthly* 265, no. 2 (February, 1990): 35–70.

Miller, Patricia H. *Theories of Developmental Psychology*. 5th ed. New York: Worth, 2011.

Nathanson, Laura Walther. *The Portable Pediatrician: A Practicing Pediatrician's Guide to Your Child's Growth, Development, Health, and Behavior from Birth to Age Five*. 2d ed. New York: HarperCollins, 2002.

Parke, Ross D., et al., eds. *A Century of Developmental Psychology*. Washington, D.C.: American Psychological Association, 1994.

Sternberg, Robert J. *Psychology: In Search of the Human Mind*. 3d ed. Fort Worth, Tex.: Harcourt College, 2001.

Whitebread, David. *Developmental Psychology and Early Childhood Education*. London: Sage, 2011.

DIABETES MELLITUS
Disease/Disorder

Anatomy or system affected: Abdomen, blood vessels, circulatory system, endocrine system, eyes, gastrointestinal system, glands, heart, kidneys, nervous system, pancreas

Specialties and related fields: Endocrinology, family medicine, genetics, internal medicine, nephrology, neurology, pediatrics, vascular medicine

Definition: A hormonal disorder in which proper blood sugar levels are not maintained; due either to insufficient production of insulin by the pancreas or to an inability of the body's cells to use insulin efficiently. If left untreated, diabetes mellitus leads to complications such as blindness, cardiovascular disease, dementia, kidney disease, and, eventually, death.

Key terms:

beta cells: the insulin-producing cells located at the core of the islets of Langerhans in the pancreas; the alpha, or glucagon-producing, cells form an outer coat

cross-linking: a chemical reaction, triggered by the binding of glucose to tissue proteins, that results in the attachment of one protein to another and the loss of elasticity in aging tissues

glucosuria: a condition in which the concentration of blood glucose exceeds the ability of the kidney to reabsorb it; as a result, glucose spills into the urine, taking with it body water and electrolytes

hyperglycemia: excessive levels of glucose in the circulating blood

insulin-dependent diabetes mellitus (IDDM): type 1 diabetes, a state of absolute insulin deficiency in which the body does not produce sufficient insulin to move glucose into the cells

insulin resistance: a lack of insulin action; a reduction in the effectiveness of insulin to lower blood glucose concentrations; characteristic of type 2 diabetes

insulitis: the selective destruction of the insulin-producing beta cells in type 1 diabetes

islets of Langerhans: clusters of cells scattered throughout the pancreas; they produce three hormones involved in sugar metabolism: insulin, glucagon, and somatostatin

ketoacidosis: high levels of ketones in the blood that result from a lack of circulating insulin

non-insulin-dependent diabetes mellitus (NIDDM): type 2 diabetes, which is the state of a relative insulin deficiency; although insulin is released, its target cells do not adequately respond to it by taking up blood glucose

Causes and Symptoms

Diabetes mellitus is by far the most common of all endocrine (hormonal) disorders. The disorder's name is derived from the Greek word *diabetes*, meaning "siphon" or "running through," a reference to the potentially large urine volume that can accompany the condition. The Latin word *mellitus*, meaning "honey," was added to the name when physicians began to make the diagnosis of diabetes mellitus based on the

Information on Diabetes Mellitus

Causes: Genetic and environmental factors
Symptoms: Large urine output, excessive thirst, dehydration, low blood pressure, weight loss despite increased appetite, fatigue, nausea, vomiting, blurred vision
Duration: Chronic
Treatments: Insulin or oral hypoglycemic drugs, lifestyle changes (diet modification and exercise)

sweet taste of the patient's urine. The disease has been depicted as a state of starvation in the midst of plenty. Although there is plenty of sugar in the blood, without proper insulin action the sugar does not reach the cells that need it for energy. Glucose, the simplest form of sugar, is the primary source of energy for many vital functions. Deprived of glucose, cells starve and tissues begin to degenerate. The unused glucose builds up in the bloodstream, which leads to a series of secondary complications.

The most common symptoms of diabetes mellitus are related to hyperglycemia, glycosuria, and ketoacidosis. The acute symptoms of diabetes mellitus are all attributable to inadequate insulin action. The immediate consequence of an insulin insufficiency is a marked decrease in the ability of muscle, liver, and adipose (fat) tissue to remove glucose from the blood. In the presence of inadequate insulin action, a second problem manifests itself. People with diabetes continue to make the hormone glucagon. Glucagon, which raises the level of blood sugar, can be considered insulin's biological opposite. Like insulin, glucagon is released from the pancreatic islets. The release of glucagon is normally inhibited by insulin; therefore, in the absence of insulin, glucagon action elevates concentrations of glucose. For this reason, diabetes may be considered a two-hormone disease. With a reduction in the conversion of glucose into its storage forms of glycogen in liver and muscle tissue and lipids in adipose cells, concentrations of glucose in the blood steadily increase (hyperglycemia). When the amount of glucose in the blood exceeds the capacity of the kidney to reabsorb this nutrient, glucose begins to spill into the urine (glucosuria). Glucose in the urine then drags additional body water along with it so that the volume of urine dramatically increases. In the absence of adequate fluid intake, the loss of body water and accompanying electrolytes (sodium) leads to dehydration and, ultimately, death caused by the failure of the peripheral circulatory system.

Insulin deficiency also results in a decrease in the synthesis of triglycerides (storage forms of fatty acids) and stimulates the breakdown of fats in adipose tissue. Although glucose cannot enter the cells and be used as an energy source, the body can use its supply of lipids from the fat cells as an alternate source of energy. Fatty acids increase in the blood, causing hyperlipidemia. With large amounts of circulating free fatty acids available for processing by the liver, the production and release of ketone bodies (breakdown products of

fatty acids) into the circulation are accelerated, causing both ketonemia and an increase in the acidity of the blood. Since the ketone levels soon also exceed the capacity of the kidney to reabsorb them, ketone bodies soon appear in the urine (ketonuria).

Insulin deficiency and glucagon excess also cause pronounced effects on protein metabolism and result in an overall increase in the breakdown of proteins and a reduction in the uptake of amino acid precursors into muscle protein. This leads to the wasting and weakening of skeletal muscles and, in children who are diabetics, results in a reduction in overall growth. The increased level of amino acids in the blood provides an additional source of material for glucose production (gluconeogenesis) by the liver. All these acute metabolic changes in carbohydrates, lipids, and protein metabolism can be prevented or reversed by the administration of insulin.

There are three distinct types of diabetes mellitus. Type 1, or insulin-dependent diabetes mellitus (IDDM), is an absolute deficiency of insulin that accounts for approximately 5 to 10 percent of all cases of diabetes. Until the discovery of insulin, people stricken with type 1 diabetes faced certain death within about a year of diagnosis. In type 2, or non-insulin-dependent diabetes mellitus (NIDDM), the most common form of the disorder, insulin secretion may be normal or even increased, but the target cells for insulin are less responsive than normal (insulin resistance); therefore, insulin is not as effective in lowering blood glucose concentrations. Although either type can be manifested at any age, type 1 diabetes has a greater prevalence in children, whereas the incidence of type 2 diabetes increases markedly after the age of forty. Genetic and environmental factors are important in the expression of both of these types of diabetes mellitus. The third type is ges-

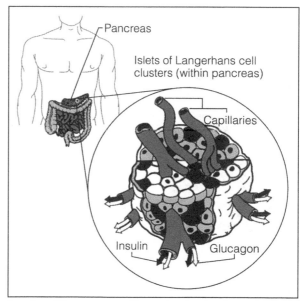

Location of the pancreas, with a section showing the specialized cells (islets of Langerhans) that produce the sugar-metabolizing hormones.

tational diabetes, which is characterized by high blood glucose during pregnancy in a person who did not previously have diabetes.

Type 1 diabetes is an autoimmune process that involves the selective destruction of the insulin-producing beta cells in the islets of Langerhans (insulitis). The triggering event that initiates this process in genetically susceptible persons is linked to environmental factors that result from an infection, a virus, or, more likely, the presence of toxins in the diet. The body's own T lymphocytes progressively attack the beta cells but leave the other hormone-producing cell types intact. T lymphocytes are white blood cells that normally attack virus-invaded cells and cancer cells. For up to ten years, there remains a sufficient number of insulin-producing cells to respond effectively to a glucose load, but when approximately 80 percent of the beta cells are destroyed, there is insufficient insulin release in response to a meal and the deadly spiral of the consequences of diabetes mellitus is triggered. Insulin injection can halt this lethal process and prevent it from recurring but cannot mimic the normal pattern of insulin release from the pancreas. It is interesting that not everyone who has insulitis actually progresses to experience overt symptoms of the disease.

Type 2 diabetes is normally associated with obesity and lack of exercise. Recently, with the reported increased rates of obesity and inactivity in children, there has also been an in-crease of type 2 diabetes at younger and younger ages. Genetic factors also play a key role in the development of the disorder. Research has shown that individuals who have a sibling or parent with type 2 diabetes are about three times as likely to develop diabetes themselves.

Because there is a reduction in the sensitivity of the target cells to insulin, people with type 2 diabetes must secrete more insulin to maintain blood glucose at normal levels. Because insulin is a storage, or anabolic, hormone, this increased secretion further contributes to obesity. In response to the elevated insulin concentrations, the number of insulin receptors on the target cell gradually decreases, which triggers an even greater secretion of insulin. In this way, the excess glucose is stored despite the decreased availability of insulin binding sites on the cell. Over time, the demands for insulin eventually exceed even the reserve capacity of the "genetically weakened" beta cells, and symptoms of insulin deficiency develop as the plasma glucose concentrations remain high for increasingly longer periods of time. This phenomenon is known as beta-cell burn out. Because the symptoms of type 2 diabetes are usually less severe than those of type 1 diabetes, many persons have the disease but remain unaware of it. By the time the diagnosis of diabetes is made in these individuals, they also exhibit symptoms of long-term complications that include atherosclerosis and nerve damage. Hence, type 2 diabetes has been called the silent killer.

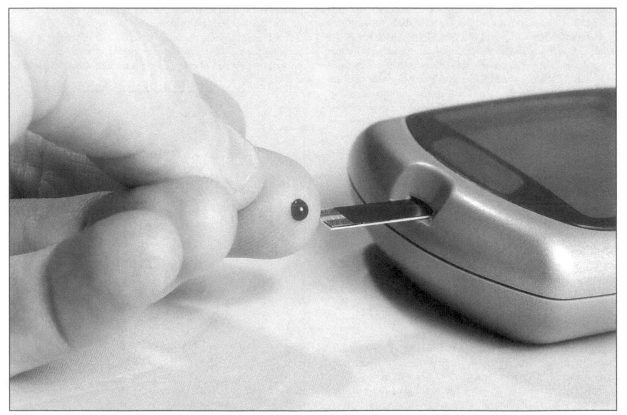

A diabetic performs a glucose level check using a finger blood test. (© Eugene Bochkarev/iStockphoto.com)

In the News:
Increase in Type 2 Diabetes in Adults and Children

There is no doubt that the United States, as well as many other countries around the world, is affected by an "obesity epidemic." Poor eating habits and sedentary lifestyles are causing higher rates of obesity across all age groups and ethnic backgrounds. Approximately 30 percent of adults in the United States are obese. The rate of obesity in children ages two to five and ages twelve to nineteen has tripled since the mid-1970s. In children ages six to eleven, this rate has quadrupled from 4 to an alarming 19 percent.

Type 2 diabetes is occurring with increasing frequency in children, adolescents, and adults. The number of people with diabetes has more than doubled in the United States, from 15 percent in 1980 to 34 percent in 2006. Type 2 diabetes accounts for 90 to 95 percent of these cases. In 2005-2006, 72 percent of adults ages twenty to seventy-four were overweight or obese.

The Centers for Disease Control and Prevention estimates that 8 to 43 percent of new cases of diabetes in children are type 2 diabetes. These young people are usually overweight or obese, have a family history of diabetes, have signs of insulin resistance such as acanthosis nigricans, are members of an ethnic group with a high risk of type 2 diabetes, and are more often girls than boys.

This increase has many causes. The serving sizes of foods sold in stores and restaurants have increased. In many neighborhoods, there are more fast food restaurants than grocery stores. Approximately 30 percent of all calories consumed by Americans are in the form of sodas and fruit-flavored drinks. Teenagers drink more soda than milk, and about half of children ages six to eleven drink soda daily. Less than 25 percent of Americans eat five or more servings of fruit and vegetables daily. To compound the problem, more than 30 percent of high school students do not exercise regularly, and more than half of adults do not get enough physical activity.

This epidemic can be stopped in a number of ways. Healthier eating habits and regular physical activity can decrease rates of obesity, diabetes, and many other chronic diseases. Breast-feeding is associated with lower rates of obesity in children. Parents can advocate for regular physical activity in schools and for healthy snacks and drinks in vending machines. Limiting television viewing and computer time, encouraging physical activity at home, and providing healthy meals and smaller portions can all contribute to controlling the "obesity epidemic" in children.

—Julie M. Slocum, R.N., M.S., C.D.E.

include the site of injection, the patient's age and health status, and the patient's level of physical activity. For a person with diabetes, however, insulin is a reprieve, not a cure.

Because of the complications that arise from chronic exposure to glucose, it is recommended that glucose concentrations in the blood be maintained as close to physiologically normal levels as possible. For this reason, it is preferable to administer multiple doses of insulin during the day. By monitoring plasma glucose concentrations, the diabetic person can adjust the dosage of insulin administered and thus mimic normal concentrations of glucose relatively closely. Basal concentrations of plasma insulin can also be maintained throughout the day by means of electromechanical insulin delivery systems. Whether internal or external, such insulin pumps can be programmed to deliver a constant infusion of insulin at a rate designed to meet minimum requirements. The infusion can then be supplemented by a bolus injection prior to a meal. Increasingly sophisticated systems automatically monitor blood glucose concentrations and adjust the delivery rate of insulin accordingly. These alternative delivery systems are intended to prevent the development of long-term tissue complications.

There are a number of chronic complications that account for the shorter life expectancy of diabetic persons. These include atherosclerotic changes throughout the entire vascular system. The thickening of basement membranes that surround the capillaries can affect their ability to exchange nutrients. Cardiovascular lesions are the most common cause of premature death in diabetic persons. Kidney disease, which is commonly found in longtime diabetics, can ultimately lead to kidney failure. For these persons, expensive medical care, including dialysis and the possibility of a kidney transplant, overshadows their lives. Diabetes is the leading cause of new blindness in the United States. Delayed gastric emptying (gastroparesis) occurs when the stomach takes too long to empty its contents; it results from damage to the vagus nerve from long-term exposure to high glucose levels. In addition, diabetes leads to a gradual decline in the ability of nerves to conduct sensory information to the brain. For example, the feet of some diabetics feel more like stumps of wood than living tissue. Consequently, weight is not distributed properly; in concert with the reduction in blood flow, this problem can lead to pressure ulcers. If not properly cared for, areas of the foot can develop gangrene, which may then lead to amputa-

Gestational diabetes develops during pregnancy in a person who did not have diabetes before becoming pregnant. It occurs in 3 to 8 percent of all pregnancies. Women with gestational diabetes have an increased risk of developing diabetes after pregnancy. Children of women with gestational diabetes have a higher risk of obesity, glucose intolerance, and diabetes in adolescence.

Prediabetes is a condition in which individuals have blood glucose levels that are high, but not high enough for them to be diagnosed with type 2 diabetes. Persons with prediabetes are at higher risk to develop diabetes in the future.

Treatment and Therapy

Insulin is the only treatment available for type 1 diabetes, and in many cases it is used to treat individuals with type 2 diabetes. Insulin is available in many formulations, which differ in respect to the time of onset of action, activity, and duration of action. Insulin preparations are classified as fast acting, intermediate acting, and long acting; the effects of fast-acting insulin last for thirty minutes to twenty-four hours, while those of long-acting preparations last from four to thirty-six hours. Some of the factors that affect the rate of insulin absorption

tion of the foot. Finally, in male patients, there are problems with reproductive function that generally result in impotence.

The mechanism responsible for the development of these long-term complications of diabetes is genetic in origin and dependent on the amount of time the tissues are exposed to the elevated plasma glucose concentrations. What, then, is the link between glucose concentrations and diabetic complications?

As an animal ages, most of its cells become less efficient in replacing damaged material, while its tissues lose their elasticity and gradually stiffen. For example, the lungs and heart muscle expand less successfully, blood vessels become increasingly rigid, and ligaments begin to tighten. These apparently diverse age-related changes are accelerated in diabetes, and the causative agent is glucose. Glucose becomes chemically attached to proteins and deoxyribonucleic acid (DNA) in the body without the aid of enzymes to speed the reaction along. What is important is the duration of exposure to the elevated glucose concentrations. Once glucose is bound to tissue proteins, a series of chemical reactions is triggered that, over the passage of months and years, can result in the formation and eventual accumulation of cross-links between adjacent proteins. The higher glucose concentrations in diabetics accelerate this process, and the effects become evident in specific tissues throughout the body.

Understanding the chemical basis of protein cross-linking in diabetes has permitted the development and study of compounds that can intervene in this process. Certain compounds, when added to the diet, can limit the glucose-induced cross-linking of proteins by preventing their formation. One of the best-studied compounds, aminoguanidine, can help prevent the cross-linking of collagen; this fact is shown in a decrease in the accumulation of trapped lipoproteins on artery walls. Aminoguanidine also prevents thickening of the capillary basement membrane in the kidney. Aminoguanidine acts by blocking glucose's ability to react with neighboring proteins. Vitamins C and B_6 are also effective in reducing cross-linking. Aminoguanidine and vitamins C and B_6 are thought to have antiaging properties and may also improve the complications resulting from the high blood-glucose levels seen in diabetes mellitus.

Alternatively, transplantation of the entire pancreas is an effective means of achieving an insulin-independent state in persons with type 1 diabetes mellitus. Both the technical problems of pancreas transplantation and the possible rejec-

---

In the News: Accord Trial

The Action to Control Cardiovascular Risk in Diabetes (Accord) trial, sponsored by the National Heart, Lung, and Blood Institute, was a large-scale clinical study of adults with type 2 diabetes who were at high risk for cardiovascular disease. More than ten thousand adults across the United States and Canada were enrolled in the study; participants were between the ages of forty and seventy, had diabetes for an average of ten years, and were at high risk for cardiovascular disease owing to at minimum two risk factors in addition to type 2 diabetes.

The Accord trial examined cardiovascular disease events in three treatment strategies compared to standard treatments: intensive lowering of blood glucose levels, treating cholesterol and triglycerides with a fibrate plus a statin, and intensive lowering of blood pressure.

In 2008, the intensive glucose control arm of the trial was stopped nearly eighteen months early because of safety concerns. After an average of 3.5 years of treatment, the intensive control group exhibited a 22 percent increased risk of death compared to the standard treatment group. The standard treatment group included 5,123 participants and aimed to lower blood-sugar levels to a hemoglobin A1C (HbA1C) of 7 to 7.9 percent. The intensive therapy group included 5,128 participants and aimed to lower HbA1C to less than 6 percent.

The causes of death were similar in both groups, and approximately half of the deaths were caused by cardiovascular events including heart attack, stroke, heart failure, or sudden cardiac death. The intensive treatment group had a 35 percent higher cardiovascular death rate than the standard treatment group. The death rates were consistent between the groups, regardless of baseline characteristics such as gender, age, race, or existing cardiovascular disease. The participants in the intensive treatment group were moved to the standard treatment arm of the study and followed to the study's planned conclusion.

Researchers have been unable to identify the exact cause of the increased risk of death, but believe it is due to a combination of factors and not a specific medication or treatment. The results underscore the importance of individualized treatment for type 2 diabetes. No changes to standard treatment guidelines are recommended. The results of the trial do not apply to people with type 1 diabetes.

The Accord trial began in 2003 and followed patients through 2009. The researchers published the final results of the study in 2010.

—*Jennifer L. Gibson, Pharm.D.*

---

tion of the foreign tissue, however, have limited this procedure as a treatment for diabetes. Diabetes is usually manageable; therefore, a pancreas transplant is not necessarily lifesaving. Success in treating diabetes has been achieved by transplanting only the insulin-producing islet cells from the pancreas or grafts from fetal pancreas tissue. It may one day be possible to use genetic engineering to permit cells of the liver to self-regulate glucose concentrations by synthesizing and releasing their own insulin into the blood.

Some of the less severe forms of type 2 diabetes mellitus can be controlled by the use of oral hypoglycemic agents that bring about a reduction in blood glucose. These drugs can be taken orally to drive the beta cells to release even more insulin than usual. These drugs also increase the ability of insulin to act on the target cells, which ultimately reduces the insulin requirement. The use of these agents remains controversial, because they overwork the already strained beta cells. If a diabetic person is reliant on these drugs for extended periods of time, the insulin cells could "burn out" and completely lose their ability to synthesize insulin. In this situation, the previously non-insulin-dependent person would have to be placed on insulin therapy for life. Other hypoglycemic agents lower blood glucose by decreasing hepatic glucose output, reducing insulin resistance, and delaying the absorption of glucose

In the News: Benefits and Risks of Diabetes Drugs

The benefits and risks of diabetes drugs have caused concern among patients and health care providers, and challenged traditional treatment options as safety concerns of new drugs mount and the effectiveness of older medications is confirmed.

Metformin is the most commonly used oral medication to treat type 2 diabetes. Metformin reduces triglycerides and LDL cholesterol and increases HDL cholesterol. According to the United Kingdom Prospective Diabetes Study, metformin reduces the risk of myocardial infarction and stroke, making it a first-choice treatment option for most patients with diabetes.

Thiazolidinediones can cause significant weight gain and fluid retention, leading to an increased risk of heart failure. Several studies suggest, but do not prove, that one agent, rosiglitazone, may increase the risk of heart attack and cardiovascular death. Conversely, another agent, pioglitazone, may reduce the risk of heart attack and stroke. Both thiazolidinediones have shown an increased risk of fractures in women. More research is needed to verify these findings.

Glucagon-like peptide-1 (GLP-1) agonists are incretin hormone-based therapies. Exenatide, a GLP-1 agonist, causes substantial gastrointestinal side effects, but these typically resolve after a few weeks of treatment. Of benefit in diabetes, exenatide leads to significant weight loss. Several cases of pancreatitis have been reported with the use of exenatide; most of the cases resolved with discontinuation of the drug. Also, several cases of kidney dysfunction have been reported with exenatide. The U.S. Food and Drug Administration (FDA) warns to use exenatide cautiously in patients with existing kidney or pancreatic disease.

Dipeptidyl peptidase-4 (DPP4) inhibitors are also incretin-based drugs. Rare cases of severe allergic reactions, including angioedema and Stevens-Johnson syndrome, have occurred with the use of DPP4 inhibitors. Sitagliptin, a DPP4 inhibitor, is also associated with several cases of severe pancreatitis; most of the cases resolved with discontinuation of the drug. In late 2009, the FDA ordered the manufacturer of sitagliptin to change the prescribing information to warn of the increased risk of pancreatitis with sitagliptin.

Many experts have questioned the urgency with which new diabetes medications have emerged, and clinicians now advocate weighing the benefits of blood glucose control with the undesirable risks associated with many diabetes drugs.

—*Jennifer L. Gibson, Pharm.D.*

from the gastrointestinal tract.

If obesity is a factor in the expression of type 2 diabetes, as it is in most cases, the best therapy is a combination of a reduction of calorie intake and an increase in activity. More than any other disease, type 2 diabetes is related to lifestyle. It is often the case that people prefer having an injection or taking a pill to improving their quality of life by changing their diet and level of activity. Attention to diet and exercise results in a dramatic decrease in the need for drug therapy in most diabetics. In some cases, the loss of only a small percentage of body weight results in an increased sensitivity to insulin. Exercise is particularly helpful in the management of both types of diabetes, because working muscle does not require insulin to metabolize glucose. Thus, exercising muscles take up and use some of the excess glucose in the blood, which reduces the overall need for insulin. Permanent weight reduction and exercise also help to prevent long-term complications and permit a healthier and more active lifestyle.

Perspective and Prospects

Diabetes mellitus is a disease of ancient origin. The first written reference to diabetes, which was discovered in the tomb of Thebes in Egypt (1500 BCE), described an illness associated with the passage of vast quantities of sweet urine and an excessive thirst.

The study of diabetes owes much to the Franco-Prussian War. In 1870, during the siege of Paris, it was noted by French physicians that the widespread famine in the besieged city had a curative influence on diabetic patients. Their glycosuria decreased or disappeared. These observations supported the view of clinicians at the time who had previously prescribed periods of fasting and increased muscular work for the treatment of the overweight diabetic individual.

It was Oscar Minkowski of Germany who, in 1889, accidentally traced the origin of diabetes to the pancreas. Following the complete removal of the pancreas from a dog, Minkowski's technician noted the animal's subsequent copious urine production. Acting on the basis of a hunch, Minkowski tested the urine and determined that its sugar content was greater than 10 percent.

In 1921, Frederick Banting and Charles Best, at the University of Toronto in Canada, successfully extracted the antidiabetic substance insulin using a cold alcohol-hydrochloric acid mixture to inactivate the harsh digestive enzymes of the pancreas. Using this substance, they first controlled the disease in a depancreatized dog and then, a few months later, successfully treated the first human diabetic patient. The clinical application of a discovery normally takes a long time, but in this case a mere twenty weeks had passed between the first injection of insulin into the diabetic dog and the first trial with a diabetic human. Three years later, in 1923, Banting and Best were awarded the Nobel Prize in physiology or medicine for their remarkable achievement.

Although insulin, when combined with an appropriate diet and exercise, alleviates the symptoms of diabetes to such an extent that a diabetic can lead an essentially normal life, insulin therapy is not a cure. The complications that arise in diabetics are typical of those found in the general population, except that they happen much earlier in the diabetic. With regard to these glucose-induced complications, it was first postulated in 1908 that sugars could react with proteins. In 1912, Louis Camille Maillard further characterized this reaction at the Sorbonne and realized that the consequences of this reaction were relevant to diabetics. Maillard suggested that sugars were destroying the body's amino acids, which then led to increased excretion in diabetics. It was not until the mid-1970s, however, that Anthony Cerami in New York introduced the concept of the nonenzymatic attachment of glucose to protein and recognized its potential role in diabetic complications. A decade later, this development led to the discovery of aminoguanidine, the first compound to limit the cross-linking of tissue proteins and thus delay the development of certain diabetic complications.

In 1974, Josiah Brown published the first report showing that diabetes could be reversed by transplanting fetal pancreatic tissue. By the mid-1980s, procedures had been devised for the isolation of massive numbers of human islets that could then be transplanted into diabetics. For persons with diabetes, both procedures represent more than a treatment; they may offer a cure for the disease.

By the turn of the twenty-first century, there was a noticeable rise in the prevalence of type 2 diabetes in both developing and developed countries. According to the World Health Organization (WHO), an estimated 347 million people worldwide have diabetes, a number expected to rise. Although the incidence of type 2 diabetes typically increases with age, the first decades of the twenty-first century have seen a dramatic rise in the number of cases in younger people.

Obesity is clearly linked to the increase of type 2 diabetes. The growing sedentary lifestyle and increase in energy-dense food intake are significant risk factors. The WHO reported that worldwide obesity nearly doubled between 1980 and 2013. By 2008, about 35 percent of adults were overweight, and 11 percent were obese. Due in large part to these factors, the WHO has predicted that diabetes will become the seventh leading cause of death by 2030.

—Hillar Klandorf, Ph.D.;
updated by Sharon W. Stark, R.N., A.P.R.N., D.N.Sc.

See also Blindness; Endocrine disorders; Endocrine glands; Endocrinology; Endocrinology, pediatric; Eye infections and disorders; Gangrene; Gastroenterology; Gastroenterology, pediatric; Gastrointestinal system; Gestational diabetes; Glands; Heart attack; Hormones; Hyperadiposis; Hypoglycemia; Internal medicine; Metabolic disorders; Metabolic syndrome; Obesity; Obesity, childhood; Pancreas; Pancreatitis.

For Further Information:

A.D.A.M. Medical Encyclopedia. "Diabetes." *MedlinePlus*, June 27, 2012.

American Diabetes Association. "Gestational Diabetes." *Diabetes Care* 26 (2003): S103–5.

American Diabetes Association. http://www.diabetes.org.

American Diabetes Association Complete Guide to Diabetes. 4th rev. ed. Alexandria, Va.: American Diabetes Association, 2006.

Becker, Gretchen. *The First Year—Type 2 Diabetes: An Essential Guide for the Newly Diagnosed*. 2d ed. New York: Marlowe, 2007.

Jovanovic-Peterson, Lois, Charles M. Peterson, and Morton B. Stori. *A Touch of Diabetes*. 3d ed. Minneapolis, Minn.: Chronimed, 1998.

Kronenberg, Henry M., et al., eds. *Williams Textbook of Endocrinology*. 11th ed. Philadelphia: Saunders/Elsevier, 2008.

McCulloch, David. *The Diabetes Answer Book: Practical Answers to More than Three Hundred Top Questions*. Naperville, Ill.: Sourcebooks, 2008.

Magee, Elaine. *Tell Me What to Eat If I Have Diabetes: Nutrition You Can Live With*. 3d ed. Franklin Lakes, N.J.: Career Press, 2008.

National Diabetes Information Clearinghouse. "Diabetes Overview." *National Institutes of Health*, April 4, 2012.

Wood, Debra. "Gestational Diabetes." *HealthLibrary*, September 10, 2012.

Wood, Debra. "Type 1 Diabetes." *HealthLibrary*, November 26, 2012.

Wood, Debra. "Type 2 Diabetes." *HealthLibrary*, July 17, 2012.

World Health Organization. "Diabetes." *World Health Organization*, March 2013.

World Health Organization. "Obesity and Overweight." *World Health Organization*, March 2013.

DIAGNOSIS

Procedure

Anatomy or system affected: All

Specialties and related fields: All

Definition: A methodical evaluation of symptoms and complaints through interview, observation, testing instruments, or procedures, including biological tests, to determine if an illness is present.

Key terms:

criteria: specific items, denoting symptoms, which are part of diagnostic decision making and rules

differential diagnosis: the process used to discern between conditions with similar or overlapping symptoms

epidemiology: the science of studying the distributions of illness across populations of people

false negative: when a specific diagnosis was ruled absent, when in fact it is actually present

false positive: when a specific diagnosis is identified as being present, when in reality it is actually absent

Indications and Procedures

When individuals see health care professionals for treatment, they are evaluated to determine the nature of their concerns. The process of evaluation usually involves a combination of assessment, screening, reassessment, and then formal diagnosis. They typically initially describe their experience, concerns, and history, and then the professional asks more questions and may follow up with screening questions.

Screening questions identify risk for any more serious conditions and for which additional assessment is needed. Screening is inexpensive and involves a small amount of time on questions that are easy to ask and answer, providing a determination of whether the person is at risk for a specific problem. If the screening result is positive, then the risk is there and further evaluation is needed; if it is negative, then the risk is deemed absent and no further evaluation is needed. Unfortunately, no screening process is perfect, and so sometimes there are false negatives. This is why it is important that if problems continue, individuals seeking care get second opinions or return for evaluation.

If a screening result is positive, then additional assessment is conducted to determine if a diagnosable condition is present. This usually involves a complete symptom history, comparing the symptoms described to known disorders, and doing differential diagnosis. If the information collected does not yield anything, then the screening process resulted in a false positive. If, on the other hand, the collection of information yields enough information to show that the criteria for a condition are satisfied, then a diagnosis is confirmed. The most common diagnostic systems in use are the *Diagnostic and Statistical Manual of Mental Disorders: DSM-5* (rev. 5th ed., 2013), and the *International Classification of Diseases* (2011).

An example of how diagnosis may work is as follows. A person comes to an emergency room, has alcohol on the breath and no other medical problems, and is screened positive for alcohol problems by a nurse asking a few questions. Additional assessment is done by a psychologist, and they determine that the individual meets the criteria for alcohol dependence. Alcohol dependence is a condition with seven criteria, and an individual who demonstrates three or more in any twelve-month period qualifies for the diagnosis. The patient might report having tolerance (using more to get the same effect), withdrawal (insomnia when stopping using), and a persistent desire to quit, all in the past year. The psychologist then diagnoses the patient with alcohol dependence, and treatment will address that problem.

Uses and Complications

Diagnoses are useful in facilitating effective and quick communications among treatment professionals and other stakeholders in the care of the client. These stakeholders include other treatment providers, insurance companies, researchers in epidemiology and other areas of science, and the clients and their families.

One complication related to diagnoses, however, is that some diagnoses have symptoms that overlap and that methods of differential diagnoses are always developing. As such, it is possible for misdiagnoses to occur. When this occurs, individuals may be treated for the wrong problem, or even overdiagnosed or underdiagnosed, and thus not properly treated. As such, it is often advised for more serious conditions that are costly to treat for patients to use multiple methods of diagnosis and even seek secondary opinions to confirm the diagnosis.

Perspective and Prospects

All forms of healers and health care providers have been involved, since the beginning human societies, in the process of diagnosis in one form or another. As science has advanced in its understanding of causes of death and illness, procedures for diagnosis have also evolved. The procedures and rules for making diagnoses in many areas of health care continue to evolve as new technology and research develop. New technologies take many forms, ranging from improved questionnaires, to new interview procedures, to automated tests and screening online, to the use of new magnetic resonance imaging (MRI), and to even the use of virtual reality-assisted robots entering the body and allowing diagnosticians to see what is happening inside specific organs. All these methods aid in quicker diagnoses and faster paths to effective treatment.

One challenge to evolving diagnostic methods is that the world has become more interconnected over the last century. As a result, it is important for diagnosticians of all types to recognize cultural differences in terms of how symptoms are experienced, expressed, and understood. This is true for both physical and mental health problems. Therefore, relevant screening, assessment, and other diagnostic technologies may need to adjust both in terms of how early symptoms are identified and in how information about diagnoses is conveyed to individuals of different backgrounds. This is the case as well because while diagnosis does involve technology, it is also a procedure involving human communication. As definitions and understandings of illness and health vary by culture, so too will communications about diagnosis need to adjust as cultures and health care providers interact more and more.

—*Nancy A. Piotrowski, Ph.D.*

See also Apgar score; Biopsy; Blood testing; Disease; Epidemiology; Hearing tests; Invasive tests; Laboratory tests; Mammography; Noninvasive tests; Pap test; Physical examination; Prognosis; Screening; Well-baby examinations.

For Further Information:
American Psychiatric Association. *Diagnostic and Statistical Manual of Mental Disorders: DSM-5.* Rev. 5th ed. Washington, DC: Author, 2013.
Doherty, Gerard M., and Lawrence W. Way. *Current Surgical Diagnosis and Treatment.* 13th ed. New York: Lange Medical/McGraw-Hill, 2010.
Helman, Cecil G., ed. *Culture, Health, and Illness.* 5th ed. London: Hodder Education, 2007.
Merck Research Laboratories. *The Merck Manual of Diagnosis and Therapy.* 19th ed. Whitehouse Station: Author, 2011.
World Health Organization. *International Statistical Classification of Diseases and Related Health Problems: 10th Revision–ICD-10.* 2010 ed. Geneva, Switzerland: Author, 2011.

DIALYSIS
Procedure
Anatomy or system affected: Abdomen, blood, circulatory system, kidneys, urinary system
Specialties and related fields: Biotechnology, hematology, internal medicine, nephrology, serology, urology
Definition: The artificial replacement of renal (kidney) function, which involves the removal of toxins in the blood by selective diffusion through a semipermeable membrane.
Key terms:
hemodialysis: the removal of toxins from blood through the process of dialysis
osmosis: the diffusion of molecules through a semipermeable membrane until there is an equal concentration on either side of the membrane
peritoneal dialysis: the removal of toxins from blood by dialysis in the peritoneal cavity
peritoneum: the membrane lining the walls of the abdominal cavity and enclosing the viscera

Indications and Procedures
The two major functions of the kidneys are to produce urine,

thereby excreting toxic substances and maintaining an optimal concentration of solutes in the blood, and to produce and secrete hormones that regulate blood flow, blood production, calcium and bone metabolism, and vascular tone. These functions can be impaired or even completely halted by kidney failure that may or may not be related to diseases such as hepatitis and diabetes. The kidney is the only human organ with a function—that is, the excretion of toxic substances from the blood—that can be artificially replaced on a reliable and chronic basis. Although dialysis cannot duplicate the intricate processes of normal renal function, it is possible to provide patients with a tolerable level of life.

The Administration of Hemodialysis

Dialysis is a method of removing wastes from the blood when the kidneys have failed to do so. Hemodialysis, which employs a machine that acts as an artificial kidney, is performed in a hospital or a local dialysis center in a session lasting two to six hours in which the blood is filtered to eliminate wastes, toxins, and excess fluid.

If a solute is added to a container of water, it will be distributed at uniform concentration through the water. This process is called diffusion and results from random movement of the solute molecules in the solvent; it can be seen as a chemical mixing of the solution. The mixing will ensure an even distribution of solute molecules throughout the solution. The time required for complete mixing depends on factors such as the nature of the solute, its molecular size, the temperature of the solution, and the size of the container. The process of dialysis is based on the diffusion of solute molecules (urea and other substances) from the blood or fluids of a patient to a sterile solution called dialysate. The artificial kidney or dialysis system is designed to provide controllable osmosis, or the transfer of solutes and water across a semipermeable membrane separating streams of blood (contaminated as a result of renal failure) and dialysate (a sterile solution). For solutes such as urea, the outflowing blood concentration is high, while the concentration in the inflowing dialysate is usually zero. The result is a concentration gradient that guarantees osmosis of urea molecules from the blood to the dialysate solution. The same process will take place for other toxins present in the blood but absent from the dialysate solution.

There are two types of clinical dialysis, hemodialysis and peritoneal dialysis. In hemodialysis, the device utilized is called a dialyzer. The three basic structural elements of all dialyzers are the blood compartment, the membrane, and the dialysate compartment. In a perfect dialyzer, diffusion equilibrium would result in the blood and dialysate streams during passage through the device, and virtually all the urea and toxins contained in the inflowing blood stream would be transferred to the dialysate stream. This level of efficiency is not achieved, however, and for maximum efficiency, dialysate flow rate should be from two to two and one-half times the actual blood flow rate.

Several fundamental material and design requirements must be met in the construction of efficient dialyzers suitable for clinical use. First, the surfaces in contact with blood and the flow geometry must not induce the formation of blood clots. The materials used must be nontoxic and free of leachable toxic substances. The ratio of membrane surface area to contained volume must be high to ensure maximum transference of substances, and the resistance to blood flow must be low and predictable.

There are three basic designs for a dialyzer: the coil, parallel plate, and hollow fiber configurations. The coil dialyzer was the earliest design. In it, the blood compartment consisted of one or two membrane tubes placed between support screens and then wound with the screens around a plastic core. This resulted in a coiled tubular membrane laminated between support screens, which was then enclosed in a rigid cylindrical case. This design had serious performance limitations, such as a high hydraulic resistance to blood flow and an increase in contained blood volume as blood flow through the device was increased.

The coil design has all but been replaced by more efficient devices. In the parallel plate dialyzer, sheets of membrane are mounted on a plastic support screen and then stacked in multiple layers, allowing for multiple parallel blood and dialysate flow channels. The original design had problems with membrane stretching and nonuniform channel performance. To minimize these problems, smaller plates and better membrane supports have been developed. The hollow fiber dialyzer is the most effective design for providing low volume and high efficiency together with modest resistance to flow. Developed in the 1970s, the membrane is composed of tiny cellulose or synthetic hollow fibers about the size of a human hair. Between seven thousand and twenty-five thousand of those fibers are enclosed in a cylindrical jacket, with the blood inlet and outlet at the top and bottom of the cylinder and the dialysate inlet and outlet being simply expanded sections of the jacket itself. This is the most commonly used geometry for hemodialysis. Extreme care must be taken to ensure that all the extra fluids that might have entered the blood during dialysis are removed. Ultrafiltration refers to the removal of water from the blood after dialysis and is a critical component of the dialysis process.

The delivery system of a dialyzer provides on-line proportioning of water with dialysate concentrate and monitors the dialysate for temperature, composition, and blood leaks. It also controls the ultrafiltration rate and regulates the dialysate flow. Normally included in the system are a blood pump, blood pressure and air monitors, and an anticoagulant pump.

The composition of the dialysate is designed to approximate the normal electrolyte concentration found in plasma and extracellular water; it contains calcium, magnesium, sodium and potassium chloride, sodium acetate, sodium carbonate, and lactic acid, kept at a pH of 7.4. The water used in this preparation is purified, heated to between 35 and 37 degrees Celsius, and deaerated to prevent air embolism. An anticoagulant must be added in the process to prevent the formation of blood clots. Heparin is the most commonly used anticoagulant, mainly because its effect is immediate, is easily measured, and can be almost immediately terminated by

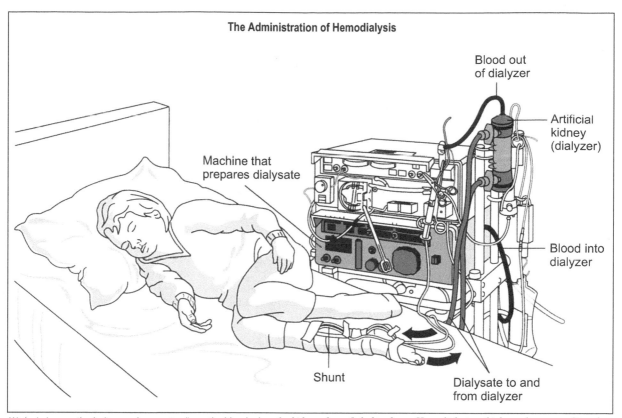

The Administration of Hemodialysis

Blood out
of dialyzer

Artificial
kidney
(dialyzer)

Machine that
prepares dialysate

Blood into
dialyzer

Shunt

Dialysate to and
from dialyzer

Dialysis is a method of removing wastes from the blood when the kidneys have failed to do so. Hemodialysis, which employs a machine that acts as an artificial kidney, is performed in a hospital or a local dialysis center in a session lasting two to six hours in which the blood is filtered to eliminate wastes, toxins, and excess fluid.

adding protamine. In addition, because of its high molecular weight and substantial protein binding, it is not dialyzable and will not be lost from the blood in the process.

Several types of polymers are commonly employed for the manufacture of the membranes utilized in hemodialysis. Cellulosic membranes, or membranes generated from the plant product cellulose, are the most commonly used polymers. (Cellophane was originally used, and later cuprophan and hemophan were introduced.) Noncellulosic artificial membranes made from synthetic polymers such as polycarbonate and polyamide are also used.

The development of efficient and more permeable synthetic membranes and ultrafiltration control delivery systems has reduced treatment time to two or three hours. Dialysis remains a potentially lethal procedure, and careful monitoring of equipment and solutions is necessary. For example, the dialysate must be monitored for hypertonic or hypotonic conditions that can result in hemolysis and death, and the flow from the dialyzer outlet back to the patient must have, among other things, an air bubble detector and filters to remove clots.

Peritoneal dialysis involves the transfer of solutes and water from the peritoneal capillary blood to the dialysate in the peritoneal cavity and the absorption of glucose and other solutes from the peritoneal fluid into the blood. The physiology of this process is less understood than that of hemodialysis. The process involves the introduction in the peritoneal cavity of a certain volume of dialysate and its removal after the dialysis process is complete. The main type of procedure is chronic intermittent peritoneal dialysis (CIPD). This process is performed three to seven times per week and takes from eight to twelve hours. It is mostly done overnight, when a pump introduces the dialysate to the peritoneal cavity and gravity removes it. Two systems are commonly used for this purpose: One is the reverse osmosis machine, which provides continuous flow through the night in a fast manner, while the other system utilizes a cycler for the cycling of the dialysate during the night. Cyclers are semiautomated systems with simple operation and a low initial expense that provide basically trouble-free performance but are expensive in the long run because they use premixed dialysates and many disposable components. Chronic ambulatory peritoneal dialysis (CAPD) is the most versatile and manageable of the techniques. In this case, the inflow and outflow of dialysate is done manually by gravity. With about two liters of dialysate used per exchange, it normally takes ten minutes for inflow and fifteen to twenty minutes for outflow. There are an average of four exchanges per day and one overnight. This is an easy, safe, and effective method of dialysis. A variation of

CAPD is continuous cycling peritoneal dialysis (CCPD), introduced in 1980. It basically reverses the CAPD cycle: Cyclers are used during the night to achieve three to four exchanges, and there is a long period without exchange during the day. This minimizes the inconvenience of scheduling exchanges during the day, and many patients can alternate between the two methods without experiencing problems.

For peritoneal dialysis, the dialysate includes dextrose, lactate, sodium, calcium, and magnesium salts. An anticoagulant such as heparin can be added when needed, such as if blood is seen in the peritoneal fluid. Other substances—such as insulin for both diabetic and nondiabetic patients, antibiotics if there is peritonitis, and bicarbonate to prevent abdominal discomfort—can also be added without major complications.

Peritoneal dialysis may be a better choice than hemodialysis for certain patients when factors such as coronary artery disease, diabetes mellitus, age, or severe hemodialysis-related symptoms are present. It is also the choice for patients whose residence is remote from a dialysis center, who wish to travel frequently, or who live alone.

Uses and Complications

Hemodialysis is used in acute and chronic renal failure patients. Some individuals, however, do not tolerate hemodialysis well, such as children, infants, geriatric patients, diabetics, and victims of traumatic injuries. Therefore, the selection of patients for this procedure must be closely monitored. The process also can be used for treatment of drug overdose (since drugs can be removed from the blood during the dialysis procedure) and hypercalcemia, an excess of calcium.

For many years, peritoneal dialysis was reserved for the treatment of acute renal failure (ARF) or for those patients awaiting transplantation or the availability of hemodialysis. Although it is used principally for the treatment of patients with end-stage renal disease, it remains a valuable tool in the management of ARF because of its simplicity and widespread availability. Essentially, it can be provided in any hospital by most internists or surgeons without the need for specially trained nephrology personnel. It also avoids the need for systematic anticoagulation, making it a good choice for patients in the immediate postoperative period with severe trauma, intracerebral hemorrhage, or hypocoagulable states. It is most suitable for the treatment of patients with an unstable cardiovascular system and for pediatric or elderly patients. It could be impossible to use, however, in postsurgical patients with many abdominal drains, with hernias, or with severe gastroesophageal reflux.

For many years, peritoneal dialysis was not used for patients with CRF (chronic renal failure) because of the problems involved in the maintenance of permanent peritoneal access, the inconvenience of manual dialysate exchanges, the high rate of peritonitis observed in these patients, and the rapid progress made in hemodialysis in the early 1960s. The advent of a safe, permanent peritoneal catheter in the late 1960s and the simultaneous development of automated re-

verse osmosis peritoneal delivery systems created new interest in the technique and resulted in safer, more effective systems. Peritoneal dialysis can also be used or is recommended in the following cases: for diabetic patients, since it provides a continuous source of insulin and also has the advantage of providing blood pressure control; for edema patients, since the process is useful in the treatment of intractable edema states such as congestive heart failure; and for pancreatitis patients or individuals who suffer from the release of pancreatic enzymes into the abdominal cavity and their subsequent absorption into the circulation. For the latter, the removal of the enzymes through peritoneal dialysis may prevent the necrotic process. Individuals exhibiting hypothermia as a consequence of accidental exposure, cold water immersion, central nervous system disorders, intoxication, or burns can be treated by performing peritoneal dialysis with dialysate solutions between 40 and 45 degrees Celsius. This will bring the body back to 34 degrees Celsius (a stable temperature) in a few hours, and, if the cause of the hypothermia is intoxication, the drugs causing the condition can be removed at the same time.

Perspective and Prospects

As early as the seventeenth century, the relationship between blood and various diseases was known. At that time, however, great difficulties existed in the transport and study of blood. By the nineteenth century, the techniques for entering the blood vessels had been refined. The dangers of air embolization (air entering the patient) and clotting were well recognized. Prior to 1850, there was no treatment for patients with renal failure, but crude methods such as applying heat, immersing in warm baths, bloodletting, or administering diaphoretic (perspiration-inducing) mixtures of nitric acid in alcohol and wine were commonly used. (In fact, diaphoretic mixtures and bloodletting for renal failure were used as late as the 1950s.)

In 1854, Thomas Graham, a Scottish chemist, presented a paper on osmotic force, which was the first reference to the process of separating a substance using a semipermeable membrane. His definitions and experimental proofs of the laws of diffusion and osmosis form the foundation upon which dialysis is based. Between 1872 and 1900, the control of membrane manufacture and the dialysis of animal blood were critical developments. One of the key turning points in the development of dialysis occurred in 1913, when John Jacob Abel, using anticoagulants, created the first extracorporeal device that could be used to diffuse a substance from blood and developed methods to quantify this diffusion. World War I brought the development of the first plate dialyzer, by Heinrich Necheles, a German-born physician. It included an air bubble trap, continuous blood flow, and an entry port for a saline solution to be used as dialysate; it was only used for animals. George Haas must be credited as the first to perform dialysis on a uremic human, in October, 1924. He used heparin, an anticoagulant discovered by William H. Howell and Luther E. Holt, two Americans. Haas had all the pieces together: a dialyzer with a large surface area, a workable membrane, a blood pump, and an anticoagulant.

The emergence of manufactured membranes in the 1930s (such as cellophane, which allows small molecules to pass through it) was crucial in the development of the technique. The lifesaving potential of an artificial kidney was shown by Willem Kolff, a physician from the Netherlands, who saved a patient from coma. His classic work *New Ways of Treating Uraemia*, published in 1947, laid out the principles that are still used and was the first manual for the treatment of patients undergoing hemodialysis. In the United States, the first clinical dialysis was performed on January 26, 1948, at Mt. Sinai Hospital in New York City, by physicians Irving Kroop and Alfred Fishman. The number of groups developing artificial kidney devices and programs between 1945 and 1950 was large. The first complete artificial kidney system commercially available came into existence in 1956, and the first home patient was treated in 1964 by Belding Scribner, from the University of Washington.

Soon the dialyzing fluid delivery systems became smaller and easier to use, the designs were simplified and made more compact, and a better understanding of the physiology of the patient was obtained. Calcium depletion, bone disease, neuropathy, dietary management, and anemia were being looked at closely in order to determine better how much dialysis was required for effective treatment. The late 1960s brought the miniaturization of the systems, in-home care, and lower prices. In fact, in 1973, legislation was enacted in the United States that provided payment through the Social Security system for the care of dialysis patients.

In the latter part of the 1970s, a shift to totally automated systems and an emphasis on negative-pressure dialysis had major impacts, resulting in a move from coil to hollow-fiber dialyzers. Some patients, however, such as diabetics, children, and older patients, did not tolerate hemodialysis well. Therefore, a closer look was taken at peritoneal and automated peritoneal dialysis delivery systems. The earliest reference to peritoneal diffusion was in 1876, and in 1895 it was formally presented as an alternative to remove toxins from the bloodstream. Nevertheless, peritoneal dialysis lay dormant until the 1940s. The basic procedure of using solutions and instilling them into the peritoneal cavity in order to reduce the toxin levels in the blood was first used in 1945 by a group of physicians in Beth Israel Hospital in Boston. The full implications of its use came in the late 1970s, with the development of reverse osmosis technology and the introduction of continuous ambulatory peritoneal dialysis. In the 1980s, the introduction of continuous intermittent peritoneal dialysis gave patients yet another treatment option.

One of the main goals of the medical community and industry is to provide the quality of care that will minimize the burden of those afflicted with renal disease. The main goal, however, remains to obtain the necessary knowledge to understand the causes of progressive renal failure and then prevent, control, or eliminate the consequences of renal disease.

—*Maria Pacheco, Ph.D.*

See also Blood and blood disorders; Circulation; Diabetes mellitus; Edema; Heart failure; Hematology; Hematology, pediatric; Hemolytic uremic syndrome; Hepatitis; Hyperthermia and hypothermia; Kidney cancer; Kidney disorders; Kidney transplantation; Kidneys; Nephrectomy; Nephritis; Nephrology; Nephrology, pediatric; Pancreatitis; Polycystic kidney disease; Renal failure; Uremia.

For Further Information:

Cameron, J. Stewart. *History of the Treatment of Renal Failure by Dialysis*. New York: Oxford University Press, 206.

Cogan, Martin G., and Patricia Schoenfeld, eds. *Introduction to Dialysis*. 2d ed. New York: Churchill Livingstone, 1991.

Fine, Leonard W., Herbert Beall, and John Stuehr. *Chemistry for Engineers and Scientists*. Fort Worth, Tex.: Saunders College, 2000.

Health Library. "Hemodialysis." *Health Library*, May 31, 2013.

Health Library. "Peritoneal Dialysis." *Health Library*, November 26, 2012.

MedlinePlus. "Dialysis." *MedlinePlus*, May 20, 2013.

National Kidney Foundation. "Dialysis." *National Kidney Foundation*, 2013.

Nissenson, Allen R., and Richard N. Fine, eds. *Clinical Dialysis*. 4th ed. New York: McGraw-Hill Medical, 2005.

Nissenson, Allen R., and Richard N. Fine, eds. *Dialysis Therapy*. 3d ed. Philadelphia: Hanley and Belfus, 2002.

Voet, Donald, and Judith G. Voet. *Biochemistry*. 4th ed. Hoboken, N.J.: John Wiley & Sons, 2011.

DIAPHRAGM

Anatomy

Anatomy or system affected: Chest, lungs, muscles, musculoskeletal system, respiratory system, spine

Specialties and related fields: Internal medicine, pulmonary medicine

Definition: The diaphragm, a dome-shaped muscle that is unique to mammals, is the major muscle of respiration and separates the thoracic and abdominal cavities. When the diaphragm contracts, it decreases the pressure within the lungs by expanding the rib cage and increasing the volume of the lungs as it flattens.

Structure and Functions

The diaphragm is attached to the spine, the ribs, and the sternum. It is pierced by the esophagus, the phrenic nerve, the aorta, and the vena cava. The human body has three types of muscles: cardiac, which is striated and under involuntary control; smooth, which is not striated and is under involuntary control; and skeletal, which is striated and under voluntary control. The diaphragm is composed of skeletal muscle and is under both voluntary and involuntary control. That is, one is able to hold the breath, take deeper breaths, or take faster breaths (panting), examples of voluntary control. However, a person normally breathes, allowing the diaphragm to contract and relax as skeletal muscle does, involuntarily—that is, without the conscious effort that is required with holding one's breath.

As skeletal muscle, the diaphragm must be innervated; that is, it must receive a nerve impulse before it will contract. The impulses that are sent to the diaphragm originate in the higher brain centers when one voluntarily controls breathing but originate in the lower brain when low oxygen concentrations or high carbon dioxide concentrations are present. The diaphragm relies on the phrenic nerve for its innervations.

When innervated, the diaphragm contracts, as all skeletal muscle does, and flattens or pulls downward. This movement serves to cause the ribs to pull outward, increasing the volume within the lungs. Air pressure inside the lungs is now lower than air pressure outside the lungs (the environment), so air rushes in. As the diaphragm muscle relaxes, it once again domes upward, allowing the ribs to move back to a resting position. The lung volume decreases, but since the lungs are filled with air, the pressure inside the lungs is now greater than the pressure outside the lungs. Air moves outward as one exhales. (This simple expansion and contraction of the lung volume is the premise behind the original iron lung machine.) This cycle of contraction and relaxation is repeated approximately twelve to fourteen times per minute; with heavy exercise, it may be repeated forty times per minute.

The diaphragm has a role in laughing, singing, crying, yawning, hiccupping, vomiting, coughing, sneezing, whistling, defecating, and urinating, as well as in childbirth.

Disorders and Diseases

The diaphragm may be affected by both neurological and anatomical processes. Common neurological problems are disorders of innervation as a result of trauma to the head or brain stem; nerve impulses to the diaphragm are disrupted and the diaphragm cannot contract and relax. These injuries are often fatal. Poliomyelitis, demyelinating diseases, and other diseases may also impair the innervation of the diaphragm. Anatomical problems may include hernias (protrusion of the stomach through the diaphragm and into the thoracic cavity). Blunt trauma from car accidents and the like may rupture the diaphragm.

—*M. A. Foote, Ph.D.*

See also Abdomen; Chest; Muscles; Pulmonary medicine; Respiration.

For Further Information:

Koch, Wijnand F. R. M., and Enrico Marani. *Early Development of the Human Pelvic Diaphragm.* New York: Springer, 2007.

Kohnle, Diana, Marcin Chwistek, and Brian Randall. "Diaphragmatic Hernia." *Health Library,* March 18, 2013.

"Lungs and Breathing." *MedlinePlus,* June 26, 2013.

Marieb, Elaine N. *Essentials of Human Anatomy and Physiology.* 10th ed. San Francisco: Pearson/Benjamin Cummings, 2012.

Sherwood, Lauralee. *Human Physiology: From Cells to Systems.* 8th ed. Belmont, Calif.: Brooks/Cole/Cengage Learning, 2013.

DIARRHEA AND DYSENTERY

Disease/Disorder

Anatomy or system affected: Abdomen, gastrointestinal system, intestines

Specialties and related fields: Family medicine, gastroenterology, internal medicine, pediatrics, public health

Definition: Intestinal disorders that may indicate minor emotional distress or a variety of diseases, some serious; diarrhea is loose, watery, copious bowel movements, whereas

dysentery is a process, usually infectious and characterized by severe diarrhea, sometimes with passage of blood, mucus, and pus.

Key terms:

electrolytes: inorganic ions dissolved in body water, including sodium, potassium, calcium, magnesium, chloride, phosphate, bicarbonate, and sulphate

functional disease: a derangement in the way that normal anatomy operates

gastroenterology: the medical subspecialty devoted to care of the digestive tract and related organs

intestines: the tube connecting the stomach and anus in which nutrients are absorbed from food; divided into the small intestine and the colon, or large intestine

mucosa: the semipermeable layers of cells lining the gut, through which fluid and nutrients are absorbed

organic disease: disease resulting from an identifiable cause, such as an enzyme deficiency, growth, hole, or organism

pathogen: an organism that causes disease

peristalsis: the wavelike muscular contractions that move food and waste products through the intestines; problems with peristalsis are called motility disorders

stool: the waste products expelled from the anus during defecation

Causes and Symptoms

A symptom of various diseases rather than a disease in itself, diarrhea is so difficult to define and can result from so many disparate causes that it is sometimes called the gastroenterologist's nightmare. Dysentery (bloody diarrhea), a more threatening symptom, presents even further complexity.

Uncontrolled, some forms of diarrhea result in dehydration, weakness, and malnutrition and quickly turn deadly. Diarrhea is implicated in more infant deaths worldwide than any other affliction. Even in mild forms, it produces so much distress in victims and has inspired so many remedies that its psychological and economic toll is monumental.

Common medical definitions of diarrhea seek to bring diagnostic precision to a nebulous complaint and to distinguish between acute and chronic forms and between organic and functional causes. Diarrhea is typically associated with increased amount and fluidity of fecal matter and frequent defecation relative to a person's usual pattern. Acute diarrhea seldom lasts more than five days, although acute dysentery may continue up to ten days; most causes are infections, that is, resulting from the presence of microorganisms (viruses, bacteria, or parasites). Physicians differ over how long the symptoms must persist before a condition is identified as chronic diarrhea, proposing from two weeks to three months. Impaired functioning of the intestinal tract (functional diarrhea) is usually responsible for such chronic cases, although persistent malfunctions may originate from pathogens that in most cases provoke only acute diarrhea.

In a single day, water intake, saliva, gastric juice, bile, pancreatic juices, and electrolyte secretions in the upper small intestine produce about 9 to 10 liters of fluid in the average per-

Information on Diarrhea and Dysentery

Causes: Bacterial, viral, or parasitic infection; laxative abuse; hormones; inflammatory bowel disease
Symptoms: Dehydration, weakness, malnutrition, nausea, bleeding, fever, bloating, persistent intestinal pain
Duration: Acute to chronic
Treatments: Oral rehydration, antibiotics if needed

son. About 1 to 2 liters of this amount empty into the colon, and 100 to 150 milligrams are excreted in the stool; the rest is absorbed through the intestinal mucosa. If for any reason more fluid enters the colon than it can absorb, diarrhea results. Schemes classifying diarrhea according to the biochemical mechanisms causing it vary considerably, although authorities generally agree on three broad types of malfunction.

The first is secretory diarrhea. The intestines, especially the small intestine, normally add water and electrolytes—principally sodium, potassium, chloride, and bicarbonate—into the nutrient load during the biochemical reactions of digestion. In a healthy person, more fluid is absorbed than is secreted. Many agents and conditions can reverse this ratio and stimulate the mucosa to exude more water than can be absorbed: toxin-producing bacteria; various organic chemicals, including caffeine and some laxatives; acids; hormones; some cancers; and inflammatory diseases of the bowel. Large stool volume (more than 1 liter a day), with little or no decrease during fasting and with normal sodium and potassium content in the body fluid, characterizes secretory diarrhea.

Second, the nutrient load in the gut may include substances that exert osmotic force but cannot be absorbed, causing osmotic diarrhea. Some laxatives (especially those containing magnesium), an inability to absorb the lactose in dairy products or the artificial fats and sweeteners in diet foods, and enzyme deficiencies are the principal causes. Stool volume tends to be less than 1 liter a day and decreases during fasting, and the sodium and potassium content of stool water is low.

Third, motility disorders occur when peristalsis, the natural wavelike contractions of the bowel wall that move waste matter toward the rectum for defecation, becomes deranged. Some drugs, irritable bowel syndrome (IBS), hyperthyroidism, and gut nerve damage (as from diabetes mellitus) may have this effect. Fluid passes through the intestines too quickly or in an uncoordinated fashion, and too little is removed from the waste matter.

These mechanisms do not conform exactly with popular names for diarrhea. For example, travelers" diarrhea, the most infamous, comprises a diverse group of microorganism infections that come from drinking polluted water or eating tainted foods. When a person is not a native to an area, and so has little or no resistance to locally abundant pathogens, these pathogens can radically alter the balance of intestinal flora or attack the mucosa, increasing secretion and disrupting absorption and motility. Similarly, terms such as "Montezuma's revenge," "the backdoor trots," and "beaver fever" can refer to a variety of organic diseases, although the last commonly refers to *Giardia lamblia* infection.

Dysentery may occur with infectious diarrhea due to certain organisms, most commonly amoebas and other unicellular or multicellular parasites, or to bacterial organisms such as *Shigella*, *Campylobacter*, and some strains of *Escherichia coli*, or *E. coli*. Any pathogen or process that injures and inflames the bowel wall—ulcerating the mucosa—may cause blood and pus to ooze into the feces. Dysentery is also seen in inflammatory diseases of the bowel, such as ulcerative colitis and Crohn's disease. Severe diarrhea, with or without dysentery, may be associated with fever, chills, nausea, and in extreme cases, delirium, convulsions, coma, and death. Dehydration is the most common complication, but systemic infection may occur. Dysentery also may be associated with significant blood loss.

Although most diarrheas result from physiological mechanisms, one relatively rare form of chronic diarrhea ultimately has a psychological origin: laxative abuse. Physicians consider this curious phenomenon a specialized manifestation of Münchausen syndrome, named after the German soldier Baron Münchausen (1720–97), who was famous for his wild tales of military exploits and injuries in battles. To be admitted to hospitals, patients mutilate themselves in such a way that the injuries mimic acute, dramatic, and convincing symptoms of serious physiological diseases. Laxative abusers secretly dose themselves with nonprescription laxatives and suffer continual diarrhea, weight loss, and weakness. When they present themselves to physicians, they lie about taking laxatives, which makes a correct diagnosis extremely difficult. Even when confronted with irrefutable evidence of the abuse, they deny it and persist in taking the laxatives.

Treatment and Therapy

Almost everyone, at one time or another, produces stools that seem somehow unusual. If the bowel movement comes swiftly and is preceded by intestinal cramps and if the stool has anything from a watery to an oatmeal-like consistency, victims are likely to believe that they have diarrhea. Such episodes seldom indicate anything except perhaps a dietary excess or a temporary motility disturbance. Normal bowel movement returns on its own, and no medical treatment is called for. When loose feces are uncontrollable, even explosive, however, and other symptoms coexist, such as nausea, bleeding, fever, bloating, and persistent intestinal pain, the distress may indicate serious illness.

Because so many organic and functional diseases can lead to diarrhea, physicians follow carefully designed algorithms when treating patients. Essentially, such an algorithm seeks to eliminate possibilities systematically. Step by step, physicians interview patients, conduct physical examinations, and, when called for, perform tests that gradually narrow the range of possible causes until one seems most likely. Only then can the physician decide upon an effective therapy. This painstaking approach is necessary because treatments for some mechanisms of diarrhea prove useless against or worsen other mechanisms. If the underlying disease is complex or uncommon, the process can be long and frustrating.

One treatment, however, always precedes a complete investigation. Because dehydration is the most immediately serious effect of diarrhea, the physician first tries to prevent or reduce dehydration in a patient through oral rehydration; that is, the patient is given fluids with electrolytes to drink. Often, mineral water or clear fruit juice with soda crackers is sufficient to restore fluid balance.

If the diarrhea lasts fewer than three days and no other serious symptoms accompany it, the physician is unlikely to recommend treatment other than oral rehydration because whatever caused the upset is already resolving itself. If the diarrhea is persistent, however, the physician queries the patient about his or her recent experience. Fever, tenesmus (the urgent need to defecate without the ability to do so satisfactorily), blood in the stool, and abdominal pain will suggest that a pathogen has infected the patient. If the patient has recently eaten seafood, traveled abroad, suffered an immune system disorder, or engaged in sexual activity without the protection of condoms, the physician has reason to suspect that viruses, bacteria, or parasites are responsible.

At that point, a stool sample is taken. If few or no white cells turn up in the stool, then the diarrhea has not caused in-flammation. Several common bacteria and parasites, usually contracted during travel, induce diarrhea without inflammation, most notably some types of *E. coli*, cryptosporidium, rotavirus, Norwalk virus, and *Giardia lamblia*. Further tests, such as the culturing and staining of stool samples and electron microscopy of stool or bowel wall tissue, will distinguish between bacterial and parasite infection. Most noninflammatory bacterial diarrheas are allowed to run their course without drug therapy; only the effects of the diarrhea (especially dehydration) are treated. If the agent responsible is a parasite, the patient is given specific antiparasite medications.

The presence of white cells in the stool is evidence of inflammatory diarrhea, and the physician considers a completely separate group of microorganisms, especially *Shigella*, *Salmonella*, amoebas, and various forms of *E. coli*. Because the inflammation may cause bleeding and pockets of pus, which in turn can lead to anemia and fever, inflammatory diarrhea often requires aggressive treatment. Cultures help identify the specific microorganism involved, and that identification enables the physician to select the proper antibiotic to kill the infecting agents.

If cultures, microscopic examination of stool samples, biopsies, or staining fails to identify a microorganism (and

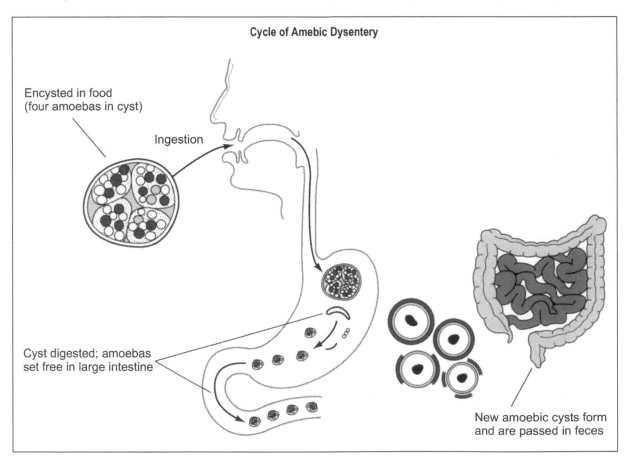

Cycle of Amebic Dysentery

Encysted in food
(four amoebas in cyst)

Ingestion

Cyst digested; amoebas
set free in large intestine

New amoebic cysts form
and are passed in feces

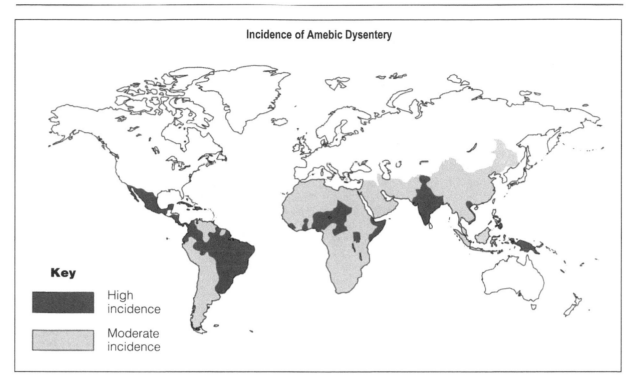

Incidence of Amebic Dysentery

Key
High incidence
Moderate incidence

some, such as the parasite *Giardia lamblia*, are difficult to spot), the physician suspects that the diarrhea derives from a source other than an infectious agent. IBS, a chronic and relapsing disorder, may be making its first appearance. Overuse of antibiotics, antacids, or laxatives is frequently the cause, in which case the cure is simple; elimination of the drugs clears up the symptom.

When neither drugs nor IBS is responsible, the physician looks for other diseases, organic or functional; these can range from the readily identifiable to the obscure, and they are often chronic. Chemical tests, for example, can show that a patient has enzyme deficiencies that produce intolerance to types of food, such as dairy products, or conditions resulting from malfunctioning organs, such as hyperthyroidism and pancreatic insufficiency. Looking through an endoscope, a long, flexible fiber-optic tube, the physician can locate diarrhea-causing tumors or the abrasions and inflammation typical of colitis and Crohn's disease. Yet neither tests nor direct examination may pin down the dysfunction. For example, diarrhea figures prominently among a group of symptoms, probably derived from assorted dysfunctions, that characterize IBS.

Cancers, Crohn's disease, and some forms of colitis can be alleviated with surgery, although in the case of Crohn's disease the relief from diarrhea may be only temporary. The surgery itself, however, may impair bowel function, worsening diarrhea rather than stopping it. Food intolerances are managed by removing the offending food from the patient's diet; similarly, some types of colitis and IBS sometimes improve after the physician and patient experiment with altering the

patient's diet. Medications are available that supplement or counteract the biochemical imbalances created by malfunctioning organs, such as treatment for hyperthyroidism. Yet, in many cases, the disease must simply be endured and the diarrhea can only be palliated with bulking agents, which often contain aluminum and bismuth, or opiates, such as morphine and codeine, which slow peristalsis.

The surest protection from diarrhea of all types is a balanced, moderate, pathogen-free diet, although diet alone seldom prevents organic diseases. When dietary control is difficult, such as when a person travels, other measures may help. Bacterial infection accounts for 80 percent of cases of travelers" diarrhea, so some physicians recommend regular doses of antibiotics or a bismuth subsalicylate preparation to kill off the pathogens before they can cause trouble. Such prophylactic treatment is controversial because the drugs, taken over long periods, can have serious side effects, including rashes, tinnitus (ringing in the ear), sensitivity to sunlight, and shock. Also, preventive doses of drugs may give travelers a false sense of security so that they fail to exercise caution in eating foreign foods. Widespread use of antibiotics for this purpose fosters the emergence of bacteria that are resistant to them, ultimately making the treatment of disease more difficult.

Perspective and Prospects

In effect, diarrhea is an urgent message from the body that something is wrong. Although it is often difficult for a physician to interpret, persistent diarrhea sends a signal that cannot be ignored without endangering the patient. Similarly, when significant numbers of people in an area suffer diarrhea, the disease is an urgent social and political message to local governments: public health is endangered, and steps must be taken to improve living conditions.

Although some endemic diarrheal diseases do exist in wealthy industrialized countries such as the United States, most severe, long-lasting plagues of diarrhea occur in impoverished nations that have inadequate sanitation systems and poor standards for food handling. Most viral, bacterial, and parasitic diarrheas are transmitted by food and water. Any food can harbor bacteria after being grown in or washed with infected water. Meat is especially vulnerable during slaughtering, but refrigerating, drying, salting, fermenting, freezing, or irradiating it prevents the bacteria from proliferating to numbers that cause illness. If the food is stored in a warm place, as is often the case in countries lacking the resources for refrigeration or other safe storage techniques, the diarrhea-causing organisms can spoil the food in hours. Spoiled food becomes a particular nuisance when served at restaurants or by street vendors, because great numbers and varieties of people are infected.

Organisms that cause many forms of diarrhea travel in human excrement. When an infected person defecates, the organism-rich stool enters the sewer system, and if that system is not well designed, the infected excrement may leak into the local water supply, spreading the infection when the water is consumed or used to wash food. Furthermore, infected persons, if they fail to wash themselves well, may have traces of excrement on their hands, and when they touch food during its preparation or touch other people directly, the organism can find a new host.

In 1989, the World Health Organization (WHO) issued ten rules for safe food preparation in an attempt to improve food-handling practices worldwide and combat diarrheal diseases. The effort, it was hoped, would reduce infant mortality in developing countries, since diarrheal dehydration kills children younger than two years of age at rates disproportionate to other age groups. The WHO advises food handlers to choose foods that are already processed, to cook foods thoroughly, to serve cooked foods immediately, to store foods carefully, to reheat foods thoroughly, to prevent raw and cooked foods from touching, to wash their hands repeatedly, to clean all kitchen surfaces meticulously, to protect foods from insects and rodents, and to use pure water.

Eliminating endemic infectious diarrheal diseases would improve general health significantly throughout the world, since diarrhea is one of the most incapacitating of afflictions even in its mild forms. International travel would also become safer. Noninfectious diarrhea from chronic functional diseases will remain a knotty problem, but it is rare in comparison to acute infectious diarrhea and cannot be transmitted, so has little or no effect on public health.

—*Roger Smith, Ph.D.*

See also Abdominal disorders; Amebiasis; Bacterial infections; Bile; *Campylobacter* infections; *Clostridium difficile* infections; Colitis; Colon; Colorectal cancer; Crohn's disease; Digestion; *E. coli* infection; Food poisoning; Gastroenteritis; Gastroenterology; Gastroenterology, pediatric; Gastrointestinal disorders; Gastrointestinal system; Giardiasis; Incontinence; Indigestion; Intestinal disorders; Intestines; Irritable bowel syndrome (IBS); Lactose intolerance; Noroviruses; Over-the-counter medications; Rotavirus; Shigellosis; Viral infections.

For Further Information:

A.D.A.M. Medical Encyclopedia. "Diarrhea." *MedlinePlus*, January 27, 2012.

Biddle, Wayne. *A Field Guide to Germs.* 2d ed. New York: Anchor Books, 2002.

Carson-DeWitt, Rosalyn. "Diarrhea." *HealthLibrary*, March 4, 2013.

DuPont, Herbert L., and Charles D. Ericsson. "Drug Therapy: Prevention and Treatment of Traveler's Diarrhea." *New England Journal of Medicine* 328 (June 24, 1993): 1821–26.

Gracey, Michael, ed. *Diarrhea.* Boca Raton, Fla.: CRC Press, 1991.

Janowitz, Henry D. *Your Gut Feelings: A Complete Guide to Living Better with Intestinal Problems.* Rev. ed. New York: Oxford University Press, 1995.

McCoy, Krisha. "Amoebic Dysentery." *HealthLibrary*, November 26, 2012.

Parker, James N., and Philip M. Parker, eds. *The Official Patient's Sourcebook on Diarrhea.* San Diego, Calif.: Icon Health, 2002.

Peikin, Steven R. *Gastrointestinal Health.* Rev. ed. New York: Quill, 2001.

Saibil, Fred. *Crohn's Disease and Ulcerative Colitis: Everything You Need to Know.* Rev. ed. Toronto, Ont.: Firefly Books, 2009.

Scarpignato, Carmelo, and P. Rampal, eds. *Traveler's Diarrhea: Recent Advances.* New York: S. Karger, 1995.

Thompson, W. Grant. *Gut Reactions: Understanding Symptoms of the Digestive Tract.* New York: Plenum Press, 1989.

DIET. *See* NUTRITION.

DIETARY DEFICIENCIES. *See* MALNUTRITION; NUTRITION; VITAMINS AND MINERALS.

DIETARY REFERENCE INTAKES (DRIs)
Biology

Anatomy or system affected: All

Specialties and related fields: Nutrition

Definition: The official U.S. guidelines for nutrient intakes in order to maintain health.

Development

The dietary reference intakes (DRIs) include four reference values that can be used in assessing and planning a healthy diet throughout the life span: estimated average requirement (EAR), recommended dietary allowance (RDA), adequate intake (AI), and tolerable upper intake limit (UL). The RDA is the amount of a nutrient needed to meet the needs of nearly all healthy individuals. In setting the RDA, an EAR is first determined. The EAR is the amount of a specific nutrient that is believed to meet the needs of half of the population. Using the assumption of a normal distribution of nutrient needs, the RDA is calculated from the EAR and the standard deviation of requirements. When data are insufficient to calculate an EAR, the available data are used to estimate an AI. The AI is similar to the RDA but acknowledges that additional research concerning nutrient requirements is needed in that area. The

UL represents the highest daily intake of a nutrient that is known to pose no health risks.

The EAR, RDA, and AI cannot be used to address the needs of those with chronic or acute disease. It can be assumed that intakes below the EAR probably need to be improved, since at this level 50 percent of the population would have inadequate intake. Intakes between the EAR for a specific nutrient and the RDA also may be improved. Intakes at or above the RDA probably are adequate, although many days of intake should be evaluated because of day-to-day variation. It is more difficult to be certain of the adequacy of intake when using AIs. However, in general, intakes below the AIs should probably be improved. Intakes at or above the UL should be lowered.

Nutrients for which EARs and RDAs have been established include phosphorus, magnesium, thiamine, riboflavin, niacin, vitamin B_6, folate, vitamin B_{12}, vitamin C, vitamin E, and selenium for adults and children over one year of age. Those for which an AI has been set include calcium, vitamin D, fluoride, pantothenic acid, biotin, and choline.

Perspective and Prospects

Although these reference values could be used for labeling and fortification guidelines, they are not yet being implemented as such. The current daily value (DV percent) on the nutrition facts labels rely on the 1968 version of the nutrient reference values. The major difficulty in applying the newer reference values for labeling purposes rests on how to choose a "reference" age group or gender. Currently the DV reflect needs for a male adult.

The first nutrient-based guidelines for healthy intake were released in 1941 in the United States, with similar guidelines released in Canada in 1938. Much research has occurred since that time concerning recording and assessing nutrient intake and in determining human requirements. However, the use of these guidelines has always been to assist in planning meals for individuals and groups, including federal assistance programs.

—*Karen Chapman-Novakofski, R.D., L.D.N., Ph.D.*

See also Antioxidants; Beriberi; Carbohydrates; Cholesterol; Digestion; Fiber; Food biochemistry; Food Guide Pyramid; Kwashiorkor; Malnutrition; Nutrition; Obesity; Obesity, childhood; Phytonutrients; Protein; Supplements; Vitamins and minerals.

For Further Information:

Insel, Paul M. *Discovering Nutrition*. 4th ed. Burlington, Mass.: Jones & Bartlett Learning, 2013.

Institute of Medicine, Food and Nutrition Board, Committee on the Use of Dietary Reference Intakes in Nutrition Labeling. *Dietary Reference Intakes. Guiding Principles for Nutrition Labeling and Fortification*. Washington, DC: National Academy Press, 2003.

Institute of Medicine, Food and Nutrition Board, Subcommittee on Interpretation and Uses of Dietary Reference Intakes and the Standing Committee on the Scientific Evaluation of Dietary Reference Intakes. *Dietary Reference Intakes: Applications in Dietary Assessment*. Washington, DC: National Academy Press, 2000.

Institute of Medicine, Food and Nutrition Board, Subcommittee on Interpretation and Uses of Dietary Reference Intakes and the Standing Committee on the Scientific Evaluation of Dietary Reference Intakes. *Dietary Reference Intakes: Applications in Dietary Planning*. Washington, DC: National Academy Press, 2003.

Ross, A. Catharine, et al., eds. *Dietary Reference Intakes for Calcium and Vitamin D*. Washington, DC: National Academies Press, 2011.

United States Department of Agriculture National Agricultural Library. "Dietary Reference Intakes." *USDA*, July 12, 2013.

DiGeorge syndrome
Disease/Disorder

Also known as: Chromosome 22 interstitial deletion, 22q11.2 deletion syndrome

Anatomy or system affected: Glands, heart, immune system, lymphatic system, mouth

Specialties and related fields: Cardiology, genetics, immunology, pediatrics, plastic surgery

Definition: A pediatric syndrome caused by a missing piece of chromosome 22 and characterized by congenital heart defects, the absence or hypoplasia of the thymus and parathyroid glands, cleft palate, and dysmorphic facial features.

Causes and Symptoms

Chromosomes possess two parts. The upper arms are called "p" arms and the lower arms are called "q" arms. Patients with DiGeorge syndrome are missing a tiny interstitial piece inside the long arm of chromosome 22. The specific region inside the long "q" arm is labeled 11.2. Thus, DiGeorge syndrome is also referred to as 22q11.2 deletion syndrome or chromosome 22 interstitial deletion.

Most microdeletions such as these cannot be observed under a microscope because they are so tiny. A molecular cytogenetic test known as fluorescence in situ hybridization (FISH) is used. It includes the use of deoxyribonucleic acid (DNA) probes made from the DiGeorge chromosomal region (DGCR). A green fluorescent probe is used to identify chromosome 22, while a red probe is specific to the DGCR. In DiGeorge syndrome, one of the chromosomes will lack the red fluorescence.

About 93 percent of patients have a spontaneous (de novo) deletion of a 22q11.2, and 7 percent have inherited the deletion from a parent. The very high de novo rate indicates that the deletion recurs with a high frequency as a result of new mutations occurring in the population. This deletion is inherited in an autosomal dominant manner. The offspring of persons with the deletion have a 50 percent chance of inheriting it. This interstitial deletion encompasses about three million base pairs of DNA in the majority of patients. About 90 percent of patients have the same three million base pair deletion, while 10 percent have a 1.5 million base pair deletion. Therefore, the deletion is large enough to contain nearly one hundred genes.

DiGeorge syndrome is initiated by defective embryonic development of the third and fourth pharyngeal pouches during the fifth week of development. These pouches normally become the thymus and the parathyroid glands. In the ab-

<table>
<tr><td colspan="2">

Information on DiGeorge Syndrome

Causes: Chromosomal abnormality resulting in absence of thymus and parathyroid glands

Symptoms: Recurrent viral infections, reduced or absent T lymphocytes, defects in antibody production, congenital heart disease, cleft palate, learning difficulties

Duration: Lifelong

Treatments: Growth hormone, speech therapy, surgery to correct heart defects and cleft palate
</td></tr>
</table>

sence of a thymus, T lymphocyte maturation is stopped at the precell stage. DiGeorge syndrome is one of the most severe forms of deficient T cell immunity. Children with DiGeorge syndrome develop recurrent viral infections and have abnormal cellular immunity, as characterized by severely reduced or absent T lymphocytes. They also have defects in T cell–dependent antibody production. A spectrum of abnormal phenotypes may develop. These defects arise from the absence of key genes that are not available for normal development when a 22q microdeletion is present. Infants with this disease may suffer from congenital heart disease of various types, palatal abnormalities (such as cleft palate), and learning difficulties.

Treatment and Therapy

Children with a 22q11.2 deletion may exhibit a wide spectrum of problems and much variation in the severity of symptoms. A patient with DiGeorge syndrome may have several organs or systems affected. DiGeorge syndrome may result in problems in different body systems, such as the heart or palate, and in cognition, such as learning style. Consequently, a multidisciplinary approach is needed for management of a specific patient.

In the neonatal period, the following clinical and laboratory studies are pursued. The serum is tested for calcium; a low concentration points to the need for supplementation. The lymphocytes are measured; a low absolute count means referral to an immunologist, who will look at T and B cell subsets. A renal ultrasound examination should be performed because of the high incidence of structural renal abnormalities. A chest X-ray is needed to identify thoracic vertebral anomalies. A cardiac evaluation is recommended for all patients with DiGeorge syndrome because possible malformations may include tetralogy of Fallot, ventricular septal defect, interrupted aortic arch, or truncus arteriosus. Pediatric cardiologists are necessary for the treatment and therapy that is needed. An endocrinologist could follow up possible growth hormone deficiencies. Since there is a high incidence of speech and language delay, speech therapy and early educational intervention are highly recommended. All children with the 22q deletion should be seen by a cleft palate team to diagnose problems and schedule surgery if necessary.

Other medical needs of children are met through evaluation by a feeding specialist, especially in the newborn period; a neurologist, for possible seizure disorders or problems with balance; a urologist, for possible kidney problems; and an otorhinolaryngologist (ear, nose, and throat doctor) for problems in this region.

Perspective and Prospects

DiGeorge syndrome is relatively frequent, occurring with a frequency of one in four thousand live births. Therefore, this disorder is a significant health concern in the general population. Since the phenotype associated with it is broad and variable, many types of clinical and laboratory specialists are needed. The medical geneticist is the most likely person to have an overview of the diagnosis. A yearly genetics evaluation is beneficial in answering questions. Parents should be tested to determine their chromosomal status. Genetic counseling could provide individuals and families with information on the nature, inheritance, and implications of DiGeorge syndrome to help them make informed medical and personal decisions. Current and future research using model organisms may help to explain the problems of phenotypic variability in DiGeorge syndrome.

—*Phillip A. Farber, Ph.D.*

See also Birth defects; Cleft lip and palate; Congenital disorders; Congenital heart disease; Genetic counseling; Genetic diseases; Genetics and inheritance; Immune system; Immunodeficiency disorders; Lymphatic system.

For Further Information:

American Academy of Allergy Asthma & Immunology. "DiGeorge Syndrome (DGS)." *AAAAI*, 2013.

Emanuel, Beverly S., et al. "The 22q11.2 Deletion Syndrome." *Advances in Pediatrics* 48 (2001): 33–73.

King, Richard A., Jerome I. Rotter, and Arno G. Motulsky, eds. *The Genetic Basis of Common Diseases*. 2d ed. New York: Oxford UP, 2002.

Maroni, Gustavo. *Molecular and Genetic Analysis of Human Traits*. Malden, Mass.: Blackwell, 2001.

McCoy, Krisha. "DiGeorge Syndrome." *Health Library*, Dec. 11, 2012.

Rimoin, David L., et al., eds. *Emery and Rimoin's Principles and Practice of Medical Genetics*. 5th ed. Philadelphia: Churchill, 2007.

Stocker, J. Thomas, and Louis P. Dehner, eds. *Pediatric Pathology*. 2d ed. Philadelphia: Lippincott, 2001.

Turnpenny, Peter, and Sian Ellard. *Emery's Elements of Medical Genetics*. 13th ed. New York: Churchill, 2007.

DIGESTION

Biology

Anatomy or system affected: Abdomen, gastrointestinal system, intestines, pancreas, stomach

Specialties and related fields: Biochemistry, family medicine, gastroenterology, internal medicine, nutrition, pharmacology

Definition: The chemical breakdown of food materials in the stomach and small intestine and the absorption into the bloodstream of essential nutrients through the intestinal walls.

Key terms:

amino acids: the product of proteins broken down by digestive enzymes; essential for the building of tissue throughout the body

cecum: the dividing passageway between the small intestine and the large intestine, or colon

chyme: partially broken-down food materials that pass from the stomach into the small intestine

dyspepsia: a general term applied to several forms of indigestion

villi: fingerlike projections on the intestinal lining that absorb essential body nutrients after enzymes break down chyme

Structure and Functions

In the most general terms, digestion is a multiple-stage process that begins by breaking down foodstuffs taken in by an organism. Some specialists consider that the actual process of digestion occurs after this breaking-down stage, when essential nutritional elements are absorbed into the body. Even after division of the digestive process into two main functions, there remains a third, by-product stage: disposal by the body of waste material in the form of urine and feces.

Several different vital organs, all contained in the abdominal cavity, contribute either directly or indirectly to the digestive process at each successive stage. Certain imbalances in the functioning of any one of these organs, or a combination, can lead to what is commonly called indigestion. Chronic imbalances in the functioning of any of the key digestive organs—the stomach, small intestine, large intestine (or colon), liver, gallbladder, and pancreas—may indicate symptoms of diseases that are far more serious than mere indigestion.

In a very broad sense, the process of digestion begins even before food that has been chewed and swallowed passes into the stomach. In fact, while chewing is underway, a first stage of glandular activity—the release of saliva by the salivary glands into the food being chewed (a process referred to as intraluminal digestion)—provides a natural lubricant to help propel masticated material down the esophagus. Although the esophagus does not perform a digestive function, its muscular contractions, which are necessary for swallowing, are like a preliminary stage to the muscular operation that begins in the stomach.

The human stomach has two main sections: the baglike upper portion, or fundus, and the lower part, which is twice as large as the fundus, called the antrum. The function of the fundus is essentially to receive and hold foods that reach the stomach via the esophagus, allowing intermittent delivery into the antrum. Here two dynamic elements of the breaking-down process occur, one physical, the other chemical. The muscular tissue surrounding the antrum acts to churn the partially liquefied food in the lower stomach, while a series of what are commonly called gastric juices flow into the mixture held by the stomach.

The most active element that is secreted from special parietal cells in the mucous membranes lining the stomach is hydrochloric acid. The possibility of damage to the stomach lining is minimized (but not removed entirely) first by the chemical reaction between the acid and the mildly alkaline chewed food and second by the presence of other gastric juices in the antrum. Primary among these is the enzyme pepsin, which is secreted by a different set of specialized cells in the gastric lining. Secretions of both hydrochloric acid and pepsin become mixed and interact chemically with food materials, while the antrum itself moves in rhythmic pulses caused by muscular contractions (peristalsis). One of the key functions of pepsin during this stage is to break down protein molecules into shorter molecular strings of less complicated amino acids, which eventually serve as building material for many body tissues.

At a certain point, food materials are sufficiently reduced to pass beyond the antrum into the duodenum, the first section of the small intestine, where a different stage in the digestive process takes place. At this juncture, the partially broken-down food material is referred to as chyme. The transfer of food from one digestive organ to another is actually monitored by a special autonomic nerve, called the vagus nerve, which originates in the medulla at the head of the spinal cord. Although the vagus nerve innervates a number of vital zones in the abdominal cavity, its function here is quite specific: It adjusts the intensity of muscular movement in the stomach wall and thus limits the amount of food passing into the small intestine.

The exact amount of food that is allowed to enter the intestinal tract represents only part of the essential question of balance between agents contributing to the digestive process. The presence of a now slightly acidic food-gastric juice mixture in the duodenum sparks what is called an enterogastric reflex. Two hormones, secretin and cholecystokinin, begin to flow from the mucous membranes of the duodenum. These hormones serve to limit the acidic strength of stomach secretions and trigger reactions in the liver, gallbladder, and pancreas—other key organs that contribute to digestion as the chyme passes through the intestines.

While in the compact, coiled mass of the small intestine (compared to the thicker, but much shorter, colon, or large intestine), food materials, especially proteins, are broken down into one of twenty possible amino acid components by the chemical action of two pancreatic enzymes, trypsinogen and chymotrypsinogen, and two enzymes produced in the intestinal walls themselves, aminopeptidase and dipeptidase. It is interesting to note that the body, which is itself in large part constructed of protein material, has its own mechanism to prevent protein-splitting enzymes from devouring the very organs that produce them. Thus, when they leave the pancreas, both trypsinogen and chymotrypsinogen are inactive compounds. They become active "protein-breakers" only when joined by another enzyme—enterokinase—which is secreted from cells in the wall of the small intestine itself.

Other nutritional components contained in chyme interact chemically with other specialized enzymes that are secreted into the small intestine. Carbohydrate molecules, especially starch, begin to break down when exposed to the enzyme amylase in saliva. This process is intensified greatly when pancreatic amylase flows into the small intestine and mixes with the chyme. The products created when carbohydrates break down are simple sugars, including disaccharides and monosaccharides, especially maltose. As these sugars are all broken down into monosaccharides, a final process that occurs in the wall of the small intestine itself (which contains more specialized enzymes such as maltase, sucrase, and lactase), they become the most rapidly assimilated body nutrients.

The process needed to break down fats is more complicated, since fats are water insoluble and enter the intestine in the form of enzyme-resistant globules. Before the fat-splitting enzyme lipase can be chemically active, bile, a fluid produced by the liver and stored in the gallbladder, must be present. Bile serves to dissolve fat globules into tiny droplets that can be broken down for absorption, like all other nutritive elements, into the body via the epithelial lining of the intestinal wall. Such absorption is locally specialized. Iron and calcium pass through the epithelial lining of the duodenum. Protein, fat, sugars, and vitamins pass through the lining of the jejunum, or middle small intestine. Finally, salt, vitamin B_{12}, and bile salts pass through the lining of the lower small intestine, or ileum.

It is this stage that many scientists consider to be the true process of digestion. Absorption occurs through enterocytes, which are specialized cells located on the surface of the epithelium. The surface of the epithelium is increased substantially by the existence of fingerlike projections called villi. These tiny protrusions are surrounded by the fluid elements of chemically altered food. Specialized enterocyte cells selectively absorb these elements into the capillaries that are inside each of the hundreds of thousands of villi. From the capillaries, the nutrients enter the blood and are carried by the portal vein to the liver. This organ carries out the essential chemical processes that prepare fats, carbohydrates, and proteins for their eventual delivery, through the main bloodstream, to various parts of the body.

Elements that are left after the enzymes in the small intestine have done their work are essentially waste material, or feces. These pass from the small intestine to the large intestine, or colon, through a dividing passageway called the cecum. The disposal of waste materials may or may not be considered to be technically part of the main digestive process.

After essential amounts of water and certain salts are absorbed into the body through the walls of the colon, the remaining waste material is expulsed from the bowels through the rectum and anus. If any prior stage in the digestive process is incomplete or if chemical imbalances have occurred, the first symptoms of indigestion may manifest themselves as bowel movement irregularities.

Disorders and Diseases

Malfunctions in any of the delicate processes that make up digestion can produce symptoms that range from what is commonly called simple indigestion to potentially serious diseases of the gastrointestinal tract. Functional indigestion, or dyspepsia, is one of the most common sources of physical discomfort experienced not only by human beings but by most animals as well. Generally speaking, dyspepsias are not the result of organic disease, but rather of a temporary imbalance in one of the functions described above. There are many possible causes of such an imbalance, including nervous stress and changes in the nature and content of foods eaten.

The most common causes of dyspepsia and their symptoms, although serious enough in chronic cases to require expert medical attention, are far less dangerous than diseases afflicting one of the digestive organs. Such diseases include gallstones, pancreatitis, peptic ulcers (in which excessive acid causes lesions in the stomach wall), and, most serious of all, cancers afflicting any of the abdominal organs.

Dyspepsia may stem from either physical or chemical causes. On the physical side, it is clear that an important part of the digestive process depends on muscular or nerve-related impulses that move partially digested food through the gastrointestinal tract. When, for reasons that are not yet fully understood, the organism fails to coordinate such physical reactions, spasms may occur at several points from the esophagus through to the colon. If extensive, such muscular contractions can create abdominal pains that are symptomatic of at least one category of functional indigestion.

Problems of motility, or physical movement of food materials through the digestive tract, may also cause one common discomfort associated with indigestion: heartburn. This condition occurs when the system fails to move adequate quantities of the mixture of food and gastric juices, including hydrochloric acid, from the stomach into the duodenum. The resultant backup of food forces part of the acidic liquid mass into the esophagus, causing instant discomfort.

Insufficient motility may also cause delays in the movement of feces through the colon, resulting in constipation. Just as the vagus nerve monitors the muscular movements that are necessary to move food from the stomach to the small intestine, an essential gastrocolic reflex, tied to the organism's nervous system, is needed to ensure a constant rhythm in the movement of feces into the rectum for elimination. If this function is delayed (as a result of nervous stress in some individuals, or because of the dilated physical state of the colon in aged persons), food residues become too tightly compressed in the bowels. As the colon continues to carry out its normal last-stage digestive function of reabsorbing essential water from waste material before it is eliminated, the feces become drier and even more compacted, making defecation difficult and sometimes painful.

Most other imbalances in digestive functions are chemical in nature. Highly spiced or unfamiliar foods frequently upset the balance in the body's chemical digestion. Symptoms may appear either in the abdomen itself (in particular, a bloated stomach accompanied by what is commonly called gas, a symptom of chemical disharmony in the digestive process) or in the stool. If the chemical breakdown of chyme is incomplete because of an imbalance in the proportion (either excessive or inadequate) of enzymes secreted into the stomach or intestines, the normal process of absorption will not take place, creating one of a number of symptoms of indigestion.

The most common symptom of indigestion is diarrhea, which can result from a variety of causes. Because movement in the bowels is affected by different nerve signals, some diarrhea attacks may be linked to nonchemical reactions, such as extreme nervousness. Relaxation of the sphincter, however, as well as the rise in the contractile pressure of the lower colon that precedes defecation (the gastroileal reflex), is also affected by the presence of gastrointestinal hormones, particularly gastrin itself. An imbalance in the amount of concentration of such components in the gastrointestinal tract (attributable to incomplete digestive chemistry) tends to relax the bowels to such a degree that elimination cannot be prevented except through determined mental resistance. It is important to note that if diarrhea continues for an extended time, its effect on the body is not simply the loss of essential body nutrients that pass through the bowels without being fully digested; the inability of the colon to reabsorb into the body an adequate proportion of the water content from the feces can lead to dehydration of the organism, especially in infants.

In most areas of the world, there is widespread consensus that treatment of indigestion is a matter of taking over-the-counter drugs whose function is to right the imbalance in some of the chemical processes described above. In theory as well as in practice, such treatments do work, since the basic chemical imbalance, if it is has not extended beyond the point of indigestion (in the case of peptic ulcers, for example), is fairly easily diagnosed, even by pharmacists. Increasingly, however, the public is becoming aware that digestion can be aided, and indigestion avoided, by paying closer attention to dietary habits, particularly the importance of increasing fiber intake to facilitate the digestive process. Critical advances are also being made in knowledge of the potentially harmful effects on digestion of chemical additives to processed foods.

Perspective and Prospects

Historical traces of the medical observation of indigestion, as well as the prescription of remedies, can be found as far back as ancient Egypt. A famous medical text from about 1600 BCE known as the Ebers Papyrus contains suggested remedies (mainly herbal drugs) for digestive ailments, as well as instructions for the use of suppositories to loosen the lower bowel. For centuries, however, such practical advice for treating indigestion was never accompanied by an adequate theoretical conception of the digestion function itself.

In the medieval Western world, many erroneous guidelines for understanding the digestive process were handed down from the works of Galen of Pergamum (129–ca. 199 CE). Galen taught that food material passed from the intestines to the liver, where it was transformed into blood. At this point, a vital life-giving spirit, or "pneuma," gave the blood power to drive the body. Similar misconceptions would continue until, following the work of William Harvey (1578–1657), medical science gained more accurate knowledge of the circulatory function of the bloodstream. By the eighteenth century, rapid advances had been made in studies of the function of the stomach and intestines, notably by the French naturalist René de Réaumur (1683–1757), who demonstrated that food is broken down by gastric juices in the stomach, and by the Italian physiologist Lazzaro Spallanzani (1729–1799), who discovered that the stomach itself is the source of gastric juices.

It was an American army surgeon, William Beaumont (1785–1853), who wrote what became, until well into the twentieth century, the most complete medical guide to digestive functions. Beaumont carried out direct clinical observations of the actions of gastric juices in humans. He also observed the way in which the anticipation of eating can spark not only the secretion of such fluids but also the muscular stimuli that promote motility in the digestive process. Soon after Beaumont's findings were published, the German physiologist Theodor Schwann (1810–1882) first isolated pepsin. Others would show that a variety of enzymes in the gastrointestinal tract are secreted by different organs in the abdomen, notably the pancreas.

—*Byron D. Cannon, Ph.D.*

See also Acid-base chemistry; Acid reflux disease; Bile; Celiac sprue; Chyme; Colitis; Constipation; Crohn's disease; Diarrhea and dysentery; Enzymes; Esophagus; Fiber; Food biochemistry; Food poisoning; Gastroenteritis; Gastroenterology; Gastroenterology, pediatric; Gastrointestinal disorders; Gastrointestinal system; Heartburn; Hirschsprung's disease; Indigestion; Intestines; Irritable bowel syndrome (IBS); Malabsorption; Metabolism; Nutrition; Over-the-counter medications; Peristalsis; Supplements; Ulcer surgery; Ulcers; Vagotomy; Vitamins and minerals.

For Further Information:

Bonci, Leslie. *American Dietetic Association Guide to Better Digestion*. New York: Wiley, 2003.

Carson-DeWitt, Rosalyn. "Diarrhea." *Health Library*, March 4, 2013.

"Indigestion." *MedlinePlus*, February 4, 2011.

Jackson, Gordon, and Philip Whitfield. *Digestion: Fueling the System*. New York: Torstar Books, 1984.

Janowitz, Henry D. *Indigestion: Living Better with Upper Intestinal Problems, from Heartburn to Ulcers and Gallstones*. New York: Oxford University Press, 1994.

Johnson, Leonard R., ed. *Gastrointestinal Physiology*. 7th ed. Philadelphia: Mosby/Elsevier, 2007.

Magee, Donal F., and Arthur F. Dalley. *Digestion and the Structure and Function of the Gut*. Basel, Switzerland: S. Karger, 1986.

Mayo Clinic. *Mayo Clinic on Digestive Health: Enjoy Better Digestion with Answers to More than Twelve Common Conditions*. 2d ed. Rochester, Minn.: Author, 2004.

Scanlon, Valerie, and Tina Sanders. *Essentials of Anatomy and Physiology*. 5th ed. Philadelphia: F. A. Davis, 2007.

Young, Emma. "Alimentary Thinking." *New Scientist* 2895 (December 15, 2012): 38–42.

DIPHTHERIA

Disease/Disorder

Anatomy or system affected: Heart, nervous system, throat

Specialties and related fields: Bacteriology, cardiology, epidemiology, family medicine, microbiology, pediatrics, toxicology

Definition: An acute, contagious disease found primarily in children, associated with toxin production by the bacterium *Corynebacterium diphtheriae*.

Causes and Symptoms

The etiological agent of diphtheria, *Corynebacterium diphtheriae*, is found in some individuals as an inhabitant of

---

Information on Diphtheria

Causes: Toxin production by bacteria
Symptoms: Sore throat, malaise, mild fever, pseudomembrane formation in throat; when systemic, damage to heart, nervous system, or other organs
Duration: Acute
Treatments: Antibiotics (penicillin, erythromycin), antitoxin

---

the nasopharynx (nose and throat). Its symptoms are associated with the production of a toxin. Only those strains of the organism carrying a bacteriophage in a lysogenic state produce the toxin. Spread of diphtheria is generally person to person through respiratory secretions or through contaminated environmental surfaces.

Following an incubation period of several days to a week, symptoms often have a sudden onset and typically include a sore throat, malaise, and a mild fever. The disease is further characterized by an exudative, pseudomembrane formation on the mucous surface of the throat, which results from replication of the organism in the pharynx or surrounding areas. The pseudomembrane can become quite thick and may cause respiratory stress through obstruction of the breathing passages. Toxin is secreted into the bloodstream, where its presence can result in damage to the heart, nervous system, or other organs. Diagnosis is based upon a combination of symptoms, as well as isolation of the organism in a throat culture.

A less common form of diphtheria may be observed on skin surfaces. It contains bacteria that can be spread through contaminated environmental surfaces. Infection generally occurs through small cuts in the skin. Cutaneous diphtheria is characterized by an ulcer that heals slowly. If the organism is a strain that produces toxin, then systemic damage may result.

Treatment and Therapy

Most diphtheria infections respond to antibiotics, either a single dose of penicillin or a seven-day or ten-day course of erythromycin. Since symptoms are associated with toxin production, the administration of antitoxin is critical to early treatment. Once toxin has been incorporated into the target, cell death is irreversible. Antibiotic treatment, however, does result in the elimination of the organism and the termination of further toxin production.

Vaccination with diphtheria toxoid, an inactivated form of the toxin, has proven effective in immunization against the disease. Prophylaxis is generally started early in childhood as part of the trivalent DPT (diphtheria, pertussis, tetanus) series. Boosters are recommended at ten-year intervals.

Perspective and Prospects

Introduction of the diphtheria vaccine in the first decades of the twentieth century served to reduce significantly the incidence of the disease in the West. The use of antibiotic therapy further reduced the fatality rate associated with this disease, which ranged from 30 to 50 percent at its peak. Diphtheria is almost unknown in the United States in the twenty-first century, with only five reported cases in the first decade, according to the Centers for Disease Control. The disease still exists as a childhood scourge in the developing world, although fewer than 5,000 cases were reported worldwide in 2011, according to the World Health Organization.

—*Richard Adler, Ph.D.*

See also Antibiotics; Bacterial infections; Bacteriology; Childhood infectious diseases; Immunization and vaccination; Sore throat.

For Further Information:
Atkinson, William, Charles Wolfe, and Jennifer Hamborsky, eds. "Diphtheria." In *Epidemiology and Prevention of Vaccine-Preventable Diseases*. 12th ed. Washington, D.C.: Centers for Disease Control and Prevention, 2011.
Grob, Gerald N. *The Deadly Truth: A History of Disease in America.* Cambridge, Mass.: Harvard University Press, 2002.
Martin, Julie J. "Diphtheria." *Health Library*, January 7, 2013.
Parker, James N., and Philip M. Parker, eds. *The Official Patient's Sourcebook on Diphtheria.* San Diego, Calif.: Icon Health, 2002.
World Health Organization. "Diphtheria." *World Health Organization*, September 27, 2012.

Disease

Disease/Disorder
Anatomy or system affected: All
Specialties and related fields: All
Definition: A morbid (pathological) process with a characteristic set of symptoms that may affect the entire body or any of its parts; the cause, pathology, and course of a disease may be known or unknown.

Key terms:
diagnosis: the art of distinguishing one disease from another
lesion: any pathologic or traumatic discontinuity of tissue or loss of function of a body part
pathology: the study of the essential nature of disease, especially as it relates to the structural and functional changes that are caused by that disease
prognosis: a forecast regarding the probable cause and result of an attack of disease
syndrome: a congregation of a set of signs and symptoms that characterize a particular disease process, but without a specific etiology or a constant lesion

Types of Disease

It is difficult to answer the question "What is disease?" To the patient, disease means discomfort and disharmony with the environment. To the treating physician or surgeon, it means a set of signs and symptoms. To the pathologist, it means one or more structural changes in body tissues, called lesions, which may be viewed with or without the aid of magnifying lenses.

The study of lesions, which are the essential expression of disease, forms part of the modern science of pathology. Pathology had its beginnings in the morgue and the autopsy room, where investigations into the cause of death led to the appreciation of "morbid anatomy"—at first by gross (naked-eye) examination and later microscopically. Much later, the investigation of disease moved from the cold autopsy room to the patient's bedside, from the dead body to the living body, on which laboratory tests and biopsies are performed for the purpose of establishing a diagnosis and addressing proper treatment.

Diagnosis is the art of determining not only the character of the lesion but also its etiology, or cause. Because so much of this diagnostic work is done in laboratories, the term "laboratory medicine" has increased in popularity. The explosion in high technology has expanded the field of laboratory medicine tremendously. The diagnostic laboratory today is highly automated and sophisticated, containing a team of laboratory technologists and scientific researchers rather than a single pathologist.

The lesions laid bare by the pathologist usually bear an obvious relation to the symptoms, as in the gross lesions of acute appendicitis, the microscopic lesions in poliomyelitis, or even the chromosomal lesions in genetically inherited conditions such as Down syndrome. Yet there may be lesions without symptoms, as in early cancer or "silent" diseases such as tuberculosis. There may also be symptoms without obvious lesions, as in the so-called psychosomatic diseases, functional disorders, and psychiatric illnesses. It is likely that future research will reveal the presence of "biochemical lesions" in these cases. The presence of lesions distinguishes organic disease, in which there are gross or microscopic pathologic changes in an organ, from functional disease, in which there is a disturbance of function without a corresponding obvious organic lesion. Although most diagnoses consist largely of naming the lesion (such as cancer of the lung or a tooth abscess), diseases should truly be considered in the light of disordered function rather than altered structure. Scientists are searching beyond the presence of obvious lesions in tissues and cells to the submicroscopic, molecular, and biochemical alterations affecting the chemistry of cells.

Not every disease has a specific etiology. A syndrome is a complex of signs and symptoms with no specific etiology or constant lesion. It results from interference at some point with a chain of body processes, causing impairment of body function in one or more systems. A specific biochemical molecular derangement caused by yet undiscovered agents is usually found. An example is acquired immunodeficiency syndrome (AIDS), for which a specific human immunodeficiency virus (HIV) agent is now accepted as the etiologic agent.

Some diseases have an acute (sudden) onset and run a relatively short course, as with acute tonsillitis or the common cold. Others run a long, protracted course, as with tuberculosis and rheumatoid arthritis; these are called chronic illnesses. The healthy body is in a natural state of readiness to combat disease, and thus there is a natural tendency to recover from disease. This is especially true in acute illness, in which inflammation tends to heal with full resolution of structure and function. Sometimes, however, healing does not occur, and the disease overwhelms the body and causes death. Therefore, a patient with acute pneumonia may have a full recovery, with complete healing and resolution of structure and function, or may die. The outcome of disease can vary between the extremes of full recovery and death and can run a chronic, protracted course eventually leading to severe loss of function. The accurate diagnosis of disease is essential for its treatment and prognosis, a forecast of what may be expected to happen.

There are four aspects to the study of disease. The first is etiology, or cause; for example, several viruses cause the common cold. The second is pathogenesis, or course, which refers to the sequence of events in the body that occurs in response to injury and the method of the lesion's production and development. The relation of an etiologic agent to disease, of cause to effect, is not always as simple a matter as it is in most acute illnesses; for example, a herpesvirus causes the development of fever blisters. In many illnesses, indeed in most chronic illnesses, the concept of one agent causing one disease is an oversimplification. In tuberculosis, for example, the causative agent is a characteristic slender microbe called tubercle bacillus (*Mycobacterium tuberculosis*). Many people may be exposed to and inhale the tuberculosis bacteria, but only a few will get the disease; also, the bacteria may lurk in the body for years and become clinically active only as a result of an unrelated, stressful situation that alters the body's immunity, such as prolonged strain, malnutrition, or another infection. In investigating the causation and pathogenesis of disease, several factors—such as heredity, sex, environment, nutrition, immunity, and age—must be considered. That is why there is no simple answer to questions such as "Does cigarette smoking cause cancer?" and "Does a cholesterol-rich diet cause hardening of the blood vessels (atherosclerosis)?" The third aspect to the study of disease relates to morphologic and structural changes associated with the functional alterations in cells and tissues that are characteristic of the disease. These are the gross and microscopic findings that allow the pathologist to establish a diagnosis. The fourth aspect to disease study is the evaluation of functional abnormalities and their clinical significance; the nature of the morphologic changes and their distribution in different organs or tissues influence normal function and determine the clinical features, signs and symptoms, and course and outcome (prognosis) of disease.

All forms of tissue injury start with molecular and structural changes in cells. Cells are the smallest living units of tissues and organs. Along with their substructural components, they are the seat of disease. Cellular pathology is the study of disease as it relates to the origins, molecular mechanisms, and structural changes of cell injury.

The normal cell is similar to a factory. It is confined to a fairly narrow range of function and structure dictated by its genetic code, the constraints of neighboring cells, the availability of and access to nutrition, and the disposal of its waste products. It is said to be in a "steady state," able to handle normal physiologic demands and to respond by adapting to other excessive or strenuous demands (such as the muscle enlargement seen in bodybuilders) to achieve a new equilibrium with a sustained workload. This type of adaptive response is called hypertrophy. Conversely, atrophy is an adaptive response to decreased demand, with a resulting diminished size and function.

If the limits of these adaptive responses are exceeded, or if no adaptive response is possible, a sequence of events follows that results in cell injury. Cell injury is reversible up to a certain point, but if the stimulus persists or is severe, then the cell suffers irreversible injury and eventual death. For example, if the blood supply to the heart muscle is cut off for only a few minutes and then restored, the heart muscle cells will experience injury but can recover and function normally. If the blood flow is not restored until one hour later, however, the cells will die.

Whether specific types of stress induce an adaptive response, a reversible injury, or cell death depends on the nature and severity of the stress and on other inherent, variable qualities of the cell itself. The causes of cell injury are many and range from obvious physical trauma, as in automobile accidents, to a subtle, genetic lack of enzymes or hormones, as in diabetes mellitus. Broadly speaking, the causes of cell injury and death can be grouped into the following categories: hypoxia, or a decrease in the delivery of available oxygen; physical agents, as with mechanical and thermal injuries; chemical poisons, such as carbon monoxide and alcohol, tobacco, and other addictive drugs; infectious agents, such as viruses and bacteria; immunological and allergic reactions, as with certain sensitivities; genetic defects, as with sickle cell disease; and nutritional imbalances, such as severe malnutrition and vitamin deficiencies or nutritional excesses predisposing a patient to heart disease and atherosclerosis.

Causes of Disease

By far the most common cause of disease is infection, especially by bacteria. Certain forms of animal life known as animal parasites may also live in the body and produce disease; parasitic diseases are common in low-income societies and countries. Diseases can also be caused by viruses, forms of living matter so minute that they cannot be seen with the most powerful light microscope; they are visible, however, with the electron microscope. Viruses have attracted much attention for their role in many diseases, including cancer.

Bacteria, or germs, can be divided into three morphologic groups: cocci, which are round; bacilli, which are rod-shaped; and spirilla or spirochetes, which are spiral-shaped, like a corkscrew. Bacteria produce disease either by their presence in tissues or by their production of toxins (poisons). They cause inflammation and either act on surrounding tissues, as in an abscess, or are carried by the bloodstream to other distant organs. Strep throat is an example of a local infection by cocci—in this case, streptococci. Some dysenteries and travelers" diarrheas are caused by coliform bacilli. Syphilis is an example of a disease caused by a spirochete. The great epidemics of history, such as bubonic plague and cholera, have been caused by bacteria, as are tuberculosis, leprosy, typhoid, gas gangrene, and many others. Bacterial infections are treatable with antibiotics, such as penicillin.

Viruses, on the other hand, are not affected by antibiotics; they infect and live within the cell itself and are therefore protected. Viruses cause a wide variety of diseases. Some, such as many childhood diseases, the measles, and the common cold, run a few days" course. Others, such as poliomyelitis and AIDS, can cause serious body impairment. Still others are probably involved in causing cancer and such diseases as multiple sclerosis.

Of the many physical agents causing injury, trauma is the most obvious; others relate to external temperatures that are either too high or too low. A high temperature may produce local injury, such as a burn, or general disease, such as heatstroke. Heatstroke results from prolonged direct exposure to the sun (sunstroke) or from very high temperatures, so that the heat-regulating mechanism of the body becomes paralyzed. The internal body temperature shoots up to alarming heights, and collapse, coma, and even death may result. Low temperatures can cause local frostbite or general hypothermia, which can also lead to death.

Other forms of physical agents causing injury are radiation and atmospheric pressure. Increased atmospheric pressure can cause the "bends," a decompression sickness that can affect deep-sea divers. The pressure of the water causes inert gases, such as nitrogen, to be dissolved in the blood plasma. If the diver passes too rapidly from a high to a normal atmospheric pressure, the excessive nitrogen is released, forming gas bubbles in the blood. These tiny bubbles can cause the blockage of small vessels of the brain and result in brain damage. The same problem can occur in high-altitude aviators unless the airplane is pressurized.

The study of chemical poisoning, or toxicology, as a cause of disease is a large and specialized field. Poisons may be introduced into the body by accident (especially in young children), in the course of suicide or homicide, and as industrial pollution. Lead poisoning is a danger because of the use of lead in paints and soldering. Acids and carbon monoxide are emitted into the atmosphere by industry, and various chemicals are dumped into the ground and water. Such environmental damage will eventually affect plants, livestock, and humans.

Hypoxia (lack of oxygen) is probably the most common cause of cell injury, and it may also be the ultimate mechanism of cell death by a wide variety of physical, biological, and chemical agents. Loss of adequate blood and oxygen supply to a body part, such as a leg, is called ischemia. If the blood loss is very severe, the result is hypoxia or anoxia. This condition may also result from narrowing of the blood vessels, called atherosclerosis. If this narrowing occurs in the artery of the leg, as may be seen in patients with advanced diabetes, then the tissues of the foot will eventually die, a condition known as gangrene. An even more critical example of ischemia is blockage of the coronary arteries of the heart, resulting in a myocardial infarction (heart attack), with damage to the heart muscle. Similarly, severe blockage of arteries to the brain can cause a stroke.

Nutritional diseases can be caused either by an excessive intake and storage of foodstuffs, as in extreme obesity, or by a deficiency. Obesity is a complex condition often associated with hereditary tendencies and hormonal imbalances. The deficiency conditions are many. Starvation and malnutrition can occur because of intestinal illnesses that prevent the delivery of food to the blood (malabsorption) or because of debilitating diseases such as advanced cancer. Even more important than general malnutrition as a cause of disease is a deficiency of essential nutrients such as minerals, vitamins, and other trace elements. Iron deficiency causes anemia, and calcium deficiency causes osteoporosis (bone fragility). Vitamin deficiencies are also numerous, and deficiency of the trace element iodine causes a thyroid condition called goiter.

Genetic defects as a cause of cellular injury and disease are of major interest to many researchers. The results of genetic disorders may be as visible as the physical characteristics seen in patients with Down syndrome or as subtle as molecular alterations in the coding of the hemoglobin molecule that causes sickle cell disease.

Cellular injuries and diseases can be induced by immune mechanisms. The anaphylactic reaction to a foreign protein, such as a bee sting or drug, can actually cause death. In the autoimmune diseases, such as lupus erythematosus, the immune system turns against the cellular components of the very body that it is supposed to protect.

Finally, neoplastic diseases, or cancers, are presently of unknown etiology. Some are innocuous growths, while others are highly lethal. Diagnosing cancer and determining its precise nature can be an elaborate, and elusive, process. The methods involve clinical observations and laboratory tests; a biopsy of the involved organ may be taken and analyzed.

Perspective and Prospects

It is sometimes said that the nature of disease is changing and that more people are dying of heart failure and cancer than was once the case. This does not mean that these diseases have actually become more common, although more people do die from them. This increase is attributable to a longer life span and vastly improved diagnostic methods.

For primitive humans, there were no diseases, only patients stricken by evil; therefore, magic was the plausible recourse. Magic entails recognition of the principle of causality—that, given the same predisposing conditions, the same results will follow. In a profound sense, magic is early science. In ancient Egypt, priests assumed the role of healers. Unlike magic, religion springs from a different source. Here the system is based on the achievement of results against, or in spite of, a regular sequence of events. Religion heals with miracles and antinaturals that require the violation of causality. The purely religious concept of disease, as an expression of the wrath of gods, became embodied in many religious traditions.

The ancient Greeks are credited with attempts at introducing reason to the study of disease by asking questions about the nature of things and considering the notion of health as a harmony, as the adjustment of such opposites as high and low, hot and cold, and dry and moist. Disease, therefore, was a disharmony of the four elements that make up life: earth, air, fire, and water. This concept was refined by Galen in the second century and became dogma throughout the Dark Ages until the Renaissance, when the seat of disease was finally assigned to organs within the body itself through autopsy studies. Much later, in the nineteenth century, the principles espoused by French physiologist Claude Bernard were introduced, whereby disease was considered not a thing but a process that distorts normal physiologic and anatomic features. The nineteenth-century German pathologist Rudolf Virchow emphasized the same principle—that disease is an alteration of life's processes—by championing the concept of cellular pathology, identifying the cell as the smallest unit of life and as the seat of disease.

As new diseases are discovered and old medical mysteries deciphered, as promising new medicinal drugs and vaccines are tested and public health programs implemented, the age-old goal of medicine as a healing art seems to be closer at hand.

—*Victor H. Nassar, M.D.*

See also Centers for Disease Control and Prevention (CDC); Childhood infectious diseases; Dental diseases; Diagnosis; Environmental diseases; Gallbladder diseases; Genetic diseases; Infection; Insect-borne diseases; Motor neuron diseases; National Institutes of Health (NIH); Parasitic diseases; Pathology; Prion diseases; Prognosis; Protozoan diseases; Pulmonary diseases; Sexually transmitted diseases (STDs); Signs and symptoms; Syndrome; Zoonoses; *specific diseases.*

For Further Information:
Biddle, Wayne. *A Field Guide to Germs.* 2d ed. New York: Anchor Books, 2002.
Bliss, Michael. *The Making of Modern Medicine: Turning Points in the Treatment of Disease.* Chicago: University of Chicago Press, 2011.
Boyd, William. *Boyd's Introduction to the Study of Disease.* 11th ed. Philadelphia: Lea & Febiger, 1992.
Frank, Steven A. *Immunology and Evolution of Infectious Disease.* Princeton, N.J.: Princeton University Press, 2002.
Grist, Norman R., et al. *Diseases of Infection: An Illustrated Textbook.* 2d ed. New York: Oxford University Press, 1992.
Hart, Michael N., and Agnes G. Loeffler. *Introduction to Human Disease.* Burlington, Mass.: Jones & Bartlett, 2011.
Kumar, Vinay, Abul K. Abbas, and Nelson Fausto, eds. *Robbins and Cotran Pathologic Basis of Disease.* 8th ed. Philadelphia: Saunders/Elsevier, 2010.
McCance, Kathryn L., and Sue M. Huether. *Pathophysiology: The Biologic Basis for Disease in Adults and Children.* 6th ed. St. Louis, Mo.: Mosby/Elsevier, 2010.
Shaw, Michael, ed. *Everything You Need to Know About Diseases.* Springhouse, Pa.: Springhouse Press, 1996.
Strauss, James, and Ellen Strauss. *Viruses and Human Disease.* 2d ed. Boston: Academic Press/Elsevier, 2008.
World Health Organization. "Disease Outbreaks." *World Health Organization,* 2013.

DISK REMOVAL

Procedure

Anatomy or system affected: Back, bones, nervous system, spine

Specialties and related fields: General surgery, neurology, orthopedics, physical therapy

Definition: A surgical procedure used to remove intervertebral disks that are compressing nerves that enter and exit the spinal cord.

Key terms:

cervical vertebrae: the first seven bones of the spinal column, located in the neck

disk prolapse: the protrusion (herniation) of intervertebral disk material, which may press on spinal nerves

intervertebral disks: flattened disks of fibrocartilage that separate the vertebrae and allow cushioned flexibility of the spinal column

lumbar vertebrae: the five bones of the spinal column in the lower back, which experience the greatest stress in the spine

spinal cord: a column of nervous tissue housed in the vertebral column that carries messages to and from the brain

Indications and Procedures

A relatively common disorder that causes lower back and sometimes leg pain is the herniation or prolapse of an intervertebral disk in the lower back. These disks are made of cartilage and serve to separate the bones that make up the vertebral column. The spinal cord is located within the bony structure of the vertebrae and has nerves which enter and exit between these bones. These sensory and motor nerves must pass alongside the intervertebral disks. When a disk's jellylike center bulges out through a weakened area of the firmer outer core, the disk is said to be herniated or prolapsed. This may compress the spinal cord or the nerve roots and yield such symptoms as interference with muscle strength or pain and numbness of the lower back and leg.

More than 90 percent of disk prolapses occur in the lumbar region of the back, but they may also occur in the cervical vertebrae. Occasionally, disk herniation is caused by improper lifting of heavy objects, sudden twisting of the spinal column, or trauma to the back or neck. More typically, however, a prolapsed disk develops gradually as the patient ages and the intervertebral disks degenerate.

To diagnose a prolapsed disk, a physician will likely want to visualize the vertebrae and spinal cord using X rays, computed tomography (CT) scans, or magnetic resonance imaging (MRI). Once diagnosed, most cases can be treated with analgesics, muscle relaxants (such as cyclobenzaprine and methocarbamol), and physical therapy. If the symptoms recur, however, it may be necessary to have the protruding portion of the disk or the whole disk surgically removed. This procedure usually requires that the patient have general anesthesia and remain hospitalized for several days.

For a lumbar procedure, the patient is anesthetized and placed on the operating room table in a modified kneeling position, with the abdomen suspended and the legs placed over the end of the table. The lower back is then prepared for a sterile procedure, and the surgeon makes an incision in the middle of the back along the spine. The surrounding tissues are retracted, and the vertebrae are exposed. At this time, the surgeon must make a careful dissection of the tissues in order to identify the affected nerves and intervertebral disk. Once the prolapsed disk is found, the physician will cut away the fragment of the disk impinging on the nerve. It is important that all free fragments be removed, as these could cause symptoms at a later time. Often, the surgeon must remove some of the vertebrae to gain access to the disk. This is known as a laminectomy.

Uses and Complications

Because the vertebral column houses the spinal cord, any surgical manipulation of this area must be approached with extreme caution. Very large arteries (the aorta) and veins (the vena cava) lie adjacent to the spinal column, and accidental cuts can lead to rapid blood loss. The spinal cord is surrounded by a covering called the meninges, which helps to protect the cord and which contains the cerebral spinal fluid. Trauma to the meninges may cause the fluid to leak out or lead to meningitis (inflammation of the meninges). One surgical approach to reduce the adverse affects of a lesion on the meninges is to use some of the patient's fat to pack the leak and help prevent scarring. Patients with operative trauma to the meninges may complain of headache, which usually decreases in severity as the lesion heals.

Other complications that may arise include infections in approximately 3 percent of patients, thromboembolism in less than 1 percent, and death in about one patient per 1,000. Unfortunately, one of the major long-term complications reported in the study involved a worsening of symptoms after surgery.

Perspective and Prospects

Even with some potential complications, disk removal typically has a favorable outcome, although this varies somewhat depending on the patient, the treatment method, and what the patient and physician consider to be a good result. Typically, favorable outcomes range from 50 to 95 percent. The number of patients who need a second operation ranges from 4 to 25 percent.

Health care professionals are beginning to emphasize the importance of prevention of back pain. Educating patients on proper lifting techniques, such as bending the legs rather than the back and avoiding twisting, will reduce the potential for damage to the intervertebral disks. Individuals who are overweight are also at risk for developing lower back pain because of the added stress to the lumbar spine, as well as because of their relatively weak abdominal muscles. The abdominal muscles are important in stabilizing and supporting the lower back. Exercises that help strengthen these muscles are recommended for a weight-reducing exercise and diet program. Patients who must sit for long periods of time are also at risk for lower back pain. These people should take several quick breaks to stand and stretch, which reduces the constant stress on the lumbar spine.

—Matthew Berria, Ph.D.,
and Douglas Reinhart, M.D.

See also Back pain; Bone disorders; Bones and the skeleton; Braces, orthopedic; Laminectomy and spinal fusion; Meningitis; Orthopedic surgery; Orthopedics; Slipped disk; Spinal cord disorders; Spine, vertebrae, and disks.

For Further Information:

Aminoff, Michael J. "Nervous System." In *Current Medical Diagnosis and Treatment 2007*, edited by Lawrence M. Tierney, Jr., Stephen J. McPhee, and Maxine A. Papadakis. New York: McGraw-Hill Medical, 2006. Print.

Bradford, David S., and Thomas A. Zdeblick, eds. *The Spine*. 2d ed. Philadelphia: Lippincott Williams & Wilkins, 2004. Print.

Canale, S. Terry, ed. *Campbell's Operative Orthopaedics*. 11th ed. 4 vols. St. Louis, Mo.: Mosby/Elsevier, 2008. Print.

"Diskectomy." *MedlinePlus*, June 7, 2012.

Filler, Aaron G. *Do You Really Need Back Surgery? A Surgeon's Guide to Back and Neck Pain and How to Choose Your Treatment*. Rev. ed. New York: Oxford University Press, 2007. Print.

Haldeman, Scott, William H. Kirkaldy-Willis, and Thomas N. Bernard, Jr. *Atlas of Back Pain*. Boca Raton, Fla.: Parthenon, 2002. Print.

Leikin, Jerrold B., and Martin S. Lipsky, eds. *American Medical Association Complete Medical Encyclopedia*. New York: Random House Reference, 2003. Print.

Poppert, Elizabeth M., and Kornelia Kulig. "Rehabilitation Following Lumbar Diskectomy." *Physical Therapy* 93, no. 5 (May 2013): 591–96.

Scholten, Amy. "Herniated Disc." *Health Library*, September 30, 2011.

DISLOCATION. *See* FRACTURE AND DISLOCATION.

DISSEMINATED INTRAVASCULAR COAGULATION (DIC)

Disease/Disorder

Also known as: Consumption coagulopathy

Anatomy or system affected: Blood, blood vessels, circulatory system, immune system

Specialties and related fields: Hematology, internal medicine, neonatology, obstetrics, oncology

Definition: A hemorrhagic disorder that occurs as a complication of several different disease states and results from abnormally initiated and accelerated blood clotting.

Key terms:

acute DIC: a disorder of the blood-clotting mechanism that develops within hours of an initial attack on an underlying body system

chronic DIC: a disorder of the blood-clotting mechanism that persists in a suppressed state until a coagulation disorder worsens

coagulation: the process of blood clot formation

coagulation cascade: the series of steps starting with the activation of the intrinsic or extrinsic pathways of coagulation and proceeding through the common pathway of coagulation leading to the formation of fibrin clots

ecchymosis: bleeding into the skin, subcutaneous tissue, or mucous membranes, resulting in bruising

hemostasis: the stopping of blood flow through the blood vessels, usually as a result of blood clotting

petechiae: round pinpoint hemorrhages in the skin

platelets: cells, found in the blood of all mammals, that are involved in the coagulation of blood and the contraction of blood clots

---

Information on Disseminated Intravascular Coagulation (DIC)

Causes: Accelerated blood clotting that may be a complication of bacterial, fungal, parasitic, or viral infections; inflammatory bowel disease; pregnancy; cancer; surgery; major trauma; burns; heatstroke; shock; transplant rejection; drug use; snakebite

Symptoms: Hemorrhaging, bruising, bleeding of mucosa, depletion or absence of platelets and clotting factors in blood

Duration: Acute or chronic, depending on cause

Treatments: Dependent on underlying condition; anticoagulants (heparin, antithrombin III), antifibrinolytics (Amicar, Cykokapron), blood products (fresh frozen plasma, cryoprecipitate, red blood cells, platelets)

---

thrombocytopenia: a markedly decreased number of platelets in the blood

thromboembolism: the obstruction of a blood vessel with a clot that has broken loose from its site of origin

Causes and Symptoms

Disseminated intravascular coagulation (DIC) is a disorder that occurs as a life-threatening complication of many different conditions. It is most commonly seen as a complication of bacterial, fungal, parasitic, or viral infections; inflammatory bowel disease; pregnancy; cancer; surgery; major trauma; burns; heatstroke; shock; transplant rejection; toxicity resulting from recreational drug use; or snakebite. It can occur as either an acute or a chronic condition, depending on the underlying cause.

In both forms, DIC involves the systemic activation of the hemostasis system. In its acute form, DIC involves hemorrhaging, the development of ecchymoses, bleeding of the mucosa, and depletion or absence of platelets and clotting factors in the blood. In the most severe cases, it is accompanied by extensive consumption of the proteins involved in coagulation, significant deposits of fibrin in the vasculature and organs, and bleeding that may lead to organ failure and death. In its chronic form, it is more subtle and usually includes thromboembolism along with activation of the coagulation system.

In acute DIC, the introduction of tissue factors into the circulation (from injury, surgery, or tissue necrosis), stagnant blood flow (from shock or cardiac arrest), or the presence of infectious agents leads to systemic activation of the coagulation system. A massive clotting cascade is triggered and leads to the formation of blood clots, possibly compromising the blood supply to major organs, and simultaneously to the exhaustion of platelets and coagulation factors, resulting in hemorrhaging.

Thus, DIC occurs when endothelial cells or monocytes are damaged by toxic substances. When these cells are injured, they release tissue factor on the surface of the cell, which in turn triggers the hemostasis system, activating a coagulation cascade. Thrombin accumulates rapidly, and fibrin is produced in large quantities and is deposited in the microvasculature, leading to blood clots throughout the capillary system. This clot formation leads rapidly to the depletion of platelets and coagulation factors throughout the body. Simultaneously, thrombin activates fibrinolytic pathways that release anticoagulants and dissolve the clots by turning them into fibrin split products, further contributing to uncontrollable bleeding. In chronic DIC, these events occur more slowly, allowing compensation to take place.

The diagnosis of DIC is based on clinical signs and laboratory findings. In acute DIC, the symptoms include multiple bleeding sites, the development of petechiae on the skin, ecchymoses of the skin and mucous membranes, visceral hemorrhaging, and the development of ischemic tissue. In chronic DIC, symptoms will include deep vein or arterial thrombosis or embolism, superficial venous thrombosis (especially in the absence of varicose veins), multiple and simultaneous thrombus sites, or serial thrombotic episodes. Laboratory findings indicative of DIC are decreased platelet count, prolonged prothrombin time (PT), activated partial thromboplastin time (APTT), and thrombin time along with decreased fibrinogen levels and increased fibrin-fibrinogen degradation product (FDP) levels. Peripheral smears will show the presence of schistocytes (fragments of red blood cells).

Treatment and Therapy

The treatment of either the acute or the chronic form of DIC is based on the etiology and pathophysiology of the underlying clinical condition. Aside from the treatment of the underlying disorder, acute DIC requires aggressive treatment of the bleeding through the use of anticoagulants (such as heparin or antithrombin III) and antifibrinolytics (aminocaproic acid or tranexamic acid) as well as the administration of blood products, including fresh frozen plasma, cryoprecipitate, red blood cells, and platelets. The prognosis is determined by the underlying condition that led to DIC as well as the severity of the DIC. Follow-up care for those who survive is provided by a primary physician, for the underlying disorder, and by a hematologist.

Perspective and Prospects

Historically, disseminated intravascular coagulation has always been considered a secondary disease resulting as a consequence of some underlying disorder. Thus, DIC has always referred to the secondary activation of the coagulation system as a result of an underlying problem. The condition occurs with equal frequency in males and females and does not appear to be related to age.

While DIC is generally categorized, treated, and evaluated based on the pathophysiology of the underlying disorder, researcher Rodger L. Bick has proposed a DIC scoring system to assess the severity of the coagulation disorder as well as the effectiveness of the treatment modalities. New treatment modalities, such as the use of recombinant activated protein C, are being investigated in large multicenter clinical trials.

—*Robin Kamienny Montvilo, R.N., Ph.D.*

See also Bleeding; Blood and blood disorders; Circulation; Hematology; Hematology, pediatric; Hemorrhage; Ischemia; Thrombosis and thrombus.

For Further Information:

A.D.A.M. Medical Encyclopedia. "Bleeding Disorders." *MedlinePlus*, February 28 2011.

Bick, Roger L. "Disseminated Intravascular Coagulation: Objective Criteria for Diagnosis and Management." *Medical Clinics of North America* 78 (1994): 511–43.

Kasper, Dennis L., et al., eds. *Harrison's Principles of Internal Medicine.* 16th ed. New York: McGraw-Hill, 2005.

Kellicker, Patricia Griffin. "Disseminated Intravascular Coagulation." *HealthLibrary*, April 11, 2013.

Lichtman, Marshall A., et al., eds. *Williams Hematology.* 7th ed. New York: McGraw-Hill, 2006.

National Heart, Lung, and Blood Institute. "What Is Disseminated Intravascular Coagulation?" *National Institutes of Health*, November 2, 2011.

Diuretics

Treatment

Also known as: Water pill

Anatomy or system affected: Bladder, blood, blood vessels, cells, circulatory system, heart, kidneys, urinary system

Specialties and related fields: Cardiology, critical care, internal medicine, nephrology, nursing, pharmacology, urology

Definition: Prescription medications used to prevent passive reabsorption of water in the kidney unit (nephron), resulting in an increased urinary output.

Key terms:

acid-base balance: the balance between acids (proton donors) and bases (proton acceptors) in the blood that normally maintains the blood pH (hydrogen ion concentration) between 7.35 and 7.45; components of the acid-base system include the lungs, blood buffer system, and kidneys

aldosterone: a hormone produced by the adrenal gland that helps regulate the salt (sodium) and water balance in the body by increasing both sodium and water retention

diuresis: increased formation and excretion of urine

electrolyte: minerals (sodium, potassium, calcium, magnesium, chloride, bicarbonate) that carry an electrical charge and assist in body functions (metabolic processes, nerve conduction, heart rhythm and contraction, and muscle contraction)

filtrate: water and small solute molecules filtered from the blood by the glomerulus of the nephron

nephron: the functional unit of the kidney consisting of the glomerulus, the proximal convoluted tubule, the loop of Henle, and the distal convoluted tubule; the nephron produces urine

osmotic: an agent resulting in osmosis, the movement of a solvent (such as water) through a semipermeable membrane (such as a cell wall) from an area of lower solute concentration to an area of higher solute concentration; aim is to equalize the solvent-solute ratio (concentration) on both sides of the membrane

ototoxic: creating damage resulting in hearing loss; the loss may or may not be reversible when the damaging agent is removed

reabsorption: in the kidney, the process of reabsorbing water and electrolytes from the filtrate and returning them to the bloodstream (circulation)

solute: the dissolved particles in a solution; common solutes in humans are the electrolytes

Indications and Procedures

The basic functional unit of the kidney is the nephron. It consists of four regions: glomerulus, proximal convoluted tubule, loop of Henle, and distal convoluted tubule. The purpose of the nephron is to filter waste products from the blood and excrete these products as urine. Blood filtering occurs in the glomerulus. In the adult, approximately 180 liters of filtrate is produced daily. The purpose of the other three segments of the nephron are to reabsorb the majority of water and electrolytes from the filtrate and return these items to circulation, leaving approximately 1.8 liters to be discarded as urine.

In certain disease states it becomes necessary to enhance urine production to relieve symptoms and prevent morbidity (illness) or mortality (death). Increased urine production can be accomplished by the administration of a category of drugs known as diuretics. Diuretics are prescription medications that work by blocking the reabsorption of solutes, especially salt (sodium) and water, which passively follows sodium. Thus, solutes and water are excreted from the body rather than being returned to circulation. Diuretics are prescribed for conditions such as high blood pressure (hypertension), heart failure, pulmonary edema, kidney (renal) failure, and liver (hepatic) failure or cirrhosis with accompanying fluid in the abdominal cavity (ascites). Diuresis results in a lower blood volume and reduces blood pressure and the work of the heart. By removing fluid from the lungs breathing is less labored. Diuretics also maintain urine production in shock states. This prevents acute renal failure. Removing abdominal fluid makes it easier to breathe and comfort of the individual is increased.

The care provider will prescribe diuretic therapy after examining a patient and obtaining supporting information such as blood pressure, radiological examinations, and laboratory tests. The patient's lifestyle, preferences, and the cost of medications are considered in the decision to prescribe diuretics and which type of diuretics to prescribe.

Uses and Complications

There are four major types of diuretics: high-ceiling, thiazide, potassium-sparing, and osmotic diuretics. The most potent are high-ceiling agents (for example, furosemide). These drugs are commonly referred to as loop diuretics because they exert effects on the loop of Henle portion of the nephron. Administration of loop diuretics may result in

profound fluid and electrolyte loss. This can lead to serious side effects such as low blood volume (hypovolemia), low blood pressure (hypotension), and electrolyte and acid-base disturbances requiring treatment. Loop diuretics are ototoxic and can lead to hearing loss. Hearing loss may be reversed if reported to the care provider and the medication is stopped. An advantage of loop diuretics is that they continue to work even if renal blood flow is decreased. This is not true with other types of diuretics.

Another class of diuretic agents is the thiazides (for example, hydrochlorothiazide). Thiazides exert their effects on the proximal portion of the distal convoluted tubule. Although not as potent as high-ceiling diuretics they produce losses of electrolytes and water. Thiazide diuretics do not cause as much calcium excretion as loop diuretics and are useful in patients prone to calcium kidney stones. They suppress insulin production and glycogen storage resulting in higher blood glucose levels. This requires diabetic patients receiving thiazide diuretics to monitor blood glucose closely. Thiazides also decrease the excretion of uric acid. As uric acid blood levels rise, gout may develop. This class of diuretics is relatively inexpensive and well tolerated and is often used as first-line therapy for hypertension.

Potassium-sparing diuretics exert only a modest increase in urine output. There are two types of potassium-sparing agents: aldosterone antagonists (for example, spironalactone) and non-aldosterone antagonists (for example, amiloride). Aldosterone, a hormone secreted by the adrenal gland, increases sodium and water reabsorption in the nephron. By blocking aldosterone the reuptake of sodium and water is prohibited. Aldosterone antagonists require approximately forty-eight hours to demonstrate an effect. Non-aldosterone antagonists directly inhibit sodium and water reabsorption and effects begin without delay. Potassium-sparing diuretics cause minimal amounts of potassium to be lost in the urine. This class of diuretics is frequently used with loop or thiazide diuretics, not for diuresis, but to prevent potassium depletion. Side effects include too much potassium in the body (hyperkalemia) resulting in fatal heart rhythms, and endocrine effects. Because aldosterone antagonists are steroid hormones gynecomastia, menstrual irregularities, impotence, hirsutism, and deepening of the voice may occur. Potassium-sparing diuretics should not be taken with other drugs which are potassium sparing

(angiotensin-converting enzyme inhibitors, angiotensin receptor blockers, or direct renin inhibitors), potassium supplements, or salt substitutes containing potassium.

Osmotic diuretics are the final class of diuretic agents (for example, mannitol). Osmotic agents differ from other diuretic groups in their mechanism of action and indications for use. Osmotic drugs work by creating an osmotic force. When utilized to maintain urine production and prevent renal failure in patients suffering from shock, the drug is administered intravenously. In the kidney, the osmotic agent is freely filtered from the blood into the filtrate. It remains in the filtrate and holds water close to it in an attempt to maintain a normal solute-solvent ratio. The degree of diuresis is directly proportional to the concentration of osmotic agent in the filtrate. In treating increased pressure within the eye (intraocular pressure) as in glaucoma, osmotic eye drops work the same way—they create an osmotic force thus reducing pressure within the eye.

Diuretic drugs should be used with caution in patients with diabetes, gout, or renal impairment; during pregnancy; and when taking other drugs such as digoxin, lithium, ototoxic medications, nonsteroidal anti-inflammatory drugs (NSAIDs), or additional antihypertensive agents. Individuals should weigh daily in the morning before eating or drinking and keep a weight record that should be shared with the care provider. Also, they should check and record the blood pressure as instructed and remain alert to side effects of dehydration (dry mouth, thirst, low urine output), low potassium levels (irregular heartbeat, muscle weakness, cramping), or high potassium levels (slow or irregular heartbeat, high muscle tone, tingling).

Perspective and Prospects

Control of fluid and electrolytes to treat pathologic conditions such as hypertension, heart failure, pulmonary edema, and ascites is not new. Historical references go back to ancient Egypt. Throughout the centuries various medications to control these pathologies have been utilized including plants and herbs, and in the 1940s, mercury compounds. Thiazide diuretics were introduced in 1958 followed by the loop diuretic furosemide in 1966. Since that time additional diuretics have been invented. As the rate of obesity, type 2 diabetes mellitus, and hypertension continue to rise in the United States the need for diuretic agents will increase. Pharmaceutical companies consider new compounds that may show benefit as the next diuretic agent.

—*Wanda Todd Bradshaw,
M.S.N., N.N.P., P.N.P., C.C.R.N.*

See also Hypertension; Kidney disorders; Kidneys; Nephrectomy; Nephritis; Nephrology; Pharmacy; Renal failure; Urinalysis; Urinary system; Urology.

For Further Information:
Adams, Michael, and Robert Koch. "Diuretic Therapy and the Pharmacotherapy of Renal Failure." In *Pharmacology: Connections to Nursing Practice.* Upper Saddle River, N.J.: Pearson, 2010.

Broyles, Bonita, Barry Reiss, and Mary Evans, eds. *Pharmacological Aspects of Nursing Care.* 8th ed. Clifton Park, N.Y.: Cengage Learning, 2013.

Herbert-Ashton, Marilyn, and Nancy Clarkson, eds. *Pharmacology.* 2d ed. Sudbury, Mass.: Jones and Bartlett, 2008.

Mayo Clinic. "Diuretics." *Mayo Clinic,* December 16, 2010.

Will, Julie. "Diuretic Therapy and Drugs for Renal Failure." In *Pharmacology for Nurses: A Pathophysiologic Approach,* edited by Michael Adams, Leland Holland, Jr., and Paula Bostwick. Upper Saddle River, N.J.: Pearson-Prentice Hall, 2008.

DIVERTICULITIS AND DIVERTICULOSIS
Disease/Disorder

Anatomy or system affected: Abdomen, gastrointestinal system, intestines

Specialties and related fields: Gastroenterology, internal medicine, proctology

Definition: Diverticulosis is a disease involving multiple outpouchings, or diverticuli, of the wall of the colon; these diverticuli may become inflamed, leading to the painful condition called diverticulitis.

Key terms:

colon: the portion of the large intestine excluding the cecum and rectum; it includes the ascending, transverse, descending, and sigmoid colon

dietary fiber: indigestible plant substances that humans eat; fiber may be soluble, meaning that it dissolves in water, or insoluble, meaning that it does not dissolve in water

hernia: the bulging out of part or all of an organ through the wall of the cavity that usually contains it

infection: multiplication of disease-causing microorganisms in the body; the body normally also contains microorganisms that do not cause disease

inflammation: a tissue response to injury involving local reactions that attempt to destroy the injurious material and begin healing

lumen: the channel within a hollow or tubular organ

mucosa: the inner lining of the digestive tract; in the colon, the major function of the mucosal cells is to reabsorb liquid from feces, creating a semisolid material

perforation: an abnormal opening, such as a hole in the wall of the colon

peritoneal cavity: the cavity in the abdomen and pelvis that contains the internal organs

prevalence: the frequency of disease cases in a population, often expressed as a fraction (such as cases per 100,000)

Information on Diverticulitis and Diverticulosis

Causes: Aging, low-fiber diet

Symptoms: Abdominal pain; rectal bleeding; sudden urge to defecate followed by passage of red blood, clots, or maroon-colored stool; sometimes fever

Duration: Chronic, with acute episodes

Treatments: Increased dietary fiber, intravenous fluids, antispasmodic drugs, antibiotics, blood transfusions, surgery

---

Causes and Symptoms

Diverticulosis is an acquired condition of the colon that involves a few to hundreds of blueberry-sized outpouchings of its wall, called diverticuli. Diverticular disease is usually manifested by the presence of multiple diverticuli that are at risk of causing abdominal pain, inflammation, or bleeding.

Although the wall of the colon is thin, microscopically it has four layers. The innermost layer is called the mucosa. Its main function is to absorb fluids from the substance entering the colon, turning it into a semisolid material called feces. Outside the mucosa is the submucosa, a layer that contains blood vessels as well as nerve cells that control the functions of mucosal cells. Outside the submucosa is the muscularis, which contains muscle cells that are able to contract, pushing feces along the colon and eventually out through the rectum. Outside the muscularis is the serosa, which forms a wrap around the colon and helps prevent infections in this organ from spreading beyond its walls.

The diverticuli that form in the colon are not true diverticuli, in that the entire wall is not present in the outpouching. Only the mucosal and submucosal layers pouch out through weakened areas in the muscularis layer. When examined by the naked eye, however, it appears as if the entire wall of the colon is involved in the tiny outpouching. The mucosa bulges out in the part of the colonic wall that is weakened; this is where arteries penetrate through clefts in the muscularis.

The large intestine begins with the cecum, which is connected to the small intestine. The cecum is a pouch leading to the colon, whose components are the ascending, transverse, descending, and sigmoid colon. The sigmoid colon leads to the rectum, which is connected to the outside of the body by the anal canal. Although diverticuli can appear at a variety of locations in the gastrointestinal (GI) tract, they are usually located in the colon, most commonly in the sigmoid colon.

The most common form of diverticulosis is called spastic colon diverticulosis, which is a condition involving diverticuli that develop when the lumen (cavity) of the sigmoid colon is abnormally narrowed. Since the circumference of the colon alternately narrows and widens along its length, muscle contractions may result in local occlusions of the lumen at the narrowed sections. Occlusion may cause the lumen of the colon to become multiple, separate chambers. When this happens, the pressure within the chambers can increase to the point where the mucosa herniates out through small clefts in the muscularis, creating diverticuli.

Most people with diverticulosis never notice it. When abdominal pain related to painful diverticular disease develops, it is felt in the lower abdomen and may last for hours or days. Eating usually makes it worse, whereas passing gas or having a bowel movement may relieve it.

Besides causing abdominal pain, diverticuli may cause rectal bleeding, which may vary from mild to life threatening. Usually, there is a sudden urge to defecate followed by passage of red blood, clots, or maroon-colored stool. If the stool is black, the bleeding is probably from the upper GI tract.

Since the colon may be studded with multiple diverticuli, and the bleeding may stop by the time of evaluation, it is often difficult to tell which one bled. Diverticulosis is most common in elderly people, who may have other conditions of the colon that are associated with bleeding. Therefore, it is often impossible to confirm that the cause of bleeding was diverticular disease—even if the colon is lined with hundreds of diverticuli.

What is most important is to establish what part of the GI tract is bleeding. To find out if the bleeding could have come from the upper GI tract, a tube is passed through the nose into the stomach, and the contents are aspirated. If blood is not present, this suggests lower GI bleeding. In addition, the esophagus, stomach, and upper small intestine can be visualized with a flexible, snakelike instrument called an endoscope to exclude a source such as a bleeding ulcer.

It is more difficult to examine the lower GI tract. The simplest procedure is anoscopy, by which the physician can examine the inside of the anal canal for hemorrhoids. Proctosigmoidoscopy, a procedure similar to endoscopy, offers a view of the rectum and part of the sigmoid colon. It may reveal diverticuli or other lesions such as a bleeding growth called a polyp. Colonoscopy is most easily performed after bleeding has stopped. It requires cleaning out the contents of the colon and then inserting a long, flexible instrument called a colonoscope all the way to the cecum. The entire lining of the colon can be visualized while withdrawing the colonoscope.

Angiography is a test done in the radiology department; it involves injecting dye into the vessels that lead to the colon. If there is active bleeding, it can help localize the source. Even if the bleeding has stopped, this procedure can sometimes identify abnormal blood vessel formations suggestive of cancer or a blood vessel abnormality called angiodysplasia.

Between 10 and 25 percent of people with diverticulosis suffer from one or more episodes of diverticulitis, which is an inflammatory condition that may progress to an infection. Initially, feces may become trapped and inspissated (thickened) in a diverticulum, irritating it and leading to inflammation. Inflammation is a tissue response to injury that involves local reactions that attempt to destroy the injurious material and begin the healing process. It is usually the first step in the body's attempt to prevent infection and involves the migration of white blood cells out of blood vessels and into tissues, where they begin to fight off bacteria. The white blood cells release enzymes that cause tissue destruction. Because it is thin, the wall of the diverticulum may develop a tiny perforation.

Feces are made up of waste material and bacteria that normally do not cause problems when confined within the lumen of the colon. When a diverticulum perforates, however, they travel outside the colon and into other regions such as the peritoneal cavity, causing an infection. This infection along the outside of the colon is often limited, because many adjacent structures are able to wall off the bacteria, limiting their ability to extend through the peritoneal cavity. Although they become sealed off, they often form a pus-filled lesion called an abscess.

Fever and abdominal pain are the most common symptoms of diverticulitis. The fever may be high and associated with shaking chills. The pain is often sudden in onset, is often continuous, and may radiate from the left lower abdomen to the back. Laboratory findings usually include an elevated white blood cell count, a nonspecific finding that occurs with a variety of infections.

Radiographic studies are helpful for diagnosing and assessing the severity of diverticulitis. For example, a computed tomography (CT) scan can detect diverticuli or a thickening of the bowel wall associated with diverticulitis and can help assess whether abscesses are present.

Treatment and Therapy

There are two treatment goals in treating uncomplicated, painful diverticular disease: prevention of further development of diverticuli and pain relief. It is important to understand that the pressure that is able to develop inside the lumen of the colon is inversely related to the radius of the lumen. Therefore, if the lumen's radius can be increased, the pressures within the lumen will lessen, theoretically decreasing the chance of diverticuli formation. One key to increasing the radius of the lumen of the colon is to increase the bulk of the stool by the addition of dietary fiber.

A Western diet tends to be high in fiber-free animal products, and many foods that would ordinarily contain fiber, such as bread, lose much of their fiber during processing. This low-fiber diet may contribute to diverticulosis, which is prevalent in countries that have low-fiber diets. The typical American diet contains an average of ten to fifteen grams of fiber per day, whereas diets from regions such as Africa and Asia contain significantly more fiber. A high-fiber diet can increase stool bulk by 40 to 100 percent. Fiber adds bulk to the stool because it acts like a sponge, retaining water that would normally be reabsorbed by the colonic mucosa. Fiber also in-

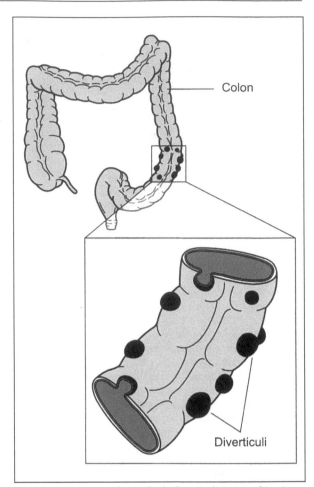

Diverticulosis occurs when multiple diverticuli (outpouchings) appear on the colon wall.

creases stool bulk because 50 to 70 percent of the fiber is degraded by the bacteria in the colon, and the products of degradation attract water by a process called osmosis.

The main fibers that increase stool bulk are the water-insoluble fibers, such as cellulose, hemicellulose, and lignin; they are derived from plants such as vegetables and whole-grain cereals. Diets high in these fibers have been shown to decrease the intraluminal pressure in the sigmoid colon as well as to relieve the pain associated with uncomplicated diverticular disease. Some research has suggested that adding ten to twenty-five grams per day of coarse, unprocessed wheat bran to various liquid and semisolid foods may provide the best results. The sudden addition of large amounts of bran to one's diet, however, may cause bloating. Commercial preparations such as methylcellulose may be better tolerated during the first few weeks of therapy; their use may then be tapered off as bran is added to the diet. There are also various antispasmodic drugs available for inhibiting the muscle spasms of the colon, but many are not very effective for decreasing symptoms.

For diverticular bleeding, the most effective therapy is patience. Most episodes stop on their own, and conservative treatments such as maintaining the patient's blood volume with intravenous fluids and possibly performing blood transfusions are all that is necessary. In those patients with continued active bleeding and in whom the source of the bleeding can be identified with angiography, a drug called vasopressin may be administered into the artery over several hours. This causes constriction of the vessel and stops bleeding most of the time. Once the vasopressin is stopped, however, patients may resume bleeding.

If vasopressin fails, surgery may be necessary. Surgery is most often successful if the bleeding site has been well localized before the operation. In that case, only the involved segment of the colon needs to be removed. If the bleeding site cannot be identified, it may be necessary to remove a majority of the colon; this procedure is associated with a higher rate of postoperative complications.

Diverticulitis that warrants hospitalization is initially treated with intravenous antibiotics for seven to ten days. Antibiotics help prevent many patients from needing surgery. Most of those who respond to antibiotics will not have future attacks severe enough to warrant hospitalization.

Other measures may be necessary for the care of someone with diverticulitis, because the inflammation around the colon may be associated with problems such as narrowing of the bowel lumen to the point where it causes a partial or complete colonic obstruction. In this case, nothing should be given by mouth, and a tube should be passed through the nose into the stomach in order to suck out air and the stomach contents. This suction helps to reduce the amount of material that can pass through the colon and worsen the dilation of the colon that occurs proximal to the obstruction.

If the fever persists for more than a few days, the diverticulitis may be associated with complications. One complication is the formation of a large abscess outside the colon, which may be detected by a CT scan. An abscess has a rim around it that makes it difficult for antibiotics to penetrate the liquid center. If it does not go away despite antibiotic therapy, surgery may be necessary. If the abscess is small, it is possible to remove the involved segment of bowel and reattach the two free ends. If the abscess is very large, it may be necessary first to drain the abscess and then to cut across the colon proximal to the diseased segment, attaching the free end of the proximal segment to the abdominal wall, a procedure called a diverting colostomy. Later, the diseased segment of colon can be removed, and the remaining two free ends of colon can be joined. Another option is to drain the abscess with the aid of visual guidance by the CT scan and then operate on the colon. Draining the abscess in this manner helps get the infection under control before surgery is performed. Other indications for surgery in diverticulitis include complications such as a persistent bowel obstruction. In this case, it is often necessary to use a two-stage approach rather than cure the problem in one operation.

Another complication of diverticulitis is a generalized infection of the peritoneal cavity, called peritonitis. Surgery for

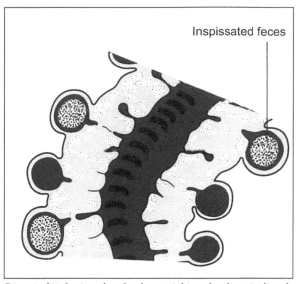

Inspissated feces

Diverticulitis begins when fecal material invades diverticuli and thickens (inspissated feces); when a diverticulum perforates, bacteria travel outside the colon into other regions and cause serious symptoms, including lower abdominal pain, fever, chills, and abscesses.

peritonitis involves removing the leaking segment of bowel and attaching the remaining two free ends of the colon to the abdominal wall. In addition, the peritoneal cavity is rinsed with a sterile solution in an attempt to clean out the contaminating materials.

Diverticulitis may also be complicated by the presence of a perforation of a diverticulum leading to a fistula, an abnormally existing channel connecting two hollow organs. When there is a fistula between the colon and the bladder, stool can travel into the bladder. The bacteria in the stool can cause severe, recurrent urinary tract infections. Another symptom is that bowel gas gets into the bladder; when the patient urinates, there is an intermittent stream because of colonic gas being passed along with the urine. When a fistula exists, it is necessary to remove the diseased segment of colon, the fistula tract, and a small portion of the bladder where the tract entered it.

Even if a patient with diverticulitis seems to improve and is able to return home from the hospital without needing surgery, there is still a chance that surgery will be necessary in the future. Surgery may be needed if the patient continues to have repeated, severe attacks of diverticulitis or if a fistula between the colon and bladder causes recurring urinary tract infections. Another reason for surgery is persistent partial colonic obstruction and no possibility of inspecting the narrowed region of colon to exclude a constricting cancerous lesion as the cause of the obstruction.

Perspective and Prospects

Diverticuli are quite common in the United States and other countries in which much of the population tends to eat processed, low-fiber foods. Although residents of countries where a high-fiber diet is common tend to have a low prevalence of diverticulosis, their risk of developing this disease increases within ten years of moving to a country with a low-fiber diet. The prevalence of diverticulosis and diverticulitis appears to be increasing. For example, before 1900, colonic diverticuli were considered a curiosity in the United States, whereas by the early twenty-first century, they were found in more than half of Americans over the age of sixty. There are a few possible explanations for why this increasing prevalence is seen.

First, the change in the American diet probably plays a large part in the pathogenesis of diverticular disease. Fiber consumption may have fallen off by as much as 30 percent during the twentieth century. Many people in the United States eat foods such as quick-cooking rice, highly processed cereals, and processed flour, all of which contain less fiber than their unprocessed counterparts. In addition, the population tends to eat more fats and proteins and fewer carbohydrates. Many fibers are from food sources rich in carbohydrates and are carbohydrates themselves.

The increasing prevalence of diverticular disease may also be attributable to the changing survival pattern. The average life expectancy in the United States rose significantly over the course of the twentieth century, and the proportion of people over sixty-five has likewise risen. Thus, the American population is not only growing but also getting older. Since diverticulosis is seen in increasing frequencies with aging, it is understandable that more of it was seen in the late twentieth century and early twenty-first century than during the early twentieth century.

Another reason for the increase in the prevalence of diverticular disease could be improvements in detection. Now it is detected not only at autopsy but also by barium enema, during sigmoidoscopy, and during surgery. Thus, there are more opportunities for discovering diverticulosis.

—*Marc H. Walters, M.D.*

See also Colon; Colon therapy; Colonoscopy and sigmoidoscopy; Colorectal cancer; Colorectal polyp removal; Colorectal surgery; Constipation; Digestion; Gastroenterology; Gastroenterology, pediatric; Gastrointestinal disorders; Gastrointestinal system; Intestinal disorders; Intestines; Irritable bowel syndrome (IBS); Nutrition; Peritonitis.

For Further Information:

Achkar, Edgar, Richard G. Farmer, and Bertram Fleshler, eds. *Clinical Gastroenterology*. 2d ed. Philadelphia: Lea & Febiger, 1992.

A.D.A.M. Medical Encyclopedia. "Diverticulitis." *MedlinePlus*, April 16, 2012.

A.D.A.M. Medical Encyclopedia. "Fiber." *MedlinePlus*, August 14, 2012.

Feldman, Mark, Lawrence S. Friedman, and Lawrence J. Brandt, eds. *Sleisenger and Fordtran's Gastrointestinal and Liver Disease: Pathophysiology, Diagnosis, Management*. New ed. 2 vols. Philadelphia: Saunders/Elsevier, 2010.

Ganong, William F. *Review of Medical Physiology*. 23d ed. New York: Lange Medical Books/McGraw-Hill Medical, 2009.

International Foundation for Functional Gastrointestinal Disorders. "Diverticula, Diverticulosis, Diverticulitis: What's the Difference?" *International Foundation for Functional Gastrointestinal Disorders*, January 17, 2013.

Kapadia, Cyrus R., James M. Crawford, and Caroline Taylor. *An Atlas of Gastroenterology: A Guide to Diagnosis and Differential Diagnosis*. Boca Raton, Fla.: Pantheon, 2003.

Kumar, Vinay, et al., eds. *Robbins Basic Pathology*. 8th ed. Philadelphia: Saunders/Elsevier, 2007.

National Digestive Diseases Information Clearinghouse. "Diverticulosis and Diverticulitis." *National Institutes of Health*, February 21, 2012.

Peikin, Steven R. *Gastrointestinal Health*. Rev. ed. New York: Quill, 2001.

Tortora, Gerard J., and Bryan Derrickson. *Principles of Anatomy and Physiology*. 12th ed. Hoboken, N.J.: John Wiley & Sons, 2009.

Wood, Debra. "Diverticulitis." *HealthLibrary*, March 5, 2013.

DIZZINESS AND FAINTING

Disease/Disorder

Anatomy or system affected: Blood vessels, brain, circulatory system, head, nervous system, psychic-emotional system

Specialties and related fields: Cardiology, emergency medicine, family medicine, internal medicine, neurology

Definition: Dizziness is a feeling of light-headedness and unsteadiness, sometimes accompanied by a feeling of spinning or other spatial motion; fainting is a loss of consciousness as a result of insufficient amounts of blood reaching the brain. Both are symptoms of many conditions, which may be harmless or serious.

Key terms:

cardiac output: the amount of blood that the heart can pump per unit of time (usually per minute); if the brain does not receive enough of the cardiac output, the person becomes dizzy and may faint

dizziness: a sensation of whirling, with difficulty balancing

fainting: a weak feeling followed by a loss of consciousness, usually due to a lack of blood flow to the brain; also called syncope

hypertension: a condition in which the patient's blood pressure is higher than that demanded by the body

hypotension: decrease in blood pressure to the point that insufficient blood flow causes symptoms

vasoconstriction: a reduction in the diameter of arteries, which increases the amount of work required for the heart to move blood

vasodilation: an increase in the diameter of arteries, which decreases the amount of work required for the heart to move blood

venous return: the amount of blood returning to the heart; one factor that determines the amount of blood the heart can pump out

vertigo: a sensation of moving in space or having objects move about when the patient is stationary, the most common symptom of which is dizziness; vertigo results from a disturbance in the organs of equilibrium

Causes and Symptoms

In humans, several mechanisms have evolved by which adequate blood flow to organs is maintained. Without a constant blood supply, the body's tissues would die from a lack of essential nutrients and oxygen. In particular, the brain and heart are very sensitive to changes in their blood supply as they, more than any other organs, must receive oxygen and nutrients at all times. If they do not, their cells will die and cannot be replaced.

While the heart supplies most of the force needed to propel the blood throughout the body, tissues rely on changes in the size of arteries to redirect blood flow to where it is needed most. For example, after a large meal the blood vessels that lead to the gastrointestinal tract enlarge (vasodilate) so that more blood can be present to collect the nutrients from the meal. At the same time, the blood vessels that supply muscles decrease in diameter (vasoconstrict) and effectively shunt the blood toward the stomach and intestines. During exercise, the blood vessels that supply the muscles dilate and the ones leading to the intestinal tract vasoconstrict. This mechanism allows the cardiovascular system to supply the most blood to the most active tissues.

The brain is somewhat special in that the body tries to maintain a nearly constant blood flow to it. Located in the walls of the carotid arteries, which carry blood to the brain, are specialized sensory cells that have the ability to detect changes in blood pressure. These cells are known as baroreceptors. If the blood pressure going to the brain is too low, the baroreceptors send an impulse to the brain, which in turn speeds up the heart rate and causes a generalized vasoconstriction. This reflex response raises the body's blood pressure, reestablishing adequate blood flow to the brain. If the baroreceptors detect too high a blood pressure, they send a signal to the brain, which in turn slows the heart rate and causes the arteries of the body to dilate. These reflexes prevent large fluctuations in blood flow to the brain and other tissues.

Most people have experienced a dizzy feeling or maybe even a fainting response when they have stood up too quickly from a prone position. The ability of the baroreceptors to maintain relatively constant arterial pressure is extremely important when a person stands after having been lying down. Immediately upon standing, the pressure in the carotid arteries falls, and a reduction of this pressure can cause dizziness or even fainting. Fortunately, the falling pressure at the baroreceptors elicits an immediate reflex, resulting in a more rapid heart rate and vasoconstriction, minimizing the decrease in blood flow to the brain.

Blood pressure is not the only factor that is essential in maintaining tissue viability. The accumulation of waste products and a lack of essential nutrients and gases can also have a profound effect on how much blood flows through a particular tissue and how quickly. In a region of the carotid arteries near the baroreceptors are chemoreceptors. Chemoreceptors detect the concentration of the essential gas oxygen and the concentration of the gaseous waste product carbon dioxide. When carbon dioxide concentrations increase and oxygen concentrations decrease, the chemoreceptors stimulate regions in the brain to increase the heart rate and blood pressure in an attempt to supply the tissues with more oxygen and flush away the excess carbon dioxide. If the chemoreceptors detect high levels of oxygen and low levels of carbon dioxide, an impulse is transmitted to the brain, which in turn slows the heart rate and decreases the blood pressure.

Normally, most of the blood flow to the brain is controlled by the baroreceptor and chemoreceptor reflexes. However, the brain has a backup system. If blood flow decreases enough to cause a deficiency of nutrients and oxygen and an accumulation of waste products, special nerve cells respond directly to the lack of adequate energy sources and become strongly excited. When this occurs, the heart is stimulated and blood pressure rises.

Dizziness is a sensation of light-headedness often accompanied by a sensation of spinning (vertigo). Occasionally, a person experiencing dizziness will feel nauseated and may even vomit. Most attacks of dizziness are harmless, resulting from a brief reduction in blood flow to the brain. There are several causes of dizziness, and each alters blood flow to the brain for a slightly different reason.

A person rising rapidly from a sitting or lying position may become dizzy. This is known as postural hypotension, which is caused by a relatively slow reflexive response to the reduced blood pressure in the arteries providing blood to the brain. Rising requires increased blood pressure to supply the brain with adequate amounts of blood. Postural hypotension is more common in the elderly and in individuals prescribed antihypertensive medicines (drugs used to lower high blood pressure).

If the patient experiences vertigo with dizziness, the condition is usually caused by a disorder of the inner ear equilibrium system. Two disorders of the inner ear that can cause dizziness are labyrinthitis and Ménière's disease. Labyrinthitis, inflammation of the fluid-filled canals of the inner ear, is usually caused by a virus. Since these canals are involved in maintaining equilibrium, when they become infected and inflamed, one experiences the symptom of dizziness. Ménière's disease is a degenerative disorder of the ear in which the patient experiences not only dizziness but also progressive hearing loss.

Some brain-stem disorders also cause dizziness. The brain stem houses the vestibulocochlear nerve, which transmits messages from the ear to several other parts of the nervous system. Any disorder that alters the functions of this nerve will result in dizziness and vertigo. Meningitis (inflammation of the coverings of the brain and spinal cord), brain tumors, and blood-flow deficiency disorders such as atherosclerosis may affect the function of the vestibulocochlear nerve.

Syncope (fainting) is often preceded by dizziness. Syncope is the temporary loss of consciousness as a result of an inadequate blood flow to the brain. In addition to losing consciousness, the patient may be pale and sweaty. The most common cause of syncope is a vasovagal attack, in which an overstimulation of the vagus nerve slows the heart. Often vasovagal syncope results from severe pain, stress, or fear. For example, people may faint when hearing bad news or at the sight of blood. More commonly, individuals who have received a painful injury will faint. Rarely, vasovagal syncope may be caused by prolonged coughing, straining to defecate or urinate, pregnancy, or forcing expiration. Standing still for long periods of time or standing up rapidly after lying or sitting can cause fainting. With the exception of vasovagal syncope, all the causes of syncope are attributable to inadequate blood returning to the heart. If blood pools in the lower extremities, there is a reduced amount available for the heart to pump to the brain. In vasovagal syncope and some disorders of heart rhythm such as Adams-Stokes syndrome, it is the heart itself that does not force enough blood toward the brain.

Treatment and Therapy

Short periods of dizziness usually subside after a few minutes. Deep breathing and rest will usually help relieve the symptom. Prolonged episodes of dizziness and vertigo should be brought to the attention of a physician.

Recovery from fainting likewise will occur when adequate blood flow to the brain is reestablished. This happens within minutes because falling to the ground places the head at the same level as the heart and helps return the blood from the legs. If a person does not regain consciousness within a few minutes, a physician or emergency medical team should be notified.

The most common cause of syncope is decreased cerebral blood flow resulting from the limitation of cardiac output. When the heart rate falls below its normal seventy-five beats per minute to approximately thirty-five beats per minute, the patient usually becomes dizzy and faints. Although slow heart rates can occur in any age group, they are most often found in elderly people who have other heart conditions. Drug-induced syncope can also occur. Drugs for congestive heart failure (digoxin) or antihypertensive medications that slow the heart rate (propranolol, metoprolol) may reduce blood flow to the brain sufficiently to cause dizziness and fainting.

Exertional syncope occurs when individuals perform some physical activity to which they are not accustomed. These physical efforts demand more work from the cardiovascular system, and in patients with some obstruction of the arteries which leave the heart, the cardiovascular system is overstressed. This defect, combined with the vasodilation in the blood vessels that provide blood to the working muscles, reduces the amount of blood available for use by the brain. If the person also hyperventilates during exercise, he or she will effectively reduce the amount of carbon dioxide in the blood and rid the cardiovascular system of this normal stimulus for increasing heart rate and blood flow to the brain. Some persons also hold their breath during periods of high exertion. For example, people attempting to lift something very heavy often take a deep breath just prior to exerting and then hold their breath when they lift the object. This practice, known as the Valsalva maneuver, increases the pressure within the chest cavity, which in turn reduces the amount of blood returning to the heart. A decrease in blood returning to the heart (venous return) causes a decrease in the availability of blood to be pumped out of the heart and reduces cardiac output. The reduction in cardiac output decreases the amount of blood flowing to the brain and initiates a fainting response. It is interesting to note that humans also use the Valsalva maneuver when defecating or urinating, particularly when they strain. These acts can also lead to exertional syncope.

For a physician to diagnose and treat dizziness and fainting accurately, he or she must take an accurate medical history, paying particular attention to cardiovascular and neurological problems. In addition to experiencing episodes of dizziness and fainting, patients often have a weak pulse, low blood pressure (hypotension), sweating, and shallow breathing. Heart rate and blood pressure are monitored while the patient assumes different positions. The clinician also listens to the heart and carotid arteries to determine whether there are any problems with these tissues, such as a heart valve problem or atherosclerosis of the carotid arteries. An electrocardiogram (ECG or EKG) can detect abnormal heart rates and rhythms that may reduce cardiac output. Laboratory tests are used to determine whether the patient has low blood sugar (hypoglycemia), too little blood volume (hypovolemia), too few red blood cells (anemia), or abnormal blood gases suggesting a lung disorder. Finally, if the physician suspects a neurological problem such as a seizure disorder, he or she may run an electroencephalogram (EEG) to record brain activity.

Treatment for any of these underlying disorders may cure the dizziness and fainting episodes. In patients with postural hypotension, merely being aware of the condition will allow them to change their behavior to lessen the chances of becoming dizzy and fainting. These patients should not make any sudden changes in posture that could precipitate an attack. Often, this means simply slowing down their movements and learning to assume a horizontal position if they feel dizzy. Patients also can learn to contract their leg muscles and not hold their breath when rising. This increases the amount of blood available for the heart to pump toward the brain. If these techniques do not provide an adequate solution for postural hypotension, then a physician can prescribe drugs, such as ephedrine, which increase blood pressure.

Heart rhythm disturbances that cause an abnormally fast or slow heart rate can be corrected with drug therapy such as quinidine or disopyramide (if the rate is too rapid) or a pacemaker (if the rate is too slow). It is interesting to note that even too fast a heart rate can cause dizziness and fainting. In patients with this type of arrhythmia, the heart beats at such a rapid rate that it cannot efficiently fill with blood before the next contraction. Therefore, less blood is pumped with each beat.

Other treatments for dizziness and fainting may include correcting the levels of certain blood elements. Patients with hypoglycemia often feel dizzy. The brain and spinal cord require glucose as their energy source. In fact, the brain and spinal cord have a very limited ability to utilize other substrates such as fat or protein for energy. Because of this, patients often feel light-headed when there are inadequate levels of glucose in the blood. Patients can correct this condition by eating more frequent meals, and if necessary, physicians can administer drugs such as epinephrine or glucagon. These agents liberate glucose from storage sites in the liver.

Individuals with a low blood volume are often dehydrated and upon becoming rehydrated no longer have dizziness or fainting episodes. If dehydration is not corrected and becomes worse, the patient can go into shock, a state of inadequate blood flow to tissues that will result in death if left untreated. In addition to being dizzy or fainting, the patient is often cold to the touch and has a rapid heart rate, low blood pressure, bluish skin, and rapid breathing. These patients are treated by emergency medical personnel, who keep the individual warm, elevate the legs, and infuse fluid into a vein. Drugs may be used to help bring blood pressure back to normal. The cause of the shock should be identified and corrected.

Perspective and Prospects

As humans evolved, they assumed an upright posture. This is advantageous because it allows for the use of the front limbs for other things besides locomotion. Unlike most four-legged animals, however, humans have their brains above their hearts and must continually force blood uphill to reach this vital tissue. This adaptation to the upright posture is a continuing physiological problem because the cardiovascular system must counteract the forces of gravity to provide the brain with blood. If this does not occur, the individual becomes dizzy and faints.

Another significant problem that humans face is adaptation to brain blood flow during exercise. The amount of blood flowing to a tissue is usually proportional to the metabolic demand of the tissue. At rest, various organs throughout the body receive a certain amount of the cardiac output. For example, blood flow to abdominal organs such as the spleen and the kidneys requires about 43 percent of the total blood volume. The total flow to the brain is estimated to be only 13 percent, and the skin and skeletal muscles require 21 percent and 9 percent, respectively. Other areas such as the gastrointestinal tract and heart receive the remaining 14 percent. During exercise, the skeletal muscles may receive up to 80 percent of the cardiac output while the rest of the organs are perfused at a much reduced rate.

Most data indicates that the brain receives only 3 percent of the total cardiac output during heavy exercise. Even though there is a large change in the redistribution of cardiac output, physiologists do not know the absolute amount of blood reaching the brain or the mechanism for the change in the perfusion rate.

With strenuous aerobic exercise such as jogging, there is an increase in cardiac output. During strenuous anaerobic exercise such as weight lifting, however, there may be a decrease in cardiac output, attributable to the Valsalva maneuver. Therefore, it has been difficult to predict accurately, using available techniques, the volume of blood reaching this critical tissue.

—Matthew Berria, Ph.D.

See also Anxiety; Balance disorders; Blood vessels; Brain; Brain disorders; Circulation; Ear infections and disorders; Ears; Exercise physiology; Headaches; Huntington's disease; Hypotension; Ménière's disease; Meningitis; Migraine headaches; Multiple chemical sensitivity syndrome; Narcolepsy; Nausea and vomiting; Nervous system; Neuralgia, neuritis, and neuropathy; Neurology; Neurology, pediatric; Palpitations; Unconsciousness.

For Further Information:

Babikian, Viken K., and Lawrence R. Wechsler, eds. *Transcranial Doppler Ultrasonography*. 2d ed. Boston: Butterworth-Heinemann, 1999.

"Balance Problems." *MedlinePlus*, 25 June 2013.

Brandt, Thomas. *Vertigo: Its Multisensory Syndromes*. 2d ed. New York: Springer, 2003.

"Dizziness and Vertigo." *MedlinePlus*, 29 June 2013.

"Ear Disorders." *MedlinePlus*, 3 Aug. 2013.

"Fainting." *MedlinePlus*, 23 July 2013.

Furman, Joseph M., and Stephen P. Cass. *Vestibular Disorders: A Case-Study Approach*. 3d ed. New York: Oxford University Press, 2010.

Geelen, G., and J. E. Greenleaf. "Orthostasis: Exercise and Exercise Training." *Exercise and Sport Sciences Reviews* 21 (1993): 201–30.

Guyton, Arthur C. *Human Physiology and Mechanisms of Disease*. 6th ed. Philadelphia: W. B. Saunders, 1997.

Leikin, Jerrold B., and Martin S. Lipsky, eds. *American Medical Association Complete Medical Encyclopedia*. New York: Random House Reference, 2003.

"Low Blood Pressure." *MedlinePlus*, 23 July 2013.

"Understanding Vestibular Disorders." *Vestibular Disorders Association*, 2013.

DOWN SYNDROME

Disease/Disorder

Anatomy or system affected: Brain, nervous system, psychic-emotional system

Specialties and related fields: Embryology, genetics, obstetrics, pediatrics

Definition: A congenital abnormality characterized by moderate to severe mental retardation and a distinctive physical appearance caused by a chromosomal aberration, the result of either an error during embryonic cell division or the inheritance of defective chromosomal material.

Key terms:

chromosomes: small, threadlike bodies containing the genes that are microscopically visible during cell division

gametes: the egg and sperm cells that unite to form the fertilized egg (zygote) in reproduction

gene: a segment of the DNA strand containing instructions for the production of a protein

homologous chromosomes: chromosome pairs of the same size and centromere position that possess genes for the same traits; one homologous chromosome is inherited from the father and the other from the mother

meiosis: the type of cell division that produces the cells of reproduction, which contain one-half of the chromosome number found in the original cell before division

mitosis: the type of cell division that occurs in nonsex cells, which conserves chromosome number by equal allocation to each of the newly formed cells

translocation: an aberration in chromosome structure resulting from the attachment of chromosomal material to a nonhomologous chromosome

---

Information on Down Syndrome

Causes: Genetic defect
Symptoms: Mental retardation, characteristic facial appearance, lack of musfcle tone, increased risk for heart malformations, increased disease susceptibility
Duration: Lifelong
Treatments: None

Causes and Symptoms

Down syndrome is a genetic disorder—that is, a disorder arising from an abnormality in an individual's genetic material. Down syndrome results from an incorrect transfer of genetic material in the formation of cells. Genetic information is contained in large "library" molecules of deoxyribonucleic acid (DNA). DNA molecules are formed by joining together units called nucleotides, which come in four different varieties: adenosine, thymine, cytosine, and guanine (identified by their initials A, T, C, and G). These nucleotides store hereditary information by forming "words" with this four-letter alphabet. In a gene, a section of DNA that contains the chemical message controlling an inherited trait, three consecutive nucleotides combine to specify a particular amino acid. This word order forms the "sentences" of a recipe telling cells how to construct proteins, such as those coloring the hair and eyes, from amino acids.

In living systems, tissue growth occurs through cell division processes in which an original cell divides to form two cells containing duplicate genetic material. Just before a cell divides, the DNA organizes itself into distinct, compact bundles called chromosomes. Normal human cells, diploid cells, contain twenty-three pairs (or a total of forty-six) of these chromosomes. Each pair is a set of homologues containing genes for the same traits. These chromosomes are composed of two DNA strands, chromatids, joined at a constricted region known as the centromere. The bundle is similar in shape to the letter *X*. The arms are the parts above and below the constriction, which may be centered or offset toward one end (giving arms of equal or different lengths, respectively). During mitosis, the division of nonsex cells, the chromatids separate at the centromere, forming two sets of single-stranded chromosomes, which migrate to opposite ends of the cell. The cell then splits into two genetically equivalent cells, each containing twenty-three single-stranded chromosomes that will duplicate to form the original number of forty-six chromosomes.

In sexual reproduction, haploid egg and sperm cells, each containing twenty-three single-stranded chromosomes, unite in fertilization to produce a zygote cell with forty-six chromosomes. Haploid cells are created through a different, two-step cell division process termed meiosis. Meiosis begins when the homologues in a diploid cell pair up at the equator of the cell. The attractions between the members of each pair then break, allowing the homologues to migrate to opposite ends of the cell, each twin to a different pole, without splitting at the centromere. The parent cell then divides once to form two cells containing twenty-three double-stranded chromosomes, and then divides again through the process of mitosis to form cells that contain only twenty-three single-stranded chromosomes. Thus, each cell contains half of the original chromosomes.

Although cell division is normally a precise process, occasionally an error called nondisjunction occurs when a chromosome either fails to separate or fails to migrate to the proper pole. In meiosis, the failure to move to the proper pole results in the formation of one gamete with twenty-four chromosomes and one with twenty-two chromosomes. Upon fertilization, zygotes of forty-seven or forty-five chromosomes are produced, and the developing embryo must function with either extra or missing genes. Since every chromosome contains a multitude of genes, problems result from the absence or excess of proteins produced. In fact, the embryos formed from most nondisjunctional fertilizations die at an early stage in development and are spontaneously aborted. Occasionally, nondisjunction occurs in mitosis, when a chromosome migrates before the chromatids separate, yielding one cell with an extra copy of the chromosome and no copy in the other cell.

Down syndrome is also termed trisomy 21, as it most commonly results from the presence of an extra copy of the smallest human chromosome, chromosome 21. Actually, it is not the entire extra chromosome 21 that is responsible but rather a small segment of the long arm of this chromosome. Only two other trisomies occur with any significant frequency: trisomy 13 (Patau syndrome) and trisomy 18 (Edwards syndrome). Both of these disorders are accompanied by multiple severe malformations, typically resulting in death within a few months of birth. Most incidences of Down syndrome are a consequence of a nondisjunction during meiosis. In about 75 percent of these cases, the extra chromosome is present in the egg. About 1 percent of Down syndrome cases occur after the fertilization of normal gametes from a mitosis nondisjunction, producing a mosaic in which some of the embryo's cells are normal and some exhibit trisomy. The degree of mosaicism and its location will determine the physiological consequences of the nondisjunction.

In about 4 percent of all Down syndrome cases, the individual possesses not an entire third copy of chromosome 21 but rather extra chromosome 21 material, which has been incorporated via a translocation into a nonhomologous chromosome. In translocation, pieces of arms are swapped between two nonrelated chromosomes, forming hybrid chromosomes. The most common translocation associated with Down syndrome is that between the long arm (Down gene area) of chromosome 21 and an end of chromosome 14. The individual in whom the translocation has occurred shows no evidence of the aberration, since the normal complement of genetic material is still present, only at different chromosomal locations. The difficulty arises when this individual forms gametes. A mother who possesses the 21/14 translocation, for example, has one normal 21, one normal 14, and the hybrid chromosomes. She is a genetic carrier for the disorder, because she can pass it on to her offspring even though she is clinically normal. This mother could produce three types of viable gametes: one containing the normal 14 and 21; one containing both translocations, which would result in clinical normality; and one containing the normal 21 and the translocated 14 having the long arm of 21. If each gamete were fertilized by normal sperm, two apparently normal embryos and one partial trisomy 21 Down syndrome embryo would result. Down syndrome that results from the passing on of translocations is termed familial Down syndrome and is an inherited disorder.

The presence of an extra copy of the long arm of chromosome 21 causes defects in many tissues and organs. One major effect of Down syndrome is delayed mental development. The intelligence quotients (IQs) of affected individuals are typically in the range of 40–50. The IQ varies with age, being higher in childhood than in adolescence or adult life. The disorder is often accompanied by physical traits such as short stature, stubby fingers and toes, protruding tongue, and an unusual pattern of hand creases. Perhaps the most recognized physical feature is the distinctive slanting of the eyes, caused by a vertical fold (epicanthal fold) of skin near the nasal bridge that pulls and tilts the eyes slightly toward the nostrils. For Caucasians without Down syndrome, the eye runs parallel to the skin fold below the eyebrow; for Asians, this skin fold covers a major portion of the upper eyelid. In contrast, the epicanthal fold in trisomy 21 does not cover a major part of the upper eyelid.

It should be noted that not all defects associated with Down syndrome are found in every affected individual. About 40 percent of Down syndrome patients have congenital heart defects, while about 10 percent have intestinal blockages. Affected individuals are prone to respiratory infections and contract leukemia at a rate twenty times that of the general population. Although Down syndrome children develop the same types of leukemia in the same proportions as other children, the survival rates of the two groups are markedly different. While the survival rate for patients without Down syndrome after ten years is about 30 percent, survival beyond five years is negligible in those with Down syndrome. It appears that the extra copy of chromosome 21 not only increases the risk of contracting the cancer but also exerts a decisive influence on the disease's outcome. Reproductively, males are sterile while some females are fertile. Although many Down syndrome infants die in the first year of life, the average life expectancy is about fifty years. This reduced life expectancy results from defects in the immune system, causing a high susceptibility to infectious disease. Many individuals with Down syndrome develop an Alzheimer's-like condition later in life.

Treatment and Therapy

Trisomy 21 is one of the most common human chromosomal aberrations, occurring in about one out of every eight hundred live births. Even before the chromosomal basis for the disorder was determined, the frequency of Down syndrome births was correlated with increased maternal age. For mothers at age twenty, the incidence of Down syndrome is about 0.05 percent, but the incidence increases to 0.9 percent by age thirty-five and 3 percent at age forty-five. Studies comparing the chromosomes of the affected offspring with those of both parents have shown that the nondisjunction event is maternal about 75 percent of the time. This maternal age effect is thought to result from the different manner in which the male and female gametes are produced. Gamete production in the male is a continual, lifelong process, while it is a one-time event in females.

Formation of the female's gametes begins early in embryonic life, somewhere between the eighth and twentieth weeks. During this time, cells in the developing ovary divide rapidly by mitosis, forming cells called primary oocytes. These cells then begin meiosis by pairing up the homologues. The process is interrupted at this point, and the cells are held in a state of suspended animation until needed in reproduction, when they are triggered to complete their division and form eggs. It appears that the frequency of nondisjunction events increases with the length of the storage period. Studies have demonstrated that cells in a state of meiosis are particularly sensitive to environmental influences such as viruses, x-rays, and cytotoxic chemicals. It is possible that environmental influences may play a role in nondisjunction events. Up to age thirty-two, males contribute an extra chromosome 21 as often as do females. Beyond this age, there is a rapid increase in nondisjunctional eggs, while the number of nondisjunctional sperm remains constant. Where the maternal age effect is minimal, mosaicism may be an important source of the trisomy. An apparently normal mother who possesses undetected mosaicism can produce trisomy offspring if gametes with an extra chromosome are produced. In some instances, characteristics such as abnormal fingerprint patterns have been observed in the mothers and their children with Down syndrome.

Techniques such as amniocentesis, chorionic villus sampling, and alpha-fetoprotein screening are available for prenatal diagnosis of Down syndrome in fetuses. Amniocentesis, the most widely used technique for prenatal diagnosis, is generally performed between the fourteenth and sixteenth weeks of pregnancy. In this technique, about one ounce of fluid is removed from the amniotic cavity surrounding the fetus by a needle inserted through the mother's abdomen. Although some testing can be done directly on the fluid (such as the assay for spina bifida), more information is obtained from the cells shed from the fetus that accompany the fluid. The mixture obtained in the amniocentesis is spun in a centrifuge

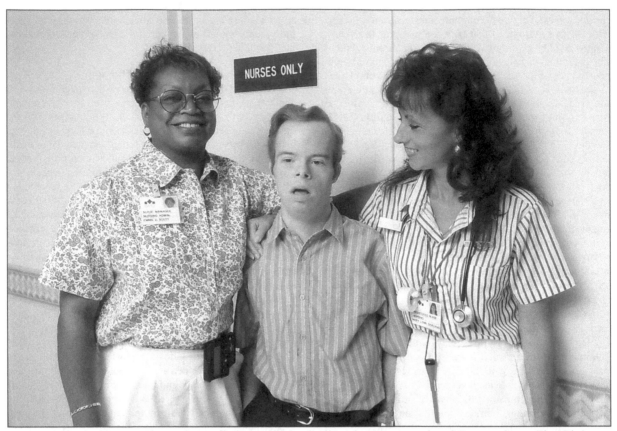

Nurses and other health care professionals can offer both medical and emotional support to people with Down syndrome. (PhotoDisc)

to separate the fluid from the fetal cells. The chromosome analysis for Down syndrome cannot be conducted directly on the amount of cellular material obtained. Although the majority of the cells collected are nonviable, some will grow in culture. These cells are allowed to grow and multiply in culture for two to four weeks, and then the chromosomes undergo karyotyping, which will detect both trisomy 21 and translocational aberration.

In karyotyping, the chromosomes are spread on a microscope slide, stained, and photographed. Each type of chromosome gives a unique, observable banding pattern when stained, which allows it to be identified. The chromosomes are then cut out of the photograph and arranged in homologous pairs, in numerical order. Trisomy 21 is easily observed, since three copies of chromosome 21 are present, while the translocation shows up as an abnormal banding pattern. Termination of the pregnancy in the wake of an unfavorable amniocentesis diagnosis is complicated, because the fetus at this point is usually about eighteen to twenty weeks old, and elective abortions are normally performed between the sixth and twelfth weeks of pregnancy. Earlier sampling of the amniotic fluid is not possible because of the small amount of fluid present.

An alternate testing procedure called chorionic villus sampling became available in the mid-1980s. In this procedure, a chromosomal analysis is conducted on a piece of placental tissue that is obtained either vaginally or through the abdomen during the eighth to eleventh week of pregnancy. The advantages of this procedure are that it can be done much earlier in the pregnancy and that enough tissue can be collected to conduct the chromosome analysis immediately, without the cell culture step. Consequently, diagnosis can be completed during the first trimester of the pregnancy, making therapeutic abortion an option for the parents. Chorionic villus sampling does have some negative aspects. One disadvantage is the slightly higher incidence of test-induced miscarriage as compared to amniocentesis. Also, because tissue of both the mother and the fetus are obtained in the sampling process, they must be carefully separated, complicating the analysis. Occasionally, chromosomal abnormalities are observed in the tested tissue that are not present in the fetus itself.

Prenatal maternal alpha-fetoprotein testing has also been used to diagnose Down syndrome. Abnormal levels of a substance called maternal alpha-fetoprotein are often associated with chromosomal disorders. Several research studies have described a high correlation between low levels of maternal alpha-fetoprotein and the occurrence of trisomy 21 in the fetus. Through correlating alpha-fetoprotein levels, the age of the mother, and specific female hormone levels, between 70 and 80 percent of fetuses with Down syndrome can be de-

In the News:
New Screening Tests for Down Syndrome

Down syndrome is the most common chromosome condition, occurring in 1 of every 750 live births. Individuals who have Down syndrome usually have an extra copy of chromosome number 21 (trisomy 21). The extra chromosome leads to a distinctive appearance, mild-to-moderate mental retardation, and sometimes additional medical complications such as a heart defect or digestive system problems.

The risk to have a pregnancy with Down syndrome increases with a women's age, but all women have a risk to have an affected pregnancy. Therefore, all pregnant women are offered screening tests for Down syndrome. These screening tests can be performed as early as the first trimester of pregnancy. The accumulation of fluid behind the fetal neck—called a nuchal translucency, or NT—can be measured on ultrasound between ten and thirteen weeks of gestation. This measurement tends to be larger in fetuses that have Down syndrome. The NT measurement can be combined with a measurement of hormones found in the maternal blood that are produced by the pregnancy as well as a woman's age, weight, and ethnicity to give a personalized risk estimate for the fetus to have Down syndrome. There are many variations of this testing, and some versions of this screening test involve an additional maternal blood sample in the second trimester.

Although these tests can detect more than 90 percent of fetuses with Down syndrome, they do not give a definitive diagnosis. Women found to be in the high-risk category on screening, also called a screen positive, are offered additional testing, such as a detailed level II ultrasound at approximately 18 weeks gestation. Half of fetuses with Down syndrome will display a marker, or soft sign on ultrasound, such as thickened skin behind the neck, short bones, or a bright spot in the heart. The presence or absence of a soft marker can be used to further refine the risk for the pregnancy to have Down syndrome, but is not diagnostic.

The only diagnostic testing for Down syndrome in the pregnancy is chorionic villus sampling (CVS) or amniocentesis. Both tests are invasive and carry a small risk of miscarriage and many women forgo this testing due to the procedure-related risk. The technology to detect fetal cells in the maternal bloodstream is rapidly evolving, and soon pregnant woman may be able to learn if their fetus has Down syndrome with a simple blood draw. This technology could certainly revolutionize the field of prenatal diagnosis for Down syndrome.

—Lauren Lichten, M.S., C.G.C.

sultant trisomy 21 is not of a hereditary nature, the abnormality can be detected only by prenatal screening, which is recommended for all pregnancies of women older than age thirty-four.

For parents of a child with Down syndrome, genetic counseling can be beneficial in determining their risk factor for future pregnancies. The genetic counselor determines the specific chromosomal aberration that occurred, using chromosome studies of the parents and affected child as well as additional information provided by the family history. If the cause was nondisjunction and the mother is young, the recurrence risk is much less than 1 percent; for mothers over the age of thirty-four, it is about 5 percent. If the cause was translocational, the Down syndrome is hereditary and risk is greater—statistically, there is a one-in-three chance that the next child will have Down syndrome. In addition, there is a one-in-three chance that offspring without Down syndrome will be carriers of the syndrome, producing it in the next generation. It is suggested that couples who come from families having a history of spontaneous miscarriages, which often result from lethal chromosomal aberrations, or incidence of Down syndrome, undergo chromosomal screening to detect the presence of a Down syndrome translocation.

Perspective and Prospects

English physician John L. H. Down is credited with recording the first clinical description of Down syndrome in 1886. Since the distinctive epicanthic fold gave children with the syndrome an appearance that Down associated with Asians, he called the condition *mongolism*—an unfortunate term implying that those affected with the condition are throwbacks to a more "primitive" racial group. Today, the inappropriate term has been replaced with the name Down syndrome.

A French physician, Jérôme Lejeune, suspected that Down syndrome had a genetic basis and began to study the condition in 1953. A comparison of the fingerprints and palm prints of affected individuals with those of unaffected individuals showed a high frequency of abnormalities in the prints of those with Down syndrome. These prints appear very early in development and serve as a record of events that take place early in embryogenesis. The extent of the changes in print patterns led Lejeune to the conclusion that the condition was

tected. Although techniques allow Down syndrome to be detected readily in a fetus, there is no effective intrauterine therapy available to correct the chromosomal abnormality.

The care of a Down syndrome child presents many challenges for the family unit. Until the 1970s, most children with Down syndrome spent their lives in institutions. With the increased support services available, however, it is now common for children to remain in the family environment. Although many children with Down syndrome have happy dispositions, a significant number have behavioral problems that can consume the energies of the parents, to the detriment of other children. Rearing a child with Down syndrome often places a large financial burden on the family; for example, they are particularly susceptible to illness, possibly necessitating extensive medical care, and also have special educational needs. Since children with Down syndrome are often conceived late in the parents" reproductive period, the parents may not be able to continue to care for these children throughout their offspring's adult years. This is problematic because many individuals with Down syndrome do not possess sufficient mental skills to earn a living or to manage their affairs without supervision.

All women in their mid-thirties have an increased risk of giving birth to an infant with Down syndrome. Since the re-the result of the action not of one or two genes but of many genes or even an entire chromosome. Upon microscopic examination, he observed that Down syndrome children possess forty-seven chromosomes instead of the forty-six chromosomes found in normal children. In 1959, Lejeune published his findings, showing that Down syndrome is caused by the presence of the extra chromosome that was later identified as a copy of chromosome 21. This first observation of a human chromosomal abnormality marked a turning point in the study of human genetics. It demonstrated that genetic defects not only were caused by mutations of single genes but also could be associated with changes in chromosome number. Although the presence of an extra chromosome allows varying degrees of development to occur, most of these abnormalities result in fetal death, with only a few resulting in live birth. Down syndrome is unusual in that the affected individual often survives into adulthood.

—*Arlene R. Courtney, Ph.D.*

See also Amniocentesis; Birth defects; Chorionic villus sampling; Congenital disorders; DNA and RNA; Genetic diseases; Genetics and inheritance; Leukemia; Mental retardation; Mutation.

For Further Information:

A.D.A.M. Medical Encyclopedia. "Down Syndrome." *MedlinePlus*, May 16, 2012.

Cohen, William, Lynn Nadel, and Myra E. Madnick, eds. *Down Syndrome: Visions for the Twenty-first Century.* New York: Wiley-Liss, 2002.

Hassold, Terry J., and David Patterson, eds. *Down Syndrome: A Promising Future, Together.* New York: Wiley-Liss, 1999.

Miller, Jon F., Mark Leddy, and Lewis A. Leavitt, eds. *Improving the Communication of People with Down Syndrome.* 2d ed. Baltimore: Paul H. Brookes, 2003.

Moore, Keith L., and T. V. N. Persaud. *The Developing Human.* 8th ed. Philadelphia: Saunders/Elsevier, 2008.

National Center on Birth Defects and Developmental Disabilities. "Facts about Down Syndrome." *Centers for Disease Control and Prevention*, June 8, 2011.

National Down Syndrome Society. http://www.ndss.org.

Pueschel, Siegfried M. *A Parent's Guide to Down Syndrome.* Rev. ed. Baltimore: Paul H. Brookes, 2001.

Pueschel, Siegfried M., ed. *Adults with Down Syndrome.* Baltimore: Paul H. Brookes, 2006.

Rondal, Jean A., et al., eds. *Down's Syndrome: Psychological, Psychobiological, and Socioeducational Perspectives.* San Diego, Calif.: Singular, 1996.

Wood, Debra. "Down Syndrome." *HealthLibrary*, May 21, 2013.

DROWNING
Disease/Disorder

Anatomy or system affected: Brain, circulatory system, heart, kidneys, lungs, nervous system, respiratory system, stomach, throat

Specialties and related fields: Critical care, emergency medicine, environmental health, nursing, pulmonary medicine

Definition: A drowning victim dies by suffocation from submersion in a liquid medium, usually water.

Key terms:

alveolar ventilation: the volume of air that ventilates all the perfused alveoli; the normal average is four to five liters per minute

asphyxia: cessation of breathing

bradycardia: a heart rate below sixty beats per minute

glottis: the opening to the larynx

hypertonic fluid: a solution that increases the degree of osmotic pressure on a semipermeable membrane

hypothermia: an abnormal and dangerous condition in which the temperature of the body is below 95 degrees Fahrenheit; usually caused by prolonged exposure to cold

hypoxia: inadequate oxygen at the cellular level

intrapulmonary shunting: a condition of perfusion without ventilation

laryngospasm: spasm of the larynx

Causes and Symptoms

Drowning is one of the leading causes of accidental death. The victim dies by suffocation from submersion in a liquid medium. Although suffocation most commonly results from the aspiration of fresh or salt water into the lungs, about 10 percent to 20 percent of victims experience a laryngospasm with subsequent glottic closure, followed by asphyxiation. Near-drowning is defined as recovery after submersion. Victims are typically children or adolescents. Males more often engage in risk-taking behavior and have a significantly greater incidence of drowning and near-drowning than do females.

Victims of near-drowning, if rescued and resuscitated quickly enough, may fully recover. In many instances, however, near-drowning victims are left with mild to severe neurologic effects. Even if the victim has been submerged in water for some time, vigorous attempts at resuscitation are indicated because of documented recovery following such incidents.

Boating and swimming accidents account for the largest number of drownings in the adult population, and many are alcohol-related. Factors that influence the extent of damage in near-drowning include the length of time submerged, the temperature of the water, and the victim's resistance to asphyxia and anoxia (oxygen deprivation). Recovery may be more successful if the victim drowns in cold water, because the induced hypothermia lowers the body's metabolic demands and, therefore, oxygen needs. Extremely cold water may decrease the victim's core body temperature so rapidly that death from hypothermia may actually occur before drowning.

Generally, there is an inverse relation between the victim's age and the victim's resistance to asphyxia and anoxia. The younger the victim, the greater the resistance. The resistance is especially strong in very young victims, usually under two or three years of age, because of the diving reflex triggered in young children when the face is immersed in very cold water. Blood is shunted to the vital organs, especially the brain and heart. Hypothermia offers some protection to the hypoxic brain by reducing the cerebral metabolic rate. Although the victim suffers severe bradycardia, the remaining oxygen supply is concentrated in the heart and brain. The diving reflex is generally not a factor in adult drownings.

Information on Drowning

Causes: Submersion in a liquid medium, resulting in aspiration or asphyxiation

Symptoms: Slow heart rate, hypoxemia, ineffective circulation, cardiac arrest, brain injury, brain death; following near-drowning, may include acute respiratory failure, cerebral and pulmonary edema, shock acidosis, electrolyte imbalance, stupor, coma, cardiac arrest

Duration: Acute and often fatal; possible permanent effects for near-drowning

Treatments: For near-drowning, cardiopulmonary resuscitation (CPR), intubation, mechanical ventilation, stomach decompression, sometimes induced coma and hypothermia

Approximately 10 percent of drowning victims develop laryngospasm concurrently with the first gulp of water and thus do not aspirate (swallow) fluid. Even in the majority of victims who do aspirate, the amount of fluid aspirated is small. In the past, salt water and freshwater drowning were differentiated. These differences are of little clinical significance in humans, primarily because so little fluid is aspirated. In both cases, drowning quickly diminishes perfusion to the alveoli, interfering with ventilation and soon leading to hypoxemia, ineffective circulation, cardiac arrest, brain injury, and brain death.

When water is aspirated into the lungs, the composition of the water is a key factor in the pathophysiology of the near-drowning event. Aspiration of freshwater causes surfactant to wash out of the lungs. Surfactant reduces surface tension within the alveoli, increases lung compliance and alveolar radius, and decreases the work of breathing. Loss of surfactant from freshwater aspiration destabilizes the alveoli and leads to increased airway resistance. Conversely, salt water—a hypertonic fluid—creates an osmotic gradient that draws protein-rich fluid from the vascular space into the alveoli. The consequences of both types of aspiration include impaired alveolar ventilation and resultant intrapulmonary shunting, which further compound the hypoxic state.

When submersion is brief, the near-drowning victim may spontaneously regain consciousness or may recover quickly following rescue. Even when victims have not aspirated fluid, they should be hospitalized for observation because respiratory symptoms may not develop for twelve to twenty-four hours. Victims who have been submerged for longer periods may show varying degrees of recovery following resuscitation. Manifestations may include acute respiratory failure, pulmonary edema, shock acidosis, electrolyte imbalance, stupor, coma, and cardiac arrest. Damage causes cerebral edema (brain swelling) and may lead to increased intracranial pressure. Care for the patient who has suffered brain damage involves careful and frequent assessment of the patient's neurologic status, including vital signs, pupil reaction, and reflexes.

Treatment and Therapy

Immediate care should focus on a safe rescue of the victim. Once rescuers gain access to the victim, priorities include safe removal from the water, while maintaining spine stabilization with a board or flotation device, and initiating airway clearance and ventilatory support measures. If hypothermia is a concern, then gentle handling of the victim is essential to prevent ventricular fibrillation. Abdominal thrusts should only be delivered if airway obstruction is suspected. Once the victim is safely removed from the water, airway and cardiopulmonary support interventions begin. Emergency care involves cardiopulmonary resuscitation (CPR), intubation, and mechanical ventilation with 100 percent oxygen.

In the clinical setting, stomach decompression using a tube down the nose or mouth is indicated to prevent the aspiration of gastric contents and to improve breathing.

Patients who experience near-drowning require complex care to support their body systems. The full spectrum of critical care technology may be needed to manage the physiological problems and effects associated with near-drowning, including lung infection, acute respiratory distress syndrome, and central nervous system impairment. Metabolic acidosis results from severe hypoxia. Arterial blood gases must be monitored frequently, and sodium bicarbonate is usually administered to correct the acidosis. Coma may be induced with barbiturates and a state of hypothermia maintained for several days following the near-drowning. These interventions reduce the metabolic and oxygen demands of the brain. Diuretics are prescribed to treat pulmonary and cerebral edema. Fluid therapy must be monitored carefully to prevent fluid overload and to promote adequate renal function.

Perspective and Prospects

Drowning is the third leading cause of preventable death worldwide, according to the World Health Organization. The Centers for Disease Control and Prevention states that drowning is the leading cause of preventable death in children. Drowning prevention recommendations warn parents to be certain that everyone caring for a child understands the need for constant supervision around water and other liquids.

—*Jane C. Norman, Ph.D., R.N., C.N.E.*

See also Accidents; Asphyxiation; Brain damage; Cardiopulmonary resuscitation (CPR); Choking; Critical care; Critical care, pediatric; Emergency medicine; Emergency medicine, pediatric; First aid; Hyperbaric oxygen therapy; Lungs; Pulmonary medicine; Pulmonary medicine, pediatric; Respiration; Resuscitation; Unconsciousness.

For Further Information:

Black, Joyce M., and Jane H. Hawks, eds. *Medical-Surgical Nursing: Clinical Management for Positive Outcomes*. 8th ed. St. Louis, Mo.: Saunders/Elsevier, 2009.

Dean, Normal L. "Drowning." *Merck Manual Home Health Handbook*, Jan. 2009.

"Drowning." *MedlinePlus*, 30 July 2013.

"Drowning." *World Health Organization*, Oct. 2012.

Heller, Jacob L., and David Zieve. "Near Drowning." *MedlinePlus*, 4 Jan. 2011.

Lewis, Sharon M., et al., eds. *Medical-Surgical Nursing: Assessment and Management of Clinical Problems*. 7th ed. St. Louis, Mo.: Mosby/Elsevier, 2007.

Smeltzer, Suzanne C., and Brenda G. Bare, eds. *Brunner and Suddarth's Textbook of Medical-Surgical Nursing*. 12th ed. Philadelphia: Wolters Kluwer/Lippincott Williams & Wilkins, 2010.

"Unintentional Drowning: Get the Facts." *Centers for Disease Control and Prevention*, 29 Nov. 2012.

DRUG ADDICTION. *See* ADDICTION.

DRY EYE
Disease/Disorder

Anatomy or system affected: Outer layers of the eye, with possible effects on clear vision through inflammation; nasal lacrimal duct

Specialties and related fields: Ophthalmology

Definition: Dry eye syndrome (DES), or keratoconjunctivitis sicca, affects the outer layers of the eye, which must be continually moistened by the liquid content of the tears. The normal flow of tears may be reduced as a result of the aging process or various external causes, including wearing contact lenses. DES occurs more among women than among men.

Key terms:

blepharospasm: increased blinking to try to compensate for a lack of moisture on the eye surface

conjunctiva: the transparent tissue that covers the surface of the eye and inner sections of the eyelid; this tissue secretes oils and mucous that, helped by the presence of tears, lubricate the eye

corneal epithelium: the transparent covering of the outer surface of the eye that serves mainly to protect the eye; the cornea can be damaged as a result of DES

lacrimal glands: located (as pairs) in recesses in the skull above each eye, these glands release liquid tears; these are then spread across the surface of the eye when the eyelids blink

tear breakup time: the time between initial tear flow onto the eye surface and the first phase of evacuation of moisture via the lacrimal fossi into the lacrimal sac

Causes and Symptoms

If the eye surface does not receive sufficient moisture and lubrication from the normal flow of tears from the lacrimal glands, a first symptom may be a feeling of scratchiness when blinking. This can be accompanied by a burning sensation. In advanced stages of DES, damage may spread, in the form of inflammation, to the cornea and the eyelids.

The essential cause of DES stems in one way or another from a reduced flow of tears from the lacrimal glands. In addition to a natural decrease in lacrimal gland activity as part of the aging process, external factors (some obvious, like extended exposure to dry wind or smoky conditions) can affect the necessary supply of tears to the surface of the eyes. Eye fatigue after long hours of television viewing, computer use, or driving can contribute directly to the onset of DES.

Several eye diseases are directly or indirectly related to keratoconjuntivitis sicca. The most common is blepharitus, a chronic inflammation of the eyelid. It begins with characteristic eyelid redness but-if not treated promptly-develops into more dangerous conditions involving flaking of the skin and crusting at the lid edges. In advanced cases cysts may develop. Inflammation of the cornea is also linked to DES.

In both moderate and more serious cases of DES, the functioning of the lacrimal drainage system (LDS) can be adversely affected. The anatomy of the LDS, which is linked to the mucosa bearing parts of the conjuctiva, consists of two apertures (lacrimal puncti) at the ends of the eyelids. Soon after the lacrimal glands have released tears onto the eye a "tear breaking point" occurs. Excess liquid tears are taken into the lacrimal puncta, passing through narrow canals into the lacrimal sac, from which liquid flows into the naso-lacrimal duct into the nose. Any malfunctioning of this transfer process linked to DES-particularly insufficient moisture moving from the eyes into and through the lacrimal puncta-may call for delicate treatments that are specific to DES (see below).

Treatment and Therapy

Many ophthalmologists favor regular consumption of dark fleshed fish (which contains omega-3 fatty acids), as a natural measure for people seeking to prevent DES. When less serious cases begin, eye dropper application of a prepared solution of artificial tears (sold over the counter at most pharmacies) can provide relief. Such solutions contain a mixture of water, salts, and one or more chemicals such as carboxymethyl cellulose, or hydroxpropyl cellulose. The latter additive has a thickening effect on the precorneal tear film, causing tears to remain longer on the surface of the eye before the draining process described above. Artificial tears lack, however, essential proteins (mainly lysozyme) found in natural tears, so they cannot be fully effective.

Several immune response reactions occurring naturally on the ocular surface, including the synthesis and release by the epithelium of cytokines (soluable proteins, peptides, and glycoproteins) and enzymes that serve as catalysts in combination with chemicals in the outer layers of the eye, are the body's way of providing soothing effects.

When DSE symptoms suggest that natural tears are being evacuated too rapidly via the lacrimal puncti, several treatments may be appropriate. These can involve insertion of specially prepared plugs into the puncta (a process which can be adjusted periodically) or actual shrinkage of the puncti apertures by cauterization and permanent scarring of the surrounding tissue.

Perspective and Prospects

Because DES is mentioned widely in the media (especially television) the general public is much more aware now than in the past of symptoms and preventive treatment. As for its more serious potential consequences, recent scientific advances have made it possible to correct eye disorders stemming from advanced keratoconjuntivitis sicca. A notable example is the (now relatively widespread) possibility of transplants to replace damaged corneas.

Ongoing research in the field of molecular cloning and gene transfer techniques suggests that, because the surface of the eye is particularly accessible for skilled surgical intervention, serious eye diseases that initially develop from DES conditions may in the future be treatable by transferring highly selective "foreign" genes into target cells in the epithelial tissue.

—*Byron Cannon, Ph.D.*

See also Vision; Vision disorders

For Further Information:

Asbell, Penny A., and Michael A. Lemp. *Dry Eye Disease: The Clinician's Guide to Diagnosis and Treatment.* New York: Thieme, 2006.

Kao, Winston W. "Particle-Mediated Gene Transfer to Ocular Surface Epithelium." *Lacrimal Gland, Tear Film, and Dry Eye Syndromes 3, Part A,* edited by David A. Sullivan, et al. New York: Kluwer Academic/Plenum Publishers, 2002.

Pflugfelder, Stephen C., and Roger W. Beuerman. *Dry Eye and Ocular Surface Disorders.* New York: Butterworth-Heineman, 2003.

Weizer, Jennifer S., and Joshua D. Stein. *Reader's Digest Guide to Eye Care: Common Vision Problems, from Dry Eye to Macular Degeneration.* Pleasantville, NY: Reader's Digest Association, 2009.

DWARFISM
Disease/Disorder

Anatomy or system affected: Back, bones, brain, endocrine system, glands, hips, legs, musculoskeletal system, nervous system, respiratory system

Specialties and related fields: Endocrinology, genetics, orthopedics, pediatrics

Definition: Underdevelopment of the body, most often caused by a variety of genetic or endocrinological dysfunctions and resulting in either proportionate or disproportionate development, sometimes accompanied by other physical abnormalities and/or mental deficiencies.

Key terms:

amino acid: the building blocks of protein

autosomal: refers to all chromosomes except the X and Y chromosomes (sex chromosomes) that determine body traits

cleft palate: a gap in the root of the mouth, sometimes present at birth and frequently combined with harelip

collagen: protein material of which the white fibers of the connective tissue of the body are composed

hypoglycemia: low blood sugar

laminae: arches of the vertebral bones

spondylosis: a condition characterized by restriction of movement of the vertebral bones; occurs naturally as a child grows

stenosis: any narrowing of a passage or orifice of the body

Causes and Symptoms

Dwarfism in humans may be caused by a number of conditions that occur either before birth or in early childhood. When short stature is the only observable feature, growth—though abnormal relative to height—is proportionate. Short stature is nearly always attributed to endocrinological dysfunction, but few cases are actually the result of endocrinopathy. If short stature is caused by endocrinopathy, it is often attributable to a deficiency in the pituitary gland (which produces growth hormone) or the thyroid gland. Those who are unusually short but have no other obvious disease are divided into two categories: those who were afflicted prenatally and those who were afflicted postnatally. Many cases are actually the result of chromosomal or skeletal aberrations; other events that may inhibit prenatal growth include magnesium deficiency (which would prohibit ribosome synthesis and, in turn, halt protein synthesis) or a uterus that is too small. Postnatal inhibition of growth may be caused by heredity if both parents are short; there is no skeletal abnormality at fault. Other short-statured children may simply mature at a much slower rate, yet grow normally. Typically, one of the parents may have had a late onset of puberty.

Unusually short-statured males are those who are shorter than sixty inches tall; in females, fifty-eight inches and below is short-statured. Children are classified as dwarfs if their height is below the third percentile for their age. When this is the case, doctors will look primarily to four major causes of dwarfism: an underactive or inactive pituitary gland, achondroplasia (failure of normal development in cartilage), emotional or nutritional deprivation, or Turner syndrome (the possession of a single, X, chromosome). If the answer is not found in one of these alternatives, then it may be found in rarer causes, either genetically based or disease induced.

Growth hormone, also called somatotropin, determines a person's height. Growth hormone does not affect brain growth but may influence the brain's functions. In addition, it may enhance the growth of nerves radiating from the brain so that they can reach their targets. Growth hormone elevates the appetite, increases metabolic rate, maintains the immune system, and works in coordination with other hormones to regulate carbohydrate, protein, lipid, nucleic acid, water, and electrolyte metabolism. Target areas for growth hormone include cell membranes as well as other cell organelles in bone, cartilage, bone marrow, adipose tissue, and the liver, kidney, heart, pancreas, mammary glands, ovaries, testes, thymus gland, and hypothalamus. Fetuses not producing growth hormone still grow normally until birth; they may even weigh more than average at birth. These babies may thrive at first, but if no growth hormone is administered, they will grow to a maximum height of thirty inches. Other telltale physical attributes include higher-than-average body fat, a high forehead, wrinkled skin, and a high-pitched voice. During childhood, there may be episodic hypoglycemia attacks. If the endocrine system is functioning properly, puberty may be delayed but will still occur. Complete reproductive maturity will be reached, and there is great likelihood that the afflicted person will develop his or her complete intellectual potential. When it is inherited, growth hormone deficiency occurs as an autosomal recessive trait. Yet the genetic basis for growth hormone deficiency may not simply be caused by a gene. The condition could, in theory, be the result of a structural defect

Information on Dwarfism

Causes: Genetic or endocrinological dysfunctions
Symptoms: Short stature, higher-than-average body fat, high forehead, wrinkled skin, high-pitched voice, episodic hypoglycemia during childhood, late onset of puberty
Duration: Lifelong
Treatments: Growth hormone

in the pituitary gland or the hypothalamus, or in the secretory mechanisms of growth hormone itself. Prenatal factors that contribute to the inhibition of growth include toxemia, kidney and heart disease, rubella, maternal malnutrition, maternal age, small uterus, and environmental influences such as alcohol and drug use.

Prenatal thyroid dysfunction that goes untreated results in congenital hypothyroidism. Children with this disorder do not undergo nervous, skeletal, or reproductive maturation; they may not grow over thirty inches tall. When administered before a child is two months of age, treatment can cause a complete reversal of symptoms. Delayed treatment, however, cannot reverse brain damage, although growth and reproductive organs can be dramatically affected.

Achondroplasia is the most common form of short-limb dwarfism. It is inherited as an autosomal dominant form of dwarfism. Achondroplasia is expressed only when one copy of the gene is present; when an offspring inherits the dominant gene from both parents, the condition is lethal. Incidence of achondroplasia increases with parental age and is more closely related to the father's age. Mutations may account for a majority of cases of achondroplasia, since there is an affected parent in only about 20 percent of cases. Achondroplasia results from abnormal embryonic development that affects bone growth; metaphyseal development is prevented, which means that cartilaginous bone growth is impaired. This is accompanied by unusually small laminae of the spine, resulting in spinal stenosis. The spinal cord may become compressed during the normal process of spondylosis. Individuals with achondroplasia may experience slowly progressing weakness of the legs as a result of the spinal cord compression. Achondroplasia is often distinguished by the presence of a disproportionately large head and dwarfed and curved limbs; in addition, an individual may have a prominent forehead and a depressed nasal bridge. A shallow thoracic cage and pelvic tilt may cause a protuberant abdomen. Bowlegs are caused by overly long fibulae. Individuals with achondroplasia who live to adulthood are typically thirty-six to sixty inches tall and have unusual muscular strength; reproductive and mental development are not affected, and neither is longevity.

Marasmus, severe emaciation resulting from malnutrition prenatally or in early infancy, may be considered a form of dwarfism. It is caused by extremely low caloric and protein intake, which causes a wasting of body tissues. Usually marasmus is found in babies either weaned very early or never breast-fed. All growth is inhibited, including head cir-

cumference. If the area housing the brain fails to grow, then it cannot house a normal-sized brain, and the individual may develop an intellectual disability. Infants with marasmus are frequently apathetic and hyperirritable. As they lie in bed, they are completely unresponsive to their environment and are irritable when moved or handled. Although the symptoms are treatable and may disappear, the inhibition of growth is permanent.

Occasionally, dwarfism may be induced by emotional starvation. This type of child abuse causes extreme growth inhibition, inhibition of skeletal growth, and delayed psychomotor development. Fortunately, it can be reversed by social and dietary changes. Children with this form of dwarfism are extremely small but perfectly proportioned; however, they have distended abdomens.

The height achieved in females with Turner syndrome is typically between fifty-four and sixty inches. Turner syndrome results when an egg has no X chromosome and is fertilized by an X-bearing sperm. The offspring are females with only one X chromosome. These individuals cannot undergo puberty; their ovaries never develop and are unable to function. Physical manifestations of Turner syndrome include short stature, stocky build, and a webbed neck.

Another cause of short stature may be as a consequence of chronic disease. Children with chronic renal (kidney) failure nearly always experience inhibition of growth because of hormonal, metabolic, and nutritional abnormalities. This occurs more often in children with congenital renal disease than in those with acquired renal disease.

With congenital heart disease, several factors may prohibit growth. Growth inhibition may be a direct result of the disease or an indirect result of other problems associated with heart disease. These babies experience stress, with periods of cardiac failure, and either caloric or protein deficiency. These conditions slow the multiplication of cells and hence growth. If surgery corrects the condition, some catching up can be expected, depending on how much time has elapsed without treatment.

Treatment and Therapy

The more a child is below the average stature, the greater the likelihood of determining the cause. A child who is short statured should be evaluated so that if an endocrine disorder is the root, the child can be treated. Time is an important consideration with hypothyroidism especially, since the longer it goes untreated, the more likely it is that mental development will be arrested.

Children born with congenital growth hormone deficiency are sometimes small for their gestational age; however, the majority of children with growth hormone deficiency acquire the disorder after birth. For the first year or two, the children grow normally, but growth then dramatically decreases. Diagnosis of growth hormone deficiency requires numerous tests and sampling. If bone age appears the same as the child's age, then growth hormone deficiency can be eliminated. A test for growth hormone secretion is performed by measuring a blood sample for growth hormone twenty minutes after ex-

ercise in a fasting child. If this test shows a hormone deficiency, then growth hormone therapy may allow the child to
continue to grow.

At first, growth hormone was harvested from human pituitary glands after persons" deaths. This process was so expensive, however, that few children with hormone deficiency
could be treated. Even worse, some of those who did undergo
this treatment were inadvertently infected with a slow-acting
virus that proved fatal. In the mid-1980s, it was found that
some men who had received human growth hormone died at
an early age of a neurological disorder called Creutzfeldt-
Jakob disease (CJD). These men were found to have contracted the disease via a growth hormone that had been obtained from pituitary glands during autopsies. Once the relationship was determined, more victims were identified. CJD
is a nervous disorder caused by a slow-acting, viruslike particle. Its symptoms include difficulty in balance while walking,
loss of muscular control, slurred speech, impairment of vision, and other muscular disorders. Behavioral and mental
changes such as memory loss, confusion, and dementia may
also occur. The symptoms appear, progress rapidly over the
next months, and usually cause death in less than a year.
There is no treatment or cure.

These unfortunate circumstances led to the development
of a synthetic growth hormone. It is made by encoding bacterial deoxyribonucleic acid (DNA) with the sequence of human growth hormone; the bacteria used are those that grow
normally in the human intestinal tract. The bacteria synthesize human growth hormone using the preprogrammed human sequence of DNA; it is then purified so that no bacteria
remain in the hormone that is used for treatment. The Food
and Drug Administration (FDA) approved the biosynthetic
hormone in 1985. The sole difference between the synthetic
and the naturally produced growth hormone was one amino
acid; in 1987, a new synthetic form without the extra amino
acid became available. This synthetic hormone works exactly
as natural growth hormone does. Moreover, it does not carry
the danger of contamination. In most cases, the patient's immune system does not interfere with the synthetic growth
hormone's effectiveness.

Those children with various forms of chondrodystrophies
(cartilage disorders), such as achondroplasia, are diagnosed
using skeletal measurements, clinical manifestations, x-rays,
laboratory study and analysis of cartilage, and observed abnormalities of the body's proteins, such as collagen and cell
membranes. In chondrodystrophies, skeletal growth is disproportionate, with shortened limbs more common than a
shortened trunk. If visual examination is not confirmation

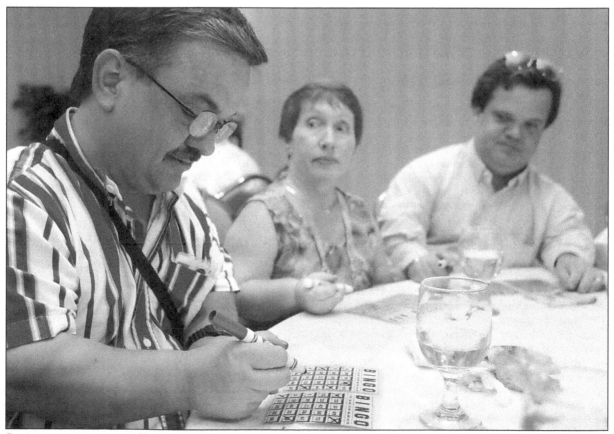

Participants at a convention of Little People of America, an organization for people with dwarfism, play bingo. (AP/Wide World Photos)

enough, the diagnosis may be assured through x-rays. Although histological studies do not necessarily enhance diagnosis, making an analysis of the patient's cartilage may lead to a better understanding of the condition. Biochemical studies of abnormal proteins in chondrodystrophies actually have little diagnostic value, but they too may lead to better understanding. Because achondroplasia is genetically inherited, prevention involves genetic counseling before conception.

A child with achondroplasia may be treated symptomatically; surgery on the fibulae to correct bowlegs may be desirable, either for cosmetic reasons or for functional reasons. Laminectomies or skull surgery may be indicated for neurological problems. Orthodontic surgery may be necessary to correct malocclusions and other dental deformities. If hearing loss occurs because of recurrent ear infections, then corrective surgery may be necessary. Individuals with achondroplasia generally enjoy a normal life span, barring complications.

Other chondrodystrophies that cause dwarfism may have more severe symptoms than achondroplasia. Cockayne syndrome, a type of progeria, is the sudden onset of premature old age in extremely young children. It is the result of inheritance of an autosomal recessive gene. Physical signs of the disease begin after a normal first year of life. In the second year, growth begins to falter, and psychomotor development becomes abnormal. As time passes, dwarfism becomes evident. Other observable characteristics that develop are a shrunken face with sunken eyes and a thin nose, optic degeneration, cavities of the teeth, a photosensitive skin rash that produces scarring, disproportionately long limbs with large hands and feet, and hair loss. The life span for children with this disease is very short.

Another chondrodystrophy inherited through autosomal recessive genes is thanotophoric dwarfism. All known individuals with this condition have died during the first four weeks of life as a result of respiratory distress; most are stillborn. Thanotophoric dwarfism is characterized by an extremely small thoracic cage with only eleven pairs of ribs present. Other physical characteristics of the disease are that the infant has a large skull relative to its face, which is often elongated with a prominent forehead. The eyes are widely spaced, and there is a broad, flat nasal bridge. Frequently, cleft palate is present. The ears are low-set and poorly formed, and the neck is short and fleshy. The limbs, particularly the legs, are bowed; clubfoot is common, as are dislocated hip joints.

A small percentage of short-statured individuals may be unusually short because of social and psychological factors. This condition is called psychosocial dwarfism. This type of nongrowth is secondary to emotional deprivation and is representative of a type of child abuse. The behavior of such children is characterized by apathy and inadequate interpersonal relationships, with inhibited motor and language development. They generally do not gain weight in spite of their extraordinary appetite and excessive thirst; such a child may steal and hoard food yet have the distended abdomen of a starving child. Diagnosis generally identifies a growth hormone deficiency, and when these children are moved to stimulating and accepting environments, their behavior becomes more normal. Their caloric intake decreases as their growth hormone secretion normalizes, and their growth undergoes a dramatic catch-up.

Perspective and Prospects

Because of the complications associated with some forms of dwarfism, medical counseling should begin early. A physical examination should take place in order to determine the type of dwarfism that the child has. If it is ascertained that the short stature cannot be treated, or if the parents and patient choose not to do so, they should be informed of the details of the patient's specific condition and cautioned regarding any future complications that may arise. The patient should be assured that intelligence will not be affected, even if the head is somewhat large. Ear infections are common, and the child should be closely monitored to prevent hearing loss. Normal fertility is the rule, but giving birth will necessitate a cesarean section. In many cases, the child will not be limited physically or mentally as he or she matures. The problems that the patient may face are usually social and emotional; for example, short-statured children may face bullying and discrimination. However, joining nonprofit groups that provide education and support to short-statured individuals may aid children and families in overcoming these difficulties.

—Iona C. Baldridge;
updated by Sharon W. Stark, R.N., A.P.R.N., D.N.Sc.

See also Congenital disorders; Congenital heart disease; Congenital hypothyroidism; Cornelia de Lange syndrome; Endocrine disorders; Endocrinology; Endocrinology, pediatric; Gigantism; Growth; Hormones; Metabolic disorders; Rubinstein-Taybi syndrome.

For Further Information:

Adelson, B., and J. Hall. *Dwarfism: Medical and Psychological Aspects of Profound Short Stature.* Baltimore: Johns Hopkins University Press, 2005.

Brooks, S. J., and Robert S. Bar. *Early Diagnosis and Treatment of Endocrine Disorders.* Totowa, N.J.: Humana Press, 2003.

Juul, Anders, and Jens O. L. Jorgensen, eds. *Growth Hormone in Adults: Physiological and Clinical Aspects.* 2d ed. New York: Cambridge University Press, 2000.

Kelly, Thaddeus E. *Clinical Genetics and Genetic Counseling.* 2d ed. Chicago: Year Book Medical, 1986.

Kronenberg, Henry M., et al., eds. *Williams Textbook of Endocrinology.* 11th ed. Philadelphia: Saunders/Elsevier, 2008.

Little People of America. http://www.lpaonline.org.

Mayo Clinic. "Dwarfism." *Mayo Foundation for Medical Education and Research*, August 27, 2011.

MedlinePlus. "Dwarfism." *MedlinePlus*, May 13, 2013.

MedlinePlus. "Growth Disorders." *MedlinePlus*, May 13, 2013.

Morgan, Brian L. G., and Roberta Morgan. *Hormones: How They Affect Behavior, Metabolism, Growth, Development, and Relationships.* Los Angeles: Price, Stern, Sloan, 1989.

Shaw, Michael, ed. *Everything You Need to Know About Diseases.* Springhouse, Pa.: Springhouse Press, 1996.

DYSENTERY. *See* **DIARRHEA AND DYSENTERY.**

DYSKINESIA

Disease/Disorder

Also known as: Hyperkinesia, levodopa-induced dyskinesia, paroxysmal dyskinesia, tardive dyskinesia

Anatomy or system affected: Arms, brain, feet, hands, head, legs, mouth, neck, nerves, nervous system, psychic-emotional system

Specialties and related fields: Geriatrics and gerontology, neurology, pharmacology, physical therapy, psychiatry

Definition: Abnormal involuntary movements with different causes and clinical presentations.

Key terms:

anticholinergic: an agent that blocks the neurotransmitter acetylcholine

anticonvulsant: an agent that prevents or relieves seizures

antiemetic: an agent that prevents or relieves nausea and vomiting

basal ganglia: a group of interconnected deep brain nuclei that includes striatum, pallidum, subthalamic nucleus, and substantia nigra

benzodiazepine: any of a group of drugs with strong sedative and hypnotic action

brain stem: a part of the brain that connects the cerebral hemispheres with the spinal cord

dopaminergic: related to the neurotransmitter dopamine; nerve terminals releasing the neurotransmitter dopamine

levodopa: a precursor to the neurotransmitter dopamine, used in treating Parkinson's disease

neuroleptic: an agent that modifies psychotic behavior; in general, synonymous with "antipsychotic"

Causes and Symptoms

There are many types of dyskinesia, with different clinical appearances, pathogenetic mechanisms, and treatment modalities. The most common manifestations are akathisia (restlessness), athetosis (slow, writhing movements), ballism (arm or leg flinging), chorea (jerky, dancelike movements), dystonia (increased muscle tone with repetitive patterned movements and distorted posturing), myoclonus (lightning-fast movements), stereotypy (repetitive, patterned, coordinated ritualistic movements), restless legs, tic, and tremor. These abnormal movements may involve the head, face, mouth, limbs, or trunk. Depending on the specific clinical type, the disease mechanism includes damage to cerebral cortex or subcortical structures such as basal ganglia, brain stem, and cerebellum. In adults, multiple neurodegenerative diseases, inherited conditions, vascular disorders (stroke), tumors, infections, malformations, and drug treatments can lead to dyskinesia. In children, abnormal involuntary movements can be caused by genetic conditions, hypoxia, and excessive bilirubin in the nervous system (kernicterus).

Huntington's disease, an autosomal dominant neurodegenerative disorder, is a common genetic cause of chorea and ballism. Cerebral palsy, overactive thyroid, pregnancy, metabolic abnormalities, and drug-induced disorders are some of the nongenetic causes of choreic motions.

Information on Dyskinesia

Causes: Neurologic, vascular, genetic, or metabolic disorders; pharmacotherapy

Symptoms: Abnormal involuntary movements

Duration: Acute, chronic

Treatments: Pharmacotherapy, drug treatment modification, deep brain stimulation

Combinations of various involuntary movements occur in a group of conditions called paroxysmal dyskinesias, characterized by the sudden occurrence of dyskinetic movements (dystonia, chorea, athetosis, ballism), either spontaneous or triggered by an unexpected stimulus.

Neuroleptic-induced tardive dyskinesia and levodopa-induced dyskinesia are two of the most common drug-induced abnormal movement syndromes. Tardive dyskinesia manifests with grimacing, masticatory motions of the mouth and tongue, and choreo-athetoid movements of the trunk and limbs. Most often it develops after months or years of neuroleptic treatment, especially with typical antipsychotic drugs (such as haloperidol). Nevertheless, it was observed in schizophrenic patients long before the advent of antipsychotic dopaminergic antagonists, which suggests that these individuals might be susceptible to involuntary movements. It is also known to occur after antiemetic treatment (metoclopramide). The pathophysiology of tardive dyskinesia is not completely understood, but dopaminergic hypersensitivity and oxidative stress are believed to be involved.

Dyskinesia can occur after years of levodopa, or L-dopa, therapy for Parkinson's disease. Some movements appear at the peak blood levels of medication (peak-dose dyskinesia), others when the drug level is peaking and falling (biphasic dyskinesia) and even at low drug levels. Young age, longer disease duration, and high levodopa dosage are known risk factors for these complications. The intricate mechanism generating levodopa-induced dyskinesia involves an interplay between the loss of dopaminergic nerve terminals and long-term drug treatment with pulsatile stimulation of receptors.

Treatment and Therapy

Therapeutic approaches vary, depending on the type of movement and etiology of dyskinesia. Recommended pharmacologic treatments include benzodiazepines (myoclonus, tremor, dystonia), tetrabenazine (chorea, stereotypy, tremor), anticholinergic agents (dystonia), dopaminergic drugs (restless legs), anticonvulsants (tremor, myoclonus), botulinum toxin (tremors, tics, dystonia), antipsychotics, and brain metabolism enhancers. Deep brain stimulation and repetitive transcranial magnetic stimulation are effective procedures. Stress and activity often aggravate dyskinesia, while relaxation and sleep alleviate it. Physical therapy and self-help groups should be employed as necessary.

In drug-induced dyskinesia, prevention is crucial. Once

the levodopa-induced dyskinesia occurs, modification of the Parkinson's disease treatment regimen becomes necessary. Deep brain stimulation and pharmacotherapy (dopaminergic agents, amantadine) are beneficial in certain categories of patients.

Patients treated with neuroleptics should be examined for involuntary movements before commencing therapy and subsequently maintained on the lowest effective dose. If symptoms develop, then dosage reduction is advised. No agent is truly effective in treating tardive dyskinesia, but vitamin E, tetrabenazine, and botulinum toxin have been shown to alleviate the symptoms. Mild tardive dyskinesia may improve with benzodiazepines and cholinergic agents. Atypical antipsychotic drugs (clozapine, olanzapine, risperidone) are less prone to inducing dyskinesia and may even be beneficial in patients who develop the symptoms.

Perspective and Prospects

In the sixteenth century, Andrea Vesalius and Francisco Piccolomini distinguished subcortical nuclei from cerebral cortex and white matter, and Paracelsus introduced the concept of chorea. The nineteenth century brought the recognition of striatal lesions as causes of chorea and athetosis. Classifications and descriptions for myoclonic movements were introduced. In the late nineteenth century, Gilles de la Tourette and Jean M. Charcot presented cases of tic disorders. A relationship between subthalamic nucleus lesions and ballism was demonstrated in the first half of the twentieth century. Since then, the important role played by this nucleus in hyperkinetic disorders has become evident. In the late twentieth century, genetic mutations were identified in families with dystonia. Therapeutic strategies for levodopa-induced dyskinesia were implemented. Physicians and neuroscientists continue to make significant progress in elucidating the physiology of basal ganglia and the pathogenesis of hyperkinetic movement disorders. Brain imaging, animal models, and molecular techniques are widely used. New modalities of delivering levodopa are being explored. Tardive dyskinesia remains a source of concern as a result of its drug-induced nature. The available data suggest a lower risk of dyskinesia with newer medications. However, more studies of relative risk and appropriate doses are needed.

While attempting to find pathogenesis-targeted therapies, it is imperative to achieve a good understanding of the clinical syndromes and to use comprehensive rating systems. This will allow for more effective patient management, with the goal of improving the quality of life by reducing disability and reliance on caregivers.

—*Mihaela Avramut, M.D., Ph.D.*

See also Cerebral palsy; Huntington's disease; Muscle sprains, spasms, and disorders; Muscles; Nervous system; Neuroimaging; Neurology; Palsy; Parkinson's disease; Seizures; Tics; Tourette's syndrome; Trembling and shaking.

For Further Information:

Bradley, Walter G., et al., eds. *Neurology in Clinical Practice.* 5th ed. Philadelphia: Butterworth Heinemann/Elsevier, 2007.

Dystonia Medical Research Foundation. "Paroxysmal Dystonia and Dyskinesias." *Dystonia Medical Research Foundation*, 2010.

Jankovic, Joseph. "Treatment of Hyperkinetic Movement Disorders." *Lancet Neurology* 8, no. 9 (September, 2009): 844–56.

MedlinePlus. "Movement Disorders." *MedlinePlus*, April 19, 2013.

Parker, James N., and Philip M. Parker, eds. *The Official Patient's Sourcebook on Tardive Dyskinesia: A Revised and Updated Directory for the Internet Age.* San Diego, Calif.: Icon Health, 2002.

Wood, Debra. "Tardive Dyskinesia." *HealthLibrary*, March 15, 2013.

DYSLEXIA

Disease/Disorder

Anatomy or system affected: Brain, ears, eyes, nervous system, psychic-emotional system

Specialties and related fields: Audiology, neurology, psychology, speech pathology

Definition: Severe reading disability in children with average to above-average intelligence.

Key terms:

auditory dyslexia: the inability to perceive individual sounds that are associated with written language

cognitive: relating to the mental process by which knowledge is acquired

computed tomography (CT) scan: a detailed X-ray picture that identifies abnormalities of fine tissue structure

dysgraphia: illegible handwriting resulting from impaired hand-eye coordination

electroencephalogram: a graphic record of the brain's electrical activity

imprinting: training that overcomes reading problems by use of repeated, exaggerated language drills

kinesthetic: related to sensation of body position, presence, or movement, resulting mostly from the stimulation of sensory nerves in muscles, tendons, and joints

phonetics: the science of speech sounds; also called phonology

visual dyslexia: the inability to translate observed written or printed language into meaningful terms

Causes and Symptoms

The term *dyslexia* was first introduced by the German ophthalmologist Rudolf Berlin in the nineteenth century. Berlin defined it as designating all those individuals who possessed average or above-average intelligence quotients (IQs) but who could not read adequately because of their inability to process language symbols. At the same time as Berlin and later, others reported on dyslexic children. These children saw everything perfectly well but acted as if they were blind to all written language. For example, they could see a bird flying but were unable to identify the word *bird* in a written sentence.

The problem involved in dyslexia has been defined and redefined many times since its introduction. The modern definition of the disorder, which is close to Berlin's definition, is based on long-term, extensive studies of dyslexic children. These studies have identified dyslexia as a complex syndrome composed of a large number of associated behavioral dysfunctions that are related to visual-motor brain immaturity and brain dysfunction. These problems include a poor memory for details, easy distractibility, poor motor skills, visual letter and word reversal, and the inability to distinguish between important elements of the spoken language.

Understanding dyslexia in order to correct this reading disability is crucial and difficult. To learn to read well, an individual must acquire many basic cognitive and linguistic skills. First, it is necessary to pay close attention, to concentrate, to follow directions, and to understand the language spoken in daily life. Next, one must develop an auditory and visual memory, strong sequencing ability, solid word decoding skills, the ability to carry out structural-contextual language analysis, the capability to interpret the written language, a solid vocabulary that expands as quickly as is needed, and speed in scanning and interpreting written language. These skills are taught in good developmental reading programs, but some or all are found to be deficient in dyslexic individuals.

Two basic explanations have evolved for dyslexia. Many physicians propose that it is caused by brain damage or brain dysfunction. Evolution of the problem is attributed to accident, disease, or hereditary faults in body biochemistry. Here, the diagnosis of dyslexia is made by the use of electroencephalograms (EEGs), computed tomography (CT) scans, and related neurological technology. After such evaluation is complete, medication is often used to diminish hyperactivity and nervousness, and a group of physical training procedures called patterning is used to counter the neurological defects in the dyslexic individual.

In contrast, many special educators and other researchers believe that the problem of dyslexia is one of dormant, immature, or undeveloped learning centers in the brain. Many proponents of this concept strongly encourage the correction of dyslexic problems through the teaching of specific reading skills. While such experts agree that the use of medication can be of great value, they attempt to cure dyslexia mostly through a process called imprinting. This technique essentially trains dyslexic individuals and corrects their problems via the use of exaggerated, repeated language drills.

Another interesting point of view, expressed by some experts, is the idea that dyslexia may be the fault of the written languages of the Western world. For example, Rudolph F. Wagner argues that Japanese children exhibit a lower incidence of dyslexia. The explanation for this, say Wagner and others, is that unlike Japanese, Western languages require both reading from left to right and phonetic word attack. These characteristics—absent in Japanese—may make the Western languages either much harder to learn or much less suitable for learning.

A number of experts propose three types of dyslexia. The most common type and the one most often identified as dyslexia is called visual dyslexia, the lack of ability to translate the observed written or printed language into meaningful terms. The major difficulty is that afflicted people see certain words or letters backward or upside down. The resultant problem is that to the visual dyslexic, any written sentence is a jumble of many letters whose accurate translation may require five or more times as much effort as is needed by an unafflicted person. The other two problems viewed as dyslexia are auditory dyslexia and dysgraphia. Auditory dyslexia is the inability to perceive individual sounds of spoken language. Despite having normal hearing, auditory dyslexics are deaf to the differences between certain vowel or consonant sounds, and what they cannot hear they cannot write. Dysgraphia is the inability to write legibly. The basis for this problem is a lack of the hand-eye coordination that is required to write clearly.

Many children with visual dyslexia also exhibit elements of auditory dyslexia. This complicates the issue of teaching many dyslexic students because only one type of dyslexic symptom can be treated at a time. Also, dyslexia appears to be a sex-linked disorder, being much more common in boys than in girls.

Treatment and Therapy

The early diagnosis and treatment of dyslexia is essential to its eventual correction. The preliminary identification of a dyslexic child can be made from symptoms that include poor written schoolwork, easy distractibility, clumsiness, poor coordination, poor spatial orientation, confused writing and spelling, and poor left-right orientation. Because numerous nondyslexic children also show many of these symptoms, a second step is required for such identification: the use of written tests designed to identify dyslexics. These tests include the Peabody Individual Achievement Test and the Halstead-Reitan Neuropsychological Test Battery.

EEGs and CT scans are often performed in the hope of pinning down concrete brain abnormalities in dyslexic patients. There is considerable disagreement, however, regarding the value of these techniques, beyond finding evidence of tumors or severe brain damage—both of which may indicate that the condition observed is not dyslexia. Most researchers agree that children who seem to be dyslexic but who lack tumors or damage are no more likely to have EEG or CT scan abnormalities than nondyslexics. An interesting adjunct to EEG use is a technique called brain electrical activity mapping (BEAM). BEAM converts an EEG into a brain map. Viewed by some workers in the area as a valuable technique, BEAM is contested by many others.

Once conclusive identification of a dyslexic child has been made, it becomes possible to begin corrective treatment. Such treatment is usually the preserve of special education programs. These programs are carried out by the special education teacher in school resource rooms. They also involve special classes limited to children with reading disabilities and schools that specialize in treating learning disabilities.

An often-cited method used is that of Grace Fernald, which utilizes kinesthetic imprinting, based on combined language experience and tactile stimulation. In this popular method or adaptations of it, a dyslexic child learns to read in the following way. First, the child tells a spontaneous story to the teacher, who transcribes it. Next, each word that is unrecognizable to the child is written down by the teacher, and the child traces its letters repeatedly until he or she can write the word without using the model. Each word learned becomes part of the child's word file. A large number of stories are handled this way. Though the method is quite slow, many reports praise its results. Nevertheless, no formal studies of its effectiveness have been made.

A second common teaching technique used by special educators is the Orton-Gillingham-Stillman method, which was developed in a collaboration between two teachers and a pediatric neurologist, Samuel T. Orton. The method evolved from Orton's conceptualization of language as developing from a sequence of processes in the nervous system that ends in its unilateral control by the left cerebral hemisphere. He proposed that dyslexia arises from conflicts between this cerebral hemisphere and the right cerebral hemisphere, which is usually involved in the handling of nonverbal, pictorial, and spatial stimuli.

Consequently, the corrective method that is used is a multisensory and kinesthetic approach, like that of Fernald. It

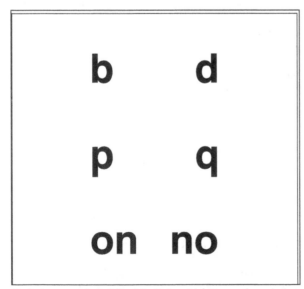

Dyslexia may make it difficult to distinguish letters and words that are mirror images of each other, thus making it difficult for an otherwise intelligent child to learn to read.

begins, however, with the teaching of individual letters and phonemes. Then, it progresses to dealing with syllables, words, and sentences. Children taught by this method are drilled systematically, to imprint them with a mastery of phonics and the sounding out of unknown written words. They are encouraged to learn how the elements of written language look, how they sound, how it feels to pronounce them, and how it feels to write them down. Although the Orton-Gillingham-Stillman method is as laborious as that of Fernald, it is widely used and appears to be successful.

Another treatment aspect that merits discussion is the use of therapeutic drugs in the handling of dyslexia. Most physicians and educators propose the use of these drugs as a useful adjunct to the special education training of those dyslexic children who are restless and easily distracted and who have low morale because of continued embarrassment in school in front of their peers. The drugs that are used most often are amphetamine, dextroamphetamine, and methylphenidate.

These stimulants, given at appropriate dose levels, will lengthen the time period during which certain dyslexic children function well in the classroom and can also produce feelings of self-confidence. Side effects of their overuse, however, include loss of appetite, nausea, nervousness, and sleeplessness. Furthermore, there is also the potential problem of drug abuse. When they are administered carefully and under close medical supervision, however, the benefits of these drugs far outweigh any possible risks.

A proponent of an entirely medical treatment of dyslexia is psychiatrist Harold N. Levinson. He proposes that the root of dyslexia is in inner ear dysfunction and that it can be treated with the judicious application of proper medications. Levinson's treatment includes amphetamines, antihistamines, drugs used against motion sickness, vitamins, and nutrients mixed in the proper combination for each patient. Critics of Levinson's work pose several questions, including whether the studies reported were well controlled and whether the patients treated were actually dyslexic. A major basis for the latter criticism is Levinson's statement that many of his cured patients were described to him as outstanding students. The contention is that dyslexic students are never outstanding students and cannot work at expected age levels.

An important aspect of dyslexia treatment is parental support. Such emotional support helps dyslexics cope with their problems and with the judgment of their peers. Useful aspects of this support include a positive attitude toward an afflicted child, appropriate home help that complements efforts at school, encouragement and praise for achievements, lack of recrimination when repeated mistakes are made, and positive interaction with special education teachers.

Perspective and Prospects

The identification of dyslexia by German physician Rudolf Berlin and England's W. A. Morgan began the efforts to solve this unfortunate disorder. In 1917, Scottish eye surgeon James Hinshelwood published a book on dyslexia, which he viewed as being a hereditary problem, and the phenomenon became much better known to many physicians. Attempts at educating dyslexics were highly individualized until the endeavors of Orton and his coworkers and of Fernald led to more standardized and widely used methods. These procedures, their adaptations, and several others had become the standard treatments for dyslexia by the late twentieth century.

Many famous people—including Hans Christian Andersen, Winston Churchill, Albert Einstein, George Patton, and Woodrow Wilson—had symptoms of dyslexia, which they subsequently overcame. This was fortunate for them, because adults who remain dyslexic are very often at a great disadvantage. Job opportunities open to dyslexics of otherwise adequate intelligence are quite limited.

With the development of a more complete understanding of the brain and its many functions, better counseling facilities, and the conceptualization and actualization of both parent-child and parent-counselor interactions, the probability of success in dyslexic training has improved greatly. Moreover, while environmental and socioeconomic factors contribute relatively little to the occurrence of dyslexia, they strongly affect the outcome of its treatment.

The endeavors of special education have so far made the greatest inroads in the treatment of dyslexia. It is hoped that many more advances in the area will be made as the science of the mind grows and diversifies and the contributions of psychologists, physicians, physiologists, and special educators mesh even more effectively. Perhaps BEAM or the therapeutic methodology suggested by Levinson may provide or contribute to definitive understanding of and treatment of dyslexia.

—*Sanford S. Singer, Ph.D.*

See also Brain; Brain disorders; Developmental disorders; Developmental stages; Learning disabilities.

For Further Information:

Bucciarelli, Alia. "Dyslexia." *HealthLibrary*, January 2, 2013.
Huston, Anne Marshall. *Understanding Dyslexia: A Practical Approach for Parents and Teachers*. Rev. ed. Lanham, Md.: Madison Books, 1992.
International Dyslexia Association. http://www.interdys.org.
Jordan, Dale R. *Overcoming Dyslexia in Children, Adolescents, and Adults*. 3d ed. Austin, Tex.: Pro-Ed, 2002.
Levinson, Harold N. *Smart but Feeling Dumb: The Challenging New Research on Dyslexia—and How It May Help You*. Rev. ed. New York: Warner Books, 2003.
Mayo Clinic. "Dyslexia." *Mayo Foundation for Medical Education and Research*, August 23, 2011.
National Institute of Neurological Disorders and Stroke. "NINDS Dyslexia Information Page." *National Institutes of Health*, September 30, 2011.
Reid, Gavin, and Jane Kirk. *Dyslexia in Adults: Education and Employment*. New York: John Wiley & Sons, 2001.
Snowling, Margaret. *Dyslexia: A Cognitive Developmental Perspective*. 2d ed. Malden, Mass.: Blackwell, 2002.
Wolraich, Mark L., ed. *Disorders of Development and Learning: A Practical Guide to Assessment and Management*. 3d ed. Hamilton, Ont.: B. C. Decker, 2003.

DYSMENORRHEA
Disease/Disorder
Anatomy or system affected: Reproductive system, uterus
Specialties and related fields: Gynecology
Definition: A common menstrual disorder characterized by painful menstrual flow that is more severe than the usual cramps experienced by women with menstruation.

Causes and Symptoms

Dysmenorrhea is classified into primary and secondary dysmenorrhea. In primary dysmenorrhea, no organic cause of the menstrual pain is found, although multiple theories exist in the medical literature as to why pain occurs. Dysmenorrhea is associated with a number of psychological symptoms, including depression, irritability, and insomnia, although it is not clear whether these psychological symptoms are causes or effects.

Secondary dysmenorrhea is painful menstruation that occurs in the setting of a known pelvic disease, such as endometriosis or adenomyosis; an infection such as endometritis, pelvic inflammatory disease (PID), or a sexually transmitted disease; or anatomic abnormalities, such as uterine fibroids, ovarian cysts, or developmental abnormalities of the uterus, cervix, or vagina. Other potential factors include inflammatory bowel disease (IBD), use of a copper intrauterine device (IUD), and scar tissue from surgery.

The symptoms of dysmenorrhea involve dull lower abdominal pain or cramping at the midline. The discomfort may radiate to the lower back or thighs. It can be associated with a number of other symptoms, most commonly nausea and vomiting or fatigue. Dysmenorrhea can occur up to one to two days before the onset of menstrual flow and usually lasts for forty-eight to seventy-two hours. The most severe pain usually occurs on the first day of menstrual flow.

Treatment and Therapy

Treatment is recommended if dysmenorrhea interferes with the activities of daily living. The two most common treatments are hormones and nonsteroidal anti-inflammatory drugs (NSAIDs). Ibuprofen is particularly effective and commonly prescribed in doses of 600 and even 800 milligrams every six hours, which exceeds the over-the-counter limits of 400 milligrams every six hours. Ibuprofen should never be taken on an empty stomach or by women with gastric conditions that are contraindications to the drug. In women who do not desire pregnancy, combined hormonal contraception, either in the form of birth control pills, patches, vaginal rings, or hormone-containing IUDs, are an effective method of controlling dysmenorrhea, as they can reduce the volume of blood flow. A progestin-only birth control injection or implant may also be effective. If combined hormonal contraception is utilized, dosing in a continuous or extended fashion can help to reduce symptoms.

In women nearing menopause, hormones that artificially induce menopause can serve as a bridge until natural menopause occurs. In women with primary dysmenorrhea whose symptoms do not improve after six to twelve months of medi-

---

Information on Dysmenorrhea

Causes: Primary type unknown but associated with psychological symptoms (depression, irritability, insomnia); secondary type caused by pelvic disease (endometriosis or adenomyosis), infection (endometritis or pelvic inflammatory disease), or anatomic abnormalities (uterine fibroids or developmental abnormalities of uterus, cervix, or vagina)

Symptoms: Dull lower abdominal pain or cramping radiating to lower back or thighs; associated with nausea, vomiting, fatigue

Duration: Two or three days

Treatments: Hormones, prostaglandin synthetase inhibitors, treatment of underlying condition

---

cal treatment, laparoscopy may be considered to search for organic causes of pain.

In secondary dysmenorrhea, the treatment of any underlying pelvic disease may ameliorate the symptoms. For instance, anatomic abnormalities may be amenable to surgery. Endometriosis may be treated with hormones or removal procedures.

Pain from either primary or secondary amenorrhea is often responsive to prostaglandin synthetase inhibitors, such as ibuprofen. These drugs decrease the levels of prostaglandins (which cause uterine cramping) in the menstrual blood. Patients with psychological symptoms accompanying their dysmenorrhea may benefit from psychological counseling and therapy. In cases of dysmenorrhea that resist standard treatment, a number of alternate treatments have been tried, with varying levels of success. They include nonspecific analgesics (such as opiates), acupuncture, and even surgical procedures such as presacral neurectomy, the interruption of the nerves going to the uterus. Relaxation techniques, application of heat (such as through a heating pad or hot shower), and exercise provide relief to some women.

—*Anne Lynn S. Chang, M.D.*

See also Contraception; Endometriosis; Genital disorders, female; Gynecology; Hormones; Menstruation; Pain; Pain management; Pelvic inflammatory disease (PID); Premenstrual syndrome (PMS); Reproductive system; Uterus; Women's health.

For Further Information:

A.D.A.M. Medical Encyclopedia. "Painful Menstrual Periods." *MedlinePlus*, July 23, 2012.

American College of Obstetricians and Gynecologists. "Dysmenorrhea: Frequently Asked Questions." *American Congress of Obstetricians and Gynecologists*, July 2012.

Golub, Sharon. *Periods: From Menarche to Menopause*. Newbury Park, Calif.: Sage, 1992.

Kasper, Dennis L., et al., eds. *Harrison's Principles of Internal Medicine*. 18th ed. New York: McGraw-Hill, 2012.

Minkin, Mary Jane, and Carol V. Wright. *The Yale Guide to Women's Reproductive Health: From Menarche to Menopause*. New Haven, Conn.: Yale University Press, 2003.

Shannon, Diane W., and Andrea Chisholm. "Painful Menstrual Periods." *Health Library*, September 27, 2012.

Stenchever, Morton A., et al. *Comprehensive Gynecology*. 5th ed. St. Louis, Mo.: Mosby/Elsevier, 2007.

Mackay, H. Trent. "Gynecologic Disorders." In *Current Medical Diagnosis and Treatment 2013*, edited by Maxine A. Papadakis, Stephen J. McPhee, and Michael W. Rabow. 52d ed. New York: McGraw-Hill, 2013.

DYSPHASIA. *See* APHASIA AND DYSPHASIA.

DYSTONIA

Disease/Disorder

Anatomy or system affected: Neuromuscular system

Specialties and related fields: Movement disorders, Parkinsonism, writer's cramp, musician's dystonia, performing arts medicine

Definition: Dystonia is the term used to describe an array of movement disorders characterized by repetitive muscle spasms, tremor, or excessive muscle activation. Dystonia is generally intermittent in nature, often leading to twisting, abnormal contraction patterns in skeletal muscles. It affects men, women, and children of all ages, and is present in about 300,000 people in the United States alone. It is a chronic, nonfatal condition that in most cases does not affect longevity, cognition, or intelligence.

Key terms:

basal ganglia: an area of the inner brain responsible for integrating sensory and motor activity to insure appropriate levels of muscle activation

co-contraction: the tendency for nontask-specific muscles to contract during the execution of a motor skill, often disrupting or opposing normal motor patterns

dysphonia: abnormal function of the larynx or voice box leading to thin, airy speech (abduction dysphonia) or difficulty in having the vocal cords initiate sound (adduction dysphonia)

focal dystonia: a form of dystonia where only specific, localized muscles are susceptible to dystonic symptoms

task-specific focal dystonia: a form of dystonia whereby localized dystonic contractions are present only during the execution of very specific actions

motor neuron: a nerve cell that is responsible for initiating skeletal muscle activity

motor activity or patterns: the characteristics of muscle contraction that result from motor neuron stimulation

motor cortex: that part of the cerebral cortex of the brain responsible for the activation of specific motor neurons to create movement

primary dystonia: forms of dystonia that occur without the presence of other neurologic or metabolic disease

secondary dystonia: forms of dystonia that occur in response to the presence of another neurologic or metabolic disease, to specific trauma, or to exposure to specific medication

sensory neuron: a nerve cell that is responsible for conveying sensory information from various parts of the body back to the brain and spinal cord

somatosensory cortex: that part of the cerebral cortex that is responsible for receiving and interpreting sensory information from various parts of the body

Types of Dystonia

Early-onset generalized dystonia (DYT 1 and Non-DYT 1). This nonfatal, chronic form of dystonia begins in childhood. Difficulties in the limbs are often the initial signs, but it often spreads to other body parts in such a way as to lead to twisting types of contractions. It may be due to a mutation of the DYT 1 gene, although mutation of the DYT 1 gene is not always a prerequisite (non-DYT 1). It is often referred to by different names including Oppenheim's dystonia, early onset dystonia, idiopathic torsion dystonia, or child-onset dystonia.

Myoclonic dystonia. This is a hereditary form of dystonia, and it includes jerking muscular contractions in combination with more sustained postural abnormalities. Depression, anxiety, obsessive-compulsive disorders, and panic attacks may accompany its expression.

Paroxysmal dystonia (dyskinesia). This is an episodic form of dystonia where abnormal movements are only present during attacks. The movements may be jerky and ballistic, or in other cases, may involve quick motions of the hands and feet (referred to as choreic movements). Between episodes, victims experience normal movement.

Rapid-onset dystonia parkinsonism. This term has recently been used to describe a wide-ranging set of disorders having sudden onset where Parkinson-like movements are accompanied by dystonic symptoms. It is thought to be hereditary, with numerous forms including autosomal-dominant, recessive, and x-linked varieties. Symptoms may develop over hours or a few days, and will usually stabilize in four weeks without further deterioration. It is also hereditary.

Focal dystonia. This category includes several adult-onset forms that affect various parts of the body. These include the eyes (blepherospasm characterized by excessive squinting and blinking), the neck and shoulders (cervical dystonia, otherwise known as spasmodic torticollis, characterized by a twisted torso posture), the face, mouth, or jaw (oromandibular dystonia), the vocal chords (laryngeal dystonia or spasmodic dysphonia), or the hands (writer's cramp). These all may have primary or secondary origins.

Task-specific focal dystonia. Task-specific dystonia describes forms of dystonia where dystonic symptoms occur only during selective motor activities that often involve highly skilled, repetitive movements. The same muscles that show dystonic activity under such conditions are very often normal when used for other activities.

Musician's dystonia. Musician's dystonia is a subcategory of task-specific dystonia in which key muscle functions required to play a given instrument are subjected to dystonic symptoms, but only during the use of the instrument. The symptoms typically appear in the hands or fingers of pianists or plucked instrument players (guitar and harp, for example), in the facial muscles of brass players (particularly muscles controlling the lips), but may affect muscles of the jaw as well, typically leading to a clamping effect due to over-activation of the masseter muscle. Co-contraction of nontask-specific muscles is common as well.

Psychogenic dystonia. This occurs when dystonic symptoms are secondary to some preexisting psychological disorder. The type of disorder may vary from patient to patient, and the unwanted movements that result are not under conscious control.

Causes and Symptoms

The symptoms of the various forms of dystonia have been addressed above. With respect to the causes of this disorder, several varieties of dystonia have clear genetic origins, as has been previously noted in the cases of early-onset generalized dystonia, myoclonic dystonia, X-linked dystonia Parkinsonism, and rapid-onset dystonia Parkinsonism. However, genetic causes are not always the case. Many forms of dystonia are idiopathic, with no known specific cause. Precise biochemical mechanisms for developing this organic disorder remain elusive to scientists. Nonetheless, numerous factors have been implicated. Among these are physical trauma to the affected body part, secondary responses to medication, and various toxins that specifically can affect the basal ganglia. Whatever the cause, it appears that alterations in sensory-motor processing occurring at various levels within the brain (particularly in the basal ganglia) are involved. These alterations result in the loss of appropriate inhibition of nontask-specific muscles which, in turn, leads to an overactivation of motor activity, including co-contractions of nontask-specific muscles. In the task-specific varieties in particular, personality traits such as anxiety and perfectionism have been suggested as possible co-factors, along with overuse through repetitive activities, particularly those requiring very rapid and fine movements. Most likely, the cause is multifactorial.

Treatment and Therapy

To date, there is no cure for dystonia that restores function to 100 percent of normal capacity. Because of the wide variety of types of dystonia, treatment and therapy is highly specialized. For some forms of secondary dystonia, oral medications may be helpful. Among the drugs often used with varied success are levodopa, trihexyphenidyl, clonazepam, and baclofen. In focal dystonia where the offending muscles can be isolated, botulinum toxin (BOTOX) is frequently injected with fairly good success, although chronic use can lead to atrophy (wasting and weakness) of the injected muscles. BOTOX essentially blocks transmission of motor neurons in the sites where it is injected. Other approaches, particularly in task-specific focal dystonia such as writer's cramp and the varied forms of musician's dystonia, sensory-motor retraining or splinting techniques may be employed to attempt to reestablish a level of control, though these efforts are typically unable to restore function completely.

In some drastic cases where oral medications, BOTOX injections, or other treatments are ineffective (usually severe generalized dystonia), surgical techniques have been employed. Among these are very precisely targeted ablation surgeries where areas of the brain are physically disrupted or removed. Careful identification of target tissues is imperative. Modern three-dimensional imaging techniques as well as microelectrode brain mapping make these procedures much more precise than in previous years, and the outcomes have been modestly favorable. Target areas that have shown some success in severe cases include the globus pallidus or the thalamus, both substructures of the basal ganglia. These procedures are not without risk, however, including a one to two percent chance of stroke or hemorrhage. In procedures targeting the globus pallidus, a risk is that vision may be adversely affected. Additionally, deep brain stimulation techniques have shown some promise. In these procedures, electrodes are implanted deep within the brain in very precise locations and a pulse generator is implanted under the collarbone. Through careful testing, a correct amount of electrical pulse stimulation can be identified that helps to ameliorate symptoms.

Perspective and Prospects

Dystonia, and particularly task-specific focal dystonia (like musician's dystonia) is a relative newcomer to medicine and research. In the past 15-20 years, there has been an exponential rise in the number of peer-reviewed publications that have been investigating the causes and treatment of this movement disorder. Numerous national and international organizations exist that are devoted to helping understand and treat dystonia. The Dystonia Medical Research Foundation (DMRF), founded in 1976, supports a wide array of research efforts, providing seed money for initiatives aimed at ameliorating the far-reaching effects of this disorder. To date, it has provided 26 million dollars in support of some 492 research projects. In many cases, this seed money has led to more widely-funded projects supported by the National Institutes of Health. The major areas where emphasis has most recently been placed have been (1) research that has identified dystonia as a disorder primarily brought on by aberrant brain circuitry; (2) studies identifying various triggers for dystonia; (3) studies identifying and isolating no fewer than nineteen genes and gene markers thought to be implicated in dystonia; and (4) papers that have an examined and evaluated various treatment strategies. The DMRF recently joined forces with two other organizations, the Dystonia Coalition and the European Dystonia Federation, to sponsor the Fifth International Dystonia Symposium in Barcelona, Spain, held in the fall of 2011. Additionally, the International Parkinson and Movement Disorders Society as well as the Performing Arts Medical Association have dedicated many of their resources into publicizing dystonia research. The ongoing efforts of these organizations, coupled with the work of neurologists and physicians who are dedicated to working with dystonia, provide much hope for future.

—*Peter Iltis, Ph.D.*

See also Motor neuron diseases; Muscle sprains, spasms, and disorders

For Further Information:
In addition to the following references, an excellent source of information is the Dystonia Medical Research Foundation. Their website address is http://www.dystonia-foundation.org.
Altenmuller, E., and H.C. Jabusch. "Focal Dystonia in Musicians: Phenomenology, Pathophysiology and Triggered Factors." European Journal of Neurology 17 (July, 2010): 31-36.
Aranguiz, R., P. Chana-Cuevas, D. Alburquerque, and M. Leon. "Focal Dystonia in Musicians." Neurologia 26, no. 1 (January-February, 2011): 45-52.
Candia, V., T. Schafer, E. Taub, H. Rau, E. Altenmuller, B. Rockstroh, and T. Elbert. "Sensory Motor Retuning: A Behavioral Treatment for Focal Hand Dystonia of Pianists and Guitarists." Archives of Physical Medicine and Rehabilitation 83, no. 10 (October, 2002): 1342-1348.
Fonoff, E.T., W.K. Campos, M. Mandel, E.J. Alho, and M.J. Teixiera. "Bilateral Subthalamic Nucleus Stimulation for Generalized Dystonia after Bilateral Pallidotomy." Movement Disorders 27, no. 12 (October, 2012): 1559-1563.
Ford, B. "Pallidotomy for Generalized Dystonia." Advances in Neurology 94 (2004): 287-299.
Garcia-Ruiz, P.J. "Task-Specific Dystonias: Historical Review: A New Look at the Classics." Journal of Neurology 260, no. 3 (March, 2013): 750-753.
Geyer, H.L., and S.B. Bressman. "Rapid-Onset Dystonia-Parkinsonism." Handbook of Clinical Neurology 100 (2011): 559-562.
Hashimoto, T., K. Naito, K. Kitazawa, S. Imai, and T. Goto. "Pallidotomy for Severe Tardive Jaw-Opening Dystonia." Stereotactic and Functional Neurosurgery 88, no. 2 (2010): 105-108.
Jabusch, H.C., D. Zschucke, A. Schmidt, S. Schuele, and E. Altenmuller. "Focal Dystonia in Musicians Treatment Strategies and Long-Term Outcome in 144 Patients." Movement Disorders 20, no. 12 (December, 2005): 1623-1626.
Kinugawa, K., M. Vidailhet, F. Clot, E. Apartis, D. Grabli, and E. Roze. "Myoclonus-Dystonia: An Update." Movement Disorders 24, no. 4 (March 15, 2009): 479-489.
Robottom, B.J., W.J. Weiner, and C.L. Comella. "Early-Onset Primary Dystonia." Handbook of Clinical Neurology 100 (2011): 465-479.
Schuele, S., H.C. Jabusch, R.J. Lederman, and E. Altenmuller. "Botulinum Toxin Injections in the Treatment of Musician's Dystonia. Neurology 64, no. 2 (January 25, 2005): 341-343.
Torres-Russotto, D., and J.S. Perlmutter. "Task-Specific Dystonias: A Review." Annals of the New York Academy of Sciences 1142 (October, 2008): 179-199.
Waln, O., and J. Jankovic. "Bilateral Globus Pallidus Internus Deep Brain Stimulation after Bilateral Pallidotomy in a Patient with Generalized Early-Onset Primary Dystonia." Movement Disorders 28, no. 8 (July, 2013): 1162-1163.

E. COLI INFECTION
Disease/Disorder

Anatomy or system affected: Blood, gastrointestinal system, intestines, nervous system, urinary system

Specialties and related fields: Bacteriology, epidemiology, family medicine, gastroenterology, internal medicine, microbiology, neonatology, nephrology, pediatrics, public health, urology

Definition: Infection by a gram-negative bacillus that normally colonizes the gastrointestinal tract of humans and other mammals.

Key terms

conjugation: a process in which two bacteria come together and the donor transfers genetic material (plasmid) to the recipient via tubular bridges called fimbriae

facultative anaerobe: a bacterium that prefers to live and grow in oxygen-rich conditions but can also grow in reduced-oxygen concentration

fimbriae: small hairlike projections on the outside of *E. coli* that enable attachment to human or animal cells; also called pili

plasmids: small, double-stranded loops of deoxyribonucleic acid (DNA) inside bacteria that are independent of the chromosome and capable of autonomous replication

Causes and Symptoms

Escherichia coli (*E. coli*) is a rod-shaped, gram-negative bacterium and a member of the Enterobacteriaceae family. Its cytoplasm is enclosed by an inner membrane, a periplasmic space, a peptidoglycan layer, an outer membrane, and, finally, a capsule. Most strains produce two types of projections, flagellae for motility and fimbriae (pili) for cellular adhesion and genetic transfer. There is no nucleus. The genome consists of a single circular chromosome that is usually complemented by multiple plasmids. There are no intracellular organelles, and respiratory processes occur at the cellular membrane.

E. coli are found as normal flora in the gastrointestinal tracts of mammals and are the most common facultative anaerobes in the human intestinal tract. The traits that transform these benign inhabitants into disease-causing pathogens are called virulence factors. The virulence factors of *E. coli* may be divided into adhesins, toxins, and capsules. Adhesins consist of fimbriae or outer membrane proteins that allow the bacteria to bind to host cells and exert their disease-causing effects. Toxins are proteins made by *E. coli* that can be released to damage, or even kill, host cells. Capsules can enable the bacteria to elude the immune system and invade host tissues.

Plasmids can be transmitted between various strains of *E. coli* and other bacteria by a process called conjugation. In order for a bacterium to conjugate, it must possess F (fertility) factor, which is a specific type of plasmid that contains genes for plasmid DNA replication and pili construction. A bacterium with F factor can use its F factor–generated pili to hold onto another bacterium and inject selected portions of genetic

material into the bacterial partner. This genetic material can add new virulence factors or antibiotic resistance attributes to the recipient bacterium.

The diseases caused by *E. coli* may be divided into intestinal and extraintestinal. The *E. coli* strains causing intestinal diseases are of several different types. Enteropathogenic *E. coli* (EPEC) cause disease by adhering to intestinal epithelial cells with an outer membrane adhesin (intimin) and special pili, both of which are plasmid-mediated. The exact mechanism by which these virulence factors alter the intestine—resulting in watery diarrhea, low-grade fever, and vomiting—is unclear. Enterotoxigenic *E. coli* (ETEC) cause illness using a combination of mucosal adherence and toxin production. The enterotoxin is similar to cholera toxin and alters ionic transfer in the intestinal cells, producing copious amounts of watery diarrhea. The illness can vary greatly, from a lack of symptoms to severe diarrhea with cramps, nausea, and dehydration. The adhesins and toxins appear to be mediated by both chromosomal and plasmid genes. Some *E. coli* have acquired genes from *Shigella dysenteriae* via conjugation, and these strains can produce Shiga toxins (STEC). The toxins permit intestinal invasion, resulting in painful, bloody diarrhea indistinguishable from shigellosis; such strains are referred to as enterohemorrhagic (EHEC). In about 5 percent of cases, Shiga toxins enter the bloodstream, causing damage to red blood cells, endothelial cells, and kidney cells; this is called the hemolytic-uremic syndrome (HUS). The life-threatening HUS is usually associated with the O157:H7 strain of *E. coli* and is seen more often in children than in adults. The O157:H7 strain often colonizes cattle, and humans may then acquire the infection from eating beef or fresh vegetables contaminated by cattle manure.

The extraintestinal diseases caused by *E. coli* vary widely. *E. coli* is the most common cause of urinary tract infections (UTIs). The strains that cause UTIs are different from those strains that colonize healthy individuals. These uropathogenic *E. coli* possess fimbriae the bind to cells lining the urinary tract. They are also encapsulated and produce a toxin (hemolysin). The *E. coli* may ascend the urinary tract through the urethra to the bladder and kidney. The route is more common in women because of a shorter urethra and can be facilitated in both men and women by the use of a urinary catheter. Infection of the kidney can also occur via the bloodstream. *E. coli* infection can follow surgery, especially when the intestinal tract is violated. Surgical wound infection, ab-

---

Information on *E. coli* Infection

Causes: Bacterial infection

Symptoms: Stomach cramping, fever, watery or bloody diarrhea, bowel wall inflammation, difficulty urinating, platelet and red blood cell destruction, organ damage

Duration: Acute

Treatments: None; symptom management and supportive therapy

scesses, and peritonitis are possible. Because ducts connect the gallbladder and pancreas directly with the intestinal lumen (cavity), *E. coli* often play a prominent role in cholecystitis and pancreatitis. Newborns with undeveloped immune systems may experience ear infections, bacteremia, or meningitis caused by *E. coli*. The strains producing neonatal meningitis have a K1 capsule, which may facilitate passage into the brain. Because *E. coli* are so common and possess many virulence factors, they can produce many additional types of infection.

Treatment and Therapy

Mild cases of diarrhea caused by EPEC strains usually can be managed with fluids and other supportive therapies, but the duration of illness may be made shorter with the use of antibiotic therapy. ETEC diarrhea is treated with loperamide and oral antibiotics. STEC and HUS are treated with supportive care. HUS may require renal dialysis.

Extraintestinal infection is treated by antibiotic therapy. Since *E. coli* are becoming increasingly resistant to antibiotics, susceptibility testing on the particular strain of *E. coli* causing the infection, isolated from diagnostic cultures, must be performed.

Perspective and Prospects

Escherichia coli is named after Theodore Escherich, who described the bacterium in a paper published in 1885. Frederich Blattner of the University of Wisconsin completed the sequencing of the 4,288 genes of the *E. coli* genome in 1997. Nearly half of these genes were newly identified.

Epidemiological studies have assisted in the understanding of the origins of *E. coli* infections. Intestinal illness can be prevented with improved farming methods, better food processing and handling, expanded sewage and sanitation facilities, purification of drinking water, and hand washing. The prevalence of hospital-acquired infections, such as UTIs, can be reduced by limiting the use of urinary catheters and the employment of closed drainage systems when catheters are necessary.

The treatment of extraintestinal *E. coli* infection, and some intestinal infections, depends upon the use of one or more effective antibiotics. Resistance is a rapidly growing problem and can be controlled only through reduction of the inappropriate use of antibiotics and the development of new agents.

—*H. Bradford Hawley, M.D.*

See also Antibiotics; Bacterial infections; Bacteriology; Centers for Disease Control and Prevention (CDC); Colitis; Diarrhea and dysentery; Drug resistance; Food poisoning; Gastroenteritis; Gastroenterology; Gastroenterology, pediatric; Gastrointestinal disorders; Gastrointestinal system; Hemolytic uremic syndrome; Infection; Intestinal disorders; Intestines; Meningitis; Microbiology; Mutation; Renal failure.

For Further Information:

A.D.A.M. Medical Encyclopedia. "*E. coli* Enteritis." *MedlinePlus*, January 10, 2011.
Alcamo, I. Edward. *Fundamentals of Microbiology.* 6th ed. Sudbury, Mass.: Jones and Bartlett, 2001.
Centers for Disease Control and Prevention. "*E. coli.*" *Centers for Disease Control and Prevention*, August 3, 2012.
Forbes, Betty A., Daniel F. Sahm, and Alice S. Weissfeld. *Bailey & Scott's Diagnostic Microbiology.* 12th ed. Saint Louis: Mosby Elsevier, 2007.
Koneman, Elmer W. *The Other End of the Microscope: The Bacteria Tell Their Own Story.* Washington, D.C.: ASM Press, 2002.
Mandell, Gerald L., John E. Bennett, and Raphael Dolin, eds. *Principles and Practice of Infectious Diseases.* 7th ed. 2 vols. Philadelphia: Churchill Livingstone Elsevier, 2010.
McCoy, Krisha. "*Escherichia coli* Infection." *HealthLibrary*, March 20, 2013.

EAR INFECTIONS AND DISORDERS
Disease/Disorder
Anatomy or system affected: Ears
Specialties and related fields: Audiology, neurology, otorhinolaryngology
Definition: Infections or disorders of the outer, middle, or inner ear, which may result in hearing impairment or loss.
Key terms:
conductive loss: a hearing loss caused by an outer-ear or middle-ear problem which results in reduced transmission of sound
frequency: the number of vibrations per second of a source of sound, measured in hertz; correlates with perceived pitch
intensity of sound: the physical phenomenon that correlates approximately with perceived loudness; measured in decibels
otitis: any inflammation of the outer or middle ear
sensorineural loss: a hearing loss caused by a problem in the inner ear; this impairment is caused by a hair cell or nerve problem and is usually not amenable to surgical correction

Causes and Symptoms

The hearing mechanism, one of the most intricate and delicate structures of the human body, consists of three sections: the outer ear, the middle ear, and the inner ear. The outer ear converts sound waves into the mechanical motion of the eardrum (tympanic membrane), and the middle ear transmits this mechanical motion to the inner ear, where it is transformed into nerve impulses sent to the brain.

The outer ear consists of the visible portion, the ear canal, and the eardrum. The middle ear is a small chamber containing three tiny bones—the auditory ossicles, termed malleus (hammer), incus (anvil), and stapes (stirrup)—which transmit the vibrations of the eardrum (attached to the hammer) into the inner ear. The chamber is connected to the back of the throat by the Eustachian tube, which allows equalization with the external air pressure. The inner ear, or cochlea, is a fluid-filled cavity containing the complex structure necessary to convert the mechanical vibrations of the cochlear fluid into nerve pulses. The cochlea, shaped something like a snail's shell, is divided lengthwise by a slightly flexible partition into upper and lower chambers. The upper chamber begins at the oval window, to which the stirrup is attached. When the oval window is pushed or pulled by the stirrup, vibrations of the eardrum are transformed into cochlear fluid vibrations.

The lower surface of the cochlear partition, the basilar membrane, is set into vibration by the pressure difference between the fluids of the upper and lower ducts. Lying on the basilar membrane is the organ of Corti, containing tens of thousands of hair cells attached to the nerve transmission lines leading to the brain. When the basilar membrane vibrates, the cilia of these cells are bent, stimulating them to produce electrochemical impulses. These impulses travel along the auditory nerve to the brain, where they are interpreted as sound.

Although well protected against normal environmental exposure, the ear, because of its delicate nature, is subject to various infections and disorders. These disorders, which usually lead to some hearing loss, can occur in any of the three parts of the ear.

The ear canal can be blocked by a buildup of waxy secretions or by infection. Although earwax serves the useful purpose of trapping foreign particles that might otherwise be deposited on the eardrum, if the canal becomes clogged with an excess of wax, less sound will reach the eardrum, and hearing will be impaired.

Swimmer's ear, or otitis externa, is an inflammation caused by contaminated water that has not been completely drained from the ear canal. A moist condition in a region with little light favors fungal growth. Symptoms of swimmer's ear include an itchy and tender ear canal and a small amount of foul-smelling drainage. If the canal is allowed to become clogged by the concomitant swelling, hearing will be noticeably impaired.

A perforated eardrum may result from a sharp blow to the side of the head, an infection, the insertion of objects into the ear, or a sudden change in air pressure (such as a nearby explosion). Small perforations are usually self-healing, but larger tears require medical treatment.

Inflammation of the middle ear, acute otitis media, is one of the most common ear infections, especially among children. Infection usually spreads from the throat to the middle ear through the Eustachian tube. Children are particularly susceptible to this problem because their short Eustachian tubes afford bacteria in the throat easy access to the middle ear. When the middle ear becomes infected, pus begins to accumulate, forcing the eardrum outward. This pressure stretches the auditory ossicles to their limit and tenses the ligaments so that vibration conduction is severely impaired. Untreated, this condition may eventually rupture the eardrum or permanently damage the ossicular chain. Furthermore, the pus from the infection may invade nearby structures, including the facial nerve, the mastoid bones, the inner ear, or even the brain. The most common symptom of otitis is a sudden severe pain and an impairment of hearing resulting from the reduced mobility of the eardrum and the ossicles.

Secretory otitis media is caused by occlusion of the Eustachian tube as a result of conditions such as a head cold, diseased tonsils and adenoids, sinusitis, improper blowing of the nose, or riding in unpressurized airplanes. People with allergic nasal blockage are particularly prone to this condition. The blocked Eustachian tube causes the middle-ear cavity to

---

Information on Ear Infections and Disorders

Causes: Infection, buildup of earwax, fluid retention, injury, fungal growth, allergies, exposure to loud noise, sudden change in air pressure, certain drugs

Symptoms: Hearing impairment or loss, itchiness, pain, inflammation, discharge, tinnitus

Duration: Temporary to chronic

Treatments: Wide ranging; can include flushing ear with a warm solution under pressure, antibiotics, surgery

---

fill with a pale yellow, noninfected discharge which exerts pressure on the eardrum, causing pain and impairment of hearing. Eventually, the middle-ear cavity is completely filled with fluid instead of air, impeding the movement of the ossicles and causing hearing impairment.

A mild, temporary hearing impairment resulting from airplane flights is termed aero-otitis media. This disorder results when a head cold or allergic reaction does not permit the Eustachian tube to equalize the air pressure in the middle ear with atmospheric pressure when a rapid change in altitude occurs. As the pressure outside the eardrum becomes greater than the pressure within, the membrane is forced inward, while the opening of the tube into the upper part of the throat is closed by the increased pressure. Symptoms are a severe sense of pressure in the ear, pain, and hearing impairment. Although the pressure difference may cause the eardrum to rupture, more often the pain continues until the middle ear fills with fluid or the tube opens to equalize pressure.

Chronic otitis media may result from inadequate drainage of pus during the acute form of this disease or from a permanent eardrum perforation that allows dust, water, and bacteria easy access to the middle-ear cavity. The main symptoms of this disease are fluids discharging from the outer ear and hearing loss. Perforations of the eardrum result in hearing loss because of the reduced vibrating surface and a buildup of fibrous tissue that further induces conductive losses. In some cases, an infection may heal but still cause hearing loss by immobilizing the ossicles. There are two distinct types of chronic otitis, one relatively harmless and the other quite dangerous. An odorless, stringy discharge from the mucous membrane lining the middle ear characterizes the harmless type. The dangerous type is characterized by a foul-smelling discharge coming from a bone-invading process beneath the mucous lining. If neglected, this process can lead to serious complications, such as meningitis, paralysis of the facial nerve, or complete sensorineural deafness.

The ossicles may be disrupted by infection or by a jarring blow to the head. Most often, a separation of the linkage occurs at the weakest point, where the anvil joins the stirrup. A partial separation results in a mild hearing loss, while complete separation causes severe hearing impairment.

Disablement of the mechanical linkage of the middle ear may also occur if the stirrup becomes calcified, a condition known as otosclerosis. The normal bone is resorbed and replaced by very irregular, often richly vascularized bone. The increased stiffness of the stirrup produces conductive hearing loss. In extreme cases, the stirrup becomes completely immobile and must be surgically removed. Although the exact cause of this disease is unknown, it seems to be hereditary. About half of the cases occur in families in which one or more relatives have the same condition, and it occurs more frequently in females than in males. There is also some evidence that the condition may be triggered by a lack of fluoride in drinking water and that increasing the intake of fluoride may retard the calcification process.

Tinnitus is characterized by ringing, hissing, or clicking noises in the ear that seem to come and go spontaneously without any sound stimulus. While tinnitus is not a disease of the ear, it is a common symptom of various ear problems. Possible causes of tinnitus are earwax lodged against the eardrum, a perforated or inflamed eardrum, otosclerosis, high aspirin dosage, or excessive use of the telephone. Tinnitus is most serious when caused by an inner-ear problem or by exposure to very intense sounds, and it often accompanies hearing loss at high frequencies.

Ménière's disease is caused by production of excess cochlear fluid, which increases the pressure in the cochlea. This condition may be precipitated by allergy, infection, kidney disease, or a number of other causes, including severe stress. The increased pressure is exerted on the walls of the semicircular canals as well as on the cochlear partition. The excess pressure in the semicircular canals (the organs of balance) is interpreted by the brain as a rapid spinning motion, and the victim experiences abrupt attacks of vertigo and nausea. The excess pressure in the cochlear partition has the same effect as a very loud sound and rapidly destroys hair cells. A single attack causes a noticeable hearing loss and could result in total deafness without prompt treatment.

Of all ear diseases, damage to the hair cells in the cochlea causes the most serious impairment. Cilia may be destroyed by high fevers or from a sudden or prolonged exposure to intensely loud sounds. Problems include destroyed or missing hair cells, hair cells that fire spontaneously, and damaged hair cells that require unusually strong stimuli to excite them. At the present time, there is no means of repairing damaged cilia or of replacing those that have been lost.

Viral nerve deafness is a result of a viral infection in one or both ears. The mumps virus is one of the most common causes of severe nerve damage, with the measles and influenza viruses as secondary causes.

Ototoxic (ear-poisoning) drugs can cause temporary or permanent hearing impairment by damaging auditory nerve tissues, although susceptibility is highly individualistic. A temporary decrease of hearing (in addition to tinnitus) accompanies the ingestion of large quantities of aspirin or quinine. Certain antibiotics, such as those of the mycin family, may also cause permanent damage to the auditory nerves.

Repeated exposure to loud noise (in excess of 90 decibels) will cause a gradual deterioration of hearing by destroying cilia. The extent of damage, however, depends on the loudness and the duration of the sound. Rock bands often exceed 110 decibels; farm machinery averages 100 decibels.

Presbycusis (hearing loss with age) is the inability to hear high-frequency sounds because of the increasing deterioration of the hair cells. By age thirty, a perceptible high-frequency hearing loss is present. This deterioration progresses into old age, often resulting in severe impairment. The problem is accelerated by frequent unprotected exposure to noisy environments. The extent of damage depends on the frequency, intensity, and duration of exposure, as well as on the individual's predisposition to hearing loss.

Treatment and Therapy

The simplest ear problems to treat are a buildup of earwax, swimmer's ear, and a perforated eardrum. A large accumulation of wax in the ear canal is best removed by having a medical professional flush the ear with a warm solution under pressure. One should never attempt to remove wax plugs with a sharp instrument. A small accumulation of earwax may be softened with a few drops of baby oil left in the ear overnight and then washed out with warm water and a soft rubber ear syringe. Swimmer's ear can usually be prevented by thoroughly draining the ears after swimming. The disease can be treated with an application of antibiotic ear drops after the ear canal has been thoroughly cleaned. A small perforation of the eardrum will usually heal itself. Larger tears, however, require an operation, tympanoplasty, that grafts a piece of skin over the perforation.

Fortunately, the bacteria that usually cause acute otitis respond quickly to antibiotics. Although antibiotics may relieve the symptoms, complications can arise unless the pus is

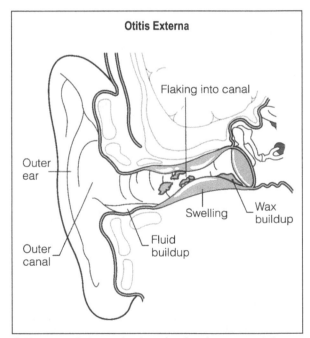

Otitis Externa

Flaking into canal

Outer ear

Outer canal

Fluid buildup

Swelling

Wax buildup

Otitis externa (swimmers' ear) results when the outer ear is inflamed by contaminated water that has not been completely drained from the ear canal.

thoroughly drained. The two-part treatment—draining the fluid from the middle ear and antibiotic therapy—resolves the acute otitis infection within a week. Secretory otitis is cured by finding and removing the cause of the occluded Eustachian tube. The serous fluid is then removed by means of an aspirating needle or by an incision in the eardrum so as to inflate the tube by forcing air through it. In some cases, a tiny polyethylene tube is inserted through the eardrum to aid in reestablishing normal ventilation. If the Eustachian tube remains inadequate, a small plastic grommet may be inserted. The improvement in hearing is often immediate and dramatic. The pain and hearing loss of aero-otitis is usually temporary and disappears of its own accord. If, during or immediately after flight, yawning or swallowing does not allow the Eustachian tube to open and equalize the pressure, medicine or surgical puncture of the eardrum may be required. The harmless form of chronic otitis is treated with applied medications to kill the bacteria and to dry the chronic drainage. The eardrum perforation may then be closed to restore the functioning of the ear and to recover hearing. The more dangerous chronic form of this disease does not respond well to antibacterial agents, but careful x-ray examination allows diagnosis and surgical removal of the bone-eroding cyst.

Ossicular interruption can be surgically treated to restore the conductive link by repositioning the separated bones. This relatively simple operation has a very high success rate. Otosclerosis is treated by operating on the stirrup in one of several ways. The stirrup can be mechanically freed by fracturing the calcified foot plate or by fracturing the foot plate and one of the arms. Although this operation is usually successful, recalcification often occurs. Alternatively, the stirrup can be completely removed and replaced with a prosthesis of wire or silicon, yielding excellent and permanent results.

Since tinnitus has many possible, and often not readily identifiable, causes, few cases are treated successfully. The tinnitus masker has been invented to help sufferers live with this annoyance. The masker, a noise generator similar in appearance to a hearing aid, produces a constant, gentle humming sound that masks the tinnitus.

Ménière's disease, usually treated with drugs and a restricted diet, may also require surgical correction to relieve the excess pressure in severe cases. If this procedure is unsuccessful, the nerves of the inner ear may be cut. In drastic cases, the entire inner ear may be removed.

Presently there is no cure for damaged hair cells; the only treatment is to use a hearing aid. It is more advantageous to take preventive measures, such as reducing noise at the source, replacing noisy equipment with quieter models, or using ear-protection devices. Recreational exposure to loud music should be severely curtailed, if not completely eliminated.

Perspective and Prospects

For many centuries, treatment of the ear was associated with that of the eye. In the nineteenth century, the development of the laryngoscope (to examine the larynx) and the otoscope (to examine the ears) enabled doctors to examine and treat

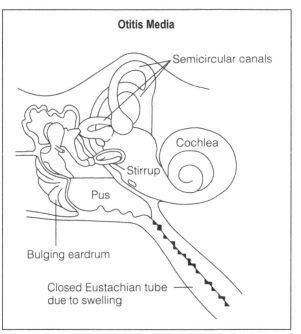

Otitis media occurs when infection spreads from the throat to the middle ear via the Eustachian tube; it is a serious condition which, left untreated, may lead to permanent ear damage and even infection of the brain.

disorders such as croup, sore throat, and draining ears, which eventually led to the control of these diseases. As an offshoot of the medical advances made possible by these technological devices, the connection between the ear and throat became known, and otologists became associated with laryngologists.

The study of ear diseases did not develop scientifically until the early nineteenth century, when Jean-Marc-Gaspard Itard and Prosper Ménière made systematic investigations of ear physiology and disease. In 1853, William R. Wilde of Dublin published the first scientific treatise on ear diseases and treatments, setting the field on a firm scientific foundation. Meanwhile, the scientific investigation of the diseased larynx was aided by the laryngoscope, invented in 1855 by Manuel Garcia, a Spanish singing teacher who used his invention as a teaching aid. During the late nineteenth century, this instrument was adopted for detailed studies of larynx pathology by Ludwig Türck and Jan Czermak, who also adapted this instrument to investigate the nasal cavity, which established the link between laryngology and rhinology. Friedrich Voltolini, one of Czermak's assistants, further modified the instrument so that it could be used in conjunction with the otoscope. In 1921, Carl Nylen pioneered the use of a high-powered binocular microscope to perform ear surgery. The operating microscope opened the way for delicate operations on the tiny bones of the middle ear. With the founding of the American Board of Otology in 1924, otology (later otolaryngology) became the second medical specialty to be formally established in North America.

Prior to World War II, the leading cause of deafness was

the various forms of ear infection. Advances in technology and medicine have now brought ear infections under control. Today the leading type of hearing loss in industrialized countries is conductive loss, which occurs in those who are genetically predisposed to such loss and who have had lifetime exposure to noise and excessively loud sounds. In the future, protective devices and reasonable precautions against extensive exposure to loud sounds should reduce the incidence of hearing loss to even lower levels.

—*George R. Plitnik, Ph.D.*

See also Altitude sickness; Audiology; Balance disorders; Deafness; Decongestants; Ear surgery; Ears; Earwax; Hearing; Hearing aids; Hearing loss; Hearing tests; Ménière's disease; Motion sickness; Myringotomy; Nasopharyngeal disorders; Neurology; Neurology, pediatric; Otoplasty; Otorhinolaryngology; Sense organs; Sinusitis; Speech disorders; Tinnitus; Tonsillitis.

For Further Information:

Canalis, Rinaldo, and Paul R. Lambert, eds. *The Ear: Comprehensive Otology*. Philadelphia: Lippincott Williams & Wilkins, 2000.

Dugan, Marcia B. *Living with Hearing Loss*. Washington, D.C.: Gallaudet University Press, 2003.

Ferrari, Mario. *PDxMD Ear, Nose, and Throat Disorders*. Philadelphia: PDxMD, 2003.

Friedman, Ellen M., and James M. Barassi. *My Ear Hurts! A Complete Guide to Understanding and Treating Your Child's Ear Infections*. Darby, Pa.: Diane, 2004.

Greene, Alan R. *The Parent's Complete Guide to Ear Infections*. Reprint. Allentown, Pa.: People's Medical Society, 2004.

Jerger, James, ed. *Hearing Disorders in Adults: Current Trends*. San Diego, Calif.: College-Hill Press, 1984.

Kemper, Kathi J. *The Holistic Pediatrician: A Pediatrician's Comprehensive Guide to Safe and Effective Therapies for the Twenty-five Most Common Ailments of Infants, Children, and Adolescents*. Rev. ed. New York: Quill, 2002.

"Lack of Consensus About Surgery for Ear Infections." *Health News* 18, no. 3 (June/July, 2000): 11.

MedlinePlus. "Ear Disorders." *MedlinePlus*, April 1, 2013.

MedlinePlus. "Ear Infections." *MedlinePlus*, April 1, 2013.

National Center for Immunization and Respiratory Diseases, Division of Bacterial Diseases. "Ear Infections." *Centers for Disease Control and Prevention*, May 23, 2011.

Pender, Daniel J. *Practical Otology*. Philadelphia: J. B. Lippincott, 1992.

Roland, Peter S., Bradley F. Marple, and William L. Meyerhoff, eds. *Hearing Loss*. New York: Thieme, 1997.

EAR, NOSE, AND THROAT MEDICINE. *See* **OTORHINOLARYNGOLOGY.**

EAR SURGERY

Procedure

Anatomy or system affected: Bones, ears, musculoskeletal system, nervous system

Specialties and related fields: Audiology, general surgery, otorhinolaryngology, speech pathology

Definition: An invasive procedure to correct structural problems of the ear that produce some degree of hearing loss.

Key terms:

cochlea: a structure in the inner ear that receives sound vibrations from the ossicles and transmits them to the auditory nerve

myringotomy: incision of the tympanic membrane used to drain fluid and reduce middle-ear pressure

ossicles: tiny bones located between the eardrum and the cochlea

otosclerosis: a condition in which the stapes becomes progressively more rigid, and hearing loss results

stapedectomy: a surgical procedure in which the stapes is replaced with an artificial substitute

stapes: the ossicle that makes contact with the cochlea

tympanic membrane: the eardrum, which separates the external ear canal from the middle ear and ossicles and which transmits sound vibration to the ossicles

tympanoplasty: a surgical procedure to repair the tympanic membrane

Indications and Procedures

Humans are able to detect sound because of the interaction between the ears and the brain. When sound waves strike the tympanic membrane (eardrum), it vibrates. The movement of the tympanic membrane then causes the movement of the ossicles, the three tiny bones within the middle ear (malleus, incus, and stapes). These moving bones transfer the vibrations to the cochlea of the inner ear, which stimulates the auditory nerve and eventually the brain.

Hearing problems may result when any part of the ear is damaged. Hearing difficulties can be categorized into two main areas: conductive and sensorineural hearing loss. In conductive hearing loss, the ear loses its ability to transmit sound from the external ear to the cochlea. Common causes include earwax buildup in the outer ear canal; otosclerosis, in which the stapes loses mobility and cannot stimulate the cochlea effectively; and otitis media, in which the middle ear becomes infected and a sticky fluid is produced, which causes the ossicles to become inflexible. Otitis media is the most common cause of conductive hearing loss and typically occurs in children. If antibiotics such as amoxicillin or ampicillin fail to clear the ear of infection, surgery may be required. Sensorineural hearing loss results from damage to the cochlea or auditory nerve. Common causes include loud noises, rubella (a type of viral infection) during embryonic development, and certain drugs such as gentamicin and streptomycin. Occasionally, a tumor (neuroma) of the auditory nerve may cause sensorineural hearing loss.

Myringotomy is a surgical procedure in which an incision is made in the tympanic membrane to allow drainage of fluid (effusion) from the middle ear to the external ear canal. The surgeon usually performs this operation to treat recurrent otitis media, a condition in which pressure builds in the middle ear and pushes outward on the tympanic membrane. The patient, usually a child, is given general anesthesia. An incision is made in the eardrum so that a small tube can be inserted to allow continuous drainage of the pus. The tube usually falls out in a few months, and the tympanic membrane heals rapidly.

Otosclerosis, the overgrowth of bone that impedes the

movement of the stapes, can be treated by stapedectomy (surgical removal of the stapes). General anesthesia is used to prevent pain or movement when an incision is made in the ear canal and the tympanic membrane is folded to access the ossicles. The stapes can then be removed and a metal or plastic prosthesis inserted in its place. The eardrum is then repaired.

Tympanoplasty is an operation to repair the tympanic membrane or ossicles. Sudden pressure changes in an airplane or during deep-sea diving may perforate the tympanic membrane (barotrauma) and require tympanoplasty. The procedure is similar to stapedectomy. With the patient under general anesthesia, an incision is made next to the eardrum to provide access to the tympanic membrane and ossicles. The tympanic membrane may need to be repaired if the perforated eardrum does not heal on its own. An operating microscope is employed for optimal visualization of the middle ear. If the tympanoplasty involves the ossicles, microsurgical instruments are used to reposition, repair, or replace the damaged bones. They are then reset in their natural positions, and the eardrum is repaired.

Auditory neuromas are benign tumors of the supporting cells surrounding the auditory nerve. Although rare, these tumors can cause deafness. Once neuromas are confirmed by computed tomography (CT) scanning, surgical removal is necessary. With the patient under general anesthesia, the surgeon must make a hole in the skull and attempt to remove the tumor carefully without damaging the auditory nerve or adjacent nerves.

Uses and Complications

More than 90 percent of the patients undergoing stapedectomy experience improved hearing. Approximately 1 percent, however, show deterioration of hearing or total hearing loss postoperatively. For this reason, most surgeons perform stapedectomy on one ear at a time.

Occasionally, the surgical removal of auditory neuromas causes total deafness because of damage to the auditory nerve itself. In rare cases, damage to nearby nerves may cause weakness and/or numbness in that part of the face. Depending on the extent of nerve damage, the symptoms may or may not lessen with time.

Perspective and Prospects

Improvements in technology promise new methods of treating hearing loss. For example, cochlear implants have been developed for the treatment of total sensorineural hearing loss. These implants are surgically inserted into the inner ear. Electrodes in the cochlea receive sound signals transmitted to them from a miniature receiver implanted behind the skin of the ear. Directly over the implant, the patient wears an external transmitter that is connected to a sound processor and microphone. As the microphone picks up sound, the sound is eventually conducted to the electrodes within the cochlea.

—*Matthew Berria, Ph.D.,*
and Douglas Reinhart, M.D.

See also Audiology; Deafness; Ear infections and disorders; Ears; Hearing; Hearing loss; Ménière's disease; Myringotomy; Neurol-ogy; Neurology, pediatric; Otoplasty; Otorhinolaryngology; Plastic surgery; Sense organs.

For Further Information:

Brunicardi, F. Charles, et al., eds. *Schwartz's Principles of Surgery.* 9th ed. New York: McGraw-Hill, 2010.

Ferrari, Mario. *PDxMD Ear, Nose, and Throat Disorders.* Philadelphia: PDxMD, 2003.

Kassir, Kari. "Myringotomy." *Health Library,* Sept. 10, 2012.

Leikin, Jerrold B., and Martin S. Lipsky, eds. *American Medical Association Complete Medical Encyclopedia.* New York: Random House Reference, 2003.

Nadol, Joseph B., Jr., and Michael J. McKenna. *Surgery of the Ear and Temporal Bone.* 2nd ed. Philadelphia: Lippincott Williams & Wilkins, 2005.

O'Reilly, Robert C. "Middle Ear Infections and Ear Tube Surgery." *KidsHealth.* Nemours Foundation, Oct. 2011.

Pender, Daniel J. *Practical Otology.* Philadelphia: J. B. Lippincott, 1992.

Schwartz, Seth, and David Zieve. "Ear Tube Insertion." *MedlinePlus,* July 30, 2012.

Tierney, Lawrence M., Stephen J. McPhee, and Maxine A. Papadakis, eds. *Current Medical Diagnosis and Treatment 2007.* New York: McGraw-Hill Medical, 2006

EARS

Anatomy

Anatomy or system affected: Bones, musculoskeletal system, nervous system

Specialties and related fields: Audiology, neurology, otorhinolaryngology, speech pathology

Definition: The organs responsible for both hearing and balance.

Key terms:

auditory nerve: the nerve that conducts impulses originating in hair cells of cochlea to the brain for processing as the sensation of sound

cochlea: the fluid-filled coil of the inner ear containing hair cells that change vibrations in the fluid into nerve impulses

eardrum: the membrane separating the outer ear canal from the middle ear that changes sound waves into movements of the ossicles; also called the tympanic membrane

Eustachian tube: the tube connecting the middle ear to the back of the throat; air exchange through this tube equalizes air pressure in the middle ear with the outside air pressure

inner ear: an organ that includes the cochlea (for detection of sound) and the labyrinth (for detection of movement)

labyrinth: a structure consisting of three fluid-filled, semicircular canals at right angles to one another in the inner ear; they monitor the position and movement of the head

middle ear: the air-filled cavity in which vibrations are transmitted from the eardrum to the inner ear via the ossicles

ossicles: three small bones in the middle ear that transmit vibrations from the eardrum to the fluid of the inner ear

otoscope: an instrument for viewing the ear canal and the eardrum

outer ear: the visible, fleshy part of the ear and the ear canal; transmits sound waves to the eardrum

tympanic membrane: another term for the eardrum

Structure and Functions

The ear is composed of three parts: the outer ear, the middle ear, and the inner ear. All three parts are involved in hearing, while only the inner ear is involved in balance.

Sound can be thought of as pressure waves that travel through the air. These waves are collected by the fleshy part of the outer ear and are funneled down the ear canal to the eardrum. The eardrum, being a thin membrane, vibrates as it is hit by the sound waves. Attached to the eardrum is the first of the ossicles (the hammer or malleus), which moves when the eardrum moves. The second ossicle (the anvil or incus) is attached to the first, and the third to the second. Therefore, as the first bone moves, the others move also. The base of the third bone (the stirrup or stapes) is in contact with the oval window at the beginning of the inner ear. Movement of the oval window sets up vibrations in the fluid of the cochlea. These vibrations are detected by hair cells. Depending on their position in the cochlea, the hair cells are sensitive to being moved by vibrations of different frequencies. When the hair of a hair cell is bent by the fluid, an impulse is generated. The impulses are transmitted to the brain via the auditory nerve. The nerve impulses are processed in the brain, and the result is the sensation of sound, in particular the sense of pitch. Thus the three parts of the ear turn sound waves into "sound" by changing air vibrations into eardrum vibrations, then ossicle movement, then fluid vibrations, and finally nerve impulses.

Disorders and Diseases

Each of the three parts of the ear can be affected by diseases that can lead to temporary or, in some cases, permanent hearing loss. Damage to the eardrum, ossicles, or any part of the ear before the cochlea results in conductive hearing loss, as these structures conduct the sound or vibrations. Damage to the hair cells or to the auditory nerve results in sensorineural hearing loss. Sound may be conducted normally but cannot be detected by the hair cells or transmitted as nerve impulses to the brain.

Disorders of the outer ear include cauliflower ear, blockage by earwax, otitis externa, and tumors. Cauliflower ear is a severe hematoma (bruise) to the outer ear. In some cases, the blood trapped beneath the skin does not resorb and instead turns into fibrous tissue that may become cartilaginous or even bonelike.

Earwax is secreted by the cells in the lining of the ear canal. Its function is to protect the eardrum from dust and dirt, and it normally works its way to the outer opening of the ear. The amount secreted varies from person to person. In some people, or in people who are continually exposed to dusty environments, excessive amounts of wax may be secreted and may block the ear canal sufficiently to interfere with its transmission of sound waves to the eardrum.

Otitis externa can take two forms, either localized or generalized. The localized form, a boil or abscess, is a bacterial infection that results from breaks in the lining of the ear canal and is often caused by attempts to scratch an itch in the ear or to remove wax. The generalized form can be a bacterial or fungal infection, known as otomycosis. Generalized otitis externa is also called swimmer's ear because it often results from swimming in polluted waters or from chronic moisture in the ear canal.

Tumors of the ear can be benign (noncancerous) or malignant (cancerous) growths of either the soft tissues or the underlying bone. Bony growths, or osteomas, can cause sufficient blockage, by themselves or by leading to the buildup of earwax, to result in hearing loss.

The middle ear consists of the eardrum, three small bones called the ossicles, and the eustachian tube. The bones of the middle ear move in an air-filled cavity. Air pressure within this cavity is normally the same as the outside air pressure because air is exchanged between the middle ear and the outside world via the eustachian tube. When this tube swells and closes, as it often does with a head cold, one experiences a stuffy feeling, decreased hearing, mild pain, and sometimes ringing in the ears (tinnitus) or dizziness. The middle ear is susceptible to infection, such as otitis media, because bacteria and viruses can sometimes enter via the eustachian tube. Young children are especially prone to middle-ear infections because a child's eustachian tubes are shorter and more directly in line with the back of the throat than those of adults. Untreated ear infections can sometimes spread into the surrounding bone (mastoiditis) or into the brain (meningitis).

Fluid in the middle ear during an ear infection interferes with the free movement of the ossicles, causing hearing loss that, although significant while it lasts, is temporary. In other instances, there is the prolonged presence of clear fluid in the middle ear, resulting from a combination of infection or allergy and eustachian tube dysfunction, which itself can result from swelling caused by an allergy. This condition, known as glue ear or persistent middle-ear effusion, can last long enough to cause detrimental effects on speech, particularly in young children. Middle-ear infections can sometimes become chronic, as in chronic otitis media; permanent damage to the hearing can result from the ossicles being dissolved away by the pus from these chronic infections.

During a middle-ear infection, fluid can build up and increase pressure within the middle-ear cavity sufficiently to rupture (perforate) the eardrum. Very loud noises are another form of increased pressure, in this case from the outside. If a loud noise is very sudden, such as an explosion or gunshot, then pressure cannot be equalized fast enough and the eardrum can rupture. Scuba diving without clearing one's ears (that is, getting the eustachian tube to open and allow airflow) can also result in ruptured eardrums. Other causes of ruptured eardrums include puncture by a sharp object inserted into the ear canal to remove wax or relieve itching, a blow to the ear, or a fractured skull. Some hearing is lost when the eardrum is ruptured, but if the damage is not too severe, the eardrum heals itself and hearing returns.

The middle ear does not always fill with fluid if the eustachian tube is blocked. In some instances, the middle-ear cavity remains filled with trapped air. This trapped air is taken up by the cells lining the middle-ear cavity, decreasing the air pressure inside the middle ear and allowing the eardrum to

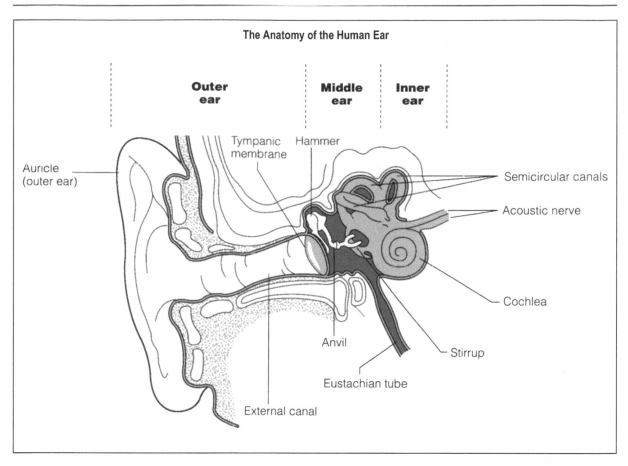

The Anatomy of the Human Ear

Outer ear

Middle ear

Inner ear

Tympanic membrane   Hammer

Auricle (outer ear)

Semicircular canals

Acoustic nerve

Cochlea

Anvil

Stirrup

Eustachian tube

External canal

push inward. Cells that are constantly shed from the eardrum collect in this pocket and form a ball that can become infected. This infected ball, or cholesteatoma, produces pus, which can erode the ossicles. If left untreated, the erosion can continue through the roof of the middle-ear cavity (causing brain abscesses or meningitis) or through the walls (causing abscesses behind the ear). The symptoms of a cholesteatoma go beyond the symptoms of an earache to include headache, dizziness, and weakness of the facial muscles.

Permanent conductive hearing loss can also result from calcification of the ossicles, a condition called osteosclerosis. Abnormal spongy bone can form at the base of the stirrup bone, interfering with its normal movement against the oval window. Hearing loss caused by osteosclerosis occurs gradually over ten to fifteen years, although it may be accelerated in women by pregnancy. There is a hereditary component.

The inner ear begins at the oval window, which separates the air-filled cavity at the middle ear from the fluid-filled cavities of the inner ear. The inner ear consists of the cochlea, which is involved in hearing, and the labyrinth, which maintains balance.

Disorders of the cochlea result in permanent sensorineural hearing loss. Hair cells can be damaged by the high fever accompanying some diseases such as meningitis. They may also be damaged by some drugs. The largest, and most pre-

ventable, sources of damage to the hair cells are occupational and recreational exposure to loud sounds, particularly if they are prolonged. In some occupations, the hearing loss from working without ear protection may be confined to certain frequencies of sounds, while other occupations lead to general loss at all sound frequencies. Prolonged exposure to overamplified music will likewise cause permanent hearing loss at all frequencies. This is more severe and has much earlier onset than presbycusis—the progressive loss of hearing, particularly in the high frequencies, that occurs with normal aging.

The labyrinth is the part of the ear that maintains one's balance; therefore the major system of disorders of the labyrinth is vertigo (dizziness). Labyrinthitis is an infection, generally viral, of the labyrinth. The vertigo can be severe but is temporary.

With Ménière's disease, there is an increase in the volume of fluid in the labyrinth and a corresponding increase in internal pressure, which distorts or ruptures the membrane lining. The symptoms, which include vertigo, noises in the ear, and muffled or distorted hearing especially of low tones, flare up in attacks that may last from a few hours to several days. The frequency of these attacks varies from one individual to another, with some people having episodes every few weeks and others having them every few years. This condition, which may be accompanied by migraine headaches, usually clears spontaneously but in some people may result in deafness.

Diagnostic and Treatment Techniques

The most common ear disorders, outer-ear or middle-ear infections, are diagnosed visually with an otoscope. This handheld instrument is a very bright light with a removable tip. Tips of different sizes can be attached so that the doctor can look into ear canals of various sizes. Infections or obstructions in the outer ear are readily visible. Middle-ear infections can often be discerned by the appearance of the eardrum, which may appear red and inflamed. Fluid in the middle ear can sometimes be seen through the eardrum, or its presence can be surmised if the eardrum is bulging toward the ear canal. In other cases, the eardrum will be seen to be retracted or bulging inward toward the middle-ear cavity. Holes in the eardrum can also be seen, as can scars from previous ruptures that have since healed.

Impedance testing may be used in addition to the otoscope for the diagnosis of middle-ear problems. Impedance testing is based on the fact that, when sound waves hit the eardrum, some of the energy is transmitted as vibrations of the drum, while some of the energy is reflected. If the eardrum is stretched tight by fluid pushing against it or by being retracted, it will be less mobile and will reflect more sound waves than a normal eardrum. In the simplest form, the mobility of the eardrum is tested with a small air tube and bulb attached to an otoscope. The doctor gently squeezes a puff of air into the ear canal while watching through the otoscope to see how well the eardrum moves.

A far more quantitative version of impedance testing can be done in cases of suspected hearing loss. This type of impedance testing is generally administered by an audiologist, a professional trained in administering and interpreting hearing tests. The ear canal is blocked with an earplug containing a transmitter and receiver. The transmitter releases sounds of known frequency and intensity into the ear canal while also changing the pressure in the ear canal by pumping air into it. The receiver then measures the amount of energy reflected back. The machine analyzes the efficiency of reflection at various pressures and prints out a graph. By comparison of the graph to that from an eardrum with normal mobility, conclusions can be drawn about the degree of immobility and, consequently, about the stage of the middle-ear infection. Many pediatricians or family physicians have handheld versions of this instrument, which resembles an otoscope but is capable of transmitting sound and measuring reflected sound intensity.

When an ear infection has been diagnosed, the treatment is generally with antibiotics. For outer-ear infections, drops containing antibiotic or antifungal agents are prescribed. For middle-ear infections, antibiotics are prescribed that can be taken by mouth. The patient is rechecked in about three weeks to ensure that the ear has healed.

In some cases, the ear does not heal, or the fluid in the middle ear does not go away. This can occur if a new infection starts before the ear is fully recovered or if the infecting microorganisms are resistant to the antibiotic used for treatment. In cases of chronic or repeated otitis media, a surgical procedure called a myringotomy can be performed in which a small slit is made in the eardrum to release fluid from the middle ear. Often, a small tube is inserted into the slit. These ear tubes, or tympanostomy tubes, keep the middle ear ventilated, allowing it to dry and heal. In most cases, these tubes are spontaneously pushed out by the eardrum as healing takes place, usually within three to six months. Patients must be cautious to keep water out of their ears while the tubes are in place.

A permanently damaged eardrum—from an explosion, for example—can be replaced by a graft. This procedure is called tympanoplasty, and the tissue used for the graft is generally taken from a vein from the same person. If the ossicles are damaged, they too can be replaced, in this case by metal copies of the bones. For example, when otosclerosis has damaged the stapes (stirrup) bone, hearing can often be restored by replacing it with a metal substitute.

Tumors, osteomas in the ear canal, or cholesteatomas on the eardrum may need to be removed surgically. Surgery may also be needed if infections have spread into the surrounding bone. Bone infections or abnormalities of the inner ear are diagnosed by X-rays or by computed tomography (CT) scans.

For some persons who have complete sensorineural hearing loss, some awareness of sound can be restored with a cochlear implant. This electronic device is surgically implanted and takes the place of the nonexistent hair cells in detecting sound and generating nerve impulses.

Problems of balance may sometimes be treated successfully with drugs to limit the swelling in the labyrinth. Ringing in the ears (tinnitus) is usually resolved when the underlying condition is resolved. In some cases, tinnitus is caused by drugs (large doses of aspirin, for example) and will cease when the drugs are stopped. However, it is difficult to identify the cause of most tinnitus cases, and there is no specific cure.

Doctors who specialize in the diagnosis and treatment of disorders of the ear and who do these surgeries are called otorhinolaryngologists (ear, nose, and throat doctors; also called otolaryngologists). They are medical doctors who have several years of training beyond medical school in surgery and in problems of the ear, nose, and throat.

Perspective and Prospects

The basic anatomy of the ear has been known for some time. Bartolommeo Eustachio (1520–1574), an Italian anatomist, first described the eustachian tube as well as a number of the nerves and muscles involved in the functioning of the ear. An understanding of how the ear functions to discriminate the pitch of sounds, however, was not arrived at until the twentieth century. Georg von Békésy won the Nobel Prize in Physiology or Medicine in 1961 for his work on the acoustics of the ear and how it functions to analyze sounds of varying frequencies (pitch).

Treatment of diseases of the ear has been radically changed by the advent of antibiotics. Older texts describe rupture of the eardrum by middle-ear fluid as a desired outcome of middle-ear infection, one which would ensure that the infection drained and healed, rather than becoming chronic.

Chronic ear infections used to be associated with diseases such as tuberculosis, measles, and syphilis, which themselves became far less common with the widespread use of antibiotics or vaccines. In the past, chronic ear infections were much more likely to result in mastoiditis, or infection of the air spaces of the mastoid bone, requiring surgical removal of the infected portions of the mastoid bone.

Adenoids and tonsils were frequently removed from patients with recurrent ear infections, as these were thought to be the source of the reinfection. It is now known that these tissues are involved in the formation of immunity to infectious bacteria and viruses. Their removal is not advocated in most circumstances—except, for example, when they are large enough to block the opening of the eustachian tube.

Reconstructive surgery began in the 1950s with the development by Samuel Rosen and others of the operation to free up the calcified stapes bone in cases of otosclerosis. Today, virtually all components of the middle ear can be replaced.

While ear infections used to be much more dangerous, perhaps there is an equal danger today of taking threats to the ears too lightly. Chronic ear infections can still cause permanent hearing loss and may even become life-threatening infections if left untreated. Damage involving the inner ear remains untreatable, as do many cases of tinnitus and loss of balance. Because the largest source of inner ear damage is prolonged exposure to noise, the prevention of damage is far more effective than treatment.

—*Pamela J. Baker, Ph.D.*

See also Altitude sickness; Anatomy; Audiology; Balance disorders; Biophysics; Deafness; Dyslexia; Ear infections and disorders; Ear surgery; Earwax; Hearing; Hearing loss; Hearing tests; Ménière's disease; Motion sickness; Myringotomy; Nervous system; Neurology; Neurology, pediatric; Otoplasty; Otorhinolaryngology; Plastic surgery; Sense organs; Speech disorders; Systems and organs; Tinnitus.

For Further Information:
Carson-DeWitt, Rosalyn, and Kari Kassir. "Middle Ear Infection." *Health Library*, September 30, 2012.
"Ear Disorders." *MedlinePlus*, June 12, 2013.
"Ears, Nose, and Throat." *MedlinePlus*, January 7, 2013.
Gelfand, Stanley A. *Essentials of Audiology*. 3d ed. New York: Thieme, 2009.
Katz, Jack, ed. *Handbook of Clinical Audiology*. 6th ed. Philadelphia: Wolters Kluwer/Lippincott Williams & Wilkins, 2009.
Leikin, Jerrold B., and Martin S. Lipsky, eds. *American Medical Association Complete Medical Encyclopedia*. New York: Random House Reference, 2003.
Mendel, Lisa Lucks, Jeffrey L. Danhauer, and Sadanand Singh. *Singular's Illustrated Dictionary of Audiology*. San Diego, Calif.: Singular, 1999.
Nettina, Sandra M., ed. *The Lippincott Manual of Nursing Practice*. 9th ed. Philadelphia: Lippincott Williams & Wilkins, 2010.
Pender, Daniel J. *Practical Otology*. Philadelphia: J. B. Lippincott, 1992.
"Tinnitus." *MedlinePlus*, June 7, 2013.
Zuckerman, Barry S., and Pamela A. M. Zuckerman. *Child Health: A Pediatrician's Guide for Parents*. New York: Hearst Books, 1986.

EARWAX
Anatomy
Also known as: Cerumen
Anatomy or system affected: Ears
Specialties and related fields: Audiology, family medicine, otorhinolaryngology
Definition: A normal, waxy product with antibacterial properties that forms in the outer third of the ear canal. It protects the ear from water and helps to prevent infection.

Structure and Functions
Earwax is made of a combination of dead skin cells, sebum (an oily substance produced by sebaceous glands), and a wax that is secreted by special glands in the outer third of the ear canal. There are two basic types of earwax, described as wet or dry; a gene has been identified that determines this characteristic: wet earwax contains more fat.

The function of earwax is to protect the ear by trapping dust, bacteria, and foreign particles. Earwax moves out of the ear canal to the ear opening, where it becomes dry and falls out. This action is assisted by the motion of the jaw during chewing and speaking.

Disorders and Diseases
Too much or too little earwax can both increase the possibility of infection. Too little earwax compromises the protection of the ear from bacteria and foreign particles. Too much earwax can trap bacteria in the ear and cause infection, plug the ear and cause some loss in hearing, or cause a blockage that does not allow a doctor to adequately see the outer and middle ear canal during examination.

Symptoms of a wax blockage, called cerumen impaction, can be a decrease in hearing, an earache, a feeling of fullness in the ear, or a feeling that the ear is plugged. When individuals probe or try to clean out their own ears using a cotton swab or other device, such as a hairpin, this often pushes the wax deeper into the ear and can cause wax blockage against the eardrum and possible perforation of the eardrum.

The best method for earwax removal is by a doctor using a device, a microscope or an otoscope, to see a lighted and magnified view of the outer and middle ear; earwax can then be removed using a cerumen spoon or with forceps or mild suction. Other methods of earwax removal by a doctor include use of a cerumenolytic agent (a wax softener) or by irrigation of the ear with water. Over-the-counter irrigation products for individuals to use at home are available, but some studies have shown that water is as effective as these products. Other do-it-yourself products for earwax removal, including vacuum kits and "candling," where a cone-shaped device is put in the ear canal and lighted at the outside end to draw wax and impurities from the ear, are strongly discouraged.

—*Vicki J. Miskovsky*

See also Audiology; Ear infections and disorders; Ears; Hearing;

Hearing loss; Host-defense mechanisms; Otorhinolaryngology; Sense organs.

For Further Information:
"Earwax." *American Academy of Otolaryngology–Head and Neck Surgery*, 2013.
"Ear Disorders." *MedlinePlus*, June 12, 2013.
Gelfand, Stanley A. *Essentials of Audiology*. 3d ed. New York: Thieme, 2009.
Harkin, H. "A Nurse-Led Ear Care Clinic: Sharing Knowledge and Improving Patient Care." *British Journal of Nursing* 14, no. 5 (March 10–23, 2005): 250–254.
Katz, Jack, ed. *Handbook of Clinical Audiology*. 6th ed. Philadelphia: Wolters Kluwer/Lippincott Williams & Wilkins, 2009.
Kraszewski, Sarah. "Safe and Effective Ear Irrigation." *Nursing Standard* 22, no. 43 (July, 2008): 45–48.
Roland, P. S., et al. "Clinical Practice Guideline: Cerumen Impaction." *Archives of Otolaryngology—Head and Neck Surgery* 139, no. 3, supp. 2 (September, 2008): S1–S21.
Safer, Diane A., and Kari Kassir. "Cerumen Impaction." *Health Library*, February 1, 2013.

EATING DISORDERS

Disease/Disorder

Anatomy or system affected: Abdomen, bones, gastrointestinal system, intestines, mouth, psychic-emotional system, reproductive system, stomach, teeth, throat

Specialties and related fields: Dentistry, family medicine, pediatrics, psychiatry, psychology

Definition: A group of conditions characterized by disordered eating patterns, preoccupation with body size and weight, and distorted body image. Eating disorders can cause serious medical complications and even death. The causes of eating disorders are complex and involve biological, psychological, and societal factors.

Key terms:

amenorrhea: the absence of menstruation

antidepressant: medication used to treat depression

cardiomyopathy: disease of the heart muscle

diuretic: an agent that promotes the secretion of urine

fast: to abstain from food

laxative: an agent that promotes evacuation of the bowel

neurotransmitters: chemicals in the brain that stimulate activity

osteopenia: reduced bone mass

osteoporosis: demineralization of the bone

pharmacotherapy: the treatment of disease with medication

satiety: the state of feeling full or fed and free from hunger

serotonin: the neurotransmitter associated with pain perception, sleep, impulsivity, and aggression; implicated in disorders associated with anxiety, depression, and migraines

Causes and Symptoms

Identified eating disorders include anorexia nervosa, bulimia nervosa, and binge-eating disorder. These disorders are not always distinct, and many individuals exhibit symptoms of more than one. Their prevalence has increased during the past several decades. Anorexia nervosa and bulimia nervosa predominantly affect adolescent and young adult females.

However, they can also occur in males and the elderly, and binge-eating disorder occurs more frequently in males. Approximately 4 percent of females have eating disorders, although the number of those who do not meet the full criteria for diagnosing any specific disorder is much higher. There is an approximately nine to one ratio of females to males with eating disorders. The incidence of eating disorders in males is rising, however, and they are most commonly associated with sports (such as wrestling), bodybuilding, and the performing arts (such as dance). The disorders can be chronic and recur across the life span of an individual. Recognition of eating disorders in the elderly has increased, as have the negative health affects of the conditions on this population.

Anorexia nervosa is characterized by refusal to maintain normal body weight (less than 85 percent of expected weight), extreme fear of becoming fat, and relentless pursuit of thinness. Individuals with anorexia nervosa have a distorted perception of body weight and size and consider themselves to be overweight even when the opposite is true. Their view of themselves is heavily dependent on factors such as their level of adherence to a restrictive diet or the fit of their clothes. They often deny the negative aspects of low weight even in the face of serious health problems.

Two types of anorexia nervosa have been identified: the restricting type, involving dieting, fasting, or skipping meals, but not bingeing/purging; and the binge-eating/purging type, involving binge eating and purging (self-induced vomiting or misusing laxatives, enemas, or diuretics). The latter type is primarily distinguished from bulimia nervosa by refusal to maintain 85 percent of normal body weight. Dieting regimens may be severe, with intake reduced to between three hundred and six hundred kilocalories (Calories) per day and strict habits regarding food selection and eating.

Individuals with anorexia nervosa commonly display a set of personality and behavioral characteristics including being goal driven, perfectionistic, and overtly competent at school or work. Underlying these tendencies is often a lack of confidence and low sense of self-worth. As dieting increases, individuals may become depressed and fatigued, causing school or work to suffer and further eroding self-perception. Rigid "all or nothing" thinking influences the severity of dieting. Thus, anorexic people might believe that if they permit themselves even one lapse in dieting, then they will become obese. As starvation develops, focus on food and weight increases, and behaviors such as hoarding food, gazing in mirrors, or seeking reassurance about appearance may be observed. Significant energy is expended to keep secret the severity of weight loss efforts. Consequently, exercise may be conducted privately, family meals and public eating avoided, or food disposed of surreptitiously. In some cases, anorexia nervosa is not discovered until after a health problem has developed consequent to malnutrition.

A number of serious health problems stemming from starvation and malnutrition are seen in people with anorexia nervosa. Among the most serious are those associated with cardiac functioning, including cardiomyopathy, arrhythmias, and altered heart rates. In rare cases, sudden death can occur as a result of irregular heart muscle contractions. Other health problems caused by anorexia nervosa involve the gastrointestinal system (bloating and constipation), the reproductive system (amenorrhea, hormonal abnormalities, and infertility), and the skeletal system (osteoporosis and osteopenia). Additional complications include lowered metabolism, cold intolerance, weakness, loss of muscle mass, low body temperature, and growth suppression. While elderly individuals with anorexia nervosa may not exhibit a drive for thinness, behaviors such as food refusal, the hoarding or hiding of food, and distorted body image are often observed. The health effects of anorexia nervosa in this population are significant and worsen coexisting illnesses, sometimes hastening death. A very serious condition known as the "female athlete triad" is a combination of factors involving athletic training: disordered eating, amenorrhea, and osteoporosis. Permanent damage to bone strength can result from this condition. Despite the numerous medical problems caused by anorexia nervosa, many with the disorder appear superficially healthy even after significant weight loss.

Bulimia nervosa is characterized by recurrent episodes of binge eating followed by purging or other inappropriate efforts to avoid weight gain. The episodes are accompanied by feelings of being out of control and subsequent self-disgust, guilt, and depression. Bingeing involves eating over a limited period of time an amount of food that is markedly larger than most people would under similar circumstances. Caloric intake during binges may range from two thousand to ten thousand. Social interruption, fear of discovery, or physical discomfort (nausea or abdominal pain) typically terminates the binge episode. The binge-purge cycle may occur several times per day, with considerable effort directed toward keeping the episodes secret. Typically, bulimics recognize that their behavior is abnormal and desire to change (as opposed to those with anorexia nervosa). The disorder is divided into two types. The purging type involves self-induced vomiting or laxative, diuretic, or enema misuse as methods to avoid weight gain. The nonpurging type involves fasting or excessive exercise to prevent weight gain.

Self-induced vomiting is the most frequent method of purging and is typically accomplished by initiating the gag reflex by placing fingers down the throat. Over time, many bulimics are able to vomit reflexively without the need to use their fingers. Though employed less frequently as the sole methods of purging, laxatives, enemas, and rarely diuretics may be used in conjunction with vomiting. Abuse of laxatives is more common among the elderly.

Individuals with nonpurging bulimia nervosa, especially males, engage in hours of exercise every day or fast following bingeing. Typically, the fast is broken by another binge episode and the cycle continues.

Those with bulimia nervosa place strong emphasis on appearance, and their mood and view of themselves are highly dependent on their weight and body shape. Most are at a normal weight, but some are underweight or overweight. Often bulimia nervosa is initiated by a restrictive diet that appears to cause many of the unusual behaviors and thinking patterns

---

Information on Eating Disorders

Causes: Psychological disorder

Symptoms: Intense preoccupation with food and weight, disordered eating; may include ingestion of laxatives, depression and suicidal feelings, nutritional deficiencies, dehydration, hormonal changes, gastrointestinal problems, changes in metabolism, heart disorders, persistent sore throat, teeth and gum damage

Duration: Chronic

Treatments: Psychotherapy, nutritional counseling, medication

---

associated with anorexia nervosa, such as secretive behavior, food hoarding, and extreme focus on food and eating. There may be signs of depression and anxiety as well as compulsive behavior. As opposed to anorexia nervosa, those with bulimia nervosa are more likely to be interested in social relations and to worry more about how others perceive them. Some engage in impulsive behaviors such as substance abuse or shoplifting.

Serious medical complications can result from bulimia nervosa. Chronic vomiting or laxative abuse and consequent loss of body fluids may cause dizziness, cardiac abnormalities, dehydration, and weakness. Tooth decay caused by repeated exposure to gastric acids from vomiting may occur. Erosion or tearing of the esophagus can result from chronic vomiting. Bingeing is associated with a variety of gastrointestinal disturbances including bloating, diarrhea, and constipation.

Binge-eating disorder is a relatively newly identified condition, and less is known about it. The disorder is similar to bulimia nervosa but does not involve efforts to avoid weight gain (such as purging). Individuals with the disorder regularly engage in binges lasting up to several hours, during which from two thousand to ten thousand Calories may be consumed. Eating during binges is typically at a rapid pace and continues in spite of feeling discomfort or pain. Bingeing may occur when an individual is not very hungry, after attempting to keep a strict diet, or as a means to reduce stress. It is usually done in private and kept secret. Feeling out of control during binges is common, followed by feelings of self-disgust and shame. Preoccupation with food and unusual food-related behaviors (such as hiding food) are common. Individuals with binge-eating disorder are typically overweight and unhappy with their body shape and size. General mood and self-perception may be dependent on their weight and size. Depression and anxiety are common coexisting conditions. Distorted body image is less likely than with anorexia nervosa and bulimia nervosa. The health problems related to obesity are seen in those with binge-eating disorder. They include high blood pressure, diabetes, high cholesterol, and heart disease. Gastrointestinal problems may also result from bingeing.

The precise causes of eating disorders are unknown; however, a number of factors involving biological, psychological, and social variables have been identified as contributing to the conditions. The primary biological influences on all eating disorders are related to hunger and starvation. Research indicates that in healthy individuals, severe dieting produces moodiness, irritability, depression, food obsessions, social isolation, and apathy. These symptoms are also found in eating disorders and become more pronounced as starvation emerges. Thus, anorexia nervosa, bulimia nervosa, or binge-eating disorder may develop after food deprivation has occurred as a result of purposeful dieting in order to lose weight or enhance athletic performance, or consequent to food restriction resulting from illness (especially in the elderly) or stress. Hunger resulting from restrictive dieting is the major stimulus for bingeing. Because a majority of those who diet do not develop eating disorders, there is likely some as yet unidentified biological or genetic predisposition in some individuals. Biological abnormalities associated with the hypothalamus and thyroid gland have been identified in some individuals with anorexia nervosa, while other research points to neurochemical or hormonal imbalances. In the elderly, medications, coexisting health problems, and even poorly fitting dentures may initiate restricted eating, leading to anorexia nervosa. Irregular levels of the neurotransmitter serotonin may influence bingeing in bulimia nervosa and binge-eating disorder since it is associated with triggering signals of satiety to the brain. Knowledge of the causes of binge-eating disorder is limited; however, as with bulimia nervosa, there often is a history of being overweight or obese prior to developing the disorder.

A number of psychological factors have been identified as causing eating disorders. Most of these are not mutually exclusive, and none has been universally accepted as the primary causative factor for the conditions. Factors proposed to account for anorexia nervosa include phobic responses to food and weight gain, conflicted feelings over adolescent development and sexual maturity, and reactions to feelings of personal ineffectiveness by "controlling" hunger and the body. Faulty thinking, known as cognitive distortions, may cause misperceptions in body image and undue emphasis on the importance of appearance. Powerful needs to demonstrate self-discipline and to develop feelings of uniqueness and independence may also contribute to anorexia nervosa. Individuals with bulimia nervosa often exhibit mood fluctuations as well as impulsive behaviors. Bulimia nervosa is thought by some to be a variant of obsessive-compulsive disorder (OCD)

in which bingeing results from irresistible urges to eat and purging is engaged in to alleviate overwhelming anxiety. Fewer psychological causes have been identified in binge-eating disorder. Some research suggests that characteristics seen in bulimia nervosa such as impulsivity and mood changes are also associated with this disorder. Depression, especially in the elderly population, appears to play a role in all eating disorders. Middle-aged and elderly individuals may employ behaviors such as extreme dieting, bingeing, and purging to reduce anxiety or to exert control in their lives.

Societal factors appear to also contribute to eating disorders. Popular media increasingly promotes physical appearance, and thinness is held up as the ideal body type. Since the 1950s, there have been steady decreases in the weights of influential persons such as actors, fashion models, and musicians. Many popular role models for females and males are underweight. Significant social approval is often associated with weight loss and disapproval with weight gain. Thus, females and males may feel pressured to attain an unhealthy weight or unrealistic body shape. A number of Web sites are devoted to promoting anorexia nervosa and bulimia nervosa as a means of personal choice and self-expression and minimizing the medical and psychological damage caused by these disorders. No reliable family characteristics have been conclusively associated with eating disorders; however, some families appear to have higher than usual levels of

In the News:
Genetic Links to Eating Disorders

A study published in the April, 2003, volume of the *International Journal of Eating Disorders* revealed substantial heritability for obesity and moderate heritability for binge eating among 2,163 female twins. The study also showed that obesity and binge eating share a moderate genetic correlation. Another study published in the same volume demonstrated that some genetic influences may be activated during puberty, suggesting that age-related development may be an important factor to consider in the study of eating disorders. This study used 530 twins who were eleven years of age and 602 twins who were seventeen years of age from the Minnesota Twins Family Study. The genetic contribution was zero in the eleven-year-olds but 55 percent in the seventeen-year-olds. The correlation of developmental stage with eating disorders was also highlighted in *Aging and Mental Health* (2001), which reported on anorexia and the elderly.

In February, 2003, *Clinical Psychology Review* presented a review of relevant literature suggesting that disorders such as anorexia nervosa and bulimia nervosa may also share relationships with other conditions that have genetic contributions. For instance, both disorders may be associated with depression, and anorexia has been associated with obsessive-compulsive disorder.

Similarly, a study of 256 female twins reported in the *Journal of Abnormal Psychology* (2002) suggested that eating disorders might be related to inherited personality characteristics. In this study, the results indicated that phenotypic associations between the Multidimensional Personality Questionnaire and the Eating Disorders Inventory were more likely to be genetic; however, their shared genetic variance was limited. Thus, personality may play a role in the expression of eating disorders, but this role may be limited.

Together, these studies suggest that genetics and environment play roles in the development of various eating disorders. They also suggest that more than one mechanism may account for these contributions related to factors such as psychiatric conditions (depression or anxiety), personality factors, and even age-related development.

—*Nancy A. Piotrowski, Ph.D.*

depression, difficulties in communication, conflict, and focus on weight and appearance.

Treatment and Therapy

Treatment of eating disorders incorporates medical, behavioral, and psychological interventions. Typically, those with anorexia nervosa believe that their diet is justified, and resistance to treatment is the norm. Males may be especially resistant. Weight restoration is the central focus of initial treatment. Hospitalization is recommended for persons with more serious medical complications or who have less than 75 percent of expected weight. During hospitalization, daily monitoring of weight and caloric intake occurs, as well as any other necessary medical management. Behavioral therapy is employed to facilitate eating habits, and privileges such as social activity or family visits are made dependent upon increased eating and daily weight gains. Individual and family therapy are introduced as malnutrition cases and irritability, depression, and preoccupation with diet diminishes. Lengths of hospital stays vary from weeks to months depending on severity of illness and treatment progress.

Outpatient treatment may be recommended with individuals who have less severe medical complications, who are motivated to cooperate with treatment, and who have families that can independently monitor diet and health status. Weight restoration is facilitated by supervision of caloric intake and regular measurements as well as behavioral therapy techniques. Individual therapy focuses on altering cognitive distortions and assumptions about diet, weight, and body image and developing more effective means of dealing with stress. Family therapy aims to improve communication patterns, eating habits, and supportive behaviors.

No medications have been identified as effective agents in treating the core symptoms of anorexia nervosa. Medications that promote hunger may be used during the initial stages of treatment to facilitate eating. Also, medications to treat coexisting conditions such as depression and anxiety are often employed in the treatment regimen.

Most patients with bulimia nervosa do not require hospitalization unless medical complications are severe. Outpatient treatment involves individual psychotherapy, family therapy, and pharmacotherapy. Individual psychotherapy addresses cognitive distortions involving appearance and body image as well as behaviors, thoughts, and emotions that lead to binge episodes. Skills for problem solving and stress reduction are also taught. Treatment methods used for obsessive-compulsive disorder may also be employed, involving exposure to stimuli that usually trigger binge-purge behaviors while preventing them from occurring. Family therapy for bulimia nervosa aims at strengthening support and communication and developing healthy eating habits. With adolescents, impulsive behaviors associated with bulimia nervosa may be addressed by helping parents develop more effective methods of discipline and behavior management.

Antidepressant medications that regulate the neurotransmitter serotonin have been found to reduce bingeing, improve mood, and lessen preoccupation with weight and size.

These same medications are useful in treating depression and anxiety, which are also commonly seen in those with bulimia nervosa.

Treatment of binge-eating disorder is similar to that of bulimia nervosa. Psychotherapy aims toward identifying and altering behaviors and feelings that lead to bingeing and developing effective methods of dealing with stress. Group therapy and weight loss programs with medical management may also be utilized. Antidepressants have also been found effective with binge-eating disorder.

Perspective and Prospects

Behaviors associated with eating disorders have been identified in the earliest writings of Western civilization, including those by the ancient Greeks and early Christians. Formal identification of eating disorders as medical illnesses occurred in the nineteenth century when case studies were first recorded. Treatment methods at that time were limited and often involved "mental hygiene" measures such as rest, fresh air, and cold or hot baths.

In the early to mid-twentieth century, psychological theories influenced by Sigmund Freud, an Austrian psychiatrist, dominated treatment methods for eating disorders. These conditions were viewed as resulting from early childhood experiences that caused problems with psychological and sexual development. Treatment involved psychoanalysis, a form of psychotherapy, often lasting several years. Limited evidence for the success of this approach caused its decline in use.

More recent and successful treatment approaches involve cognitive and behavioral therapy that aims to alter thinking and behavior contributing to eating disorders. Medications have increasingly been used in treating eating disorders since the 1980s. Identifying biological causes of the conditions and refining pharmacotherapy may offer the best hope for improving treatment in the future.

Eating disorders were once thought to occur exclusively among young Caucasian females from middle- and upper-class families. Consequently, research into the disorders has historically focused on this population. Increased awareness of the illnesses has revealed that they occur in all socioeconomic classes and races, as well as in males and the elderly. Additional research into these groups is needed.

Awareness of eating disorders and their dangers has expanded among the general public since the 1970s. Nevertheless, rates of these disorders are rising. The media publicizes celebrities" struggles with these conditions, which may glamorize the illnesses even when negative aspects are reported. Establishing healthy eating habits and identifying potential problems early constitute the current focus of prevention efforts in medicine and education.

—Paul F. Bell, Ph.D.

See also Addiction; Amenorrhea; Anorexia nervosa; Anxiety; Appetite loss; Bariatric surgery; Bulimia; Depression; Diuretics; Enemas; Hyperadiposis; Malnutrition; Nausea and vomiting; Nutrition; Obesity; Obesity, childhood; Obsessive-compulsive disorder; Psychiatric disorders; Psychiatry; Psychiatry, child and adolescent; Puberty and adolescence; Sports medicine; Stress; Vitamins and minerals; Weight loss and gain; Weight loss medications; Women's health.

For Further Information:

American Psychiatric Association. *Diagnostic and Statistical Manual of Mental Disorders: DSM-IV-TR.* 5th ed. Arlington, Va.: American Psychiatric Publishing, 2013.

"Anorexia Nervosa." *MedlinePlus*, February 13, 2012.

Duyff, Roberta Larson, ed. *365 Days of Healthy Eating from the American Dietetic Association.* Hoboken, N.J.: John Wiley & Sons, 2006.

McCoy, Krisha. "Binge Eating Disorder." *Health Library*, March 15, 2013.

National Association of Anorexia Nervosa and Associated Disorders. http://www.anad.org.

Parker, James M., and Philip M. Parker, eds. *The 2002 Official Patient's Sourcebook on Binge Eating Disorder.* San Diego, Calif.: Icon Health, 2002.

Paterson, Anna. *Fit to Die: Men and Eating Disorders.* Thousand Oaks, Calif.: Sage, 2004.

Sackler, Ira M., and Marc A. Zimmer. *Dying to Be Thin: Understanding and Defeating Anorexia Nervosa and Bulimia—A Practical, Lifesaving Guide.* New York: Warner Books, 2001.

Thompson, Ron A., and Roberta Trattner Sherman. *Helping Athletes with Eating Disorders.* Champaign, Ill.: Human Kinetics, 1993.

Wood, Debra. "Bulimia Nervosa." *Health Library*, September 10, 2012.

EBOLA VIRUS
Disease/Disorder

Anatomy or system affected: Blood, circulatory system, gastrointestinal system, muscles, skin

Specialties and related fields: Epidemiology, public health, virology

Definition: A virus responsible for a severe and often fatal hemorrhagic fever.

Key terms:

Filoviridae: the family to which the Ebola virus belongs

maculopapular rash: a discolored skin rash observed in patients with Ebola fever

Causes and Symptoms

The Ebola virus is named after the Ebola River in northern Zaire (now the Democratic Republic of the Congo), Africa. The virus was first detected in 1976, when hundreds of deaths were recorded in Zaire as well as in neighboring Sudan. Four subtypes of the virus cause human disease: Zaire, Sudan, Côte d'Ivoire (or Ivory Coast), and Bundibugyo. A fatal disease among cynomolgus laboratory monkeys that were imported from the Philippines to Texas in 1996 was caused by the Reston subtype of the virus, which causes disease in non-human primates and in pigs but is not believed to cause symptoms in humans. Another devastating outbreak among humans took place in early 1995 in Kikwit, Zaire, claiming the

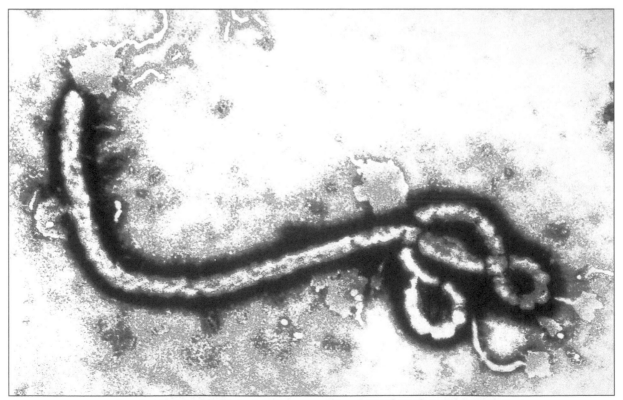

An enlarged view of the Ebola virus that causes African hemorrhagic fever. (Digital Stock)

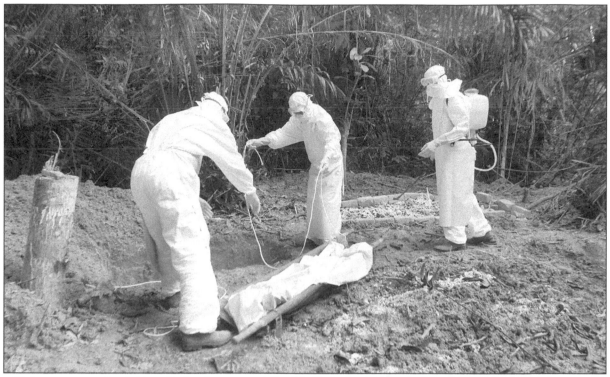

Workers wear protective clothing when burying a young victim of the Ebola virus in Gabon in 2001. (AP/Wide World Photos)

lives of 250 patients out of 315 reported cases, an 88 percent fatality rate. It is interesting to note that the epidemic ended within a few months, as suddenly as it began; this puzzled scientists, who are still not fully aware of the causes and nature of the virus. Despite the dreadful speed with which the disease killed its victims, scientists were able to contain it with a relatively small number of fatalities. Outbreaks in Africa have continued to occur, some of them severe; a 2007 outbreak in the Democratic Republic of the Congo resulted in 264 cases and 187 deaths.

The Ebola virus appears to have an incubation period of two to twenty-one days, after which time the impact is devastating. The patient develops appetite loss, increasing fever, headaches, and muscle aches. The next stage involves disseminated intravascular coagulation (DIC), a condition characterized by both blood clots and hemorrhaging. The clots usually form in vital internal organs such as the liver, spleen, and brain, with subsequent collapse of the neighboring capillaries. Other symptoms include vomiting, diarrhea with

---

Information on Ebola Virus

Causes: Viral infection
Symptoms: Severe blood clotting and hemorrhaging, fever, lethargy, appetite loss, headaches, muscle aches, skin rash
Duration: Acute
Treatments: None

---

blood and mucus, and conjunctivitis. An unusual type of skin irritation known as maculopapular rash first appears in the trunk and quickly covers the rest of the body. The final stages of the disease involve a spontaneous hemorrhaging from all body outlets, coupled with shock and kidney failure and often death within eight to seventeen days.

Treatment and Therapy

The Ebola virus is classified as a ribonucleic acid (RNA) virus and is closely related to the Marburg virus, first discovered in 1967. The Marburg and the Ebola viruses are the only two identified members of the Filoviridae family, which was first established in 1987. Electron microscope studies show the Ebola virus as long filaments, 650 to 14,000 nanometers in length, that are often either branched or intertwined. Its virus part, known as the virion, contains one single noninfectious minus-strand RNA molecule and an endogenous RNA polymerase. The lipoprotein envelope contains a single glycoprotein, which behaves as the type-specific antigen. Spikes are approximately seven nanometers in length, are spaced at approximately ten-nanometer intervals, and are visible on the virion surface. It is believed that once in the body, the virus produces proteins that suppress the organism's immune system, thus allowing its uninhibited reproduction. In 2002, researchers announced a new discovery about how Ebola makes entry into and subverts human cells. Findings show that the virus targets a "lipid raft," tiny fat platforms that float atop the membranes of human cells. These rafts act as gateways for the virus, the assembly platform for making new virus particles, and the exit point where new particles bud. This research is a significant step toward one day creating drugs that would stop viruses from replicating.

The Ebola virus can be transmitted through contact with body fluids, such as blood, semen, mucus, saliva, and even urine and feces. It is thought that the first person in an outbreak acquires the virus through contact with an infected animal, including carcasses of dead animals.

The level of infectivity of the Ebola virus is quite stable at room temperature. Its inactivation is accomplished via ultraviolet or gamma irradiation, 1 percent formalin, beta propiolactone, and an exposure to phenolic disinfectants and lipid solvents, such as deoxycholase and ether. The virus isolation is usually achieved from acute-phase serum of appropriate cell cultures, such as the Ebola-Sudan virus MA-104 cells from a fetal rhesus monkey kidney cell line. Satisfactory results have been accomplished using tissues obtained from the liver, spleen, lymph nodes, kidneys, and heart during autopsy. The virus isolation from brain and other nervous tissues, however, has been rather unsuccessful so far. Neutralization tests have been inconsistent for all filoviruses. Ebola strains, however, show cross-reactions in tests of immunofluorescence assays.

There appears to be no known or standard treatment for Ebola fever. No chemotherapeutic or immunization strategies are available, and no antiviral drug has been shown to provide positive results, even under laboratory conditions. Human interferon, human convalescent plasma, and anticoagulation therapy have been used with unconvincing results.

At this stage, therapy involves sustaining the desired fluid and electrolyte balance by the frequent administration of fluids. Bleeding may be fought off with blood and plasma transfusion. Sanitary conditions to avoid further contact with the disease are required. Proper decontamination of medical equipment, isolation of the patients from the rest of the community, and prompt disposal of infected tissues, blood, and even corpses limit the spread of the disease.

Perspective and Prospects

The puzzling characteristics of the Ebola virus are the location of its primary natural reservoir, its sudden eruption and quick end, and the unusual discovery of the virus in the organs of people who have survived it.

In the past, experimental work on the virus has been slow because of its high pathogenicity. The progress of recombinant deoxyribonucleic acid (DNA) technology has shed the first light on the molecular structure of this virus. It is hoped that further work using this technique as well as the results of viruses of lower pathogenicity (such as the Reston virus) will provide the desired information on replication and virus-host interactions. Finally, the improvement of the various diagnostic tools will allow more accurate virus identification and assessment of transmission modes.

In 1995, the World Health Organization (WHO) investigators and epidemiologists captured about three thousand birds, rodents, and other animals and insects that are suspected of spreading the disease in order to investigate the source of the virus. The results, however, were obscure and inconclusive, and the main facts about the disease are still a mystery, with the exception of the established link between primates and Ebola virus infection in humans. This conclusion was reached after the fatal infection of a French researcher in Côte d'Ivoire who performed an autopsy on a chimpanzee that had died from a disease with the same symptoms as Ebola fever. Yet, the human outbreaks in the Democratic Republic of the Congo and the Sudan have not been traced to primates. As long as these puzzling questions linger, the disease should be contained, with particular emphasis on the improvement of sanitary conditions and the control of body fluid contact.

—*Soraya Ghayourmanesh, Ph.D.;*
updated by H. Bradford Hawley, M.D.

See also Bleeding; Centers for Disease Control and Prevention (CDC); Dengue fever; Epidemiology; Hemorrhage; Marburg virus; Tropical medicine; Viral hemorrhagic fevers; Viral infections; Zoonoses.

For Further Information:

A.D.A.M. Medical Encyclopedia. "Ebola Hemorrhagic Fever." *MedlinePlus*, August 24, 2011.

Balter, Michael. "On the Trail of Ebola and Marburg Viruses." *Science* 290, no. 5493 (November 3, 2000): 923–25.

Biddle, Wayne. *A Field Guide to Germs.* 2d ed. New York: Anchor Books, 2002.

Dyer, Nicole. "Killers Without Cures." *Science World* 57, no. 3 (October 2, 2000): 8–12.

Global Alert and Response. "Ebola Haemorrhagic Fever." *World Health Organization*, 2013.

Jaax, Nancy. *Lethal Viruses, Ebola, and the Hot Zone: Worldwide Transmission of Fatal Viruses.* Lincoln: University of Nebraska Foundation, 1996.

Jahrling, Peter B., et al. "Filoviruses and Arenaviruses." In *Manual of Clinical Microbiology*, edited by Patrick R. Murray et al. 8th ed. Washington, D.C.: ASM Press, 2007.

McGraw-Hill Encyclopedia of Science and Technology. 10th ed. 20 vols. New York: McGraw-Hill, 2007.

Peters, C. J., and J. W. LeDuc. "An Introduction to Ebola: The Virus and the Disease." *Journal of Infectious Diseases* 179, supp. 1 (1999): ix–xvi.

Special Pathogens Branch. "Ebola Hemorrhagic Fever" *Centers for Disease Control and Prevention*, December 21, 2012.

Special Pathogens Branch. "Known Cases and Outbreaks of Ebola Hemorrhagic Fever, in Chronological Order." *Centers for Disease Control and Prevention*, July 31, 2012.

Strauss, James, and Ellen Strauss. *Viruses and Human Disease.* 2d ed. Boston: Academic Press/Elsevier, 2008.

ECG OR EKG. *See* ELECTROCARDIOGRAPHY (ECG OR EKG).

ECHOCARDIOGRAPHY

Procedure

Also known as: Cardiac ultrasound, 2-D echo, stress echo

Anatomy or system affected: Circulatory system, heart

Specialties and related fields: Cardiology, critical care, emergency medicine, family medicine, internal medicine

Definition: A diagnostic technique that uses ultrasound to display anatomical and physiological characteristics of the heart and related structures.

Key terms:

stress echocardiography: echocardiography procedure performed while the heart is stressed, either with medications or by exercising on a treadmill

transducer: the tip of the ultrasound probe

transesophageal echocardiography: the method of performing echocardiography with the ultrasound probe inserted via the esophagus (food pipe)

transthoracic echocardiography: the routine method of performing echocardiography by placing the ultrasound probe on the chest

Indications and Procedures

Echocardiography is a technique that uses ultrasound waves to detect the structures of the heart. The most common indication for echocardiography is to evaluate chamber size, thickness of the heart muscle, valve abnormalities, and the flow of blood through the heart. The procedure is usually performed to evaluate the functioning of the heart in a patient with heart failure and can detect any damage to the heart muscles after a heart attack. In addition, valvular abnormalities of any of the four heart valves, such as thickening or leakage, can be detected. Other indications include evaluation of congenital or birth defects of the heart and fluid collection in the sac covering the heart (pericardial effusion). The use of a color Doppler further helps in assessing the velocity of blood flow through the heart.

Transthoracic echocardiography (TTE) is a simple outpatient, noninvasive procedure. While undergoing echocardiography, the patient lies down on his or her back and turns a little toward to the left so that the heart can be better visualized. The area on the left side of chest is wiped dry (no shaving is necessary), and a gel is applied over the skin for better conduction of the ultrasound waves. The operator then applies the transducer or the ultrasound probe over the chest, and two-dimensional images of the heart are seen on the attached monitor. Multiple still and motion pictures of the heart are recorded, which are then read by a cardiologist. The procedure takes about thirty minutes, and the patient is able to go home immediately after the procedure.

Special types of echocardiography include trans-esophageal echocardiography (TEE) and stress echocardiography. In TEE, the ultrasound probe is mounted on an endoscope and introduced into the esophagus. The structures at the back of the heart and valves are better visualized with this procedure. Stress echocardiography includes performing echocardiography while the patient is undergoing a stress test (while exercising on a treadmill or after medications such as dobutamine have been given). Both these procedures take a longer time and require experienced operators. Patients may be observed for a few hours after the procedure.

Uses and Complications

Echocardiography helps in identifying congenital heart defects such as tetralogy of Fallot, atrial and ventricular septal defects, valvular abnormalities such as stenosis (narrowing) or regurgitation (leaking) of the four heart valves, the functioning of the heart muscle after a heart attack, the collection of fluid in the sac covering the heart, the rupture of heart muscle, and the progression of heart failure.

Different modes of echocardiography are used in clinical practice. The most common is two-dimensional echocardiography (2-D echo), as described above, which detects cardiac structure and function and displays results in two dimensions. A newer, more expensive three-dimensional echocardiography is gaining popularity, as it displays the findings in a three-dimensional form and localizes specific lesions more accurately. Stress echocardiography is used to detect areas in the heart that have a reduced blood flow, especially during exercise or stress. This enables cardiologists to locate the diseased artery and correct it by stenting or by surgery. TEE specifically looks for blood clots in one of the heart chambers called the left atrium and also looks closely at infections of the valves (endocarditis).

TTE is a safe procedure without any known complications. Patients undergoing TEE or stress echocardiography are carefully screened before undergoing the procedure. Rare complications of stress echocardiography are chest pain and heart attack in patients with very poor circulation to the heart, and this procedure should not be performed in persons with ongoing heart attack symptoms. TEE rarely can cause rupture of the esophagus because of the invasive nature of the procedure. Occasionally, aspiration of food contents into the lungs can occur, and hence patients are required to have an empty stomach before the procedure. If complications do occur, then patients are hospitalized and treated appropriately.

Perspectives and Prospects

The term *echo* was first coined by the Roman architect Vesuvius during the rule of the Roman Empire. Karl Dussik first used ultrasound in medicine to outline the ventricles of the brain. The first use of ultrasound to examine the heart was by W. D. Keidel in the 1940s. Clinical echocardiography was initiated by Helmut Hertz and Inge Edler of Sweden using a commercial ultrasonoscope to examine the heart. Though echocardiography was introduced in the United States by John J. Wild, H. D. Crawford, and John Reid in the 1960s, most of the credit for its further development and popularity goes to Harvey Feigenbaum at Indiana University.

Echocardiography is a great tool for assessing cardiac function. Recent echocardiography machines are portable and allow physicians to do bedside evaluation of the heart. Newer models are handheld, further enhancing ease of use. A role for echocardiography has been proposed in other systemic diseases such as diabetes, hypertension, pregnancy, kidney disease, and thyroid disease and also in the screening of athletes. Echocardiography is a cost-effective, versatile procedure that has a significant role in clinical medicine.

—*Venkat Raghavan Tirumala, M.D., M.H.A.*

See also Angiography; Arrhythmias; Arteriosclerosis; Cardiac rehabilitation; Cardiology; Cardiology, pediatric; Circulation; Congenital heart disease; Diagnosis; Electrocardiography (ECG or EKG); Endocarditis; Exercise physiology; Heart; Heart attack; Heart disease; Heart failure; Hypertension; Imaging and radiology; Magnetic resonance imaging (MRI); Mitral valve prolapse; Noninvasive tests; Pacemaker implantation; Palpitations; Sports medicine; Ultrasonography; Vascular medicine; Vascular system.

For Further Information:

Fauci, Anthony S., et al., eds. *Harrison's Principles of Internal Medicine*. 18th ed. New York: McGraw-Hill, 2012.

Feigenbaum, Harvey, William F. Armstrong, and Thomas Ryan. *Feigenbaum's Echocardiography*. 7th ed. Philadelphia: Lippincott Williams & Wilkins, 2010.

Health Library. "Echocardiogram." *Health Library*, March 5, 2013.

NIH National Heart, Lung, and Blood Institute. "What Is Echocardiography?" *NIH National Heart, Lung, and Blood Institute*, October 31, 2011.

Papadakis, Maxine, et. al., eds. *Current Medical Diagnosis and Treatment 2013*. [N. p.]: McGraw-Hill, 2012.

ECLAMPSIA. *See* PREECLAMPSIA AND ECLAMPSIA.

ECTOPIC PREGNANCY
Disease/Disorder
Also known as: Tubal pregnancy
Anatomy or system affected: Reproductive system
Specialties and related fields: Embryology, gynecology
Definition: The implantation of an embryo outside the uterine endometrium, most commonly in the Fallopian tube.

Causes and Symptoms

Although ectopic pregnancies can occur without any known cause, several factors increase a woman's risk. Studies have shown an increase in ectopic pregnancies in women with previous pelvic inflammatory disease (PID). Intrauterine devices (IUDs), so effective at preventing pregnancies, do not increase the risk of ectopic pregnancy. However, when a woman with an IUD does get pregnant, the risk for an ectopic pregnancy is increased, especially for women using an IUD containing progestin at the time of conception. There is also an increased risk in women who have had tubal ligations and other surgeries of the Fallopian tubes.

Endometriosis, multiple induced abortions, fertility treatments, anatomical abnormalities in the uterus or Fallopian tubes, and pelvic adhesions also may increase a woman's chance of ectopic pregnancy. In general, women whose Fallopian tubes are damaged for any reason have a higher risk. The risk is heightened because damage slows the progress of the developing embryo through the tube, allowing the embryo to be mature enough to implant itself before reaching the uterus. Another factor that may increase the chances of ectopic pregnancy is smoking. Nicotine slows the movement of cilia in the Fallopian tubes, thus slowing the progress of the embryo.

The symptoms of an early ectopic pregnancy are similar to those of any early pregnancy, except that spotting, cramping, and pain, especially on only one side of the abdomen, may occur as the embryo grows. Hormone levels mimic early pregnancy but usually do not rise as high as in a normal intrauterine implantation. If the tube ruptures, bleeding, severe pain, low blood pressure, and fainting may occur.

Information on Ectopic Pregnancy

Causes: Unknown; factors may include previous pelvic inflammatory disease, IUD use, tubal ligation, endometriosis, multiple abortions, pelvic adhesions

Symptoms: Similar to those of early pregnancy, followed by spotting, cramping, abdominal pain (especially on one side); if Fallopian tube ruptures, bleeding and severe pain

Duration: Acute

Treatments: Only in early cases, methotrexate to end pregnancy; usually surgical removal of embryo and Fallopian tube

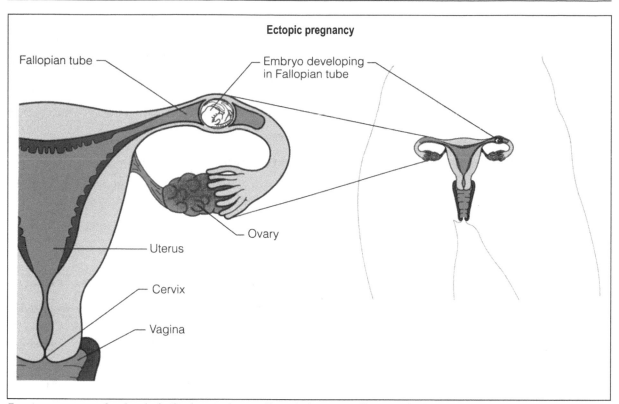

Ectopic pregnancy

Fallopian tube

Embryo developing in Fallopian tube

Ovary

Uterus

Cervix

Vagina

Ectopic pregnancy results when the fertilized egg implants itself outside the uterus and begins to develop; surgical intervention is usually required.

Transvaginal ultrasounds and blood tests, along with physical examination, are often used to determine the presence of an ectopic pregnancy.

Treatment and Therapy

If a tubal ectopic pregnancy is diagnosed early enough, methotrexate, a chemical that attacks quickly growing cells, may be administered via injection, and surgery may be avoided. The drug causes the death of the embryo. Surgical removal is now less common than is management with methotrexate; when surgery is performed, however, it is usually done through laparoscopy. In conservative surgery, the Fallopian tube is preserved, while in radical surgery, it is removed. Following surgery, methotrexate may be administered to help remove any remaining tissues from the pregnancy. Because there is no known way to implant the removed embryo in the uterus, surgical removal also results in the death of the embryo. For shock associated with tubal rupture, treatments may include intravenous fluids, oxygen, and blood transfusion.

—*Richard W. Cheney, Jr., Ph.D.*

See also Conception; Contraception; Genital disorders, female; Miscarriage; Obstetrics; Pregnancy and gestation; Women's health.

For Further Information:

A.D.A.M. Medical Encyclopedia. "Ectopic Pregnancy." *MedlinePlus*, February 26, 2012.
American Academy of Family Physicians. "Ectopic Pregnancy." *FamilyDoctor.org*, January 2011.
Carson, Sandra Ann, ed. *Ectopic Pregnancy*. Philadelphia: Lippincott-Raven, 1999.
Carson-DeWitt, Rosalyn, and Andrea Chisholm. "Ectopic Pregnancy." *Health Library*, September 10, 2012.
Hey, Valerie, et al., eds. *Hidden Loss: Miscarriage and Ectopic Pregnancy*. 2d ed. London: Women's Press, 1997.
Leach, Richard E., and Steven J. Ory, eds. *Management of Ectopic Pregnancy*. Malden, Mass.: Blackwell Science, 2000.
Preidt, Robert. "Ultrasound Best Detector of Dangerous Ectopic Pregnancies, Study Finds." *HealthDay*, April 23, 2013.
Stabile, Isabel. *Ectopic Pregnancy: Diagnosis and Management*. New York: Cambridge University Press, 1996.

ECZEMA

Disease/Disorder

Also known as: Dermatitis

Anatomy or system affected: Skin

Specialties and related fields: Dermatology, pediatrics

Definition: An inflammation of the skin.

Causes and Symptoms

The term *eczema* refers to a noncontagious inflammation of the skin. Several types of eczema exist, resulting in a range of symptoms that vary in appearance, duration, and severity. The common characteristic, however, is red, dry, and itchy skin. Other symptoms may include scaling, thickening, or

---

Information on Eczema

Causes: Genetic sensitivity to irritants (soaps, detergents, rough clothes), allergens (certain foods, pollen, animal dander), and climate or temperature changes

Symptoms: Red, dry, and itchy skin; scaling, thickening, or cracking of skin

Duration: Often chronic

Treatments: Minimal exposure to irritants, drugs (corticosteroid creams and ointments, antihistamines, antibiotics); in severe cases, oral corticosteroids or phototherapy

---

cracking of the skin, leading to infections and severe discomfort.

Atopic dermatitis, the most common form of eczema, is characterized by itchy and cracked skin of the cheeks, arms, and legs. The onset of this chronic type of eczema occurs most often during infancy or childhood, although symptoms may continue into adulthood. The cause of atopic dermatitis is thought to be a hereditary predisposition to skin sensitivities to various environmental factors. These factors include irritants such as soaps, detergents, and rough clothes; allergens such as certain foods, pollen, or animal dander; and changes in climate or temperature. Other forms of eczema, such as contact dermatitis, have similar environmental causes. Seborrheic eczema, nummular eczema, and dishydrotic eczema may result from a combination of several possible causes. Emotional factors, such as stress or frustration, may aggravate the symptoms.

The diagnosis of eczema requires a careful and detailed observation of symptoms. Family and personal medical histories are often useful to determine the presence of allergies or exposure to allergens or irritants. Dermatologists may also use skin biopsies or blood tests to determine a tendency toward elevated allergic or immune response.

Treatment and Therapy

The treatment of eczema involves minimizing exposure to possible causes while at the same time managing symptoms to maintain a high quality of life. Identifying known allergens and irritants specific to the individual is an important first step. Lifestyle changes aimed at avoiding exposure to these possible causes can lower the frequency and duration of symptoms dramatically. Proper skin care to avoid excessive drying of the skin, including the use of moisturizers or creams and minimizing exposure to water, may also help reduce skin irritation. Avoiding scratching of existing irritations and eliminating sources of emotional stress are other ways that patients can lessen the severity of their symptoms. Dermatologists may prescribe additional treatments, such as corticosteroid creams and ointments, antihistamines, or antibiotics. In more severe cases, systemic corticosteroid treatments or phototherapy, the use of ultraviolet (UV) light, may be tried.

The approval of a new type of treatment for eczema called topical immunomodulators has changed the way eczema is treated in recent years. This new class of drug counteracts the inflammation of the skin without interfering in the body's normal immune response. This treatment has been successful in preventing and even eliminating symptoms of eczema.

—*Paul J. Frisch*

See also Allergies; Dermatitis; Dermatology; Dermatology, pediatric; Itching; Lesions; Rashes; Skin; Skin disorders; Wiskott-Aldrich syndrome.

For Further Information:

Fry, Lionel. *An Atlas of Atopic Eczema.* New York: Parthenon, 2004.

Hellwig, Jennifer. "Eczema." *Health Library*, Mar. 11, 2013.

MedlinePlus. "Eczema." *MedlinePlus*, May 6, 2013.

National Eczema Society. *National Eczema Society*, n. d.

Rakel, Robert E., and Edward T. Bope, eds. *Conn's Current Therapy.* Philadelphia: Saunders, 2007.

Ring, J., B. Przybilla, and T. Ruzicka, eds. *Handbook of Atopic Eczema.* 2d ed. New York: Springer, 2006.

Turkington, Carol A., and Jeffrey S. Dover. *Skin Deep: An A-Z of Skin Disorders, Treatments, and Health.* 3d ed. New York: Checkmark, 2007.

Westcott, Patsy. *Eczema: Recipes and Advice to Provide Relief.* New York: Welcome, 2000.

EDEMA

Disease/Disorder

Anatomy or system affected: Blood vessels, circulatory system, liver, lungs, lymphatic system, respiratory system, skin

Specialties and related fields: Internal medicine, nephrology, pulmonary medicine

Definition: Accumulation of fluid in body tissues that may indicate a variety of diseases, including cardiovascular, kidney, liver, and medication problems.

Key terms:

extracellular fluid: the fluid outside cells; includes the fluid within the vascular system and the lymphatic system and the fluid surrounding individual cells

hydrostatic pressure: the physical pressure on a fluid, such as blood; it tends to push fluids across membranes toward areas of lower pressure

interstitial fluid: the fluid between the vascular system and cells; nutrients from the vascular compartment must diffuse across the interstitial compartment to enter the cells

intracellular fluid: the fluid within cells

intravascular fluid: the fluid carried within the blood vessels; it is in a constant state of motion because of the pumping action of the heart

osmotic pressure: the ability of a concentrated fluid on one side of a membrane to draw water away from a less concentrated fluid on the other side

Process and Effects

Edema is not a disease but a condition that may be caused by a number of diseases. It signals a breakdown in the body's fluid-regulating mechanisms. The body's water can be envisioned as divided into three compartments: the intracellular

Information on Edema

Causes: Wide ranging; includes disease, heart failure, deep vein thrombosis, inadequate blood levels of albumin

Symptoms: Varies; may include accumulated fluid, shortness of breath, pain and tenderness, impacted mobility

Duration: Acute to chronic

Treatments: Dependent on cause; may include frequent elevation of feet to heart level, support stockings, avoidance of prolonged standing or sitting, dietary changes, medications (e.g., diuretics)

compartment, the interstitial compartment, and the vascular compartment. The intracellular compartment consists of the fluid contained within the individual cells. The vascular compartment consists of all the water that is contained within the heart, the arteries, the capillaries, and the veins. The last compartment, and in many ways the most important for a discussion of edema, is called the interstitial compartment. This compartment includes all the water not contained in either the cells or the blood vessels. The interstitial compartment contains all the fluids between the intracellular compartment and the vascular compartment and the fluid in the lymphatic system. The sizes of these compartments are approximately as follows: intracellular fluid at 66 percent, interstitial fluid at 25 percent, and vascular fluid at only 8 percent of the total body water.

When the interstitial compartment becomes overloaded with fluid, edema develops. To understand the physiology of edema formation, it may be helpful to follow a molecule of water as it travels through the various compartments, beginning when the molecule enters the aorta soon after leaving the heart. The blood has just been ejected from the heart under high pressure, and it speedily begins its trip through the body. It passes from the great vessel, the aorta, into smaller and smaller arteries that divide and spread throughout the body. At each branching, the pressure and speed of the water molecule decrease. Finally, the molecule enters a capillary, a vessel so small that red blood cells must flow in a single file. The wall of this vessel is composed only of the membrane of a single capillary cell. There are small passages between adjacent capillary cells leading to the interstitial compartment, but they are normally closed.

The hydrostatic pressure on the water molecule is much lower than when it was racing through the aorta, but it is still higher than that of the surrounding interstitial compartment. At the arterial end of the capillary, the blood pressure is sufficient to overcome the barrier of the capillary cell's membrane. A fair number of water and other molecules are pushed through the membrane into the interstitial compartment.

In the interstitial compartment, the water molecule is essentially under no pressure, and it floats amid glucose molecules, oxygen molecules, and many other compounds. Glucose and oxygen molecules enter the cells, and when the water molecule is close to a glucose molecule it is taken inside a cell with that molecule. The water molecule is eventually expelled by the cell, which has produced extra water from the metabolic process.

Back in the interstitial compartment, the molecule floats with a very subtle flow toward the venous end of the capillary. This occurs because, as the arterial end of the capillary pushes out water molecules, it loses hydrostatic pressure, eventually equaling the pressure of the interstitial compartment. Once the pressure equalizes, another phenomenon that has been thus far overshadowed by the hydrostatic pressure takes over—osmotic pressure. Osmotic pressure is the force exercised by a concentrated fluid that is separated by a membrane from a less concentrated fluid. It draws water molecules across the membrane from the less concentrated side. The more concentrated the fluid, the greater the drawing power. The ratio of nonwater molecules to water molecules determines concentration.

The fluid that stays within the capillary remains more concentrated than the interstitial fluid for two reasons. First, the plasma proteins in the vascular compartment are too large to be forced across the capillary membrane; albumin is one such protein. These proteins stay within the vascular compartment and maintain a relatively concentrated state, compared to the interstitial compartment. At the same time, the concentration of the fluid in the interstitial compartment is being lowered constantly by the cellular compartment's actions. Cells remove molecules of substances such as glucose to metabolize, and afterward they release water—a by-product of the metabolic process. Both processes conspire to lower the total concentration of the interstitial compartment. The net result of this process is that water molecules return to the capillaries at the venous end because of osmotic pressure.

The water molecule is caught by this force and is returned to the vascular compartment. Back in the capillary, the molecule's journey is not yet complete. Now in a tiny vein, it moves along with blood. On the venous side of the circulatory system, the process of branching is reversed, and small veins join to form increasingly larger ones. The water molecule rides along in these progressively larger veins. The pressure surrounding the molecule is still low, but it is now higher than the pressure at the venous end of the capillary. One may wonder how this is possible if the venous pressure at the beginning of the venous system is essentially zero, and there is only one pump, the heart, in the body. As the molecule flows through the various veins, it occasionally passes one-way valves that allow blood to flow only toward the heart. The action of these valves, combined with muscular contractions from activities such as walking or tapping the foot, force blood toward the heart. Without these valves, it would be impossible for the venous blood to flow against gravity and return to the heart; the blood would simply sit at the lowest point in the body. Fortunately, these valves and contractions move the molecule against gravity, returning it to the heart to begin a new cycle.

In certain disease states, there is marked capillary dilation and excessive capillary permeability, and excessive amounts of fluid are allowed to leave the intravascular compartment.

The fluid accumulates in the interstitial space. When capillary permeability is increased, plasma proteins also tend to leave the vascular space, reducing the intravascular compartment's osmotic pressure while increasing the interstitial compartment's osmotic pressure. As a result, the rate of return of fluid from the interstitial compartment to the vascular compartment is lowered, thus increasing the interstitial fluid levels.

Another route of return of interstitial fluid to the circulation is via the lymphatic system. The lymphatic system is similar to the venous system, but it carries no red blood cells. It runs through the lymph nodes, carrying some of the interstitial fluid that has not been able to return to the vascular compartment at the capillary level. If lymphatic vessels become obstructed, water in the interstitial compartment accumulates, and edema may result.

Causes and Symptoms

Heart failure is a major cause of edema. When the right ventricle of the heart fails, it cannot cope with all the venous blood returning to the heart. As a consequence, the veins become distended, the interstitial compartment is overloaded, and edema occurs. If the patient with heart failure is mostly upright, the edema collects in the legs; if the patient has been lying in bed for some time, the edema tends to accumulate in the lower back. Other clinical signs of right heart failure include distended neck veins, an enlarged and tender liver, and a "galloping" sound on listening to the heart with a stethoscope.

When the left ventricle of the heart fails, the congestion affects the pulmonary veins instead of the neck and leg veins. Fluid accumulates in the same fashion within the interstitial compartment of the lungs; this condition is termed pulmonary edema. Patients develop shortness of breath with minimal activity, upon lying down, and periodically through the night. They may need to sleep on several pillows to minimize this symptom. This condition can usually be diagnosed by listening to the lungs and heart through a stethoscope and by taking an x-ray of the chest.

Deep vein thrombosis is another common cause of edema of the lower limbs. When a thrombus (a blood clot inside a blood vessel) develops in a large vein of the legs, the patient usually complains of pain and tenderness of the affected leg. There is usually redness and edema as well. If the thrombus affects a small vein, it may not be noticed. The diagnosis can be made by several specialized tests, such as ultrasound testing and impedance plethysmography. Other tests may be needed to make the diagnosis, such as injecting radiographic dye in a vein in the foot and then taking x-rays to determine whether the flow in the veins has been obstructed or using radioactive agents that bind to the clot. Risks for developing venous thrombosis include immobility (even for relatively short periods of time such as a long car or plane ride), injury, a personal or family history of venous thrombosis, the use of birth control pills, and certain types of cancer. Elderly patients are at particular risk because of relative immobility and an increased frequency of minor trauma to the legs.

When repeated or large thrombi develop, the veins deep inside the thigh (the deep venous system) become blocked, and blood flow shifts toward the superficial veins. The deep veins are surrounded by muscular tissue, and venous flow is assisted by muscular contractions of the leg (the muscular pump), but the superficial veins are surrounded only by skin and subcutaneous tissue and cannot take advantage of the muscular pump. As a consequence, the superficial veins become distended and visible as varicose veins.

When vein blockage occurs, the valves inside become damaged. Hydrostatic pressure of the venous system below the blockage then rises. The venous end of the capillary is normally where the osmotic pressure of the vascular compartment pulls water from the interstitial compartment back into the vascular compartment. In a situation of increased hydrostatic pressure, however, this process is slowed or stopped. As a result, fluid accumulates in the interstitial space, leading to the formation of edema.

A dangerous complication of deep vein thrombosis occurs when part of a thrombus breaks off, enters the circulation, and reaches the lung; this is called a pulmonary embolus. It blocks the flow of blood to the lung, impairing oxygenation. Small emboli may have little or no effect on the patient, while larger emboli may cause severe shortness of breath, chest pain, or even death.

Another potential cause of edema is the presence of a mass in the pelvis or abdomen compressing the large veins passing through the area and interfering with the venous return from the lower limbs to the heart. The resulting venous congestion leads to edema of the lower limbs. The edema may affect either one or both legs, depending on the size and location of the mass. This diagnosis can usually be established by a thorough clinical examination, including rectal and vaginal examinations and x-ray studies.

Postural (or gravitational) edema of the lower limbs is the most common type of edema affecting older people; it is more pronounced toward the end of the day. It can be differentiated from the edema resulting from heart failure by the lack of signs associated with heart failure and by the presence of diseases restricting the patient's degree of mobility. These diseases include Parkinson's disease, osteoarthritis, strokes, and muscle weakness. Postural edema of the lower limbs results from a combination of factors, the most important being diminished mobility. If a person stands or sits for prolonged periods of time without moving, the muscular pump becomes ineffective. Venous compression also plays an important role in the development of this type of edema. It will occur when the veins in the thigh are compressed between the weight of the body and the surface on which the patient sits, or when the edge of a reclining chair compresses the veins in the calves. Other factors that aggravate postural edema include varicose veins, venous thrombi, heart failure, some types of medication, and low blood albumin levels.

Albumin is formed in the liver from dietary protein. It is essential to maintaining adequate osmotic pressure inside the blood vessels and ensuring the return of fluid from the interstitial space to the vascular compartment. When edema is caused by inadequate blood levels of albumin, it tends to be quite extensive. The patient's entire body and even face are often affected. The liver may be unable to produce the necessary amount of albumin for several reasons, including malnutrition, liver impairment, the aging process, and excessive protein loss.

In cases of malnutrition, the liver does not receive a sufficient quantity of raw material from the diet to produce albumin; this occurs when the patient does not ingest enough protein. Healthy adults need at least 0.5 grams of protein for each pound of their body weight. Infants and children of poor families who cannot afford to prepare nutritious meals often suffer from malnutrition. The elderly, especially men living on their own, are also vulnerable, regardless of their income.

A liver damaged by excessive and prolonged consumption of alcohol, diseases, or the intake of some types of medication or other chemical toxins will be unable to manufacture albumin at the rate necessary to maintain a normal concentration in the blood. Clinically, the patient shows other evidence of liver impairment in addition to edema. For example, fluid may also accumulate in the abdominal cavity, a condition known as ascites. The diagnosis of liver damage is made by clinical examination and supporting laboratory investigations. The livers of older people, even in the absence of disease, are often less efficient at producing albumin.

The albumin also can be deficient if an excessive amount of albumin is lost from the body. This condition may occur in certain types of diseases affecting the kidneys or the gastrointestinal tract. An excessive amount of protein also may be lost if a patient has large, oozing pressure ulcers, extensive burns, or chronic lung conditions that produce large amounts of sputum.

Patients with strokes and paralysis sometimes develop edema of the paralyzed limb. The mechanism of edema formation in these patients is not entirely understood. It probably results from a combination of an impairment of the nerves controlling the dilation and a constriction of the blood vessels in the affected limb, along with postural and gravitational factors.

Severe allergic states, toxic states, or local inflammation are associated with increased capillary permeability that results in edema. The amount of fluid flowing out to the capillaries far exceeds the amount that can be returned to the capillaries at the venous end. A number of medications, including steroids, estrogens, some arthritis medications, a few blood pressure medications, and certain antibiotics, can induce edema by promoting the retention of fluid. Salt intake tends to cause retention of fluid as well. Obstruction of the lymphatic system often leads to accumulation of fluid in the interstitial compartment. Obstruction can occur in certain types of cancer, after radiation treatment, and in certain parasitic infestations.

Treatment and Therapy

The management of edema depends on the specific reason for its presence. To determine the cause of edema, a thorough history, including current medications, dietary habits, and activity level, is of prime importance. Performing a detailed physical examination is also a vital step. It is frequently necessary to obtain laboratory, ultrasound, and x-ray studies before a final diagnosis is made. Once a treatable cause is found, therapy aimed at the cause should be instituted.

If no treatable, specific disease is responsible for the edema, conservative treatment aimed at reducing the edema to manageable levels without inducing side effects should be initiated. Frequent elevation of the feet to the level of the heart, use of support stockings, and avoidance of prolonged standing or sitting are the first steps. If support stockings are ineffective or are too uncomfortable, then custom-made, fitted stockings are available. A low-salt diet is important in the management of edema because a high salt intake worsens the fluid retention. If all these measures fail, then diuretics in small doses may be useful.

Diuretics work by increasing the amount of urine produced. Urine is made of fluids removed from the vascular compartment by the kidneys. The vascular compartment then replenishes itself by drawing water from the interstitial compartment. This reduction in the amount of interstitial fluid improves the edema. There are various types of diuretics, which differ in their potency, duration of action, and side effects. Potential side effects include dizziness, fatigue, sodium and potassium deficiency, excessively low blood pressure, dehydration, sexual dysfunction, the worsening of a diabetic's blood sugar control, increased uric acid levels, and increased blood cholesterol levels. Although diuretics are a convenient and effective means of treating simple edema, it is important to keep in mind that the cure should not be worse than the disease. When the potential side effects of diuretic therapy are compared to the almost total lack of complications of conservative treatment, one can see that mild edema that is not secondary to significant disease is best managed conservatively. Edema caused by more serious diseases, however, calls for more intensive measures.

Perspective and Prospects

The prevalence of edema could decrease as people become more health conscious and medical progress is made. Nutritious diets, avoidance of excessive salt, and an increased awareness of the dangers of excessive alcohol intake and of the benefits of regular physical exercise all contribute to decreasing the incidence of edema. Improved methods for the early detection, prevention, and management of diseases that may ultimately result in edema could also significantly reduce the scope of the problem. It is also expected that safer and more convenient methods of treating edema will become available.

—*Ronald C. Hamdy, M.D., Mark R. Doman, M.D., and Katherine Hoffman Doman*

See also Arteriosclerosis; Circulation; Diuretics; Elephantiasis; Embolism; Heart; Heart disease; Heart failure; Kidney disorders; Kidneys; Kwashiorkor; Liver; Liver disorders; Lungs; Malnutrition; Nutrition; Phlebitis; Protein; Pulmonary diseases; Pulmonary medicine; Pulmonary medicine, pediatric; Respiration; Signs and symptoms; Thrombosis and thrombus; Varicose vein removal; Varicose veins; Vascular medicine; Vascular system; Venous insufficiency.

For Further Information:

Andreoli, Thomas E., et al., eds. *Andreoli and Carpenter's Cecil Essentials of Medicine.* 8th ed. Philadelphia: Saunders/Elsevier, 2010.

Cleveland Clinic. "Edema." *Cleveland Clinic Foundation*, April 26, 2012.

Guyton, Arthur C., and John E. Hall. *Human Physiology and Mechanisms of Disease.* 6th ed. Philadelphia: W. B. Saunders, 1997.

Hosenpud, Jeffrey D., and Barry H. Greenberg, eds. *Congestive Heart Failure.* 3d ed. Philadelphia: Lippincott Williams & Wilkins, 2007.

Marieb, Elaine N., and Katja Hoehn. *Human Anatomy and Physiology.* 9th ed. San Francisco: Pearson/Benjamin Cummings, 2010.

Mayo Clinic. "Edema." *Mayo Foundation for Medical Education and Research*, October 13, 2011.

MedlinePlus. "Edema." *MedlinePlus*, January 22, 2013.

EEG. *See* Electroencephalography (EEG).

Ehrlichiosis
Disease/Disorder

Anatomy or system affected: Immune system, musculoskeletal system, nervous system

Specialties and related fields: Family medicine, pediatrics

Definition: Infection by one of a group of intracellular bacteria transmitted to humans through tick bites.

Causes and Symptoms

Human ehrlichiosis is a group of tick-borne bacterial infections caused by *Anaplasma phagocytophilum* (formerly *Ehrlichia phagocytophilum*), *Ehrlichia chaffeensis*, and *Ehrlichia ewingii.* These bacteria are transmitted by the bite of *Ixodes spp.* or *Amblyomma americanum* ticks and subsequently infect circulating white blood cells (leukocytes).

After an incubation period of five to ten days, the disease is typically characterized by fever, chills, and other nonspecific symptoms. A percentage of asymptomatic infections have also been documented. Confirmation of ehrlichiosis infection is accomplished via laboratory methods, including blood-smear examination, polymerase chain reaction, culture, and serologic analysis for the presence of anti-ehrlichia antibodies.

Treatment and Therapy

Ehrlichiosis is effectively treated with a tetracycline antibiotic, most commonly doxycycline. With the increased number of diagnoses, more significant cases requiring hospitalization and condition-appropriate treatment have been documented. Significant complications include respiratory distress, myocarditis, neurological complications, hepatitis, septicemia, and opportunistic infections. Despite clinical similarities between the causative agents, a higher percentage of opportunistic infection has been documented with human granulocytic anaplasmosis (HGA), caused by *A. phagocytophilum*, whereas increased disease severity and higher mortality has been associated with human monocytic ehrlichiosis (HME), caused by *E. chaffeensis.* Death resulting from complications may occur in up to 3 percent of cases.

Information on Ehrlichiosis

Causes: Bite of an infected tick

Symptoms: Fever, chills, headache, muscle aches and weakness, joint pain, nausea

Duration: Acute

Treatments: Antibiotics

Perspective and Prospects

The reported prevalence and incidence of human ehrlichiosis has been on the rise in regions where specified tick vectors are found. Although historically considered an acute infection conferring long-term immunity, one study found a percentage of HME patients experienced a significantly higher than expected rate of fever, chills, sweats, and fatigue one to three years after the initial illness. Because these symptoms did not correlate with the severity or duration of the initial episode, nor did serological tests confirm the presence of ehrlichia, determination of whether these findings are attributed to a persistent/recurrent infection or a type of postinfection syndrome is still under investigation.

—*Pam Conboy*

See also Bacterial infections; Bacteriology; Bites and stings; Insect-borne diseases; Lice, mites, and ticks; Lyme disease; Parasitic diseases.

For Further Information:

Beltz, Lisa A. "Human Ehrlichiosis." In *Emerging Infectious Diseases: A Guide to Diseases, Causative Agents, and Surveillance*, by Lisa A. Beltz. San Francisco: John Wiley & Sons, 2011.

Dumler, J. Stephen. "Anaplasma and Ehrlichia Infection." *Annals of the New York Academy of Sciences* 1063 (December, 2005): 361–73.

Dumler, J. Stephen, John E. Madigan, Nicola Pusterla, and Johan S. Bakken. "Ehrlichioses in Humans: Epidemiology, Clinical Presentation, Diagnosis, and Treatment." *Clinical Infectious Diseases* 45, suppl. 1 (July 15, 2007): S45–51.

Ganguly, S., and S. K. Mukhopadhayay. "Tick-Borne Ehrlichiosis Infection in Human Beings." *Journal of Vector Borne Diseases* 45, no. 4 (December, 2008): 273–80.

Thomas, R. J., J. S. Dumler, and J. A. Carlyon. "Current Management of Human Granulocytic Anaplasmosis, Human Monocytic Ehrlichiosis, and *Ehrlichia ewingii* Ehrlichiosis." *Expert Review of Anti-Infective Therapy* 7, no. 6 (August, 2009): 709–22.

Electrical shock
Disease/Disorder

Anatomy or system affected: Heart, nervous system, skin

Specialties and related fields: Critical care, emergency medicine, neurology

Definition: The physical effect of an electrical current entering the body and the resulting damage.

Causes and Symptoms

Electrical shock ranges from a harmless jolt of static electricity to a power line's lethal discharge. The severity of the shock depends on the current flowing through the body, and the current is determined by the skin's electrical resistance. Dry skin has a very high resistance; thus, 110 volts produces a small, harmless current. The resistance for perspiring hands, however, is lower by a factor of one hundred, resulting in potentially fatal currents. Currents traveling between bodily extremities are particularly dangerous because of their proximity to the heart.

Electrical shock causes injury or death in one of three ways: paralysis of the breathing center in the brain, paralysis of the heart, or ventricular fibrillation (extremely rapid and uncontrolled twitching of the heart muscle).

The threshold of feeling (the minimum current detectable) ranges from 0.5 to 1.0 milliamperes. Currents up to five milliamperes, the maximum harmless current, are not hazardous, unless they trigger an accident by involuntary reaction. Currents in this range create a tingling sensation. The minimum current that causes muscular paralysis occurs between ten and fifteen milliamperes. Currents of this magnitude cause a painful jolt. Above eighteen milliamperes, the current contracts chest muscles, and breathing ceases. Unconsciousness and death follow within minutes unless the current is interrupted and respiration resumed. A short exposure to currents of fifty milliamperes causes severe pain, possible fainting, and complete exhaustion, while currents in the one hundred" to three hundred–milliampere range produce ventricular fibrillation, which is fatal unless quickly corrected. During ventricular fibrillation, the heart stops its rhythmic pumping and flutters uselessly. Since blood stops flowing, the victim dies from oxygen deprivation in the brain in a matter of minutes. This is the most common cause of death for victims of electrical shock.

Relatively high currents (above three hundred milliamperes) may produce ventricular paralysis, deep burns in the body's tissue, or irreversible damage to the central nervous system. Victims are more likely to survive a large but brief current, even though smaller, sustained currents are usually lethal. Burning or charring of the skin at the point of contact may be a contributing factor to the delayed death that often follows severe electrical shock. Very high voltage discharges of short duration, such as a lightning strike, tend to disrupt the body's nervous impulses, but victims may survive. On the other hand, any electric current large enough to raise body temperature significantly produces immediate death.

Treatment and Therapy

Before medical treatment can be applied, the current must be stopped or the shock victim must be separated from the current source without being touched. Nonconducting materials such as dry, heavy blankets or pieces of wood can be used for this purpose. If the victim is not breathing, artificial respiration immediately applied provides adequate short-term life support, though the victim may become stiff or rigid in reaction to the shock. Victims of electrical shock may suffer from severe burns and permanent aftereffects, including eye cataracts, angina, or disorders of the nervous system.

Electrical shock can usually be prevented by strictly adhering to safety guidelines and using commonsense precautions. Careful inspection of appliances and tools, compliance with manufacturers" safety standards, and the avoidance of unnecessary risks greatly reduce the chance of an electrical

---

Information on Electrical Shock

Causes: Electrical current entering the body
Symptoms: Unconsciousness, moderate to severe pain, ventricular fibrillation, burning or charring of skin
Duration: Acute
Treatments: Resuscitation, emergency care

---

shock. Electrical appliances or tools should never be used when standing in water or on damp ground, and dry gloves, shoes, and floors provide considerable protection against dangerous shocks from 110-volt circuits.

Electrical safety is also provided by isolation, guarding, insulation, grounding, and ground-fault interrupters. Isolation means that high-voltage wires strung overhead are not within reach, while guarding provides a barrier around high voltage devices, such as those found in television sets.

Old wire insulation may become brittle with age and develop small cracks. Defective wires are hazardous and should be replaced immediately. Most modern power tools are double-insulated; the motor is insulated from the plastic insulating frame. These devices do not require grounding, as no exposed metal parts become electrically live if the wire insulation fails.

In a home, grounding is accomplished by a third wire in outlets, connected through a grounding circuit to a water pipe. If an appliance plug has a third prong, it will ground the frame to the grounding circuit. In the event of a short circuit, the grounding circuit provides a low resistance path, resulting in a current surge that trips the circuit breaker.

In some instances the current may be inadequate to trip a circuit breaker (which usually requires fifteen or twenty amperes), but currents in excess of ten milliamperes could still be lethal to humans. A ground-fault interrupter ensures nearly complete protection by detecting leakage currents as small as five milliamperes and breaking the circuit. This relatively inexpensive device operates very rapidly and provides an extremely high degree of safety against electrocution in the household. Many localities now have codes that require the installation of ground-fault interrupters in bathrooms, kitchens, and other areas where water is used.

—George R. Plitnik, Ph.D.

See also Burns and scalds; Cardiac arrest; Critical care; Critical care, pediatric; Emergency medicine; First aid; Intensive care unit (ICU); Resuscitation; Shock; Unconsciousness.

For Further Information:

Atkinson, William. "Electric Injuries Can Be Worse than They Seem." *Electric World* 214, no. 1 (January/February, 2000): 33–36.

Bridges, J. E., et al., eds. *International Symposium on Electrical Shock Safety Criteria.* New York: Pergamon Press, 1985.

Cooper, Mary Ann. "Electrical Injuries." *Merck Manual Home Health Handbook,* Jan. 2009.

Dugdale, David C., Michael A. Chen, and David Zieve. "Ventricular Fibrillation." *MedlinePlus,* 22 June 2012.

"Electric Shock." *HealthyChildren.org.* American Academy of

Pediatrics, 10 July 2013.

Heller, Jacob L., and David Zieve. "Electrical Injury." *MedlinePlus*, 5 Jan. 2011.

Hewitt, Paul G. *Conceptual Physics*. 11th ed. San Francisco: Pearson Addison Wesley, 2010.

"Home Electrical Safety Checklist." *US Consumer Product Safety Commission*, July 2008. PDF.

Hogan, David E., and Jonathan L. Burstein. *Disaster Medicine*. 2d ed. Philadelphia: Lippincott Williams & Wilkins, 2007.

Liu, Lynda. "Pullout Emergency Guide: Electric Shock." *Parents* 75, no. 1 (January, 2000): 65–66.

Mayo Clinic Staff. "Electrical Shock: First Aid." *Mayo Clinic*, 15 Mar. 2012.

US Department of Labor. Occupational Safety and Health Administration. *Controlling Electrical Hazards*. Rev. ed. Washington, D.C.: Author, 2002.

ELECTROCARDIOGRAPHY (ECG OR EKG)

Procedure

Anatomy or system affected: Chest, circulatory system, heart

Specialties and related fields: Biotechnology, cardiology, critical care, emergency medicine, exercise physiology, preventive medicine

Definition: A noninvasive procedure that provides insight into the rate, rhythm, and general health of the heart.

Key terms:

ECG waves: the repeated deflections of an electrocardiogram; one complete wave consists of a P wave, followed by a QRS complex, and then a T wave and represents one complete cardiac cycle, or heartbeat

electrocardiogram (ECG or EKG): a record of the waves produced by the rhythmically changing electrical conduction within the heart; often recorded by a strip chart recorder

Indications and Procedures

Electrocardiography is a useful medical diagnostic and evaluative procedure that reveals much information about the function or malfunction of a person's heart. ECG is a noninvasive, easy-to-use, and economical tool that is an essential part of diagnosing chest pain. It serves an important role in both cardiology and emergency medicine. ECG is also commonly used in preventive medicine to monitor heart health. For this purpose, ECG is frequently used in a format known as a stress test. Athletes often have ECG analysis performed as a part of their training and cardiovascular conditioning.

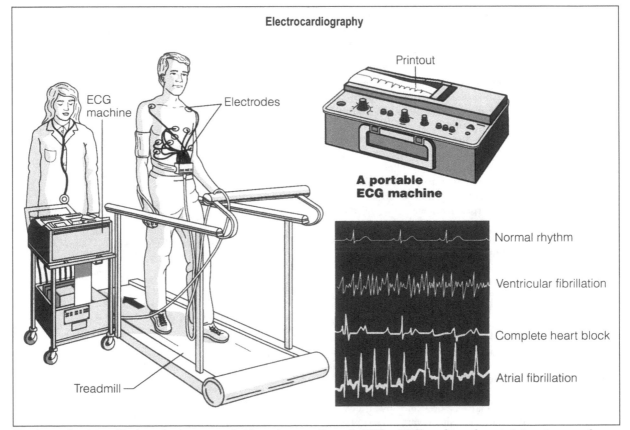

The electrical activity of the heart can be measured with an electrocardiograph (ECG or EKG) machine; characteristic patterns can be used to diagnose arrhythmias (irregular heartbeats). The patient may also be asked to walk on a treadmill while the heart is monitored in order to gauge its function during exercise.

Electrocardiography

The electrical activity of the heart can be measured with an electrocardiograph (ECG or EKG) machine; characteristic patterns can be used to diagnose arrhythmias (irregular heartbeats). The patient may also be asked to walk on a treadmill while the heart is monitored in order to gauge its function during exercise.

In a stress test, a person is studied for regularity of rhythm, rate, and unimpeded flow of electrical conduction within the heart. ECG recordings are first made while the person is at rest, then during light exercise, and, finally, if healthy enough, during rigorous exercise. Such exercise causes the heart to work harder and allows a physician to determine whether a person has a heart that beats with a regular, repetitive rhythm and at an appropriate pace for the level of rest or exercise. The stress of exercise can also help in assessing whether the heart muscle masses contract in the proper sequence: atrial contraction followed by ventricular contraction. An irregularity of electrical conduction, poor muscle contraction, dead regions of heart tissue (from a recent or old heart attack), and other maladies can be revealed.

To obtain an electrocardiogram, small metallic contact points are taped to the patient's skin via an electrically conductive adhesive or gel. The electric impulses travel across the skin to these contact points; from there, leads (plastic-coated wires) are attached to the recording device so that a complete circuit is made. Either a monitor screen or a strip chart recorder traces the electrical impulses. The waves are plotted in units of millivolts (on the y-axis) versus time in units of seconds (on the x-axis).

A twelve-lead ECG has replaced the original four-lead type. A twelve-lead ECG allows the physician to explore the performance of the heart from twelve different orientations, or angles, so that much more of the heart mass can be evaluated. Ten electrodes are placed on the body as follows: one on the right leg, which serves as the ground electrode; one on each of the other extremities; and six on the precordium, which is the area around the sternum and on the left chest wall (over the heart). The leads are explored in different combinations.

Uses and Complications

Healthy people, including athletes or certain members of the armed services, may take stress tests in order to have their health and cardiovascular conditioning monitored during training. Some professionals are required to take stress tests on a regular basis, such as commercial airline pilots and astronauts. In addition, people who have a family history of cardiovascular disease, or who are concerned about their heart health for other reasons, may have a stress test performed to find early warning signs and allow intervention before a crisis occurs. Finally, it should be noted that some insurance companies require stress tests of their applicants in order to determine insurability before issuing or rejecting a policy.

Treatment for chest pain is highly dependent on the electrical patterns seen on the ECG. Drugs may be administered or withheld depending on the shape or duration reported for the P-wave, QRS-complex, and T-wave patterns. Left-sided ver-

sus right-sided heart disease can be discerned from the traces, and infarction (heart attack) can be distinguished from angina. Although the waves in the electrocardiogram for an infarcted or anginal heart are abnormal, the patterns become abnormal in a predictable, and therefore diagnostic, manner.

Diagnostic patterns can also be seen for arrhythmias (unusual and abnormal beating patterns), such as ectopic foci, in which some part of the heart other than the sinoatrial (S-A) node (the natural pacemaker) is abnormally in control of determining when the heart contracts, or heart block, whereby electrical conduction is interrupted.

ECG is routinely used to keep close tabs on heart patients and in the postsurgery monitoring of patients who have had open heart or thoracic surgery. Certain kinds of neonatal or infant malformations or malfunctions may also be evaluated with ECG.

Because ECG is a superficial and noninvasive technique, there are no real risks associated with having this procedure performed.

Perspective and Prospects

Electrocardiography was once a wet, messy, and awkward procedure to perform: A patient dangled one arm in a huge jar filled with a conducting salt solution and placed the left leg in another saline-filled container. Changing the leads to include other limbs required the patient to take a good amount of soaking. Although it was a clumsy procedure, the basic premise of ECG remains unchanged: the heart exhibits regular patterns of electrical activity that can be useful diagnostically.

Advances in electrocardiography have involved the use of multiple electrode systems along with computers and recorders that allow rapid and simultaneous multiple-lead input and output. In addition, modern electronic instrumentation allows continuous ECG monitoring so that patients in intensive care units, coronary care units, or emergency rooms can be assessed on a second-by-second basis when seconds count. Undoubtedly, modern ECG systems, coupled with thoughtful and informed interpretation by medical doctors and emergency medical technicians (EMTs), save many lives.

—*Mary C. Fields, M.D.*

See also Angina; Arrhythmias; Biofeedback; Cardiac arrest; Cardiology; Cardiology, pediatric; Cardiopulmonary resuscitation (CPR); Critical care; Critical care, pediatric; Diagnosis; Echocardiography; Emergency medicine; Emergency medicine, pediatric; Exercise physiology; Heart; Heart attack; Paramedics; Stress; Stress reduction.

For Further Information:

Brady, William, John Camm, and June Edhouse. *ABC of Clinical Electrocardiography*. 2d ed. Malden, Mass.: Blackwell Science, 2008.

Conover, Mary Boudreau. *Understanding Electrocardiography*. 8th ed. St. Louis, Mo.: Mosby, 2003.

Dugdale, David C. III, and David Zieve. "Electrocardiogram." *MedlinePlus*, June 3, 2012.

"Electrocardiogram." *National Heart, Lung, and Blood Institute*, Oct. 1, 2010.

Phibbs, Brendan. *The Human Heart: A Complete Text on Function and Disease*. 5th ed. St. Louis, Mo.: G. W. Manning, 1992.

Scholten, Amy, Michael J. Fucci, and Brian Randall. "Electrocardiogram." *Health Library*, May 20, 2013.

Surawicz, Borys, and Timothy K. Knilans. *Chou's Electrocardiography in Clinical Practice: Adult and Pediatric.* 6th ed. Philadelphia: Saunders/Elsevier, 2008.

Thaler, Malcom S. *The Only EKG Book You'll Ever Need.* 7th ed. Philadelphia: Lippincott Williams & Wilkins, 2012.

Wellens, Hein J. J., and Mary Conover. *The ECG in Emergency Decision Making.* 2d ed. St. Louis, Mo.: Saunders/Elsevier, 2006.

Wiederhold, Richard. *Electrocardiography: The Monitoring and Diagnostic Leads.* 2d ed. Philadelphia: W. B. Saunders, 1999.

ELECTROCAUTERIZATION

Procedure

Anatomy or system affected: Blood vessels, cells, circulatory system, joints, ligaments, muscles, skin, uterus

Specialties and related fields: Cardiology, critical care, dermatology, emergency medicine, family medicine, general surgery, gynecology, internal medicine, vascular medicine

Definition: The surgical control of bleeding from small blood vessels or the removal of unwanted tissue using a controlled electric current.

Indications and Procedures

Electrocauterization is a procedure used in many surgical operations. As a surgeon's scalpel penetrates layers of skin and tissue, numerous tiny blood vessels are cut open. To stop the associated bleeding, an assisting surgeon can seal these vessels immediately using an electrical instrument to burn just enough of the tissue to produce a tiny scar. Electrocauterization is also used to destroy unwanted tissue, such as skin lesions.

Prior to any surgery involving electrocautery, local anesthesia is applied by injection. Electrocauterization is carried out with a small needle probe that is heated with an electrical current. Enough current is applied to heat the probe to temperatures at which blood will coagulate. To prevent electrical shock, a grounding pad is placed on the patient and a small electrode is attached to the skin near the surgery site to direct any excess current away from the body. Depending on the surgery site and the size and shape of unwanted tissue, the cautery pattern may be circular, dotted, or linear. In some applications, a temperature sensor near the electrical probe allows a microprocessor-based control unit to regulate the delivered electrical power as a function of tissue temperature.

Uses and Complications

Electrocauterization is commonly used to destroy unwanted tissue. It has been applied to remove growths in the nasal passage, noncancerous polyps in the colon, canker sores, and lesions on or around the skin, muscles, ligaments, blood vessels, joints, and bones. It is used to stop bleeding during surgery and also when biopsies are performed. It has been used in women to remove abnormal tissue from the cervix and to stop abnormal bleeding from the uterus that is not caused by menstruation.

The healing time after electrocauterization procedures is usually two to three weeks. After electrocautery, a patient may experience pain, swelling, redness, drainage, bleeding, bruising, scarring, or itching at or around the surgery site. Headache, muscle aches, dizziness, fever, tiredness, and a general ill feeling may also occur following electrocauterization. The most serious complication can be the onset of infection. Antibiotics are typically administered if this occurs. Acetaminophen is used to diminish pain.

Excessive electrocautery can produce superficial to deep burns, which can be treated with cold packs. Electrocauterization of the cervix may lead to the misinterpretation of future Pap tests. When electrocauterization is performed multiple times to stop the occurrence of frequent nosebleeds, scar tissue can build up in the nose, leading to increased nosebleeds because of the lack of elasticity of scar tissue.

—*Alvin K. Benson, Ph.D.*

See also Biopsy; Bleeding; Blood vessels; Canker sores; Cervical procedures; Colorectal polyp removal; Cryosurgery; Dermatology; Dermatopathology; Genital disorders, female; Healing; Laser use in surgery; Lesions; Nosebleeds; Skin; Skin disorders; Skin lesion removal; Surgery, general; Surgical procedures; Tumor removal; Tumors.

For Further Information:

Bland, Kirby I., ed. *The Practice of General Surgery.* Philadelphia: W. B. Saunders, 2002.

Brunicardi, F. Charles, et al., eds. *Schwartz's Manual of Surgery.* 8th ed. New York: McGraw-Hill Medical, 2006.

Dagtekin, Ahmet, et al. "Comparison of the Effects of Different Electrocautery Applications to Peripheral Nerves: An Experimental Study." *Acta Neurochirurgica* 153, no. 10 (October 2011): 2031–39.

Morreale, Barbara, David L. Roseman, and Albert K. Straus. *Inside General Surgery: An Illustrated Guide.* New Brunswick, N.J.: Johnson & Johnson, 1991.

Ohtsuka, Takashi, et al. "Dissection of Lung Parenchyma Using Electrocautery is a Safe and Acceptable Method for Anatomical Sublobar Resection." *Journal of Cardiothoracic Surgery* 7, no. 1 (2012): 42–45.

Peter, Neena M., Pura Ribes, and Ramona Khooshabeh. "Cardiac Pacemakers and Electrocautery in Ophthalmic Surgery." *Orbit* 31, no. 6 (December 2012): 408–11.

Pollack, Sheldon V. *Electrosurgery of the Skin.* New York: Churchill Livingstone, 1991.

ELECTROENCEPHALOGRAPHY (EEG)

Procedure

Anatomy or system affected: Brain, head, nervous system, psychic-emotional system

Specialties and related fields: Biotechnology, critical care, emergency medicine, neurology, pathology, psychiatry, psychology, speech pathology

Definition: The tracing of the electrical potentials produced by brain cells on a graphic chart, as detected by electrodes placed on the scalp.

Key terms:

brain stem: the medulla oblongata, pons, and mesencephalon portions of the brain, which perform motor, sensory, and reflex functions and contain the corticospinal and reticulospinal tracts

cerebrum: the largest and uppermost section of the brain, which integrates memory, speech, writing, and emotional responses

epilepsy: uncontrollable excessive activity in either all or part of the central nervous system

lesion: a visible local tissue abnormality such as a wound, sore, rash, or boil which can be benign, cancerous, gross, occult, or primary

neurological: dealing with the nervous system and its disorders

seizure: a sudden, violent, and involuntary contraction of a group of muscles; may be paroxysmal and episodic

Indications and Procedures

Clinical electroencephalography (EEG) uses from eight to sixteen pairs of electrodes called derivations. The "international 10-20" system of electrode placement provides coverage of the scalp at standard locations denoted by the letters F (frontal), C (central), P (parietal), T (temporal), and O (occipital). Subscripts of odd for left-sided placement, even for right-sided placements, and z for midline placement further define electrode location. During the procedure, the patient remains quiet, with eyes closed, and refrains from talking or moving. In some circumstances, however, prescribed activities such as hyperventilation may be requested. An EEG test is used to diagnose seizure disorders, brain-stem disorders, focal lesions, and impaired consciousness.

Electrical potentials caused by normal brain activity have atypical amplitudes of 30 to 100 millivolts and irregular, wavelike variations in time. The main generators of the EEG are probably postsynaptic potentials, with the largest contribution arising from pyramidal cells in the third cortical layer. The ongoing rhythms on an EEG background recording are classified according to the frequencies that they produce as delta (less than 3.5 hertz), theta (4.0 to 7.5 hertz), alpha (8.0 to 13.0 hertz), and beta (greater than 13.5 hertz). In awake but relaxed normal adults, the background consists primarily of alpha activity in occipital and parietal areas and beta activity in central and frontal areas. Variations in this activity can occur as a function of behavioral state and aging. Alpha waves disappear during sleep and are replaced by synchronous beta waves of higher frequency but lower voltage. Theta waves can occur during emotional stress, particularly during extreme disappointment and frustration. Delta waves occur in deep sleep and infancy and with serious organic brain disease.

Uses and Complications

During neurosurgery, electrodes can be applied directly to the surface of the brain (intracranial EEG) or placed within brain tissue (depth EEG) to detect lesions or tumors. Electrical activity of the cerebrum is detected through the skull in the same way that the electrical activity originating in the heart is detected by an electrocardiogram (ECG or EKG) through the chest wall. The amplitude of the EEG, however, is much smaller than that of the ECG because the EEG is generated by

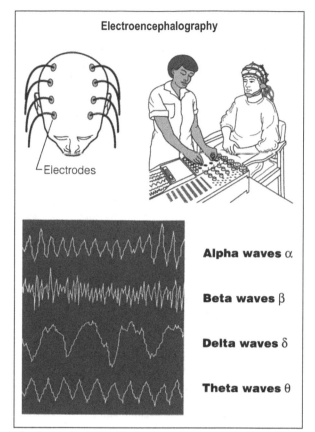

Electroencephalography

Electrodes

Alpha waves α

Beta waves β

Delta waves δ

Theta waves θ

The electrical activity of the brain can be measured with an electroencephalograph (EEG) machine; characteristic patterns can be used to diagnose some brain disorders and to determine levels of consciousness.

cells that are not synchronously activated and are not geometrically aligned, whereas the ECG is generated by cells that are synchronously activated and aligned. Variations in brain wave activity correlate with neurological conditions such as epilepsy, abnormal psychopathological states, and level of consciousness such as during different stages of sleep.

The two general categories of EEG abnormalities are alterations in background activity and paroxysmal activity. An EEG background with global abnormalities indicates diffuse brain dysfunction associated with developmental delay, metabolic disturbances, infections, and degenerative diseases. EEG background abnormalities are generally not specific enough to establish a diagnosis—for example, the "burst-suppression" pattern may indicate severe anoxic brain injury as well as a coma induced by barbiturates. Some disorders do have characteristic EEG features: An excess of beta activity suggests intoxication, whereas triphasic slow waves are typical of metabolic encephalopathies, particularly as a result of hepatic or renal dysfunction. Psychiatric illness is generally not associated with prominent EEG changes. Therefore, a normal EEG helps to distinguish psychogenic unresponsiveness from neurologic disease. EEG silence is an adjunctive test in the determination of brain death, but it is not a definitive one because it may be produced by reversible conditions such as hypothermia. Focal or lateralized EEG abnormalities in the background imply similarly localized disturbances in brain function and thus suggest the presence of lesions.

Paroxysmal EEG activity consisting of spikes and sharp waves reflects the pathologic synchronization of neurons. The location and character of paroxysmal activity in epileptic patients help clarify the disorder, guide rational anticonvulsant therapy, and assist in determining a prognosis. The diagnostic value of an EEG is often enhanced by activation procedures, such as hyperventilation, photic (light) stimulation, and prolonged ambulatory monitoring, or by using special recording sites, such as nasopharyngeal leads, anterior temporal leads, and surgically placed subdural and depth electrodes. During a seizure, paroxysmal EEG activity replaces normal background activity and becomes continuous and rhythmic. In partial seizures, paroxysmal activity begins in one brain region and spreads to uninvolved regions.

Perspective and Prospects

One of the most important uses of EEGs has been to diagnose certain types of epilepsy and to pinpoint the area in the brain causing the disturbance. Epilepsy is characterized by uncontrollable excessive activity in either all or part of the central nervous system and is classified into three types: grand mal epilepsy, petit mal epilepsy, and focal epilepsy. Additionally, EEGs are often used to localize tumors or other space-occupying lesions in the brain. Such abnormalities may be so large as to cause a complete or partial block in electrical activity in a certain portion of the cerebral cortex, resulting in reduced voltage. More frequently, however, a tumor compresses the surrounding nervous tissue and thereby causes abnormal electrical excitation in these areas.

Some researchers predict new uses of EEG technology in the future, although many of these applications appear dubious. Attempts to interpret thought patterns so that an EEG could serve as a lie detector or measurement of intellectual ability, for example, have proven unsuccessful.

—*Daniel G. Graetzer, Ph.D.*

See also Brain; Brain damage; Brain disorders; Brain tumors; Critical care; Critical care, pediatric; Diagnosis; Emergency medicine; Epilepsy; Headaches; Neuroimaging; Neurology; Neurology, pediatric; Neurosurgery; Positron emission tomography (PET) scanning; Seizures; Tumor removal; Tumors.

For Further Information:

Daube, Jasper R., ed. *Clinical Neurophysiology*. 3d ed. New York: Oxford University Press, 2009.

Ebersole, John S., and Timothy A. Pedley, eds. *Current Practice of Clinical Electroencephalography*. 3d ed. Philadelphia: Lippincott Williams & Wilkins, 2003.

Evans, James R., and Andrew Abarbanel, eds. *Introduction to Quantitative EEG and Neurofeedback*. San Diego, Calif.: Academic Press, 2004.

Hayakawa, Fumio, et al. "Determination of Timing of Brain Injury in Preterm Infants with Periventricular Leukomalacia with Serial Neonatal Electroencephalography." *Pediatrics* 104, no. 5 (November, 1999): 1077–1081.

Health Library. "Electroencephalogram." *Health Library*, May 21, 2013.

Jasmin, Luc. "EEG." *MedlinePlus*, February 16, 2012.

Mayo Clinic. "EEG (Electroencephalogram)." *Mayo Clinic*, May 19, 2011.

Powledge, Tabitha M. "Unlocking the Secrets of the Brain: Part II." *Bioscience* 47, no. 7 (July/August, 1997): 403–408.

Ricker, Joseph H., and Ross D. Zafonte. "Functional Neuroimaging and Quantitative Electroencephalography in Adult Traumatic Head Injury: Clinical Applications and Interpretive Cautions." *Journal of Head Trauma Rehabilitation* 15, no. 2 (April, 2000): 859.

ELECTROLYTES. *See* FLUIDS AND ELECTROLYTES.

ELECTROMYOGRAPHY

Procedure

Anatomy or system affected: Muscles, nerves, nervous system
Specialties and related fields: Neurology, physical therapy
Definition: A procedure used to evaluate the electrical activity of nerves when muscles are both contracting and at rest.

Key terms:

carpal tunnel syndrome: excessive compression of the median nerve located in the wrist that leads to irritation and eventually nerve damage

muscle: tissue that provides power to help the body function

myasthenia gravis: a disorder in which the nicotinic acetylcholine receptors located in junctions between nerve cells and muscles are attacked by the immune system, causing exhaustion of the muscles

nerve: a bundle of fibers that can transmit sensory and motor information among body parts

nerve compression: excessive pressure causing a nerve to be pinched

sciatica: pain related to the sciatic nerve; a herniated disc in the lower back can cause this pain, as well as several other types of inflammation

Indications and Procedures

The term "electromyography" originated in 1890, but the process of measuring and recording the electrical signals conducted by nerves as muscles move was first studied as early as the seventeenth century by such scientists as Francesco Redi, Luigi Galvani, and Emil duBois-Reymond. It was not until 1922 that an oscilloscope, which looks like a small television set, was used to show these electrical signals on a screen, making visual monitoring possible. In the 1960s, electromyography (EMG) began to be used in medical clinics and doctors" offices to diagnose muscular and nerve injuries and disorders, such as carpal tunnel syndrome.

Today, the electrical activity measured by EMG is displayed on a computer monitor and can also be printed out or recorded as an electromyogram. The results can also be heard through an audio speaker. This electrical activity can be recorded because an electrode detects any electrical activity of the muscles. When a patient does not move the muscle, no signal is detected, but when a patient contracts a muscle by

In the News:
Wireless EMG Applied to Studies Involving Backpacks and Text Messages

A portable surface electromyography (EMG) device has been developed by researchers at Johns Hopkins University and also by Portuguese investigator Joao Eduardo Castro Ribeiro. According to the September, 2004, issue of *Engineering in Medicine and Biology*, this portable EMG uses a wireless acquisition module to measure electric potentials of the muscles in the vertebral column. These muscles are subjected to a large amount of stress from heavy backpacks. Children carrying these heavy backpacks can develop scoliosis and lordosis because the weight of these backpacks can cause muscles to be affected by an altered center of gravity for the body, thus exerting unnecessary pressure on the vertebrae. The wireless acquisition module of the EMG uses two 1.5 volt class AA batteries to monitor the impact of heavy backpacks on children.

Another application of this EMG technology is the measurement of hand-applied forces important for training and rehabilitation. Muscle contractions in the upper arm and forearm when gripping an object by using the hands produce biopotentials that generate voltage. These voltage readings of a patient are then compared to the normal pull and clenching force readings of a person in a variety of movements.

Ergonomist Ewa Gustafsson at the Sahlgrenska Academy has applied this EMG technology to study the thumb movements of fifty-six young adults while typing messages on cell phones. The results of her study, reported in June, 2009, indicate that nearly 50 percent of the young people studied experienced pain in the neck, arm, and hand after typing messages on the keypads of their mobile phones because of the use of one thumb instead of both thumbs. Subjects who used both thumbs did not experience pain in these areas. Additional differences were also measured by the EMG, thus confirming Gustafsson's hypothesis regarding the improper use of just one thumb to type text messages.

—Jeanne L. Kuhler, Ph.D.

raising a leg or finger, then the nerve cells produce a smooth, wavy line. The exact size and shape of this wave form shown on the computer monitor gives information about the specific muscle's response to the nerve cells. This wave form is called the action potential. The EMG technician may also use a small electrical stimulus to cause a specific muscle to twitch, and this twitching produces an action potential that can be measured and recorded using electromyography as well.

Uses and Complications

The EMG is very safe, and most patients find that only the insertion of the needles or pins and the mild electrical voltage are somewhat uncomfortable. Any bruises heal within a few days. Very little preparation is required, but a patient does need to follow some guidelines to prevent complications. Cream and lotion should not be used before the EMG test, and smoking as well as caffeine-containing drinks and foods should be avoided for at least three hours prior to the test to avoid inaccurate results. A patient should also avoid taking any muscle relaxant medications such as anticholinergics for at least three to six days prior to the EMG testing. A pacemaker could also cause complications.

Other tests performed along with EMG include the nerve conduction velocity test, often abbreviated as the nerve conduction test. It can also be completed by the same EMG technician in the same location but does not require any needles or

small pins. Instead, small electrodes can be taped to the skin, and as the name implies, the nerve conduction velocity test can measure the speed of electrical signals, thus allowing additional disorders that affect the peripheral nervous system to be diagnosed, such as post-polio syndrome, which can develop even years after a human has suffered from polio. An EMG cannot evaluate brain or spinal cord diseases. Thus an EMG and a nerve conduction test are often completed together to more completely diagnose a range of disorders, such as carpal tunnel syndrome, sciatica (nerve root injury), muscular dystrophy, myasthenia gravis, ruptured spinal disks, spinal cord injuries, and various other nerve disorders.

Perspective and Prospects

EMG has evolved extensively since the observation by Redi in the year 1666 that the muscle of an electric ray fish could produce electricity. It only takes thirty to sixty minutes for an EMG to record the data. Because the waves can be transmitted through a loudspeaker as well, a patient's physician can instantly hear them broadcast from a speaker, or recorded on a video that the physician can see instantly.

There is no risk of infection from an EMG because the needles used are sterile and the electrical pulse is of very low voltage and is used for less than a second. Once the testing has been completed, the EMG technician removes the electrodes and cleans the patient's skin. Some patients may experience bruising or tenderness of the muscles for a few days, but this minor discomfort should disappear within a week.

Research continues to expand the useful scope of conditions that can be diagnosed using EMG. Urination problems can now be diagnosed by recording the electrical signals of the external urinary sphincter, which is a group of muscles that surround the urethra. Also, myasthenia gravis can be diagnosed by using a special type of single fiber EMG that is able to monitor the contraction of a single fiber contraction.

—Jeanne L. Kuhler, Ph.D.

See also Carpal tunnel syndrome; Electroencephalography (EEG); Motor neuron diseases; Muscle sprains, spasms, and disorders; Muscles; Nervous system; Neuralgia, neuritis, and neuropathy; Neurology; Neurology, pediatric; Poliomyelitis.

For Further Information:

Chernecky, C., and B. Berger. *Laboratory Tests and Diagnostic Procedures*. 4th ed. Philadelphia: Saunders, 2004.
"Electromyography." *MedlinePlus*, August 27, 2010.
"Electromyography (EMG)." *Health Library*, September 26, 2011.
"Electromyography (EMG)." *Mayo Clinic*, March 7, 2013.
Fischbach, F., and M. Dunning. *Manual of Laboratory and Diagnostic Tests*. 7th ed. Philadelphia: Lippincott Williams & Wilkins, 2004.

Pagana, K., and T. Pagana. *Mosby's Manual of Diagnostic and Laboratory Tests*. 3d ed. St. Louis: Mosby/Elsevier, 2006.

ELEPHANTIASIS

Disease/Disorder
Also known as: Bancroft's filariasis
Anatomy or system affected: Lymphatic system
Specialties and related fields: Environmental health, epidemiology, public health
Definition: A grossly disfiguring disease caused by a roundworm parasite; it is the advanced stage of the disease Bancroft's filariasis, contracted through roundworms.

Key terms:

acute disease: a disease in which symptoms develop rapidly and which runs its course quickly

chronic disease: a disease that develops more slowly than an acute disease and persists for a long time

host: any organism on or in which another organism (called a parasite) lives, usually for the purpose of nourishment or protection

inflammation: a response of the body to tissue damage caused by injury or infection and characterized by redness, pain, heat, and swelling

lymph nodes: globular structures located along the routes of the lymphatic vessels that filter microorganisms from the lymph

lymphatic system: a body system consisting of lymphatic vessels and lymph nodes that transports lymph through body tissues and organs; closely associated with the cardiovascular system

lymphatic vessels: vessels that form a system for returning lymph to the bloodstream

parasite: an organism that lives on or within another organism, called the host, from which it derives sustenance or protection at the host's expense

Causes and Symptoms

Elephantiasis is characterized by gross enlargement of a body part caused by the accumulation of fluid and connective tissue. It most frequently affects the legs but may also occur in the arms, breasts, scrotum, vulva, or any other body part. The disease starts with the slight enlargement of one leg or arm (or other body part). The limb increases in size with recurrent attacks of fever. Gradually, the affected part swells, and the swelling, which is soft at first, becomes hard following the growth of connective tissue in the area. In addition, the skin over the swollen area changes so that it becomes coarse and thickened, looking almost like elephant hide. The elephant-like skin, along with the enlarged body parts, gave the disease the name elephantiasis.

Elephantiasis is found worldwide, mostly in the tropics and subtropics. About 90 percent of cases of elephantiasis are a result of infection with a parasitic worm called *Wuchereria bancrofti* (*W. bancrofti*). *W. bancrofti* belongs to a group of worms called filaria, or roundworms, and infection with a filarial worm is called filariasis. Filariasis caused by *W.*

Information on Elephantiasis

Causes: Infection from roundworm parasite
Symptoms: Recurrent fever, inflammation of lymph vessels, swollen and painful lymph nodes, possible gross enlargement of body part
Duration: Acute to chronic
Treatments: Bed rest, supportive measures (e.g., hot and cold compresses to reduce swelling), drug diethylcarbamazine (DEC)

---

bancrofti is the most common and widespread type of human filarial infection and is often called Bancroft's filariasis; filarial infections that can cause elephantiasis are known in general as lymphatic filariasis. Elephantiasis is the advanced, chronic stage of lymphatic filariasis, and only a small percentage of persons with the infection will develop elephantiasis. During Bancroft's filariasis, adult forms of *W. bancrofti* live inside the human lymphatic system, and it is the person's reaction to the presence of the worm that causes the symptoms of the disease. The worm's life cycle is important in understanding how the disease is transmitted from one person to another, how the symptoms develop, and how to prevent and reduce the incidence of the disease.

The adult worms live in human lymphatic vessels and lymph nodes and measure about 4 centimeters in length for the male and 9 centimeters in length for the female. Both are threadlike and about 0.3 millimeters in diameter. After mating, the female releases large numbers of embryos or microfilariae (microscopic roundworms), which are more than one hundred times smaller in length and ten times thinner than their parents. They make their way from the lymphatic system into the bloodstream, where they can circulate for two years or longer. Interestingly, most strains of microfilariae exhibit a nocturnal periodicity, in which they appear in the peripheral blood system (the outer blood vessels, such as those in the arms, legs, and skin) only at night, mostly between the hours of 10 p.m. and 2 a.m., and spend the remainder of the time in the blood vessels of the lungs and other internal organs. This nighttime cycling into the peripheral blood is somehow related to the patient's sleeping habits, and although it is unknown exactly how or why the microfilariae do this, it is necessary for the survival of the worms. The microfilariae must develop through at least three different stages (called the first, second, and third larval stages) before they are ready to mature into adults; these stages take place not within humans but within certain types of mosquitoes, which bite at night. Thus, the microfilariae appear in the peripheral blood just in time for the mosquitoes to bite an infected human and extract them so that they can continue their life cycle. It is important to note, therefore, that both humans and the proper type of mosquito are needed to keep a filariasis infection going in a particular area.

Female night-feeding mosquitoes of the genera *Culex*, *Aedes*, and *Anopheles* serve as intermediate hosts for *Wuchereria bancrofti*. The mosquitoes bite an infected person and ingest microfilariae from the peripheral blood. The microfilariae pass into the intestines of the mosquito, invade the intestinal wall, and within a day find their way to the thoracic muscles (the muscles in the middle part of the mosquito's body). There they develop from first-stage to third-stage larvae in about two weeks, and the new third-stage larvae move from the thoracic muscles to the head and mouth of the mosquito. Only the third-stage larvae are able to infect humans successfully, and the third stage can mature only inside humans. When the mosquito takes a blood meal, infective larvae make their way through the proboscis (the tubular sucking organ with which a mosquito bites a person) and enter the skin through the puncture wound. After they enter the skin, the larvae move by an unknown route to the lymphatic system, where they develop into adult worms. It takes about one year or longer for the larvae to grow into adults, mate, and produce more microfilariae.

A person contracts Bancroft's filariasis by being bitten by an infected mosquito. Various forms of the disease can occur, depending on the person's immune response and the number of times the person is bitten. The period of time from when a person is first infected with larvae to the time microfilariae appear in the blood can be between one and two years. Even after this time some persons, especially young people, show no symptoms at all, yet they may have numerous microfilariae in their blood. This period of being a carrier of microfilariae without showing any signs of disease may last several years, and such carriers act as reservoirs for infecting the mosquito population.

In those patients showing symptoms from the infection, there are two stages of the disease: acute and chronic. In acute disease, the most common symptoms are a recurrent fever and lymphangitis or lymphadenitis in the arms, legs, or genitals. These symptoms are caused by an inflammatory response to the adult worms trapped inside the lymphatic system. Lymphangitis, an inflammation of the lymph vessels, is characterized by a hard, cordlike swelling or a red superficial streak that is tender and painful. Lymphadenitis is characterized by swollen and painful lymph nodes. The attacks of fever and lymphangitis or lymphadenitis recur at irregular intervals and may last from three weeks up to three months. The attacks usually become less frequent as the disease becomes more chronic. In the absence of reinfection, there is usually a steady improvement in the victim, each relapse being milder. Thus, without specific therapy, this condition is self-limiting and presumably will not become chronic in those acquiring the infection during a brief visit to an area where the disease is endemic.

The most obvious symptoms caused as a result of *W. bancrofti* infection, such as elephantiasis, are noted in the chronic stage. Chronic disease occurs only after years of repeated infection with the worms. It is seen only in areas where the disease is endemic and only occurs in a small percentage of the infected population. The symptoms are the result of an accumulation of damage caused by inflammatory reactions to the adult worms. The inflammation causes tissue death and a buildup of scar tissue that eventually results in the blockage

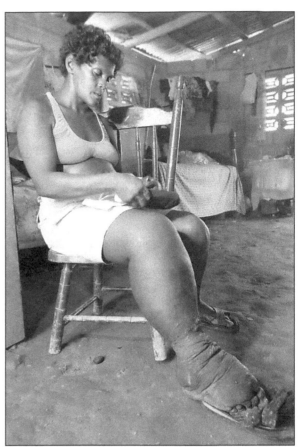

A woman in the Dominican Republic whose leg and foot have become crippled with elephantiasis, which affects many people in developing countries. (AP/Wide World Photos)

of the lymphatic vessels in which the worms live. One of the functions of lymphatic vessels is to carry excess fluid away from tissues and bring it back to the blood, where it enters the circulation again as the fluid portion of the blood. If the lymphatic vessels are blocked, the excess fluid stays in the tissues, and swelling occurs. When this swelling is extensive, grotesque enlargement of that part of the body occurs.

Treatment and Therapy

One way in which doctors can tell whether a person has Bancroft's filariasis is by taking a sample of peripheral blood at night and looking at the blood under a microscope to try to find microfilariae. Sometimes, the ability to find microfilariae is enhanced by filtering the blood to concentrate the possible microfilariae in a smaller volume of liquid. Many persons infected with *W. bancrofti* have no detectable microfilariae in their blood, so other methods are available. In the absence of microfilariae, a diagnosis can be made on the basis of a history of exposure, symptoms of the disease, positive antibody or skin tests, or the presence of worms in a sample of lymph tissue. It is important to note that in addition to *W. bancrofti*, a few other filarial worms and at least one bacteria can also cause elephantiasis; therefore, if symptoms of elephantiasis are observed, it is important to discover the correct cause so that the proper treatment can be given. Since chronic infection occurs after prolonged residence in areas where the disease occurs, patients with acute disease should be removed from those areas. They also should be reassured that elephantiasis is a rare complication that is limited to persons who have had constant exposure to infected mosquitoes for years. The best way to avoid contracting filariasis when traveling to an affected area is to avoid being bitten by mosquitoes. Insect repellent, mosquito netting, and other methods are helpful in this regard.

The World Health Organization (WHO) recommends treating lymphatic filariasis through mass drug administration to at-risk populations. The preferred regimen consists of a single dose of two combined drugs: albendazole and either ivermectin or diethylcarbamazine citrate (DEC). These drugs kill the parasites with the body. Generally, in the treatment of acute disease, excellent results are obtained when the proper dosages of the drugs are given. Side effects include nausea or vomiting, usually relatively mild, and fever and dizziness, the severity of which depends on the number of microfilariae a person has in his or her blood; the more microfilariae, the more severe the reaction. Other drugs have been used in the treatment of filariasis, including suramin, metrifonate, and levamisole, but they are generally less effective or more toxic than the WHO's recommended regimen. Additional treatment measures include bed rest and supportive measures, such as using hot and cold compresses to reduce swelling. The administration of antibiotics for patients with secondary bacterial infections and painkillers as well as anti-inflammatory agents during the painful, acute stage is helpful. Sometimes, swollen limbs can be wrapped in pressure bandages to force the lymph from them. If the distortion is not too great, this method is successful. It should also be noted that although drugs such as DEC, albendazole, and ivermectin might be effective in killing *W. bancrofti*, the chronic lesions resulting from the infection are mostly incurable. Signs of chronic filariasis, such as elephantiasis of the limbs or the scrotum, are usually unaffected or only incompletely cured by medication, and it sometimes becomes necessary to apply surgical or other symptomatic treatments to relieve the suffering of the patients. Chronic obstruction in less advanced stages is sometimes improved by surgery. The surgical removal of an elephantoid breast, vulva, or scrotum is sometimes necessary.

Theoretically, it should be possible first to control and eventually to eliminate Bancroft's filariasis. Conditions that are highly favorable for continued propagation of the infection include a pool of microfilariae carriers in the human population and the right species of mosquitoes breeding near human habitations. Thus, control can be effected by treating all microfilariae carriers in an affected area and eliminating the necessary mosquitoes. It is important to note that eliminating the mosquitoes alone will not control the disease, especially in tropical areas, since the breeding period and season in which the disease can be transmitted is so extensive. In some

temperate areas, where Bancroft's filariasis used to be endemic, measures that removed the mosquitoes alone aided in the elimination of the disease from that area, since in temperate areas the breeding period and thus the season for transmission is so short. In tropical areas, both drug therapy and mosquito control must be applied in order to control the disease.

The mosquito population can be controlled in four ways. First, general sanitation measures such as draining swamps can be carried out in order to reduce the areas where the mosquitoes are breeding. Second, insecticides can be used to kill the adult mosquitoes. Third, larvacides can be applied to sources of water where mosquitoes breed in order to kill the mosquito larvae. Finally, natural mosquito predators, such as certain species of fish, can be introduced into waters where mosquitoes breed to eat the mosquito larvae. Numerous problems stand in the way of eradication, such as poor sanitation, persons who do not cooperate with medical intervention, mosquitoes that become resistant to all known insecticides, increasing technology that yields increasing water supplies and therefore places for mosquitoes to breed, large populations, ignorance of the cause of the disease, and lack of medicine and distribution channels.

Perspective and Prospects

Dramatic symptoms of elephantiasis, especially the enormous swelling of legs or the scrotum, were recorded in much of the ancient medical literature of India, Persia, and the Far East. The embryonic form of microfilariae was first discovered and described in Paris in 1863. The organism was named for O. Wucherer, who also discovered microfilariae in 1866, and Joseph Bancroft, who discovered the adult worm in 1876. Two important facts about *W. bancrofti*—namely, its development in mosquitoes and the nocturnal periodicity of the microfilariae—were discovered by Patrick Manson between 1877 and 1879. This was the first example of a disease being transmitted by a mosquito, and its discovery earned for Manson the title of founder of tropical medicine. These and most of the other essential facts of the disease were discovered before the end of the nineteenth century. Progress in the epidemiology and control of filariasis came after World War II. In 1947, DEC was shown to kill filariae in animals, and this result was followed by the successful use of DEC in the treatment of humans. The first promising results in the control of Bancroft's filariasis by mass administration of DEC were reported in 1957 on a small island in the South Pacific. Through subsequent studies, it has become clear that effective control of the infection can be achieved if sufficient dosages of DEC and related drugs are administered to infected populations.

Filariasis is a serious health hazard and public health problem in many tropical countries. Infection with *W. bancrofti* has been recorded in nearly all countries or territories in the tropical and subtropical zones of the world. The infection occurs primarily in coastal areas and islands that experience long periods of high humidity and heat. Infections have also been noted in some temperate zone districts, such as mainland Japan, central China, and some European countries. In early 2013, the WHO estimated that more than 120 million people worldwide were infected and more than 1.4 billion were at risk

—Vicki J. Isola, Ph.D.

See also Bites and stings; Edema; Inflammation; Insect-borne diseases; Lymphadenopathy and lymphoma; Lymphatic system; Parasitic diseases; Roundworms; Tropical medicine; Worms; Zoonoses.

For Further Information:

Beaver, Paul C., and Rodney C. Jung. *Animal Agents and Vectors of Human Disease*. 5th ed. Philadelphia: Lea & Febiger, 1985.

Biddle, Wayne. *A Field Guide to Germs*. 2d ed. New York: Anchor Books, 2002.

Frank, Steven A. *Immunology and Evolution of Infectious Disease*. Princeton, N.J.: Princeton University Press, 2002.

Global Health, Division of Parasitic Diseases and Malaria. "Lymphatic Filariasis." *Centers for Disease Control and Prevention*, February 1, 2012.

Joklik, Wolfgang K., et al. *Zinsser Microbiology*. 20th ed. Norwalk, Conn.: Appleton and Lange, 1997.

MedlinePlus. "Lymphatic Diseases." *MedlinePlus*, April 23, 2013.

Ransford, Oliver. *"Bid the Sickness Cease.â€□* London: John Murray, 1983.

Roberts, Larry S., and John Janovy, Jr., eds. *Gerald D. Schmidt and Larry S. Roberts" Foundations of Parasitology*. 7th ed. Boston: McGraw-Hill Higher Education, 2005..

Salyers, Abigail A., and Dixie D. Whitt. *Bacterial Pathogenesis: A Molecular Approach*. 2d ed. Washington, D.C.: ASM Press, 2002.

World Health Organization. "Lymphatic Filariasis." *World Health Organization*, March 2013.

EMBOLISM

Disease/Disorder

Anatomy or system affected: Blood vessels, brain, circulatory system, lungs, lymphatic system

Specialties and related fields: Cardiology, internal medicine, neurology, vascular medicine

Definition: A mass of undissolved matter traveling in the blood or lymphatic current.

Causes and Symptoms

An embolism is a mass of undissolved matter traveling in the vascular or lymphatic system. Although an embolism can be solid, liquid, or gaseous, the majority of emboli are solid. Likewise, emboli may consist of air bubbles, bits of tissue, globules of fat, tumor cells, or many other materials. The majority of emboli, however, are blood clots (thrombi) that originate in one portion of the body, break loose and travel, and eventually lodge in another part of the body. Where the traveling blood clot lodges will determine what kind of damage is done.

If the thrombus starts in the veins of the legs, it may break loose, travel up the veins of the leg and abdomen, pass through the right side of the heart, and lodge in the arteries in the lungs. This condition, called a pulmonary embolism, is often fatal. If the embolism is small, it may cause only shortness of breath and chest pain. If it is even smaller, the embolism may produce no symptoms at all.

If a blood clot forms in the chambers of the heart, breaks

Information on Embolism

Causes: Blood clot, air bubble, tissue, fat globules, tumor cells, or other material lodging in part of the body

Symptoms: If in the lung, shortness of breath and chest pain; if in the heart, symptoms of heart attack; if in the brain, symptoms of stroke; if in the leg, pain, cold, numbness

Duration: Acute

Treatments: Depends on system affected; may include blood-thinners (heparin), thrombolytic drugs, bypass surgery

---

loose, and eventually lodges in an artery in the brain, then the patient will experience a stroke. If a clot breaks loose and lodges in an artery in the leg, then the patient will experience pain, coldness, or numbness in that leg. A blood clot that lodges in the coronary arteries, the arteries that feed the heart muscle, may cause a heart attack.

Treatment and Therapy

Treatment will vary depending on what system has been affected by the embolus. If the clot lodges in the lungs, then the patient will likely be placed on a blood-thinning drug such as heparin. In severe cases, thrombolytic drugs, which dissolve clots, may be used. If the clot lodges in a coronary artery, then open-heart surgery may be performed to bypass the occluded artery. If the clot lodges in the leg, a surgeon may remove the clot from the artery. This procedure is possible only when the clot is discovered early, when it has not yet formed a strong attachment to the vessel wall. Another approach to this problem may be to bypass the occluded artery using an artificial artery or a graft.

Perspective and Prospects

The prevention and treatment of emboli are constantly improving. Venous thrombosis, the most common cause of pulmonary emboli, is becoming easier to diagnose thanks to major advances in ultrasound imaging. Also, magnetic resonance imaging (MRI) is being used to make the identification of emboli in the lungs more accurate and safer. Procedures for imaging the chambers of the heart, a common spot where emboli form, are improving as well, making prevention easier.

—Steven R. Talbot, R.V.T.

See also Arteriosclerosis; Blood and blood disorders; Blood vessels; Cholesterol; Circulation; Embolization; Heart; Heart attack; Lungs; Phlebitis; Pulmonary diseases; Pulmonary medicine; Pulmonary medicine, pediatric; Respiration; Strokes; Thrombolytic therapy and TPA; Thrombosis and thrombus; Varicose vein removal; Varicose veins; Vascular medicine; Vascular system.

For Further Information:

A.D.A.M. Medical Encyclopedia. "Blood Clots." *MedlinePlus*, June 5, 2012.

Bick, Roger L. *Disorders of Thrombosis and Hemostasis: Clinical and Laboratory Practice* . 3d ed. Philadelphia: Lippincott

Williams & Wilkins, 2002.

Kroll, Michael H. *Manual of Coagulation Disorders*. Malden, Mass.: Blackwell Science, 2001.

MedlinePlus. "Pulmonary Embolism." *MedlinePlus*, May 16, 2013.

National Center on Birth Defects and Developmental Disabilities, Division of Blood Disorders. "Deep Vein Thrombosis (DVT)/ Pulmonary Embolism (PE)—Blood Clot Forming in a Vein." *Centers for Disease Control and Prevention*, September 25, 2012.

Verstrate, Marc, Valentin Fuster, and Eric Topol, eds. *Cardiovascular Thrombosis: Thrombocardiology and Thromboneurology.* 2d ed. Philadelphia: Lippincott-Raven, 1998.

Virchow, Rudolf L. K. *Thrombosis and Emboli*. Translated by Axel C. Matzdorff and William R. Bell. Canton, Mass.: Science History, 1998.

EMBOLIZATION

Procedure

Also known as: Catheter or coil embolization, endovascular embolization, embolotherapy

Anatomy or system affected: Blood vessels, brain, gastrointestinal system, genitals, liver, uterus

Specialties and related fields: Critical care, emergency medicine, gynecology, oncology, pathology, radiology, vascular medicine

Definition: A procedure used to block specific blood vessels in order to stop blood flow to a certain region—for example, to a tumor—by way of introducing special substances called emboli.

Key terms:

arteriovenous malformation (AVM): a genetic disorder in which the capillary beds that connect the arteries and the veins are abnormal or defective, resulting in malnourishment of tissues, especially in the brain and spinal cord

catheter: a thin tube that is inserted into the groin area and pushed through arteries during embolization procedure

emboli: substances that are released into the blood vessel for the purpose of their occlusion

interventional radiology: the specialty of radiology in which techniques such as X-ray imaging, computed tomography (CT) scans, ultrasounds, or magnetic resonance imaging (MRI) are used for guidance to navigate and introduce catheters or electrodes for various purposes

uterine fibroid embolization (UFE): embolization procedure to stop blood supply for uterine fibroids (benign tumors in the uterus)

varicocele: the condition in which the varicose vein of the scrotum enlarges and causes extreme pain; this condition is also associated with infertility

Indications and Procedures

Embolization is used in a variety of circumstances. In cases such as uterine fibroids, where the tumor is rarely malignant, uterine fibroid embolization (UFE) is preferred over invasive surgery. The procedure stops blood supply to the fibroids, which eventually shrink and disintegrate. In cerebral or brain aneurysms, the cerebral artery inflates or ruptures due to dilations of its wall, resulting in bleeding into the brain or in the space between the brain and the membrane. Embolization of an aneurysm using a platinum coil is performed to block the blood flow to it and to prevent its rupture.

In conditions such as varicocele, embolization is used to occlude the abnormal blood vessel and divert the blood flow from that region. Other cases where this procedure can be used are arteriovenous malformation (AVM), arteriovenous fistula, or hemangiomas, all of which concern abnormalities in blood vessels. When there are a number of small tumors, such as in cases of liver cancer, arterial embolization is the most effective treatment option. In these cases, either the artery is occluded by the embolization procedure or the procedure is used to deliver drugs into the tumors. The latter process is called chemoembolization.

Embolization involves the insertion of a small catheter from the groin area, navigation through the vascular system to the appropriate region, and the delivery of emboli, which block the desired blood vessel. In general, a fluoroscope or an x-ray camera, in combination with a tracking dye or contrasting agent, is used to help the physician guide the movement of emboli and ensure delivery to the correct location. A variety of particles are used as emboli, including polyvinyl alcohol, gelatin-coated microspheres, absolute alcohol, N-butyl-2-cyanoacrylate (NBCA), gelfoam, and platinum coils. These particles are pushed through the catheter and delivered to the affected region under anesthesia. The emboli are delivered by the application of a very small voltage current once the catheter reaches its destination. The procedure is usually performed at the doctor's office by an interventional radiologist, and the patient may be required to stay overnight after the procedure.

Uses and Complications

As with any procedure, there are both advantages and risks associated with embolization. Embolization of uterine fibroids is less invasive and complicated than surgical removal. Damage to blood vessels because of the insertion of the catheter is a possible complication, as is infection of the punctured site. Allergic reactions to the tracking dye are also a risk. Discharge of submucosal fibroids has been observed in a small percentage of women. However, the benefits associated with this procedure outweigh the risks, and therefore UFE has been widely adopted around the world.

Embolization is also used in emergency situations, such as in cases of traumatic hemorrhage, where there is severe blood loss. Embolization provides a viable solution when the problem is in a region that cannot be operated upon, as in the cases of some deep AVMs or tumors that cannot be surgically removed. Coil embolization for brain aneurysms is another commonly used procedure. After the procedure, some patients might experience pain, numbness, or strokelike symptoms. With larger aneurysms, a complete cure is not achieved through this procedure, and the chances of recurrence increase. Sometimes this procedure might have to be followed by surgery.

Perspective and Prospects

Embolization has been practiced since the 1960s, and the

medical field has witnessed many advances in this procedure over the years. Interventional radiology was established by Charles Dotter in the 1960s; though it was originally used in cardiac procedures, it has subsequently been adopted in several other fields. UFE was developed in the 1990s and is now used worldwide with great success. Many different emboli, such as microspheres and platinum coils, have been developed since and have been approved by the Food and Drug Administration (FDA) for use in patients. In a breakthrough development in the treatment of brain aneurysms, detachable coils called Guglielmi coils were developed in the early 1990s and are widely used today. Portal vein embolization, a procedure to shrink a liver affected by cancer before its surgical removal, has gained enormous acceptance in the medical field in recent years.

The embolization procedure is a viable and safe alternative to surgery and is less invasive. Side effects and recurrence rates have been reported to be quite low. Embolization is growing in its applicability in the medical field, and its usefulness is increasing with the advent of new technologies.

—*Geetha Yadav, Ph.D.*

See also Aneurysms; Blood vessels; Embolism; Liver cancer; Testicular surgery; Tumors; Uterus; Vascular medicine; Vascular systems.

For Further Information:

Bradley, L. D. "Uterine Fibroid Embolization: A Viable Alternative to Hysterectomy." *American Journal of Obstetrics and Gynecology* 201, no. 2 (August, 2009): 127–135.

Cooper, Matthew M., et al. "Endovascular Embolization." *MedlinePlus*, February 6, 2013.

Golzarian, Jafar, Sun Shiliang, and Sharfuddin Melhelm, eds. *Vascular Embolotherapy: A Comprehensive Approach.* Vol. 1. New York: Springer, 2006.

Neff, Deanna M., and Rosalyn Carson-DeWitt. "Endovascular Embolization." *Health Library*, June 5, 2012.

Ravina, Jacques. "History of Embolization of Uterine Myoma." In *Uterine Fibroids: Embolization and Other Treatments*, edited by Tulandi Togas. New York: Cambridge University Press, 2003.

EMBRYOLOGY

Specialty

Anatomy or system affected: All

Specialties and related fields: Genetics, neonatology, obstetrics, perinatology

Definition: The study of prenatal development from conception until the moment of birth.

Key terms:

blastocyst: a small, hollow ball of cells which typifies one of the early embryonic stages in humans

cleavage: the process by which the fertilized egg undergoes a series of rapid cell divisions, which results in the formation of a blastocyst

congenital malformation: any anatomical defect present at birth

embryo: the developing human from conception until the end of the eighth week

fetus: the developing human from the end of the eighth week until the moment of birth

neural tube: the embryonic structure that gives rise to the central nervous system

teratogens: substances that induce congenital malformations when embryonic tissues and organs are exposed to them

zygote: the fertilized egg; the first cell of a new organism

Science and Profession

The study of human embryology is the study of human prenatal development. The three stages of development are cleavage (the first week), embryonic development (the second through eighth weeks), and fetal development (the ninth through thirty-eighth weeks).

After an egg is fertilized by sperm in the uterine, or fallopian tube, the resulting zygote begins to divide rapidly. This period of rapid cell division is known as cleavage. By the third day, the zygote has divided into a solid ball containing twelve to sixteen cells. The small ball of cells resembles a mulberry and is called the morula, which is Latin for "mulberry." The morula moves from the uterine tube into the uterus.

The morula develops a central cavity as spaces begin to form between the inner cells. At this stage, the developing human is called a blastocyst. The ring of cells on the outer edge of the hollow ball is called the trophoblast and will form a placenta, while the cluster of cells within becomes the inner cell mass and will form the embryo. By the end of the first week, the surface of the inner cell mass has flattened to form an embryonic disc, and the blastocyst has attached to the lining of the uterus and begun to embed itself.

During the second week of development, the trophoblast makes connections with the uterus into which it has burrowed to form the placenta. Blood vessels from the embryo link it to the placenta through the umbilical cord, through which the embryo receives food and oxygen and releases wastes. Two sacs develop around the embryo: the fluid-filled amniotic sac that surrounds and cushions the embryo and the yolk sac that hangs beneath to provide nourishment. Finally, a large chorionic sac develops around the embryo and the two smaller sacs.

During the third week, the cells of the embryo are arranged in three layers. The outer layer of cells is called the ectoderm, the middle layer is the mesoderm, and the inner layer is the endoderm. The ectoderm gives rise to the epidermis (outer layer) of the skin and to the nervous system; the mesoderm gives rise to blood, bone, cartilage, and muscle; and the endoderm gives rise to body organ linings and glands.

Other significant events of the third week are the development of the primitive streak and notochord. The primitive streak is a thickened line of cells on the embryonic disk indicating the future embryonic axis. Development of the primitive streak stimulates the formation of a supporting rod of tissue beneath it called the notochord. The presence of the notochord triggers the ectoderm in the primitive streak above it to thicken, and the thickened area will give rise to the brain and spinal cord. Later, when vertebrae and muscles develop

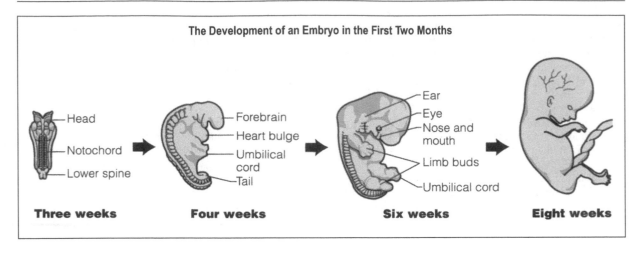

The Development of an Embryo in the First Two Months

Head — Notochord — Lower spine
Three weeks

Forebrain — Heart bulge — Umbilical cord — Tail
Four weeks

Ear — Eye — Nose and mouth — Limb buds — Umbilical cord
Six weeks

Eight weeks

around the neural tissue, the notochord will disappear, leaving the center of the vertebral disk as its remnant.

The important event of the fourth week is the formation of the neural tube. After the thickened neural plate tissue has formed, an upward folding forms a groove, finally closing to form a neural tube. Closure begins at the head end and proceeds backward. The neural tube then sinks beneath surrounding ectodermal surface cells, which will become the skin covering the embryo.

Blocks of mesoderm cells line up along either side of the notochord and neural tube. These blocks are called somites, and eventually forty-two to forty-four pairs will form. They give rise to muscle, the cartilage of the head and trunk, and the inner layer of skin. At the same time, embryonic blood vessels develop on the yolk sac. Because the human embryo is provided little yolk, there is need for the early development of a circulatory system to provide nutrition and gas exchange through the placenta.

The heart is formed and begins to beat in the fourth week, though it is not yet connected to many blood vessels. During the fourth through eighth weeks, all the organ systems develop, and the embryo is especially vulnerable to teratogens (environmental agents that interfere with normal development). A noticeable change in shape is seen during the fourth week because the rapidly increasing number of cells causes a folding under at the edges of the embryonic disk. The flattened disk takes on a cylindrical shape, and the folding process causes curvature of the embryo and it comes to lie on its side in a C-shaped position.

The beginnings of arms and legs are first seen in the fourth week and are called limb buds, appearing first as small bumps. The lower end of the embryo resembles a tail, and the swollen cranial part of the neural tube constricts to form three early sections of the brain. The eyes and ears begin to develop from the early brain tissue.

During the fifth through eighth weeks, the head enlarges as a result of rapid brain development. The head makes up almost half the embryo, and facial features begin to appear. Sexual differences exist but are difficult to detect. Nerves and muscles have developed enough to allow movement. By the

end of the eighth week the limb buds have grown and differentiated into appendages with paddle-shaped hands and feet and short, webbed digits. The tail disappears, and the embryo begins to demonstrate human characteristics. By convention, the embryo is now called a fetus.

The fetal stage of development is the period between the ninth and thirty-eighth weeks, until birth. Organs formed during the embryonic stage grow and differentiate during the fetal stage. The body has the largest growth spurt between the ninth and twentieth weeks, but the greatest weight gain occurs during the last weeks of pregnancy.

In the third month, the difference between the sexes becomes apparent, urine begins to form and is excreted into the amniotic fluid, and the fetus can blink its eyelids. The fetus nearly doubles in length during the fourth month, and the head no longer appears to be so disproportionately large. Ossification of the skeleton begins, and by the end of the fourth month, ovaries are differentiated in the female fetus and already contain many cells destined to become eggs.

During the fifth month, fetal movements are felt by the mother, and the heartbeat can be heard with a stethoscope. Movements until this time usually go unnoticed. The average length of time that elapses between the first movement felt by the mother and delivery is twenty-one weeks.

During the sixth month, weight is gained by the fetus, but it is not until the seventh month that a baby usually can survive premature birth, when the body systems, particularly the lungs, are mature enough to function. During the eighth month, the eyes develop the ability to control the amount of light that enters them. Fat accumulates under the skin and fills in wrinkles. The skin becomes pink and smooth, and the arms and legs may become chubby. In the male fetus, the testes descend into the scrotal sac. Growth slows as birth approaches. The usual gestation length is 266 days, or thirty-eight weeks, after fertilization.

Diagnostic and Treatment Techniques

Knowledge of normal embryonic development is very important both in helping women provide optimal prenatal care for their children and in promoting scientific research for improved prenatal treatment, better understanding of malignant growths, and insight into the aging process.

Environmental stress to the embryo during the fourth through eighth weeks can cause abnormal development and result in congenital malformation, which may be defined as any anatomical defect present at birth. Environmental agents that cause malformations are known as teratogens. Malformations may develop from genetic or environmental factors, but most often they are caused by a combination of the two. Some of the common teratogens are viral infections, drug use, a poor diet, smoking, alcohol consumption, and irradiation.

The genetic makeup of some individuals makes them particularly sensitive to certain agents, while others are resistant. The abnormalities may be immediately apparent at birth or hidden within the body and discovered later. Embryos with severe structural abnormalities often do not survive, and such abnormalities represent an important cause of miscarriages. In fact, up to half of all conceptions spontaneously abort, with little or no notice by the prospective mother.

Genetic birth defects are passed on from one generation to another and result from a gene mutation at some time in the past. Mutations are caused by the accidental rearrangement of deoxyribonucleic acid (DNA), the material of which genes are made, and range in severity from mild to life-threatening. They may cause such conditions as extra fingers and toes, cataracts, dwarfism, albinism, and cystic fibrosis. Gene mutations on a sex chromosome are described as sex-linked and are usually passed from mother to son; these include hemophilia, hydrocephalus (an excessive amount of cerebrospinal fluid), color blindness, and a form of baldness.

Abnormalities in the embryo may result because of an unequal distribution of chromosomes in the formation of eggs or sperm. This imbalance can cause a variety of problems in development, such as Down syndrome and abnormal sexual development. The normal human cell contains twenty-three chromosomes, twenty-two pairs of which are nonsex chromosomes, or autosomes. The last pair consists of the two sex chromosomes. Females normally have two X chromosomes, and males have an X and a Y chromosome.

When females have only one X, a set of conditions known as Turner syndrome results. The embryo will develop as a normal female, though ovaries will not fully form and there may be congenital heart defects. Because the single X chromosome does not cause enough estrogen to be produced, sexual maturity will not occur. If a male embryo should receive only the Y chromosome, it cannot survive. Sometimes a male will receive two (or more) X chromosomes along with a Y chromosome (XXY), producing Klinefelter syndrome. The appearance of the child is normal, but at puberty the breasts may enlarge and the testes will not mature, causing sterility. Males receiving two Y chromosomes (XYY) develop normally, but they may be quite tall and find controlling their impulses to be difficult.

Viral infections in the mother during the embryonic stages can cause problems in organ formation by disturbing normal cell division, fetal vascularization, and the development of the immune system. The organs most vulnerable to infection will be those undergoing rapid cell division and growth at the time of infection. For example, the lens of the eye forms during the sixth week of development, and infection at this time could cause the formation of cataracts.

While most microorganisms cannot pass through the placenta to reach the embryo or fetus, those that can are capable of causing major problems in embryonic development. Rubella, the virus that causes German measles, often causes birth defects in children should infection occur shortly before or during the first three months of pregnancy. The developing ears, eyes, and heart are especially susceptible to damage during this time. When a rubella infection occurs during the first five weeks of pregnancy, interference with organ development is most pronounced. After the fifth week, the risks of infection are not as great, but central nervous system impairment may occur as late as the seventh month.

The most common source of fetal infection may be the cytomegalovirus (CMV), a form of herpes that causes abortion during the first three months of pregnancy. If infection occurs later, the liver and brain are especially vulnerable and impairment in vision, hearing, and mental ability may result. Evidence has also suggested that the immune system of the fetus is adversely affected.

Other viruses may affect fetal development as well. When herpes simplex infects the fetus several weeks before birth, blindness or developmental disabilities may result. Toxoplasma gondii, a parasite of animals often kept as pets, may adversely affect eye and brain development without the mother having known that she had the infection. Syphilis infection in the mother leads to death or serious fetal abnormalities unless it is treated before the sixteenth week of pregnancy; if it is untreated, the fetus may possess hearing impairment, hydrocephalus, facial abnormalities, and developmental disabilities. Women infected with human immunodeficiency virus (HIV) and acquired immunodeficiency syndrome (AIDS) may transmit the virus to their infants before or during birth.

Certain chemicals can cross the placenta and produce malformation of developing tissues and organs. During an embryo's first twenty-five days, damage to the primitive streak can cause malformation in bone, blood, and muscle. While bones and teeth are being formed, they may be adversely affected by antibiotics such as tetracycline.

At one time, thalidomide was widely used as an antinauseant in Great Britain and Germany and to some extent in the United States. Large numbers of congenital abnormalities began to appear in newborns, and the drug was withdrawn from the market after two years. Thalidomide caused the failure of normal limb development and was especially damaging during the third to seventh weeks.

Exposure to other chemicals causes central nervous system disorders when the neural tube fails to close. When the anterior end of the tube does not close, development of the brain and spinal cord will be absent or incomplete and anencephaly results. Babies can live no more than a few days with this condition because the higher control centers of the brain are undeveloped. If the posterior end of the tube fails to close, one or more vertebrae will not develop completely, exposing the spinal cord; this condition is called spina bifida. This condition varies in severity with the level of the defect and the amount of neural tissue that remains exposed, because exposed tissue degenerates.

It has been long believed that neural tube disorders accompany maternal depletion of folic acid, one of the B vitamins, and research has substantiated that relationship. Anencephaly and spina bifida rarely occur in the infants of women taking folic acid supplements. One of the harmful effects of alcohol and anticonvulsants is their depletion of the body's natural folic acid. A decrease in the mother's folic acid levels in the first through third months of pregnancy can cause abortion or growth deformities.

Maternal smoking is strongly implicated in low infant birth weights and higher fetal and infant mortality rates. Cigarette smoke may cause cardiac abnormalities, cleft lip and palate, and a missing brain. Nicotine decreases blood flow to the uterus and interferes with normal development, allowing less oxygen to reach the embryo.

Alcohol use may be the number one cause of birth defects. Exposure of the fetus to alcohol in the blood results in fetal alcohol syndrome. Symptoms may include growth deficiencies, an abnormally small head, facial malformation, and damage to the heart and the nervous and reproductive systems. Behavioral disorders such as hyperactivity, attention deficit, and an inability to relate to others may accompany fetal alcohol syndrome.

Radiation treatments given to pregnant women may cause cell death, chromosomal injury, and growth retardation in the developing embryo. The effect is proportional to the dosage of radiation. Malformations may be visible at birth, or a condition such as leukemia may develop later. Abnormalities caused by radiation include cleft palate, an abnormally small head, developmental disabilities, and spina bifida. Diagnostic X-rays are not believed to emit enough radiation to cause abnormalities in embryonic development, but precautions should be taken.

Oxygen deficiency to the embryo or fetus occurs when mothers use cocaine. Maternal blood pressure fluctuates with the use of this drug, and the embryonic brain is deprived of oxygen, resulting in vision problems, lack of coordination, and developmental disabilities. Too little oxygen to the fetus may also cause death from lung collapse soon after birth.

Obvious physical malformations resulting from embryonic exposure to drugs have been recognized for a number of years, but recent investigators have found that there are more subtle levels of effect that may show up later as behavioral problems. Physical abnormalities have been easily documented, but more attention is needed regarding the behavioral effects caused by teratogens.

Perspective and Prospects

The first recorded observations of a developing embryo were performed on a chick by Hippocrates in the fifth century BCE. In the fourth century BCE, Aristotle wondered whether

a preformed human unfolded in the embryo and enlarged with time, or whether a very simple embryonic structure gradually became more and more complex. This question was debated for nearly two thousand years until the early nineteenth century, when microscopic studies of chick embryos were carefully conducted and described.

Understanding human embryology is foundational for recognizing the relationships that exist between the body systems and congenital malformations in newborns. This field of study takes on new importance in light of advances in modern technology, which have made prenatal diagnosis and treatment a reality.

The study of embryology is also making contributions toward finding the causes of malignant growth. Malignancy is a breakdown in the mechanisms for normal growth and differentiation first seen in the early embryo. Questions about uninhibited malignant growth may be answered by studying embryonic tissues and organs.

The study of old age is another area in which embryological research is valuable. Understanding the clock mechanisms of embryonic cells has led to greater understanding of the "winding down" of cells in old age. It is also important that researchers discover how environmental conditions modify rates of growth and affect the cell's clock. The degree to which the human life span can be expanded remains one of the most challenging questions in the area of aging.

In addition to the health benefits that may be derived from embryological research, this field is an important source of insight into some of the moral and ethical dilemmas facing humankind. Artificial insemination, contraception, and abortion regulations are some of the problems that should require close collaboration between ethicists and scientists, especially embryologists.

—*Katherine H. Houp, Ph.D.;*
updated by Alexander Sandra, M.D.

See also Abortion; Amniocentesis; Assisted reproductive technologies; Birth defects; Brain disorders; Cerebral palsy; Cesarean section; Chorionic villus sampling; Cloning; Conception; Down syndrome; Fetal alcohol syndrome; Fetal surgery; Gamete intrafallopian transfer (GIFT); Genetic counseling; Genetic diseases; Genetics and inheritance; Growth; Gynecology; In vitro fertilization; Miscarriage; Multiple births; Neonatology; Obstetrics; Perinatology; Placenta; Pregnancy and gestation; Premature birth; Reproductive system; Rh factor; Rubella; Sexual differentiation; Spina bifida; Stillbirth; Teratogens; Toxoplasmosis; Ultrasonography; Uterus.

For Further Information:
"Birth Defects." *MedlinePlus*, 23 July 2013.
"Fetal Health and Development." *MedlinePlus*, 23 July 2013.
"How Your Baby Grows During Pregancy." *American College of Obstetricians and Gynecologists*, Aug. 2011.
Mader, Sylvia S. *Inquiry into Life.* 14th ed. New York: McGraw-Hill, 2014.
Marieb, Elaine N. *Essentials of Human Anatomy and Physiology.* 10th ed. San Francisco: Pearson/Benjamin Cummings, 2012.
Moore, Keith L., and T. V. N. Persaud. *The Developing Human.* 9th ed. Philadelphia: Saunders/Elsevier, 2013.
Riley, Edward P., and Charles V. Vorhees, eds. *Handbook of Behavioral Teratology.* New York: Plenum Press, 1986.
Tortora, Gerard J., and Bryan Derrickson. *Principles of Anatomy and*

Physiology. 13th ed. Hoboken, N.J.: John Wiley & Sons, 2012.
Tsiaras, Alexander, and Barry Werth. *From Conception to Birth: A Life Unfolds*. New York: Doubleday, 2002.

EMERGENCY MEDICINE

Specialty

Anatomy or system affected: All

Specialties and related fields: Cardiology, critical care, gastroenterology, geriatrics and gerontology, neurology, nursing, obstetrics, pediatrics, pharmacology, psychiatry, public health, pulmonary medicine, radiology, sports medicine, toxicology

Definition: The care of patients who are experiencing immediate health crises, a field defined by twenty-four-hour availability, the management of multiple patients simultaneously, and the need for broad-based skills and interventions.

Key terms:

diagnostic: relating to the determination of the nature of a disease

emergency medical services: the complete chain of human and physical resources that provides patient care in cases of sudden illness or injury

heuristics: methods used to aid and guide in the discovery of a disease process when incomplete knowledge exists

paramedic: a person trained and certified to provide prehospital emergency medical care

pathologic: pertaining to the study of disease and the development of abnormal conditions

pathophysiology: an alteration in function as seen in disease

patient assessment: the systematic gathering of information in order to determine the nature of a patient's illness

triage: the medical screening of patients to determine their relative priority for treatment

Science and Profession

The field of emergency medicine is defined as care to acutely ill and injured patients, both in the prehospital setting and in the emergency room. It is practiced as patient-demanded and continuously accessible care and is defined by the location of its practice rather than by an anatomical concern. Emergency medicine encompasses all medical specialties and physical systems. The commitment to rapid, prudent intervention under stressful and often chaotic conditions is of paramount importance to the critically ill patient. This branch of medicine is characterized by its complexity of problems, its twenty-four-hour availability to a variety of patients, and its effective and broad-based understanding of disease and injury. These features are used to orchestrate the response of multiple hands with the ultimate goal of referring the patient to ongoing care.

The hourglass is an appropriate symbol of the nature of this medical division. It not only portrays the importance of time and the need for quick intervention, but its shape—wide at either end and narrowing in the middle—also is an appropriate visualization of the pattern of emergency medical treatment. A large number of patients converge on a single area, the emergency room, where they are diagnosed, treated, and eventually released to other appropriate care, diverging on a wide range of follow-up options.

Unique to the field of emergency medicine is the importance of rapid definition and comprehension of the pathophysiology of the critically ill patient. Emergency care physicians must have a unique understanding of the practice of medicine, and the nature of disease and injury, availing themselves of a host of clinical skills needed for the treatment of the variety of physical and psychological problems that require treatment. Emergency rooms are a melting pot of problems; most are medical, many are not. All of them reflect some person's perception of an emergency. Success in the emergency medical field often depends on the ability of personnel to use not only their medical knowledge but also their knowledge of people as well.

Most often those seeking the assistance of emergency medical providers are people suffering from pain of illness or trauma; however, any patient may seek treatment at the emergency room. Often loneliness, disability, or homelessness serves as the motivation to seek treatment. Regardless of what brought the patient, the emergency physician strives to recognize and deal with the patient's "emergency," remembering that not all patients are as ill as they might think and that not all are as well as they might appear. Physicians of this specialty sift through a multitude of information. It is necessary to know the patient's pertinent medical history and the history of the present illness or complaint before appropriate and effective treatment can be prescribed. Patients rarely follow a preconceived plan. Emergency medicine works best, therefore, when its practitioners follow heuristics—that is, incomplete guides that lead to greater knowledge, a holistic approach.

Emergency medicine is primarily a hospital-based specialty; however, it also involves extensive prehospital responsibilities. Many times, patients seeking emergency care are first the responsibility of police, fire, or ambulance personnel. In these situations, the role of emergency medicine must be viewed under the wider context of the emergency medical system. This system—beginning with the first aid administered by bystanders; leading to initial treatment and transportation by trained certified emergency medical technicians, paramedics, or flight nurses; and culminating with care at an emergency room or a highly equipped trauma center—forms a uniquely structured unit. The emergency medical system is designed to provide rapid quality intervention regardless of prehospital conditions. The emergency medical physician is best viewed as a central part of a team whose knowledge and understanding of the whole allow the best possible care to patients undergoing health crises.

Emergency physicians are charged with the responsibility of providing the highest standard of care in the hospital setting. They ensure that both staff members and equipment are maintained at their utmost level of quality. Trends, breakthroughs, and advances are monitored via journals and other medical publications. Training of personnel must keep pace with medical advancement. Developing an overall program depends as much on its planning as its dissemination. The emergency physician often plays the role of teacher, actively influencing the overall quality of the program through education and skills development. Thus, the exercise of emergency medicine is truly a team effort, with all members acting in accordance with their training and level of competence in order to minimize further injury or discomfort.

In practice, emergency medicine encompasses any person or structure involved in the immediate decision making and/or actions necessary to prevent death or further disability of a patient in the midst of a health crisis. It represents a chain of human and physical resources brought together for the purpose of providing total patient care. In this respect, everyone has a part to play in the delivery of emergency care. The bottom line of emergency medicine is the welfare of the patient. Thus, it is most appropriate to view the practice of emergency medicine in the context of the entire emergency medical system.

The components of the emergency medical system include recognition of the emergency, initiation of emergency medical response, treatment at the scene, transport by members of an emergency medical team to the appropriate facility, treatment in the emergency room or trauma center, and release of the patient. These components are only as strong as the weakest link.

Diagnostic and Treatment Techniques

Recognition of an emergency is the first step in emergency care. Often this step is complicated by the patient's own denial and ignorance of basic symptoms. "Emergency" is in part defined by the patient's ability to identify, accept, and respond to a given situation. Regardless of the nature of the illness or injury, the sooner an emergency is defined, the sooner care can be provided. The typical heart attack victim, for example, waits an average of three hours after experiencing symptoms before seeking help. In such cases, treatment by bystanders who have been trained in first aid and cardiopulmonary resuscitation (CPR) has proven effective.

In the United States, the response of emergency medical personnel has been aided by the implementation of the 911 emergency system. Similar systems exist in other countries as well. While not all communities have this capability, its use is increasing. It has been documented that patients who receive treatment at an appropriate facility within sixty minutes of the onset of a life-threatening emergency are more likely to survive. This "golden hour" is precious time.

Operating under protocols developed and approved by the emergency medical director and emergency medical councils of a given locale, emergency medical technicians (EMTs) and paramedics are trained and authorized to deliver care to the patient in need at the scene. EMTs and paramedics are

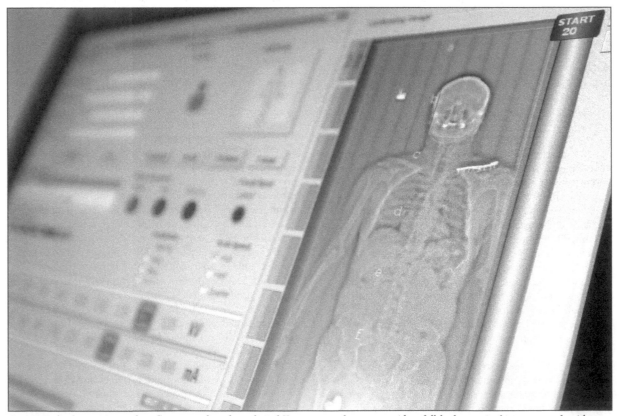

A monitor displays an image from Statscan, a low-dose, digital X-ray system that can provide a full-body scan in thirteen seconds without movement required from the patient. Such technology could prove lifesaving in emergency rooms. (AP/Wide World Photos)

charged with the initial assessment of the patient's condition, immediate stabilization prior to transport, delivery of care as far as their training allows, and the transport of the patient.

Unique to the field of emergency medicine is the special relationship of the paramedic with the doctor. Many people in need of emergency care are first treated outside the hospital. In these cases, emergency caregivers on the scene act as the eyes, ears, and hands of the physician. Through the EMT or paramedic, using telecommunications, an emergency doctor can speed the process of diagnosis. Signs and symptoms relayed through these trained professionals enable a doctor to make an accurate assessment of the patient's condition and to request a variety of treatments for a patient whom they cannot see or touch. Linked by telephone or radio, the medic and doctor can capitalize on the golden hour with the initiation of quality care.

In the United States, paramedics operate under the medical license of a medical command physician who has met all criteria set forth by the US Department of Health and has been approved to provide medical directives to prehospital and interhospital providers. Protocols are the recognized practices that are within the training of the EMT and paramedic. They serve as standard procedures for prehospital treatment. While it is recognized that situations will arise that call for deviation from particular aspects of a given protocol, they are the standards under which the doctor and emergency personnel on the scene operate.

Treatment at the scene is followed by transport with advanced life support by members of the emergency medical system in 85 percent of all emergency cases. This requires much-needed equipment for the further treatment of patients. Deficiencies in the vehicle, equipment, or training of medical personnel can seriously endanger a patient. Thus, government agencies have been designated to grant permission for ambulance services and hospitals to engage in the practice of emergency medicine. This licensure process is designed to demand a level of competency for health care providers and ensure the public's protection.

Since many emergency department admissions do not constitute life-threatening situations, not all facilities stand at the same level of readiness for a given emergency. Transportation to the appropriate facility, therefore, requires a matching of the patient's need to the hospital's capabilities. Hospitals are categorized according to their ability to render emergency intensive care, as well as to provide needed support services on a patient-demand basis. In general, they are viewed as emergency facilities and trauma centers designed

---

In the News:
Exemption from Informed Consent
Requirements for Emergency Research

Informed consent is a patient's competent, voluntary permission to undergo a proposed treatment plan or procedure. To obtain a patient's informed consent, the physician or clinician must provide the patient with sufficient information to assist the patient in making an informed decision. The information provided should include indications for the procedure, any risks, and any available alternatives. The patient should be given an opportunity to ask questions and to deny consent if, after a thorough explanation, the patient feels that denying consent is the best option.

Federally mandated Institutional Review Boards (IRBs) must approve any research involving human subjects, including research in emergency departments. The IRBs aim to protect patients by ensuring that people who participate in research give adequate informed consent. In a medical emergency, however, it is unclear whether consent is sufficiently informed. So that critically ill and injured patients are not denied an opportunity to participate in beneficial research trials, the Food and Drug Administration (FDA) and the U.S. Department of Health and Human Services issued regulations that allow "emergency research" without informed consent. These regulations create an exception to the informed consent requirement when subjects are in a life-threatening situation, when obtaining informed consent is not feasible, when the research offers possible direct therapeutic benefit to the subjects, when the investigation could not be carried out without the waiver, and when additional protections of the rights and welfare of the subjects are provided. Because a waiver of informed consent undermines one of the most significant protections of human subjects, the guidelines attempt to compensate by providing additional precautions, including community consultation, public disclosure, and intensive oversight by an independent data and monitoring committee. The basis for these regulations is the premise that if the proposed research is not harmful, and particularly if it is potentially helpful, most "reasonable" patients would give their consent. Another instance in which consent may be waived involves minimal risk research, provided that the waiver will not adversely affect the rights and welfare of the subjects.

—*Marcia J. Weiss, M.A., J.D.*

---

to provide twenty-four-hour, comprehensive emergency intensive care, including operating rooms and intensive care nurses.

When the patient reaches the emergency facility, during the first five to fifteen minutes of care, many important decisions are made by the physician on duty. The process continues to overlap with needed diagnostic tests and consultations in an effort to provide quality care directed at the source of the illness or injury. The patient's immediate needs are cared for by emergency department staff until the patient is moved to a site of continued care or released to his or her own care.

Questions correctly phrased and sharply directed are effective tools for the rapid diagnosis needed in emergency medicine. The key to this field is the ability to triage, stabilize, prioritize, treat, and refer.

Triage is the system used for categorizing and sorting patients according to the severity of their problems. Emergency practitioners seek to ascertain the nature of the patient's problem and consider any life-threatening consequences of the present condition. This stage of triage allows for immediate care to the more seriously endangered person, relegating the more stable, less seriously ill or wounded patients to a waiting period. The emergency room, in other words, does not operate on a first come, first served basis.

Secondary to triage is stabilization. This term refers to any immediate treatment or intervening steps taken to alleviate conditions that would result in greater pain or defect and/or lead to irreversible or fatal consequences. Primary stabilization steps include ensuring an unobstructed airway and providing adequate ventilation and cardiovascular function.

Once patients have been stabilized, all illnesses must be looked at on the scale of their hierarchical importance. Life-threatening diseases or injuries are treated before more moderate or minor conditions. This system of prioritization can be illustrated from patient to patient: A heart attack victim, for example, is treated prior to the patient with an ankle sprain. It can also be applied for multiple conditions within the same patient. The heart attack victim with a sprained ankle receives treatment first for the life-threatening cardiovascular incident.

Treatment of the critically ill patient often poses a series of further questions. What is the primary disorder? Is there more than one active pathologic process present? How does the patient appear? Is the patient's presentation consistent with the initial diagnosis? Is a hospital stay warranted? What consultations are needed to diagnose and treat this patient?

The emergency physician's approach is to consider the most serious disease consistent with the patient's presentation and chief complaint. By rule of thumb, thinking the worst and hoping for the best is often the psychological stance of the emergency care provider. Only when more severe conditions have been ruled out are more minor processes considered. Often too, this broad view of patient assessment allows for multiple diagnoses. Through continued probing, alternate and additional conditions are often uncovered. It is not unlikely that the patient who seeks treatment for a head injury after a fall is diagnosed with a more serious condition that caused the fall. Focusing only on the immediate condition would endanger the patient. Success in this medical field therefore demands broad-based medical knowledge and diagnostic tools.

Emergency medicine is not practiced in a vacuum. Its very nature necessitates its interfacing with a variety of medical specialties. The emergency room is often only the first step in patient recovery. Initial diagnosis and stabilization must be coupled with plans for ongoing treatment and evaluation. Consultations and referrals play important roles in the overall care of a patient.

Perspective and Prospects

Historians are unable to document specific systems for emergency patients before the 1790s. The need to provide care to the battlefield wounded is seen as the first implementation of emergency response. Early wartime treatment did not, however, include prehospital treatment. Clara Barton is credited with providing the first professional-level prehospital emergency care for the wounded as part of the American Red Cross. Ambulance services began in major cities of the United States at the beginning of the twentieth century, but it was not until 1960 that the National Academy of Sciences"

National Research Council actually studied the problem of emergency care.

Emergency medicine as a specialty is relatively new. Not until 1975, when the House of Delegates of the American Medical Association defined the emergency physician, did the US medical community even recognize this branch of medicine. In 1981, the American College of Emergency Physicians added further recognition through the development of the definition of emergency medicine. Since then, growth and changes have enabled this field to develop as a major specialty, evolving to accept greater responsibility in both education and practice. The development of emergency medicine and the increasing number of health care providers in this field have since then been dramatic.

Emergency medicine developed at a time when both the general public and the medical community recognized the need for quality accessible care in the emergency situation. It has grown to include a gamut of services provided by a community. In addition to responding to the acutely ill or injured, emergency medicine has grown to accept responsibilities of education, administration, and advocacy.

Included in the role of today's emergency medical providers is the administration of the entire emergency medical system within a community. This system includes the development of public education programs such as CPR instruction, poison control education, and the introduction of the 911 system. Emergency management systems and coordinators are now part of every state and local government. Disaster planning for both natural and human-made accidents also comes under the heading of emergency medicine.

Research, too, plays an important role in emergency medicine. The desire to identify, understand, and disseminate scientific rationale for basic resuscitative interventions, as well as the need to improve preventive medical techniques, are often driving forces in scientific research.

Finally, emergency medicine plays a key role in many of society's problems. Homelessness, drug use and abuse, acquired immunodeficiency syndrome (AIDS), and rising health costs have all contributed to the increase in the number of patients seen in the emergency room. In response, those administering emergency medical care have tried to communicate such problems to the general public and legislative bodies, as well as educate them regarding preventive measures. Being on the front line of medicine brings a special obligation to improve laws and services to ensure public safety and well-being.

—*Mary Beth McGranaghan*

See also Abdominal disorders; Altitude sickness; Amputation; Aneurysms; Antibiotics; Appendectomy; Appendicitis; Asphyxiation; Avian influenza; Biological and chemical weapons; Bites and stings; Bleeding; Botulism; Burns and scalds; Cardiac arrest; Cardiology; Cardiology, pediatric; Cardiopulmonary resuscitation (CPR); Catheterization; Cesarean section; Choking; Coma; Concussion; Critical care; Critical care, pediatric; Drowning; Electrical shock; Electrocardiography (ECG or EKG); Electroencephalography (EEG); Emergency medicine, pediatric; Emergency rooms; First aid; Fracture and dislocation; Fracture repair; Frostbite; Grafts and grafting; Head and neck disorders; Heart attack; Heat exhaustion and heatstroke; Hospitals; Hyperbaric oxygen therapy; Hyperthermia and hypothermia; Intensive care unit (ICU); Intoxication; Intravenous (IV) therapy; Laceration repair; Meningitis; Nursing; Obstetrics; Paramedics; Peritonitis; Pneumonia; Poisoning; Radiation sickness; Resuscitation; Reye's syndrome; Salmonella infection; Shock; Snakebites; Spinal cord disorders; Splenectomy; Sports medicine; Staphylococcal infections; Streptococcal infections; Strokes; Thrombolytic therapy and TPA; Tracheostomy; Transfusion; Unconsciousness; Veterinary medicine; Wounds.

For Further Information:

Bledsoe, Bryan E., Robert S. Porter, and Bruce R. Shade. *Brady Paramedic Emergency Care*. 3d ed. Upper Saddle River, N.J.: Brady/Prentice Hall, 1997.

Caroline, Nancy L. *Emergency Care in the Streets*. 7th ed. Sudbury, Mass.: Jones and Bartlett, 2013.

"Emergency Medical Services." *MedlinePlus*, 6 Aug. 2013.

Hamilton, Glenn C., et al. *Emergency Medicine: An Approach to Clinical Problem-Solving*. 2d ed. New York: W. B. Saunders, 2003.

Heller, Jacob L., and David Zieve. "Recognizing Medical Emergencies." *MedlinePlus*, 5 Jan. 2011.

Limmer, Daniel, et al. *Emergency Care*. 12th ed. Upper Saddle River, N.J.: Pearson Brady, 2012.

Markovchick, Vincent J., and Peter T. Pons, eds. *Emergency Medicine Secrets*. 5th ed. Philadelphia: Mosby/Elsevier, 2011.

Marx, John A., et al., eds. *Rosen's Emergency Medicine: Concepts and Clinical Practice*. 7th ed. Philadelphia: Mosby/Elsevier, 2010.

"Meet the Medical Emergency Team." *Emergency Care for You*. American College of Emergency Physicians, n.d.

Tintinalli, Judith E., ed. *Emergency Medicine: A Comprehensive Study Guide*. 7th ed. New York: McGraw-Hill, 2011.

"When Should I Go to the Emergency Department?" *Emergency Care for You*. American College of Emergency Physicians, n.d.

EMERGENCY ROOMS

Health care system

Also known as: ERs, trauma centers

Anatomy or system affected: All

Specialties and related fields: All

Definition: Sites that provides twenty-four-hour emergency medical care. Metropolitan trauma centers often have more than fifty patient care areas and treat hundreds of patients daily. Rural or community hospital ERs may be as small as several rooms but usually have many treatment areas available.

Key terms:

American Board of Emergency Medicine (ABEM): the agency certifying medical doctors as emergency medicine specialists; sets criteria for training and knowledge to become board certified in emergency medicine

American College of Emergency Physicians (ACEP): supports quality emergency care and promotes the interests of emergency physicians

emergency medicine: one of twenty-four medical specialties recognized by the American Board of Medical Specialties

trauma center: an ER that meets certain criteria for the delivery of emergent care to those suffering severe injuries

triage: from French word meaning "to pick or cull"; in ER triage, health care personnel, usually nurses, make an initial determination regarding the severity of a person's illness

Background

Emergency medicine is one of twenty-four medical specialties recognized by the American Board of Medical Specialties (ABMS). A board-certified specialist in emergency medicine meets training and certification requirements established by the American Board of Emergency Medicine (ABEM). Emergency medicine became a medical specialty in 1979 and is well established as a recognized body of medical specialists and knowledge.

After World War II, emergency rooms became primary health care access points for an increasing number of people. Many factors contributed to this change, including increasing specialization among physicians along with decreasing numbers of primary care and general practitioners. The resultant decrease in hospital on-call physicians available to treat ER patients fostered the concept of full-time ER specialists, whose primary duties involve treating patients coming to ERs.

The first plans for full-time emergency room physician coverage originated in the 1960s. A model featuring dedicated ER doctors proved to be the most attractive among hospitals and patients. Emergency physicians limit their practice to the emergency department while providing 24–7 coverage. Emergency physicians treat all patients, regardless of ability to pay, while establishing contractual relationships with hospitals. This model for emergency care fostered the development of emergency medicine, setting standards of care for the new specialty. (Michael T. Rapp and George Podgorny provide a detailed consideration of the many factors in the developmental history of emergency medicine in their 2005 article "Reflections on Becoming a Specialist and Its Impact on Global Emergency Medical Care: Our Challenge for the Future" in *Emergency Medicine Clinics of North America*.)

The National Academy of Sciences and the National Research Council raised concern with a 1966 report titled *Accidental Death and Disability: The Neglected Disease of Modern Society*. More rapid prehospital response along with better emergency care standards were needed to improve emergency care in the United States. Emergency physicians from Michigan, including John Wiegenstein, founded an organization fostering the national development of Emergency Medicine, the American College of Emergency Physicians (ACEP), in 1968.

Emergency physicians integrate medical care in a variety of settings, including military, disaster, community, and academic settings. Emergency physicians are experts in emergent cardiovascular care, including resuscitative medicine and the various highly specialized procedures that accompany that care. Accident and trauma stabilization is another area of ER expertise. Emergency medicine residency training is three to four years in length. This training occurs after a doctor has completed medical school and undergraduate education. During that time, a well-trained ER doctor becomes proficient in many complex, lifesaving procedures, such as thoracotomies (opening the chest to correct emergent heart and lung problems), pacemaker placement (correcting heart rate and rhythm problems), intubation (allowing airway access), chest tube insertion (draining blood and fluid from the lungs), and lumbar puncture (assessing neurological problems). Rapid recognition, prompt emergent care, and effective triage are emergency medicine physician characteristics.

Emergency physicians treat life-threatening and severe emergent medical problems, such as myocardial infarctions (heart attacks), strokes, drug overdoses, and diabetic ketoacidosis. Traumatic injuries, such as stabbings, shootings, industrial accidents, and automobile accidents, are also treated and stabilized in the emergency department, which is the major care location for disaster care. Emergency physicians treat all age groups and all conditions, at all hours of the day, simultaneously. This ability to treat the variety and breadth of emergent problems stands ER doctors out as the group of specialists best suited to assess and properly treat the greatest number of acutely ill patients.

Features and Procedures

Emergency rooms vary in size, but most share uniform characteristics. The first ER assessment is triage, a term with French roots meaning "to pick or cull." In triage, health care personnel, usually nurses, determine the severity of a patient's injury or illness and record the patient's chief complaint or medical problem. They measure and record vital signs, including pulse, temperature, respiratory rate, and blood pressure. If the patient's condition is stable, then triage personnel obtain other important information, such as medications taken, a brief medical history, and any patient allergies.

The most important triage duty determines the severity of an illness. Usually, there are three main categories: critical and immediately life threatening, such as a myocardial infarction; urgent but not immediately life threatening, such as most abdominal pain; and less urgent, such as a minor leg laceration, known as the "walking wounded" in military triage. ER personnel often refer to these categories as Cat I, Cat II, or Cat III. After assessing the patient's condition, triage personnel advance patients to appropriate care areas. A new category I patient may be wheeled on a gurney directly to the critical area, with the nurse announcing to any doctors on the way, "new Cat I patient in 101." These patients need immediate emergency care.

A stable patient is registered by front-desk personnel. Registration clerks obtain insurance and contact information. New medical charts are generated for new patients, or old records are requested if they already exist at that hospital. Patients arriving by ambulance or critically ill category I patients bypass this step until after treatment or stabilization in the critical care area of the emergency room.

Most emergency departments have many patient care areas, reflecting the wide variety of patients seen in the ER. These areas include resuscitation rooms for patients needing cardiopulmonary resuscitation; trauma care areas for patients with severe injuries like gunshot wounds or accident victims; critical care areas for patients needing cardiac monitoring along with ongoing critical care; pediatric ERs for the care of children; chest-pain evaluation areas; and suture rooms for the repairs of lacerations (cuts). Rooms for the examination of women with gynecological problems are available. ERs usually have a fast track or urgent care area for minor illness (such as sore throats) and an observation unit for patients waiting for hospital admission or diagnostic tests.

Many personnel contribute to the wide variety of care provided in emergency departments. Emergency physicians, nurses, physician assistants, medical technologists, and medical assistants have specified health care roles. Unit clerks help with the paperwork, and laboratory personnel assist with radiological and laboratory procedures. Administrative people help with staffing issues, equipment purchasing, facility maintenance, and scheduling of workers. These are some of the important roles necessary to deliver emergency care. To a varying degree, ERs will also have social workers, psychological care providers, and patient advocates available as fulltime ER personnel.

Perspective and Prospects

Many agencies promote effective, more standardized emergency and trauma care. In addition to the American Board of Emergency Medicine and the American College of Emergency Physicians, many other agencies promote effective emergency care, such as the American Academy of Emergency Medicine. The American Heart Association takes a lead in cardiopulmonary resuscitation (CPR) guidelines. The American College of Surgeons (ACS) develops standards for trauma care. Nursing organizations, emergency medical technician (EMT) agencies, and other professional organizations develop standards for improving emergency care.

The American College of Surgeons provides trauma center designation guidelines. Trauma center designation requires various important resources and characteristics. Although the ACS provides consultants and guidelines for this process, other agencies designate trauma centers, such as local or state governments. Three main trauma center levels exist in ACS guidelines.

In level I, comprehensive 24–7 trauma care specialists are available in the hospital, including emergency medicine, general surgery, and anesthesiology. Various surgical specialists are available, including neurosurgery, orthopedic surgery, and plastic surgery. Level I designation requires intensive care units (ICUs) along with operating rooms staffed and ready to go twenty-four hours daily all year round. These are major referral centers, often known as tertiary care facilities.

Level II offers comprehensive trauma and critical care, but the full array of specialists may not be as readily available as those found in a level I trauma center. Trauma volume levels are usually lower than the level I trauma centers.

In level III, resources are available for critical care and stabilization of trauma victims. Patient volume, array of specialists, and 24–7 availability vary. Transfer protocols with level II and I trauma centers allow comprehensive care after stabilization. Community or rural hospitals may have this designation.

The efforts of all these groups enhance emergency care, in

all of its various forms. Emergency medicine is at the front lines of medical care. Like any forward-moving group, backup and support improve the ultimate goal—available and effective emergency care delivered when needed the most.

—*Richard P. Capriccioso, M.D.*

See also Accidents; Critical care; Emergency medicine; Hospitals; Intensive care unit (ICU).

For Further Information:

American Board of Emergency Medicine, 2013.

American College of Emergency Physicians, 2013.

Arnold J. L. "International Emergency Medicine and the Recent Development of Emergency Medicine Worldwide." *Annals of Emergency Medicine* 33 (1999): 97–103.

"Emergency Medical Services." *MedlinePlus*, 6 Aug. 2013.

"FAQ for Resources for Optimal Care of the Injured Patient: 2006." *American College of Surgeons Trauma Programs*, 5 Oct. 2011.

Heller, Jacob L., and David Zieve. "Recognizing Medical Emergencies." *MedlinePlus*, 5 Jan. 2011.

"Meet the Medical Emergency Team." *Emergency Care for You.* American College of Emergency Physicians, n.d.

National Academy of Sciences and the National Research Council. *Accidental Death and Disability: The Neglected Disease of Modern Society.* Washington, D.C.: Government Printing Office, 1966.

Rapp, Michael T., and George Podgorny. "Reflections on Becoming a Specialist and Its Impact on Global Emergency Medical Care: Our Challenge for the Future." *Emergency Medicine Clinics of North America* 23, no. 1 (February, 2005): 259–269.

"Verified Trauma Centers." *American College of Surgeons Trauma Programs*, 5 Aug. 2013.

"When Should I Go to the Emergency Department?" *Emergency Care for You.* American College of Emergency Physicians, n.d.

EMERGING INFECTIOUS DISEASES

Disease/Disorder

Anatomy or system affected: All

Specialties and related fields: All

Definition: First introduced by Nobel laureate Joshua Lederberg, the phrase "emerging infectious diseases" applies to those diseases that newly appear in a populace or have been in existence for some time but are rapidly increasing in incidence, geographic range, or surface as new drug-resistant strains of viruses, bacteria, or parasitic species.

Key terms:

endemic: a disease that is constantly present in a particular region or country and is usually under control

epidemic: a contagious disease that is prevalent and rapidly spreading in a community

pandemic: rapidly spreading disease over a whole area, country, continent or the globe

vector: an animal, especially an insect, that transmits a pathogenic organism from a host to a noninfected animal

zoonosis: a disease or infection transmitted to humans by vertebrate animals

Background

Throughout history, populations have been afflicted by major outbreaks of emerging infectious diseases such as the bubonic plague or Black Death, a zoonosis caused by the bacterium *Yersinia pestis* that is spread by fleas that feed off rodents. The Black Plague emerged in the fourteenth century, obliterating a third of the European population within a few years. More deadly than *Y. pestis*, however, was the variola virus, the etiologic agent of smallpox, which evolved from poxviruses in cattle and emerged into human populations thousands of years ago. Between the fourteenth and the sixteenth centuries, the Spanish conquered Central America, aided in large part by the deadly smallpox epidemic that arose when the disease, previously unknown in the Americas, entered the indigenous populations. In 1980, the World Health Organization (WHO) declared that smallpox had been eradicated. However, in 2003, as the United States entered into war with Iraq, US president George W. Bush decreed that the armed forces be vaccinated against smallpox in anticipation of a bioterrorism attack. This pronouncement came on the heels of similar attacks in the United States wherein anthrax infection caused by *Bacillus anthracis* was intentionally spread in Florida and New York. In 2009, another bacterial infection, methicillin-resistant *Staphylococcus aureus* (MRSA), continued to emerge due to the apparent overuse of the antibiotic methicillin.

Influenza, known as a human disease for hundreds of years, emerged in the pandemic of 1918 that killed 20 to 40 million persons, more than died in World War I. Other influenza pandemics included the Asian flu in 1957, the Hong Kong flu in 1968, and swine flu in 1977. Avian influenza, or bird flu, previously rare in humans, emerged in 2004. The H1N1 influenza (formerly called swine flu) emerged in Mexico in 2009 and rapidly spread throughout the Northern hemisphere, infecting millions in the United States alone and countless others across the globe, sickening and killing a disproportionate number of young children and pregnant women and rarely affecting those over age sixty-five. Human immunodeficiency virus (HIV), a retrovirus, is the causative agent of acquired immunodeficiency syndrome (AIDS), one the world's deadliest infectious diseases; according to the WHO, about 2 million people die from AIDS-related diseases each year, more than from non-AIDS-related tuberculosis or malaria. Multidrug-resistant tuberculosis (MDR-TB) and extensively drug-resistant tuberculosis (XDR-TB) continued to emerge in the early twenty-first century, especially in those living with HIV infection. Malaria, a parasitic scourge, causes between 600,000 and 700,000 deaths every year, with 90 percent of deaths occurring in sub-Saharan Africa. Malaria continues to emerge with strains of its most lethal species, *Plasmodium falciparum*, which is resistant to antimalarial drugs.

Examples

Three diseases serve as important recent examples of emerging infectious diseases: H1N1 influenza, HIV/AIDS, and resistant tuberculosis.

H1N1 influenza. A zoonotic disease resulting from a mix of swine, avian, and human flu viruses, H1N1 influenza emerged in the United States following the regular 2008–2009 flu season, during which influenza A (H1), A (H3), and B viruses all circulated. In mid-April 2009, the Centers for Disease Control and Prevention (CDC) documented the first two cases of influenza A pandemic (H1N1) in the United States; after September 1, 2009, the CDC characterized the antigens of collected flu viruses: 412 2009 influenza A (H1N1); 4 influenza B; 3 influenza A (H3N2); and 1 seasonal influenza A (H1N1). In December 2009, 99 percent of flu strains were composed of pandemic H1N1 2009. According to the WHO, as of November 22, 2009, there were more than 40,617 "confirmed and probable" cases of pandemic H1N1 2009, and 7,826 deaths worldwide; by May of 2010, the estimated number of deaths had risen to more than 18,000. However, these statistics are significantly lower than the actual morbidity and mortality because they are based on limited data. Moreover, pandemic H1N1 2009 infections in which the virus mutated to a strain more virulent were identified across the globe. In addition, a number of patients developed strains of H1N1 resistant to the antiviral oseltamivir (Tamiflu). In August 2010, the WHO announced that the pandemic period had ended; although outbreaks were expected to continue to occur, the virus was no longer considered a major threat.

HIV and AIDS. Since HIV, the virus that causes AIDS, was first isolated in the early 1980s, the virus has continued to emerge into new populations and new geographic locations while morphing into new strains and variants, becoming resistant to available antiretroviral therapies (ART). Therefore, new drugs and combinations of old and new therapies must continually be produced to help keep alive the more than 34 million people living with HIV and AIDS. Moreover, while HIV infection is now treated like a chronic disease in many developed countries, many developing nations continue to struggle to obtain adequate drugs and preventive programs to treat all those infected with the virus. Despite the advent of highly active antiretroviral therapy (HAART) in 1996, a range of comorbidities continues to plague those living with HIV and AIDS, including liver disease (hepatitis B and C), non-Hodgkin's lymphoma, neurological illnesses, malignancy, malnutrition, and increased susceptibility to TB and MDR-TB. Nevertheless, according to the Joint United Nations Programme on HIV/AIDS (UNAIDS), the number of HIV/AIDS-related deaths decreased by more than 500,000 between 2005 and 2011, and the number of new HIV infections decreased by 700,000 between 2001 and 2011.

MDR-TB/XDR-TB. *Mycobacterium tuberculosis* strains resistant to multiple drugs represent an emerging threat to the global control of both tuberculosis and HIV, which often coinfect patients. The WHO estimates that between 220,000 and 400,000 cases of MDR-TB emerged in 2011. MDR-TB is defined as resistance to a minimum of the anti-TB drugs isoniazid and rifampin. While HIV may or may not be directly associated with the risk of developing MDR-TB, nosocomial outbreaks in individuals living with HIV and AIDS have been noted. HIV/AIDS has also been linked to an increased risk for rifampin-monoresistant TB. In addition,

new cases of XDR-TB, defined as MDR-TB resistant to a fluoroquinolone and a minimum of one second-line injectable agent, have been widely reported across the globe. Treatment of MDR-TB is complex, sometimes requiring the use of less effective and more toxic drugs that mandate treatment over longer periods of time, thereby lessening the chance of successful outcomes and posing serious problems for developing countries, especially those with a high prevalence of HIV-1 infection. MDR-TB and XDR-TB are also of concern in wealthier countries where massive immigration and global travel is commonplace.

—*Cynthia F. Racer, M.A., M.P.H.*

See also Acquired immunodeficiency syndrome (AIDS); Antibiotics; Avian influenza; Bacterial infections; Centers for Disease Control and Prevention (CDC); Drug resistance; Ebola virus; Epidemics and pandemics; Epidemiology; H1N1 influenza; Human immunodeficiency virus (HIV); Immunization and vaccination; Influenza; Insect-borne diseases; Malaria; National Institutes of Health (NIH); Parasitic diseases; Plague; Severe acute respiratory syndrome (SARS); Tuberculosis; Viral infections; West Nile virus; World Health Organization; Zoonoses.

For Further Information:

Garrett, Laurie. *Betrayal of Trust: The Collapse of Global Public Health*. New York: Hyperion Books, 2001.

Global Alert and Response. "Pandemic and Epidemic Diseases." *World Health Organization*, 2013.

Global Alert and Response. "Pandemic (H1N1) 2009—Update 103." *World Health Organization*, June 4, 2010.

Hill, Stuart. *Emerging Infectious Diseases*. San Francisco: Benjamin Cummings, 2005.

Leslie, T., et al. "Epidemic of *Plasmodium falciparum* Malaria Involving Substandard Anti-malarial Drugs, Pakistan, 2003." *Emerging Infectious Diseases* 15 (2009): 1753–59.

MacPherson, D. W., et al. "Population Mobility, Globalization, and Antimicrobial Drug Resistance." *Emerging Infectious Diseases* 15 (2009): 1727–32.

National Center for Emerging and Zoonotic Infectious Diseases. "Fighting Emerging Infectious Diseases." *Centers for Disease Control and Prevention*, March 12, 2012.

National Institute of Allergy and Infectious Diseases. "Emerging and Re-Emerging Infectious Diseases." *National Institutes of Health*, August 24, 2010.

UNAIDS. "World AIDS Day Report 2012." *Joint United Nations Programme on HIV/AIDS*, November 2012.

World Health Organization. "Factsheet on the World Malaria Report 2012." *World Health Organization*, December 2012.

World Health Organization. "HIV/AIDS." *World Health Organization*, 2013.

World Health Organization. "Multidrug-Resistant Tuberculosis (MDR-TB) 2012 Update." *World Health Organization*, November 2012.

EMPHYSEMA

Disease/Disorder

Anatomy or system affected: Chest, lungs, respiratory system

Specialties and related fields: Internal medicine, pulmonary medicine

Definition: A disease of the lung characterized by enlargement of the small bronchioles or lung alveoli, the destruction of alveoli, decreased elastic recoil of these structures, and the trapping of air in the lungs, resulting in shortness of breath, reduced oxygen to the body, and a variety of serious and eventually fatal complications.

Key terms:

alveoli: tiny, delicate, balloonlike air sacs composed of blood vessels that are supported by connecting tissue and enclosed in a very thin membrane; these sacs are found at the ends of the bronchioles

bronchioles: small branches of the bronchi, which are extensions of the trachea (the central duct that conducts air from the environment to the pulmonary system)

bullous emphysema: localized areas of emphysema within the lung substance

centrilobular (centriacinar) emphysema: a type of emphysema that destroys single alveoli, entering directly into the walls of terminal and respiratory bronchioles

diffusion: the passage of oxygen into the bloodstream from the alveoli and the return or exchange of carbon dioxide across the membrane between the blood vessels and the alveoli

panlobular (panacinar) emphysema: a type of emphysema that involves weakening and enlargement of the air sacs, which are clustered at the end of respiratory bronchioles

perfusion: the flow of blood through the lungs or other vessels in the body

ventilation: the transport of air from the mouth through the bronchial tree to the air sacs and back through the nose or mouth to the outside; ventilation includes both inspiration (breathing in) and expiration (breathing out)

Causes and Symptoms

Emphysema is a lung disease in which damage to the lungs causes shortness of breath and can lead to heart or respiratory failure. A discussion of the structure and function of the normal lung can illuminate the nature and effects of this damage.

Emphysema

In emphysema, the body releases enzymes in response to inhaling irritants in the air, such as cigarette smoke; these enzymes reduce the lungs" elasticity, compromising the bronchioles" ability to expand and contract normally. Air becomes trapped in the alveoli upon inhalation (top) and cannot escape upon exhalation (bottom). Over time, breathing becomes extremely difficult.

Air—along with gases, smoke, germs, allergens, and environmental pollutants—passes from the nose and mouth into a large duct called the trachea. The trachea branches into smaller ducts, the bronchi and bronchioles (small branches of the bronchi), which lead to tiny air sacs called alveoli. The respiratory system is like an upside-down tree: The trachea is the trunk, the bronchi and bronchioles are similar to the branches, and the alveoli are similar to the leaves. The blood vessels of the alveoli carry red blood cells, which pick up oxygen and transport it to the rest of the body. The cellular waste product, carbon dioxide, is released to the alveoli from the bloodstream and then exhaled. The alveoli are supported by a framework of delicate elastic fibers and give the lung a very

---

Information on Emphysema

Causes: Long-term exposure to dry air, smoke, or other environmental toxins; infection; allergies

Symptoms: Shortness of breath, labored breathing, discolored skin, wheezing, difficulty coughing and talking

Duration: Chronic

Treatments: Eliminating causes of irritation, cleaning out airways via nebulizers and intermittent positive pressure breathing machine, medications (theophylline, antibiotics, steroids)

---

distensible quality and the ability to "snap back," or recoil.

The lungs and bronchial tubes are surrounded by the chest wall, composed of bone and muscle and functioning like a bellows. The lung is elastic and passively increases in size to fill the chest space during inspiration and decreases in size during expiration. As the lung (including the alveoli) enlarges, air from the environment flows in to fill this space. During exhalation, the muscles relax, the elasticity of the lung returns it to a normal size, and the air is pushed out. Air must pass through the bronchial tree to the alveoli before oxygen can get into the bloodstream and carbon dioxide can get out, because it is the alveoli that are in contact with blood vessels. The bronchial tree has two kinds of special lining cells. The first type can secrete mucus as a sticky protection against injury and irritation. The second type of cell is covered with fine, hairlike structures called cilia. These cells are supported by smooth muscle cells and elastic and collagen fibers. The cilia wave in the direction of the mouth and act as a defense system by physically removing germs and irritating substances. The cilia are covered with mucus, which helps to trap irritants and germs.

When alveoli are exposed to irritants such as cigarette smoke, they produce a defensive cell called an alveolar macrophage. These cells engulf irritants and bacteria and call for white blood cells, which aid in the defense against foreign bodies, to come into the lungs. The lung tissue also becomes a target for the enzymes or chemical substances produced by the alveolar macrophages and leukocytes (white blood cells). In a healthy body, natural defense systems inhibit the enzymes released by the alveolar macrophages and leukocytes, but it seems that this inhibiting function is impaired in smokers. In some cases, an individual may inherit a deficiency in an enzyme inhibitor. The enzymes vigorously attack the elastin and collagen of the lungs, the lung loses its elastic recoil, and air is trapped.

Emphysema and a related disease, bronchitis, often work in concert. They are often lumped under the term "chronic obstructive pulmonary disease" (COPD). Chronic bronchitis weakens and narrows the bronchi. Often, bronchial walls collapse, choking off the vital flow of air. Air is also trapped within the bronchial walls. Weakened by enzymes, the walls of the alveoli rupture and blood vessels die. Lung tissue is replaced with scar tissue, leaving areas of destroyed alveoli that appear as "holes" on an X ray. Small areas of destroyed alveoli are called blebs, and larger ones are called bullae.

As emphysema progresses, the patient develops a set of large, overexpanded lungs with a weakened and partially plugged bronchial tree subject to airway collapse and air trapping with blebs and bullae. Breathing, especially exhalation, becomes a slow and difficult process. The patient often develops a "barrel chest" and is known, in medical circles, as a "blue bloater." The scientific world calls the mismatching of breathing to blood distribution a ventilation-to-perfusion imbalance; that is, when air arrives in the alveolus, there are no blood vessels there to transport the vital gaseous cargo to the cells (as a result of enzymatic damage). A person with chronic obstructive pulmonary disease has a bronchial tree with a

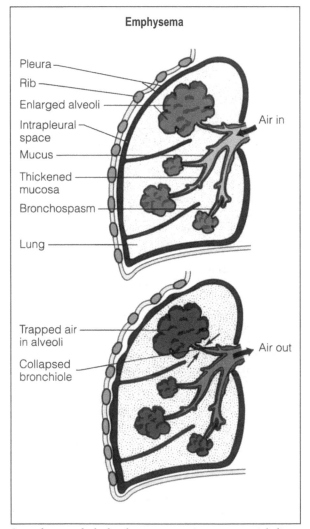

Emphysema

Pleura
Rib
Enlarged alveoli
Intrapleural space
Mucus
Thickened mucosa
Bronchospasm
Lung

Air in

Trapped air in alveoli
Collapsed bronchiole

Air out

In emphysema, the body releases enzymes in response to inhaling irritants in the air, such as cigarette smoke; these enzymes reduce the lungs' elasticity, compromising the bronchioles' ability to expand and contract normally. Air becomes trapped in the alveoli upon inhalation (top) and cannot escape upon exhalation (bottom). Over time, breathing becomes extremely difficult.

narrow, defective trunk and sparse leaves.

The loss of elasticity of the lung and alveoli is a critical problem in the emphysemic patient. About one-half of the lungs" elastic recoil force comes from surface tension. The other half comes from the elastic nature of certain fibers throughout the lungs" structure. Emphysema weakens both of these forces because it destroys the elastic fibers and interferes with the surface tension. Fluid, a saline solution, bathes all the body's cells and surfaces. In the lung, this fluid contains a surfactant, a substance that interferes with water's tendency to form a spherical drop with a pull into its center (and ultimate collapse). The tissue that gives shape to the lungs is composed of specialized fibers which contain a protein called elastin. These elastic fibers are also found in the alveolar walls and in the elastic connective tissue of the airways and air sacs. The amount of elastin in lung tissue determines its behavior. Healthy lungs maintain a proper balance between destruction of elastin and renewal. (Other parts of the body, such as bones, do this as well.) If too little elastin is destroyed, the lungs have difficulty expanding. If too much is destroyed, the lungs overexpand and cannot recoil properly.

The process of elastin destruction and renewal involves complex regulation. Specialized lung cells produce new elastin protein. Others produce elastase, an enzyme that destroys elastin. The liver plays a role in the production of a special enzyme known as alpha-1-antitrypsin, which controls the amount of elastase so that too much elastin is not digested. In emphysema, these regulatory systems fail: Too much elastin is destroyed because elastase production is no longer controlled, apparently because alpha-1-antitrypsin production has been reduced to a trickle.

The loss of elastin (and thus elastic recoil) means that the lungs expand beyond the normal range during inspiration and cannot resume their resting size during expiration. Thus, alveoli overinflate and rupture. This further reduces elasticity, because the loss of each alveolus further impairs the surface tension contribution to the lungs" ability to recoil. Thus, a state of hyperinflation is assumed in the emphysemic patient. This leads to stretched and narrowed alveolar capillaries, loss of elastic tissue, and dissolution of alveolar walls. The lungs increase in size, the thoracic (chest) cage assumes the inspiratory position, and the diaphragm becomes low and flat instead of convex. The patient becomes short of breath with any type of exertion. As the disease worsens, the patient's skin takes on a cyanotic (bluish) color, as a result of poor oxygenation and perfusion. Wheezing is often present, and coughing is difficult and tiring. In the worst cases, even talking is enough exertion to produce a spasmodic cough. The hyperinflated chest causes inspiration to become a major effort, and the entire chest cage lifts up, resulting in considerable strain. The head moves with each inspiration while the chest remains relatively fixed.

Emphysema may be diagnosed by the early symptom of dyspnea (shortness of breath) on exertion. In advanced cases, the distended chest, depressed diaphragm, increased blood carbon dioxide content, and severe dyspnea clearly point to the disease.

Treatment and Therapy

The initial step in treating emphysema is to eliminate the causes of irritation: smoke, polluted air, infection, and allergies. The second treatment is to clean out the airways. There are several techniques and medicines for loosening airway mucus and expelling it. In most chronic obstructive lung diseases, including emphysema, the mucus becomes thick and purulent; coughing up mucus of this type is difficult. In addition, in emphysema the natural cleansing action of the cilia and lung elasticity are impaired. Thus, treatment is aimed at the patient consciously taking over the function of cleaning out the lungs. Coughing is nature's way of bringing up mucus (phlegm), and the emphysemic patient is urged to cough. Since the mucus is thick, one needs to do whatever is necessary to thin it out and to lubricate the airways so that the mucus slips up easily with coughing. The cough must come from deep within the chest in order to be "productive" (to raise mucus).

Moisture is helpful in loosening up thick mucus; hence, drinking large amounts of fluid is encouraged. Adding a humidifier or a vaporizer to a home is often helpful to the emphysemic patient. There are also machines known as nebulizers and intermittent positive pressure breathing (IPPB) machines that can help to add moisture to the airway of the patient with emphysema. Nebulizers are more effective in getting moisture beyond the throat and major airways than cold vaporizers. Nebulizers, which get their name from the Latin word *nebula*, meaning cloud or mist, create a mist that is a profusion of tiny droplets that keep themselves apart, even as they bump into one another. Nebulizers release only the smallest droplets—those which can penetrate far down into air passages, where thick mucus is likely to be. (Atomizers produce small droplets as well, but they also spray large droplets.) IPPBs have a special kind of valve that opens when one begins to breathe and allows the air to move into the lungs under mild pressure. As soon as the patient has come to the end of the inhalation, the valve closes and allows the patient to exhale freely.

When phlegm cannot be brought up by breathing mist, a technique called postural drainage is often combined with chest wall percussion or vibration. The idea is to move one's body to a position such that airways are perpendicular to the floor, or at least tilted down, so that gravity can help pull the mucus toward the larger airways, from which the phlegm can be coughed up. Percussion, or clapping the chest, is another way to loosen the mucus in the airways so that it can be coughed up.

A number of medications are useful in the treatment of emphysema. The many bronchodilator drugs relieve bronchospasms, reduce wheezing and dyspnea, and improve respiratory muscle function. Theophylline is a bronchodilator that is similar chemically to caffeine; both are in a category of drugs known as xanthines. Whereas caffeine stimulates the skeletal muscles and the central nervous system, however, theophylline is potent as a cardiac stimulant and a smooth muscle relaxer. It stimulates mucociliary clearance of the airways, meaning it helps get rid of mucus. An-

other category of bronchodilator are the beta$_2$-adrenergic agonists, or beta-agonists, which generally fall into two categories, short-acting and long-acting. Examples of short-acting beta-agonists include albuterol (Ventolin), pirbuterol (Maxair), and metaproterenol (Alupent). Among the long-acting beta-agonists are salmeterol (Serevent) and formoterol (Foradil). Some side effects of beta-agonists include nervousness, headache, nausea, and muscle cramps.

Antibiotics are sometimes prescribed for emphysemic patients to combat bacterial infections that can dramatically worsen the effects of their condition. The steroid hormones, such as prednisone, decrease swelling, inflammation, and bronchospasms; they also relieve wheezing.

Treatment options other than drugs include pulmonary rehabilitation, in which the patient may be taught exercises to strengthen the chest muscles as well as breathing and coughing techniques to improve air flow into the lungs. Sometimes emphysema patients are given supplemental oxygen, also called oxygen therapy, if their lung function is too impaired to keep the oxygen levels in their blood sufficiently high. Portable oxygen tanks that deliver oxygen through a tube and a mask can give patients greater mobility to carry out tasks of daily living. In rare cases, surgery is an option for severe cases of emphysema. The two kinds of surgery available are lung volume reduction surgery (LVRS) and, as a last resort, a lung transplant. The aim of LVRS is to remove the most diseased portions of the lung to give the healthier portion more room to function. A lung transplant may be considered if a patient's lungs are in danger of failing entirely, and if the patient is determined to be strong enough to endure the procedure and the recovery period.

The emphysemic patient should avoid both excessive heat and excessive cold. If body temperature rises above normal, the heart works faster, as do the lungs. Excessive cold stresses the body to maintain its normal temperature. Smog, air pollution, dusts, powders, and hairspray should be avoided. Finally, a healthy diet consisting of foods high in calcium, vitamins, complex carbohydrates, proteins, and fiber is advised for the patient with lung disease.

A healthy core diet is high in complex carbohydrates; is low in sugars, fats, and cholesterol; and has adequate protein for moderate stress. It should be high in fiber and contain approximately 1,000 milligrams of calcium, 15,000 milligrams of vitamin A, and 250 milligrams of vitamin C. Snack foods can include skim milk, fruit, popcorn, and fresh salads. The respiratory distress of the emphysemic patient uses vast amounts of energy, and the patient should eat several small meals a day so as not to distend the stomach and limit movement of the diaphragm. Liquids are important in keeping airways clear. Good nutrition is helpful in maintaining strength and improving the quality of life for the patient with lung disease.

Perspective and Prospects

According to the Centers for Disease Control and Prevention, chronic obstructive pulmonary disease (chronic bronchitis and emphysema) was the third leading cause of death in the

United States in 2011. The CDC reported that in 2011, 6.3 percent of American adults had been diagnosed with COPD. In males over forty, COPD is second only to heart disease as a cause of disability. Although the death rates from COPD have declined slightly among men from 1999 to 2010, they have stayed about the same for women, and the overall average has barely changed. Aside from death, a disease such as emphysema can cause long years of disability, joblessness, loss of income, depression, hospitalization, and an inability to perform normal activities.

Smoking is, by far, the single most important risk factor for emphysema. In the United States especially, social acceptance of women smokers began after World War II and has increased the number of women being diagnosed with COPD, to the point where, according to the CDC study, more women have COPD than men (6.7 percent compared to 5.2 percent). Socioeconomic status also influences rates of COPD, with lower-income workers experiencing higher rates of the disease. COPD also correlates negatively with level of education: The rate in 2011 among those without a high school diploma was 9.5 percent; 6.8 percent among those with a high school diploma; and 4.6 percent among those with some college.

A number of economic pressures are likely to move COPD treatment from the hospital to the home. When effectively carried out by a well-trained health team, home care can lower medical costs. The COPD patient who finds a knowledgeable doctor and who begins a comprehensive rehabilitation program is the one who can look forward to a life that is more productive and more comfortable

—*Jane A. Slezak, Ph.D.*

See also Asbestos exposure; Aspergillosis; Bronchi; Chronic obstructive pulmonary disease (COPD); Coughing; Cyanosis; Environmental diseases; Lungs; Oxygen therapy; Pulmonary diseases; Pulmonary medicine; Respiration; Smoking; Wheezing.

For Further Information:
American Lung Association. http://www.lungusa.org.
Bates, David V. *Respiratory Function in Disease*. 3d ed. Philadelphia: W. B. Saunders, 1989.
Centers for Disease Control and Prevention. "Chronic Obstructive Pulmonary Disease (COPD)." *Centers for Disease Control and Prevention*, April 25, 2013.
Decker, Caroline D. "Room to Breathe." *Saturday Evening Post* 266, no. 6 (November/December, 1994): 48–49.
"Emphysema." *InteliHealth*, November 21, 2011.
Haas, François, and Sheila Sperber Haas. *The Chronic Bronchitis and Emphysema Handbook*. Rev. ed. New York: John Wiley & Sons, 2000.
Hedrick, Hannah L., and Austin K. Kutscher, eds. *The Quiet Killer: Emphysema, Chronic Obstructive Pulmonary Disease*. Lanham, Md.: Scarecrow Press, 2002.
Matthews, Dawn D. *Lung Disorders Sourcebook*. Detroit, Mich.: Omnigraphics, 2002.
National Emphysema Foundation. http://www.emphysemafoundation.org.
West, John B. *Pulmonary Pathophysiology: The Essentials*. 7th ed. Philadelphia: Wolters Kluwer/Lippincott Williams & Wilkins, 2008.
Wolff, Ronald K. "Effects of Airborne Pollutants on Mucociliary Clearance." *Environmental Health Perspectives* 66 (April, 1986): 223–237.
Wood, Debra. "Emphysema." *Health Library*, March 29, 2013.

ENCEPHALITIS
Disease/Disorder
Anatomy or system affected: Brain, circulatory system, neck, nerves, nervous system, psychic-emotional system
Specialties and related fields: Bacteriology, epidemiology, internal medicine, neurology, public health, virology
Definition: A disease that involves inflammation of the brain.
Key terms:
arbovirus: a virus transmitted by the bite of an arthropod, particularly a mosquito or a tick
central nervous system (CNS): in vertebrates, consisting of the brain and spinal cord
enterovirus: a virus that tends to multiply in the intestinal tract

Causes and Symptoms

Encephalitis is sometimes classified according to the causative agent or the anatomic structures affected. Limbic encephalitis, for example, affects structures in the brain known as the limbic system. Exposure to lead often produces cerebral inflammation and edema (swelling) and is referred to as lead encephalitis. If the agent is bacterial, then the disease is referred to as bacterial encephalitis. In amebic encephalitis, patients with weakened immune systems become infected through certain protozoa (*Acanthamoeba*) found in water and moist soil.

The principal cause of encephalitis, however, is viral. In primary encephalitis, the virus directly invades the brain and spinal cord. Secondary encephalitis occurs as an aftereffect of such airborne diseases as measles and influenza (postinfectious) or of certain vaccinations (postvaccinal).

Though many viruses can produce encephalitis, only a limited number tend to recur. They fall into three major groups: enteroviruses, arboviruses, and nonarthropod viruses.

Information on Encephalitis

Causes: Viral infection, complications from another disease
Symptoms: Headache, fever, stiff neck, loss of consciousness, seizures, sleep disturbances, blurred or double vision, vomiting, body aches
Duration: Acute or chronic
Treatments: Alleviation of symptoms

Nonarthropod viruses, transmitted without an insect vector, include the very common herpes simplex virus 1 (HSV-1).

Enteroviruses infect the gastrointestinal tract and are spread by a fecal-oral route. Hands come into contact with feces or bodily fluids in which the virus is present. If unwashed, the hands can transfer the virus to the mouth. Once ingested, the virus replicates in the intestines and then moves to the nervous system.

Arboviruses, which are responsible for epidemics, are spread by mosquitoes (such as in eastern equine encephalitis) and ticks (as in Powassan encephalitis). For natural reasons related to their vectors (carriers), these infections, at least in northerly climes, peak in late summer.

If a mosquito ingests a blood meal from an infected vertebrate, over a period of one to three weeks, the virus replicates in the mosquito's gut and then moves to its salivary glands. When the mosquito bites a human, the virus lurks in the person's visceral organs and then passes by means of the blood to the nervous system. A possible route to the central nervous system (CNS) is through the brain capillaries. Infection of neurons, and glial cells, which constitute the non-nervous tissue of the brain and spinal cord, follows, leading to cell dysfunction and death. The body's own immune response, which includes infusing white blood cells into the cerebrospinal fluid, contributes to the brain edema and inflammation.

In diagnosis, physicians use blood and deoxyribonucleic acid (DNA) tests and analyze the cerebrospinal fluid for a too-high count of white blood cells and elevated protein levels and fluid pressure. Neuroimaging and electroencephalograms (EEGs), which record electrical activity in the brain, are used to eliminate other possibilities, such as clotting because of the rupture of a blood vessel (hematoma). Isolation of the virus itself, with some exceptions, is difficult. Biopsy of brain tissue for evidence of the virus has largely been replaced by less invasive procedures.

Symptoms may occur within a few hours or over the course of several days and initially are nonspecific, which complicates the diagnosis. Although they vary depending on the virus and the extent and length of infection, symptoms generally include fever, headache, muscle ache, stiff neck, respiratory symptoms, sensitivity to light, abdominal pain, vomiting, dizziness, an altered level of consciousness that may range from lethargy to coma, personality changes that may progress to behavior that appears psychotic, intellectual deficit, and a host of neurological deficiencies, such as tremors, loss of muscular coordination, partial paralysis, and ocular (eye) fixation.

Treatment and Therapy

For some types of encephalitis, such as Japanese encephalitis, effective vaccines exist. In bacterial cases, antibiotics are prescribed. In patients in whom the herpes simplex virus is implicated, the antiviral acyclovirin is useful. In general, however, treatment, often initially in an intensive care unit (ICU), is supportive and designed to control complications. For example, steroids are sometimes administered to reduce brain swelling and anticonvulsants, if seizures occur.

The disease runs its course in one to two weeks. Mortality rates depend on the type of virus and the age of the patient, the very young and elderly being more vulnerable. Most cases of encephalitis are mild. In eastern equine encephalitis, the mortality rate is about 33 percent; in western equine encephalitis, it is about 3 percent in older patients and as high as 30 percent in younger patients. Residual symptoms after recovery vary, again according to the agent and extent of infection. In eastern equine encephalitis, 80 percent of patients suffer neurologic aftereffects.

Perspective and Prospects

Some historians of medicine believe that viral encephalitis appeared early in the Mediterranean area. The evidence is indirect, with the mention in the *Hippocratic corpus* (fifth century BCE and later) of genital and labial lesions consistent with the herpes virus, a leading cause of the disease. It was not until the nineteenth and twentieth centuries that the numerous agents and vectors for encephalitis were successfully identified, such as the rabies virus (isolated by Louis Pasteur's dog experiments), the spirochete of syphilis, and more recently human immunodeficiency virus (HIV).

A firm connection between the great influenza pandemic of 1918 and the repeated global outbreaks of encephalitis lethargica in the 1920s was not established until 1982. In the 1990s, aspirin therapy in children's influenza was implicated in the sometimes fatal brain edema known as Reye syndrome.

Research has focused on oral antiviral drug therapy. Interferon alpha-2b therapy and ribovarin, related to the vitamin B complex, have been tested on patients with West Nile virus, but their value has not been conclusively established. Emphasis therefore has remained on prevention: proper vaccinations and, for arboviruses, mosquito spraying campaigns, application of effective insect repellents, and limited outside exposure during the early evening hours.

—*David J. Ladouceur, Ph.D.*

See also Bites and stings; Brain; Brain damage; Brain disorders; Dementias; Hemiplegia; Inflammation; Insect-borne diseases; Lice, mites, and ticks; Nervous system; Neuroimaging; Neurology; Neurology, pediatric; Parasitic diseases; Sleeping sickness; Viral infections; West Nile virus.

For Further Information:

American Medical Association. *American Medical Association Family Medical Guide.* 4th rev. ed. Hoboken, N.J.: John Wiley & Sons, 2004.

Bloom, Ona, and Jennifer Morgan. *Encephalitis.* Philadelphia: Chelsea House, 2006.

Carson-DeWitt, Rosalyn, and Rimas Lukas. "Encephalitis." *Health Library,* Sept. 30, 2012.

"Encephalitis." *MedlinePlus,* Mar. 4, 2013.

Fauci, Anthony S., et al., eds. *Harrison's Principles of Internal Medicine.* 18th ed. New York: McGraw-Hill, 2012.

Goldman, Lee, and Dennis Ausiello, eds. *Cecil Textbook of Medicine.* 23d ed. Philadelphia: Saunders/Elsevier, 2007.

Professional Guide to Diseases. 9th ed. Philadelphia: Lippincott Williams & Wilkins, 2009.

END-STAGE RENAL DISEASE
Disease/Disorder

Anatomy or system affected: Blood, blood vessels, circulatory system, endocrine system, heart, kidneys, urinary system

Specialties and related fields: Cardiology, endocrinology, geriatrics and gerontology, internal medicine, nephrology, vascular medicine

Definition: Stage 5 of chronic kidney disease, which causes irreversible damage to and near-complete failure of the kidneys.

Key terms:

creatinine clearance: a test that measures levels of the waste product creatinine in blood and in a twenty-four-hour urine sample

diabetic nephropathy: a kidney disease associated with long-standing diabetes

dialysis: a mechanical means of cleansing the blood; an exchange of water and solute filters waste products out through diffusion

fistula: a surgically created opening that joins an artery and vein

glomerular filtration rate: the amount of glomerular filtrate formed each minute in nephrons of both kidneys; calculated from the rate of creatinine clearance and adjusted for body-surface area

renal osteodystrophy: a bone disease of chronic renal failure

uremia: a syndrome occurring with deteriorating renal function and characterized by combination of metabolic, fluid, electrolyte, and hormone imbalances

Causes and Symptoms

End-stage renal disease (ESRD) is stage 5 of chronic kidney disease, defined as kidney function at less than 10 percent of normal and a glomerular filtration rate of less than 15 milliliters per minute. Both diseases are characterized by the inability to remove wastes and concentrate urine, have poor outcomes, and are usually the result of long-standing diabetes and/or uncontrolled hypertension.

ESRD is a serious, life-threatening systematic disease characterized by renal failure, decreased production of red blood cells and active vitamin D_3, and excess excretion of acid, potassium, salt, and water. Many metabolic abnormalities and imbalances occur, causing complications, such as anemia, acidemia or acidosis, hyperkalemia, hyperphosphatemia, hyperparathyroidism, and hypocalcemia. Symptoms include swollen feet and ankles, fatigue, lethargy or weakness, itching, skin color changes, loss of mental alertness, shortness of breath, and recurrent or chronic heart failure.

Tests that measure the level of creatinine and urea in blood and urine are conducted to determine the extent of kidney damage and the filtration capacity of the kidneys. High levels of these waste products found in the blood but not in the urine are signs of kidney damage. ESRD may be suspected when very high levels of protein are detected in the urine (proteinuria). The results of a creatinine clearance are used to determine the glomerular filtration rate, the standard measurement used to assess kidney function.

Diabetes mellitus is the most common cause of ESRD, due to its underlying kidney disease—diabetic nephropathy. Approximately 20 to 40 percent of patients with diabetes develop the disease, and nearly half of them progress to ESRD within five to ten years. Diabetic nephropathy develops with changes in the microvasculature (tiny blood vessels) of the glomerulus and is characterized by a progressive and aggressive disease course: wastes increase, building up in the blood; kidneys leak larger amounts of albumin, causing proteinuria; and nodular glomerulosclerosis lesions proliferate and

---

Information on End-Stage Renal Disease

Causes: Diabetes and hypertension

Symptoms: Swollen feet and ankles, fatigue/lethargy/weakness, itching, pale skin, loss of mental alertness, shortness of breath, recurrent or chronic heart failure

Duration: Variable, fatal if not treated

Treatments: Dialysis or kidney transplant

---

destroy the glomeruli.

Hypertension (high blood pressure) is a major cause of ESRD, estimated at approximately 30 percent of all cases. Although arteries are elastic, they can become overstretched from hypertension and narrow, weaken, or harden. This is especially deadly in the kidneys, which are highly vascular and carry large volumes of blood. Damaged blood vessels and filters prevent the kidneys from functioning adequately, including reducing the hormone that they normally produce to help the body regulate its own blood pressure. Thus, hypertension is both a cause and a symptom of ESRD.

Uremia is a syndrome that develops with ESRD when metabolic, fluid, electrolyte, and hormone imbalances emerge concurrently. Clinical symptoms include nausea or vomiting, fatigue, weight loss, muscle cramps, pruritus (itching), mental status changes, visual disturbances, and increased thirst.

Renal osteodystrophy is a degenerative bone disease that develops with metabolic imbalances in the minerals phosphorus and calcium. High levels of phosphorus in the blood draw calcium out of the bones, causing them to become brittle and break. The excess of phosphorus and calcium salts in the blood deposit and harden, forming metastatic calcifications in the skin, blood vessels, and other soft tissues.

Treatment and Therapy

Dialysis and kidney transplantation are the only treatments for ESRD and provide a means of prolonging a patient's life span and maintaining quality of life.

Dialysis is a means of cleansing the blood when the kidneys do not function and is done by the process of diffusion, in which blood is passed through a filter in contact with a dialysate (salt solution), separating the smaller molecules (solute particles) from the larger molecules (colloid particles). There are two types of dialysis—hemodialysis and peritoneal dialysis—each of which has several variants.

In hemodialysis, blood is filtered by diverting it outside the body through a fistula and flows across a semipermeable membrane in the dialysis unit in a direction countercurrent to the dialysate. Hemodialysis takes three to four hours to complete and must be done three to five times a week, usually in a dialysis clinic. In peritoneal dialysis, blood is filtered internally through the peritoneum, a thin membrane inside the abdomen and peritoneal dialysis fluid is infused into the cavity via a catheter. Exchanges are repeated four to six times a day by the patient, and the process must be done every day.

Kidney transplants are another option for most ESRD patients. The United Network for Organ Sharing recommends that patients be put on the cadaveric renal transplant list when their glomerular filtration rate is less than 18 milliliters per minute. Improvements in their policies provide for a more equitable allocation system, broaden the classification of expanded donor criteria, and are expected to increase the donor pool. Unfortunately, thousands of patients die each year waiting for an available kidney.

Perspective and Prospects

Chronic kidney disease and ESRD represent a growing public health problem and reflect the disturbing health profile of present-day society—rising numbers of people with obesity, diabetes, hypertension, cardiovascular disease, and metabolic syndrome. The prevalence of chronic kidney disease has risen steadily since the 1980s. Changes in lifestyle and increased awareness of disease risk—including the monitoring of one's blood sugar levels and blood pressure—are key to preventing chronic kidney disease and reducing the number of patients who progress to ESRD.

—Barbara Woldin

See also Diabetes mellitus; Dialysis; Hypertension; Kidney disorders; Kidney transplantation; Kidneys; Nephrology; Polycystic kidney disease; Proteinuria; Pyelonephritis; Renal failure; Transplantation; Uremia.

For Further Information:
"Chronic Kidney Disease." *MedlinePlus*, Apr. 23, 2013.
"Kidney Failure." *MedlinePlus*, Apr. 23, 2013.
Offer, Daniel, Marjorie Kaiz Offer, and Susan Offer Szafir. *Dialysis Without Fear: A Guide to Living Well on Dialysis for Patients and Their Families*. New York: Oxford University Press, 2007.
Savitsky, Diane, and Adrienne Carmack. "Kidney Failure." *Health Library*, Oct. 31, 2012.
Townsend, Raymond R., and Debbie Cohen. *One Hundred Q&A About Kidney Disease and Hypertension*. Sudbury, Mass.: Jones & Bartlett, 2008.
Walser, Mackenzie, and Betsy Thorpe. *Coping with Kidney Disease: A Twelve-Step Treatment Program to Help You Avoid Dialysis*. Hoboken, N.J.: John Wiley & Sons, 2004.
Wein, Alan, et al., eds. *Campbell-Walsh Urology*. 10th ed. Philadelphia: Saunders/Elsevier, 2012.

ENDARTERECTOMY

Procedure

Anatomy or system affected: Blood vessels, circulatory system, neck

Specialties and related fields: General surgery, vascular medicine

Definition: A surgical procedure used to remove plaque from the lining of the carotid arteries in the neck.

Indications and Procedures

The internal carotid artery lies in the side of the neck, slightly in front of and beneath the sternocleidomastoid muscle. A skin incision is made anterior to this muscle. The branches of the carotid artery, adjacent blood vessels, and nerves are freed and inspected. A clamp is applied to the common carotid artery. Two additional clamps are applied to the external and

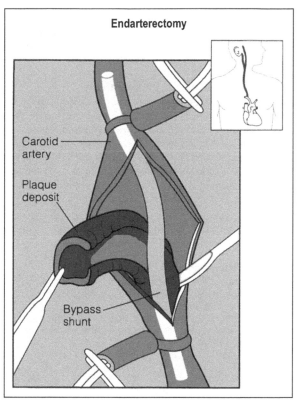

Endarterectomy

Carotid artery

Plaque deposit

Bypass shunt

The excision of plaque deposits from the carotid artery in the neck is called endarterectomy; the inset shows the location of the carotid artery.

internal carotid arteries to prevent bleeding and to prevent emboli from migrating to the brain during the procedure.

A lengthwise incision is made in the internal carotid artery from a point about 3.8 centimeters (1.5 inches) above the beginning of the vessel into the common carotid artery, about 2.5 centimeters (1 inch) below the beginning of the vessel. The edges of the artery are retracted, and the interior is exposed. The plaque can usually be scraped off the walls of the artery. The internal lining of the artery is carefully closed, and any tears are sutured. The carotid artery is then sewed together with fine suture material. If the underlying disease has been extensive or if the lining of the artery is damaged, a portion of the saphenous vein in the patient's leg is used to repair the arterial wall.

Restoring blood flow is crucial; it is important to avoid both leaks in the artery and the formation of emboli. The clamp on the external carotid artery is briefly released, and a small amount of blood is allowed to flow back into the repaired area to check for leaks under low pressure. This clamp is reapplied. The clamp on the common carotid artery is removed to check for leaks under high pressure. The clamp to the external carotid artery is removed next. Blood is allowed to flow, flushing any emboli from the operative site and away from the brain. If all is well, the clamp on the internal carotid artery is removed.

The structures that were pulled away from the carotid artery are released and briefly inspected to ensure that no damage has been done. The edges of the skin are then brought together and closed with sutures. The patient returns in about a week for a checkup and removal of the sutures.

Uses and Complications

Endarterectomy is used to restore adequate blood flow to the brain, thus preventing periods of ischemia that can result in loss of consciousness or strokes. However, complications can include emboli, which can also cause strokes by blocking important blood vessels. Endarterectomy is successful in most patients and restores more normal circulation. It has decreased the incidence of strokes in younger patients.

—*L. Fleming Fallon, Jr., M.D., Ph.D., M.P.H.*

See also Angioplasty; Arteriosclerosis; Blood vessels; Bypass surgery; Carotid arteries; Circulation; Embolism; Strokes; Vascular medicine; Vascular system.

For Further Information:

Ancowitz, Arthur. *Strokes and Their Prevention: How to Avoid High Blood Pressure and Hardening of the Arteries*. New York: Jove, 1980.

Browse, Norman L., A. O. Mansfield, and C. C. R. Bishop. *Carotid Endarterectomy: A Practical Guide*. Boston: Butterworth-Heinemann, 1997.

Loftus, Christopher M. *Carotid Endarterectomy: Principles and Technique*. 2d ed. New York: Informa Healthcare, 2007.

Loftus, Christopher M., and Timothy F. Kresowik. *Carotid Artery Surgery*. New York: Thieme, 2000.

NIH National Heart, Lung, and Blood Institute. "What Is Carotid Endarterectomy?" *NIH National Heart, Lung, and Blood Institute*, December 1, 2010.

Polsdorfer, Ricker. "Endarterectomy." *Health Library*, May 6, 2013.

Rutherford, Robert B. et al., eds. *Rutherford's Vascular Surgery*. 7th ed. Philadelphia: Saunders/Elsevier, 2010.

Topiwala, Shehzad. "Carotid Artery Surgery." *MedlinePlus*, June 4, 2012.

ENDOCARDITIS

Disease/Disorder

Anatomy or system affected: Circulatory system, heart

Specialties and related fields: Bacteriology, cardiology, internal medicine, vascular medicine

Definition: Inflammatory lesions of the endocardium, the lining of the heart.

Causes and Symptoms

The lesions of endocarditis may be noninfective, as in some autoimmune conditions, or infective. The latter are characterized by direct invasion of the endocardium by microorganisms, most often bacteria. Bacterial endocarditis may occur on normal or previously damaged heart valves and also on artificial (prosthetic) heart valves. Rarely, endocarditis may occur on the wall (mural surface) of the heart or at the site of an abnormal hole between the pumping chambers of the heart, called a ventricular septal defect.

In areas of turbulent blood flow, platelet-fibrin deposition can occur, providing a nidus for subsequent bacterial colonization. Transient bacteremia may accompany infection else-

---

> **Information on Endocarditis**
>
> **Causes:** Bacterial infection
> **Symptoms:** Fever, malaise, fatigue, dyspnea, chest pain, heart murmurs
> **Duration:** Temporary
> **Treatments:** Antibiotics

where in the body or some medical and dental procedures, and these circulating bacteria can adhere to the endocardium, especially at platelet-fibrin deposition sites, and produce endocarditis. Intravenous drug abusers using unsterile equipment and drugs often inject bacteria along with the drugs, which can result in endocarditis. The lesions produced by these depositions plus bacteria are called vegetations. Clinical symptoms and signs usually begin about two weeks later.

Bacterial endocarditis usually involves either the mitral or the aortic heart valve. In intravenous drug abusers, the tricuspid heart valve is more commonly affected because it is the first valve to be reached by the endocardium-damaging drugs and contaminating bacteria. The pulmonic valve is only rarely the site of endocarditis. Occasionally, more than one heart valve is infected; this occurs most often in intravenous drug abusers or patients with multiple prosthetic heart valves.

Gram-positive cocci are the most common cause of bacterial endocarditis. Different species predominate in various conditions or situations: *Streptococcus viridans* in native valves, *Staphylococcus aureus* in the valves of intravenous drug abusers, and *Staphylococcus epidermidis* in prosthetic heart valves. Gram-negative bacilli are found in association with prosthetic heart valves or intravenous drug addiction.

The clinical manifestations of endocarditis are varied and often nonspecific. Early symptoms are similar to those encountered in most infections: fever, malaise, and fatigue. As the disease progresses, more cardiovascular and renal-related symptoms may appear: dyspnea, chest pain, and stroke. Fever and heart murmurs are found in most patients. Enlargement of the spleen, skin lesions, and evidence of emboli are commonly present.

The key to the diagnosis of bacterial endocarditis is to suspect the presence of the illness and obtain blood cultures. Febrile patients who have a heart murmur, cardiac failure, a prosthetic heart valve, history of intravenous drug abuse, preexisting valvular disease, stroke (especially in young adults), multiple pulmonary emboli, sudden arterial occlusion, unexplained prolonged fever, or multiple positive blood cultures are likely to have endocarditis. The hallmark of bacterial endocarditis is continuous bacteremia; thus, nearly all blood cultures will be positive. Other nonspecific blood tests, such as an erythrocyte sedimentation rate, or specific blood tests, such as tests for teichoic acid antibodies, may be helpful in establishing a diagnosis.

Treatment and Therapy

Endocarditis may be prevented by administering prophylactic antibiotics to patients with preexisting heart abnormalities

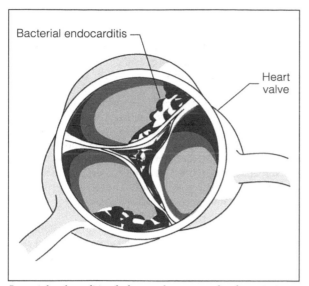

Bacterial endocarditis of a heart valve occurs when bacteria invade and cause inflammatory lesions; untreated, the condition is usually fatal.

that predispose them to endocarditis when they are likely to have transient bacteremia. An example would be a patient with an artificial heart valve scheduled to have a dental cleaning.

Endocarditis is one of the few infections that is nearly always fatal if mistreated. Antibacterial therapy with agents capable of killing the offending bacteria, along with supportive medical care and cardiac surgery when indicated, cures most patients.

Perspective and Prospects

The first demonstration of bacteria in vegetations associated with endocarditis was by Emmanuel Winge of Oslo, Norway, in 1869. Fifty years later, a fresh section was cut from the preserved heart valve described by Winge, and staining by modern methods revealed a chain of streptococci verifying his discovery. It was not until 1943, when Leo Loewe successfully treated seven cases of bacterial endocarditis with penicillin, that the era of modern therapy of this serious illness began.

While the incidence of endocarditis remained fairly constant between the 1960s and the early 1990s, the patient profile changed: heroin addicts, the elderly, and those with prosthetic heart valves. Since the late 1990s there has been a steady increase in the number of heart valve infections. Recent studies have found that 40 percent of those who end up with endocarditis acquire their infections in health care facilities. Most of these patients are elderly, are suffering from other illnesses, and have received cardiac implants such as prosthetic heart valves, pacemakers, and defibrillators.

—*H. Bradford Hawley, M.D.*

See also Bacterial infections; Cardiac arrest; Cardiology; Cardiology, pediatric; Circulation; Echocardiography; Heart; Heart disease;

Heart valve replacement; Mitral valve prolapse; Rheumatic fever; Vascular medicine; Vascular system.

For Further Information:
"What is Infective Endocarditis?" *American Heart Association*, 2012. PDF.
Carson-DeWitt, Rosalyn, and Michael J. Fucci. "Endocarditis." *Health Library*, Mar. 20, 2013.
Crawford, Michael, ed. *Current Diagnosis and Treatment—Cardiology*. 3d ed. New York: McGraw-Hill Medical, 2009.
Durack, David T., and Michael H. Crawford, eds. *Infective Endocarditis*. Philadelphia: W. B. Saunders, 2003.
Eagle, Kim A., and Ragavendra R. Baliga, eds. *Practical Cardiology: Evaluation and Treatment of Common Cardiovascular Disorders*. 2d ed. Philadelphia: Lippincott Williams & Wilkins, 2008.
"Endocarditis." *MedlinePlus*, Apr. 16, 2013.
Giessel, Barton E., Clint J. Koenig, and Robert L. Blake, Jr. "Information from Your Family Doctor: Bacterial Endocarditis, a Heart at Risk." *American Family Physician* 61, no. 6 (March 15, 2000): 1705.
Magilligan, Donald J. Jr., and Edward L. Quinn, eds. *Endocarditis: Medical and Surgical Management*. New York: Marcel Dekker, 1986.
Muirhead, Greg. "Targeting Therapy for Infective Endocarditis." *Patient Care* 33, no. 16 (October 15, 1999): 127–149.
Preidt, Robert. "Steady Rise in Heart Valve Infections Noted in US." *HealthDay. MedlinePlus*, Mar. 22, 2013.
"What is Endocarditis?" *National Heart, Lung, and Blood Institute*, Oct. 1, 2010.

ENDOCRINE DISORDERS
Disease/Disorder

Anatomy or system affected: Endocrine system, glands
Specialties and related fields: Endocrinology
Definition: The endocrine system controls the metabolic processes of the body. Endocrine disorders occur when the normal function of the endocrine system is disrupted.

Key terms:

cyclic AMP: a chemical that acts as a second messenger to bring about a response by the cell to the presence of some hormones at their receptors

endocrine: the secretion of hormones directly into the bloodstream, rather than by way of a duct

feedback: the mechanism whereby a hormone inhibits its own production; often involves the inhibition of the hypothalamus and tropic hormones

hypothalamohypophysial: relating to the hypothalamus and the hypophysis (pituitary gland)

target cell or organ: a cell or organ possessing the specific hormone receptors needed to respond to a given hormone

tropic: hormones that feed a particular physiological state

tropin: hormones that cause a "turning toward" a particular physiological state

Process and Effects

Endocrine disorders include disturbances in the production of hormones that result from either insufficient or excessive activity and tissues unable to respond to hormones. To understand endocrine disorders, it is necessary to review briefly the location of the principal endocrine glands, the hormones secreted, and the normal functions of the hormones. The hormones are released into the bloodstream and are carried throughout the body, where they affect target cells or organs that have receptors for the given hormone.

The pituitary gland, or hypophysis, is sometimes called the master gland because of its widespread influences on many other endocrine glands and the body as a whole. It is located in the midline on the lower part of the brain just above the posterior part of the roof of the mouth. The pituitary has three lobes: the posterior lobe, the intermediate lobe, and the anterior lobe.

The posterior lobe does not synthesize hormones, but it does have nerve fibers coming into it from the hypothalamus of the brain. The ends of these axons release two hormones that are synthesized in the hypothalamus, oxytocin and antidiuretic hormone (ADH). Oxytocin causes the contraction of the smooth muscles of the uterus during childbirth and the contraction of tissues in the mammary glands to release milk during nursing. ADH causes the kidneys to reabsorb water and thereby reduce the volume of urine to normal levels when necessary.

The intermediate lobe of the pituitary secretes melanocyte-stimulating hormone (MSH), a hormone with an uncertain role in humans but known to cause the darkening of melanocytes in animals. Sometimes, the intermediate lobe is considered to be a part of the anterior lobe.

The anterior lobe of the pituitary is under the control of releasing hormones produced by the hypothalamus and carried to the anterior lobe by special blood vessels. In response to these releasing hormones, some stimulatory and some inhibitory, the anterior lobe produces thyroid-stimulating hormone (TSH), adrenocorticotropic hormone (ACTH), follicle-stimulating hormone (FSH), luteinizing hormone (LH), prolactin, and somatotropin or growth hormone (GH). TSH stimulates the thyroid to produce thyroxine, ACTH stimulates the adrenal cortex to produce some of its hormones, FSH stimulates the growth of the cells surrounding eggs in the ovary and causes the ovary to produce estrogen, LH induces ovulation (the release of an egg from the ovary) and stimulates the secretion of progesterone by the ovary, prolactin is essential for milk production and various metabolic functions, and GH is needed for normal growth.

The pineal gland, or epiphysis, is a neuroendocrine gland attached to the roof of the diencephalon in the brain. It produces melatonin, which is released into the bloodstream during the night and has important functions related to an individual's biological clock.

The thyroid gland is located below the larynx in the front of the throat. It produces the hormones triiodothyronine (T_3) and thyroxine (T_4), which are essential for maintaining a normal level of metabolism and heat production, as well as enabling normal development of the brain in young children. Specialized cells called C cells are scattered throughout the thyroid, parathyroid, and thymus glands. These cells secrete the hormone calcitonin, which is involved in maintaining the correct blood levels of calcium. The thymus, located under the breast bone or sternum, produces the hormone thymosin that stimulates the immune system. Even the heart is an endocrine gland: It produces atrial natriuretic factor, which stimulates sodium excretion by the kidneys. The pancreas, located near the stomach and small intestine,

produces digestive enzymes that pass to the duodenum, but also it produces insulin and glucagon in special cells called pancreatic islets. Insulin causes blood sugar (glucose) to be taken up from the blood into the tissues of the body, and glucagon causes stored glycogen to be broken down in the liver and thereby increases blood glucose levels.

The pair of adrenal glands, located on the kidneys, are made up of two components: first, a cortex that produces glucocorticoids, mineralocorticoids, and sex steroids or androgens; and second, a medulla, or inner part, that secretes adrenaline and noradrenaline. The gonads, testes or ovaries, are located in the pelvic region and produce several hormones, including the estrogen and progesterone that are essential for reproduction in females and the testosterone that is essential for reproduction in males. The kidneys and digestive tract also produce hormones that regulate red blood cell formation and the functioning of the digestive tract, respectively.

Complications and Disorders

A wide variety of endocrine disorders can be treated successfully. In fact, the ability to restore normal endocrine function with replacement therapy has long been one of the techniques for showing the existence of hypothesized hormones.

The posterior pituitary releases both oxytocin and ADH. Chemicals similar to oxytocin are sometimes given to induce contractions in pregnant women so that birth will occur at a predetermined time. The other hormone released from the posterior pituitary, ADH, normally causes the reabsorption of water within the tubules of the kidney. A deficiency of ADH leads to diabetes insipidus, a condition in which many liters of water a day are excreted by the urinary system; the patient must drink huge quantities of water simply to stay alive. A synthetic form of ADH, desmopressin acetate, can be given in the form of a nasal spray that diffuses into the bloodstream and thus restores the reabsorption of water by the kidneys.

The anterior lobe of the pituitary produces six known hormones. The production of these hormones is stimulated and/ or inhibited by special releasing hormones secreted by the hypothalamus and carried to the anterior lobe by the hypothalamohypophysial portal system of blood vessels. Thus, the source of some anterior pituitary disorders can reside in the hypothalamus. Tumors of anterior pituitary cells can result in the overproduction of a hormone, or if the tumor is destructive, the underproduction of a hormone. Radiation or surgery can be used to destroy tumors and thereby restore normal pituitary functioning.

Anterior pituitary hormones can be the basis of a variety of disorders. As with other hormones, there may be below-normal production of the hormone (hyposecretion) or overproduction of the hormone (hypersecretion). Because the pituitary hormones are often supportive of hormone secretion by the target organ or tissue, hyposecretion or hypersecretion of the tropic or supportive hormone leads to a similar change in the production of hormones by the target organ or tissue.

For example, hyperthyroidism, or Graves' disease, can be caused by excessive secretion of TSH by the pituitary, leading to hypersecretion of thyroxine, or by nodules within the thyroid that produce excessive thyroxine. In the diagnosis process, blood levels of both TSH and thyroxine are usually measured to determine the specific cause of the disorder. Similarly, hypothyroidism can be induced by deficits at several levels. The lack of iodine in the diet can prevent the production of thyroxine, which requires iodide as part of its molecular composition. The production of thyroxine usually has a negative feedback effect on the hypothalamus and pituitary, reducing TSH production. The failure to produce thyroxine causes high blood levels of TSH and an abnormal growth of the thyroid that results in a greatly enlarged thyroid, called a goiter. The addition of iodine to salt has eliminated the incidence of goiter in developed countries. Even with an adequate supply of iodine in the diet, however, hypothyroidism can still develop from other sources. The usual treatment is to ingest a dose of thyroxine daily.

Other examples of anterior pituitary disorders include those involving changes in GH secretion. Undersecretion of GH can lead to short stature or even a type of dwarfism called pituitary dwarfism, in which an individual has normal body proportions but is smaller than normal. Now it is possible to obtain human GH from bacteria genetically engineered to produce it. Replacement GH can be given during the normal growth years to enhance growth. A tumor sometimes develops in the pituitary cells that produce GH, and this can cause abnormally increased growth or gigantism. If the tumor develops during the adult years, only a few areas of abnormal growth can occur, such as in the facial bones and the bones of the hands and feet. This condition is called acromegaly. Abraham Lincoln is thought to have had abnormal levels of GH that caused gigantism in his youth and then acromegaly in his later years. Acromegaly can be treated by radiation or surgery of the anterior pituitary.

Pineal gland tumors have been associated with precocious puberty, in which children become sexually developed in early childhood. It is thought that melatonin normally inhibits sexual development during this period. The pineal gland is influenced by changes in the daily photo-period, so that the highest levels of melatonin appear in the blood during the night, especially during the long nights of winter. Seasonal affective disorder (SAD), a mental depression that occurs during the late fall and winter, has been linked to seasonally high melatonin levels. Daily exposure to bright lights to mimic summer has been used to treat SAD. The pineal gland and melatonin are also being studied with regard to jet lag and disorders associated with shift work. The pineal gland thus seems to be involved in the functioning of the body's biological clock.

The pancreatic islets, also called the islets of Langerhans, produce insulin and glucagon. Diabetes mellitus is caused by insufficient insulin production (type 1 or juvenile-onset diabetes) or by the lack of functional insulin receptors on body cells (type 2 diabetes). Type 1 diabetes can be treated with insulin injections, an implanted insulin pump, or even a transplant of fetal pancreatic tissue. Type 2 diabetes is treated with diet and weight loss. Weight loss induces an increase in insulin receptors. Long-term complications resulting from high blood-sugar levels include damage to the kidneys, to the blood vessels in the retina (diabetic retinopathy), to the legs and feet, and to the nerves (diabetic neuropathy).

Changes in the levels of steroid hormones (glucocorticoids, mineralocorticoids, or androgens) secreted by the adrenal cortex can lead to disease. For example, hypersecretion of the glucocorticoid cortisol results in Cushing's syndrome and hyposecretion of cortisol results in Addison disease. Similar to the thyroid, the hormones produced by the adrenal cortex participate in a feedback loop mechanism with the pituitary and hypothalamus. Thus, when levels of hormones released by the adrenal glands are low, the pituitary and hypothalamus try to compensate by secreting higher levels of their own hormones. In Addison disease, low levels of adrenal glucocorticoids causes increased ACTH release from the pituitary. Addison disease is characterized by low blood pressure and a poor physiological response to stress: It can be treated by the administration of exogenous glucocorticoids. Extreme cases of adrenal insufficiency can bring about an "adrenal crisis." In this situation, an immediate injection of glucocorticoid hormone is given to prevent death.

In addition to treating Addison disease, glucocorticoids, particularly cortisone, are used to treat inflammation; however, overuse can lead to adrenal cortex suppression by the negative feedback mechanism. When athletes abuse the androgen sex hormones for the purpose of increasing muscle mass, adrenal suppression can develop along with sterility and damage to the heart. Masculinization is observed in women who have tumors of the androgen-producing cells of the adrenal glands. These women display several changes associated with increased male sex hormones, changes that include beard growth and increased muscle development.

Perspective and Prospects

The early history of endocrinology noted that boys who were castrated failed to undergo the changes associated with puberty. A. A. Berthold in 1849 described the effects of castration in cockerels. The birds failed to develop large combs and wattles and failed to show male behavior. He noted that these effects could be reversed if testes were transplanted back into the cockerels. W. M. Bayliss and E. H. Starling in 1902 first introduced the term "hormone" to refer to secretin. They found that secretin is produced by the small intestine in response to acid in the chyme and that secretin causes the pancreas to release digestive enzymes into the small intestine. Most important, F. G. Banting and G. H. Best in 1922 reported their extraction of insulin from the pancreas of dogs and their success in alleviating diabetes in dogs by means of injections of the insulin. Frederick Sanger in 1953 established the amino acid sequence for insulin and later won a Nobel Prize for this achievement.

Another Nobel Prize was awarded to Earl W. Sutherland, Jr., in 1971, for his demonstration in 1962 of the role of cyclic AMP as a second messenger in the sequence involved in the stimulation of cells by many hormones. Andrew V. Schally and Roger C. L. Guillemin in 1977 received a Nobel Prize for their work in isolating and determining the structures of hypothalamic regulatory peptides.

More recent achievements in endocrinological research have centered on the identification of receptors that bind with the hormone when the hormone stimulates a cell and on the genetic engineering of bacteria to produce hormones such as human growth hormone. The use of fetal tissues in endocrinological research and therapy—the host usually does not reject fetal implants—continues to be an area for future research.

—John T. Burns, Ph.D.;
updated by Sharon W. Stark, R.N., A.P.R.N., D.N.Sc.

See also Addison's disease; Adrenalectomy; Amenorrhea; Corticosteroids; Cushing's syndrome; Diabetes mellitus; Dwarfism; Dysmenorrhea; Endocrine glands; Endocrinology; Endocrinology, pediatric; Endometriosis; Fructosemia; Gigantism; Glands; Goiter; Growth; Hashimoto's thyroiditis; Hormone therapy; Hormones; Hyperhidrosis; Hyperparathyroidism and hypoparathyroidism; Hypoglycemia; Infertility, female; Infertility, male; Insulin resistance syndrome; Liver; Menopause; Menorrhagia; Metabolic disorders; Ovarian cysts; Pancreas; Pancreatitis; Parathyroidectomy; Pregnancy and gestation; Prostate gland; Prostate gland removal; Puberty and adolescence; Steroids; Testicular surgery; Thyroid disorders; Thyroid gland; Thyroidectomy.

For Further Information:

Griffin, James E., and Sergio R. Ojeda, eds. *Textbook of Endocrine Physiology.* 6th ed. New York: Oxford University Press, 2012.

Hadley, Mac E., and Jon E. Levine. *Endocrinology.* 6th ed. Upper Saddle River, N.J.: Pearson/Prentice Hall, 2007.

Henry, Helen L., and Anthony W. Norman, eds. *Encyclopedia of Hormones.* 3 vols. San Diego, Calif.: Academic Press, 2003.

Jameson, J. Larry, and Tinsley Randolph Harrison. *Harrison's Endocrinology.* New York: McGraw-Hill, 2013.

Koch, Christian A., George P. Chrousos. *Endocrine Hypertension: Underlying Mechanisms and Therapy.* New York: Humana Press, 2013.

Kronenberg, Henry M., et al., eds. *Williams Textbook of Endocrinology.* 12th ed. Philadelphia: Saunders/Elsevier, 2011.

Laws, Edward R., et al. *Pituitary Disorders: Diagnosis and Management.* Hoboken, N.J.: Wiley, 2013.

Martini, Frederic. *Fundamentals of Anatomy and Physiology.* 9th ed. Upper Saddle River, N.J.: Prentice Hall, 2012.

Radovick, Sally, and Margaret H. MacGillivray. *Pediatric Endocrinology: A Practical Clinical Guide.* New York: Humana Press, 2013.

Scanlon, Valerie, and Tina Sanders. *Essentials of Anatomy and Physiology.* 6th ed. Philadelphia: F. A. Davis, 2011.

Shaw, Michael, ed. *Everything You Need to Know About Diseases.* Springhouse, Pa.: Springhouse Press, 1996.

Wells, Ken R. "Endocrine System." In *Gale Encyclopedia of Nursing and Allied Health,* edited by Kristine Krapp. Detroit, Mich.: Gale Group, 2002.

ENDOCRINE GLANDS
Anatomy

Anatomy or system affected: Brain, endocrine system, glands, pancreas, reproductive system

Specialties and related fields: Biochemistry, endocrinology, internal medicine

Definition: Organs that send chemical messages through the blood to target cells. They are responsible for maintaining homeostasis by tightly regulating physiological processes.

Key terms:

exocrine gland: a gland that releases its secretions via ducts to external surfaces

homeostasis: the process by which a constant internal environment is maintained

hormones: signaling molecules secreted into the blood by endocrine glands

negative feedback: the mechanism whereby the output of a process acts on the original input, resulting in a dampening of the process

Structure and Function

Endocrine glands produce chemical messenger molecules called hormones. Hormones bind to receptors on the cells of the target organ, which causes the cells to respond internally by modifying their biochemical pathways. Unlike exocrine glands, which secrete their products via ducts, endocrine glands secrete hormones directly into the bloodstream: they are ductless. Together, the endocrine glands form the endocrine system.

The glands of the endocrine system and their target organs work in concert; many target organs of endocrine glands are, themselves, endocrine glands. In this way, relatively small signals can be amplified until the desired response takes place in the target organs. This response often leads to a signal being sent to the initiating endocrine gland, which reduces secretion of the original hormone, dampening the entire pathway. This process is called negative feedback.

The hypothalamus and the pituitary gland are located next to each other at the base of the brain. They are the master regulators of the endocrine system. The hypothalamus receives input from nerves in the brain. This triggers the hypothalamus to secrete hormones that act directly on the pituitary, causing it to secrete its own hormones. Depending on the original stimulus, the output of the hypothalamus and pituitary regulates the thyroid gland, adrenal glands, or the gonads.

The thyroid gland is in the neck wrapped around the trachea. The thyroid maintains control of metabolism, the rate at which the body uses energy. Associated with the thyroid gland are four parathyroid glands. These secrete parathyroid hormone, which is important for maintaining correct calcium levels in the blood.

There are two adrenal glands, one on top of each kidney. They are responsible for the secretion of glucocorticoids, mineralocorticoids, and androgens. Adrenal glands are important in fluid and electrolyte homeostasis and in the stress response.

The gonads (ovaries and testes) are located in the pelvic region. In addition to producing the gametes (eggs and sperm), these glands secrete androgens and estrogens, hormones that are essential for the development and maintenance of sexual characteristics.

The pancreas is in the abdominal cavity, underneath the stomach, closely associated with the digestive tract. A majority of the pancreas acts as an exocrine gland secreting digestive enzymes. However, scattered throughout the pancreas are groups of endocrine cells called islets of Langerhans. The two major hormones secreted by these islets are insulin and glucagon; they are crucial for the maintenance of constant glucose levels in the body.

The pineal gland is located in the center of the brain. It secretes melatonin, a hormone that regulates sleep patterns.

Disorders and Diseases

Endocrinology is the medical field in which endocrine glands are studied. The diagnosis of endocrine gland disorders involves testing the levels of hormones in the blood of the patient. This can be difficult, because most hormones are secreted in pulses. Testing must be performed over hours, days, or weeks, depending on the hormone.

Most diseases that involve the endocrine glands are a result of either the oversecretion or undersecretion of hormones. This upsets the optimal physiological homeostasis and forces negative feedback loops to work inappropriately. Three examples of endocrine disorders are diabetes mellitus, hyperthyroidism, and hypothyroidism.

Diabetes mellitus is the most common endocrine disorder in the United States. The pancreas of an individual suffering from diabetes mellitus produces either too little insulin or insulin that cannot be used by the target cells. The result is abnormally high levels of glucose in the blood. Symptoms of diabetes mellitus include increased thirst and urination, fatigue, and blurred vision. Long-term complications of high blood-glucose levels include blindness, numbness in the feet, kidney failure, and heart disease. Treatment for diabetes mellitus

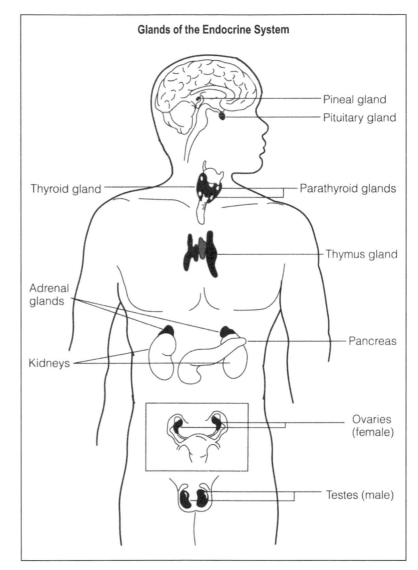

Glands of the Endocrine System

Pineal gland
Pituitary gland
Thyroid gland
Parathyroid glands
Thymus gland
Adrenal glands
Pancreas
Kidneys
Ovaries (female)
Testes (male)

includes insulin injection, drugs that improve the ability of target cells to react to glucose, and drugs that lower glucose levels in the blood.

Thyroid disorders are the second most common endocrine gland problem. Hyperthyroidism is the oversecretion of thyroid hormones caused, for example, by an enlarged thyroid gland (Graves' disease), or by nodules on the thyroid. Symptoms include a fast heart rate, weight loss, and intolerance of heat. Treatment includes drugs that reduce thyroid hormone production, surgery, or radiation therapy.

Hypothyroidism, insufficient thyroid hormone production, is more common. It is usually caused by inflammation of the thyroid (for example, Hashimoto's thyroiditis), or by over-compensatory medical treatment (for example, too much thyroid being removed during surgery to treat thyroid nodules). Symptoms include weight gain, cold intolerance, and hair loss. Hypothyroidism is usually treated with levothyroxine, a synthetic form of thyroxine which is one of the major thyroid hormones.

Perspective and Prospects

Carvings from ancient Egyptian times have been identified that show people with enlarged thyroid glands (goiter) and acromegaly (a disorder in which the pituitary gland produces too much growth hormone). However, it was in the eighteenth century that scientists and clinicians really began to understand the concept of endocrine glands and identified them as ductless glands that secrete hormones.

The revolution in the treatment of endocrine gland dysfunction came with the ability to synthesize human hormones in the laboratory. A few examples of synthetic hormones now available are insulin, growth hormone, and thyroxine. Previously, these hormones were purified from animal, or even cadaver, organs. Synthetic hormones are cheaper and safer and the doses are more easily regulated than the hormones available previously.

New testing methods and treatments for endocrine disorders are being researched. One example is the possibility of an insulin drug that can be administered orally instead of by injection. An exciting prospect for the future is the use of stem cell therapy to provide replacement hormones within the affected individual's own body.

—*Claire L. Standen, Ph.D.*

See also Addison's disease; Adrenalectomy; Corticosteroids; Cushing's syndrome; Diabetes mellitus; Endocrine disorders; Endocrinology; Endocrinology, pediatric; Gestational diabetes; Glands; Goiter; Growth; Hair loss and baldness; Hashimoto's thyroiditis; Hormone therapy; Hormones; Hyperparathyroidism and hypoparathyroidism; Obesity; Obesity, childhood; Pancreas; Pancreatitis; Parathyroidectomy; Thyroid disorders; Thyroid gland; Thyroidectomy; Weight loss and gain.

For Further Information:

Carmichael, Kim. "Hyperthyroidism." *Health Library*, November 26, 2012.

"Endocrine System." *MedlinePlus*, April 8, 2013.

Gardner, Dave, and Delores Shoback. *Greenspan's Basic and Clinical Endocrinology*. 9th ed. New York: McGraw-Hill Medical, 2011.

Koeppen, Bruce, and Bruce Stanton. *Berne and Levy Physiology*. UPdated 6th ed. Philadelphia: Elsevier, 2010.

Neal, Matthew. *How the Endocrine System Works*. Malden, Mass.: Blackwell Science, 2001.

Wood, Debra, and Kim Carmichael. "Type 1 Diabetes." *Health Library*, November 26, 2012.

Wood, Debra, and Lawrence Frisch. "Type 2 Diabetes." *Health Library*, July 17, 2012.

ENDOCRINOLOGY

Specialty

Anatomy or system affected: Brain, endocrine system, glands, immune system, nervous system, pancreas, psychic-emotional system, reproductive system, uterus

Specialties and related fields: Biochemistry, genetics, gynecology, immunology

Definition: The science dealing with how the internal secretions from ductless glands in the body act both in normal physiology and in disease states.

Key terms:

adrenal gland: an endocrine gland situated immediately above the upper pole of each kidney; it consists of an inner part or medulla, which produces epinephrine and norepinephrine, and an outer part or cortex, which produces steroid hormones

endocrine pancreas: specialized secretory tissue dispersed within the pancreas called islets of Langerhans, which are responsible for the secretion of glucagon and insulin

hypothalamus: the region of the brain called the diencephalon, forming the floor of the third ventricle, including neighboring associated nuclei

metabolism: the process of tissue change, which may be synthetic (anabolic) or degradative (catabolic)

parathyroid gland: one of four small endocrine glands situated underneath the thyroid gland, whose main product is parathyroid hormone, which regulate serum calcium levels

pituitary gland: a small (0.5-gram), two-lobed endocrine gland that is attached by a stalk to the brain at the level of the hypothalamus

thyroid gland: a 20-gram endocrine gland that sits in front of the trachea and consists of two lateral lobes connected in the middle by an isthmus

Science and Profession

The rates of metabolic pathways in the body are controlled mainly by the endocrine system, in conjunction with the nervous system. These two systems are integrated in the neuroendocrine system, which controls the secretion of hormones by the endocrine glands. The study of endocrinology deals with the normal physiology and pathophysiology of endocrine glands. The endocrine glands that are typically the main focus of clinical endocrinologists are the hypothalamus, pituitary gland, thyroid, parathyroid, adrenal glands, endocrine pancreas, ovaries, and testes. The endocrine system regulates virtually all activities of the body, including growth and development, homeostasis, energy production, and reproduction.

The hypothalamus is a highly specialized endocrine organ that sits at the base of the brain and that functions as the master gland of the endocrine system. It is the main integrator for the endocrine and nervous systems. The hypothalamus produces a number of chemical mediators that have direct control over the pituitary gland. These chemicals are made in the cells of the hypothalamus and reach the pituitary gland, which sits just below it, by a special hypophyseoportal blood system. In adult humans, the pituitary is divided into two lobes: the anterior lobe (adenohypophysis) and the posterior lobe (neural lobe).

Vasopressin and oxytocin are the two main hormones that are made in the hypothalamus but stored in the posterior lobe of the pituitary for release when needed. Vasopressin (also known as antidiuretic hormone, or ADH) is a hormone that maintains a normal water concentration in the blood and is a regulator of circulating blood volume. Oxytocin is a hormone that is involved in lactation and obstetrical labor.

The hypothalamic-pituitary-thyroid axis is important in the control of basal metabolic rate. There are a number of releasing hormones secreted from the hypothalamus that control the release of anterior pituitary hormones, which then cause the release of hormones at the end organ. Most of these hormones have the chemical structures of peptides. Thyrotropin-releasing hormone (TRH) was the first hypothalamic releasing hormone that was synthesized and used clinically. TRH, secreted in nanogram quantities, is a cyclic tripeptide that causes the release of thyrotropin-stimulating hormone (TSH) from the thyrotropic cells of the anterior pituitary gland. The release of TSH is in microgram quantities and leads to an increase in thyroid hormone release by the thyroid gland. The amount of thyroid hormone synthesized is on the order of milligrams. Therefore, the secretion of minute amounts of TRH allows for the production of thyroid hormone that is a millionfold greater than the amount of TRH itself. This is an example of an amplifying cascade, a system by which the central nervous system can control all metabolic processes with the secretion of very small amounts of hypothalamic releasing hormones. This intricate system possesses controls to stop the production of too much hormone as well. Such negative feedback is an important concept in endocrinology.

In the case of the thyroid, an increased amount of thyroid hormone produced by the thyroid gland will cause the pituitary and hypothalamus to decrease the amounts that they produce of TSH and TRH, respectively. Many hormones are subject to the laws of negative feedback control. TRH also causes potent release of the anterior pituitary hormone called prolactin. Thyroid hormone is important in determining basal metabolism and is needed for proper development in the newborn child. The thyroid gland produces both thyroxine (T_4), also called tetraiodothyronine) and triiodothyronine (T_3), both of which it synthesizes from iodine and the amino acid tyrosine.

The hypothalamic-pituitary-adrenal axis is critical in the reaction to stress, both physical and emotional. Corticotropin-releasing hormone (CRH) is a polypeptide, consisting of forty-one amino acids, that causes the production of the proopiomelanocortin molecule by the corticotropic cells of the anterior pituitary. The proopiomelanocortin molecule is cleaved by proteolytic enzymes to yield adrenocorticotropic hormone (ACTH, also called corticotropin), melanocyte-stimulating hormone, and lipotropin. It is ACTH made by the anterior pituitary, which then stimulates the adrenal cortex to produce steroid hormones. The main stress hormone produced by the adrenal cortex in response to ACTH is the glucocorticoid cortisol. ACTH also has some control over the production of the mineralocorticoid aldosterone and the androgens dehydroepiandrosterone and testosterone. These steroids are synthesized from cholesterol. The production of cortisol (also known as hydrocortisone) is subject to negative feedback by CRH and ACTH.

The hypothalamic-pituitary-gonadal axis is involved in the control of reproduction. Gonadotropin-releasing hormone (GnRH), also known as luteinizing hormone-releasing hormone (LHRH), is produced by the hypothalamus and stimulates the release of luteinizing hormone (LH) and follicle-stimulating hormone (FSH) from the gonadotrophic cells of the anterior pituitary. LH and FSH have different effects in men and women. In men, LH controls the production and secretion of testosterone by the Leydig cells of the testes. The release of LH is regulated by negative feedback from testosterone. FSH along with testosterone acts on the Sertoli cells of the seminiferous tubule of the testis at the time of puberty to start sperm production. In women, LH controls ovulation by the ovary and also the development of the corpus luteum, which produces progesterone. Progesterone is a steroid hormone that is critically important for the maintenance of pregnancy. FSH in women stimulates the development and maturation of a primary follicle and oocyte. The ovarian follicle in the nonpregnant woman is the main site of production of estradiol. Estradiol is the principal estrogen made in the reproductive years by the ovary and is responsible for the development of female secondary sexual characteristics.

Growth hormone-releasing hormone (GHRH) is a polypeptide with forty-four amino acids that stimulates the release of growth hormone (GH) from the somatotrophic cells of the anterior pituitary. The regulation of GH secretion is under dual control. While GHRH positively releases GH, somatostatin (a polypeptide with fourteen amino acids, also released from the hypothalamus) inhibits the release of GH. Somatostatin has a wide variety of functions, including the suppression of insulin, glucagon, and gastrointestinal hormones. GH released from the pituitary circulates in the bloodstream and stimulates the production of somatomedins by the liver. Several somatomedins are produced, all of which have a profound effect on growth, with the most important one in humans being somatomedin C, also called insulin-like growth factor I (IGF I). Molecular biological techniques have shown that many cells outside the liver also produce IGF I; in these cells, IGF I acts in autocrine or paracrine ways to cause the growth of the cells or to affect neighboring cells.

Prolactin is a peptide hormone that is secreted by the lactotrophs of the anterior pituitary. It is involved in the differentiation of the mammary gland cells and initiates the production of milk proteins and other constituents. Prolactin may also have other functions, as a stress hormone or growth hormone. Prolactin is under tonic negative control. The inhibition of prolactin release is caused by dopamine, which is produced by the hypothalamus. Thus, while dopamine is normally considered to be a neurotransmitter, in the case of prolactin release it acts as an inhibitory hormone. Serotonin, also classically thought of as a neurotransmitter, may cause the stimulation of prolactin release from the anterior pituitary.

Diagnostic and Treatment Techniques
One of the most common medical problems seen by specialists in the field of endocrinology is a patient with type 1

diabetes mellitus, sometimes also called juvenile-onset or insulin-dependent diabetes mellitus. "Insulin-dependent" is probably more appropriate, as not all patients with type 1 diabetes mellitus develop the disease in childhood. Type 1 diabetes is an autoimmune disease in which antibodies to different parts of the pancreatic beta cell, the cell that normally produces insulin, are produced. Some of these antibodies are cytotoxic; that is, they actually destroy the pancreatic beta cell. The most striking characteristic of patients with type 1 diabetes is that they produce very little insulin. The symptoms of type 1 diabetes include increased thirst, increased urination, blurring of vision, and weight loss. A doctor would confirm the diagnosis by running blood tests for glucose and insulin. The glucose level would be high, and the insulin level would be low. The treatment includes controlled diet, exercise, insulin therapy, and self-monitoring of blood glucose. With proper control of blood glucose, patients with type 1 diabetes can lead normal, productive lives.

Graves' disease is another autoimmune disease that is commonly seen by endocrinologists. Graves' disease is caused by the production of thyroid-stimulating immunoglobulin antibodies that bind to and activate TSH receptors. As a result, the thyroid gland produces too much thyroid hormone and the thyroid gland enlarges in size. The antibodies also commonly affect the eyes, causing a characteristic bulging. The clinical symptoms of hyperthyroidism include increased heart rate, anxiety, heat sensitivity, sleeplessness, diarrhea, and abdominal pain. Patients often lose considerable weight, despite having a great appetite and eating large amounts of food. Sometimes, the diagnosis is missed, leading to an extensive evaluation for a variety of other diseases. Often, a family history of thyroid disease or other endocrine disease can be found.

The usual method of screening for Graves' disease is with a simple blood test for thyroid function, which includes testing for T_4, T_3, and TSH. In patients with Graves' disease, both T_4 and T_3 will be elevated, and TSH will be very low. If the blood test reveals this pattern, the next usual step is to proceed to a radioactive iodine uptake and scan test, which involves giving a very small amount of radioactive iodine by mouth and having the patient return twenty-four hours later for a scan. The thyroid gland normally accumulates iodine and thus will accumulate the radioactive iodine as well. The radioactive iodine emits a gamma-ray energy that can be picked up by a solid-crystal scintillation counter placed over the thyroid gland. With this device, one can determine the percentage of iodine uptake and also obtain a picture of the thyroid gland. The normal radioactive iodine uptake is about 10 to 30 percent of the dose, depending somewhat on the amount of total body iodine, which is derived from the diet. Patients with Graves' disease will have high radioactive iodine uptakes.

Those who suffer from Graves' disease can be treated by three different means, depending on the circumstances. The first treatment that is often tried is antithyroid drugs, either propylthiouracil or methimazole. These drugs belong to the class of sulfonamides and inhibit the production of new thyroid hormone by blocking the attachment of iodine to the amino acid tyrosine. Another mode of therapy is the use of radioactive iodine. A dose of radioactive iodine (on the order of five to ten millicuries) is used to destroy part of the thyroid gland. The gamma-ray energy emitted from the iodine molecule that has traveled to the thyroid gland is enough to kill some thyroid cells. An alternative way to destroy the thyroid gland is to remove it surgically (thyroidectomy). Endocrinologists rarely send patients for surgery, as the other therapies are often effective. The goal of all treatments is to bring the level of thyroid hormone into the normal range, as well as to shrink the thyroid gland. After treatment, the patient's level of thyroid hormone sometimes falls to levels that are below normal. The symptoms of hypothyroidism are the opposite of hyperthyroidism and include fatigue, weight gain, cold sensitivity, constipation, and dry skin. If this happens, the patient is treated with thyroid hormone replacement. The dose is adjusted for each individual to produce normal levels of T_4, T_3, and TSH.

A less common but important endocrine disorder is the existence of a pituitary tumor that secretes prolactin, called a prolactinoma. Prolactinomas are diagnosed earlier in women than in men, as women with the disorder often complain of a lack of menstrual periods and spontaneous milk production from the breasts, known as galactorrhea. These tumors, which can be quite small, are called microadenomas because they are less than ten millimeters in size. They can affect men as well, causing decreased sex drive and impotence. Macroadenomas are tumors greater than ten millimeters in size. When the tumors increase in size, they can cause symptoms such as headache and decreased vision. It is important to note that most microadenomas never progress to macroadenomas. Vision loss and/or decreased eye movement can be seen with a macroadenoma and are reason for immediate treatment.

Doctors screen patients for a prolactinoma by running a blood test for prolactin. There are other reasons for mild elevations in prolactin levels, including the use of certain psychiatric drugs such as phenothiazines or the antihypertensive drugs reserpine and methyldopa, primary hypothyroidism, cirrhosis, and chronic renal failure. If a pituitary tumor is suspected, then other biochemical tests of pituitary function are conducted to determine if the rest of the gland is functioning normally. At that time, imaging tests are often done to get a picture of the hypothalamic-pituitary area; this can be done with either computed tomography (CT) scanning or magnetic resonance imaging (MRI). Patients with macroadenomas will require treatment. In patients with little neurological involvement, medical therapy may be initiated. Bromocriptine, a semisynthetic ergot alkaloid that is an inhibitor of prolactin secretion, may be used. It has been shown that patients treated with this drug have a reduction in tumor size. Patients can be maintained on the drug indefinitely because prolactin levels return to pretreatment levels when the drug is stopped. If there is severe neurologic involvement, with loss of vision and other eye problems, immediate surgery may be indicated. There is a very high incidence of tumor recurrence after surgery, requiring medical and/or radiation therapy.

Perspective and Prospects

The field of endocrinology is a continuously evolving one. Advances in biomedical technology, including molecular biology and cell biology, have made it a demanding job for the clinician to keep up with all the breakthroughs in the field. The challenge for endocrinology will be to apply many of these new technologies to novel treatments for patients with endocrine diseases.

An example of the progression of the field of endocrinology can be seen in the history of pituitary diseases. The start of pituitary endocrinology is ascribed to Pierre Marie, the French neurologist who in 1886 first described pituitary enlargement in a patient with acromegaly (enlargement of the skull, jaw, hands, and feet) and linked the disease to a pituitary abnormality. During the first half of the twentieth century, many of the hypothalamic and pituitary hormones were isolated and characterized. The field of endocrinology was revolutionized by the development of radioimmunoassay, which allows sensitive and specific measurements of hormones. Radioimmunoassay replaced bioassay techniques, which were laborious, time-consuming, and not always precise. This technique has allowed for rapid measurement of hormones and improved screening for endocrine diseases involving hormone deficiency or hormone excess.

The development of new hormone assays has been complemented by the development of noninvasive imaging techniques. Before the advent of CT scanning in the late 1970s, it was an ordeal to diagnose a pituitary tumor. Pneumoencephalography was often performed, which involved injecting air into the fluid-containing structures of the brain, with associated risk and discomfort to the patient. In the 1980s, with new generations of high-resolution CT scanners that were more sensitive than early scanners, smaller pituitary lesions could be detected and diagnosed. That decade also ushered in the use of MRI to diagnose disorders of the hypothalamic-pituitary unit. MRI has allowed doctors to evaluate the hypothalamus, pituitary, and nearby structures very precisely; it has become the method of choice for evaluating patients with pituitary disease. MRI can easily visualize the optic chiasm in the forebrain and the vascular structures surrounding the pituitary.

In patients who require surgery, advances have helped decrease mortality rates. Harvey Cushing pioneered the transsphenoidal technique in 1927 but abandoned it in favor of the transfrontal approach. This involves reaching the pituitary tumor by retracting the frontal lobes to visualize the pituitary gland sitting underneath. The modern era of transsphenoidal pituitary surgery was developed by Gérard Guiot and Jules Hardy in the late 1960s. Transsphenoidal surgery done with an operating microscope to visualize the pituitary contents allows for selective removal of the tumor, leaving the normal pituitary gland intact. The advantage of this approach from below, instead of from above, includes minimal movement of the brain and less blood loss. This technique requires a neurosurgeon with much skill and experience. There are also new drug treatments for patients with pituitary diseases, such as bromocriptine for use in patients with prolactinomas and octreotide (a somatostatin analogue) to lower growth hormone levels in patients with acromegaly.

—*RoseMarie Pasmantier, M.D.*

See also Addison's disease; Adrenalectomy; Chronobiology; Corticosteroids; Cushing's syndrome; Diabetes mellitus; Dwarfism; Endocrine disorders; Endocrine glands; Endocrinology, pediatric; Enzymes; Fructosemia; Gender reassignment surgery; Gestational diabetes; Gigantism; Glands; Goiter; Growth; Gynecology; Hair loss and baldness; Hashimoto's thyroiditis; Hormone therapy; Hormones; Hot flashes; Hyperhidrosis; Hyperparathyroidism and hypoparathyroidism; Hypoglycemia; Hysterectomy; Melatonin; Menopause; Menstruation; Metabolic disorders; Obesity; Obesity, childhood; Paget's disease; Pancreas; Pancreatitis; Parathyroidectomy; Pharmacology; Pharmacy; Prostate gland; Prostate gland removal; Puberty and adolescence; Sexual differentiation; Steroids; Thyroid disorders; Thyroid gland; Thyroidectomy; Weight loss and gain.

For Further Information:

Bar, Robert S., ed. *Early Diagnosis and Treatment of Endocrine Disorders*. Totowa, N.J.: Humana Press, 2003.

Braverman, Lewis E., and David S. Cooper, eds. *Werner and Ingbar's The Thyroid: A Fundamental and Clinical Text*. 10th ed. Philadelphia: Lippincott Williams & Wilkins, 2013.

"Diabetes." *MedlinePlus*, 7 Aug. 2013.

"Endocrine Diseases." *MedlinePlus*, 16 July 2013.

Harmel, Anne Peters, and Ruchi Mathur. *Davidson's Diabetes Mellitus: Diagnosis and Treatment*. 5th ed. Philadelphia: W. B. Saunders, 2004.

Imura, Hiroo, ed. *The Pituitary Gland*. 2d ed. New York: Raven Press, 1994.

Lebovitz, Harold E., ed. *Therapy for Diabetes Mellitus and Related Disorders*. 5th ed. Alexandria, Va.: American Diabetes Association, 2009.

Melmed, Shlomo, et al. *Williams Textbook of Endocrinology*. 12th ed. Philadelphia: Saunders/Elsevier, 2011.

"Pituitary Tumors." *MedlinePlus*, 23 July 2013.

Speroff, Leon, and Marc A. Fritz. *Clinical Gynecologic Endocrinology and Infertility*. 8th ed. Philadelphia: Lippincott Williams & Wilkins, 2011.

"Thyroid Diseases." *MedlinePlus*, 5 Aug. 2013.

Vorvick, Linda J., and David Zieve. "Endocrine Glands." *MedlinePlus*, 1 May 2011.

ENDOCRINOLOGY, PEDIATRIC

Specialty

Anatomy or system affected: Brain, endocrine system, glands, immune system, nervous system, pancreas, psychic-emotional system

Specialties and related fields: Biochemistry, genetics, immunology, neonatology, pediatrics

Definition: The study of the normal and abnormal function of the endocrine (ductless) glands in children and adolescents.

Key terms:

hormone: a chemical molecule produced in either the hypothalamus or one of the endocrine glands that is secreted and travels (usually via the bloodstream) to a target organ or to specific receptor cells, causing a specific response

insulin: a hormone that is essential in regulating blood glucose, as well as in assimilating carbohydrates for growth and energy

pancreas: a large gland near the stomach which has both exocrine and endocrine functions and which produces insulin

pituitary gland: a very small gland at the base of the brain that is referred to as the master gland; with the hypothalamus, it regulates most of the endocrine systems

thyroid: a gland in the anterior neck which regulates the level of the body's metabolism and which is instrumental in normal physical and mental growth

Science and Profession

Pediatric endocrinology is a major subspecialty, limited to children and adolescents, which involves the study of normal as well as abnormal functions of the endocrine system, which comprises the glands of internal or ductless secretions. These practitioners, referred to as endocrinologists or pediatric endocrinologists, are doctors of medicine or osteopathy who have completed three years of pediatric residency training and an additional two to three years of fellowship training in endocrinology.

Endocrinology is one of the most interesting and challenging fields in pediatrics because it requires a blend of basic science and technology in the clinical setting. Some of the diagnoses are very difficult, yet they are almost always completely logical. Endocrinology is tightly related to other areas of pediatrics, such as adolescent medicine, genetics, growth, development, nutrition, and metabolism. These relationships make this field even more complex and intellectually stimulating.

Pediatric endocrinology and adult endocrinology are relatively young fields, probably beginning with the discovery in 1888 that "myxedema" (hypothyroidism) could be improved by feeding the patient thyroid extract. Both fields deal with the major endocrine glands and their disorders, such as diabetes mellitus or hypothyroidism, but there are several key differences, most related to growth (both physical and mental), potential, and genetics. Some major areas of specific emphasis in pediatric endocrinology include diabetes mellitus (which presents very differently in children), disorders of growth, disorders of sexual maturation and differentiation, genetic disorders, and adolescent medicine.

Diagnostic and Treatment Techniques

In pediatric endocrinology, as in all medical fields, history taking and physical examination are the starting points and usually the most useful tools for diagnosis. Endocrinology is a specialty that is particularly aided by science. Blood and urine chemistries, hormone assays, chromosomal analyses, X-rays, computed tomography (CT) scans, magnetic resonance imaging (MRI), and a host of other sophisticated tests have advanced diagnoses and treatments and have made this specialty one of the favorites for physicians who like science. Virtually all the known hormones can be assayed accurately and quickly.

Since insulin was first available for injection in 1922, there have been amazing advances in treatment. Many of the treatments in endocrinology involve hormone therapy. In 1985, recombinant growth hormone was synthesized for the first time. This development has allowed endocrinologists to treat not only pituitary dwarfism but also other kinds of growth deficiencies, such as Turner syndrome.

Turner syndrome is a relatively common chromosomal abnormality affecting females and resulting in short stature and lack of sexual development. While these girls will never become fertile, the combination of growth hormone for stature and other hormonal therapy for the development of secondary sexual characteristics enables them to have a normal female body. Studies have shown that normal body image and the presence of menstruation is essential for the self-esteem of these patients.

Diabetes mellitus is the most common significant endocrine disorder in both adults and children. What was commonly referred to as juvenile diabetes years ago is now called diabetes mellitus, type 1. Unlike type 2, which usually presents insidiously in middle-aged and older adults, type 1 presents rapidly, and the patient will need daily injectable insulin treatments. Diabetes in children is complex to manage not only because of the insulin treatment but also because of the patients" growth, metabolism, fluctuating activity levels, and physiologic and psychological changes that occur, especially in adolescence.

Now small portable and quite accurate glucometers allow patients to measure blood glucose (sugar) at home, making diabetes management much simpler. Tighter control of blood glucose will decrease or delay the onset of long-term complications of the disease, such as blindness, heart disease, and kidney disease. In the United States, newborn screening, which is now performed in all fifty states, has virtually eliminated cretinism, which tragically resulted when congenital hypothyroidism was not diagnosed until later in childhood. These children were irreversibly developmentally disabled.

Enhanced techniques in pediatric surgery and neurosurgery, greatly aided by scans, play a role in the treatment of some endocrine disorders. Very small tumors and masses can be identified and often removed successfully. Often, endocrinologists and oncologists work together in concert with the surgeon.

Although this subspecialty is one of the most scientific and laboratory-based in pediatrics, it is also a field where emotional support, counseling, and often mental health care are given. Children do not like being "different," and body image is very important in children and particularly in teenagers. Even when a child appears absolutely normal, the frustration of ongoing monitoring and treatment is resented and can result in rebellion, especially in children with diabetes. Often, a team approach is needed, which involves professionals, teachers, family, and peers.

Perspective and Prospects

The future promises ever-advancing and dramatic tools for the diagnosis and treatment of endocrine disorders, as well as for their prevention. An implantible glucose pump, which can serve as a substitute pancreas, can change the lives of diabetic patients dramatically. A method for rapidly analyzing blood glucose using the surface of the skin has been developed. In addition, genetic engineering may revolutionize the approaches to treating many of these diseases.

—*C. Mervyn Rasmussen, M.D.*

See also Addison's disease; Adrenalectomy; Chronobiology; Corticosteroids; Diabetes mellitus; Dwarfism; Endocrine disorders; Endocrine glands; Endocrinology; Enzymes; Fructosemia; Gigantism; Glands; Growth; Gynecology; Hormone therapy; Hormones; Hyperparathyroidism and hypoparathyroidism; Hypoglycemia; Melatonin; Menstruation; Metabolic disorders; Obesity; Obesity, childhood; Pancreas; Pancreatitis; Parathyroidectomy; Pediatrics; Pharmacology; Pharmacy; Puberty and adolescence; Steroids; Thyroid disorders; Thyroid gland; Thyroidectomy; Weight loss and gain.

For Further Information:

Bar, Robert S., ed. *Early Diagnosis and Treatment of Endocrine Disorders.* Totowa, N.J.: Humana Press, 2003.

"Diabetes in Children and Teens." *MedlinePlus*, 24 July 2013.

Dowshen, Steven. "Endocrine System." *KidsHealth*. Nemours Foundation, Mar. 2012.

"Growth Disorders." *MedlinePlus*, 2 Aug. 2013.

Handwerger, Stuart, ed. *Molecular and Cellular Pediatric Endocrinology.* Totowa, N.J.: Humana Press, 1999.

Harmel, Anne Peters, and Ruchi Mathur. *Davidson's Diabetes Mellitus: Diagnosis and Treatment.* 5th ed. Philadelphia: W. B. Saunders, 2004.

Little, Marjorie. *Diabetes.* New York: Chelsea House, 1991.

Melmed, Shlomo, et al. *Williams Textbook of Endocrinology.* 12th ed. Philadelphia: Saunders/Elsevier, 2011.

Sperling, Mark A., ed. *Pediatric Endocrinology.* 3d ed. Philadelphia: Saunders/Elsevier, 2008.

"Thyroid Diseases." *MedlinePlus*, 5 Aug. 2013.

Wales, Jeremy K. H., and Jan Maarten Wit. *Pediatric Endocrinology and Growth.* 2d ed. Philadelphia: W. B. Saunders, 2004.

ENDODONTIC DISEASE

Disease/Disorder

Anatomy or system affected: Mouth, teeth

Specialties and related fields: Dentistry

Definition: Disease of the dental pulp and sometimes also the soft tissues and bone around the tip of the root.

Causes and Symptoms

The most common cause of endodontic disease is infection of the dental pulp by the bacteria that cause tooth decay. The pulp is composed of connective tissue, nerves, blood vessels, and tooth regenerative cells. It fills the root canal, a narrow channel in the center of the tooth root, which is embedded in the jawbone. Teeth usually contain one to four root canals. Decay-causing bacteria reach the pulp after dissolving their way through the two, hard outer layers of the tooth—the enamel and dentin. Bacteria may also reach the pulp through a crack or fracture in a tooth and through tooth wear or abrasion. Many kinds of bacteria can infect the pulp.

Pulp infected by bacteria becomes inflamed and has no place to swell because it is surrounded by dentin, which is rigid. Pain may result. Eventually, the entire pulp may become infected and die. If not treated, the infection can spread to the soft tissue and bone surrounding the tip of the root and form an abscess, which often produces severe pain.

Information on Endodontic Disease

Causes: Bacterial infection of dental pulp

Symptoms: Gum inflammation and pain, which is severe if abscess forms

Duration: Chronic if untreated

Treatments: Root canal treatment

Treatment and Therapy

To treat damaged or dead pulp tissue and preserve the tooth, endodontic therapy, or root canal treatment, is required. Endodontists specialize in this procedure. One or two visits are usually required. A small hole is made in the top (crown) of the infected tooth, and all the pulp tissue is removed. Then an inert material, usually a piece of rubberlike gum called gutta percha, is inserted in place of the pulp and secured in place with a sealer or cement. A tooth that has had root canal treatment is commonly considered to be dead, but the fibers of the periodontal ligament that hold the tooth in the jawbone are still alive. Following this procedure, additional dental treatments are necessary to preserve the weakened tooth.

Perspective and Prospects

Historically, the only remedy for endodontic disease was tooth extraction. Since the mid-twentieth century, endodontic research has yielded treatments that preserve infected teeth. Furthermore, there has been an increased appreciation of the role of dental hygiene in preventing tooth decay and the endodontic infections that can result from it. Research on the causes and prevention of endodontic disease, and treatments for it, is being conducted at dental schools and at the National Institute of Dental and Cranio-Facial Research.

—*Jane F. Hill, Ph.D.*

See also Bacterial infections; Cavities; Dental diseases; Dentistry; Gingivitis; Gum disease; Periodontal surgery; Periodontitis; Root canal treatment; Teeth; Tooth extraction; Toothache.

For Further Information:

Alan, Rick, and Michael Woods. "Tooth Abscess." *Health Library*, Mar. 18, 2013.

Christensen, Gordon J. *A Consumer's Guide to Dentistry.* 2d ed. St. Louis, Mo.: Mosby, 2002.

Chwistek, Marcin. "Root Canal Treatment." *Health Library*, Mar. 15, 2013.

Fotek, Paul, and David Zieve. "Root Canal." *MedlinePlus*, Feb. 22, 2012.

"Gum Disease." *MedlinePlus*, Apr. 25, 2013.

Healthnet: Connecticut Consumer Health Information Network. "Your Dental Health: A Guide for Patients and Families." *UConn Health Center*, Nov. 27, 2012.

Ingle, John Ide, LEif K. Bakland, and J. Craig Baumgartner. *Ingle's Endodontics.* 6th ed. Hamilton, Ont.: McGraw-Hill, 2008.

Kim, Syngcuk, ed. *Modern Endodontic Practice.* Philadelphia: W. B. Saunders, 2004.

Porter, Robert S., et al., eds. *The Merck Manual Home Health Handbook.* 3d ed. Whitehouse Station, N.J.: Merck Research Laboratories, 2009.

Smith, Rebecca W. *The Columbia University School of Dental and Oral Surgery's Guide to Family Dental Care.* New York: W. W. Norton, 1997.

ENDOMETRIAL BIOPSY

Procedure

Anatomy or system affected: Genitals, reproductive system, uterus

Specialties and related fields: Gynecology, histology, obstetrics, preventive medicine

Definition: A procedure in which a tissue sample is taken from the lining of the uterus and then examined.

Key terms:

cervix: the entrance to the uterus

dilation and curettage (D&C): a procedure in which the cervix is stretched and the lining of the uterus is scraped

endometrium: tissue lining the inside of the uterus

hysteroscopy: a procedure using a thin, lighted tube with a camera and tool to examine visually and remove part of the endometrium

uterus: the part of the reproductive tract that supports the development and nourishment of a developing fetus; also called the womb

vagina: the tube leading from the uterus to the outside of the body

Indications and Procedures

An endometrial biopsy is usually performed to identify the cause of abnormal uterine bleeding. Abnormal bleeding is that which is excessive in duration, frequency, or amount for the particular woman, and it includes bleeding at the wrong times (between menstrual periods) or after menopause. The biopsy may also be performed when there is no bleeding (or menstruation) or if a woman is having difficulty becoming pregnant.

Most women who have endometrial cancer have abnormal bleeding, so the biopsy is performed to rule out both cancer and hyperplasia, an excessive growth of tissue that could become cancerous. Women who are perimenopausal (prior to the actual end of menstrual cycles) may experience changes in their cycle that make it difficult to determine if there is abnormal bleeding or simply normal changes. Perimenopause varies in length but usually begins six to eight years before menopause, and then women become menopausal when menstrual cycles end. Women on hormone therapy are at greater risk of endometrial cancer, because they usually take the hormones estrogen and progesterone that their body is no longer producing at sufficient levels. Women who take estrogen but cannot take progesterone are at an even greater risk of endometrial cancer.

The biopsy may also be used as part of an infertility examination to determine whether there are problems with the development of the endometrium. If the endometrium does not thicken in time to accept and support a fertilized egg, then the egg cannot implant properly, a condition called "luteal phase defect" (LPD). The biopsy can show whether the uterine lining is thickening and maturing by developing more blood vessels before menstruation, a definite sign that ovulation (the maturation and release of an egg by the ovary) has occurred and that the lining can support a pregnancy. Additionally, the biopsy may be performed to help evaluate the problem of repeated early miscarriages. Another use of the procedure is to obtain a sample for patients with suspected endometritis or polycystic ovary disease.

An obstetrician or gynecologist (or, in some cases, a nurse practitioner or nurse midwife) will perform the procedure, which is usually done in an office setting. The procedure takes a few minutes, and no anesthesia is needed, although a mild over-the-counter painkiller such as ibuprofen is often recommended about one hour before the procedure to ease discomfort. In cases of cervical stenosis, cervical softening may be accomplished by administration of the medication misoprostol. Additionally, a local anesthetic may occasionally be injected into the cervix to decrease pain and discomfort.

After a pelvic examination, the clinician will insert a speculum into the vagina to hold the walls open. After the cervix is cleaned with antiseptic, a tiny hollow plastic tube is inserted into the vagina, through the cervix, and into the uterus. A plunger attached to the tube will suction out a sample of the inner layer of tissue in the uterine wall. The tube is turned clockwise or counterclockwise while being moved in and out of the uterine cavity in order to obtain specimens. The cells are then sent to a laboratory for testing and microscopic examination.

Uses and Complications

Mild cramping may occur during and after the procedure. Cramping, pressure, and discomfort may also occur when the instruments are inserted and the samples collected. A small amount of bleeding, or spotting, may occur afterward, although normal activities can be resumed immediately.

After the procedure, there are slight risks of infection or heavy bleeding. Heavy bleeding, severe pain or cramping, or a fever over 100 degrees Fahrenheit (about 38 degrees Celsius) requires immediate medical attention. Extremely rarely, the uterus may be injured or punctured by the tool or the cervix may be torn during the procedure. The procedure should not be performed if the patient is pregnant or suffers from acute pelvic inflammatory disease or acute cervical or vaginal infections.

Abnormal cells may indicate endometrial cancer, LPD, the presence of fibroids (benign, or noncancerous, excessive growths of the smooth muscle wall of the uterus), or polyps (a usually benign growth of normal tissue attached to the lining of the uterus). Surgery and/or medication may be necessary to treat these conditions.

Ultrasound is often utilized along with endometrial sampling for initial evaluation. Patients with persistent symptoms may need additional tests and procedures. Because an endometrial biopsy often misses polyps and fibroids, alternative procedures such as dilation and curettage (D&C) or hysteroscopy may be used for further diagnostic purposes.

Perspective and Prospects

The use of endometrial sampling to diagnose and treat problems has been practiced since at least 1843. The earliest tools were wide and required scraping the uterine lining. Later devices, such as the stainless-steel Novak (or Kevorkian) curette or Vabra aspirator, cause significant discomfort. The Novak curette requires a syringe to apply suction. The Vabra aspirator is a disposable device that uses an electric suction pump to obtain the sample.

By 2006, the most used tool for endometrial biopsies was the Pipelle curette, developed in France. The curette is narrower, more flexible, and easier to insert through the cervix, and it removes the sample by suction. This device is relatively inexpensive, causes little to no discomfort to the patient, and has been shown to obtain adequate specimens in 87 to 100 percent of patients.

—*Virginia L. Salmon*

See also Biopsy; Cancer; Cervical, ovarian, and uterine cancers; Cervical procedures; Diagnosis; Genital disorders, female; Gynecology; Infertility, female; Oncology; Polyps; Reproductive system; Uterus; Women's health.

For Further Information:

A.D.A.M. Medical Encyclopedia. "Endometrial Biopsy." *MedlinePlus*, September 13, 2011.

Berek, Jonathan S., ed. *Berek and Novak's Gynecology*. 15th ed. Philadelphia: Lippincott Williams & Wilkins, 2012.

Cherath, Lata. "Endometrial Biopsy." In *The Gale Encyclopedia of Medicine*, edited by Jacqueline L. Longe. 3d ed. Farmington Hill, Mich.: Thomson Gale, 2006.

Cunningham, F. Gary, et al., eds. *Williams Obstetrics*. 23d ed. New York: McGraw-Hill, 2010.

"Endometrial Biopsy: Finding the Cause of Uterine Bleeding." *Mayo Clinic Health Letter* 19, no. 8 (August, 2001): 6.

Minkin, Mary Jane, and Carol V. Wright. *The Yale Guide to Women's Reproductive Health: From Menarche to Menopause*. New Haven, Conn.: Yale University Press, 2003.

National Cancer Institute. "Endometrial Cancer Screening (PDQ)." *National Institutes of Health, US Department of Health and Human Services*, June 6, 2013.

Puzanov, Ivan, ed. "Endometrial Biopsy." *Health Library*, September 10, 2012.

Willacy, Hayley. "Endometrial Sampling." *Patient.co.uk*, June 22, 2011.

ENDOMETRIOSIS
Disease/Disorder
Anatomy or system affected: Reproductive system, uterus
Specialties and related fields: Gynecology
Definition: Growth of cells of the uterine lining at sites outside the uterus, causing severe pain and infertility.

Key terms:
cervix: an oval-shaped organ that separates the uterus and the vagina

dysmenorrhea: painful menstruation

dyspareunia: painful sexual intercourse

endometrium: the tissue that lines the uterus, builds up, and sheds at the end of each menstrual cycle; when it grows outside the uterus, endometriosis occurs

Fallopian tubes: two tubes extending from the ovaries to the uterus; during ovulation, an egg travels down one of these tubes to the uterus

hysterectomy: surgery that removes part or all of the uterus

Information on Endometriosis

Causes: Unknown
Symptoms: Painful menstrual periods, discomfort during sexual intercourse, localized pain, infertility
Duration: Chronic
Treatments: Chemotherapy, surgery

---

implant: an abnormal endometrial growth outside the uterus

laparoscopy: a surgical procedure in which a small incision made near the navel is used to view the uterus and other abdominal organs with a lighted tube called a laparoscope

laparotomy: a surgical procedure, often exploratory in nature, carried out through the abdominal wall; it may be used to correct endometriosis

laser: a concentrated, high-energy light beam often used to destroy abnormal tissue

oophorectomy (or ovariectomy): removal of the ovaries, which is often necessary in cases of severe endometriosis

prostaglandins: fatlike hormones that control the contraction and relaxation of the uterus and other smooth muscle tissue

Causes and Symptoms

Endometriosis is the presence of endometrial tissue outside its normal location as the lining of the uterus . It can be asymptomatic, mild, or a disabling disease causing severe pain. The classic symptoms of endometriosis are very painful menstruation (dysmenorrhea), painful intercourse (dyspareunia), and infertility. Some other common endometriosis symptoms include nausea, vomiting, diarrhea, and fatigue.

It has been estimated that endometriosis affects between five million and twenty-five million American women. Often, it is incorrectly stereotyped as being a disease of upwardly mobile, professional women. According to many experts, the incidence of endometriosis worldwide and across most racial groups is probably very similar. They propose that the reported occurrence rate difference for some racial groups, such as a lower incidence in African Americans and a higher diagnosis rate among Caucasians, has been a socioeconomic phenomenon attributable to the social class of women who seek medical treatment for the symptoms of endometriosis and to the highly stratified responses of many health care professionals who have dealt with the disease.

The symptoms of endometriosis arise from abnormalities in the effects of the menstrual cycle on the endometrial tissue lining the uterus. The endometrium normally thickens and becomes engorged (swollen with blood) during the cycle, a process controlled by female hormones called "estrogens" and "progestins." This engorgement is designed to prepare the uterus for conception by optimizing conditions for implantation in the endometrium of a fertilized egg, which enters the uterus via one of the Fallopian tubes leading from the ovaries.

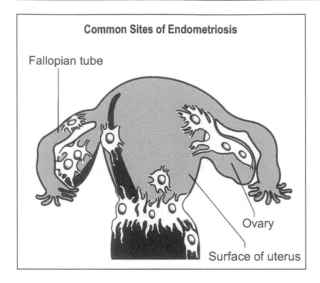

Common Sites of Endometriosis

Fallopian tube

Ovary

Surface of uterus

By the middle of the menstrual cycle, the endometrial lining is normally about ten times thicker than at its beginning. If the egg that is released into the uterus is not fertilized, pregnancy does not occur and decreases in production of the female sex hormones result in the breakdown of the endometrium. Endometrial tissue mixed with blood leaves the uterus as the menstrual flow, and a new menstrual cycle begins. This series of uterine changes occurs repeatedly, as a monthly cycle, from puberty (which usually occurs between the ages of twelve and fourteen) to menopause (which usually occurs between the ages of forty-five and fifty-five).

In women who develop endometriosis, some endometrial tissue begins to grow ectopically (in an abnormal position) at sites outside the uterus. The ectopic endometrial growths may be found attached to the ovaries, the Fallopian tubes, the urinary bladder, the rectum, other abdominal organs, and even the lungs. Regardless of body location, these implants behave as if they were still in the uterus, thickening and bleeding each month as the menstrual cycle proceeds. Like the endometrium at its normal uterine site, the ectopic tissue responds to the hormones that circulate through the body in the blood. Its inappropriate position in the body prevents this ectopic endometrial tissue from leaving the body as menstrual flow; as a result, some implants grow to be quite large.

In many cases, the endometrial growths that form between two organs become fibrous bands called "adhesions." The fibrous nature of adhesions is attributable to the alternating swelling and breakdown of the ectopic tissue, which yields fibrous scar tissue. The alterations in size of living portions of the adhesions and other endometrial implants during the monthly menstrual cycle cause many afflicted women considerable pain. Because the body location of implants varies, the site of the pain may be almost anywhere, including the back, chest, thighs, pelvis, rectum, or abdomen. For example, dyspareunia occurs when adhesions hold a uterus tightly to the abdominal wall, making its movement during intercourse painful. Many women report significant pain on a monthly

basis with ovulation as well.

The presence of endometriosis is usually confirmed by laparoscopy, viewed as being the most reliable method for its diagnosis. Laparoscopy is carried out after a physician makes an initial diagnosis of probable endometriosis from a combined study including an examination of the patient's medical history and careful exploration of the patient's physical problems over a period of at least six months. During prelaparoscopy treatment, the patient is very often maintained on pain medication and other therapeutic drugs that will produce symptomatic relief.

For laparoscopy, the patient is anesthetized with a general anesthetic, a small incision is made near the navel, and a laparoscope (flexible lighted tube) is inserted into this incision. The laparoscope, equipped with fiber optics, enables the examining physician to search the patient's abdominal organs for endometrial implants. Visibility of the abdominal organs in laparoscopic examination can be enhanced by pumping harmless carbon dioxide gas into the abdomen, causing it to distend. Women who undergo laparoscopy usually require a day of postoperative bed rest, followed by seven to ten days of curtailed physical activity. After a laparoscopic diagnosis of endometriosis is made, a variety of surgical and therapeutic drug treatments can be employed to manage the disease.

Between 30 and 50 percent of all women who have endometriosis are infertile; contemporary wisdom evaluates this relationship as one of cause and effect, which should make this disease the second most common cause of fertility problems. The actual basis for this infertility is not always clear, but it is often the result of damage to the ovaries and Fallopian tubes, scar tissue produced by implants on these and other abdominal organs, and hormone imbalances.

Because the incidence of infertility accompanying endometriosis increases with the severity of the disease, all potentially afflicted women are encouraged to seek early diagnosis. Many experts advise all women with abnormal menstrual cycles, dysmenorrhea, severe menstrual bleeding, abnormal vaginal bleeding, and repeated dyspareunia to seek the advice of a physician trained in identifying and dealing with endometriosis. Because the disease can begin to present symptoms at any age, teenagers are also encouraged to seek medical attention if they experience any of these symptoms.

John Sampson coined the term "endometriosis" in the 1920s. Sampson's theory for its causation, still widely accepted, is termed "retrograde menstruation." Also called "menstrual backup," this theory proposes that the backing up of some menstrual flow into the Fallopian tubes and then into the abdominal cavity, forms the endometrial implants. Evidence supporting this theory, according to many physicians, is the fact that such backup is common. Others point out, however, that the backup is often found in women who do not have the disease. A surgical experiment was performed on female monkeys to test this theory. Their uteri were turned upside down so that the menstrual flow would spill into the abdominal cavity. Sixty percent of the animals developed endometriosis postoperatively—an inconclusive result.

Complicating the issue is the fact that implants are also found in tissues (such as in the lung) that cannot be reached by menstrual backup. It has been theorized that the presence of these implants results from the entry of endometrial cells into the lymphatic system, which returns body fluid to the blood and protects the body from many other diseases. This transplantation theory is supported by the occurrence of endometriosis in various portions of the lymphatic system and in tissues that could not otherwise become sites of endometriosis.

A third theory explaining the growth of implants is the iatrogenic, or nosocomial, transmission of endometrial tissue. These terms both indicate an accidental creation of the disease through the actions of physicians. Such implant formation is viewed as occurring most often after cesarean delivery of a baby when passage through the birth canal would otherwise be fatal to mother and/or child. Another proposed cause is episiotomy—widening of the birth canal by an incision between the anus and vagina—to ease births.

Any surgical procedure that allows the spread of endometrial tissue can be implicated, including surgical procedures carried out to correct existing endometriosis, because of the ease with which endometrial tissue implants itself anywhere in the body. Abnormal endometrial tissue growth, called "adenomyosis," can also occur in the uterus and is viewed as a separate disease entity.

Other theories regarding the genesis of endometriosis include an immunologic theory, which proposes that women who develop endometriosis are lacking in antibodies that normally cause the destruction of endometrial tissue at sites where it does not belong, and a hormonal theory, which suggests the existence of large imbalances in hormones such as the prostaglandins that serve as the body's messengers in controlling biological processes. Several of these theories—retrograde menstruation, the transplantation theory, and iatrogenic transmission—all have support, but none has been proved unequivocally. Future evidence will identify whether one cause is dominant, whether they all interact to produce the disease, or whether endometriosis is actually a group of diseases that simply resemble one another in the eyes of contemporary medical science.

Treatment and Therapy

Laparoscopic examination most often identifies endometriosis as chocolate-colored lumps (chocolate cysts) ranging from the size of a pinhead to several inches across or as filmy coverings over parts of abdominal organs and

---

In the News:
Link Between Endometriosis and Other Diseases

In the October, 2002, issue of *Human Reproduction*, the Endometriosis Association and the National Institutes of Health (NIH) announced the results of a study involving 3,680 women who were members of the Endometriosis Association and who had been diagnosed with endometriosis. The study suggested that women with endometriosis are significantly more likely than other women to contract a number of serious autoimmune diseases including lupus, Sjögren's syndrome, rheumatoid arthritis, and multiple sclerosis.

Although a study conducted in 1980 established a link between endometriosis and immune dysfunctions, the new study sought to identify specific diseases for which women with endometriosis are at higher risk. In addition to the connection between endometriosis and autoimmune diseases, researchers found that the women in the study were more than one hundred times more likely than women in the general population to suffer from chronic fatigue syndrome; twice as likely to suffer from fibromyalgia (recurrent debilitating pain in the muscles, tendons, and ligaments), and seven times as likely to suffer from hypothyroidism (which can also be an autoimmune disorder). Researchers also found that the women studied reported higher rates of allergies and asthma than women in the general population.

Researchers warn that the study may not be representative of all patients with endometriosis, both because members of the Endometriosis Association are most probably those patients suffering pain from their condition and because the survey was completed predominantly by white, educated women. Even so, this new information provides more light on an enigmatic disease and should help health care professionals treat patients.

—*Cassandra Kircher, Ph.D.*

---

ligaments. Once a diagnosis of the disease is confirmed by laparoscopy, endometriosis is treated by chemotherapy, surgery, or a combination of both methods. The only permanent contemporary cure for endometriosis, however, is the onset of the biological menopause at the end of a woman's childbearing years. As long as menstruation continues, implant development is likely to recur, regardless of its cause. Nevertheless, a temporary cure of endometriosis is better than no cure at all.

The chemotherapy that many physicians use to treat mild cases of endometriosis (and for prelaparoscopy periods) is analgesic painkillers, including aspirin, acetaminophen, and ibuprofen. The analgesics inhibit the body's production of prostaglandins, and the symptoms of the disease are merely covered up. Therefore, analgesics are of quite limited value except during a prelaparoscopy diagnostic period or with mild cases of endometriosis. In addition, the long-term administration of aspirin will often produce gastrointestinal bleeding, and excess use of acetaminophen can lead to severe liver damage. In some cases of very severe endometriosis pain, narcotic painkillers are given, such as codeine, Percodan (oxycodone and aspirin), or morphine. Narcotics are addicting and should be avoided unless absolutely necessary.

More effective for long-term management of the disease is hormone therapy. Such therapy is designed to prevent the monthly occurrence of menstruation—that is, to freeze the body in a sort of chemical menopause. The hormone types used, made by pharmaceutical companies, are chemical cousins of female hormones (estrogens and progestins), male hormones (androgens), and a brain hormone that controls ovulation (gonadotropin-releasing hormone, or GnRH). Appropriate hormone therapy is often useful for years, although each hormone class produces disadvantageous side effects in many patients.

The use of estrogens stops ovulation and menstruation, freeing many women with endometriosis from painful symptoms. Numerous estrogen preparations have been prescribed, including the birth control pills that contain them. Drawbacks of estrogen use can include weight gain, nausea, breast soreness, depression, blood-clotting abnormalities, and elevated risk of vaginal cancer. In addition, estrogen administration may cause endometrial implants to enlarge.

The use of progestins arose from the discovery that pregnancy—which is maintained by high levels of a natural progestin called progesterone—reversed the symptoms of many suffering from endometriosis. This realization led to the utilization of synthetic progestins to cause prolonged false pregnancy. The rationale is that all endometrial implants will die off and be reabsorbed during the prolonged absence of menstruation. The method works in most patients, and pain-free periods of up to five years are often observed. In some cases, however, side effects include nausea, depression, insomnia, and a very slow resumption of normal menstruation (such as lags of up to a year) when the therapy is stopped. In addition, progestins are ineffective in treating large implants; in fact, their use in such cases can lead to severe complications.

In the 1970s, studies showing the potential for heart attacks, high blood pressure, and strokes in patients receiving long-term female hormone therapy led to a search for more advantageous hormone medications. An alternative developed was the synthetic male hormone danazol (Danocrine), which is very effective. Danazol works by decreasing the amount of estrogen that is produced by the ovaries on a monthly basis to close to that which is present at menopause. The lack of estrogen prevents endometrial cells from growing, thereby eliminating most of the symptoms associated with endometriosis. One of its advantages over female hormones is the ability to shrink large implants and restore fertility to those patients whose problems arise from nonfunctional ovaries or Fallopian tubes. Danazol has become the drug of choice for treating millions of endometriosis sufferers. Problems associated with danazol use, however, can include weight gain, masculinization (decreased bust size, increased muscle mass, muscle cramping, facial hair growth, and deepened voice), fatigue, depression, and baldness. Those women contemplating danazol use should be aware that it can also complicate pregnancy.

Because of the side effects of these hormones, other chemotherapy was sought. Another valuable drug that has become available is GnRH, which suppresses the function of the ovaries in a fashion equivalent to surgical oophorectomy (removal of the ovaries). This hormone produces none of the side effects of the sex hormones, such as weight gain, depression, or masculinization, but some evidence indicates that it may lead to osteoporosis.

Thus, despite the fact that hormone therapy may relieve or reduce pain for years, contemporary chemotherapy is flawed by many undesirable side effects. Perhaps more serious, however, is the high recurrence rate of endometriosis that is observed after the therapy is stopped. Consequently, it appears that the best treatment of endometriosis combines chemotherapy with surgery.

The extent of the surgery carried out to combat endometriosis is variable and depends on the observations made during laparoscopy. In cases of relatively mild endometriosis, conservative laparotomy surgery removes endometriosis implants, adhesions, and lesions. This type of procedure attempts to relieve endometriosis pain, to minimize the chances of postoperative recurrence of the disease, and to allow the patient to have children. Even in the most severe cases of this type, the uterus, an ovary, and its associated Fallopian tube are retained. Such surgery will often include removal of the appendix, whether diseased or not, because it is very likely to develop implants. The surgical techniques performed are the conventional excision of diseased tissue or the use of lasers to vaporize it. Many physicians prefer lasers because it is believed that they decrease the chances of recurrent endometriosis resulting from retained implant tissue or iatrogenic causes. In a new procedure, following the removal of endometrial tissue by surgical means, an intrauterine device containing levonogestrel (a hormone that will decrease estrogen levels) is placed in order to prevent recurrence of endometriosis.

In more serious cases, hysterectomy is carried out. All visible implants, adhesions, and lesions are removed from the abdominal organs, as in conservative surgery. In addition, the uterus and cervix are taken out, but one or both ovaries are retained. This allows female hormone production to continue normally until the menopause. Uterine removal makes it impossible to have children, however, and may lead to profound psychological problems that require psychiatric help. Women planning to elect for hysterectomy to treat endometriosis should be aware of such potential difficulties. In many cases of conservative surgery or hysterectomy, danazol is used, both preoperatively and postoperatively, to minimize implant size.

The most extensive surgery carried out on the women afflicted with endometriosis is radical hysterectomy, also called "definitive surgery," in which the ovaries and/or the vagina are also removed. The resultant symptoms are menopausal and may include vaginal bleeding atrophy (when the vagina is retained), increased risk of heart disease, and the development of osteoporosis. To counter the occurrence of these symptoms, hormone replacement therapy is suggested. Paradoxically, this hormone therapy can lead to the return of endometriosis by stimulating the growth of residual implant tissue.

Recently, more women have turned to complementary and alternative medicine in an attempt to relieve the symptoms of endometriosis. Acupuncture, homeopathy, and herbal therapy are currently being explored as means of treatment for endometriosis.

Perspective and Prospects

Modern treatment of endometriosis is viewed by many physicians as beginning in the 1950s. A landmark development in this field was the accurate diagnosis of endometriosis via the laparoscope, which was invented in Europe and introduced into the United States in the 1960s. Medical science has progressed greatly since that time. Physicians and researchers have recognized the wide occurrence of the disease and accepted its symptoms as valid; realized that hysterectomy will not necessarily put an end to the disease; utilized chemotherapeutic tools, including hormones and painkillers, as treatments and as adjuncts to surgery; developed laser surgery and other techniques that decrease the occurrence of formerly ignored iatrogenic endometriosis; and understood that the disease can ravage teenagers as well and that these young women should be examined as early as possible.

Research into endometriosis is ongoing, and the efforts and information base of the proactive American Endometriosis Association, founded in 1980, have been very valuable. As a result, a potentially or presently afflicted woman is much more aware of the problems associated with the disease. In addition, she has a source for obtaining objective information on topics including state-of-the-art treatment, physician and hospital choice, and both physical and psychological outcomes of treatment.

Many potentially viable avenues for better endometriosis diagnosis and treatment have become the objects of intense investigation. These include the use of ultrasonography and radiology techniques, such as magnetic resonance imaging (MRI), for the predictive, nonsurgical examination of the course of growth or the chemotherapeutic destruction of implants; the design of new drugs to be utilized in the battle against endometriosis; endeavors aimed at the development of diagnostic tests for the disease that will stop it before symptoms develop; and the design of dietary treatments to soften its effects.

Regrettably, because of the insidious nature of endometriosis—which has the ability to strike almost anywhere in the body—some confusion about the disease still exists. New drugs, surgical techniques, and other aids are expected to be helpful in clarifying many of these issues. Particular value is being placed on the study of the immunologic aspects of endometriosis. Scientists hope to explain why the disease strikes some women and not others, to uncover its etiologic basis, and to solve the widespread problems of iatrogenic implant formation and other types of endometriosis recurrence.

—Sanford S. Singer, Ph.D.;
updated by Robin Kamienny Montvilo, R.N., Ph.D.

See also Amenorrhea; Cervical, ovarian, and uterine cancers; Childbirth complications; Dysmenorrhea; Endometrial biopsy; Genital disorders, female; Gynecology; Hormone therapy; Hysterectomy; Infertility, female; Menorrhagia; Menstruation; Pregnancy and gestation; Reproductive system; Uterus; Women's health.

For Further Information:

American Society for Reproductive Medicine. "Endometriosis and Infertility: Can Surgery Help?" *ReproductiveFacts.org*, 2012.

Berek, Jonathan S., ed. *Berek and Novak's Gynecology*. 14th ed. Philadelphia: Lippincott Williams & Wilkins, 2007.

Endometriosis.org. http://www.endometriosis.org.

"Endometriosis." *Mayo Foundation for Medical Education and Research*, April 2, 2013.

Fernandez, I., C. Reid, and S. Dziurawiec. "Living with Endometriosis: The Perspective of Male Partners." *Journal of Psychosomatic Research* 61, no. 4 (October, 2006): 433–438.

Henderson, Lorraine, and Ros Wood. *Explaining Endometriosis*. 2d ed. St. Leonards, N.S.W.: Allen and Unwin, 2000.

National Institute of Child Health and Human Development. "Endometriosis: Condition Information." *National Institutes of Health*, April 3, 2012.

Phillips, Robert H., and Glenda Motta. *Coping with Endometriosis*. New York: Avery, 2000.

Physicians" Desk Reference. 64th ed. Montvale, N.J.: PDR Network, 2009.

Shaw, Michael, ed. *Everything You Need to Know about Diseases*. Springhouse, Pa.: Springhouse Press, 1996.

Sherwood, Lauralee. *Human Physiology: From Cells to Systems*. 7th ed. Pacific Grove, Calif.: Brooks/Cole, 2010.

Weinstein, Kate. *Living with Endometriosis*. Reading, Mass.: Addison-Wesley, 1991.

Weschler, Toni. *Taking Charge of Your Fertility*. Rev. ed. New York: Collins, 2001.

Wood, Debra, and Andrea Chisholm. "Endometriosis." *Health Library*, September 10, 2012.

Endoscopic retrograde cholangiopancreatography (ERCP)

Procedure

Anatomy or system affected: Abdomen, gallbladder, gastrointestinal system, liver, pancreas, stomach

Specialties and related fields: Gastroenterology, internal medicine, radiology

Definition: A procedure combining elements of an X ray with an endoscope to look into the digestive system.

Key terms:

duodenum: the first part of the small intestine

endoscope: a hollow, flexible, telescope-like tube about the size of a pen in diameter and about 2.5 feet long with a lens, light, and holes on the end

gastroenterologist: a doctor specializing in the digestive system

sphincterotomy: a small cut made in a muscle surrounding the opening of a duct, usually made by cauterization

stent: a small, hollow device left in a duct or tube to keep it open

Indications and Procedures

Endoscopic retrograde cholangiopancreatography (ERCP) is usually performed if a patient is experiencing jaundice, unexplained pain in the upper abdomen, or unexplained weight loss. It is used to determine the sources of these conditions. ERCP can be used to find tumors, blockages, cysts, tissue irregularities, or gallstones. It may also be used to discover the source of inflammation in the liver, bile ducts (which drain the liver, gallbladder, and pancreas), gallbladder, or pancreas. If imaging or blood tests are confusing or inconclusive, this procedure may be used to clarify those inconsistencies. ERCP may also help to plan surgery for a patient who is already known to be suffering from gallbladder or pancreatic disease or who has a mass or tumor shown in imaging processes.

ERCP is usually performed by a gastroenterologist who has had further training specifically in ERCP procedures. It may be performed in a hospital or a clinic. The patient lies down on a radiology bed and is sedated, usually through an IV, to relax the involuntary muscles. An anesthetic is sprayed in the patient's throat to counteract any gag reflex, and a guard may be placed over the teeth and gums to protect them during the procedure. The endoscope is inserted into the throat, and the patient is asked to swallow to help the endoscope into the correct position. The endoscope is then guided through the digestive system to the duodenum. Then a small catheter is inserted into the hollow endoscope until it reaches the duct system. Iodine or another type of contrast solution (dye) is put into the catheter so that the duct system can be shown on x-rays. X-rays are then taken and examined while the endoscope remains in place. The patient may be asked to change positions so the doctor can view different structures.

Usually, this procedure is performed in an outpatient setting, and the patient is released to go home (with a designated driver) after the sedative wears off. Occasionally, a patient may stay in the hospital for a longer period, particularly when further procedures, as described below, are performed at the time of the ERCP or when complications develop.

Uses and Complications

Some problems can be identified and solved during the ERCP procedure. Depending what is shown on the x-rays taken during this procedure, the doctor may be able to perform further procedures, such as removing gallstones (which may involve crushing the stones and removing them or simply leaving them in the intestines to pass through the digestive system naturally), taking tissue biopsies, dilating a duct with a balloon, performing a sphincterotomy, or inserting a stent. Other problems, such as possible cancers, will need to be identified through tissue samples and treated later.

Serious complications from ERCP are rare. One possible serious complication is aspiration (inhaling) of saliva, which may lead to pneumonia. Other serious complications may include perforation, inflammation, bleeding, injury, or infection of any of the organs examined or the stomach, esophagus, or intestines. Complications from sedation and contrast dyes, such as allergies, are also possible. More common complications are nausea and stomach pain. One may feel discomfort (such as a sore throat), tenderness, or bloating, depending on whether air is blown into the endoscope during the process to open up the structures that the doctor wishes to view.

Factors that complicate this procedure include obesity, allergies, diabetes, hypertension, or certain drugs, especially anticlotting drugs. Another complicating factor may be that the patient has not fasted for at least six hours prior to this procedure as instructed.

Perspective and Prospects

Endoscopic procedures were first reported in 1968. Improvements to the procedure, then called endoscopic cholangiopancreatography (ECPG), occurred throughout the early 1970s, when Japanese doctors worked with engineers to develop better instruments to use during the procedure. The procedure spread through Europe during the 1970s and soon became known as a valuable diagnostic tool despite its potential for serious complications in its early stages. From the mid-1970s, it was recognized as a cost-saving alternative to surgical procedures with a much quicker recovery time for the patient. With the addition of x-ray technology, it became an often used diagnostic and therapeutic tool.

With improvements in imaging technology, such as high-quality ultrasound, computed tomography (CT) scans, endoscopic ultrasonography, and magnetic resonance imaging (MRI), the use of this procedure for solely diagnostic purposes has diminished somewhat. Its use as a therapeutic tool is still acknowledged, however, and it is still an alternative diagnostic procedure when noninvasive procedures result in inconclusive diagnosis.

—*Marianne M. Madsen, M.S.*

See also Abdomen; Abdominal disorders; Arthritis; Arthroscopy; Biopsy; Cholecystectomy; Colon and rectal polyp removal; Colon cancer; Colonoscopy and sigmoidoscopy; Cystoscopy; Endoscopy; Gallbladder diseases; Gastrointestinal disorders; Gastrointestinal system; Invasive tests; Laparoscopy; Pulmonary diseases; Stone removal; Stones.

For Further Information:

Aronson, Naomi. *Endoscopic Retrograde Cholangiopancreatography.* Washington, D.C.: Department of Health and Human Services, Public Health Service, Agency for Healthcare Research & Quality, 2002.

Cotton, P. B., and J. W. Leung, eds. *Advanced Digestive Endoscopy: ERCP.* Hoboken, N.J.: Wiley-Blackwell, 2006.

Longstreth, George F. "ERCP." *MedlinePlus*, August 8, 2011.

Mahnke, Daus. "Endoscopic Retrograde Cholangiopancreatography." *Health Library*, May 30, 2013.

National Digestive Diseases Information Clearinghouse. "ERCP (Endoscopic Retrograde Cholangiopancreatography)." *National Digestive Diseases Information Clearing House*, June 29, 2012.

Seigel, J. H., J. Delmont, and A. G. Harris. *Endoscopic Retrograde Cholangiopancreatography: Technique, Diagnosis, and Therapy.* New York: Raven Press, 1991.

Talley, N. J.*Clinical Gastroenterology: A Practical Problem-Based Approach.* 3d ed. New York: Churchill-Livingstone/Elsevier, 2011.

ENDOSCOPY

Procedure

Anatomy or system affected: Abdomen, anus, bladder, gastrointestinal system, intestines, joints, knees, lungs, stomach, urinary system

Specialties and related fields: Gastroenterology, gynecology, obstetrics, orthopedics, proctology, pulmonary medicine, urology

Definition: The use of a flexible tube to look into body structures in order to inspect and sometimes correct pathologies.

Key terms:

biopsy: the collection and study of body tissue, often to determine whether it is cancerous

fiber optics: the transmission of light through thin, flexible tubes

pathology: a disease condition; also the study of diseases

Indications and Procedures

Early endoscopes were simply rigid hollow tubes with a light source. They were inserted into body orifices, such as the anus or the mouth, to allow the physician to look directly at structures and processes within. Modern instruments are more sophisticated. They often use fiber optics in flexible cables to penetrate deep into body structures. For example, one form of colonoscope can be threaded though the entire lower intestine,

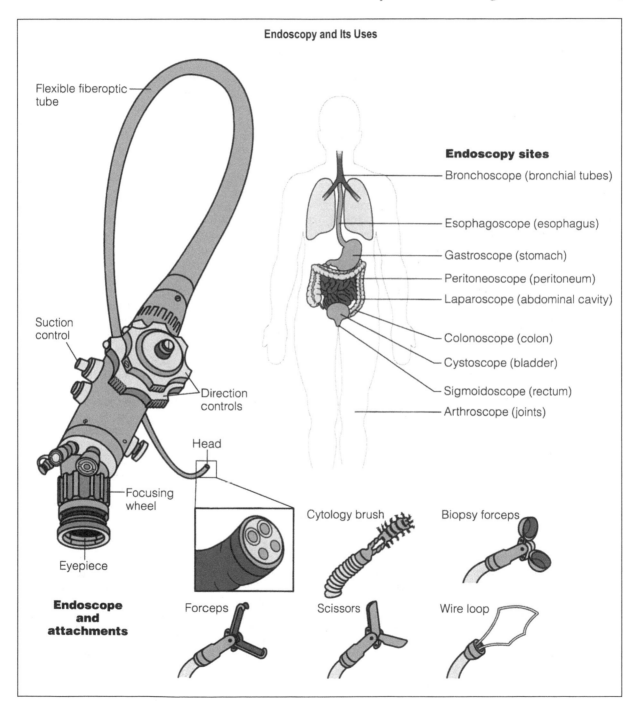

Endoscopy and Its Uses

Flexible fiberoptic tube

Suction control

Direction controls

Head

Focusing wheel

Eyepiece

Endoscope and attachments

Endoscopy sites

Bronchoscope (bronchial tubes)

Esophagoscope (esophagus)

Gastroscope (stomach)

Peritoneoscope (peritoneum)

Laparoscope (abdominal cavity)

Colonoscope (colon)

Cystoscope (bladder)

Sigmoidoscope (rectum)

Arthroscope (joints)

Cytology brush

Biopsy forceps

Forceps

Scissors

Wire loop

allowing the physician to search for pathologies all the way from the anus to the cecum of the colon (large intestine).

There are eight basic types of endoscope: gastroscope, colonoscope, bronchoscope, cystoscope, laparoscope, colposcope, arthroscope, and amnioscope. Their primary uses are diagnostic; however, they can be fitted with special instruments to perform many different tasks, including taking bits of tissue for biopsy and carrying out surgical procedures.

Uses and Complications

The gastroscope and its variants are used to inspect structures of the gastrointestinal system. The name of one class of procedure gives an idea of how sophisticated the gastroscope has become: esophagogastroduodenoscopy. As the term implies, this technique can be used to investigate the esophagus (the tube leading to the stomach), the stomach itself, and the intestines all the way into the duodenum (the first link of the small intestine). Furthermore, in a procedure called "endoscopic retrograde cholangiopancreatography," the endoscope can be used to investigate processes in the gallbladder, the cystic duct, the common hepatic duct, and the common bile duct. By far the most common use of the gastroscope is in the diagnosis and management of esophageal and stomach problems. The gastroscope is used to confirm the suspicion of stomach ulcers and other gastroesophageal conditions and to monitor therapy.

The colonoscope and its variants are critical in the diagnosis of diseases in the lower intestine and in some aspects of therapy. The long, flexible fiber-optic tube can be threaded through the anus and rectum into the S-shaped sigmoid colon (flexible fiber-optic sigmoidoscopy). The tube can be made to rise up the descending colon, across the transverse colon, and down the ascending colon to the cecum. With the colonoscope, the physician can discover abnormalities such as polyps, diverticula, and blockages and the presence of cancer, Crohn's disease, ulcerative colitis, and many other diseases. The physician can also use the colonoscope to remove polyps; this is the major therapeutic use of colonoscopy.

Like most other forms of endoscopy, bronchoscopy is used for both diagnosis and treatment. The bronchoscope allows direct visualization of the trachea (the tube leading from the throat to the lungs) and the bronchi (the two main air ducts leading into the lungs). It will show certain forms of lung cancer, various infectious states, and other pathologies. The bronchoscope can also be used to remove foreign objects, excise local tumors, remove mucus plugs, and improve bronchial drainage.

The cystoscope is used for visual inspection of the urethra and bladder. The bladder stores urine; the urethra is the tube through which it is eliminated. Cystoscopy discovers many of the conditions that can afflict these organs: obstruction, infection, cancer, and other disorders.

The laparoscope is used to look into the abdominal cavity for evidence of a wide variety of conditions. It can inspect the liver, help evaluate liver disease, and take tissue samples for biopsy. Laparoscopy can confirm the diagnosis of ectopic pregnancy (a condition in which a fetus develops outside the uterus, usually in one of the Fallopian tubes). It can confirm the presence or absence of abdominal and female reproductive cancers and diagnose disease conditions in the gallbladder, spleen, peritoneum (the membrane that surrounds the abdomen), diaphragm, ovaries, and uterus, as well as give some views of the small and large intestine. Importantly, the laparoscope is commonly used to remove gallbladders (cholecystectomy). This procedure is far less traumatic than the old surgery, often permitting release of the patient a day or two after the operation rather than requiring weeks of recuperation. Likewise, many other surgeries, such as appendectomies, gastric bypasses, hysterectomies, and colectomies, are also now performed laparoscopically.

The colposcope is used to inspect vaginal tissue and adjacent organs. Common reasons for colposcopy include abnormal bleeding and suspicion of tumors.

Arthroscopy, the investigation of joint structures by endoscopy, is now the most common invasive technique used on patients with arthritis or joint damage. In addition to viewing the area, the arthroscope can be fitted with various instruments to perform surgical procedures.

The term "amnioscope" comes from the amnion, the membrane that surrounds a fetus. This type of endoscope is used to enter the uterus and inspect the growing fetus in the search for any visible abnormalities.

Endoscopy is one of the most useful and most used techniques for diagnosis because it permits the investigation of many internal body organs without surgery. It is extraordinarily safe in the hands of experienced practitioners and is relatively free of pain and discomfort for patients, although there are risks of bleeding, pain, infection, and rarely, perforation of the tissue wall. In addition, specialized endoscopes are assuming greater roles in therapy. Many procedures that once involved major surgery can now be conducted through endoscopy, saving the patient pain, trauma, and expense.

Perspective and Prospects

Endoscopes have become highly sophisticated instruments with enormous range throughout the body and enormous potential. Colonoscopy, for example, promises to revolutionize the treatment of cancerous and precancerous polyps by helping physicians attain a clearer understanding of the polyp-to-cancer progression. The laparoscope has revolutionized gallbladder removal, as the arthroscope has revolutionized joint surgery. The gastroscope gives the physician new security and control in the management of gastrointestinal conditions, and the bronchoscope facilitates many lung procedures.

Similarly throughout the entire range of endoscopy, new opportunities are opening and leading to significant improvements in therapy, and these improvements will continue. Wireless electronic and video techniques are being introduced into endoscopy, and this new technology promises to widen the applications and therapeutic range of endoscopy still further.

—*C. Richard Falcon*

See also Abdomen; Abdominal disorders; Arthritis; Arthroscopy; Biopsy; Cholecystectomy; Colonoscopy and sigmoidoscopy;

Colorectal cancer; Colorectal polyp removal; Cystoscopy; Endoscopic retrograde cholangiopancreatography (ERCP); Gallbladder diseases; Gastrointestinal disorders; Gastrointestinal system; Invasive tests; Laparoscopy; Pulmonary diseases; Stone removal; Stones.

For Further Information:
A.D.A.M. Medical Encyclopedia. "Endoscopy." *MedlinePlus*, February 20, 2011.
American Cancer Society. "What Is Endoscopy?." *Cancer.org*, February 6, 2013..
Classen, Meinhard, G. N. J. Tytgat, and C. J. Lightdale, eds. *Gastroenterological Endoscopy.* 2d ed. New York: Thieme Medical, 2010.
Emory, Theresa S., et al. *Atlas of Gastrointestinal Endoscopy and Endoscopic Biopsies.* Washington, D.C.: Armed Forces Institute of Pathology, 2000.
Litin, Scott C., ed. *Mayo Clinic Family Health Book.* 4th ed. New York: HarperResource, 2009.
Scott-Conner, Carol E. H., ed. *The SAGES Manual: Fundamentals of Laparoscopy, Thoracoscopy, and GI Endoscopy.* 2d ed. New York: Springer, 2006.

ENEMAS
Procedure
Anatomy or system affected: Abdomen, anus, gastrointestinal system, intestines
Specialties and related fields: Gastroenterology
Definition: A procedure to assist the body in evacuating fecal material from the bowel.

Indications and Procedures

Enemas are used primarily for two purposes: cleansing and retention. Many solutions have been used to promote cleansing. The most commonly used is made up of mild soapsuds and tap water. Commercially prepared solutions containing premeasured mild soap and water are also available.

To receive an enema, the patient should lie on the left side of the body with the upper thigh drawn up to the abdomen. The solution should be slightly above body temperature. The source of the enema fluid should be 30 to 45 centimeters (12 to 18 inches) above the anus. All air should be removed from the tubing that connects the enema reservoir and the tip. The tip is warmed in the hands, lubricated with a commercial preparation or a bit of soapy water, and gently inserted into the anus with a combination of soft pressure and a twisting motion. The tip should not be inserted more than 10 centimeters (4 inches) into the rectum. The solution is allowed to flow slowly into the rectum to prevent cramping.

A towel may be held gently against the rectum to prevent leakage. If cramping does occur, the flow should be interrupted by pinching the tubing. For an adult, approximately 1 liter (1 quart) of solution is probably sufficient; the patient should hold the solution for two to three minutes. The enema tube is tightly clamped and slowly withdrawn; a towel is again held against the anus to catch any leakage. A readily available bedpan or toilet stool is used while the patient evacuates the bowel. Depending on the need for the enema, the procedure may be repeated.

The procedure for administering a retention enema is simi-lar except that the solution is instilled very slowly to promote retention. Lubricants or medicines are administered in this fashion. The patient holds the instilled solution as long as possible before evacuating the bowel.

Uses and Complications

Cleansing enemas are used to promote bowel evacuation by softening fecal material and stimulating the movement by bowel walls (peristalsis). Retention enemas are used to lubricate or soothe the mucosal lining of the rectum, to apply medication to the bowel wall or for absorption by the colon, and to soften feces.

There is no physiological need to have a bowel movement every day; normality is defined as from three to ten per week. Enemas should not be used routinely for cleansing because the bowel quickly becomes dependent on them. This problem is especially common among older individuals.
—*L. Fleming Fallon, Jr., M.D., Ph.D., M.P.H.*

See also Anus; Colon; Colonoscopy and sigmoidoscopy; Colorectal cancer; Colorectal polyp removal; Colorectal surgery; Gastroenterology; Gastrointestinal disorders; Gastrointestinal system; Hemorrhoid banding and removal; Hemorrhoids; Internal medicine; Intestines; Peristalsis; Proctology; Rectum; Surgery, general.

For Further Information:
Heuman, Douglas M., A. Scott Mills, and Hunter H. McGuire, Jr. *Gastroenterology.* Philadelphia: W. B. Saunders, 1997.
Icon Health. *Enemas: A Medical Dictionary, Bibliography, and Annotated Research Guide to Internet References.* San Diego, Calif.: Author, 2003.
Mitsuoka, Tomotari. *Intestinal Bacteria and Health: An Introductory Narrative.* Translated by Syoko Watanabe and W. C. T. Leung. Tokyo: Harcourt Brace Jovanovich, 1978.
Peikin, Steven R. *Gastrointestinal Health: The Proven Nutritional Program to Prevent, Cure, or Alleviate Irritable Bowel Syndrome (IBS), Ulcers, Gas, Constipation, Heartburn, and Many Other Digestive Disorders.* 3d ed. New York: Perennial Currents, 2004.

ENTEROCOLITIS
Disease/Disorder
Also known as: Acute infectious diarrhea
Anatomy or system affected: Gastrointestinal system, intestines
Specialties and related fields: Family medicine, gastroenterology, pediatrics
Definition: Inflammation of the small and large intestines, which may be caused by a severe bacterial infection.

Causes and Symptoms

Enterocolitis is characterized by copious and sometimes bloody diarrhea, abdominal pain, vomiting, and dehydration. A high fever usually exists in young children. Cultures of the stool and blood can establish the exact organism involved.

Campylobacter enterocolitis, resulting from infection with *Campylobacter* bacteria, is the most common bacterial cause of diarrhea. It is endemic in developing countries, and epidemics are seen in Western countries in daycare centers. Salmonella enterocolitis is an infection in the lining of the

---

Information on Enterocolitis

Causes: Bacterial infection; unknown for necrotizing enterocolitis

Symptoms: For bacterial infection, copious and sometimes bloody diarrhea, abdominal pain, vomiting, dehydration, high fever in young children; for necrotizing enterocolitis, poor feeding, abdominal distention or tenderness, decreased bowel sounds, apnea, lethargy, shock, cardiovascular collapse

Duration: Acute

Treatments: For bacterial infection, intravenous fluids and antibiotics; for necrotizing enterocolitis, surgery (intestinal resection)

---

small intestine caused by *Salmonella* bacteria acquired through the ingestion of contaminated food or water or exposure to reptiles. This type of enterocolitis can range from mild to severe and lasts from one to two weeks.

A different type of enterocolitis is necrotizing enterocolitis (NEC), the most common gastrointestinal medical emergency occurring in newborns. It is more prevalent in premature infants. NEC may begin with poor feeding, abdominal distention or tenderness, and decreased bowel sounds. If it becomes systemic, then symptoms can include apnea, lethargy, shock, and cardiovascular collapse. Outbreaks of NEC seem to follow an epidemic pattern, suggesting an infectious disease, but a specific causative organism has not been identified. Research suggests that several factors may be involved.

Treatment and Therapy

The treatment of bacterial enterocolitis involves rehydration and, in some cases, antibiotics. In underdeveloped countries, where medical care is poor, enterocolitis causes more than 60 percent of all deaths in children under age five.

Infants with NEC cannot take food by mouth and often must be fed through a central venous catheter. Those with severe disease may require surgical intervention such as intestinal resection. The mortality rate for NEC approaches 50 percent in infants weighing less than 1,500 grams.

—Connie Rizzo, M.D., Ph.D.;
updated by Tracy Irons-Georges

See also Antibiotics; Bacterial infections; *Campylobacter* infections; Dehydration; Diarrhea and dysentery; Fever; Gastroenterology, pediatric; Gastrointestinal disorders; Gastrointestinal system; Intestinal disorders; Intestines; Nausea and vomiting; Salmonella infection.

For Further Information:

"*Campylobacter* Infections." *MedlinePlus*, Mar. 4, 2013.

Carson-DeWitt, Rosalyn, and Daus Mahnke. "Diarrhea." *Health Library*, Mar. 4, 2013.

Denning, Patricia Wei, and Akhil Maheshwari. *Necrotizing Enterocolitis*. Philadelphia: Elsevier, 2013.

"Diarrhea." *MedlinePlus*, Apr. 15, 2013.

Gilchrist, Brian F., ed. *Necrotizing Enterocolitis*. Georgetown, Tex.: Landes Bioscience, 2000.

Janowitz, Henry D. *Your Gut Feelings: A Complete Guide to Living Better with Intestinal Problems*. Rev. and updated ed. New York:

Oxford University Press, 1995.

"Necrotizing Enterocolitis." *National Institute of Child Health and Human Development*, Apr. 3, 2013.

Ochoa, Blanca, and Christina M. Surawicz. "Diarrheal Diseases " Acute and Chronic." *American College of Gastroenterology*, Dec. 2012.

"*Salmonella* Infections." *MedlinePlus*, Apr. 19, 2013.

Stoll, Barbara J., and Robert M. Kliegman, eds. *Necrotizing Enterocolitis*. Philadelphia: W. B. Saunders, 1994.

Thompson, W. Grant. *Gut Reactions: Understanding Symptoms of the Digestive Tract*. New York: Plenum Press, 1989.

ENTEROVIRUSES
Disease/Disorder

Anatomy or system affected: Brain, eyes, heart, nervous system, skin

Specialties and related fields: Cardiology, dermatology, environmental health, internal medicine, microbiology, neurology, virology

Definition: A class of viruses capable of infecting multiple organ systems, such as the central nervous system, the skin, the eyes, and the heart.

Key terms:

lesion: an abnormal area of tissue

meningitis: the inflammation of the protective tissues surrounding the brain and spinal cord

syndrome: a constellation of different symptoms or signs that are associated with a certain illness

vesicle: a fluid-filled blister

wild type: the form of species that occurs in nature

Causes and Symptoms

Enteroviruses are a class of viruses that include the well-known poliovirus and also coxsackieviruses, echoviruses, and other enteroviruses. Genetically, they are small, nonenveloped, single-stranded deoxyribonucleic acid (DNA) viruses that belong to the family *Picornaviridae*. These viruses are ubiquitous and infections occur year-round.

Enteroviruses cause a variety of clinical syndromes with different clinical manifestations depending on the specific viruses involved. Typically, transmission is through direct contact with fecal matter and contaminated food or water. The virus usually replicates initially in the throat and the small intestine, from where it then spreads to other organs.

Rash is a symptom common in all enterovirus infections. A maculopapular rash (mixture of flat and raised spots) can be seen in echovirus and poliovirus infections. Coxsackieviruses can cause the hand-foot-mouth syndrome in children, which presents as fever and vesicles in the oral cavity, hands, feet, buttocks, and sometimes genitalia. Transmission is through direct contact, and the illness usually resolves in two to three days. Herpangina is another syndrome caused by coxsackieviruses; it presents with painful vesicular lesions on the tonsils and soft palates in children. Echovirus and coxsackievirus can both cause a petechial rash (small, red or purple spots), which sometimes may be confused with a meningococcal infection.

The central nervous system (CNS) is a well-known site of

enteroviral infections. Enteroviruses as a group is the most common cause of viral meningitis in adults, which is usually due to echoviruses and coxsackieviruses. Because infants are not able to verbalize, they usually exhibit signs of irritability and fever, whereas in adults the common complaints are fever, headache, stiff neck, nausea, and vomiting. Encephalitis, the swelling and inflammation of the brain, is usually also the result of coxsackieviruses and echoviruses. It can develop either as a complication of meningitis or as an isolated event. Encephalitis typically presents as fever, lethargy, headache, seizures, or confusion. Paralytic poliomyelitis is the well-known syndrome due to polioviruses, but this presentation is the least common, since most people who have been infected with poliovirus do not have symptoms and only a minority of

patients develop meningitis. Those who do develop paralysis usually present with a progressive, asymmetric weakness. The legs are commonly involved, followed by the arms and abdominal, chest, or throat muscles. It is the involvement of respiratory and throat muscles that may be life threatening since these patients are prone to respiratory failure. While muscle paralysis is the hallmark of poliovirus infection, a similar picture may also be seen with echovirus infections, although the symptoms are not as severe or persistent.

Enterovirus and coxsackievirus are also capable of causing eye infections, commonly known as acute hemorrhagic conjunctivitis (AHC), with red eyes, pain, and swelling of the eyelids.

Coxsackieviruses can affect the chest and abdominal muscles, causing what is known as pleurodynia, which presents as fever and spasms of the chest and abdominal muscles. Coxsackievirus infection of the heart muscles and its surrounding tissues, known as myopericarditis, can present with mild symptoms such as chest pain or severe and rapid progression to heart failure and death.

Treatment and Therapy

Because most enteroviral infections are self-limited and resolve spontaneously, specific treatments are not warranted. In cases of severe infections—such as paralytic disease, meningitis, or myocarditis—supportive therapies are needed as life preservation measures. Even in such severe cases, no specific antiviral agents are available. Serum intravenous immunoglobulin has been tested in patients with certain immunodeficiencies and in neonates, although results have been mixed.

As in most infections, prevention is just as important as treatment. Because enteroviral infections are transmitted

through contaminated sources, it is imperative to exercise good judgment regarding handwashing and hygienic practices.

Perspective and Prospects

As one of the most recognized members of the enteroviral class, poliovirus has come a long way since its isolation in 1909 by Karl Landsteiner and Erwin Popper. The development of polio vaccines along with implementation of polio eradication programs have largely eliminated the disease due to wild-type poliovirus. The virus has been largely eradicated in the United States and other developed countries, and it is targeted for imminent global eradication.

The first polio vaccine was developed in 1952 by Jonas Salk. It was developed as an injectable vaccine using dead virus and is known as the inactivated polio vaccine (IPV). Doses are given at two, four, and six to eighteen months and at four to six years of age. Albert Sabin subsequently developed an oral polio vaccine (OPV) in 1962 that utilizes an attenuated but live poliovirus. Dosing is the same as that for the inactivated polio vaccine. A major concern of the oral polio vaccine is its ability to cause vaccine-induced polio, although the likelihood is very low, with rates of approximately 1 in 2.5 million vaccine recipients. Since most wild-type poliovirus have been eradicated, most cases of poliomyelitis in the twenty-first century are attributed to vaccine-induced poliomyelitis.

—*Andrew Ren, M.D.*

See also Childhood infectious diseases; Encephalitis; Epidemiology; Hand-foot-and-mouth disease; Immunization and vaccination; Meningitis; Paralysis; Poliomyelitis; Viral infections.

For Further Information:
Dugdale, David C. III, and David Zieve. "ECHO Virus." *MedlinePlus*, Oct. 6, 2012.
Fauci, Anthony, et al., eds. "Enteroviruses and Reoviruses." In *Harrison's Principles of Internal Medicine*. 18th ed. New York: McGraw-Hill, 2012.
Mandell, Gerald, eds. *Mandell, Douglas, and Bennett's Principles and Practice of Infectious Diseases*. 7th ed. Philadelphia: Churchill Livingstone, 2010.
"Non-Polio Enterovirus." *Centers for Disease Control and Prevention*, May 10, 2013.
Richman, Douglas, eds. *Clinical Virology*. 3d ed. Washington, D.C.: ASM Press, 2009.
"Viral Infections." *MedlinePlus*, Apr. 19, 2013.
Vorvick, Linda J., and David Zieve. "Hand-Foot-Mouth Disease." *MedlinePlus*, Aug. 10, 2012.

ENURESIS. *See* BED-WETTING.

ENVIRONMENTAL DISEASES
Disease/Disorder
Anatomy or system affected: All
Specialties and related fields: All
Definition: Sicknesses caused or exacerbated by human exposure to physical, chemical, biological, or social environmental conditions, the duration and intensity of the exposure typically affecting the manifestation of symptoms

and fatality-case ratios. Acute environmental diseases may result in rapid decline of health status and warrant emergency response, while chronic conditions often result from long-term exposures to low levels of environmental risk factors.

Key terms:

acute: referring to exposure to hazardous environmental agents or conditions that occur once or over a short period of time (typically fourteen days or less); environmental disease symptoms that appear rapidly

chronic: referring to exposure to environmental risk factor or agent occurring over a long period of time, typically more than one year; symptoms of environmental diseases that take a long time to appear after first contact with the causative agent

dose-response: the relationship between the dose (a quantitative measurement of exposure usually expressed in terms of concentration and duration) and the quantitative expression of change to the status of human health and well-being resulting in disease

environmental epidemiology: the systematic study of the distribution and determinants of environmental diseases in a population

environmental infection: human exposure to infectious agents of diseases (including bacteria, fungi, parasites, and viruses) through contact with environmental media such as contaminated water, air, food, and soil

environmental radiation: human exposure to electromagnetic radiation at doses and durations that can produce adverse impacts on human health

environmental toxicity: human exposure to chemical or biochemical substances at doses that produce harmful modification to the body's physiological mechanisms, leading to diseases

exposure assessment: a systematic process of discovering the pathway through which humans are exposed to specific environmental agents and risk factors, and of ascertaining the quantity and duration of that exposure

Causes and Symptoms

The modern word "miasma" comes from the Greek *miasma* or *miainein,* meaning "pollution" or "to pollute." Before scientific theories of disease became entrenched in medical practice, miasma was used to connote bad environments in which human exposure led to various diseases. Even today, one of the most devastating human diseases, malaria, draws its name from references to "bad air." There is clearly a rich historical record of human recognition of the intimate connection between environmental quality and diseases. It is now known that serious human diseases are caused by numerous chemical, physical, and biological agents (risk factors) that occur naturally or as a result of human actions that modify the environment. In fact, the more that is learned about disease etiology, the more the complex interplay between environmental conditions and root causes of diseases within the body are recognized. Furthermore, some people are more sensitive to environmental risk factors because of

their age, sex, occupation, culture, or genetic characteristics.

Environmental diseases are those illnesses for which cause and effect can be reasonably associated through epidemiological studies, preferably verified through laboratory experiments. Therefore, the recognition of environmental diseases draws upon two traditional postulates regarding causation in the study of human diseases, one ascribed to Robert Koch (1843–1910) and the other ascribed to Austin Bradford Hill (1897–1991). The more important set of guidelines for environmental diseases is generally known in epidemiology as Hill's criteria of causation, based on his landmark 1965 publication entitled "The Environment and Disease: Association or Causation?" Hill warned that cause-effect decisions should not be based on a set of rules. Instead, he supported the view that cost-benefit analysis is essential for policy decisions on controlling environmental quality in order to avoid diseases. It is arguable that Hill's treatise initiated current trends characterized by the precautionary principle in environmental health science. Nevertheless, Hill's nine viewpoints for exploring the relationship between environment and disease are worth emphasizing. They are precedence, correlation, dose-response relationship, consistency, plausibility, alternatives, empiricism, specificity, and coherence.

According to the precedence viewpoint, exposure must always precede the outcome in every case of the environmental disease. One of the most famous examples here is the classic epidemiological study of John Snow (1813–58) on the spread of cholera and its association with exposure to contaminated water in the densely populated city of London.

According to the correlation viewpoint, a strong association or correlation should exist between the exposure and the incidence of the environmental disease. The clustering of diseases within neighborhoods or among workers at a specific occupation is frequently the beginning of investigations into environmental diseases. Clusters can provide strong evidence of correlations. Bernardino Ramazinni (1633–1714), considered by many to be one of the founders of the discipline of occupational and environmental health sciences, published his treatise *De Morbis Artificum* in 1700 following critical observations regarding the correlation between environmental exposures of and diseases in workers.

According to the dose-response viewpoint, the relationship between exposure and the severity of environmental disease should be characterized by a dose-response relationship, in which an increase in the intensity and/or duration of exposure produces a more severe disease outcome. "The dose makes the poison" is one of the central tenets of environmental toxicology. This phrase is attributed to Paracelsus (1493–1541). This tenet has proven difficult to interpret for formulating health policy in the case of environmental diseases because the variation in human genetics and physiology means that, in many situations, a single threshold of toxicity cannot be established as safe for every person. Exposure to ionizing radiation is an example of a situation in which it is difficult to establish dose-response relationships that are useful for setting uniformly applicable preventive health policy.

According to the consistency viewpoint, there should be consistent findings in different populations, across different studies, and at different times regarding the association between exposure and environmental disease. This means that the relationship should be reproducible. For example, exposure of people to mercury across civilizations, occupations, and age groups has been consistently associated with certain health effects that allowed the recognition of the special hazards posed by this toxic metal. Mercury was used in various manufacturing processes for several centuries, and where precautions are not taken to prevent human exposure, disease invariably results.

Consistency should cut across not only generations but also occupations and different doses of exposure. For example, "mad hatter's" disease was associated with the use of mercury in the production of fur felt, in which mercurous nitrate was used to add texture to smooth fibers such as rabbit fur to facilitate matting (the process is called "carroting" because of the resulting orange color). More recently, the exposure of pregnant women to fish contaminated with methyl mercury from industrial sources in Japan produced developmental diseases in fetuses. The societal repercussions of the so-called Minamata Bay disease are still not completely settled after more than fifty years. Mercury is now widely recognized as a cumulative toxicant with systemic effects and organ damage, with symptoms including trembling, dental problems, blindness, ataxia, depression, and anxiety.

According to the plausibility viewpoint, compelling evidence of "biological plausibility" should exist that a physiological pathway leads from exposure to a specific environmental risk factor to the development of a specific environmental disease. This does not exclude the possibility of multiple causes, some acquired through environmental exposures and others through genetic processes. For example, lead poisoning has been recognized since the 1950s as a pervasive and devastating environmental disease. The symptoms of lead poisoning vary, from specific organ effects, such as kidney disease, to systemic effects, such as anemia, and to cognitive effects, such as intelligence quotient (IQ) deficiency. How a single environmental toxicant can produce such wide-ranging diseases was a puzzle until the molecular mechanisms underpinning lead poisoning and the pharmacokinetic distribution of lead in the human body was understood. Lead is temporarily stored in the blood, where it binds to a key enzyme, aminolevulinate dehydratase, which participates in the synthesis of heme. The by-products of that reaction produce anemia and organ effects, including kidney and brain diseases. Long-term storage of lead in the body occurs in bony tissue, where other effects are possible. These biological understandings have helped activists and scientists agitate for environmental policy to reduce lead exposure worldwide.

According to the alternatives viewpoint, alternative explanations for the development of diseases should be considered alongside the plausible environmental causes. These alternative explanations should be ruled out before conclusions are reached about causal relationships between environmental exposures and disease. For example, the typically low doses to which populations are exposed to pesticides and the long time period between exposure and the typical chronic disease outcomes, such as cancers and neurodegenerative disorders, make it difficult to reconstruct the disease pathways and pinpoint causative agents. This is where it is important to consider all alternatives and to eliminate them before compelling arguments can be made about the effects of pesticide toxicity. Sometimes observing wildlife response to environmental risk factors help narrow down alternative explanations, as Rachel Carson taught in her timeless book *Silent Spring* (1962).

According to the empiricism viewpoint, the course of environmental disease should be alterable by appropriate intervention strategies verifiable through experimentation. In other words, the disease can be preventable or curable following manipulation of the environment and/or human physiology. For acute exposures, the emergency response is to eliminate the source of exposure. However, this is not always

---

In the News:
Iraq War Increases Disease Risks

Throughout the history of warfare, diseases have often caused more casualties among both soldiers and civilians than weaponry itself. The conflict in Iraq is no exception. A rare type of lung infection, acute eosinophilic pneumonia (AEP), is occurring at a higher rate among U.S. soldiers in Iraq than in any other segment of the population. The illness, characterized by fever, serious lung impairment, and eventually respiratory failure, has killed a number of soldiers since the war began in 2003. Of the individuals who contracted this pneumonia, all reported exposure to fine sand and dust particles, a common hazard in the desert environments of the Middle East. Administration of corticosteroids proved life-saving for most patients, but many who have recovered complain of residual lung problems.

Veterans of Operation Iraqi Freedom are not alone in fighting disabling illnesses. Brain cancer, amyotrophic lateral sclerosis (ALS), fibromyalgia, and multiple sclerosis are among the serious ailments plaguing the earlier Gulf War veterans from 1991. The demolition of weapons dumps in Iraq in March, 1991, released the deadly nerve agents sarin and cyclosarin. Many Gulf War veterans claim that this incident is to blame for the diseases from which they now suffer. A U.S. Department of Defense-sponsored study conducted by the Institute of Medicine of the National Academy of Sciences and published in the *American Journal of Public Health* (August, 2005), focused on the nerve gas release event at Al Khamisiyah and subsequent increase in neurological illnesses in those exposed to the chemical contamination that followed.

Inflamed joints, heat and chemical sensitivities, severe headaches, hair loss, and recurrent skin rashes are just a few of the symptoms endured by affected troops who have returned from both Iraq conflicts. Thousands of Gulf War veterans are currently receiving disability payments from the Veterans Administration, and many of those payments are for battle-related illness rather than for injury.

Lenola Glass-Godwin, M.WS.

possible in cases where patients are unconscious or otherwise unable to articulate clearly the source of exposure, as is the case for many children. Nevertheless, standardized procedures exist for responding to environmental exposure beyond eliminating the source. For example, therapy based on chelation (from the Greek *chele*, meaning "claw") works for toxic metal exposure because the mode of action of the therapeutic agent, ethylene diamine tetra-acetic acid (EDTA), is well understood. It is possible to establish empirically the relative effectiveness of EDTA in dealing with various forms of toxic metal exposures. For example, under normal physiological conditions, EDTA binds metals in the following order: iron (ferric ion), mercury, copper, aluminum, nickel, lead, cobalt, zinc, iron (ferrous ion), cadmium, manganese, magnesium, and calcium. Based on this information, it is possible to design therapeutic processes that minimize adverse side effects.

According to the specificity viewpoint, when an environmental disease is associated with only one environmental agent, the relationship between exposure and environmental disease is said to be specific. This strengthens the argument for causality, but this situation is extremely rare. For example, the rarity of mesothelioma, a lung disease that afflicts people who have been exposed to asbestos fibers, made it possible to use epidemiological evidence quickly to support policy in restricting the use of asbestos in commercial products and to protect employees from occupational exposures.

The recognition of new diseases often leads to speculation about causative agents or conditions. Occasionally, new ideas about causation challenge orthodox theories. According to the coherence viewpoint, it is important to conduct a rigorous assessment of coherence with existing information and scientific ideas before such causes are accepted in the case of environmental diseases. For example, the origin of neurodegenerative diseases associated with exposure to prion protein remains mysterious, and some environmental causes have been proposed, including exposure to toxic metal ions. Another example is the current concern with the introduction of oxy_comment_start author="clacerte" timestamp="20130523T100220-0400" comment="http://www.niehs.nih.gov/health/topics/agents/sya-nano/index.cfm"?nanoparticlesoxy_comment_end? into commercial products, with concomitant environmental dissemination. Although much has been learned from an understanding of the human health effects of respirable particulate matter, researchers should be sufficiently open-minded to the possibility that nanoparticles will behave differently in the environment and in the human body.

Hill's nine viewpoints were presented in the context of pitfalls associated with overreliance on statistical tests of "significance" as a justification to base health policy on epidemiological observations. Hill's viewpoints have been debated extensively, and it is worth noting the following caveats presented in the 2004 article "The Missed Lessons of Sir Austin Bradford Hill," by Carl V. Phillips and Karen J. Goodman: statistical significance should not be mistaken for evidence of substantial association; association does not prove causation; precision should not be mistaken for validity; evidence that a causal relationship exists is not sufficient to suggest that action should be taken; and uncertainty about causation or association is not sufficient to suggest that action should not be taken.

The second set of guidelines regarding causality derives from what is generally known as Koch's postulates, but it is perhaps only useful for precautionary approaches to proactive assessment of potential health impacts of new agents about to be introduced into the environment. This approach complements the epidemiology-based inferences described by Hill, but further refinement is warranted to deal with complicated issues such as interactions between multiple environmental agents, which could have additive, neutral, or canceling effects. The question of dose is also difficult to subject to simple conclusions because of phenomena such as hormesis, in which small doses may show beneficial effects.

For environmental diseases, a modified version of Koch's postulates can be expressed as follows. First, exposure to an environmental agent must be demonstrable in all organisms suffering from the disease but not in healthy organisms (assuming predisposition factors). Second, the identity, concentrations in different environmental and physiological compartments, and transformation pathways of the agent must be known as much as possible. Third, the agent should cause disease when introduced into healthy organisms. Fourth, biomarkers showing modification of the physiological target affected by the environmental agent must be observable in experimentally exposed organisms.

Treatment and Therapy

The symptoms of environmental diseases vary widely, and physiological, anatomical, and behavioral characteristics can succumb to the effects of environmental agents. In evaluating treatment and therapy, it is useful to consider two categories of symptoms. Acute symptoms are exhibited in response to human exposure to high doses of toxic agents within a short period of time. Essentially, the body is overwhelmed, and emergency therapy is necessary to avoid death or permanent disability. For toxic air contaminants, respiratory distress is a common symptom, and mortality can occur rapidly. Conversely, chronic symptoms of human exposures to low levels of environmental (particularly air) pollutants are difficult to diagnose, as in the case of cancers attributable to secondhand tobacco smoke or ambient exposure to respirable particulate matter. Similarly, exposure of the skin to rapidly absorbed toxins can produce rapid mortality, but the development of skin cancer due to ultraviolet (UV) light exposure may take decades to manifest. Ingestion of contaminated liquids or food may take minutes to provoke distress and vomiting, whereas it may take years for chronic symptoms to manifest in cases of carcinogenic water pollutants.

Treatment and therapy of environmental diseases requires accurate diagnosis of the causative agent. The first line of response is to limit exposure through flushing the body with clean air or liquids. Chelation therapy can be used to reduce the body burden of certain toxic metals. Curative measures follow the established procedures developed for specific organs. For example, chemotherapy, radiotherapy, and surgery are used to treat cancers regardless of the involvement of known environmental factors in their etiology. Skin diseases such as chloracne associated with exposure to chlorinated aromatic hydrocarbon pollutants, including dioxins and polychlorinated biphenyls (PCBs), are managed to reduce the severity of lesions and enhance natural healing processes. Cognitive deficits associated with exposure to metals and other environmental pollutants are believed to be reversible as long further exposures are avoided. Finally, environmental diseases associated with infectious agents such as bacteria can be controlled through a combination of source disinfection and antibiotic therapy.

Perspective and Prospects

There has been a resurgence of interest in environmental diseases because of societal changes at regional and international levels. Industrialization demands the use of thousands of potentially hazardous chemicals that ultimately end up polluting human environments and remain an important source of causative agents for environmental diseases. Recent threats associated with global environmental change, bioterrorism, and chemical warfare have all contributed to the need for rapid detection of hazardous environmental agents and tougher laws to protect air, water, soil, and food resources. Prevention is still the crucial solution to reducing the human burden of environmental diseases worldwide.

On June 16, 2006, the World Health Organization (WHO) issued a landmark report estimating that environmental risk factors play a role in more than 80 percent of diseases regularly reported by WHO across fourteen regions globally. The environment has an impact on human health through exposures to physical, chemical, and biological risk factors and through changes in human behavior in response to environmental change at local and global levels. Globally, nearly 25 percent of all deaths and of the total disease burden (measured in disability-adjusted life years, or DALYs) can be attributed to environmental quality. The situation is more dire for children aged fourteen and younger, with environmental risk factors accounting for more than 33 percent of the disease burden. These discoveries have important implications for national and international health policy, because many of the implicated environmental risk factors can be modified by established interventions. The lack of understanding on how to deploy these interventions globally has inspired the involvement of well-funded organizations and institutions in environmental health issues.

—*Oladele A. Ogunseitan, Ph.D., M.P.H.*

See also Allergies; Asbestos exposure; Aspergillosis; Asthma; Bronchitis; Cancer; Carcinogens; Carpal tunnel syndrome; Chronic obstructive pulmonary disease (COPD); Coccidioidomycosis; Dengue fever; *E. coli* infection; Emerging infectious diseases; Emphysema; Environmental health; Epidemics and pandemics; Epidemiology; Food poisoning; Gulf War syndrome; Lead poisoning; Lung cancer; Melanoma; Mercury poisoning; Mesothelioma; Multiple chemical sensitivity syndrome; Occupational health; Poisoning; Pulmonary diseases; Radiation sickness; Respiration; Rocky Mountain spotted fever; Skin cancer; Skin lesion removal; Teratogens; Toxicology; Tularemia.

For Further Information:

Carson, Rachel. *Silent Spring*. 50th anniversary ed. London: Penguin Classics, 2012.

"Health Effects of Exposure to Substances and Carcinogens." *Agency for Toxic Substances and Disease Registry*, March 3, 2011.

Hill, Austin Bradford. "The Environment and Disease: Association or Causation?" *Proceedings of the Royal Society of Medicine* 58 (1965): 295–300.

McMichael, Tony. *Human Frontiers, Environments, and Disease.* New York: Cambridge University Press, 2003.

National Institute of Environmental Health Sciences (NIEHS). "Environmental Diseases from A to Z." 2d ed. Research Triangle Park, N.C.: U.S. Department of Health and Human Services, National Institutes of Health, June 2007.

National Institute of Environmental Health Sciences (NIEHS). "Advancing Science, Improving Health: A Plan for Environmental Health Research—2012–2017 Strategic Plan." Research Triangle Park, N.C.: U.S. Department of Health and Human Services, National Institutes of Health, 2012.

National Toxicology Program.*Report on Carcinogens*. 12th ed. Research Triangle Park, N.C.: U.S. Department of Health and Human Services, Public Health Service, 2011.

Phillips, Carl V., and Karen J. Goodman. "The Missed Lessons of Sir Austin Bradford Hill." *Epidemiologic Perspectives and Innovations* 1, no. 3 (October 4, 2004). http://www.epi-perspectives.com/content/1/1/3.

Pruss-Ustun, A., and C. Corvalan, eds. *Preventing Disease Through Healthy Environments: Towards an Estimate of the Environmental Burden of Disease*. Geneva: World Health Organization, 2006.

Solomon, Gina, Oladele A. Ogunseitan, and Jan Kirsch. *Pesticides and Human Health: A Resource for Health Care Professionals*. San Francisco: Physicians for Social Responsibility, 2000.

ENZYME THERAPY

Treatment

Also known as: Enzyme replacement therapy

Anatomy or system affected: All

Specialties and related fields: Alternative medicine, biochemistry, genetics

Definition: The use of enzymes as drugs to treat specific medical problems.

Indications and Procedures

Enzymes are large, complex protein molecules that catalyze chemical reactions in living organisms. The phrase *enzyme therapy* is sometimes used to refer to enzyme preparations given as dietary supplements, often as digestive aids. Such treatment is of questionable value because enzymes, like all proteins, are degraded in the stomach. Legitimate enzyme therapy is an innovative procedure based on emerging technology. Enzymes used to treat various medical conditions are delivered intravenously.

Enzyme therapy is used to dissolve clots in stroke and cardiac patients. Enzymes such as streptokinase, plasmin, and human tissue plasminogen activator (TPA) are able to dissolve clots when injected into the bloodstream.

Some types of adult leukemia can be treated by injection of

the enzyme asparaginase, which destroys asparagine. Tumors in these patients require asparagine, and the asparaginase removes it from the blood, thus inhibiting the ability of these tumors to grow.

Enzyme therapy can also be used to treat certain inherited diseases. One of these is Fabry's disease. Patients with this disease are deficient in an enzyme called alpha-galactosidase A. Without this enzyme, harmful levels of a substance called ceremide trehexoside accumulate in the heart, brain, and kidneys. If left untreated, patients usually die in their forties or fifties after a lifetime of pain. On the other hand, patients injected with alpha-galactosidase A once every two weeks lead nearly normal lives.

Gaucher's disease is another severe inherited disease characterized by a deficiency in an enzyme that normally prevents the buildup of a chemical to injurious levels. It can be treated by injections of the enzyme glucocerebrosidase.

Uses and Complications

The use of enzymes to treat clotting problems and genetic diseases started in the early 1990s; thus, the long-term effects are unknown. Enzyme therapy does not cure genetic disease, so the therapy must be lifelong.

Some people are encouraged to swallow enzyme preparations to aid digestion. For example, the enzyme papain is promoted as a digestive aid. Although papain is very effective at breaking down proteins in the laboratory or as a meat tenderizer in the kitchen, it does not function well in the stomach. Papain is most effective at a nearly neutral pH of 6.2, whereas the stomach is highly acidic with a pH of about 2.0. On the other hand, papain is active in the more neutral esophagus. Although normally little or no food is found in the esophagus, papain has the potential to damage the esophageal lining, especially in people with esophageal disorders.

—*Lorraine Lica, Ph.D.*

See also Blood and blood disorders; Digestion; Enzymes; Fatty acid oxidation disorder; Fructosemia; Galactosemia; Gaucher's disease; Genetic diseases; Glycogen storage diseases; Heart attack; Leukemia; Metabolism; Mucopolysaccharidosis (MPS); Niemann-Pick disease; Oncology; Pharmacology; Strokes; Tay-Sachs disease; Thrombolytic therapy and TPA; Thrombosis and thrombus; Tumors.

For Further Information:

Cichoke, Anthony J. *The Complete Book of Enzyme Therapy.* Garden City Park, N.Y.: Avery, 1999.

Devlin, Thomas M., ed. *Textbook of Biochemistry: With Clinical Correlations.* 7th ed. Hoboken, N.J.: Wiley-Liss, 2010.

Rimoin, David L., et al., eds. *Emery and Rimoin's Principles and Practice of Medical Genetics.* 5th ed. Philadelphia: Churchill Livingstone/Elsevier, 2007.

Scriver, Charles R., et al., eds. *The Metabolic and Molecular Bases of Inherited Disease.* 8th ed. New York: McGraw-Hill, 2001.

EPIDEMICS AND PANDEMICS
Disease/Disorder

Anatomy or system affected: All

Specialties and related fields: Bacteriology, critical care, epidemiology, gastroenterology, hematology, immunology, internal medicine, microbiology, nursing, otorhinolaryngology, pathology, pharmacology, public health, pulmonary medicine, serology, virology

Definition: An epidemic is a widespread, rapid occurrence of an infectious disease in a community or region at a particular time. A pandemic is an epidemic prevalent throughout a country, a continent, or the world.

Key terms:

coronavirus: a member of the family Coronaviridae, characterized by a viral envelope that looks like a crown and has a positive-sense single-stranded ribonucleic acid (RNA) genome

filovirus: a member of the family Filoviridae, characterized by a filamentous form of the virus and causing severe hemorrhagic fever in humans; it has a negative-sense single-stranded RNA genome; these viruses are so pathological that they require biosafety level four (BSL-4) containment

hemorrhagic fever: a disease in humans or other animals characterized by a high fever and a bleeding disorder, affecting multiple organ systems and, if severe, leading to death

negative-sense RNA virus: a virus in which the virion-enclosed genome is a single strand of RNA that requires transcription to a positive messenger RNA strand before protein synthesis can occur; these viruses enclose a RNA-dependent RNA polymerase to carry this out

orthomyxovirus: a member of the family Orthomyxoviridae, characterized by a spherical (or occasionally filamentous) form and having two major surface glycoproteins, N (neuraminidase) and H (hemagglutinin), that vary from strain to strain; it has a negative-sense single-stranded RNA genome of seven to eight segments

pathogen: an agent that is capable of causing a disease, including viruses, bacteria, protozoa, rickettsia, or parasitic worms

positive-sense RNA virus: a virus in which the virion-enclosed genome is a single strand of RNA that acts directly as a messenger RNA and can be translated directly into protein

Causes and Symptoms

Epidemics, those caused by old diseases that have been around for centuries or newly identified diseases, break out regularly in the human population. Whether they become full-scale pandemics depends on several factors, including how contagious the pathogen; the number of pathogens needed to initiate a disease; how the pathogen is transmitted;

Information on Epidemics and Pandemics

Causes: Often viruses or bacteria

Symptoms: Depend upon particular disease

Duration: Some pandemics run their course in three to four months; others last for years

Treatments: Depend upon individual disease; antibiotics for bacterial infections, antiviral medications for viral diseases

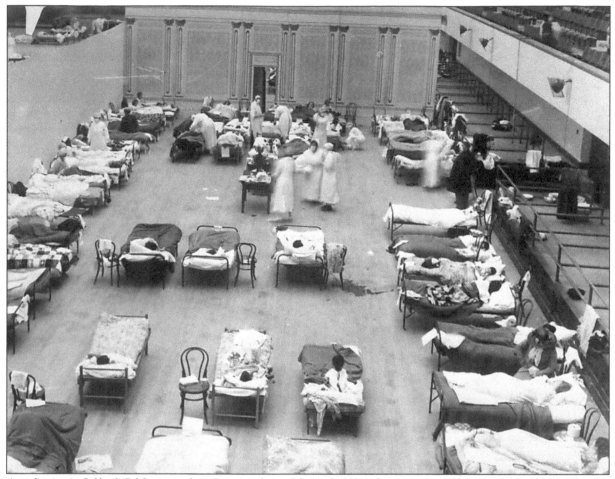

An auditorium in Oakland, California, used as a temporary hospital during the 1918 influenza pandemic. (Courtesy, Oakland Public Library)

the period during which a person is infectious before and after symptoms appear; how long the pathogen can survive in the environment; if an intermediate or alternate host for the pathogen exists; whether vaccines are available, effective, and have been widely used; whether there are any drugs or medications to treat the disease; and whether the contagion can be isolated and contained. Some examples can illustrate these points.

Ebola, one of the most deadly diseases known, is a hemorrhagic fever first identified in 1976 along the Ebola River in the Democratic Republic of the Congo (formerly Zaire). It is caused by a filovirus, a negative-sense single-stranded RNA virus that, in the electron microscope, looks like string, or thread, or filament. Infection leads to a disruption of connective tissues, including that of the blood vessel wall. This results in hemorrhaging from all orifices of the body and rapid death. The death rate for Ebola hemorrhagic fever is greater than 80 percent. There is no treatment or cure. Fortunately, the virus is not airborne; it is transmitted only by direct contact with contaminated bodily fluids. There is an alternate host, believed to be another mammal, possibly bats. Thus pe-

riodic, local outbreaks occur. However, despite it being extremely deadly, Ebola can be contained by isolation. It has never led to a widespread epidemic or pandemic.

Severe acute respiratory syndrome (SARS) is another example of a recent disease that did lead to an epidemic. SARS was first identified in Guangdong Province, China, in 2003. It is caused by a coronavirus, a positive-sense RNA virus that, in the electron microscope has a ring of viral spikes somewhat like a crown, from which this type of virus gets its name. The virus infects the epithelia of the upper respiratory tract. The symptoms are similar to influenza (fever, headache, muscle ache, fatigue, coughing, sneezing). However, in a significant number of cases, the lungs become involved. This causes severe respiratory distress. There is no cure for SARS, and the disease needs to run its course. The body will produce antibodies against the virus. Antivirals can reduce the severity, and when appropriate, antibiotics are used to treat secondary bacterial infections. Nevertheless, the death rate is estimated at about 10 percent, but more than 50 percent in those over sixty-five.

The disease is spread by virus-containing droplets from

coughing or sneezing. Unlike influenza, however, fairly close contact is needed, and the virus does not remain viable in the environment for more than a few hours. SARS quickly spread to twenty-nine countries in 2003 because of air travel, but a rapid and effective global public health response with isolation of SARS cases prevented the disease from becoming a severe pandemic. Although SARS was widespread, a total of only 8,096 cases worldwide were reported to the World Health Organization (WHO); the organization declared SARS to be eradicated in 2005. Because the virus can infect mammals and birds, however, some scientists believed that new outbreaks of the disease could occur in the future.

In 2009, a pandemic of the H1N1 influenza virus broke out. Initially believed to have begun in Mexico, later reports indicated that it most likely developed in Asia. The swine flu, as it was called, claimed 18,500 lives, according to the World Health Organization, which declared an official end to the outbreak in August, 2010.

In contrast, a disease becomes a pandemic when it is both widespread and affects a significant percentage of the population. The best example is the seasonal influenza (flu). The well-known symptoms are fever (often elevated), head and general body aches, sore throat, cough, nasal congestion, and fatigue. It may or may not be accompanied by diarrhea and/or vomiting, symptoms more often seen in young children. It usually runs its course in a week to ten days. Influenza is caused by orthomyxoviruses, which in the electron microscope appear as a spherical or ovoid particles, or occasionally as a filament. These viruses have a negative-sense, single-stranded RNA genome, but it is segmented into several RNA molecules. Infection reaches a peak during the winter months (December through March in the Northern Hemisphere, June through September in the Southern Hemisphere). Estimates indicate that 5 to 30 percent of the world population may become infected in any given year. The reasons that flu pandemics are so common is because flu viruses are highly contagious, survive in the environment for long periods, and frequently mutate so that immunity to one strain of influenza virus does not protect against the same but mutated virus in the future. Moreover, influenza viruses can infect other organisms, which act as a reservoir and in which the virus can mutate or recombine with other coinfected influenza viruses, producing a new strain. The mortality rate for seasonal influenza is about 0.1 percent, usually in the very young, the elderly, and those with other underlying medical conditions such as asthma, diabetes, or cardiovascular disease. Flu vaccines are effective in preventing or reducing the severity of the disease, if they have been made against the type of influenza virus circulating in the world that year. Antiviral medications such as Tamiflu reduce severity of the disease.

Treatment and Therapy

Treatment and therapies for various contagions will depend on the specific disease, but they usually includes antibiotics for bacterial infections and antiviral medications for viral diseases.

Perspective and Prospects

Epidemics and pandemics have plagued humans throughout history. Approximately forty thousand years ago, humans began to domesticate plants and animals for food. Clearing land for crops exposed them to new pathogens, and the close proximity to domesticated animals allowed for transmission of animal pathogens to people. Ancient diseases including smallpox, tuberculosis, measles, and influenza probably arose from animal pathogens adapting to humans. In more recent times, human immunodeficiency virus (HIV) probably adapted to humans in the past fifty years and can be traced to similar simian viruses (SIV) of the chimpanzee and the sooty mangebey monkey. Monkeys are common pets in Africa. Chimpanzees have been used as bush meat, and the transmission of SIV probably occurred during butchering of the animal. The gathering of ancient peoples into larger groups and forming villages with close proximity of inhabitants allowed for pathogens to spread easily. Later, diseases spread along trade routes from Asia and Africa to Europe. Wars have always contributed to the spread of disease as a result of unsanitary conditions, malnutrition, rape, susceptibility of the new population to the pathogen, and lack of sufficient medical care.

History records many epidemics and pandemics. Homer wrote of pestilence devastating the Greeks in the siege of Troy. Thucydides described the Athenian plague of 430-427 BCE Hippocrates, the so-called father of medicine, has one of the earliest descriptions of an influenza epidemic in 412 BCE The Bible records pestilences in the books of Numbers and in Exodus, the latter most likely being an epidemic of Black Plague in Egypt. In Rome, the physician Pliny the Elder described epidemics of smallpox (165–85 CE) and measles (251–66). Probably the best-known pandemic is the Black Plague that devastated Europe in the fourteenth century. In December, 1347, three spice ships from China disembarked at Messina, Italy, carrying plague-infected rats. The plague spread quickly throughout Europe. Ultimately an estimated 25 million died of plague by 1355, amounting to as much as 42 percent of the European population. This pandemic led to great social changes, including the end of the feudal system and the rise of the middle class. Lesser epidemics of plague reappeared in the seventeenth century in Europe and each century since, including one of pneumonic plague in India in the 1990s.

The greatest pandemic in recorded history is that of the influenza pandemic of 1918. Indeed, 80 percent of all Americans who died in Europe during World War I died of influenza, not in direct combat. The 50 to 100 million people worldwide died of what has been called the Spanish flu not because it originated in Spain but because Spain was particularly hard hit by the pandemic. This virus, a mixture of avian and human influenza components, was one hundred times more lethal than the typical seasonal flu. This has caused concern over a reemergence of a highly contagious form of avian flu.

Since about 1980, many new or reemerging diseases, or old pathogens that have developed drug resistance, have been identified. They include Lyme disease; Ebola hemorrhagic fever; Marburg hemorrhagic fever; Lassa fever; Legionnaires' disease; toxic shock syndrome; acquired immunodeficiency syndrome (AIDS), caused by HIV; hantavirus pulmonary syndrome; *E. coli* O157:H7, a Shigella toxin-producing strain of *E. coli*; variant Creutzfeldt-Jakob disease (vCJD), the human equivalent of mad cow disease; hepatitis C; cryptosporidiosis; cyclospiridosis; Whitewater arroyo virus; enterovirus 71; hendra virus; West Nile virus; Malaysian Nipah virus; human monkeypox; pneumonic plague; SARS; avian flu; methicillin-resistant *Staphlococcus aureus* (MRSA); vancomycin-resistant *Staphlococcus aureus*; drug-resistant malaria; and multi-drug resistant tuberculosis.

Finally, there is great concern that many of these highly contagious and deadly agents could be "weaponized" and used as biological agents for bioterrorism. Moreover, using biotechnology, new viruses with the contagion of smallpox or influenza along with the lethality of something like Ebola could be developed.

—*Ralph R. Meyer, Ph.D.*

See also Acquired immunodeficiency syndrome (AIDS); Antibiotics; Avian influenza; Bacterial infections; Centers for Disease Control and Prevention (CDC); Drug resistance; Ebola virus; Emerging infectious diseases; Epidemiology; H1N1 influenza; Human immunodeficiency virus (HIV); Immunization and vaccination; Influenza; Insect-borne diseases; Malaria; National Institutes of Health (NIH); Parasitic diseases; Plague; Severe acute respiratory syndrome (SARS); Tuberculosis; Viral infections; West Nile virus; World Health Organization; Zoonoses.

For Further Information:

Barry, John M. *The Great Influenza: The Story of the Deadliest Pandemic in History*. New York: Penguin Books, 2005.

Doherty, P. C. *Pandemics*. New York: Oxford University Press, 2013.

Killingray, David. *The Spanish Influenza Pandemic of 1918-1919: New Perspectives*. New York: Routledge 2013.

Krause, Richard M. "The Origin of Plagues: Old and New." *Science* 257 (August 21, 1992): 1073–1078.

Morens, David M., Gregory K. Folkers, and Anthony S. Fauci. "The Challenge of Emerging and Re-emerging Infectious Diseases." *Nature* 430 (July 8, 2004): 242–249.

Oldstone, Michael B. A. *Viruses, Plagues, and History: Past, Present, and Future*. New York: Oxford University Press, 2010.

Sherman, Irwin W. *Twelve Diseases That Changed Our World*. Washington, D.C.: ASM Press, 2007.

Tucker, Jonathan B. *Scourge: The Once and Future Threat of Smallpox*. New York: Atlantic Monthly Press, 2001.

EPIDEMIOLOGY

Specialty

Anatomy or system affected: All

Specialties and related fields: Public health

Definition: The study of distributions and patterns of disease, injury, and death in populations. Epidemiology involves investigating determinants, causes, and exacerbating factors of health risks.

Key terms:

case series: an observational study design that arranges affected persons in the order in which they were affected and their relationships to previously affected persons.

case-control study: an observational study design which organizes individuals into groups by their outcomes, and attempts to retroactively uncover which preceding factors may have been linked to those outcomes.

cohort study: an observational study design that organizes study participants into groups by common possible risk factors, and follows those groups over a period and evaluates their collective outcomes.

epidemiological triangle: a theory of infectious disease transmission which emphasizes the interactions of the host, a disease agent, and the environment in which they meet; also known as the "chain of transmission."

incidence: the rate at which new cases of a disease develop in a population.

observational study: a research model that relies on collecting data from participants without experimentally controlling their environment, as opposed to a randomized trial.

prevalence: the proportion of a population affected by a selected disease or disability.

surveillance: a consistent, periodic collection and review of population health statistics, that attempts to determine the presence of disease and uncover abnormal disease activity.

Science and Profession

Epidemiologists distinguish themselves from traditional medical practice in two ways: their focus is on understanding diseases rather than treating them, and their priority lies not with the individual patient, but the whole population. This distinction allows the epidemiologist to focus on improving medical screening and methods and contributing to the understanding of disease, injury, disability, and death. The major concern of an epidemiologist is in determining how a patient became sick, investigating factors that may make a patient even sicker, and improving medical doctors' understanding of what will allow a patient to improve.

In essence, epidemiology is used to understand two crucial measures of disease and injury: prevalence and incidence. Prevalence gives a current picture of how many individuals in a population at risk are afflicted with disease. This measure is given as a fraction, with the number of diseased individuals in the numerator, and the total number of individuals at risk for disease (the population at risk) in the denominator (e.g., the prevalence of cancer in this population is 12 per 1000 persons at risk, or 1.2 percent). In determining incidence, the epidemiologist is concerned with the rate at which new cases of a disease develop. This is also expressed as a fraction, but with an element of time added into the denominator (e.g., the incidence of cancer in this population is 3 per 1000 persons at risk per year). The measure of prevalence can give a quick indication of the burden a disease places upon a population, while the incidence provides a measure of risk that any given person in that population may develop the disease.

Using the tools of prevalence and incidence, the epidemiologist is able to approach the heart of understanding infectious disease transmission, the epidemiological triangle. The triangle consists of three entities that all interact with each other in the transmission of disease-host, agent, and environment. In order for a disease to take hold in the host, the agent must be able to persist both in the host and in the environment where the agent meets the host. Using this model, infection control professionals can take the findings of epidemiological studies of infectious diseases and agents and focus preventive efforts on disrupting one or several parts of the triangle (referred to as "breaking the chain of transmission").

However, the triangle does not apply as cleanly to chronic diseases as it does to infectious diseases. The relative decline of infectious disease (contagious diseases like polio and smallpox) as a result of public health initiatives, such as sanitation and immunization, has created a greater concern for the mitigation of chronic diseases, such as heart disease and cancer. Instead of being spurred by specific disease-causing agents, chronic diseases tend to develop over a long period of time under the influence of genetics, behavior, and the environment. Because of the relative cost of following a population over the number of years it takes to develop these diseases, it is generally more difficult to uncover the causes of these conditions.

In terms of formal training and education, an epidemiologist comprises one part of a very diverse disciplinary field. For example, the Epidemic Intelligence Service (EIS), a premier team of epidemiologists at the Centers for Disease Control and Prevention (CDC), has accepted into their ranks medical doctors, veterinarians, nurses, engineers, dentists, scientists, and even lawyers. While many epidemiologists have completed doctorates-a great many of those medical doctorates in a wide range of specialties-a master's level training in epidemiology is adequate for performing the necessary responsibilities of a typical epidemiologist. Since the public health profession encompasses epidemiology as one of its core disciplines, an epidemiologist may be fully prepared with a Master's in Public Health (M.P.H.) or a Master's of Science in Public Health (M.S.P.H.).

Diagnostic and Treatment Techniques

The epidemiologist assumes responsibility for two distinct public health activities: surveillance and investigation. Surveillance involves collecting and analyzing population morbidity and mortality data on a scheduled basis. These surveillance systems may be automated, as is often the case with potentially serious infectious diseases (a medical claim for anthrax poisoning, for example, may send an automatic alert to authorities). In broader health surveillance, surveys and databases with de-identified data-such as the CDC's National Health and Nutrition Examination Survey (NHANES)-can provide a snapshot of that population's health outcomes and exposures. Statistical reports from surveillance data help epidemiologists understand baselines and outbreaks, which inform professionals when direct corrective action may be necessary to address a community health threat.

Investigations are outright expeditions to answer questions about factors that impose health risks. These risks may be temporary, as in the case of an outbreak investigation. In special cases, the risks of disease may be more stable or per-

manent. The conclusions resulting from studies of recurring health problems often lead to better methods of treating and preventing the problem in the future. When an investigation or study is necessary in order to learn more about a certain interaction, epidemiologists have several study designs at their disposal. These studies range in cost and strength of evidence, but they are typically in the vein of an observational study. An observational study involves collecting data from study participants (or even data that have been collected previously and stored for future use) without changing their surroundings. This style of study is easier to manage, since participants do not need to be artificially divided into experimental groups with controlled exposures or treatments. Helpful observational study designs in epidemiology include (but are not confined to) case-control studies, cohort studies, and case series. These studies range in their strength of evidence as well as their general resource cost.

The case-control study is tailored to quick collection and analysis of data pertaining to an event that has already occurred. When conducting a case-control study, the epidemiologist finds study participants and organizes them into groups based on their outcomes. Then, participants provide data on different factors to which they had been exposed before the event. Once the data have been collected, an appropriate analysis-usually a 2x2 table-arranges the participants by outcome status (e.g., "sick" or "not sick") and exposure status (e.g., "ate potato salad" or "did not eat potato salad").

As this study is the most appropriate choice for investigating a foodborne disease outbreak, an excellent illustration is available in the classic "church potluck" example. Around 48 hours after a church potluck, several parishioners complained of a sudden onset of gastrointestinal illness. An epidemiologist contacts the parishioners who ate at the potluck and asks them to describe their symptoms, if any (placing them in "sick" and "not sick" categories). Next, the epidemiologist asks each parishioner to describe what they ate at the potluck, if they can. After collecting the data, the epidemiologist finds that nearly all the parishioners who ate a matriarch's "famous" potato salad developed the illness, while the group who chose to pass on the potato salad exhibited almost no symptoms at all. The epidemiologist then concludes the odds are that the potato salad, though famously delicious, was also infamously contaminated with a disease agent.

In contrast to case-control studies, cohort studies choose to organize the participants by exposure first, and then follow them to their health outcomes. Cohort studies can be more expensive to conduct, but often provide stronger evidence for an association between an exposure and a health effect. Cohort studies can be both prospective (organizing the study and following participants as time goes on) and retrospective (historically grouping persons and following available records to their outcomes). Another major benefit of the cohort study is that their outcomes are not determined at the beginning of their time in the study, allowing unforeseen associations to possibly rise to the surface during analysis.

Examples of excellent cohort studies can be found in the history of epidemiology and in common understanding. A very famous cohort was carried out by Richard Doll and A. Bradford Hill with British medical doctors as a population, examining the outcomes of those who smoked tobacco versus those who did not smoke from 1951 to 1954. The results, which associated risk of dying from lung cancer to increasing frequency of tobacco smoking, prompted a public health awareness campaign that brought the dangers of smoking to light. Other cohorts, such as the Dutch Famine cohort and the Whitehall study, have led to historic insights on the influence of environmental and occupational hazards to health (prenatal nutrition and occupational stress, respectively). Famous cohorts continue to provide data to this day, like the Framingham Heart Study cohort and the Nurses' Health Study cohort.

Finally, the case series is a study that attempts to identify persons who have been affected by a particular condition, then diagram these persons in order of their disease onset and their relationships to previously affected persons. This type of study can be particularly time-sensitive, as the participants' memories are the primary sources of data. In addition, it can be very difficult to describe any kind of links between exposures and the development of disease without the formal organization of comparative study groups. However, the case series is a very useful method for determining the first person to develop a disease in an outbreak, often referred to as "patient zero." It can also be helpful in attempting to understand how a disease may be transmitted.

For example, a case series which proves a timeline of disease onsets similar to the development of romantic encounters between subjects suggests that the disease may be transmitted sexually. This was indeed the case during the investigation of a disease outbreak in the early 1980s, which came to be known as acquired immunodeficiency syndrome, or AIDS. Further inquiry over several years gave evidence that AIDS is caused by a blood-borne virus (specifically, human immunodeficiency virus, or HIV) that attacks immune system cells, allowing other opportunistic infections to take hold of the host without resistance. The original case series in the investigation gave epidemiologists the clues they needed to describe the dangerous new disease.

Perspective and Prospects

The epidemiological discipline has been present throughout the development of human medicine, as humans employed methods of understanding the forces of disease and their causes. The ancient Greeks, most notably Hippocrates, sought a physical system of disease causation, and therefore a practical means of controlling or curing disease. Over time, many medical practitioners and scientists have offered up causes of diseases. Some have proven correct, such as Percival Pott's inference in 1775 that English chimney sweeps were prone to scrotal cancer due to their exposure to massive amounts of soot. On the other hand, some early epidemiological assertions have been woefully incorrect-such was the hypothesis that the bubonic plague seeped into the pores of infected persons, which were opened to the "plague air" by water. The subsequent avoidance of baths led to more

flea infestations, which tragically happened to be the true source of the bubonic plague.

John Snow, the English physician who uncovered a link between contaminated drinking water and an 1854 cholera outbreak in London in his publication, On the Mode of Communication of Cholera (1855), is commonly cited as the father of epidemiology. At that time, the commonly accepted theory of causation for cholera was the "miasma" theory-that "bad air" caused by rotting flesh, low altitude, and putrid odors carried diseases that seeped into the body through pores. Snow was a skeptic of this theory, and favored instead a "germ" theory of disease. His study proved to be a major piece of evidence in support of the idea that exposure to microscopic organisms, such as bacteria, caused disease.

In his study, Snow systematically plotted each affected person on a map centered on a water pump. After noticing that deaths congregated around the pump, Snow hypothesized that cholera was being caused by drinking water from this pump and removed the pump handle, preventing anyone from drawing water. Cholera cases around the pump then fell dramatically. Since Snow's groundbreaking study, germ theory has become the prevailing understanding of infectious disease. This relatively new understanding aids epidemiologists in understanding "life cycles" of disease with respect to the epidemiological triangle: where disease agents persist in the environment, how they are able to infect hosts, and how hosts interact with these disease agents. Armed with this knowledge, public health efforts, such as water sanitation and immunization programs, have reduced the burden of diseases that were once terrifyingly common-or, in the case of smallpox, eliminated entirely. Still, infectious diseases persist, and new diseases with mysterious origins remain to be investigated.

With the prolonged lifespan offered by these barriers to infectious disease, the field of epidemiology has turned to investigate health problems with more persistent causes and effects, such as chronic diseases, injury, and violence. The development of computerized tools-such as statistical analysis software, web-based data repositories, and geographic information systems (GIS)-has further improved an epidemiologist's ability to work with vast arrays of data, collaborate with other professionals, and condense results for policymakers and community stakeholders. Epidemiologists now have a wide arena in which to apply their methods, talents, and expertise in providing insight on modern health problems.

—Kimberly Y. Z. Forrest, Ph.D.;
updated by James E. Grant, M.P.H.

See also Acquired immunodeficiency syndrome (AIDS); Anthrax; Avian influenza; Bacterial infections; Bacteriology; Biological and chemical weapons; Biostatistics; Centers for Disease Control and Prevention (CDC); Childhood infectious diseases; Cholera; Creutzfeldt-Jakob disease (CJD); Department of Health and Human Services; Disease; E. coli infection; Ebola virus; Elephantiasis; Environmental diseases; Environmental health; Epidemics and pandemics; Epstein-Barr virus; Food poisoning; Forensic pathology; Hanta virus; Hepatitis; H1N1 influenza; Human papillomavirus (HPV); Influenza; Insect-borne diseases; Kawasaki disease; Laboratory tests;

Legionnaires' disease; Leprosy; Lice, mites, and ticks; Malaria; Marburg virus; Measles; Mercury poisoning; Microbiology; National Institutes of Health; Necrotizing fasciitis; Noroviruses; Occupational health; Parasitic diseases; Pathology; Plague; Poisoning; Poliomyelitis; Prion diseases; Pulmonary diseases; Rabies; Salmonella infection; Severe acute respiratory syndrome (SARS); Sexually transmitted diseases (STDs); Stress; Teratogens; Tropical medicine; Tularemia; Veterinary medicine; Viral infections; World Health Organization; Yellow fever; Zoonoses.

For Further Information

Gordis, Leon. *Epidemiology.* 4th ed. Philadelphia: Saunders Elsevier, 2009. Provides an excellent primer on the basic terminology and methods of epidemiology, including foundational concepts, study designs, and necessary explanation of the statistics.

Pendergrast, Mark. *Inside the Outbreaks: The Elite Medical Detectives of the Epidemic Intelligence Service.* New York: Houghton Mifflin, 2010. Pendergrast offers an approachable history and profile of the EIS, an American hallmark of epidemiology, along with its associated investigations.

Johnson, Steven. *The Ghost Map: The Story of London's Most Terrifying Epidemic-and How It Changed Science, Cities, and the Modern World.* New York: Penguin, 2006. Gives an in-depth presentation of John Snow's groundbreaking cholera investigation and a discussion on the resultant historical implications of the study and germ theory.

Barzilay, Ezra, et al. "Cholera Surveillance during the Haiti Epidemic-The First 2 Years." *New England Journal of Medicine* 368, no.7 (February, 2013): 599-609. Describes the development of a disease surveillance system built from the ground up to serve a specific purpose and provides an example of findings from a surveillance report.

EPIDERMAL NEVUS SYNDROMES

Disease/Disorder

Also known as: Feuerstein and Mims syndrome, Solomon's syndrome

Anatomy or system affected: All

Specialties and related fields: All

Definition: A group of systemic diseases that have in common pigmented spots on the skin.

Key terms:

dysdiadochokinesis: inability to perform rapid movements

hamartoma: a benign tumor that results from overgrowth of mature tissues

hemiparesis: weakness on one side of the body

hypertrichosis: excessive hair growth

hypoplasia: incomplete development or underdevelopment of an organ

keratinocytes: predominant cell type in the epidermis of the skin

nevus: a pigmented spot on the skin

phacomatosis: any condition characterized by hamartomas

Causes and Symptoms

Approximately one in one thousand people have birthmarks or beauty marks. Birthmarks, or nevi (singular: nevus), are noncancerous growths (hamartomas) of pigmented skin cells. They appear flat or raised, smooth or velvety, and tend to thicken and darken and they age. Nevi appear at birth or develop during childhood, and typically form along the routes

---

cells take during development (lines of Blaschko).

Many different types of skin cells can form nevi: cells from hair follicles, sebaceous glands (glands in the skin that secrete oils that protect the skin and hair), and epidermal skin cells (keratinocytes). Nevi that consist solely of keratinocytes are called nonorganoid nevi, but nevi that consist of hair follicle or sebaceous gland cells are organoid epidermal nevi.

Often, people have epidermal nevi and no other associated conditions. However, some people with epidermal nevi also have problems in other body systems. Epidermal nevus syndromes are a group of nine disorders that affect multiple organs, but all of these conditions have epidermal nevi in common. Epidermal nevus syndromes include Congenital Hemidysplasia with Ichthyosiform erythroderma and Limb Defects (CHILD syndrome), Nevus comedonicus syndrome, Schimmelpenning syndrome (also known as nevus sebaceous syndrome), Angora hair nevus syndrome (also known as Schauder syndrome), Proteus syndrome, phacomatosis pigmentokeratotica, Type 2 segmental Cowden nevus, García-Hafner-Happle syndrome (also known as Fibroblast Growth Factor Receptor 3 epidermal nevus syndrome), and Becker nevus syndrome.

Proteus syndrome shows patchy overgrowth of multiple tissues, blood vessel malformations, nevi in the lower layer of the skin (dermis) and connective tissue, asymmetric growth of the limbs, skull, vertebrae, and ears, lung cysts, fatty tumors, ovarian cysts, and salivary gland tumors. The genetic cause of Proteus syndrome remains unknown, but it occurs in

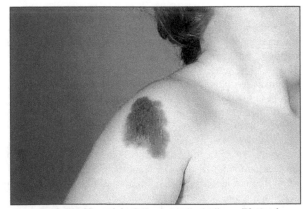

Congenital nevi (Copyright © Bart's Medical Library/Phototake. All rights reserved.)

one per one million people.

Patients with phacomatosis pigmentokeratotica have a sebaceous gland nevus in combination with a peculiar epidermal nevus that resembles sesame seeds scattered on a dirty table cloth (papular nevus spilus). Other symptoms include mental deficiency, seizures, weakness on one side of the body (hemiparesis), abnormal sensation, heart abnormalities, scoliosis, hearing loss, misalignment of the eyes (strabismus), and excessive sweating. Patients with this disease are prone to develop vitamin D-resistant rickets (hypophosphatemic rickets). This condition is caused by mutations in the HRAS gene that occur after conception. The sebaceous nevi in the case of phacomatosis pigmentokeratotica can develop into basal cell carcinomas. The incidence of phacomatosis pigmentokeratotica is unknown.

The CHILD syndrome results from mutations in the X-linked NSDHL gene, which encodes an enzyme involved in cholesterol synthesis (3ß-hydroxysteroid dehydrogenase). Patients with CHILD syndrome have inflammatory epidermal nevi that have a tendency to form at skin folds and may resemble psoriasis in their appearance. These lesions also tend to only form on one side of the body. The nails of the fingers and toes thicken and may form large strawberry-like lesions. Skeletal, heart, limb, and neurological defects can also occur. Approximately 60 cases of CHILD syndrome have been reported in the United States.

Spontaneous mutations in the PTEN gene that occur after conception cause Type 2 segmental Cowden disease (also known as linear PTEN nevus). The PTEN gene encodes a tumor suppressor protein that down-regulates cell proliferation. Besides a thick, wart-like nevus (linear Cowden nevus), the symptoms and signs of linear Cowden nevus include limb overgrowth, scarring in the kidneys, an abnormally large head (macrocephaly), seizures, intestinal polyps, ballooning of the toes, lymphatic tumors, vascular and connective tissue nevi, varicose veins in the legs, breast and thyroid cancer, a slow-growing tumor of the cerebellum (Lhermitte-Duclos disease), and fatty tumors. The prevalence of this disease is unknown.

Nevus comedonicus syndrome causes atrophy of skin follicles and a pitted, acne-like appearance. Additional symptoms include cataracts and erosion of the corneas, hand skeleton deformities, scoliosis and other vertebral deformities, and neurological abnormalities. The molecular basis of this disease and its incidence are unknown.

Schimmelpenning syndrome characteristically shows sebaceous gland nevi (nevus sebaceous). Additionally, these patients have face and skull defects, spine deformities, dislocation of the hips and limb deformities, hypophosphatemic rickets, mental deficiencies, seizures, brain abnormalities, optic nerve defects, and eye defects. The incidence of malignancy of sebaceous nevi in the case of Schimmelpenning syndrome is low. No known molecular basis for this condition is presently known, but infection of the early embryo with papilloma virus remains a possible cause. The prevalence is unknown.

Becker nevus syndrome manifests differently in males and females because the organoid nevus in males show excessive hair growth at the site of the nevi (hypertrichosis) whereas the same nevi in females do not. However, females characteristically show poor growth (hypoplasia) of one their breasts. The nevi in Becker nevus syndrome also show a kind of checkerboard distribution throughout the body. Other symptoms include extra nipples, extra scrotum in males, skeletal defects, tooth abnormalities, and poor growth of the muscles of the shoulder girdle. One study showed that 0.52 percent of men have Becker nevus syndrome.

Angora hair nevus syndrome shows broad, band-like areas covered with long, smooth, white hair. Additional symptoms with this condition include a larger than normal head, epileptic seizures, mental deficiency, brain structural anomalies, weakness, inability to perform rapid movements (dysdiadochokinesis), facial defects, and eye abnormalities. The incidence of this disease is unknown.

Gain-of-function mutations in the FGFR3 gene, which encodes one of the receptors for fibroblast growth factor, cause García-Hafner-Happle syndrome. The specific mutation in the FGFR3 gene (R248C) has been identified in biopsies of epidermal nevi. In fact, one-third of nevi harbor this mutation. In the case of García-Hafner-Happle syndrome, large portions of the patient's body harbor this mutation and not just small skin patches. The symptoms of this disease include soft, velvety nevi, brain defects, seizures, and facial defects. The incidence of this disease is unknown.

Treatment and Therapy

Diagnosis of epidermal nevus syndromes remains as much an art as a science. Magnetic resonance imaging (MRI) studies of the brain and other internal organs can properly evaluate brain anomalies, internal growths, and other abnormalities. Electroencephalogram (EEG) readings of the brain can be helpful, since they tend to be abnormal in the majority of epidermal nevus syndrome patients. Skin biopsies of the nevi followed by histological studies of the nevus tissue can also provide diagnostic information. Genetic testing of abnormal tissue can give definitive answers as to the diagnosis of these conditions in particular cases.

Treating these diseases is challenging. Epidermal nevi tend to not respond to topical steroids, retinoids, and other agents. Topical calcipotriol may be effective in some cases, but this agent is not approved for children under the age of 12 in the United States. Calcipotriol works as a vitamin D_3 analog and inhibits epidermal proliferation and promotes the differentiation of keratinocytes. Surgical excision of epidermal nevi is an option in some cases, but removal by cryosurgery or electrodesiccation show high rates of recurrence.

In those who suffer seizures, antiseizure medicines can quell epileptic episodes. In some cases, the seizures may not respond to medication and the only option left may be to surgically sever the connection between the two cerebral hemispheres (hemispherectomy).

Nevus comedonicus patients with cataracts require consultation with an ophthalmologist as will all patients with eye defects.

Phacomatosis pigmentokeratotica and patients should consult an oncologist if diagnosed with basal cell carcinoma. All epidermal nevus syndrome patients should be under the care of a dermatologist.

Perspective and Prospects

In 1957, Gustav Schimmelpenning, while training in psychiatry and neurology at the University of Kiel, described in some detail a case of a 17-year old patient who had a "phacomatosis," which refers to any disease characterized by benign tumors derived from mature cells. In 1962, two California physicians, R.C. Feuerstein and L.C. Mims reported two cases of what they referred to as "linear nevus sebaceus with convulsions and mental retardation." Unfortunately, they were unaware of Schimmelpenning's earlier precise clinical description. From that time, a host of published cases describing similar syndromes led to a morass of different names for very similar conditions or the same names for extremely different conditions. In 1968, Solomon coined the phrase "epidermal nevus syndrome" as an umbrella for all these related but distinct conditions.

In order to better understand the epidermal nevus syndromes, further embryological and molecular genetic studies must uncover the precise cause of each particular disease. Better diagnosis and treatments should proceed from a greater understanding of the mechanisms behind these diseases.

-Michael A. Buratovich, Ph.D.

See also Cutis Marmorata Telangiectatica Congenita; Dermatology; Dermopathology; Genetic counseling; Moles; Nephrology; Neurology; Oncology; Ophthalmology; Surgery; general

For Further Information:

Barnhill, Raymond L., Michael Piepkorn, and Klaus J, Busam, eds. *Pathology of Melanotic Nevi and Melanoma.* New York: Springer, 2013.

del Carmen Boente, María, Raúl Asial, Norma Beatriz Primc, and Rudolf Happle. "Angora Hair Nevus: A Further Case of an Unusual Epidermal Nevus Representing a Hallmark of Angora Hair Nevus Syndrome." *Journal of Dermatological Case Reports* 7, no. 2 (June, 2013): 49-51.

Happle, Rudolf. "The Group of Epidermal Nevus Syndromes. Part I. Well-Defined Phenotypes." *Journal of the American Academy of Dermatology* 63, no. 1 (July, 2010): 1-22.

Newkirk, Maria. *Julia's Special Mark: A Birthmark Story.* Seattle: Create Space Independent Publishing Platform, 2013.

EPIGLOTTITIS

Disease/Disorder

Also known as: Supraglottitis

Anatomy or system affected: Respiratory system, throat

Specialties and related fields: Bacteriology, emergency medicine, family medicine, internal medicine, pediatrics

Definition: An acute, life-threatening inflammation of the epiglottis.

Causes and Symptoms

Epiglottitis is an acute, severe infection that most often affects children between ages two and six. It is most commonly

---

> ## Information on Epiglottitis
>
> **Causes:** Usually bacterial infection; sometimes fungal or viral infection
>
> **Symptoms:** Sore throat, fever, inability to eat, drooling, stridor
>
> **Duration:** Acute
>
> **Treatments:** Hospitalization, humidified oxygen, antibiotics, intravenous fluids, corticosteroids, emergency tracheostomy if needed

caused by the bacterium *Haemophilus influenzae* type B, but it can also be caused by other bacteria such as *Staphylococcus aureus* or *Streptococcus pneumoniae*, fungi such as *Candida albicans*, and viruses.

Epiglottitis presents classically with a fever and sore throat in a young child, who progresses rapidly within a few hours to an inability to eat and drooling, with signs of respiratory obstruction such as stridor (an abnormal high-pitched sound when breathing). The epiglottis is a thin flap of cartilage at the back of the tongue that closes the respiratory tract while swallowing. When it is inflamed, respiratory obstruction results. Drooling can occur, as the child may be unable to swallow his or her own saliva. This is an emergency situation, as the respiratory distress can progress rapidly and become life-threatening within minutes.

It is strongly advised that the mouth and larynx not be examined using a tongue depressor, as this could precipitate a spasm of the epiglottis and exacerbate respiratory distress. Epiglottitis is diagnosed by a clinician through laryngoscopy, with efforts made to secure the airway first. Neck x-rays reveal a characteristic "thumbprint" sign caused by an enlarged epiglottis. A blood culture may reveal the causative organism, and an elevated white blood cell count may be observed.

Treatment and Therapy

In most cases of epiglottitis, hospitalization is required, and the patient is usually admitted to the intensive care unit (ICU). The foremost concern is to secure and maintain the airway as soon as possible. Humidified oxygen, oxygen that has been moistened to help the patient breathe better, is administered. If the airway obstruction is severe enough, a tracheal intubation, in which a plastic tube is inserted into the windpipe through the mouth or nose, may be necessary. If the swelling is too severe to allow for intubation, a cricothyrotomy, or emergency airway puncture, may be needed to secure the airway; this is a less intensive procedure than a conventional tracheotomy, although a tracheotomy may be undertaken in some cases too. Antibiotics, intravenous fluids, and corticosteroids may also be administered to decrease the swelling. With proper and prompt treatment, the prognosis is very good.

Perspective and Prospects

Epiglottitis is an acute inflammation of the epiglottis that should be distinguished from laryngotracheobronchitis or croup. Also, children ingesting hot liquids may present with similar symptoms. The disease must be managed efficiently and in a clinical setting only. Since the causative agent of the disease is infectious, family members must also be screened and treated for the disease. In the United States, the aggressive immunization of children against *Haemophilus influenzae* type B with the Hib vaccine, starting in the 1980s, has resulted in the near-elimination of the incidence of epiglottitis.

—*Venkat Raghavan Tirumala, M.D., M.H.A.*

See also Antibiotics; Bacterial infections; Cartilage; Childhood infectious diseases; Choking; Croup; Otorhinolaryngology; Pulmonary medicine, pediatric; Respiration; Sore throat; Tracheostomy.

For Further Information:

"Epiglottitis." *Mayo Clinic*, October 2, 2012.

"Epiglottitis." *MedlinePlus*, February 2, 2012.

Kasper, Dennis L., et al., eds. *Harrison's Principles of Internal Medicine*. 16th ed. New York: McGraw-Hill, 2005.

Rakel, Robert E., ed. *Textbook of Family Practice*. 6th ed. Philadelphia: W. B. Saunders, 2002.

Rymaruk, Jen. "Epiglottitis." *Health Library*, March 15, 2013.

Tapley, Donald F., et al., eds. *The Columbia University College of Physicians and Surgeons Complete Home Medical Guide*. Rev. 3d ed. New York: Crown, 1995.

EPILEPSY

Disease/Disorder

Anatomy or system affected: Brain, head, nerves, nervous system

Specialties and related fields: Neurology

Definition: A serious neurologic disease characterized by seizures, which may involve convulsions and loss of consciousness.

Key terms:

anticonvulsant: a therapeutic drug that prevents or diminishes convulsions

aura: a sensory symptom or group of such symptoms that precedes a grand mal seizure

clonic phase: the portion of an epileptic seizure that is characterized by convulsions

electroencephalogram (EEG): a graphic recording of the electrical activity of the brain, as recorded by an electroencephalograph

grand mal: a type of epileptic seizure characterized by severe convulsions, body stiffening, and loss of consciousness during which victims fall down; also called tonic-clonic seizure

idiopathic disease: a disease of unknown origin

petit mal: a mild type of epileptic seizure characterized by a very short lapse of consciousness, usually without convulsions; the epileptic does not fall down

psychomotor epilepsy: condition of impairment of consciousness with amnesia of the episode which may include movements of the arms and legs and hallucinations

seizure: a sudden convulsive attack of epilepsy that can involve loss of consciousness and falling down

seizure discharges: characteristic brain waves seen in the EEGs of epileptics; their strength and frequency depend upon whether a seizure is occurring and its type

status epilepticus: a rare, life-threatening condition in which many sequential seizures occur without recovery between them

tonic-clonic seizure: another term for a grand mal seizure

tonic phase: the portion of an epileptic seizure characterized by loss of consciousness and body stiffness

Causes and Symptoms

Epilepsy is characterized by seizures, which may involve convulsions and the loss of consciousness. It was called the "falling disease" or "sacred disease" in antiquity and was mentioned in 2080 BCE in the laws of the famous Babylonian king Hamurabi. Epilepsy is a serious neurologic disease that usually appears between the ages of two and fourteen. It does not affect intelligence, as shown by the fact that the range of intelligence quotients (IQs) for epileptics is quite similar to that of the general population.

In 400 BCE, Hippocrates of Cos proposed that epilepsy arose from physical problems in the brain. This origin of the disease is now known to be unequivocally true. Despite many centuries of exhaustive study and effort, however, only a small proportion (20 percent) of cases of epilepsy caused by brain injuries, brain tumors, and other diseases are curable. This type of epilepsy is called symptomatic epilepsy. In contrast, 80 percent of epileptics can be treated to control the occurrence of seizures but cannot be cured of the disease, which is therefore a lifelong affliction. In these cases, the basis of the epilepsy is not known, although the suspected cause is genetically programmed brain damage that still evades discovery. Most epilepsy is, therefore, an idiopathic disease (one of unknown origin), and such epileptics are thus said to suffer from idiopathic epilepsy.

A common denominator in idiopathic epilepsy, and also in symptomatic epilepsy, is that it is evidenced by unusual electrical discharges, or brain waves, seen in the electroencephalograms (EEGs) of epileptics. These brain waves are called seizure discharges. They vary in both their strength and their frequency, depending on whether an epileptic is having a seizure and what type of seizure is occurring. Seizure discharges are almost always present and recognizable in the EEGs of epileptics, even during sleep.

There are four types of common epileptic seizures. Two of these are partial (local) seizures called focal motor and temporal lobe seizures, respectively. The others, grand mal and petit mal, are generalized and may involve the entire body. A

Information on Epilepsy

Causes: Brain injury, brain tumors, disease, possible genetic factors
Symptoms: Seizures, loss of consciousness
Duration: Typically chronic
Treatments: Surgery to remove tumor or causative brain tissue abnormality, anticonvulsant drugs

focal motor seizure is characterized by rhythmic jerking of the facial muscles, an arm, or a leg. As with other epileptic seizures, it is caused by abnormal electrical discharges in the portion of the brain that controls normal movement in the body part that is affected. This abnormal electrical activity is always seen as seizure discharges in the EEG of the affected part of the brain.

In contrast, temporal lobe seizures (also known as psychomotor epilepsy), again characterized by seizure discharges in a distinct portion of the cerebrum of the brain, are characterized by sensory hallucinations and other types of consciousness alteration, a meaningless physical action, or even a babble of some incomprehensible language. Thus, for example, temporal lobe seizures may explain some cases of people "speaking in tongues" in religious experiences or in tales of the Delphic oracles of ancient Greece.

The term "grand mal" refers to the most severe type of epileptic seizure. Also called tonic-clonic seizures, grand mal attacks are characterized by very severe EEG seizure discharges throughout the entire brain. A grand mal seizure is usually preceded by sensory symptoms called an aura (probably related to temporal lobe seizures), which warn an epileptic of an impending attack. The aura is quickly followed by the grand mal seizure itself, which involves the loss of consciousness, localized or widespread jerking and convulsions, and severe body stiffness.

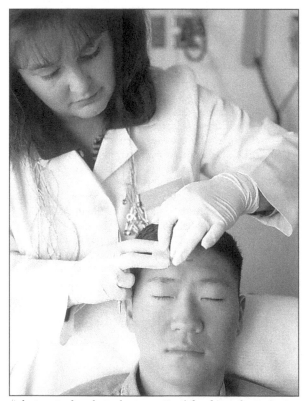

A doctor attaches electrodes to a patient's head in order to monitor his epilepsy. (PhotoDisc)

Epileptics suffering a grand mal seizure usually fall to the ground, may foam at the mouth, and often bite their tongues or the inside of their cheeks unless something is placed in the mouth before they lose consciousness. In a few cases, the victim will lose bladder or bowel control. In untreated epileptics, grand mal seizures can occur weekly. Most of these attacks last for only a minute or two, followed quickly by full recovery after a brief sense of disorientation and feelings of severe exhaustion. In some cases, however, grand mal seizures may last for up to five minutes and lead to temporary amnesia or to other mental deficits of a longer duration. In rare cases, the life-threatening condition of status epilepticus occurs, in which many sequential tonic-clonic seizures occur over several hours without recovery between them.

The fourth type of epileptic seizure is petit mal, which is often called generalized nonconvulsive seizure or, more simply, absence. A petit mal seizure consists of a brief period of loss of consciousness (ten to forty seconds) without the epileptic falling down. The epileptic usually appears to be daydreaming (absent) and shows no other symptoms. Often a victim of a petit mal seizure is not even aware that the event has occurred. In some cases, a petit mal seizure is accompanied by mild jerking of hands, head, or facial features and/or rapid blinking of the eyes. Petit mal attacks can be quite dangerous if they occur while an epileptic is driving a motor vehicle.

Diagnosing epilepsy usually requires a patient history, a careful physical examination, blood tests, and a neurologic examination. The patient history is most valuable when it includes eyewitness accounts of the symptoms, the frequency of occurrence, and the usual duration of the seizures observed. In addition, documentation of any preceding severe trauma, infection, or episodes of addictive drug exposure provides useful information that will often differentiate between idiopathic and symptomatic epilepsy.

Evidence of trauma is quite important, as head injuries that caused unconsciousness are often the basis for later symptomatic epilepsy. Similarly, infectious diseases of the brain, including meningitis and encephalitis, can cause this type of epilepsy. Finally, excessive use of alcohol or other psychoactive drugs can also be a causative agent for symptomatic epilepsy.

Blood tests for serum glucose and calcium, electroencephalography, and computed tomography (CT) scanning are also useful diagnostic tools. The EEG will nearly always show seizure discharges in epileptics, and the location of the discharges in the brain may localize problem areas associated with the disease. CT scanning is most useful for identifying tumors and other serious brain damage that may cause symptomatic epilepsy. Other tests that may be used to diagnose epilepsy include magnetic resonance imaging (MRI), magnetoencephalography (MEG) imaging, and a lumbar puncture or spinal tap. When all tests are negative except for abnormal EEGs, the epilepsy is considered idiopathic.

It is thought that epileptic symptoms occur because of a malfunction in nerve impulse transport in some of the billions of nerve cells (neurons) that make up the brain and link it to the body organs that it innervates. This nerve impulse transport is an electrochemical process caused by the ability of the neurons to retain substances (including potassium) and to excrete substances (including sodium). This ability generates the weak electrical current that makes up a nerve impulse and that is registered by electroencephalography.

A nerve impulse leaves a given neuron via an outgoing extension (or axon), passes across a tiny synaptic gap that separates the axon from the next neuron in line, and enters an incoming extension (or dendrite) of that cell. The process is repeated until the impulse is transmitted to its site of action. The cell bodies of neurons make up the gray matter of the brain, and axons and dendrites (white matter) may be viewed as connecting wires.

Passage across synaptic gaps between neurons is mediated by chemicals called neurotransmitters, and it is believed that epilepsy results when unknown materials cause abnormal electrical impulses by altering neurotransmitter production rates and/or the ability of sodium, potassium, and related substances to enter or leave neurons. The various nervous impulse abnormalities that cause epilepsy can be shown to occur in the portions of the gray matter of the cerebrum that control high-brain functions. For example, the frontal lobe—which controls speech, body movement, and eye movements—is associated with temporal lobe seizures.

Treatment and Therapy

Idiopathic epilepsy is viewed as the expression of a large group of different diseases, thought to stem from genetic abnormalities, all of which present themselves clinically as seizures. This is extrapolated from the various types of symptomatic epilepsy observed, which have causes that include faulty biochemical processes (such as inappropriate calcium levels), brain tumors or severe brain injury, infectious diseases (such as encephalitis), and the chronic overuse of addictive drugs.

Symptomatic epilepsy is treated with medication and either by the extirpation of the tumor or other causative brain tissue abnormality that was engendered by trauma or disease or by the correction of the metabolic disorder involved. The more common, incurable idiopathic disease is usually treated entirely with medication that relieves symptoms. This treatment is essential, because without it most epileptics cannot attend school successfully, maintain continued employment, or drive a motor vehicle safely.

A large number of anticonvulsant drugs are available for epilepsy management. However, no one therapeutic drug will control all types of seizures. In addition, some patients require several such drugs for effective therapy, and the natural history of a given case of epilepsy may often require periodic changes from drug to drug as the disease evolves. Furthermore, many antiepilepsy drugs have dangerous side effects that may occur when present in the body above certain levels or after they are used beyond some given time period. Therefore, each epileptic patient must be monitored at frequent intervals to ascertain that no dangerous physical symptoms are developing and that the drug levels in the body (monitored by the measurement of drug content in blood samples) are within a tolerable range.

Dozens of antiepilepsy drugs are widely used. Phenytoin (Dilantin) is very effective for grand mal seizures. Because of its slow metabolism, phenytoin can be administered relatively infrequently, but this slow metabolism also requires seven to ten days before its anticonvulsant effects occur. Side effects include cosmetically unpleasant hair overgrowth, swelling of the gums, and skin rash. These symptoms are particularly common in epileptic children. More serious are central nervous effects including ataxia (unsteadiness in walking), drowsiness, anemia, and marked thyroid deficiency. Most such symptoms are reversed by decreasing the drug doses or by discontinuing it. Phenytoin is often given together with other antiepilepsy drugs to produce optimum seizure prevention. In those cases, great care must be taken to prevent dangerous synergistic drug effects from occurring. High phenytoin doses also produce blood levels of the drug that are very close to toxic 25 micrograms per milliliter values.

Carbamazepine (Tegretol) is another frequently used antiepileptic drug. Chemically related to the drugs used as antidepressants, it is useful against both psychomotor epilepsy and grand mal seizures. Common carbamazepine side effects are ataxia, drowsiness, and double vision. A more dangerous, and fortunately less common, side effect is the inability of bone marrow to produce blood cells. Again, very serious and unexpected complications occur in mixed-drug therapy that includes carbamazepine, and at high doses toxic blood levels of the drug may be exceeded.

Phenobarbital (Luminal), a sedative hypnotic also used as a tranquilizer by nonepileptics, is a standby for treating epilepsy. It too can have serious side effects, including a lowered attention span, hyperactivity, and learning difficulties. In addition, when given with phenytoin, phenobarbital will speed up the excretion of that drug, lowering its effective levels.

A newer generation of antiepileptic medications that act by various mechanisms became available starting in the 1990s. These drugs, which include gabapentin, lamotrigine, topiramate, tiagabine, levetiracetam, zonisamide, oxcarbazepine, and pregabalin, are often better tolerated, safer, and faster acting than the older generation of antiepileptics, which have been available since the mid-twentieth century. However, the efficacy of both the newer and older drugs to prevent seizures remains highly dependent on the individual patient.

About 20 percent of idiopathic epileptics do not achieve adequate seizure control after prolonged and varied drug therapy. Another option for some—but not all—such people is brain surgery. This type of brain surgery is usually elected after two conditions are met. First, often-repeated EEGs must show that most or all of the portion of the brain in which the seizures develop is very localized. Second, these affected areas must be in a brain region that the patient can lose without significant mental loss (often in the prefrontal or temporal cerebral lobes). When such surgery is carried out, it is reported that 50 to 75 percent of the patients who are treated and given chronic, postoperative antiepilepsy drugs become able to achieve seizure control.

The most frequent antiepilepsy surgery is anterior temporal lobectomy. The brain has two temporal lobes, one of which is dominant in the control of language, memory, and thought expression. An anterior temporal lobectomy is carried out by removing a portion of the front part of the temporal lobe, when it is the site of epilepsy. About 6 percent of temporal lobectomies lead to a partial loss of temporal lobe functions, which may include impaired vision, movement, memory, and speech. However, better than 60 percent of patients become completely seizure-free following the procedure, making this surgery the standard approach for patients with temporal lobe epilepsy who are resistant to drug therapy.

Another common type of antiepilepsy surgery is called corpus callosotomy. This procedure involves partially disconnecting the two cerebral hemispheres by severing some of the nerves in the corpus callosum that links them. This surgery is performed when an epileptic has frequent, uncontrollable grand mal attacks that cause many dangerous falls. The procedure usually results in reduced numbers of seizures and decreases in their severity.

Other treatments for epilepsy include vagus nerve stimulation (VNS), in which a device similar to a pacemaker is implanted in the patient to deliver regular electrical currents to the vagus nerve in the neck, which has been shown to reduce the number of seizures for about half of patients. In a limited number of cases, the rate of seizures may also be reduced by a special dietary regimen called a ketogenic diet, which is high in fat and low in carbohydrates.

Physicians also believe that many cases of epilepsy may be prevented by methods aimed at avoiding head injury (especially in children) and the use of techniques such as amniocentesis to identify potential epileptics and treat them before birth. Furthermore, the prophylactic administration of antiepilepsy drugs to nonepileptic people who are afflicted with encephalitis and other diseases known to produce epilepsy is viewed as wise.

Perspective and Prospects

A great number of advances have occurred in the treatment of epilepsy via therapeutic drugs and surgical techniques. Drug therapy has been the method of choice, because it is less drastic than surgery, is easier to manage, and rarely has the potential for the irreversible damage to patients that can be caused by the removal of a portion of the brain. A tremendous variety of chemical therapies has been developed and utilized successfully.

In addition to antiepileptic drugs, alternative nonsurgical treatments that have been tried include high doses of vitamins, injections of muscle relaxants, and changes in diet. The variety is unsurprising, considering the vast number of disease states that can cause seizures. Readers are encouraged to investigate the many epilepsy treatments that have not been noted. Such an examination may be quite valuable, as there are about 2 million epileptics in the United States alone, and some estimates indicate that four of every thousand humans are likely to develop some epileptic symptoms during their lifetime.

Modern surgical treatment of epilepsy reportedly began in 1828, with the efforts of Benjamin Dudley, who removed epilepsy-causing blood clots and skull fragments from five patients, who all survived despite primitive and nonsterile operating rooms. The next landmark in such surgery was the removal of a brain tumor by the German physician R. J. Godlee, in 1884, without the benefit of X rays or EEG techniques, which did not then exist.

By the 1950s, EEGs were used to locate epileptic brain foci, and physicians such as the Canadians Wilder Penfield and Herbert Jasper pioneered their use to locate brain regions to remove for epilepsy remission without damaging vital functions. After considerable evolution, antiepilepsy surgery had by the 1990s become widespread, commonplace, and relatively safe.

Nevertheless, because of the imperfections of all available methodologies, 5 to 8 percent of epileptics cannot achieve seizure control by any method or method combination, and even the "well-managed" epilepsy treatment regimen has its flaws. There is still much to be learned about curing epilepsy. Clinical and experimental perioperative studies are now possible during epilepsy surgery to examine the bioelectrical activity and molecular events of the affected neurons. It is hoped that the efforts of ongoing biomedical research, both in basic science and in clinical settings, will drastically reduce or eliminate epilepsy through the development of new therapeutic drugs and advances in surgery and other nondrug methods.

—*Sanford S. Singer, Ph.D.;*
updated by W. Michael Zawada, Ph.D.

See also Auras; Brain; Brain damage; Brain disorders; Brain tumors; Computed tomography (CT) scanning; Electroencephalography (EEG); Nervous system; Neuroimaging; Neurology; Neurology, pediatric; Neurosurgery; Phenylketonuria (PKU); Seizures; Unconsciousness.

For Further Information:
Appleton, Richard, and Anthony G. Marson. *Epilepsy: The Facts*. 3d ed. New York: Oxford University Press, 2009.
Beers, Mark H., et al., eds. *The Merck Manual of Diagnosis and Therapy*. 18th ed. Whitehouse Station, N.J.: Merck Research Laboratories, 2006.
Bloom, Floyd E., M. Flint Beal, and David J. Kupfer, eds. *The Dana Guide to Brain Health*. New York: Dana Press, 2006.
Carson-DeWitt, Rosalyn. "Seizure Disorder—Adult." *Health Library*, September 30, 2012.
Devinsky, Orrin. *Epilepsy: Patient and Family Guide*. 3d ed. New York: Demos Medical, 2008.
Epilepsy Foundation. http://www.epilepsyfoundation .org.
Freeman, John M., Eileen P. G. Vining, and Diana J. Pillas. *Seizures and Epilepsy in Childhood: A Guide*. 3d ed. Baltimore: Johns Hopkins University Press, 2002.
Gumnit, Robert J. *Living Well with Epilepsy*. 2d ed. New York: Demos Vermande, 1997.
Kohnle, Diana, and Rebecca J. Stahl. "Seizure Disorder—Child." *Health Library*, June 6, 2012.
Nolte, John. *Human Brain: An Introduction to Its Functional Anatomy*. 6th ed. Philadelphia: Mosby/Elsevier, 2009.

"Seizures and Epilepsy: Hope through Research." *National Institute of Neurological Disorders and Stroke*, April 8, 2013.

Weaver, Donald F. *Epilepsy and Seizures: Everything You Need to Know*. Toronto, Ont.: Firefly Books, 2001.

EPISIOTOMY
Procedure
Anatomy or system affected: Anus, genitals, reproductive system
Specialties and related fields: Gynecology, obstetrics
Definition: A surgical cut made in the pelvic floor to enlarge the vagina for the facilitation of childbirth.

Indications and Procedures

An episiotomy is performed to enlarge the vaginal opening and ease the delivery of a baby during childbirth. While not a routine procedure, some circumstances that indicate the need for an episiotomy include macrosomia (large fetal size), rapid delivery, breech delivery, and presentation of the baby with face to the front of the birth canal, all of which prevent the perineum (the area between the vagina and the anus) from stretching rapidly enough to prevent tearing. Scarring from vaginal surgeries also limits the ability of the vagina to expand.

During the procedure, a local anesthetic is injected into the perineum. The provider uses straight-bladed blunt scissors to snip the tissue between the vagina and anus diagonally, avoiding the anal sphincter muscle and preventing tearing into the anal sphincter. After delivery, the incision is carefully stitched together, along with any minor tears in the birth canal. Delivery by a nurse midwife as opposed to a private obstetrician is far less likely to result in an episiotomy, as episiotomies are not done routinely by nurse midwives. Furthermore, with a nurse midwife, techniques such as vaginal-perineal massage with warm oil are employed to help stretch the perineum and avoid the need for episiotomy.

Uses and Complications

The birth canal has very limited space to accommodate an infant, and situations such as feetfirst or face-forward presentation can lead to compression of the umbilical cord and interruption of the oxygen supply to the baby, or even to potential crushing of the infant. An episiotomy can facilitate a rapid delivery in these circumstances, thereby preventing serious injury to the infant. Failure of the perineum to stretch sufficiently to accommodate the child can result in severe, irregular tears of the vagina and even of the anal sphincter muscles. Ragged tears are very difficult to repair surgically and are much more prone to infection. Tearing of the anal sphincter could lead to permanent incontinence. The easily repaired incisions of episiotomy eliminate these potential difficulties.

Healing of the incisions is rapid and straightforward, but the area may itch and be somewhat painful for a few weeks. Painkilling drugs may be prescribed, and ice packs can be used to alleviate pain. Women who do not desire episiotomies and have controlled, problem-free deliveries may try to stretch the perineum gradually by massaging it with warm oil during the delivery. While in the past, episiotomies were considered a routine part of delivery, they are now done less commonly, only as necessitated for conditions like those indicated above. Additionally, maternal satisfaction is increasing as episiotomies are being done more when they are necessary and to a lesser extent when they are avoidable.

—Karen E. Kalumuck, Ph.D.;
updated by Robin Kamienny Montvilo, R.N., Ph.D.

See also Anus; Childbirth; Childbirth complications; Incontinence; Obstetrics; Women's health.

For Further Information:

Carlson, Karen J., Stephanie A. Eisenstat, and Terra Ziporyn. *The New Harvard Guide to Women's Health*. Cambridge, Mass.: Harvard University Press, 2004.

Cunningham, F. Gary, et al., eds. *Williams Obstetrics*. 23d ed. New York: McGraw-Hill, 2010.

"Episiotomy." *MedlinePlus*, April 22, 2012.

Goldberg, Roger P. *Ever Since I Had My Baby: Understanding, Treating, and Preventing the Most Common Physical After-Effects of Pregnancy and Childbirth*. New York: Crown, 2003.

Gonik, Bernard, and Renee A. Bobrowski. *Medical Complications in Labor and Delivery*. Cambridge, Mass.: Blackwell Scientific, 1996.

Lucey, Julie Rackliffe. "Vaginal Laceration." *Health Library*, September 10, 2012.

Lurie, Samuel. "Need for Episiotomy in a Subsequent Delivery Following Previous Delivery with Episiotomy." *Archives of Gynecology & Obstetrics* 287, no. 2 (February, 2013): 201–204.

Machisio, Sara, et al. "Care Pathways in Obstetrics: The Effectiveness in Reducing the Incidence of Episiotomy in Childbirth." *Journal of Nursing Management* 14, no. 7 (October, 2006): 538-543.

Reynolds, Karina, Christoph Lees, and Grainne McCarten. *Pregnancy and Birth: Your Questions Answered*. Rev. ed. New York: DK, 2007.

Sears, William, and Martha Sears. *The Birth Book: Everything You Need to Know to Have a Safe and Satisfying Birth*. Boston: Little, Brown, 1994.

Simkin, Penny, Janet Whalley, and Ann Keppler. *Pregnancy, Childbirth, and the Newborn: The Complete Guide*. 3d ed. Minnetonka, Minn.: Meadowbrook Press, 2008.

Stoppard, Miriam. *Conception, Pregnancy, and Birth*. Rev. ed. New York: DK, 2005.

Warhus, Susan. *Countdown to Baby: Answers to the One Hundred Most Asked Questions About Pregnancy and Childbirth*. Omaha, Nebr.: Addicus Books, 2003.

EPSTEIN-BARR VIRUS
Disease/Disorder
Also known as: Human herpesvirus 4 (HHV-4)
Anatomy or system affected: Blood, cells, glands, immune system, lymphatic system, mouth, muscles, nose, throat
Specialties and related fields: Cytology, hematology, immunology, microbiology, oncology, pathology, pediatrics, virology
Definition: An extensively occurring virus which infects almost all humans during their lifetime, often remaining latent in their systems but sometimes causing malignant tumors and various types of cancer.

Key terms:

antibodies: protein molecules that detect antigens and destroy infected host cells

antigens: viral proteins that attract antibodies, which the immune system designs to attack them

B cells: also known as B lymphocytes; white blood cells that create antibodies

oncoviruses: viruses causing the growth of cancerous cells

replication: the viral insertion of genetic information into host cell nuclei to create additional similar viruses

T cells: also known as cytotoxic T lymphocytes; white blood cells that destroy cells hosting antigens or infected by pathogens which eluded antibodies

virion: a viral particle that contains genetic information inside a protective structure

---

Information on Epstein-Barr Virus

Causes: Viral infection spread primarily through saliva

Symptoms: In children, usually none; in adolescents and adults, often mononucleosis; associated with a number of cancers and other diseases

Duration: Acute and then chronic

Treatments: None for viral infection; chemotherapy and radiation for resulting cancers

---

Causes and Symptoms

Present only in humans, Epstein-Barr virus was the first documented oncovirus. The virus, resembling other human herpesviruses, consists of sphere-shaped, barbed virions approximately 120 to 220 nanometers in diameter. Each Epstein-Barr virus genome contains two strands of deoxyribonucleic acid (DNA). A protein shell protects the genome, and an envelope surrounds the protein shell. Various Epstein-Barr virus strains have evolved that can infect an individual at the same time.

The Epstein-Barr virus typically infects salivary gland cells or B cells. Usually, Epstein-Barr viral infections are transmitted through saliva. Seeking host cells in order to replicate, the Epstein-Barr virus proliferates, creating approximately one hundred types of antigens, including nuclear antigen EBNA 1, which the Epstein-Barr virus uses to put its DNA into new cells created during cell division.

T cells fight Epstein-Barr virus antigens by destroying infected host cells. T cells and antibodies stay in the immune system to continue protecting against infection, regulating latency, and developing immunity. EBNA1 is necessary for the Epstein-Barr virus genomes to endure being latent. T cells cannot detect the antigen EBNA1 and attack those host cells, which results in the Epstein-Barr virus often being invisible to immune protection. Latent infections are not apparent, usually remaining passive, but they can become active, potentially resulting in tumors and diseases.

The Epstein-Barr virus usually infects throat, blood, or immune system cells. Infectious mononucleosis, also known as glandular fever, is the most widely known Epstein-Barr viral infection. Physicians determine if people have been infected by Epstein-Barr virus by performing laboratory tests analyzing blood samples to detect if any of the antibodies to combat Epstein-Barr virus antigens are present and, if so, how many are present. Such antibodies might have existed for years and are not proof of an active infection.

People can contract the virus as children, adolescents, or adults, depending on geographic location and socioeconomic factors. Some infants are born with the virus transmitted by their mothers. The Epstein-Barr virus usually infects people when they are children, without obvious signs. Often, these individuals never know that they are infected. Approximately half of the people who contract the Epstein-Barr virus as an adolescent or at an older age, however, develop infectious mononucleosis.

Activated Epstein-Barr virus can result in several serious diseases, and people with suppressed immune systems are vulnerable to developing such malignancies as cancerous tumors in smooth muscle tissue, stomach carcinomas, lymphomas, and sarcomas. Epstein-Barr virus often causes nasal and throat cancers known as nasopharyngeal carcinoma. In some individuals with acquired immunodeficiency syndrome (AIDS), Epstein-Barr virus replicates in tongue cells, resulting in oral hairy leukoplakia. Epstein-Barr virus has also been associated with leukemia.

Weak immune systems cause people to be vulnerable to Epstein-Barr virus infections, particularly after organ transplantation and the use of immunosuppressive drugs to lower the immune reaction and to encourage acceptance of the new organ. In those cases, Epstein-Barr virus sometimes causes post-transplant lymphoproliferative disease to occur.

When it infects the nodes, Epstein-Barr virus might be a factor in people affected by Hodgkin disease. Researchers have considered a possible role of Epstein-Barr virus in the development of multiple sclerosis and breast cancer. They have eliminated it as a factor in chronic fatigue syndrome.

Treatment and Therapy

Approximately 90 to 95 percent of humans globally at any time have been infected with Epstein-Barr virus, which remains latent and endures in their bodies until death. There is currently no way to eliminate the virus once infection has occurred. Treatment focuses instead on the diseases that Epstein-Barr virus causes.

Researchers have attempted to develop antiviral vaccines to stop the replication of Epstein-Barr virus. In the early twenty-first century, scientists at Queensland Institute of Medical Research developed a vaccine prototype to strengthen T cells combatting Epstein-Barr virus antigens.

Perspective and Prospects

The Epstein-Barr virus was located as a result of researchers seeking viruses possibly associated with cancer in humans, In 1961, London researcher M. Anthony Epstein attended a lecture at which Denis P. Burkitt discussed his work with tumors, later called Burkitt lymphoma, in African children's facial bones. Epstein, experienced with investigating viruses causing animal tumors, wanted to examine Burkitt lymphoma tumor tissues to detect any viruses. The British Empire Cancer Campaign funded Epstein's travel to Uganda to acquire a consistent supply of tumor samples for his Middlesex Hospital Medical School laboratory. Epstein tried unsuccessfully to locate a virus for a couple of years.

The U.S. National Cancer Institute presented Epstein $45,000 for his investigations, and he hired doctoral student Yvonne M. Barr and colleague Bert G. Achong to expand his laboratory work attempting to culture viruses. The trio successfully grew a Burkitt lymphoma cell line in culture. When cells from that sample were examined with an electron microscope, the London scientists saw viral particles with structural elements of herpesvirus. Scrutinizing the virions, the trio declared that they had isolated a previously unknown human herpesvirus. They published their results in a 1964 *Lancet* article. After Epstein-Barr virus was identified, additional investigators studied the virus to expand knowledge of its structure, replication, and the diseases associated with it, determining that it was an oncovirus.

Research into ways to fight Epstein-Barr virus is ongoing. Scientists at the European Molecular Biology Laboratory and Institut de Virologie Moléculaire et Structurale have focused on controlling a protein molecule known as ZEBRA that accompanies Epstein-Barr virus, helping activate it from the latent phase.

—*Elizabeth D. Schafer, Ph.D.*

See also Acquired immunodeficiency syndrome (AIDS); Burkitt's lymphoma; Cancer; Carcinoma; Carcinogens; Ewing's sarcoma; Herpes; Leukemia; Lymphadenopathy and lymphoma; Lymphatic system; Mononucleosis; Oncology; Sarcoma; Transplantation; Tumors; Viral infections.

For Further Information:

Cohen, Jeffrey I., et al. "The Need and Challenges for Development of an Epstein-Barr Virus Vaccine." *Vaccine* 31 (April, 2013): B194–B196.

Epstein, M. Anthony, and Bert G. Achong, eds. *The Epstein-Barr Virus*. New York: Springer, 1979.

Ford, Jodi L., and Raymond P. Stowe. "Racial-Ethnic Differences in Epstein-Barr Virus Antibody Titers Among U.S. Children and Adolescents." *Annals of Epidemiology* 23, no. 5 (May, 2013): 275–280.

Odumade, Oludare A., Kristin A. Hogquist, and Henry H. Balfour, Jr. "Progress and Problems in Understanding and Managing Primary Epstein-Barr Virus Infections." *Clinical Microbiology Review* 24, no. 1 (January, 2011): 193–209.

Jackson, Alan C. *Viral Infections of the Human Nervous System*. New York: Springer, 2013.

Robertson, Erle S., ed. *Epstein-Barr Virus*. Norfolk, England: Caister Academic Press, 2010.

Tselis, Alex C., and Hal B. Jenson, eds. *Epstein-Barr Virus*. New York: Taylor & Francis, 2006.

Umar, Constantine S., ed. *New Developments in Epstein-Barr Virus Research*. New York: Nova Science, 2006.

Wilson, Joanna B., and Gerhard H. W. May, eds. *Epstein-Barr Virus Protocols*. Totowa, N.J.: Humana Press, 2001.

ERECTILE DYSFUNCTION
Disease/Disorder
Also known as: Impotence
Anatomy or system affected: Blood vessels, cells, genitals, reproductive system
Specialties and related fields: Urology
Definition: A disorder whereby a male cannot achieve an erection suitable for sexual intercourse.
Key terms:
atherosclerosis: a condition in which the artery wall becomes thickened due to a buildup of fatty materials such as cholesterol; the arteries become less elastic because of the formation of plaques within the arteries
corpora cavernosa: two spongelike regions of erectile tissue that run the length of the penis and fill with blood during a penile erection
phosphodiesterase type 5 inhibitors: phosphodiesterases are enzymes within cells that degrade phosphodiesterase; in the penis, phosphodiesterase type 5 degrades the substance cGMP made by another enzyme, guanylate cyclase; when levels of cGMP are allowed to increase, it causes the smooth muscle cells in the penile vasculature to relax

Causes and Symptoms

When a human male is sexually aroused, the brain sends a signal through the nervous system to the penis. The signal tells the blood vessels in the penis to relax so that the vessels get larger and fill with blood. Two spongy, cylinder-shaped chambers called the corpora cavernosa run the length of the penis. It is these chambers filled with blood vessels and blood sinuses that become engorged with blood. The same nerve signals that tell the vessels entering the penis to fill with blood also slow down the rate of blood leaving the penis, such that the penis fills with blood and becomes erect. In most males with erectile dysfunction (ED), the blood flow or nerve signals to the penis are reduced or damaged such that one cannot achieve an erection suitable for sexual intercourse.

Erectile dysfunction is more common with advancing age. The prevalence of any degree (mild to complete) of erectile dysfunction in men forty years of age and older is about 40 percent. Age is strongly associated with erectile dysfunction, but men with heart disease, hypertension, diabetes, and depression are more likely to experience erectile dysfunction than are men of the same age without these health problems. Men who have surgery of the prostate gland, located near the base of the penis, might have damage to the nerves that go to the penis and might experience erectile dysfunction that is either temporary or permanent.

Erectile dysfunction seems to be associated with cardiovascular diseases, leading to speculation that vascular causes for erectile dysfunction might be due to a process similar to atherosclerosis that occurs in the penile blood vessels and keeps them from being able to relax and enlarge. Sometimes drugs taken for other disorders can cause erectile dysfunction. They include drugs taken for depression (amitriptyline, doxepin), psychosis (phenothiazines, haloperidol,

---

Information on Erectile Dysfunction

Causes: Physical (nerve damage or vascular disease), psychological

Symptoms: Inability to achieve a penile erection suitable for sexual intercourse

Duration: Chronic

Treatments: Pharmaceuticals (phosphodiesterase inhibitors), mechanical vacuum devices, intracavernous injection therapy, intraurethral suppositories, penile implants, and surgery

---

benzisoxazole), and high blood pressure (beta blockers, thiazide diuretics, methyldopa, clonidine).

Although complete erectile dysfunction, defined as no hardening of the penis with sexual stimulation, may be easily recognized as erectile dysfunction, the subtler symptoms of milder erectile dysfunction are not always identified as such by men. Additionally, despite the publicity and advertisements for ED medications, some men are still reluctant to discuss erection problems with their health care provider or are concerned that treatments for ED are unsafe.

Treatment and Therapy

Lifestyle changes such as weight loss, which can improve high blood pressure and type 2 diabetes, can also improve erectile dysfunction. Oral therapy with phosphodiesterase type 5 inhibitors (Viagra, Cialis, or Levitra) are the treatment options usually tried first in men with erectile dysfunction. These drugs act by stimulating the blood vessels in the penis to relax. Phosphodiesterase inhibitors have a good safety record, but some men experience visual or other side effects after taking these drugs. Men who take nitrates for chest pain should not take phosphodiesterase inhibitors, because the combination of nitrates and phosphodiesterase inhibitors can cause the blood pressure to drop below normal and cause blackouts.

Other treatments include mechanical vacuum devices, intracavernous injection therapy, intraurethral suppositories, penile implants, and surgery. Mechanical vacuum devices create a vacuum around the penis, which draws blood into the penis to cause an erection. The penis is placed in a plastic cylinder and then a pump pulls the air out of the cylinder. Once an erection is achieved, an elastic band is placed at the base of the penis to maintain the erection after the cylinder is removed. With intracavernous injection therapy, drugs are injected directly into the penis to cause an erection. Intraurethral suppositories are prostaglandin-containing pellets that are inserted into the urethra. Occasional side effects include pain in the penis and sometimes in the testicles, mild urethral bleeding, and dizziness. After inserting the pellet, the man must remain standing to increase blood flow to the penis. It can take about fifteen minutes to achieve an erection. This method can also have consequences for a man's female sex partner by causing vaginal itching and possibly uterine contractions. The latter reason is why men should not use this method when having intercourse with a pregnant woman unless a condom or other type of barrier device is also used.

Penile implants are inflatable inserts surgically implanted on either side of the penis. The implants are attached to a pump placed in the scrotum and a reservoir fitted just below the groin muscles. The implants are inflated with saline solution from the reservoir to make the penis erect. There is some risk of mechanical failure with these kinds of devices.

Vascular reconstructive surgery for erectile dysfunction is rarely performed and is considered experimental. The surgery involves taking a vein from the leg and attaching it so that it allows blood to bypass areas of vascular blockage in the penis. Venous ligation is performed to keep the veins going out of the penis from leaking so that enough blood stays in the penis to keep it erect.

Studies carried out at the Rambam Medical Center in Israel indicated that extracorporeal shockwave therapy, a procedure used to treat kidney stones, may be able to replace prescription medication to treat ED in some cases. The shockwave procedure increases blood flow and enables new blood vessels to be created, enhancing a man's chances of producing an erection.

Perspective and Prospects

Before the approval of Viagra, the subject of erectile dysfunction or impotence was rarely discussed. To market the drug, Pfizer, the company that produces Viagra, launched an advertising campaign that included several celebrities who acknowledged that they had ED. This advertising campaign brought the subject of erectile dysfunction into the public domain, and soon erectile dysfunction was no longer a forbidden topic of conversation. Viagra was originally developed as a medicine intended to treat the heart disease angina pectoris. Viagra was not effective as a treatment for that condition, but one of the side effects reported during clinical trials in angina was that of erections.

Phosphodiesterase inhibitors have also become drugs of abuse, because these drugs can also enhance erections in persons who do not have erectile dysfunction. Some men take a phosphodiesterase inhibitor after taking illicit recreational drugs that can cause erection problems to counteract the effect on their sexual performance.

—*Nancy E. Price, Ph.D.*

See also Alcoholism; Anxiety; Aphrodisiacs; Genital disorders, female; Genital disorders, male; Hormones; Hypertension; Men's health; Psychiatry; Psychiatry, geriatric; Psychosomatic disorders; Sexual dysfunction; Sexuality; Stress; Urinary disorders.

For Further Information:

Kirby, Michael. *Erectile Dysfunction and Vascular Disease.* Malden, Mass.: Blackwell, 2003.

Kirby, Roger S. *An Atlas of Erectile Dysfunction.* 2d ed. New York: Parthenon, 2003.

Kirby, Roger S., Culley C. Carson, and Irwin Goldstein. *Erectile Dysfunction: A Clinical Guide.* Oxford, England: Isis Medical Media, 1999.

Lalong-Muh J., T. Colm, and M. Steggall. "Erectile Dysfunction Following Retropubic Prostatectomy." *British Journal of Nursing* 22, no. 4 (February/March, 2013): S4, S7–9.

Resnick M. J., et al. "Long-Term Functional Outcomes After Treatment for Localized Prostate Cancer." *New England Journal of*

Medicine 368, no. 5 (January, 2013):436–445.

Schwarz, Ernst R. *Erectile Dysfunction*. New York: Oxford University Press, 2013.

Vardi, Yoram, et al. "Can Low-Intensity Extracorporeal Shockwave Therapy Improve Erectile Function? A Six-Month Follow-Up Pilot Study in Patients with Organic Erectile Dysfunction." *European Urology* 58, no. 2 (August, 2010): 243–248.

ERGOGENIC AIDS
Biology

Also known as: Blood doping, steroids, caffeine, growth hormone, creatine

Anatomy or system affected: Blood, brain, cells, circulatory system, endocrine system, genitals, glands, heart, joints, kidneys, liver, musculoskeletal system

Specialties and related fields: Biochemistry, endocrinology, ethics, exercise physiology, family medicine, hematology, internal medicine, nephrology, orthopedics, pharmacology, psychology, sports medicine, toxicology

Definition: Substances used by athletes in an effort to gain an advantage. Most of these substances are illegal and unethical within competitive sports.

Introduction

In the history of sport, athletes have attempted to find a competitive advantage through advanced techniques in training, nutrition, and even in ergogenic aids, such as nutritional supplements and pharmacological aids. The use of these substances—such as anabolic-androgenic steroids (AAS), testosterone precursors (such as androstenedione), and nonsteroidal aids such as human growth hormone (GH) and creatine—have become increasingly popular in recent years, even without thorough scientific data supporting their efficacy and safety.

The population using such performance-enhancing drugs ranges from collegiate to professional athletes to adolescents and high school students. Recent meta-analyses estimate that 3 to 12 percent of adolescent boys have used an anabolic steroid at least once, and 28 percent of collegiate athletes admit to taking creatine. Other studies have suggested that the number may be closer to 41 percent.

Though such ergogenic aids are thought to improve strength, endurance, agility, and overall performance, most athletic improvement is anecdotal at best. Scientific evidence supporting these ideas is scarce and incomplete. Even with aids that may improve strength and/or performance, the safety of these substances has been seriously questioned, such as with the use of AAS, GH, and ephedra.

Types of Ergogenic Aids

Anabolic-androgenic steroids (AAS) as ergogenic aids in sports are chemical compounds that resemble the structure of testosterone, the naturally occurring male sex hormone that affects muscle growth and strength. "Anabolic" refers to the growth of cells, and "androgenic" refers to the stimulation of the growth of male sex organs and masculine sex characteristics. AAS bind to cells that are used for muscle repair and that

can transform into muscle fibers.

AAS has been one of the most studied ergogenic aids, yet many of its mechanisms and adverse effects are still not well understood. Studies have shown that increased doses of testosterone can decrease total body adipose tissue in the body and can increase strength and fat-free mass. Adverse effects of AAS use include hypothalamic-pituitary dysfunction, gynecomastia, severe acne, infection as a result of sharing needles, aggressive and depressive behavior, and a possible association with premature death.

Androstenedione (andro) is a testosterone precursor produced by the adrenal glands and gonads. Its ergogenic effect occurs after it is converted to testosterone in the testes as well as in other tissues. It can also be converted to estrone and estradiol, which are steroid compounds that are primary female sex hormones (found in both men and women). The creation of testosterone is regulated by the amount of testosterone precursors in the body. Theoretically, an increase in androstenedione would increase the production of testosterone and thus can increase protein synthesis, lean body mass, and strength.

Older studies showed that andro supplementation results in increased serum testosterone levels. However, more recent studies have shown that andro supplementation fails to directly improve lean body mass, muscular strength, or serum testosterone levels. Possible side effects to andro use are suppressed testosterone production, liver dysfunction, cardiovascular disease, testicular atrophy, baldness, acne, and aggressive behavior.

Similar to androstenedione, dihydroepiandrosterone (DHEA) is a precursor of testosterone and is also formed in the adrenal glands and gonads. DHEA is the most abundant steroid hormone in circulation and is a precursor to androstenedione and other testosterone precursors (such as androstenediol). Studies of DHEA supplementation have not been shown to increase lean body mass, strength, or testosterone levels. Possible side effects are similar to andro and AAS use.

Human growth hormone (GH) is a metabolic hormone that is secreted into the blood by cells found in the anterior pituitary gland. After its secretion, GH stimulates the production of insulin-like growth factor (IGF)-1 in the liver. These hormones stimulate bone growth, protein synthesis, and the conversion of fat to energy. Athletes have been attracted to GH not only because of such theoretical benefits but also because of the limited techniques in detecting GH in the urine. GH levels vary in individuals of different, ages, sex, and activity and can vary throughout the day, so no reliable benchmark can be made to determine if illicit use has taken place.

Scientific studies have been unable to show that GH leads to increased muscle strength and exercise performance or changes in protein synthesis. Because of ethical limitations, it is difficult to study the effect of larger doses of GH on healthy individuals. Adverse effects of GH use include cosmetic damage, joint pain, muscle weakness, fluid retention, impaired glucose regulation (which may lead to diabetes mellitus), cardiomyopathy, hyperlipidemia, and possibly death.

Erythropoieten (EPO) is a hormone secreted by the kidneys that is a precursor to bone marrow. EPO increases the oxygen-carrying capacity of blood and, as a result, aids in endurance and aerobic respiration. The appeal of EPO among athletes is this endurance-enhancing effect. As a result, many users have been found to be skiers, cyclists, and other athletes who require high levels of endurance. Early use of EPO as an ergogenic aid, termed "blood doping,â€□ came in the form of autologous blood transfusions, in which athletes would harvest their own red blood cells and reintroduce them into their systems before events. A synthetic form of EPO, recombinant human erythropoietin (r-HuEPO) became available in 1988.

Scientific studies have shown that EPO and r-HuEPO treatments do increase certain blood concentrations and can aid in endurance. EPO may also have serious and dangerous side effects, however, such as hypertension, seizures, thromboembolic events, and possibly death.

Creatine monohydrate is an amine synthesized in the kidneys, pancreas, and liver, and it can also be obtained through the diet from meat and fish. Approximately 90 to 95 percent of creatine in the body is found in skeletal muscle. Creatine, which is converted to creatine phosphate (PCr), is an important limiting factor in the resynthesis of adenosine triphosphate (ATP), which plays a significant role in energy reserves within the body. Theoretically, an increase of PCr in the body would increase the regeneration of ATP, resulting in an increase in sustained maximal energy production for short-term exercise. This could lead to increased intensity and repetition frequency, and thus possible increases in skeletal muscle mass.

In 2002, A. M. Bohn and colleagues argued in an article in *Current Sports Medicine Reports* that there are "no studies demonstrating benefit with the relatively indiscriminant use of variable amounts of creatine by large numbers of athletes on a specific team." Nevertheless, creatine has been shown to enhance performance in small populations of athletes of various sports. Possible adverse effects of creatine include muscle cramping, dehydration, gastrointestinal distress, weight gain, increased risk of muscle tears, inhibited insulin and creatine production, renal damage, and possibly nephropathy.

Stimulants are drugs that increase nervous system activity. Examples of stimulants commonly used as ergogenic aids include the class of drugs called amphetamines, as well as specific chemical compounds such as caffeine and ephedrine. The use of caffeine has been shown to improve exercise time to exhaustion and may even significantly increase intestinal glucose absorption. It has been suggested that caffeine increases fat utilization for energy and delays the depletion of glycogen (the stored form of glucose). As a result, caffeine and other stimulants are popular ergogenic aids for extended aerobic activity.

Caffeine in small doses has been shown to increase performance. Possible adverse effects of caffeine may include anxiety, dependency, withdrawal, and possibly a diuretic effect (dehydration). Ephedrine may have similar adverse affects. Other stimulants, such as amphetamines or cocaine, have more serious and detrimental effects.

Perspective and Prospects

The use of ergogenic aids in the history of sport has progressively moved from primitive aids to more sophisticated performance enhancers. Crude natural concoctions and stimulants have paved the way for complex pharmacological agents (such as erythropoietin) and designer anabolic steroids (such as tetrahydrogestrinone). Athletes and trainers have utilized any and all means to gain a competitive edge, even if that results in damage to health and even a risk of death.

The biggest problem stemming from the use of such aids is the difficulty in detecting them. This is evident in recent media attention given to ergogenic aids and their popularity, as seen through the 2007 Mitchell Report, an independent congressional investigation of the use of performance-enhancing drugs in Major League Baseball, as well as the 2012 discoveries of abuse by high-profile cyclists and athletes at the Summer Olympics held in London. This media attention has also shown the difficulties among investigators, such as the International Olympic Committee, the World Anti-Doping Agency, and the United States Anti-Doping Agency, in detecting the use of new designer steroids and new ergogenic aids among elite athletes.

—Julien M. Cobert and Jeffrey R. Bytomski, D.O.

See also Blood and blood disorders; Blood testing; Caffeine; Ethics; Exercise physiology; Hormones; Hypertrophy; Metabolism; Muscles; Pharmacology; Sports medicine; Steroid use; Steroids.

For Further Information:

Bhazin, S., et al. "The Effects of Supraphysiologic Doses of Testosterone on Muscle Size and Strength in Normal Men." *New England Journal of Medicine* 335 (1996): 1–7.

Bohn, Amy Miller, Stephanie Betts, and Thomas L. Schwenk. "Creatine and Other Nonsteroidal Strength-Enhancing Aids." *Current Sports Medicine Reports* 1, no. 4 (August, 2002): 239–245.

Foster, Zoë J., and Jeffrey A. Housner. "Anabolic-Andogenic Steroids and Testosterone Precursors: Ergogenic Aids and Sport." *Current Sports Medicine Reports* 3, no. 4 (August, 2004): 234–241.

Graham, T. E. "Caffeine and Exercise: Metabolism, Endurance, and Performance." *Sports Medicine* 31, no. 11 (November 1, 2001): 785–807.

Health Library. "Sports and Fitness Support: Enhancing Performance." *Health Library*, July 25, 2012.

Juhn, Mark S. "Ergogenic Aids in Aerobic Activity." *Current Sports Medicine Reports* 1, no. 4 (August, 2002): 233–238.

Mayo Clinic. "Performance-Enhancing Drugs: Know the Risks." *Mayo Clinic*, December 12, 2012.

MedlinePlus. "Anabolic Steroids." *MedlinePlus*, June 17, 2013.

Powers, Michael E. "The Safety and Efficacy of Anabolic Steroid Precursors: What Is the Scientific Evidence?" *Journal of Athletic Training* 37, no. 3 (2002): 300–305.

Shekelle, Paul G., et al. "Efficacy and Safety of Ephedra and Ephedrine for Weight Loss and Athletic Performance: A Meta-analysis." *Journal of the American Medical Association* 289, no. 12 (March 26, 2003): 1537–1545.

Singbart, G. "Adverse Events of Erythropoietin in Long-Term and in Acute/Short-Term Treatment." *Clinical Investigation* 72 (1994): S36–S43.

Sotas, Pierre-Edouard, et al. "Prevlance of Blood Doping in Samples Collected from Elite Track and Field Athletes." *Clinical Chemistry* 57, no. 5 (May 2011): 762–769.

Stacy, Jason J., Thomas R. Terrell, and Thomas D. Armsey. "Ergogenic Aids: Human Growth Hormone." *Current Sports Medicine Reports* 3, no. 4 (August, 2004): 229–233.

Yesalis, C. E., and M. S. Bahrke. "Doping Among Adolescent Athletes." *Baillieres Best Practice and Research in Clinical Endocrinology and Metabolism* 14, no. 1 (March, 2000): 25–35.

ESOPHAGEAL CANCER. *See* MOUTH AND THROAT CANCER.

ESOPHAGUS

Anatomy

Anatomy or system affected: Gastrointestinal system, mouth, stomach, throat

Specialties and related fields: Gastroenterology, otorhinolaryngology

Definition: A muscular tube, approximately 10 inches in length, that carries food from the mouth or pharynx to the stomach.

Structure and Function

The esophagus lies between the spine and the trachea and is part of the digestive system. The esophagus, however, does not produce or secrete any digestive enzymes, and absorption of nutrients in this part of the digestive system is almost nil. The esophagus pierces the diaphragm as it moves through the thoracic cavity and into the abdominopelvic cavity, where it joins with the stomach.

All parts of the digestive system have four tunics (tissues): from superficial to deep, tunica serosa, tunica muscularis, tunica submucosa, and tunica mucosa. Tunica serosa anchors the esophagus in the mesentery. Tunica muscularis is composed of smooth muscle fibers arranged in circular and longitudinal fibers. These two layers of muscles are important as they are able to squeeze the food bolus (chewed mass of food) and move it down toward the stomach. The muscles are involuntary and perform peristaltic contractions behind the bolus, pushing it downward, as if a tennis ball were being pushed through a leg of panty hose. Tunica submucosa is a layer of loose connective tissue; blood vessels and nerves, including the important submucosa plexus, are found in this layer. The innermost layer, tunica mucosa, is comprised of epithelial cells and is the layer in contact with the bolus. Of all the tunics, tunica mucosa is the most variable along the length of the digestive system. The epithelium here is stratified squamous epithelial tissue to protect the esophagus from sharp or dangerous food items, such as bones, hot pizza, or insufficiently chewed carrots.

The esophagus has an upper and a lower sphincter. When one swallows, the upper sphincter relaxes. In a coordinated effort, the larynx pulls forward and the epiglottis clamps down to cover this opening into the respiratory system (lungs). Glands produce mucus to lubricate food as it passes along the lumen. The lower sphincter closes once the bolus has passed into the stomach. Failure to do so would allow stomach acids to leak up into the esophagus, causing what is commonly called heartburn or acid indigestion, more properly known as gastroesophageal reflux disease.

Disorders and Diseases

The most common medical problem with the esophagus is gastroesophageal reflux disease (GERD), which is caused when the lower sphincter fails to close properly. Stomach contents, which are acidic, then leak into the esophagus and irritate it. Left untreated, GERD can damage the esophagus.

Barrett's esophagus is a disease often is found in patients with GERD. In Barrett's esophagus, the tissue that lines the esophagus, tunica mucosa, is replaced by tissue that is more similar to tissue lining the intestines. The process is called intestinal metaplasia. Barrett's esophagus may lead to the development of esophageal cancer, but this is a rare event. It should be emphasized that not all patients with GERD develop Barrett's esophagus and that very few people with Barrett's esophagus develop cancer. The cause of Barrett's esophagus is unknown, as is the cause of esophageal cancer.

—*M. A. Foote, Ph.D.*

See also Acid reflux disease; Bile; Digestion; Enzymes; Gastroenterology; Gastroenterology, pediatric; Gastrointestinal disorders; Gastrointestinal system; Heartburn; Indigestion; Peristalsis.

For Further Information:

"Digestive System." *MedlinePlus*, January 14, 2013.

"Esophagus Disorders." *MedlinePlus*, June 12, 2013.

Johnson, Leonard R., ed. *Gastrointestinal Physiology*. 7th ed. Philadelphia: Mosby/Elsevier, 2007.

Mayo Clinic. *Mayo Clinic on Digestive Health: Enjoy Better Digestion with Answers to More than Twelve Common Conditions*. 2d ed. Rochester, Minn.: Author, 2004.

Scanlon, Valerie, and Tina Sanders. *Essentials of Anatomy and Physiology*. 6th ed. Philadelphia: F. A. Davis, 2012.

Wood, Debra, Daus Mahnke, and Brian Randall. "Heartburn—Overview." *Health Library*, March 18, 2013.

ESTROGEN REPLACEMENT THERAPY. *See* HORMONE THERAPY.

ETHICS

Also known as: Bioethics, medical ethics

Definition: Ethics is a code of conduct based on established moral principles. Medical ethics is the study of the conduct of professionals in the field of medicine.

Key terms:

autonomy: independence and self-reliance, especially referring to decision making

beneficence: doing good

informed consent: the dialogue between physician and patient prior to an invasive procedure

justice: the rationing of scarce resources according to a prearranged plan

nonmaleficence: avoiding evil

paternalism: acting in the manner of a father to his children

Principles

Ethics deals with a code of conduct based on established moral principles. When applied to a particular professional field, abstract theories as well as concrete principles are considered. Often the consequences of a particular course of action dictate its rightness or wrongness. Bioethics is the study of ethics by professionals in the fields of medicine, law, philosophy, or theology. Some also refer to this area as applied ethics. The term *bioethics* is often used interchangeably with *medical ethics*, but purists would define medical ethics as the study of conduct by professionals in the field of medicine. Codes of ethics promulgated by professional groups or associations define obligations governing members of a given profession.

Initial questions concerning medical ethics involve purpose, to whom a duty is owed (legal or moral), and how far that duty extends. Does it extend solely to patients, to their families, or to society as a whole? For example, public health obligations to society involve a duty to prevent disease, maintain the health of the populace, and oversee the delivery of health care.

In his 1972 article "Models for Ethical Practice in a Revolutionary Age," Robert M. Veatch proposes four models for ethical medicine. The first is the engineering model, in which the physician becomes an applied scientist interested in treating disease rather than caring for a patient. The Nazi physicians during World War II acting as so-called scientists and technicians are examples of the engineering model taken to its extreme. The second is the priestly model, in which the physician assumes a paternalistic role of moral dominance, treating the patient as a child. The main principle of this model is the traditional one of *primum non nocere*, or "first, do no harm." It neglects principles of patient autonomy, dignity, and freedom. The third is the collegial model, in which physician and patient are colleagues cooperating in the pursuit of a common goal, such as preserving health, curing illness, or easing pain. This model requires mutual trust and confidence, demanding a continued dialogue between the parties. The fourth is the contractual model, in which the relationship between health-care provider and patient is analogous to a legal contract, with rights and obligations on both sides. The contractual model can be modified to provide for shared decision making and cooperation between physician and patient and tailored to the particular physician-patient relationship involved, resulting in a collegial association.

Autonomy and informed consent. Since the Nuremberg trials, which presented horrible accounts of medical experimentation in Nazi concentration camps, the issue of consent has been one of primary importance. These basic concepts recognize an individual's uniqueness and inherent right to make decisions without coercion or undue influence from others. Respect for privacy and freedom is fundamental to human dignity. Even when people present difficult problems, such as being unconscious or in a coma, they must continue to be respected. Rational decision making by patients or their surrogates must be followed, and those with specialized knowledge or expertise are not authorized to impose their will on another person or limit that person's freedom.

Informed consent seeks to encourage open communication between patient and health-care provider, protect patients and research subjects from harm, and encourage health-care providers to act responsibly vis-à-vis patients and subjects, ultimately preserving autonomy and rational decision making. Especially applicable in invasive procedures, such as those involving surgery or treatments with serious risks, informed consent requires the presence of certain conditions, including a patient's competency or decision-making capability, in order to understand the relative consequences of a proposed course of treatment and its effect on a patient's life and health. The health-care provider must inform patients of alternative courses of action, if any, and of the fact that patients have the option to refuse treatment, even if that alternative is contrary to the recommendation of the physician. The information conveyed to the patient must include the diagnosis, the nature of the proposed treatment, the known risks and consequences (excluding those that are too remote or improbable to bear significantly on the ultimate decision whether to proceed on a course of treatment, as well as those that are so well known that they are obvious to everyone), the benefits of the proposed treatment, any alternatives, the prognosis without treatment, economic cost, and how the treatment plan will impact the patient's lifestyle. The patient should also be made aware that once given, an informed consent can be withdrawn. Hospital consent forms do not provide this type of information.

The information conveyed must be material and important to this patient, not a fictional reasonable and prudent person. Information is material if it could change the decision of that patient. Inherent problems include speculation as to what factors would have a dramatic impact on the patient's life, requiring a dialogue between patient and health-care provider. It is also important to recognize the role of the physician's time constraints and the patient's overall stress level while the information is being conveyed, including possible information overload. Not only must the information be conveyed adequately, but it must also be assimilated and understood. The ability of an individual to process information raises substantial issues about understanding. Comprehension is not always easily ascertainable. Sometimes a person's ability to make decisions is affected by problems of nonacceptance of information, even if it was comprehended. A patient may voluntarily waive informed consent and ask not to be informed, thereby relieving the physician of the obligation to obtain informed consent and ultimately delegating decision-making authority to the physician.

Medical emergencies constitute exceptions to the informed-consent requirement, provided that four conditions are met: the patient, whose wishes are unknown because no advance directive or living will exists, is incapable of giving consent because of the emergency; no surrogate is available; the medical condition poses a danger to the patient's life or seriously impairs the patient's health; and immediate treatment is required to avert the danger to life or health. This exception is justified on the grounds that consent can be assumed in cases in which a reasonable person would consent if informed. If the patient is not in imminent danger, or if consent can be obtained at a later time, the emergency exception does not apply. Another exception is the therapeutic privilege, in which health-care providers are justified in legitimately withholding information from a patient when they reasonably believe that disclosure will have an adverse effect on the patient's condition or health, as in the case of a depressed, emotionally drained, or unstable patient. Again, the decision is subjective, referring to a specific patient, decided on a case-by-case basis. The privilege does not apply if the health-care provider withholds information based on the belief that the patient will refuse consent if told all the facts. In that instance, withholding information amounts to misrepresentation or deception.

Another ethical dilemma involving intentional deception or incomplete disclosure concerns the therapeutic use of placebos. One defense is that deception is moral when it is used for the patient's welfare.

Paternalism. From the Latin word *pater*, meaning "father," paternalism refers to controlling others as a father acts in his relationship with his children. In medical ethics, paternalism involves overriding the patient's wishes in order to act to benefit or avert harm to the patient. Intervention by a health-care provider to prevent competent patients from harming themselves is called strong paternalism. Strong paternalism is generally rejected by ethicists because of the view that health-care providers do not know all the factors influencing the life of another person and therefore lack the ability to decide what is best for another person. Weak paternalism is when the health-care provider overrules the wishes of an incompetent or questionably competent patient. It is sometimes justified in nonemergencies without informed consent to relieve serious pain and suffering. Another example of weak paternalism is the temporary use of restraints, justified on the grounds that confused and disoriented patients are otherwise likely to injure themselves. When restraints are necessary, the patient's surrogate is generally asked to give consent, a recognition that restraints, albeit temporary, constitute a limitation of one's liberty.

Beneficence and nonmaleficence. The principles of beneficence (doing good) and nonmaleficence (avoiding evil) are both expressed in the Hippocratic oath: "I will use treatment to help the sick according to my ability and judgment, but I will never use it to injure or wrong them." Each principle has a bearing on the other, and each is limited by the other. The obligation to do good is limited by the obligation to avoid evil. One may perform an act that risks evil if the following conditions are present (the principle of double effects): the action is good or morally indifferent, the agent intends a good effect, the evil effect is not the means to achieving good, and proportionality exists between good and evil. The principle of proportionality states that provided an action does not go directly against the dignity of the individual, there must be a proportionate good to justify risking evil consequences. Factors to be considered include the possible existence of an alternative means with less evil or no evil, the level of good intended compared to the level of evil risked, and the certitude or probability of good or evil. The second of these factors is related to what is called the wedge principle, referring to the fact that putting the tip of a wedge into a crack in a log and striking the wedge will split the log and destroy it; by analogy, once an exception is made in a single case, it will inevitably

be made again on a larger scale, and the person making the exception must consider the effect it would have if made on that scale. The last element to be considered is the causal influence of the agent, recognizing that most effects result from many causes and that a particular agent is seldom the sole cause. For example, as noted by Thomas M. Garrett and colleagues in *Health Care Ethics: Principles and Problems* (5th ed., 2010), lung cancer can be triggered not only by smoking but also by conditions in the workplace, the environment, and heredity.

Obligations imposed on the patient demand the use of ordinary but not extraordinary means of preserving and restoring health. In other words, the patient should use means that produce more good than harm and evaluate the effects on the self, family, and society, including pain, cost, and benefits to one's health and quality of life. The health-care provider's obligation demands that the benefits outweigh the burdens on the patient. An overarching obligation to society exists to provide health-care information and leadership to ensure the equitable distribution of scarce medical resources in a way that will allow the goals of health care to be achieved. Finally, the surrogate's obligation depends on whether the wishes of the once-competent patient are known or can be ascertained. If so, the surrogate should decide accordingly (the substituted judgment principle). Overruling the person's wishes would constitute a denial of the patient's autonomy. If the person has never been competent or has never expressed his or her wishes, the surrogate should act in the best interests of the patient alone, disregarding the interests of family, society, and the surrogate. Another approach requires the surrogate to choose what the patient would have chosen if and when competent after having considered all relevant information and the interests of others.

Certain conditions justify the decision to withhold treatment, such as when treatment would be pointless or futile, especially with regard to the dead or those who are dying, and situations in which the burdens of treatment would outweigh the benefits. It should be noted that no bright line exists here because these cases are not decided easily. Neither ethicists nor those in the medical professions who debate these issues have reached a clear-cut solution that applies in every case.

Justice. Also called distributive justice, justice establishes principles for the distribution of scarce resources in circumstances where demand outstrips supply and rationing must occur. Needs are to be considered in terms of overall needs and the dignity of members of society. Aside from the biological and physiological elements, the social context of health and disease may influence a given problem and its severity. Individual prejudices and presuppositions may enlarge the nature and scope of the disease, creating a demand for health care that makes it even more difficult to distribute scarce resources to all members of society. Principles of fair distribution in society often supersede and become paramount to the concerns of the individual. Questions about who should receive what share of society's scarce resources generate controversies about a national health policy, unequal distributions of advantages to the disadvantaged, and the rationing of health care.

Similar problems occur regarding access to and distribution of health insurance, medical equipment, and artificial organs. The lack of insurance and the problem of underinsurance constitute a huge economic barrier to health-care access in the United States. In *Principles of Biomedical Ethics* (7th ed., 2012), Tom L. Beauchamp and James F. Childress point out that the acquired immunodeficiency syndrome (AIDS) crisis has presented dramatic instances of the problems of insurability and underwriting practices, in which insurers often appeal to actuarial fairness in defending their decisions while neglecting social justice. Proposals to alleviate the unfairness to those below the poverty line have been based on charity, compassion, and benevolence toward the sick rather than on claims of justice. The ongoing debate in the United States over the entitlement to a minimum of health care involves not only government entitlement programs but also complex social, political, economic, and cultural beliefs.

Decisions concerning the allocation of funds will dictate the type of health care that can be provided and for which problems. Numerous resources, supplies, and spaces in intensive care units (ICUs) have been allocated for specific patients or classes of patients. A life-threatening illness complicates this decision. In the United States, health care has often been allocated based on a patient's ability to pay rather than other criteria; rationing has at times been based on ranking a list of services or a patient's age.

Confidentiality and privacy. In the United States, the medical profession has always strived to maintain the confidentiality of physician-patient communications, as well as the privacy of a patient's medical records. While admirable, these values have not been absolute, and no uniformity exists among the fifty states regarding access to a patient's medical records. In the past, as technology improved, with computers and fax machines transmitting health-care data to distant locations and medical records themselves existing in electronic form, no laws had been created to protect medical records adequately. In the late twentieth and early twenty-first centuries, the administrations of Bill Clinton, George W. Bush, and Barack Obama sought to enact legislation that would bridge the privacy gaps and create uniform standards while also eliminating discrimination in employment and insurance coverage based on one's genetic predisposition. The Health Insurance Portability and Accountability Act (HIPAA) became law in 1996, with various aspects of the act going into effect in later years as circumstances allowed. Subsequently, when the Health Information Technology for Economic and Clinical Health (HITECH) Act was enacted in 2009, one section extended HIPAA's privacy and security provisions and requirements.

Application of Ethical Principles

Advances in medical technology have expanded the scope of what medicine can accomplish. As medicine becomes increasingly sophisticated, medical ethics seeks to resolve age-old dilemmas as well as evaluate the use of new technologies. Certain ethical dilemmas have provoked sharp disagreement.

Chief among these is the issue of death and dying, which brings into controversy two theories about the nature of health care. The "curing" approach is based on traditional medical ethical principles that date back to Hippocrates and include the principles of beneficence, nonmaleficence, and justice. The "caring" approach focuses on patient autonomy, proper bedside manner by health-care providers, the preparation of advance directives or living wills, and the hospice movement.

The curing approach to medical ethics equates medicine with healing. The sanctity of life is important because it is a gift from God and must be sustained to the extent reasonably possible. All ordinary measures must be taken to preserve life. This tradition holds that only God can decide the time of death, and even in the face of suffering, the health-care provider must not take measures to shorten life. Physicians are the primary decision makers, and they are in the best position to recommend and advise the patient and direct the treatment plan. The model is paternalistic.

In the caring approach, the health-care provider's role is to minimize pain, present alternatives and the relative consequences of various options, and ultimately proceed according to the patient's determination. This approach is subjective, as each case is decided individually. Quality of life, rather than sanctity of life, becomes the guiding principle.

Issues regarding futility of treatment arise, as well as the recognition that prolonging life does not always benefit patients. Physicians are not obligated to provide futile treatment, and in fact doing so may violate the physician's duty not to harm patients, as such treatments are often burdensome and invasive, exacerbating the patient's pain and discomfort. Patients cannot ethically compel health-care workers to provide treatment that violates the worker's own personal beliefs or the standards of the profession. Other issues in this area deal with physician-assisted suicide and whether to provide or withhold lifesaving treatments.

The transplantation of vital organs—notably the heart, liver, and kidney—raises difficult ethical questions. As organ transplantation has become routine at many medical centers, its success has opened a Pandora's box of ethical questions involving the allocation of scarce donor organs. One such question is whether the sickest person on the waiting list for an organ should be the recipient, or whether it should go to someone more robust who may live longer. Another is whether live donors should be compensated for donating an organ, just as blood donors are compensated. Many countries outside the United States and the United Kingdom condone the sale of organs; the 1984 National Organ Transplant Act makes selling organs illegal in the United States. Ethicists are debating animal-to-human organ transplants to alleviate the scarcity of human donor organs for transplantation.

Assisted reproduction in the form of in vitro fertilization (IVF), egg freezing, and sperm banking is largely an unregulated industry. Couples seeking help must make complex ethical decisions dealing with the preselection of embryos based on genetic traits through screening of a single cell. Other decisions deal with how many eggs should be fertilized and whether the remainder should be disposed of or frozen. The rights of the participants and the children created through assisted reproduction remain largely undefined. Several countries, including Sweden, Great Britain, and Australia, have banned anonymous sperm donation. The European Court of Human Rights has ruled that article 8 of the European Convention on Human Rights gives a child conceived from donor eggs or sperm the right to know the identity of his or her biological parents. In the United States, the issue is not addressed by federal statute, and laws vary widely from state to state on the matter.

The identification of human embryonic stem cells has been widely acknowledged as extremely valuable because it will assist scientists in understanding basic mechanisms of embryo development and gene regulation. It also holds the promise of allowing the development of techniques for manipulating, growing, and cloning stem cells to create designer cells and tissues. Stem cells are created in the first days of pregnancy. Scientists hope to direct stem cells to grow into replacement organs and tissues to treat a wide variety of diseases. Embryos are valued in research for their ability to produce stem cells, which can be harvested to grow a variety of tissues for use in transplantation to treat serious illnesses such as cancer, heart disease, and diabetes. In so doing, however, researchers must destroy days-old embryos, a procedure condemned by the Catholic Church, some antiabortion activists, and some women's rights organizations. Other research points to similar promise using stem cells harvested from adults, so that no embryos are destroyed.

Perspective and Prospects

Medical ethics in Western culture has its roots in ancient Greek and Roman medicine, namely the Greek physician Hippocrates and the Roman physician Galen. In ancient Greece, as in most early societies, healing wounds and treating disease first appeared as folk practice and religious ritual. The earliest statement about ethics appears in a clinical and epidemiological book entitled *Epidemics I*, attributed to Hippocrates. It is in this work that the admonition "to help and not to harm" first appeared. The book itself deals with prognosis rather than treatment, which is the approach taken by Hippocrates. Galen asserts that any worthwhile doctor must know philosophy, including the logical, the physical, and the ethical, and be skilled at reasoning about the problems presented to him and understanding the nature and function of the body within the physical world.

Between the fourth and the fourteenth centuries CE, medicine became firmly established in the universities and the public life of the emerging nations of Europe. During this time, the Roman Catholic Church had a strong influence on Western civilization. Medicine was deeply touched by the doctrine and discipline of the church, and its theological influence shaped the ethics of medicine. The early church endorsed the use of human medicine and encouraged care of the sick as a work of charity. One of the greatest physicians during this period was the Jewish Talmudic scholar Maimonides, whose writings sometimes dealt with ethical questions in medicine.

The duty to comfort the sick and dying was a moral imperative in Christianity and Judaism. As the bubonic plague swept across Europe over the following several centuries, Protestant leader Martin Luther urged doctors and ministers to fulfill the obligation of Christian charity by faithful service, but John Calvin argued that physicians and ministers could depart if the preservation of their lives was in the common interest.

The ethical debates surrounding the plague moved medical ethics ahead. As noted by Albert R. Jonsen in *A Short History of Medical Ethics* (2000), the question became, "Under what circumstances does a person who has medical skills have a special obligation to serve the community?" When syphilis emerged in epidemic proportions at the end of the fifteenth century, a similar question regarding service to the sick at the cost of danger to oneself resurfaced, and members of the medical profession struggled with the link between medical necessity and moral correctness. Not until the nineteenth century did a consensus appear, mandating that the physician should take personal risks to serve the needy without appraising the morality of a patient's behavior.

—*Marcia J. Weiss, M.A., J.D.*

See also Abortion; Aging: Extended care; Animal rights vs. research; Assisted reproductive technologies; Cloning; Contraception; Ergogenic aids; Euthanasia; Fetal tissue transplantation; Genetic engineering; Hippocratic oath; Hospice; In vitro fertilization; Law and medicine; Living will; Malpractice; Medicare; Palliative medicine; Resuscitation; Screening; Stem cells; Suicide; Terminally ill: Extended care; Transplantation; Xenotransplantation.

For Further Information:

Beauchamp, Tom L., and James F. Childress. *Principles of Biomedical Ethics*. 7th ed. New York: Oxford University Press, 2012.
Beauchamp, Tom L., Leroy Walters, Jeffrey P. Kahn, and Anna C. Mastroianni, eds. *Contemporary Issues in Bioethics*. 8th ed. Belmont, Calif.: Wadsworth, 2013.
Garrett, Thomas M., Harold W. Baillie, and Rosellen M. Garrett. *Health Care Ethics: Principles and Problems*. 5th ed. Upper Saddle River, N.J.: Prentice Hall, 2010.
Jonsen, Albert R. *A Short History of Medical Ethics*. New York: Oxford University Press, 2000.
"Medical Ethics." *American Medical Association*, 1995–2013.
"Medical Ethics." *MedlinePlus*, May 15, 2013.
Pence, Gregory E. *Re-creating Medicine: Ethical Issues at the Frontiers of Medicine*. Lanham, Md.: Rowman & Littlefield, 2007.
Resnik, David B. "What Is Ethics in Research and Why Is It Important?" *National Institute of Environmental Health Sciences*, May 1, 2011.
Torr, James D., ed. *Medical Ethics*. San Diego, Calif.: Greenhaven Press, 2000.
Veatch, Robert M. "Models for Ethical Practice in a Revolutionary Age." *Hastings Center Report* 2, no. 3 (June 1972): 5–7.

EUTHANASIA
Ethics

Definition: The intentional termination of a life, which may be active (resulting from specific actions causing death) or passive (resulting from the refusal or withdrawal of life-sustaining treatment), and voluntary (with the patient's consent) or involuntary (on behalf of infants or others who are incapable of making this decision, such as comatose patients).

Key terms:

active euthanasia: administration of a drug or some other means that directly causes death; the motivation is to relieve patient suffering

durable power of attorney: designation of a person who will have legal authority to make health care decisions if the patient becomes incapable of making decisions for himself or herself

living will: a legal document in which the patient states a preference regarding life-prolonging treatment in the event that he or she cannot choose

nonvoluntary euthanasia: a decision to terminate life made by another when the patient is incapable of making a decision for himself or herself

passive euthanasia: ending life by refusing or withdrawing life-sustaining medical treatment

voluntary euthanasia: a patient's consent to a decision which results in the shortening of his or her life

The Controversy Surrounding Euthanasia

In the past, the role of the doctor was clear: The physician should minimize suffering and save lives whenever possible. In the present, it is possible for these two goals to be at odds. Saving lives in some situations seems to prolong the misery of the patient. In other cases, procedures or treatments may only marginally postpone the time of death. Advances in medical technology enable many to live who would have died just a few years ago, and massive amounts of money are spent each year on medical research with the goal of prolonging life. Experts in US population trends indicate that by the year 2030, those over the age of sixty-five will comprise about 20 percent of the country's total population. These people will probably be healthy and alert well into their eighties; however, in the last years of their lives they will probably require significant medical care, putting financial stress on the health care system.

The complex issues surrounding death, suffering, and economics create demands for answers to difficult ethical questions. Does all life have value? Should one fight against death even when suffering is intense? Should suffering be lessened if the time of death is brought nearer? Should a patient be given the right to refuse medical treatment if the result is death? Should others be allowed to make this decision for the patient? Should other factors such as the financial or emotional burden on the family be part of the decision-making process? Once a decision has been made to terminate suffering by death, is there any ethical difference between discontinuing medical treatment and giving a lethal dosage of painkilling medication? Should laws be put into place that offer guidelines in these situations, or should each case be decided on an individual basis? And who should decide? There is a wide range of opinion and much uncertainty involving euthanasia and what constitutes a "good" death.

Euthanasia comes from a Greek word that can be trans-

lated as "good death" and is defined in several ways, depending on the philosophical stance of the one giving the definition. Tom Beauchamp, in his book *Health and Human Values* (1983), defines euthanasia as

> *putting to death or failing to prevent death in cases of terminal illness or injury; the motive is to relieve comatoseness, physical suffering, anxiety or a serious sense of burdensomeness to self and others. In euthanasia at least one other person causes or helps to cause the death of one who desires death or, in the case of an incompetent person, makes a substituted decision, either to cause death directly or to withdraw something that sustains life.*

Most patients who express a wish to die more quickly are terminally ill; however, euthanasia is sometimes considered as a solution for nonterminal patients as well. An example of the latter would be seriously deformed or retarded infants whose futures are judged to have a poor "quality of life" and who would be a serious burden on their families and society.

When discussing the ethical implications of euthanasia, the types of cases have been divided into various classes. A distinction is made between voluntary and nonvoluntary euthanasia. In voluntary euthanasia, the patient consents to a specific course of medical action in which death is hastened. Nonvoluntary euthanasia would occur in cases in which the patient is not able to make decisions about his or her death because of an inability to communicate or a lack of mental facility. Each of these classes has advocates and antagonists. Some believe that voluntary euthanasia should always be allowed, but others would limit voluntary euthanasia to only those patients who have a terminal illness. Some, although agreeing in principle that voluntary euthanasia in terminal situations is ethically permissible, nevertheless oppose euthanasia of any type because of the possibility of abuses. With nonvoluntary euthanasia, the main ethical issues deal with when such an action should be performed and who should make the decision. If a person is in an irreversible coma, most agree that that person's physical life could be ended; however, arguments based on "quality of life" can easily become widened to include persons with physical or mental disabilities. Infants with severe deformities can sometimes be saved but not fully cured with medical technology, and some individuals would advocate nonvoluntary euthanasia in these cases because of the suffering of the infants" caregivers. Some believe that family members or those who stand to gain from the decision should not be allowed to make the decision. Others point out that the family is the most likely to know what the wishes of the patient would have been. Most believe that the medical care personnel, although knowledgeable, should not have the power to decide, and many are reluctant to institute rigid laws. The possibility of misappropriated self-interest from each of these parties magnifies the difficulty of arriving at well-defined criteria.

The second type of classification is between passive and active euthanasia. Passive euthanasia occurs when sustaining medical treatment is refused or withdrawn and death is allowed to take its course. Active euthanasia involves the administration of a drug or some other means that directly causes death. Once again, there are many opinions surrounding these two types. One position is that there is no difference between active and passive euthanasia because in each the end is premeditated death with the motive of prevention of suffering. In fact, some argue that active euthanasia is more compassionate than letting death occur naturally, which may involve suffering. In opposition, others believe that there is a fundamental difference between active and passive euthanasia. A person may have the right to die, but not the right to be killed. Passive euthanasia, they argue, is merely allowing a death that is inevitable to occur. Active euthanasia, if voluntary, is equated with suicide because a human being seizes control of death; if nonvoluntary, it is considered murder.

Passive euthanasia, although generally more publicly acceptable than active euthanasia, has become a topic of controversy as the types of medical treatment that can be withdrawn are debated. A distinction is sometimes made between ordinary and extraordinary means. Defining these terms is difficult, since what may be extraordinary for one patient is not for another, depending on other medical conditions that the patient may have. In addition, what is considered an extraordinary technique today may be judged ordinary in the future. Another way to assess whether passive euthanasia should be allowed in a particular situation is to weigh the benefits against the burdens for the patient. Although most agree that there are cases in which high-tech equipment such as respirators can be withdrawn, there is a question about whether administration of food and water should ever be discontinued. Here the line between passive and active euthanasia is blurred.

Religious and Legal Implications

Decisions about death concern everyone because everyone will die. Eventually, each individual will be the patient who is making the decisions or for whom the decisions are being made. In the meantime, one may be called upon to make decisions for others. Even those not directly involved in the hard cases are affected, as taxpayers and subscribers to medical insurance, by the decisions made on the behalf of others. In a difficult moral issue such as this, individuals look to different institutions for guidelines. Two sources of guidance are the church and the law.

In 1971, the Roman Catholic Church issued *Ethical and Religious Directives for Catholic Health Facilities*. Included in this directive is the statement that

> *[I]t is not euthanasia to give a dying person sedatives and analgesics for alleviation of pain, when such a measure is judged necessary, even though they may deprive the patient of the use of reason or shorten his life.*

This thinking was reaffirmed by a 1980 statement from the Vatican that considers suffering and expense for the family legitimate reasons to withdraw medical treatment when death is imminent. Bishops from The Netherlands, in a letter to a government commission, state that

> *[B]odily deterioration alone does not have to be unworthy of a man. History shows how many people, beaten, tortured and broken in body, sometimes even grew in personality in spite of it. Dying becomes unworthy of a man, if family and friends begin to look upon the dying person as a burden, withdraw themselves from him....*

When speaking of passive euthanasia, the bishops state, "We see no reason to call this euthanasia. Such a person after all dies of his own illness. His death is neither intended nor caused, only nothing is done anymore to postpone it." Christians from Protestant churches may reflect a wider spectrum of positions. Joseph Fletcher, an Episcopal priest, defines a person as one having the ability to think and reason. If a patient does not meet these criteria, according to Fletcher, his or her life may be ended out of compassion for the person he or she once was. The United Church of Christ illustrates this view in its policy statement:

> *When illness takes away those abilities we associate with full personhood...we may well feel that the mere continuance of the body by machine or drugs is a violation of their person.... We do not believe simply the continuance of mere physical existence is either morally defensible or socially desirable or is God's will.*

These varied positions generally are derived from differing emphases on two truths concerning the nature of God and the role of suffering in the life of the believer. First is the belief that God is the giver of life and that human beings should not usurp God's authority in matters of life and death. Second, alleviation of suffering is of critical importance to God, since it is not loving one's neighbor to allow him or her to suffer. Those who give more weight to the first statement believe as well that God's will allows for suffering and that the suffering can be used for a good purpose in the life of the believer. Those who emphasize the second principle insist that a loving God would not prolong the suffering of people needlessly and that one should not desperately fight to prolong a life which God has willed to die.

C. Everett Koop, former surgeon general of the United States, differentiates between the positive role of a physician in providing a patient "all the life to which he or she is entitled" and the negative role of "prolonging the act of dying." Koop has opposed euthanasia in any form, cautioning against the possibility of sliding down a slippery slope toward making choices about death that reflect the caregivers" "quality of life" more than the patient's.

Jack Kevorkian, a Michigan physician, became the best-known advocate of assisted suicide in the United States. From 1990 to 1997, Kevorkian assisted at least sixty-six people in terminating their lives. According to Kevorkian's lawyer, many other assisted suicides have not been publicized. Kevorkian believes that physician-assisted suicide is a matter of individual choice and should be seen as a rational way to end tremendous pain and suffering. Most of the patients assisted by him spent many years suffering from extremely painful and debilitating diseases, such as multiple sclerosis, bone cancer, and brain cancer.

The American Medical Association (AMA) has criticized this view, calling it a violation of professional ethics. When faced with pain and suffering, the AMA asserts that it is a doctor's responsibility to provide adequate "comfort" care, not death. In the AMA's view, Kevorkian served as "a reckless instrument of death." Three trials in Michigan for assisting in suicide resulted in acquittals for Kevorkian before another trial delivered a guilty verdict on the charge of second-degree murder in March, 1999.

During the course of reevaluating the issues involved in terminating a life, the law has been in a state of flux. The decisions that are made by the courts act on the legal precedents of an individual's right to determine what is done to his or her own body and society's position against suicide. The balancing of these two premises has been handled legally by allowing refusal of treatment (passive euthanasia) but disallowing the use of poison or some other method that would cause death (active euthanasia). The latter is labeled "suicide," and anyone who assists in such an act can be found guilty of assisting a suicide, or of murder. Following the Karen Ann Quinlan case in 1976, in which the family of a comatose woman secured permission to withdraw life-sustaining treatment, the courts routinely allowed family members to make decisions regarding life-sustaining treatment if the patient could not do so. The area of greatest legal controversy involves the withdrawal of food and water. Some courts have charged doctors with murder for the withdrawal of basic life support measures such as food and water. Others have ruled that invasive procedures to provide food and water (intravenously, for example) are similar to other medical procedures and may be discontinued if the benefit to the patient's quality of life is negligible.

In 1994, 51 percent of the voters in Oregon passed the world's first "death with dignity" law. It allowed physician-assisted suicide. Doctors could begin prescribing fatal overdoses of drugs to terminally ill patients. The vote was reaffirmed in 1997 by 60 percent of the state's voters, despite opposition from the Catholic Church, the AMA, and various anti-abortion and right-to-life groups. The Ninth United States Circuit Court of Appeals in San Francisco then lifted a lower court order blocking implementation of the law. Doctors in Oregon became free to prescribe fatal doses of barbiturates to patients with less than six months to live. Physicians were required to file forms with the Oregon Health Division before prescribing the overdose. Then, there would be a fifteen-day waiting period between the request for suicide assistance and the approval of the prescription. Opponents of the Oregon law charged that it perverted the practice of medicine and forced many suffering people to "choose" an early death to save themselves from expensive medical care or pain that could be manageable if physicians were aware of new methods of pain control. The National Right to Life Committee indicated that it would continue to fight implementation of the law in federal courts.

Since 1999, several states, including Hawaii, Connecticut, New Hampshire, Massachusetts, and Kansas, have witnessed attempts to legalize physician-assisted suicide, but the cases have either been withdrawn or defeated by voters or in state legislature. In November 2008, Washington state passed its own death with dignity act by voter initiative, with 57.8 percent of votes cast in favor of the law. In May 2013, Vermont governor Peter Shumlin signed into law the Patient Choice and Control at End of Life Act, thereby legalizing physician-assisted suicide in the state.

Although the laws vary from state to state, most states allow residents to make their wishes known regarding terminal health care either by writing a living will or by choosing a durable power of attorney. A living will is a document in which one can state that some medical treatments should not be used in the event that one becomes incapacitated to the point where one cannot choose. Living wills allow the patient to decide in advance and protect health care providers from lawsuits. Which treatment options can be terminated and when this action can be put into effect may be limited in some states. Most states have a specific format that should be followed when drawing up a living will and require that the document be signed in the presence of two witnesses. Often, qualifying additions can be made by the individual that specify whether food and water may be withdrawn and whether the living will should go into effect only when death is imminent or also when a person has an incurable illness but death is not imminent. A copy of the living will should be given to the patient's physician and become a part of the patient's medical records. The preparation or execution of a living will cannot affect a person's life insurance coverage or the payment of benefits. Since the medical circumstances of one's life may change and a person's ethical stance may also change, a patient may change the living will at any time by signing a written statement.

A second way in which a person can control what kind of decisions will be made regarding his or her death is to choose a decision maker in advance. This person assumes a durable power of attorney and is legally allowed to act on the patient's behalf, making medical treatment decisions. One advantage of a durable power of attorney over a living will is that the patient can choose someone who shares similar ethical and religious values. Since it is difficult to foresee every medical situation that could arise, there is more security with a durable power of attorney in knowing that the person will have similar values and will therefore probably make the same judgments as the patient. Usually a primary agent and a secondary agent are designated in the event that the primary agent is unavailable. This is especially important if the primary agent is a spouse or a close relative who could, for example, be involved in an accident at the same time as the patient.

Perspective and Prospects

Although large numbers of court decision, articles, and books suggest that the issues involved in euthanasia are recent products of medical technology, these questions are not new. Euthanasia was widely practiced in Western classical culture. The Greeks did not believe that all humans had the right to live, and in Athens, infants with disabilities were often killed.

Although in general they did not condone suicide, Pythagoras, Plato, and Aristotle believed that a person could choose to die earlier in the face of an incurable disease and that others could help that person to die. Seneca, the Roman Stoic philosopher, was an avid proponent of euthanasia, stating that

> Against all the injuries of life, I have the refuge of death. If I can choose between a death of torture and one that is simple and easy, why should I not select the latter? As I choose the ship in which I sail and the house which I shall inhabit, so I will choose the death by which I leave life.

The famous Hippocratic oath for physicians acted in opposition to the prevailing cultural bias in favor of euthanasia. Contained in this oath is the statement, "I will never give a deadly drug to anybody if asked for it...or make a suggestion to this effect." The AMA has reaffirmed this position in a policy statement:

> the intentional termination of the life of one human being by another—"mercy killing"—is contrary to that for which the medical profession stands and is contrary to the policy of the American Medical Association.

The great English poet John Donne, in his *Devotions Upon Emergent Occasions*, wrote extensively on the concept of suffering in the severely ill. He wrote, "Affliction is a treasure, and scarce any man hath enough of it." In addition, Jewish and Christian theology have traditionally opposed any form of euthanasia or suicide, avowing that since God is the author of life and death, life is sacred. Therefore, a man would rebel against God if he prematurely shortens his life, because he violates the Sixth Commandment: "Thou shalt not kill." Suffering was viewed not as an evil to be avoided but as a condition to be accepted. The apostle Paul served as an example for early Christians. In 2 Corinthians, he prayed for physical healing, yet when it did not come, he accepted his weakness as a way to increase his dependence on God. This position was affirmed by Saint Augustine in his work *De Civitate Dei* (413-426; *The City of God*) when he condemned suicide as a "detestable and damnable wickedness" that was worse than murder because it left no room for repentance. These strong indictments from the Church against suicide and euthanasia were largely responsible for changing the Greco-Roman attitudes toward the value of human life. They were accepted as society's position until the advent of technologies in the late twentieth century that made it possible to extend life beyond what would have been the point of death.

Although these issues have been debated by physicians and philosophers for centuries, there remains a heightened need for thoughtful discussion and resolution. The majority of nations, as well as major medical organizations such as the AMA, oppose euthanasia as contrary to the proper role of the physician and society. However, closely related and complex issues such as the treatment of pain in the terminally ill leave much room for development in human understanding.

—*Katherine B. Frederich, Ph.D.;*
updated by Leslie V. Tischauser, Ph.D.

See also Aging: Extended care; Critical care; Critical care, pediatric; Death and dying; Ethics; Hippocratic oath; Hospice; Law and medicine; Living will; Pain management; Palliative medicine; Psychiatry; Psychiatry, geriatric; Suicide; Terminally ill: Extended care.

For Further Information:
Corr, Charles A., Clyde M. Nabe, and Donna M. Corr. *Death and Dying, Life and Living*. 7th ed. Belmont, Calif.: Wadsworth/Cengage Learning, 2013.
Dowbiggin, Ian Robert. *A Merciful End: The Euthanasia Movement in Modern America*. New York: Oxford University Press, 2003.
Fenigsen, Richard. "Other People's Lives: Reflections on Medicine, Ethics, and Euthanasia. Part Two: Medicine versus Euthanasia." *Issues in Law & Medicine* 28, 1 (2012): 71–87.
Gorovitz, Samuel. *Drawing the Line: Life, Death, and Ethical Choices in an American Hospital*. Philadelphia: Temple University Press, 1993.
Harron, Frank, John Burnside, and Tom Beauchamp. *Health and Human Values*. New Haven, Conn.: Yale University Press, 1983.
Leone, Daniel A. *The Ethics of Euthanasia*. San Diego, Calif.: Greenhaven Press, 1998.
Magnusson, Roger, and Peter H. Ballis. *Angels of Death: Exploring the Euthanasia Underground*. New Haven, Conn.: Yale University Press, 2002. Print.
Rebman, Renée C. *Euthanasia and the Right to Die: Pro/Con Issues*. Berkeley Heights, N.J.: Enslow, 2002.
Sharp, Robert. "The Dangers of Euthanasia and Dementia: How Kantian Thinking Might Be Used to Support Non-Voluntary Euthanasia in Cases of Extreme Dementia." *Bioethics* 26, 5 (June, 2012): 231–235.
Spring, Beth, and Ed Larson. *Euthanasia*. Portland, Oreg.: Multnomah Press, 1988.
Torr, James D. *Euthanasia: Opposing Viewpoints*. San Diego, Calif.: Greenhaven Press, 2000.
Wennberg, Robert N. *Terminal Choices: Euthanasia, Suicide, and the Right to Die*. Grand Rapids, Mich.: Wm. B. Eerdmans, 1989. oxy_options track_changes="on"?

EWING'S SARCOMA
Disease/Disorder
Also known as: Bone cancer
Anatomy or system affected: Bones, musculoskeletal system
Specialties and related fields: Oncology, orthopedics, pediatrics, radiology
Definition: A rare bone cancer involving any part of the skeleton but found commonly in the long bones (60 percent), the pelvis (18 percent), and the ribs (15 percent) of children and young adults.

Causes and Symptoms

The specific cause of Ewing's sarcoma is unknown, but it may be associated with recurrent trauma, metal implants, congenital anomalies, unrelated tumors, or exposure to ionizing radiation. Approximately 90 percent of patients are between five and twenty-five years of age; rarely are patients younger than five or older than forty.

The initial symptom is pain, discontinuous at first and then intense, in the long bones, vertebra, or pelvis. Swelling may follow. Neurological signs involving the nerve roots or spinal cord depression are characteristic of nearly one-half of patients with involvement of the axial skeleton. Weight loss may occur, with remittent fever and mild anemia.

Information on Ewing's Sarcoma

Causes: Unknown; possibly related to recurrent trauma, metal implants, congenital anomalies, unrelated tumors, exposure to ionizing radiation
Symptoms: Pain in long bones, vertebra, or pelvis; swelling; neurological disorders; weight loss; fever; mild anemia
Duration: Long-term
Treatments: Surgery, chemotherapy, radiation

The phases of Ewing's sarcoma are based on degree of metastasis: the local phase (a nonmetastatic tumor), the regional phase (lymph node involvement), and the distant phase (involvement of the lungs, bones, and sometimes the central nervous system).

Treatment and Therapy

Patients are of two types, those with localized tumors and those with metastasized tumors. Depending on where the tumor is located, the treatment of Ewing's sarcoma is complex in all stages of disease and requires a multidisciplinary perspective. It is best treated when diagnosed early. Obtaining a bone biopsy is recommended in nearly all cases.

Surgery may be used to remove a tumor, followed by chemotherapy administered to kill any remaining cancer cells. Radiation may be prescribed to kill cancer cells and shrink tumors.

Perspective and Prospects

Ewing's sarcoma is one of the most malignant of all tumors. It may be localized or metastasize to the lungs and other bones. The primary tumor can be controlled by irradiation, but the prognosis is poor. Often, amputation is not justifiable. Recent developments in multiagent chemotherapy, however, are encouraging. Long-term survival of patients with Ewing's sarcoma is 50 to 70 percent or more with localized disease; the rate drops to less than 30 percent for metastatic disease.

—*John Alan Ross, Ph.D.*

See also Bone cancer; Bone disorders; Bones and the skeleton; Cancer; Orthopedics, pediatric.

For Further Information:
"Bone Cancer." *MedlinePlus*, Apr. 10, 2013.
Cady, Blake, ed. *Cancer Manual*. 8th ed. Boston: American Cancer Society, 1990.
Dollinger, Malin, et al. *Everyone's Guide to Cancer Therapy*. Rev. 5th ed. Kansas City, Mo.: Andrews McMeel, 2008.
Dorfman, Howard D., and Bogdan Czerniak. *Bone Tumors*. St. Louis, Mo.: Mosby, 1998.
Dugdale, David C. III, and David Zieve. "Ewing's Sarcoma." *MedlinePlus*, Mar. 14, 2012.
"Ewing Family of Tumors." *American Cancer Society*, Jan. 18, 2013.
Eyre, Harmon J., Dianne Partie Lange, and Lois B. Morris. *Informed Decisions: The Complete Book of Cancer Diagnosis, Treatment, and Recovery*. 2d ed. Atlanta: American Cancer Society, 2002.
Grealy, Lucy. *Autobiography of a Face*. New York: Perennial, 2003.
Holleb, Arthur I., ed. *The American Cancer Society Cancer Book: Prevention, Detection, Diagnosis, Treatment, Rehabilitation,*

Cure. Garden City, N.Y.: Doubleday, 1986.
Janes-Hodder, Honna, and Nancy Keene. *Childhood Cancer: A Parent's Guide to Solid Tumor Cancers*. 2d ed. Cambridge, Mass.: O'Reilly, 2002.
Kohnle, Diana, Patricia G. Kellicker, and Igor Puzanov. "Ewing's Sarcoma." *Health Library*, Sept. 12, 2012.
Kohnle, Diana, et al. "Ewing's Sarcoma—Child." *Health Library*, June 6, 2012.
Morra, Marion, and Eve Potts. *Choices: Realistic Alternatives in Cancer Treatment*. Rev. ed. New York: Viking, 1987.

EXERCISE PHYSIOLOGY

Specialty

Anatomy or system affected: Circulatory system, heart, joints, knees, lungs, muscles, musculoskeletal system, respiratory system, tendons
Specialties and related fields: Cardiology, family medicine, nutrition, physical therapy, preventive medicine, sports medicine
Definition: The science that studies the effects on the body of various intensities and types of physical activity, including cellular metabolism, cardiovascular responses, respiratory responses, neural and hormonal adaptations, and muscular adaptations to exercise.

Key terms:

adenosine triphosphate (ATP): a high-energy compound found in the cell which provides energy for all bodily functions

aerobic: metabolism involving the breakdown of energy substrates using oxygen

anaerobic: metabolism involving the breakdown of energy substrates without using oxygen

electrocardiogram (ECG): a graphic record of electrical currents of the heart

glycogen: the form that glucose takes when it is stored in the muscles and liver

heart rate: the number of times the heart contracts, or beats, per minute

maximal oxygen uptake: the maximum rate of oxygen consumption during exercise

metabolic equivalent (MET): a unit used to estimate the metabolic cost of physical activity; 1 MET is equal to 3.5 milliliters of oxygen consumed per kilogram of body weight per minute

Science and Profession

The primary aim of research in the field of exercise physiology is to gain a better understanding of the quantity and type of exercise needed for health maintenance and rehabilitation. A major goal of professionals in exercise physiology is to find ways to incorporate appropriate levels of physical activity into the lifestyles of all individuals.

Physiology is the science of the physical and chemical factors and processes involved in the function of living organisms. The study of exercise physiology examines these factors and processes as they relate to physical exertion. The physical responses that occur are specific to the intensity, duration, and type of exercise performed.

Exercise of low or moderate intensity relies on oxygen to

The Effects of Exercise on the Body

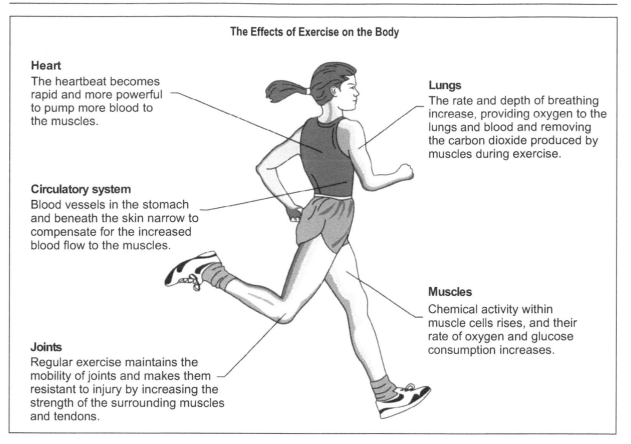

Heart
The heartbeat becomes rapid and more powerful to pump more blood to the muscles.

Circulatory system
Blood vessels in the stomach and beneath the skin narrow to compensate for the increased blood flow to the muscles.

Joints
Regular exercise maintains the mobility of joints and makes them resistant to injury by increasing the strength of the surrounding muscles and tendons.

Lungs
The rate and depth of breathing increase, providing oxygen to the lungs and blood and removing the carbon dioxide produced by muscles during exercise.

Muscles
Chemical activity within muscle cells rises, and their rate of oxygen and glucose consumption increases.

release energy for work. This process is often referred to as aerobic exercise. In the muscles, carbohydrates and fats are broken down to produce adenosine triphosphate (ATP), the basic molecule used for energy. Aerobic exercise can be sustained for several minutes to several hours.

Higher-intensity exercise is predominantly fueled anaerobically (in the absence of oxygen) and can be sustained for up to two minutes only. Muscle glycogen is broken down without oxygen to produce ATP. Anaerobic metabolism is much less efficient at producing ATP than is aerobic metabolism.

During anaerobic metabolism, a by-product called lactic acid begins to accumulate in the blood as blood lactate. The point at which this accumulation begins is called the anaerobic threshold (AT), or the onset of blood lactate accumulation (OBLA). Blood lactate can cause muscle soreness and stiffness, but it also can be used as fuel during aerobic metabolism.

A third and less often used energy system is the creatine phosphate (ATP-CP) system. Using the very limited supply of ATP that is stored in the muscles, phosphate molecules are exchanged between ATP and CP to provide energy. This system provides only enough fuel for a few seconds of maximum effort.

The type of muscle fiber recruited to perform a specific type of exercise is also dependent on exercise intensity. Skeletal muscle is composed of "slow-twitch" and two types of "fast-twitch" muscle fibers. Slow-twitch fibers are more

suited to using oxygen than are fast-twitch fibers, and they are recruited primarily for aerobic exercise. One type of fast-twitch fiber also functions during aerobic activity. The second type of fast-twitch fiber serves to facilitate anaerobic, or high-intensity, exercise.

Exercise mode is also a factor in people's physiological responses to exercise. Dynamic exercise (alternating muscular contraction and relaxation through a range of motion) using many large muscles requires more oxygen than does activity using smaller and fewer muscles. The greater the oxygen requirement of the physical activity, the greater the cardiorespiratory benefits.

Many bodily adaptations occur over a training period of six to eight weeks, and other benefits are gradually manifested over several months. The positive adaptations include reduced resting and working heart rates. As the heart becomes stronger, there is a subsequent increase in stroke volume (the volume of blood the heart pumps with each beat), which allows the heart to beat less frequently while maintaining the same cardiac output (the volume of the blood pumped from the heart each minute). Another beneficial adaptation is increased metabolic efficiency. This is partially facilitated by an increase in the number of mitochondria (the organelles responsible for ATP production) in the muscle cells.

One of the most recognized representations of aerobic fitness is the maximum volume of oxygen (VO_{2max}) an individual can use during exercise. VO_{2max} is improved through habitual, relatively high-intensity aerobic activity. After three to six months of regular training, levels of high-density lipoproteins (HDLs) in the blood increase. HDL molecules remove cholesterol (a fatty substance) from the tissues to aid in protecting the heart from atherosclerosis.

Various internal and external factors influence the metabolic processes that take place during and after exercise. Internally, nutrition, degree of hydration, body composition, flexibility, sex, and age are some of the variables that play a role in the physiological responses. Other internal variables include medical conditions such as heart disease, diabetes, and hypertension (high blood pressure). Externally, environmental conditions such as temperature, humidity, and altitude alter how the exercising body functions.

Various modes of exercise testing and data collection are used to study the physiological responses of the body to exercise. Treadmills and cycle ergometers (instruments that measure work and power output) are among the most common methods of evaluating maximum oxygen consumption. During these tests, special equipment and computers analyze expired air, heart rate is monitored with an electrocardiograph (ECG), and blood pressure is taken using a sphygmomanometer. Blood and muscle-fiber samples can also be extracted to aid in identifying the fuel system and type of muscle fibers being used. Other data sometimes collected, such as skin temperature and body-core temperature, can provide pertinent information.

Metabolic equivalent units, or METs, are often used to translate a person's capability into workloads on various pieces of exercise equipment or into everyday tasks. For every 3.5 milliliters of oxygen consumed per kilogram of body weight per minute, the subject is said to be performing at a workload of one MET. One MET is approximately equivalent to 1.5 kilocalories per minute, or the amount of energy expended per kilogram of body weight in one minute when a person is at rest.

Another factor greatly affecting the physical response to exercise is body composition. The three major structural components of the body are muscle, bone, and fat. Body composition can be evaluated using a combination of anthropometric measurements. These measurements include body weight, standard height, measurements of circumferences at various locations using a tape measure, measurements of skeletal diameters using a sliding metric stick, and measurements of skinfold thicknesses using calipers.

Body fat can be estimated using several methods, the most accurate of which is based on a calculation of body density. This method, called hydrostatic weighing, involves weighing the subject under water while taking into account the residual volume of air in the lungs. The principle underlying this measurement of body density is based on the fact that fat is less dense than water and thus will float, whereas bone and muscle, which are denser than water, will sink. One biochemical technique often used to determine levels of body fat is based on the relatively constant level of potassium-40 naturally existing in lean body mass. Another method uses ultrasound

waves to measure the thickness of fat layers. X-rays and computed tomography (CT) scanning can be used to provide images from which fat and bone can be measured. Bioelectrical impedance (BIA) is a method of estimating body composition based on the resistance imposed on a low-voltage electrical current sent through the body. The most widely used and easily assessable method, however, involves measurement of skinfolds at various sites on the body using calipers. In all cases, mathematical formulas have been devised to interpret the collected data and provide the best estimate of an individual's body composition.

Other tests have been developed to determine muscular strength, muscular endurance, and flexibility. Muscular strength is often measured by performance of one maximal effort produced by a selected muscle group. Muscular endurance of a muscle or muscle group is often demonstrated by the length of time or number of repetitions a particular submaximal workload or skill can be performed.

Two major types of flexibility have been identified. One type consists of the ability to move a muscle group or joint through its full range of motion at low speeds or hold a part of the body still at the extent of its range of motion. This is called static flexibility, and it can be measured using a metric stick or a protractor-type instrument called a goniometer. Dynamic flexibility, the other major identified type of flexibility, is the flexibility through the full range of motion of a muscle group or joint at normal or high speeds. Measuring dynamic flexibility is much more difficult.

Overlapping the science of exercise physiology are the studies of biomechanics or kinesiology (sciences dealing with human movement) and nutrition. Only through an understanding of efficient body mechanics and proper nutrition can the physiological responses of the body to exercise be identified correctly.

Diagnostic and Treatment Techniques

Exercise prescription is the primary focus in the application of exercise physiology. General health maintenance, cardiac rehabilitation, and competitive athletics are three major areas of exercise prescription.

Before making recommendations for an exercise program, an exercise physiologist must evaluate the physical limitations of the exerciser. In a normal health-maintenance setting, often called a "wellness" program, a health-related questionnaire can reveal relevant information. Such a questionnaire should include questions about family medical history and the subject's history of heart trouble or chest pain, bone or joint problems, and high blood pressure. The presence of any of these problems suggests the need for a physician's consent prior to exercising. After the individual has been deemed eligible to participate, an assessment of the level of physical fitness should be performed. Determining or estimating VO_{2max}, muscular strength, muscular endurance, flexibility, and body composition is usually part of this assessment. It is then possible to design a program best suited to the needs of the individual.

For the healthy adult participant, the American College of

Sports Medicine (ACSM), a widely recognized authoritative body on exercise prescription, recommends three to five sessions of aerobic exercise weekly. Each session should include a five- to ten-minute warm-up period, twenty to sixty minutes of aerobic exercise at a predetermined exercise intensity, and a five- to ten-minute cool-down period.

To recommend an appropriate aerobic exercise intensity, the exercise physiologist must determine an individual's maximum heart rate. The best way to obtain this maximum heart rate is to administer a maximal exercise test. Such a test can be supervised by an exercise physiologist or an exercise-test technician; it is advisable, especially for the older participant, that a cardiologist also be in attendance. An ECG is monitored for irregularities as the subject walks, runs, cycles, or performs some dynamic exercise to exhaustion or until the onset of irregular symptoms or discomfort.

Exercise prescription using heart rate as a measure can be achieved by various methods. A direct correlation exists between exercise intensity, in terms of oxygen consumption, and heart rate. From data collected during a maximal exercise test, a target heart-rate range of 40 to 85 percent of functional capacity can be calculated. Another method used to determine an appropriate heart-rate range is based on the difference between an individual's resting heart rate and maximum heart rate, called the heart-rate reserve (HRR). Values representing 60 percent and 80 percent of the HRR are calculated and added to the resting heart rate, yielding the individual's target heart-rate range. A third method involves calculating 70 percent and 85 percent of the maximum heart rate. Although this method is less accurate than the other two methods, it is the simplest way to estimate a target heart-rate range.

Intensity of exercise can also be prescribed using METs. This method relies on the predetermined metabolic equivalents required to perform activities at various intensities. Activity levels reflecting 40 to 85 percent of functional capacity can be calculated.

The rating of perceived exertion (RPE) is another method of prescribing exercise intensity. Verbal responses by the participant describing how an exercise feels at various intensities are assigned to a numerical scale, which is then correlated to heart rate. Through practice, the participant learns to associate heart rate with the RPE, reducing the necessity of frequent pulse monitoring in the healthy individual.

Adequate physical fitness can be defined as the ability to perform daily tasks with enough reserve for emergency situations. All aspects of health-related fitness direct attention toward this goal. Aerobic exercise often provides some conditioning for muscular endurance, but muscular strength and flexibility need to be addressed separately.

The ACSM recommends resistance training using the "overload principle," which involves placing habitual stress on a system, causing it to adapt and respond. For this training, it is suggested that eight to twelve repetitions of eight to ten strengthening exercises of the major muscle groups be performed a minimum of two days per week.

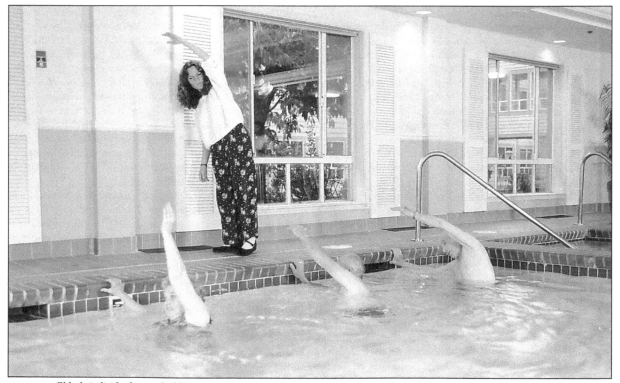

Elderly individuals may find low-impact exercise, such as swimming, to be a safer and easier way to stay fit. (PhotoDisc)

Flexibility of connective tissue and muscle tissue is essential to maximize physical performance and limit musculoskeletal injuries. At least one stretching exercise for each major muscle group should be executed three to four times per week while the muscles are warm. Three methods of stretching that have been designed to improve flexibility are ballistic stretching, static stretching, and proprioceptive neuromuscular facilitation (PNF). Ballistic stretching incorporates a bouncing motion and is generally prescribed only in sports that replicate this type of movement. During a static stretch, the muscles and connective tissue are passively stretched to their maximum lengths. PNF involves a contract-relax sequence of the muscle.

In addition to exercise prescription for cardiorespiratory fitness, muscular fitness, and flexibility, it is appropriate for the exercise physiologist to make recommendations concerning body composition. Exercise is an effective tool in fat loss. Dietary caloric restriction without exercise results in a greater loss of muscle mass along with fat than if exercise is part of a weight loss program.

For persons with special health concerns, such as diabetes mellitus or high blood pressure, the exercise physiologist works with the participant's physician. The physician prescribes necessary medications and often decides which modes of exercise are contraindicated (that is, should be avoided).

A second application, cardiac rehabilitation, takes exercise prescription a step further. Participation of a heart patient in cardiac rehabilitation is more individualized than in wellness programs. The conditions of the circulatory system, pulmonary system, and joints are only a few of the special concerns. Secondary conditions such as obesity, diabetes, and hypertension must also be considered. The responsibilities of cardiac-rehabilitation specialists include monitoring blood sugar in diabetic patients and blood pressure in all patients, especially those with hypertension. Many drugs affect heart rate or blood pressure, and most of these participants are taking more than one type of medication. Patients with heart damage caused by a heart attack may display atypical heart rhythms, which can be seen on an ECG monitor. Furthermore, the stage of recovery of the postsurgical patient is a major factor in recommending the type, frequency, intensity, and duration of exercise.

Patient education is also important. Lifestyle is usually the main factor in the development of heart disease. Cardiac patients often have never participated in a regular exercise program. They may smoke, be overweight, or have poor eating habits. Helping them to identify and correct destructive health-related behaviors is the focus of education for the heart patient.

A third application of the study of exercise physiology involves dealing with the competitive athlete. In this case, findings from the most recent research are constantly applied to yield the best athletic performance possible. A delicate balance of aerobic training, anaerobic training, strength training, endurance training, and flexibility exercises are combined with the optimum percentage of body fat, proper nutrition, and adequate sleep. The program that is designed must enhance the athletic qualities that are most beneficial to the sport in which the athlete participates.

The competitive athlete usually pushes beyond the boundaries of general exercise prescription in terms of intensity, duration, and frequency of exercise performance. As a result, the athlete risks suffering more injuries than the individual who exercises for health benefits. If the athlete sustains an injury, the exercise physiologist may work in conjunction with an athletic trainer or sports physician to return the athlete to competition as soon as possible.

Perspective and Prospects

The modern study of exercise physiology developed out of an interest in physical fitness. In the United States, the concern for development and maintenance of physical fitness was well established by the end of the twentieth century. As early as 1819, Stanford and Harvard Universities offered professional physical-education programs. At least one textbook on the physiology of exercise was published by that time.

Much of the pioneer work in this field, however, was done in Europe. Nobel Prize–winning European research on muscular exercise, oxygen utilization as it relates to the upper limits of physical performance, and production of lactic acid during glucose metabolism dates back to the 1920s.

In the early 1950s, poor performance by children in the United States on a minimal muscular fitness test helped lead to the formation of what became known as the President's Council on Physical Fitness and Sport. Concurrently, a significant number of deaths of middle-aged American males were found to be caused by poor health habits associated with coronary artery disease. A need for more research in the areas of health and physical activity was recognized by the mid-1960s. The subsequent research was facilitated by the existence of fifty-eight exercise physiology research laboratories in colleges and universities throughout the country. Organizations such as the American Physiological Society (APS), the American Alliance of Health, Physical Education, Recreation and Dance (AAHPERD), and the American College of Sports Medicine (ACSM) were established by the mid-1950s. In an effort to ensure that well-trained professionals were involved in cardiac-rehabilitation programs, the ACSM developed a certification program in 1975. Certifications for fitness personnel were added later.

Increasingly sophisticated testing equipment should lead to a better understanding of fundamental physiological mechanisms, allowing practitioners to be more effective in measuring physical fitness and prescribing exercise programs. Health maintenance has become a priority as the number of adults over the age of fifty continues to increase. Advances in medical techniques also increase the survival rate of victims of heart attacks, creating a need for more cardiac-rehabilitation programs and practitioners. Health-care professionals and the general population need to be made more aware of the benefits of exercise for the maintenance of good health and the rehabilitation of individuals with medical problems.

—Kathleen O'Boyle;
updated by Bradley R. A. Wilson, Ph.D.

See also Biofeedback; Bones and the skeleton; Braces, orthopedic; Cardiac rehabilitation; Cardiology; Electrocardiography (ECG or EKG); Ergogenic aids; Glycolysis; Heart; Hyperbaric oxygen therapy; Kinesiology; Lungs; Metabolism; Muscle sprains, spasms, and disorders; Muscles; Nutrition; Orthopedics; Orthopedics, pediatric; Overtraining syndrome; Oxygen therapy; Physical rehabilitation; Physiology; Preventive medicine; Pulmonary medicine; Respiration; Sports medicine; Steroid abuse; Sweating; Tendinitis; Vascular system.

For Further Information:

Brooks, George A., and Thomas D. Fahey. *Fundamentals of Human Performance*. New York: Macmillan, 1987.

Clarke, D. C., and P. F. Skiba. "Rationale and Resources for Teaching the Mathematical Modeling of Athletic Training and Performance." *Advances in Physiology Education* 37, no. 2 (June 2013): 134–152.

Issurin, Vladimir. "Training Transfer: Scientific Background and Insights for Practical Application." *Sports Medicine* 43, no. 8 (August 2013): 675–694.

McArdle, William, Frank I. Katch, and Victor L. Katch. *Exercise Physiology: Nutrition, Energy, and Human Performance*. 7th ed. Boston: Lippincott Williams & Wilkins, 2010.

Pescatello, Linda S., et al., eds. *ACSM's Guidelines for Exercise Testing and Prescription*. 9th ed. Philadelphia: Lippincott Williams & Wilkins, 2014.

Powers, Scott K., and Edward T. Howley. *Exercise Physiology: Theory and Application to Fitness and Performance*. 8th ed. New York: McGraw-Hill, 2012.

Swain, David P., et al., eds. *ACSM's Resource Manual for Guidelines for Exercise Testing and Prescription*. 7th ed. Baltimore: Lippincott Williams & Wilkins, 2014.

EXTENDED CARE FOR THE AGING. *See* AGING: EXTENDED CARE.

EXTENDED CARE FOR THE TERMINALLY ILL. *See* TERMINALLY ILL: EXTENDED CARE.

EXTREMITIES. *See* FEET; FOOT DISORDERS; LOWER EXTREMITIES; UPPER EXTREMITIES.

EYE INFECTIONS AND DISORDERS

Disease/Disorder

Anatomy or system affected: Blood vessels, brain, cells, eyes, glands, head, ligaments, muscles, nerves

Specialties and related fields: Bacteriology, cytology, general surgery, geriatrics and gerontology, histology, neurology, nursing, nutrition, ophthalmology, optometry, pathology, pediatrics, radiology, virology

Definition: Eye infections involve the invasion, multiplication, and colonization of microorganisms in the tissues of the eye. Eye disorders are derangement or abnormality of the functions of parts of the eye and the general impairment of function of the eye for precise and clear vision.

Key terms:

allergy: abnormal reaction or increased sensitivity to a foreign substance

infection: invasion and multiplication of microorganisms in body tissues

inflammation: localized protective response provoked by injury or destruction of tissues

laser: an extremely intense small beam producing immense heat

ocular: pertaining to the eye

ophthalmologist: a physician who specializes in diagnosing and treating eye diseases and disorders

sign: a doctor's objective evidence of disease or dysfunction

symptom: any indication of disease perceived by the patient

Causes and Symptoms

Several varieties of eye problems exist worldwide. Among the most important are corneal infections, ocular herpes, trachoma, conjunctivitis, iritis, cataracts, glaucoma, macular degeneration, diabetic retinopathy, styes, ptosis, ectropion, entropion, either watery or dry eyes, astigmatism, myopia, hyperopia, presbyopia, amblyopia, and keratoconus.

Many organisms can infect the eye. In corneal infections, bacteria, fungi, or viruses invade the cornea and cause painful inflammation and corneal infections called keratitis. Visual clarity is reduced, and the cornea produces a discharge or becomes destroyed, resulting in corneal scarring and vision impairment.

Ocular herpes is a recurrent viral infection by the herpes simplex virus. Symptoms are a painful sore on the eyelid or eye surface and inflammation of the cornea. More severe infection destroys stromal cells and causes stromal keratitis, cornea scarring, and vision loss or blindness. It is the most common infectious cause of corneal blindness in the United States.

Trachoma is a chronic and contagious bacterial disease of the conjunctiva and cornea. The eye becomes inflamed, painful, and teary. Small gritty particles develop on the cornea. Conjunctivitis is the inflammation of the conjunctiva caused by virus or bacteria infection, chemical irritations, physical factors, and allergic reactions. Inflammation of the cornea accompanies viral forms. The eyes become very sensitive to light. The infectious form is highly contagious, especially acute contagious conjunctivitis (pinkeye). Signs are red, extremely itching, and irritating eyes with a gritty feeling; tearing; nasal discharge; sinus congestion; swollen eyelids (in severe cases); and eyelids that may stick together from dry mucus formed during the night.

Iritis is inflammation of the iris. The cause is still under investigation, but it is associated with rheumatoid arthritis, diabetes mellitus, syphilis, diseased teeth, tonsillitis, trauma, and infections. Symptoms are red eyes, contracted and irregularly shaped pupil, extreme sensitivity to light, tender eyeball, and blurred vision.

A cataract is a clouding of the lens that causes a progressive, slow, and painless loss of vision. Symptoms are reduced night vision, blurriness, poor depth perception, color distortion, problems with glare, and frequent eyeglass prescription changes. Cataracts are the world's leading cause of blindness. Causes are under investigation, but it could result from eye injury, prolonged exposure to drugs such as corticosteroids or to X rays, inflammatory and infectious eye diseases, complications of diseases such as diabetes, prolonged exposure to direct sunlight, poor nutrition, and smoking. Babies can be born with congenital cataracts.

Glaucoma is an optic nerve disease caused by fluid pressure that builds up abnormally within the eye because of very slow fluid production and draining. This can damage the optic nerve, retina, or other parts of the eye and result in vision loss. Early stages have no symptoms. Side (peripheral) vision is lost at an advanced point when irreversible damage makes vision restoration impossible. Blindness results if the condition is left untreated.

In macular degeneration, often called age-related macular degeneration (AMD or ARMD), the light-sensing cells of the macula, which is responsible for sharp and clear central vision, degenerates. The result is a slow, painless loss of central vision necessary for important activities such as driving and reading. Early signs are shadowy areas in the central vision, or fuzzy, blurry, or distorted vision. About 90 percent of cases are "dry" AMD, without bleeding, and 10 percent cases a more severe "wet" type, in which new blood vessels grow and leak blood and fluid under the macula, causing the most vision loss.

Diabetic retinopathy is damage to the blood vessels of the retina caused by uncontrolled diabetes. Early signs may not be exhibited, but blurred vision, pain in the eye, floaters, and gradual vision loss are the symptoms in advanced cases.

A number of disorders can affect the eyelids. A stye, or hordeolum, is a painful localized swelling produced by infection or inflammation in a sweat gland of the eyelids or the sebaceous glands that secrete oil to stop the eyelids from sticking together. Ptosis is drooping of the upper eyelid that obstructs the upper field of vision for one or both eyes. It produces blurred vision, refractive errors, astigmatism, strabismus (in which the eyes are not properly aligned), or amblyopia (lazy eye). Symptoms include aching eyebrows, difficulty in keeping the eyelids open, eyestrain, and eye fatigue, especially during reading.

With an ectropion, the lower eyelid and eyelashes turn outward and sag, usually because of aging. Scarring of the eyelid caused by thermal and chemical burns, skin cancers, trauma, or previous eyelid surgery can also cause the problem. Symptoms are eye irritation, excessive tearing, mucus discharge, and crusting of the eyelid. With an entropion, the lower eyelid and eyelashes roll inward toward the eye and rub against the cornea and conjunctiva. This condition is also primarily the result of aging. Symptoms are irritation of the cornea, excessive tearing, mucus discharge, crusting of the eyelid, a feeling of something in the eye, and impaired vision. It can also be caused by allergic reactions, inflammatory diseases, and scarring of the inner surface of the eyelid caused by chemical and thermal burns.

Watery eyes are caused by the blockage of the lacrimal puncta (two small pores that drain tear secretions from lacrymal glands that bathe the conjunctival surfaces of the eye) or oversecretion of the lacrimal glands. Dry eyes result from inadequate tear production due to malfunction of the lacrymal (tear) glands, more common in women, especially after menopause. Symptoms are a scratchy or sandy feeling in the eye, pain and redness, excessive tearing following dry sensations, a stinging or burning feeling, discharge, heaviness of the eyelids, and blurred, changing, or decreased vision. Causes include dry air; the use of drugs such as tranquilizers, nasal decongestants, antidepressants, and antihistamines; connective tissue diseases such as rheumatoid arthritis; or the aging process.

Several refractive vision disorders are common. Astigmatism is blurred vision caused by a misshapen lens or cornea that makes light rays converge unevenly without focusing at any one point on the retina. In hyperopia (farsightedness), the eye can see distant objects normally but cannot focus at short distances because the eyeball is shorter than normal, causing the lens to focus images behind the retina. Presbyopia is farsightedness that develops with age. The lens gradually loses its ability to change shape and focus on nearby objects, creating difficulty in reading. In myopia (nearsightedness), the eye cannot focus properly on distant objects, although it can see well at short distances, because the eyeball is longer than normal. The lens cannot flatten enough to compensate and focuses distant objects in front of, instead of on, the retina.

Amblyopia, commonly called lazy eye, is a neurologic disorder in which the brain favors vision in one eye. Misalignment of the eyes (strabismus) creates two different images for the brain. If the condition goes untreated, then the weaker eye ceases to function.

Keratoconus is the progressive thinning of the cornea, producing conical protrusion of the central part of the cornea. It results in astigmatism or myopia and swelling or scarring of cornea tissue that ultimately impairs sight. Its causes are heredity, eye injury, and systemic diseases.

Treatment and Therapy

The treatment of eye infections and disorders depends on their cause and severity. Minor corneal infections are treated with antibacterial eyedrops. Intensive antibiotic, antifungal, and steroid eyedrop treatments eliminate the infection and reduce inflammation in severe cases. With ocular herpes, prompt treatment with antiviral drugs stops the herpesvirus from multiplying and destroying epithelial cells. The resulting stromal keratitis, however, is more severe and therefore difficult to treat. The primary treatment for trachoma consists of three to four weeks of antibiotic therapy. Severe cases require surgical correction.

A conjunctivitis infection can clear without medical care, but sometimes treatment is necessary to avoid long-term effects of corneal inflammation and loss of vision. Treatment includes antibiotic eyedrops or ointments, antihistamine eyedrops or pills, decongestants, nonsteroidal anti-inflammatory drugs (NSAIDs), or mast-cell stabilizers. Artificial tears and warm compresses offer some relief. Tinted glasses reduce the discomfort of bright light.

With iritis, warm compresses can lessen the inflammation and pain. Certain steroid drugs produce quick reduction of the inflammation. A protective covering enables the eye to rest, and atropine drops could be used to dilate the pupils and prevent scarring or adhesions.

For cataracts, a stronger eyeglass prescription is recommended, but surgery that replaces the clouded lens with an artificial one is the only real cure. Drugs that keep the pupil dilated may help with vision.

Glaucoma detection is challenging because the disease is asymptomatic until it is advanced. Medical therapy is the first step for treatment. Glaucoma is difficult to cure, but some medications successfully lower pressure in the eye. If medication is ineffective, then laser surgery is applied to create openings and facilitate fluid draining in the eye.

One way to diagnose macular degeneration is by viewing a chart of black lines arranged in a graph pattern (Amsler grid). Early signs can be detected through retinal examination. No outright cure has been discovered, but some drug treatments may delay its progression or even improve vision.

Some cases of diabetic retinopathy can be treated with laser surgery that shrinks or seals leaking and abnormal vessels on the retina. Vision already lost cannot be restored. A vitrectomy is recommended for some advanced cases, in which the vitreous component of the eye is surgically removed and replaced with a clear solution.

In treating a stye, applying hot compresses for fifteen minutes every two hours may help localize the infection and promote drainage. Mild antiseptics may be applied to prevent spread of the infection. A small surgical incision may be necessary in some cases.

Surgery is the treatment for congenital ptosis. The procedure tightens the levator muscle to lift the upper eyelid to the required position, allowing a full field of vision. For

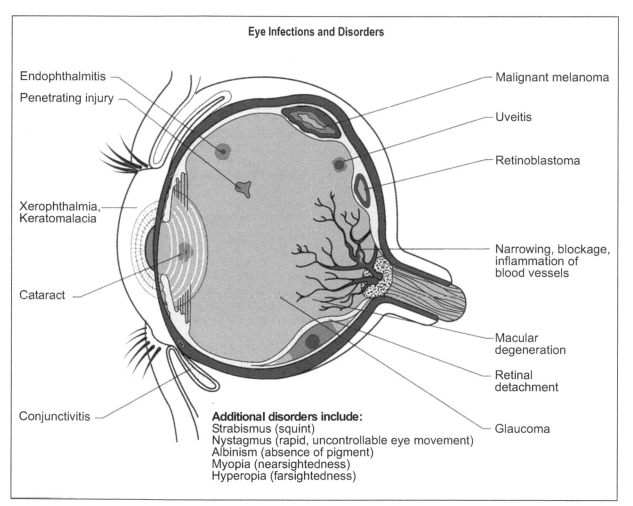

Eye Infections and Disorders

Endophthalmitis

Penetrating injury

Xerophthalmia, Keratomalacia

Cataract

Conjunctivitis

Malignant melanoma

Uveitis

Retinoblastoma

Narrowing, blockage, inflammation of blood vessels

Macular degeneration

Retinal detachment

Glaucoma

Additional disorders include:
Strabismus (squint)
Nystagmus (rapid, uncontrollable eye movement)
Albinism (absence of pigment)
Myopia (nearsightedness)
Hyperopia (farsightedness)

ectropion and entropion, surgery, under local anesthesia, is used to repair the abnormal eyelid before the cornea becomes infected and scarred. This is followed by an overnight patch and application of antibiotics for a week.

For dry eyes, lubricating artificial tears in the form of eyedrops are the usual answer. Serious cases of watery eyes may be treated by surgically closing the lacrimal puncta (tear drain) temporarily or permanently. Sterile ointments prevent the eye from drying at night.

Astigmatism is corrected with asymmetrical lenses that compensate for the asymmetry in the eye. Surgery and laser treatments are used to reshape the cornea and change its focusing power. Myopia is corrected by concave-shaped glasses or contact lenses that diverge light rays from distant objects to focus on the retina. Hyperopia and presbyopia are corrected with convex-shaped eyeglasses or contact lenses that converge light rays from nearby objects slightly before entering the eye, in order to focus on the retina. For those with amblyopia, a patch over the preferred eye forces the brain to use the other eye, but the drug atropine, which temporarily blurs vision in the preferred eye, offers a better medical alternative to eye patches.

For keratoconus, vision is corrected with eyeglasses initially, followed by special contact lenses that reduce distortion if astigmatism worsens. Corneal transplantation becomes necessary when scarring becomes too severe. Preventive measures in strong sunlight are protective eyeglasses, sunglasses, and hats with brims.

Perspective and Prospects

Ancient papyri indicate that physicians of Egypt were the first to establish clinical practices for the treatment of eye infections and disorders. Herbs and eye paints with bacteriocidal properties, such as malachite, were used to prevent infections. Medicated ointments were used by Arab and Greek physicians to treat trachoma. Leukoma (a white spot on the cornea) was treated with animal galls, especially the gall of tortoise. Antimony sulfite and copper solutions were used to treat eyelid disorders. Herbs have been used in Africa, Asia, and Latin America to treat eye problems since ancient times.

In the twenty-first century, improved antibiotics and other chemicals are widely used to treat eye diseases. Technological advances in surgical procedures and laser techniques have provided additional options for treating vision disorders. Cataract surgery that once required several days of hospitalization is performed in less than thirty minutes on an outpatient basis. Multifocal lenses are designed to provide both near and distant vision that eliminates the use of reading glasses, advanced lens technology provide more foldable and flexible lens materials, and doctors use lasers to reduce secondary opacification in lenses. Immunotherapy is used to treat allergies that cause conjunctivitis.

Innovative research provides new knowledge and treatments for eye disorders. The Collaborative Longitudinal Evaluation of Keratoconus Study by the National Eye Institute (NEI) is investigating factors that influence the progression and severity of keratoconus. The NEI supported the clinical trials of the Herpetic Eye Disease Study that investigated treatments for severe ocular herpes, the most common infectious cause of corneal blindness in the United States.

Research that explored ayurvedic herbs of India has produced the isotine eyedrop, which effectively treats different eye disorders without surgery, including early stages of cataracts.

Functional MRI (fMRI) techniques allow researchers to create images of neurological activity in real time and to obtain insight into neurological eye diseases such as amblyopia. Scientists are conducting research to obtain implanted lens material that is able to form a new lens within the eye and that works efficiently with the original eye muscles. Investigations are in progress for glaucoma medications that reduce eye pressure and also protect the optic nerve. Research shows that antioxidants and nutrients such as zeaxanthin and lutein (found in green, leafy vegetables), zinc, and vitamins A, C, and E help to control AMD, and omega-3 fatty acids (abundant in coldwater fish) have a protective and healing effect against AMD.

The Food and Drug Administration (FDA) approved Lucentis in 2006 for treating the more severe "wet" AMD by monthly injections into the eye. Macugen (pegaptanib sodium), another AMD treatment medication that improves vision with six-week interval injections, was FDA-approved in 2004. In 2006, it was reported that a team of international research scientists discovered a protein called sVEGFR-1 that prevents blood vessels from forming in the cornea; it could become the basis of new treatments for cancer and macular degeneration. In 2012, research published in the journal *Ophthalmology* indicated that monthly injections of ranibizumab into the center of the eye halts the progression of scarring and the leaking of blood vessels in "wet" AMD sufferers. Stem cell research is also advancing the potentional for cures for AMD and other eye diseases and disorders.

Also in 2006, the *HealthDay News* reported that a visual aid invented by U.S. scientists comprising a tiny camera, a pocket-sized computer, and a transparent computer display mounted on a pair of glasses provides better vision and mobility for people with tunnel vision, who have lost their peripheral vision. Such innovations are welcome, since one in two hundred Americans over age fifty-five has tunnel vision, which is caused by diseases such as retinitis pigmentosa and glaucoma.

Early detection of signs and symptoms is a primary key to the treatment of all eye infections and disorders. As preventive measures, people must avoid eyestrain, exercise their bodies, eat healthy foods, control their sugar levels and blood pressure, avoid smoking, protect the eyes from sunlight, and have regular medical checkups.

—*Samuel V. A. Kisseadoo, Ph.D.*

See also Albinos; Astigmatism; Blindness; Cataract surgery; Cataracts; Chlamydia; Color blindness; Conjunctivitis; Corneal transplantation; Diabetes mellitus; Dyslexia; Eye surgery; Eyes; Face lift and blepharoplasty; Glaucoma; Gonorrhea; Herpes; Jaundice; Keratitis; Laser use in surgery; Macular degeneration; Microscopy, slitlamp; Myopia; Ophthalmology; Optometry; Optometry, pediatric; Pigmentation; Ptosis; Refractive eye surgery; Sense organs; Sjögren's syndrome; Strabismus; Styes; Systems and organs; Trachoma; Transplantation; Vision; Vision disorders.

For Further Information:

Boron, Walter F., and Emile L. Boulpaep. *Medical Physiology: A Cellular and Molecular Approach*. Rev. 2d ed. Philadelphia: Saunders/Elsevier, 2012.

Jenkins, Gail W., Christopher P. Kemnitz, and Gerard J. Tortora. *Anatomy and Physiology: From Science to Life*. Hoboken, N.J.: John Wiley & Sons, 2009.

McKinley, Michael P., and Valerie D. O'Loughlin. *Human Anatomy*. 3d ed. Dubuque, Iowa: McGraw-Hill, 2012.

Marieb, Elaine N., Jon Mallatt, and Patricia Brady Wilhelm. *Human Anatomy*. 6th ed. San Francisco: Pearson/Benjamin Cummings, 2012.

Pollack, Andrew. "Stem Cell Treatment for Eye Diseases Shows Promise." *New York Times*, January 23, 2012.

Saladin, Kenneth S. *Human Anatomy*. 3d ed. Dubuque, Iowa: McGraw-Hill, 2011.

Samuel, Michael A. *Macular Degeneration: A Complete Guide for Patients and Their Families*. North Bergen, N.J.: Basic Health, 2013.

Sutton, Amy L. *Eye Care Sourcebook: Basic Consumer Health Information About Eye Care and Eye Disorders*. 3d ed. Detroit, Mich.: Omnigraphics, 2008.

Tortora, Gerard J., and Bryan Derrickson. *Principles of Anatomy and Physiology*. 13th ed. Hoboken, N.J.: John Wiley & Sons, 2012.

Traboulsi, Elias I. *A Compendium of Inherited Disorders and the Eye*. New York: Oxford University Press, 2006.

Van De Graaff, Kent M. *Human Anatomy*. 6th ed. New York: McGraw-Hill, 2002.

EYE SURGERY

Procedure

Anatomy or system affected: Eyes

Specialties and related fields: General surgery, geriatrics, ophthalmology, optometry

Definition: Surgical removals from or repairs to the eye.

Key terms:

choroid: the vascular, intermediate coat furnishing nourishment to parts of the eyeball

cornea: the clear, transparent portion of the eye's outer coat, forming the covering of the aqueous chamber

iris: a colored circular membrance suspended behind the cornea and in front of the lens, regulating the amount of light entering the eye by changing the size of the pupil

lens: the transparent biconvex body of the eye

retina: the innermost coat of the eye, formed from sensitive nerve elements and connected with the optic nerve

sclera: the white part of the eye; with the cornea, it forms the eye's external protective coat

trabeculae: the portion of the eye in front of the canal of Schlemm and within the angle created by the iris and cornea

Indications and Procedures

Compared to surgery performed on internal organs and any number of outpatient procedures, eye surgery can fill patients with added fears, often concerned with great suffering and the possibility of permanent sight loss. Surgery to an internal organ is usually perceived as happening in a remote location in an unseen portion of the body, and most patients have little idea of the organ's function. Often, if an internal growth or organ is removed, the body continues to function quite well. Most patients have some knowledge of the eye, unlike most internal organs, and thus are more likely to develop anxiety about even common surgical procedures involving it. Patients know what eyes are and what they are used for and that they are extremely sensitive and painful to touch. A grain of sand or a hair touching the eye is painful, so the thought of contacting the eye with a needle or making an incision in it with a scalpel or laser can be almost unimaginable. Patients with ocular problems requiring surgery fear damage to the eye and know all too well the consequences of removal. In most instances, the general public has little to no knowledge or understanding of the function and mechanics of eye surgery. Common eye surgeries include, but are not limited to, cataract surgery, corneal transplantation, vision correction, pterygium removal, retinal detachment repair, and tear duct surgery.

A cataract is an opacity on the eye's lens. A cataract may be minimal in size and low in density, so that light transmission is not appreciably affected, or it may be large and opaque so that light cannot gain entry into the interior eye. When the cataract is pronounced, the interior of the patient's eye cannot be seen with clarity, and the patient cannot see out clearly. Over time, the lens takes on a yellowish hue and begins to lose transparency. As the lens thus becomes "cloudy," the patient needs brighter and brighter lights for visual clarity. If the lens becomes completely opaque, then the patient is functionally blind. A cataract is removed when it endangers the health of the eye or interferes with a patient's ability to function. Conditions such as contrast sensitivity, glare, pupillary constriction, and ambient light may significantly affect a patient's functionality.

The objective of cataract surgery is to remove the crystalline lens of the eye that has become cloudy. Modern surgical procedures involve removing the lens, either intact or in pieces after shattering it with high-frequency sound. The surgery is usually performed under an operating microscope because magnification is necessary. Many methods are used for cataract surgery, including an extracapsular procedure, an intracapsular procedure, and phacoemulsification. Most surgeons perform cataract surgery in freestanding surgical centers on an outpatient basis.

In extracapsular surgery, an incision is made at the superior limbus and a small opening is made into the anterior chamber. A viscoelastic substance is introduced and then a small, bent needle, or cystotome, is introduced. An incision is made into the anterior capsule in a circular, triangular, or D-shaped fashion. The wound is enlarged to a diameter of 10 to 11 millimeters, allowing removal of the cataractous nucleus.

The most common cataract surgical procedure is phacoemulsification, or small-incision cataract surgery. A stair-stepped incision of between 1.5 and 4.0 millimeters is made in the front of the eye. A cystotome is inserted to cut the

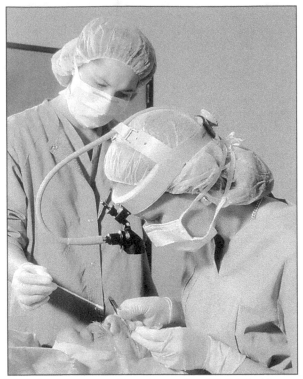

An eye surgeon performs an operation. (Digital Stock)

anterior capsule of the lens. An emulsifier and aspirator is inserted to remove the collapsed lens. The missing lens is then replaced by an artificial substitute that is folded and inserted through the incision and rotated into place. The wound is sealed with a single suture or no suture at all. This procedure has become favored because it causes less tissue destruction, less wound reaction, and less astigmatism, and patients can resume normal activities immediately after surgery. Vision is then fine-tuned with glasses or contact lenses, if needed.

Another common eye surgery is corneal transplantation. The cornea is the clear portion in the front part of that eye. When injured, degenerated, or infected, the cornea can become cloudy and vision disrupted. Corneal surgery restores lost vision by replacing a portion of the cornea with a clear window taken from a donor eye. Usually, the donor cornea is taken from a recently deceased person. However, not everyone with corneal disease can be helped by corneal transplantation.

The cornea was one of the first structures of the body to be transplanted. Because the cornea is devoid of blood vessels, it is one of the few tissues in the human body that may be transplanted from one human to another with a high degree of success. The absence of blood vessels in the donor cornea reduces immune system reactions.

Two types of corneal transplants are performed: partial penetration, in which a half thickness of the cornea is transplanted, and penetrating transplantation, which involves the full thickness of the cornea. In partial penetration, the anterior

of the eye is not entered; only the outer half or two-thirds of the cornea is transplanted. Union is made by several sutures around the periphery of the donor tissue. Depending on the extent of the disease, the donor tissue may be 6 to 10 millimeters in diameter. In a penetrating transplantation, surgery involves entering the anterior chamber of the eye, inserting the donor cornea, and establishing a tight fit with a continuous suture.

Glaucoma is an ocular disease affecting roughly 2 percent of the population over forty. The major characteristic of the condition is a sustained increase in intraocular pressure so great that the fibrous scleral coat cannot expand significantly and the eye cannot withstand the increasing pressures against surrounding soft tissue without damage to its structure and vision impairment. The results of this pressure increase include excavation of the optic disc, hardness of the eyeball, reduced vision, the appearance of colored halos around lights, visual field defects, and headaches. Surgical procedures are performed to relieve this pressure. Although many types of surgical procedures are performed to treat glaucoma, they are all basically fistulizing surgeries, attempting to create an opening between the anterior chamber and the subconjunctival space or between the surgically prepared layers of the sclera.

Glaucoma surgery involves a small incision made either directly through the cornea at the upper limbus or under a flap of conjunctival tissue. The iris is grasped with small forceps and pulled out of the eye, and a small portion of the trabecular meshwork is partially removed, allowing the aqueous fluid to filter out of the anterior chamber. The cornea is then sutured and the eye bandaged. The most popular procedure of this type is trabeculectomy. As a whole, glaucoma surgeries are performed less often today because of the success of nonsurgical treatments and management with drug therapies. A major consequence of some glaucoma surgery is the development of cataracts.

A common early stage nonincisive procedure in treating glaucoma is laser trabeculoplasty. This procedure involves lasing the middle to anterior portion of the trabecular meshwork with eighty to one hundred equally spaced burns. The argon laser reopens blocked drainage channels and reduces fluid pressure in the eye. More than 90 percent of patients experience successful outcomes from this treatment. Surgery is performed only if patients continue to lose the visual field.

A pterygium is a fibrovascular membrane that extends from the medial aspect of the bulbar conjunctiva and invades the cornea. It is a progressive growth related to overexposure to ultraviolet (UV) light. In time, it can make its way to the central portion of the cornea and interfere with vision. Pterygia are most common in southern climates, where people have greater exposure to UV light. In northern regions, people who work outdoors, especially in open fields or on open water, are most prone to developing a pterygium growth.

The purpose of removing a pterygium is to excise the membrane before it can interfere with vision. The operation requires incision into the cornea as well as the conjunctiva, then removal of the pterygium tissue or its transplantation to another position to redirect its growth.

In a normal eye, the retina lies against the choroidal layer, from which it receives part of its blood supply and nourishment. The retina is loosely attached to the choroid, but when it becomes separated from the choroid, it flaps and hangs within the eye's vitreous fluid. Retinal detachment does not allow adequate nutrients to reach the retina and thus causes poor function, and it eventually leads to vision loss. Retinal detachment may be caused by injury, myopia, or previous eye surgeries. Often, a tear or hole permits fluid to collect under the retina, causing the detachment.

Retinal detachment surgery corrects the loose retina by bringing it back to the choroid or by pushing the choroid up to the retina. To bring the retina back into place, scleral punctures are made to drain fluids that lay between the retina and the choroid. When the retina returns to lie against the choroid, either electrocoagulation or cryotherapy with a cold probe against the sclera unites the retina to the choroid. Then the retina and choroid are brought together with a silicone buckling band to exert inward pressure. If the retina is not attached at this point, then air, special gas, or oil is injected into the vitreous fluid to push the retina back against the choroid.

Surgery involving corrective procedures to tear ducts is common, especially in older patients. A blockage in the nasolacrimal passage may result in a condition called epiphora, in which the tear ducts water constantly. Such a blockage of the tear canal may result from some form of obstruction. These obstructions are cleared by a surgical procedure called dacryocystorhinostomy. In this procedure, a large incision of 8 to 10 millimeters is made in the wall of the nose, and a union is created between the mucosal lining of the nose and the lacrimal sac. In this way, the lacrimal sac opens directly into the nose. The operation is usually successful in curing the tearing and infection problems arising from stagnation in the blocked tear duct.

Elective refractive eye surgery for the purpose of vision correction began in the Soviet Union in the 1970s and gained popularity in the United States in the 1990s with the use of lasers. It is performed for the relief of myopia, hypermyopia, and astigmatism, with the goal of eliminating the need for either eyeglasses or contact lenses. It is also used to correct refractive errors caused by cataract surgery and corneal transplantation.

Two of the most common refractive surgeries are radial keratotomy (RK) and photorefractive keratectomy (PRK), also known as excimer laser surgery. Myopic patients suffer from a cornea that is either too convex or has an axial length that is too long, causing light to converge at a focal point anterior to the retina. In refractive surgery, corneal reshaping is the important concept. The surgical goal is to flatten the center of the cornea so that light will focus more posteriorly.

RK reshapes the cornea by radial incisions made with a diamond knife. This process weakens the cornea, so normal intraocular pressure pushes the center of the cornea outward, flattening the central cornea. PRK uses a laser to remove the superficial layers of the central cornea, about 50 to 100 microns of tissue, to achieve a similar reshaping of the cornea.

Uses and Complications

The introduction of lasers to eye surgery has proved both beneficial and controversial, depending on its use. An excimer laser can remove any opacifications of the superficial layers of the cornea while retaining the health and clarity of deeper corneal layers. The laser can be used to remove injury-related and surgical corneal scars and to treat astigmatism that may follow implant cataract surgery. The excimer laser also enables surgeons to treat diseases such as fungal ulcers and to smoothe out pterygium irregularities.

Patients interested in pursuing elective refractive surgeries, however, should be aware of the inherent risks of the procedures and that some ophthalmologists are hesitant to use these procedures to correct nearsightedness. The leading cause of skepticism is a reluctance to operate on an essentially healthy eye, thus putting it at risk. These operative procedures have been developed to correct only refractive vision errors. Refractive surgery does not treat glaucoma, cataracts, or other disorders that affect or damage vision.

Perspective and Prospects

As experience and long-term results from the use of laser energy as a surgical tool increase, other forms of therapy will be investigated. Noninvasive glaucoma procedures and laser disruptions of vitreous opacities and retinal traction bands are already being performed. Ablation procedures to control late-stage glaucoma and techniques to emulsify and remove cataract lenses with lasers in a noninvasive procedure have undergone positive trials.

Today, lasers share space in many clinics and operating rooms along with traditional surgical techniques. Laser technology is providing new types of therapy and is treating more challenging forms of eye disease.

—*Randall L. Milstein, Ph.D.*

See also Blindness; Blurred vision; Cataract surgery; Cataracts; Corneal transplantation; Eye infections and disorders; Eyes; Glaucoma; Keratitis; Laser use in surgery; Myopia; Ophthalmology; Optometry; Refractive eye surgery; Sense organs; Surgery, general; Vision; Vision disorders.

For Further Information:

Bartlett, Jimmy D., and Siret D. Jaanus, eds. *Clinical Ocular Pharmacology.* 5th ed. Boston: Butterworth-Heinemann/Elsevier, 2008.

Berman, Eric L. "Retinal Detachment Repair." *Health Library*, Feb. 28, 2012.

Cheyer, Christopher. "Cataract Removal." *Health Library*, Feb. 28, 2012.

Cheyer, Christopher. "Glaucoma Surgery." *Health Library*, Feb. 28, 2012.

Eden, John. *The Physician's Guide to Cataracts, Glaucoma, and Other Eye Problems.* Yonkers, N.Y.: Consumer Reports Books, 1992.

Johnson, Gordon J., et al., eds. *The Epidemiology of Eye Disease.* 3d ed. New York: Oxford University Press, 2012.

"Laser Eye Surgery." *MedlinePlus*, Dec. 27, 2012.

Lusby, Franklin W., et al. "Pterygium." *MedlinePlus*, Nov. 20, 2012.

Newell, F. W. *Ophthalmology: Principles and Concepts.* 8th ed. St. Louis, Mo.: Mosby, 1996.

Riordan-Eva, Paul, and John P. Whitcher. *Vaughan and Asbury's*

General Ophthalmology. 18th ed. New York: Lange Medical Books/McGraw-Hill, 2011.

Roche, Kelly de la, and Eric L. Berman. "Corneal Transplant." *Health Library*, Feb. 28, 2012.

Salvin, Jonathan H. "Tear-Duct Obstruction and Surgery." *KidsHealth*. Nemours Foundation, July 2011.

Stein, Harold A., Raymond M. Stein, and Melvin I. Freeman. *The Ophthalmic Assistant: A Text for Allied and Associated Ophthalmic Personnel.* 8th ed. Philadelphia: Mosby/Elsevier, 2006.

EYES

Anatomy

Anatomy or system affected: Nervous system

Specialties and related fields: Ophthalmology, optometry

Definition: The body structures that receive and transform information about objects into neural impulses that can be translated by the brain into visual images.

Key terms:

accommodation: adjustments of the crystalline lens that are necessary for clear vision at various distances

cornea: the transparent structure forming the anterior part of the fibrous tunic of the eye; light must pass through this structure to reach the retina

crystalline lens: the transparent focusing mechanism of the eye; it is a biconvex structure situated between the posterior chamber and the vitreous body of the eye

diopter: a unit of power of a lens equal to the reciprocal of the focal length of the lens in meters

iris: the circular pigmented membrane behind the cornea, perforated by the pupil; the most anterior portion of the vascular tunic of the eye

photoreceptor: a light-responsive nerve cell or receptor located in the retina of the eye

pupil: the opening at the center of the iris through which light passes

retina: the innermost of the three tunics of the eyeball, which is situated around the vitreous body and is continuous posteriorly with the optic nerve; it contains the photoreceptors

sclera: the tough outer coat or fibrous tunic of the eyeball, which covers the posterior five-sixths of its surface and is continuous anteriorly with the cornea

visual acuity: clarity or clearness in vision

Structure and Functions

The eye captures pictures from the environment and transforms them into neural impulses that are processed by the brain into visual images. The retina, with its light-sensitive cells, acts as a camera to "put the picture on film," while neural processing in the brain "develops the film" and forms a visual image that is meaningful and informative for the individual.

The human eye originates during development, that is, while the individual is being formed as an embryo in the uterus. Eye formation begins during the end of the third week of development when outgrowths of brain neural tissue, called the optic vesicles, form at the sides of the forebrain region. The optic vesicle induces overlying embryonic tissue to thicken in one region, forming a primitive lens structure called the lens placode. The lens placode, in turn, induces the optic vesicles to form a cuplike structure, the optic cup, while the brain's connection of the vesicles narrows into a slender stalk that forms the optic nerve. The inner part of the optic cup forms the neural or sensory retina, with its photoreceptors, while the outer part of the optic cup develops into the layers of tissues, or tunics, that make up the wall of the eyeball. The lens placode further condenses and solidifies by forming lens fibers that become transparent. The function of the lens will eventually be to focus light onto the retina. The major structures of the eye—the retina, lens, and eyeball coats—are initially formed by the fifth month of fetal development. During the remainder of the prenatal period, eye structures continue to enlarge, mature, and form increasingly complex neural networks with the visual processing regions of the brain.

At birth, an infant's eyes are about two-thirds the size of adult eyes. Until after their first month of life, most newborns lack complete retinal development, especially in the area that is responsible for visual acuity. As a result, infants cannot focus their eyes properly and typically have a vacant stare during their first weeks of life. Most of the subsequent eye growth occurs rapidly during the remainder of the first year of life. From the second year of life until puberty, the rate of eye growth progressively slows. After puberty, eye growth is negligible.

The adult human eye weighs approximately 7.5 grams and measures approximately 24.5 millimeters in its anterior-to-posterior diameter. All movement of the eyeball, or globe, is accomplished by six voluntary muscles attached anteriorly by ligaments to the outer coat of the globe and posteriorly to a tendinous ring located behind the globe. One voluntary muscle elevates the upper lid.

Three concentric tunics form the globe itself. The outermost fibrous tunic consists of two portions. In the small, anterior portion, the tunic fibrils are arranged in a regular pattern, forming the transparent cornea. Posteriorly, the tunic fibrils are irregularly spaced, forming the opaque, white sclera. The innermost tunic, or nervous tunic, consists of two parts: the pars optica, or retina, containing photoreceptor cells, and the pars ceca lining the iris and ciliary body. Tucked between the outer and inner tunics lies the vascular tunic, consisting of the pigmented iris, which gives the eye its distinctive color; the ciliary body, which forms the aqueous humor to provide nourishment for the anterior structures of the globe; and the highly vascular choroid, which provides nourishment for the retina and also acts as a cooling system by regulating blood flow to the chemically active retina. In the center of the circular, pigmented iris lies the pupil, which is a small opening into the posterior parts of the eyeball.

The cavity that contains the globe, circumscribed by the concentric tunics, is filled with a clear, jellylike substance called the vitreous body. This substance is anteriorly bounded in the vitreous cavity by the transparent crystalline lens that lies just posterior to the pupil. The crystalline lens is elastic in structure, allowing for variations in thickness that change the focusing power of the eye.

The Anatomy of the Human Eye

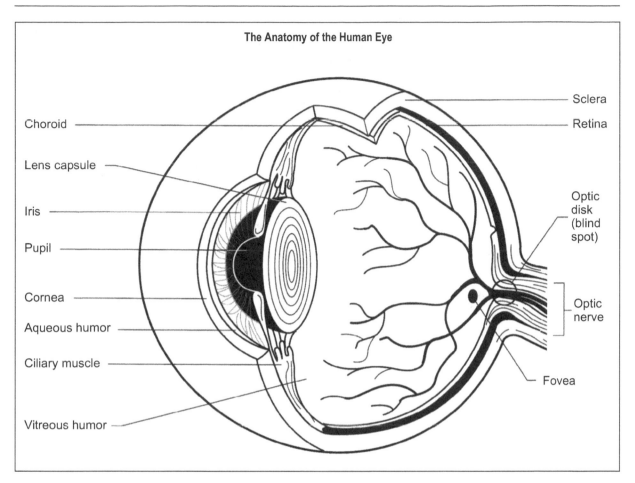

Choroid

Lens capsule

Iris

Pupil

Cornea

Aqueous humor

Ciliary muscle

Vitreous humor

Sclera

Retina

Optic disk (blind spot)

Optic nerve

Fovea

The eye can refract, or bend, light rays because of the curved surfaces of two transparent structures, thecornea and the crystalline lens, through which light rays must pass to reach the retina. Any curved surface, or lens, will refract light rays to a greater or lesser degree depending on the steepness or flatness of the surface curve. The steeper the curve, the greater the refracting power. If a curved surface refracts light rays to an intersection point one meter away from the refracting lens, this lens is defined as having one diopter of power. The human eye has approximately fifty-nine diopters of power in its constituent parts, including the cornea and crystalline lens.

Light rays emitted from a distant point of light enter the eye in a basically parallel pattern and are bent to intersect perfectly at the retina, forming an image of the distant point of light. If the point of light is near the eye, the rays that are emitted are divergent in pattern. These divergent rays must also be refracted to meet at a point on the retina, but these rays require more bending—hence, a steeper curved surface is needed. By a process called accommodation, the human eye automatically adjusts the thickness of the crystalline lens, forming a steeper curve on its surface and thereby creating a perfect image on the retina. Variations from the normal in either the length of an

eyeball or the curves of the cornea and crystalline lens will result in a refractive error or blurred image on the retina.

The major task of the eye is to focus environmental light rays on the photoreceptor cells, the rods and cones of the retina. These photoreceptors absorb the light energy, transforming it into electrical signals that are carried to the visual center of the brain. Cones are specialized for color or daylight vision and have greater visual discrimination or acuity than the rods, which are specialized for black-and-white or nighttime vision.

The fovea is a pin-sized depression in the center of the retina that contains only cone cells in high concentrations. This makes the fovea the point of the most distinct vision, or greatest visual acuity. When the eye focuses on an object, the object's image falls on the retina in the area of the fovea. Immediately surrounding the fovea is a larger area called the macula lutea that contains a relatively high concentration of cones. Macula lutea acuity, while not as great as in the fovea, is much greater than in the retina's periphery, which contains fewer cones. The concentration of cones is greatest in the fovea and declines toward the periphery of the retina. Conversely, the concentration of the rods is greater at the more peripheral areas of the retina than in the macula luteal area. The retina of each eye contains about 100 million rod cells and about 300 million cone cells.

The optic nerve carries impulses from the photoreceptors to the brain. This nerve exits the retina in a central location called the blind spot. No image can be detected in this area because it contains neither rods nor cones. Normally, an individual is not aware of the retinal blind spot because the brain's neural processing compensates for the missing information when some portion of a peripheral image falls across this part of the retina.

On a cellular level, rod and cone photoreceptors consist of three parts: an outer segment that detects the light stimulus, an inner segment that provides the metabolic energy for the cell, and a synaptic terminal that transmits the visual signal to the next nerve cell in the visual pathway leading to the brain. The outer segment is rod-shaped in the rods and cone-shaped in the cones (hence their names). This segment is made of a stack of flattened membranes containing photopigment molecules that undergo chemical changes when activated by light.

The rod photopigment, called rhodopsin, cannot discriminate between various colors of light. Thus rods provide vision only in shades of gray by detecting different intensities of light. Rhodopsin is a purple pigment (a combination of blue and red colors), and it transmits light in the blue and red regions of the visual spectrum while absorbing energy from the green region of the spectrum. The light that is absorbed best by a photopigment is called its absorption maximum. Thus at night, when rods are used for vision, a green car is seen far more easily than a red car, because red light is poorly absorbed by rhodopsin. Only absorbed light produces the photochemical reaction that results in vision.

When rhodopsin absorbs light, the photopigment dissociates or separates into two parts: retinene, which is derived from vitamin A, and opsin, a protein. This separation of retinene from opsin, called the bleaching reaction, causes the production of nerve impulses in the photoreceptors. In the presence of bright light, practically all the rhodopsin undergoes the bleaching reaction and the person is in a light-adapted state. When a light-adapted person initially enters a darkened room, vision is poor since the light sensitivity of the rod photoreceptors is very low. After some time in the dark, however, a gradual increase in light sensitivity, called dark adaptation, occurs as increased amounts of retinene and opsin are recombined by the rods to form rhodopsin. The increased level of rhodopsin occurs after a few minutes in the dark and reaches a maximum sensitivity in about twenty minutes.

Each kind of cone—red, green, and blue—is distinguished by its unique photopigment, which responds to a particular wavelength or color of light. Combinations of cone colors provide the basis for color vision. While each type of cone is most sensitive to the particular wavelength of light indicated by its color—red, green, or blue—cones can respond to other colors with varying degrees. One's perception of color rests on the differential response of each cone type to a particular wavelength of light. The extent that each cone type is activated is coded and sent in separate parallel pathways to the brain. A color vision center in the brain combines and processes these parallel inputs to create the perception of color. Color is thus a concept in the mind of the viewer.

The intricacies of the human visual system require various methods to assess eye structure and function. Visual acuity is a measure of central cone function. Clinically, the most common method for testing visual acuity is by the use of a Snellen chart, consisting of a white background with black letters. All symbols on the chart create, or subtend, a visual angle at the approximate center of the eye. The smaller the symbol, the smaller the angle and the more difficult cone recognition becomes. At the standard distance of twenty feet, the smallest letters on the Snellen chart subtend an angle of five minutes of arc at the eye's center. The larger letters on the chart are calibrated such that each consecutively larger letter subtends a multiple unit of five minutes of arc. If the eye can detect the smallest letters on the chart, the patient is said to have normal (20/20) vision. The numerator of the clinical fraction designates the test distance of twenty feet. The denominator varies with the patient's visual function, identifying the distance at which the smallest letter recognized by the patient subtends an angle of five minutes of arc. For example, if the smallest letter recognized is fifty minutes of arc in size, the fraction used to record this visual acuity is 20/200 because the letter with fifty minutes of arc is ten times as large as the smallest letters on the chart. Therefore, the distance needed for this letter to create five minutes of arc at the eye is ten times as far as the normal twenty feet. In this example, the patient is said to have a refractive error.

Disorders and Diseases

Commonly existing refractive errors are astigmatism, myopia, hyperopia, and presbyopia. Presbyopia is an anomaly that occurs with aging when the crystalline lens loses its ability to accommodate. Causes include thickening of the lens and changes in the attachment fibers that anchor the lens. Because of these alterations, the lens is not able to change its shape and the eye remains focused at a specific distance. To compensate for this problem, bifocal lenses are normally prescribed, with the upper region of the lens focused for distant vision and the lower lens focused for near vision. Hyperopia, also called farsightedness, results when an eyeball is too short. Because light rays are not bent sufficiently by the lens system, the image is focused not on the retina but behind the retina. To compensate for this problem, convex lenses are prescribed, which bring the focus point back on the retina. Conversely, myopia, or nearsightedness, results from an abnormally long eyeball. In this case, the lens system focuses in front of the retina. This abnormal vision can be corrected by concave lenses. Astigmatism results from a refractive error of the lens system, usually caused by an irregular shape in the cornea or less frequently by an irregular shape in the lens. The consequence of this anomaly is that some light rays are focused in front of the retina and some behind the retina, creating a blurred image. To correct the focusing error, a special irregular pair of glasses (or the use of a contact lens) must be made to correct the abnormal irregularity of the eye's lens system.

An examiner can assess the amount of refractive error based on a patient's verbal choice as to which of a given series of lenses sharpens the retinal image of the letters on the Snellen chart. Refractive error can also be determined when a patient is not capable of response. A retinoscope is often used to shine a light through the pupil onto the retina. An image of the light is reflected back out to the examiner who, in turn, can assess refractive error by the movement and shape of the image.

Visual field testing is a measure of the integrity of the neural pathways to the vision center in the brain. To test visual fields clinically, the patient focuses on a central target. While continuing to focus centrally, test targets are serially brought into the patient's peripheral vision, or visual field. The smaller and dimmer the test target, the more sensitive the test. The simplest visual field test technique is by confrontation. The patient and examiner sit facing each other one meter apart. If both patient and examiner cover their right eyes, the patient's left visual field is being tested. Since the patient's left visual field is congruent to the examiner's left visual field, the examiner can detect visual field defects when the patient is not responsive to a test target brought into view from the side. Lesions to some portion of the visual pathway to the brain will result in a scotoma, or blind area, in the corresponding visual field.

A biomicroscope, or slitlamp microscope, is commonly used to assess external eye structures, including the eyelids, lashes, conjunctiva, cornea, sclera, and one internal structure, the crystalline lens. The white part of the eye, or sclera, is covered with a thin, transparent covering called the conjunctiva. Infections and tumors often invade this external structure. Though the normally transparent crystalline lens is essentially free of infections and tumors, it can become cloudy or opaque and develop a cataract. Causes for cataract formation are multiple, the most common being the aging process; less frequently, trauma to the lens or a secondary symptom of systemic disease can result in cataracts. When the cataract is so dense that it obstructs vision, the crystalline lens is surgically removed and replaced with an artificial, plastic lens.

To view internal eye structures, the pupil is dilated to allow more light to be introduced into the interior and posterior regions of the eyeball. Two commonly used instruments are the handheld ophthalmoscope and the head-mounted indirect ophthalmoscope. Diseases of the retina include retinal tears, detachments, artery or vein occlusions, degenerations, and retinopathies secondary to systemic disease.

Glaucoma is an eye disease characterized by raised pressure inside the eye. Normal eye pressure is stabilized by the balance between the production and removal of the aqueous humor, the solution that bathes the internal, anterior structures of the eye. Abnormal pressures are often associated with defects in the visual, or optic, nerve and in the visual field. Approximately 300 people per 100,000 are affected by glaucoma. Clinically, intraocular pressure is assessed by numerous methods in a process called tonometry.

Abnormalities of the eye muscles constitute a significant portion of visual problems. Binocular vision and good depth perception are present when both eyes are aligned properly toward an object. A weakness in any of the six rotatory eye muscles will result in a tendency for that eye to deviate away from the object, resulting in an obvious or latent eye turn called strabismus. Associated signs are eye fatigue, abnormal head postures, and double vision. To alleviate objectionable double vision, a patient often suppresses the retinal image at the brain level, resulting in functional amblyopia (often called lazy eye), in which visual acuity is deficient.

Color blindness, a trait that occurs more frequently in men than in women, is caused by a hereditary lack of one or more types of cones. For example, if the green-sensitive cones are not functioning, the colors in the visual spectral range from green to red can stimulate only red-sensitive cones. This person can perceive only one color in this range, since the ratio of stimulation of the green-red cones is constant for the colors in this range. Thus this individual is considered to be green-red color-blind and will have difficulty distinguishing green from red.

Perspective and Prospects

Early physicians recognized the importance of good eyesight, but because of limited understanding they had minimal means to treat major eye disorders. During the Middle Ages, surgeons performed eye operations, including ones for cataracts in which the lens was pushed down and out of the way with a needle inserted into the eyeball. In the eighteenth century, this operation was improved when cataract lenses were extracted from the eye. In the early seventeenth century, Johannes Kepler described how light was focused by the lens of the eye on the retina, thus providing insight into why spectacles are valuable in cases of poor eyesight. In 1801, Thomas Young published a foundational text entitled *On the Mechanics of the Eye*. Hermann von Helmholtz in the nineteenth century invented the first ophthalmoscope, which allowed inspection of the interior structures of the eye. Young and Helmholtz also developed theories to explain the phenomenon of color vision. From the invention of the ophthalmoscope, the range of clinical observation was extended to the inside of the eyeball, allowing the diagnosis of eye disorders. The modern understanding of eyesight and vision is increasing with contributions from ongoing research.

Ophthalmology is the study of the structure, function, and diseases of the eye. An ophthalmologist is a physician who specializes in the diagnosis and treatment of eye disorders and diseases with surgery, drugs, and corrective lenses. An optometrist is a specialist with a doctorate in optometry who is trained to examine and test the eyes and treat defects in vision by prescribing corrective lenses. An optician is a technician who fits, adjusts, and dispenses corrective lenses that are based on the prescription of an ophthalmologist or optometrist.

Vision care personnel are vital to industry, public health, recreation, highway safety, education, and the community. Since 85 percent of learning is visual-based, good vision is extremely important in education, work, and play. Good vision enhances the production and morale of workers, and athletic performance is improved when vision problems are corrected. Vision care specialists work to promote the prevention of eye injuries and diseases while supporting practices that enhance good health and vision. Vision therapy may be used to correct many disorders of the eye such as amblyopia, reduced visual perception, reading disorders, poor eye coordination, and reduced visual acuity.

—Elva B. Miller, O.D., and Roman J. Miller, Ph.D.

See also Albinos; Astigmatism; Blindness; Cataract surgery; Cataracts; Chlamydia; Color blindness; Conjunctivitis; Corneal transplantation; Diabetes mellitus; Dyslexia; Eye infections and disorders; Eye surgery; Face lift and blepharoplasty; Glaucoma; Gonorrhea; Jaundice; Keratitis; Laser use in surgery; Macular degeneration; Microscopy, slitlamp; Myopia; Ophthalmology; Optometry; Optometry, pediatric; Pigmentation; Ptosis; Refractive eye surgery; Sense organs; Sjögren's syndrome; Strabismus; Styes; Systems and organs; Trachoma; Transplantation; Vision; Vision disorders.

For Further Information:

Badash, Michelle, and Eric L. Berman. "Nearsightedness and Farsightedness." *Health Library*, September 1, 2011.

Buettner, Helmut, ed. *Mayo Clinic on Vision and Eye Health: Practical Answers on Glaucoma, Cataracts, Macular Degeneration, and Other Conditions*. Rochester, Minn.: Mayo Foundation for Medical Education and Research, 2002.

"The Eye and How We See." *Prevent Blindness America*, 2011.

"Eyes and Vision." *MedlinePlus*, June 26, 2013.

Guyton, Arthur C., and John E. Hall. *Human Physiology and Mechanisms of Disease*. 6th ed. Philadelphia: W. B. Saunders, 1997.

Litin, Scott C., ed. *Mayo Clinic Family Health Book*. 4th ed. New York: HarperResource, 2009.

Riordan-Eva, Paul, and John P. Whitcher. *Vaughan and Asbury's General Ophthalmology*. 18th ed. New York: Lange Medical Books/McGraw-Hill, 2011.

Tortora, Gerard J., and Bryan Derrickson. *Principles of Anatomy and Physiology*. 14th ed. Hoboken, N.J.: John Wiley & Sons, 2013.

Vorvick, Linda J., Franklin W. Lusby, and David Zieve. "Standard Ophthalmic Exam." *MedlinePlus*, February 10, 2011.

FACE LIFT AND BLEPHAROPLASTY

Procedures

Anatomy or system affected: Eyes, skin
Specialties and related fields: General surgery, plastic surgery
Definition: Techniques used to remove unwanted wrinkles and other indicators of aging from the face.

Indications and Procedures

Aging may create serious problems for individuals whose success in their occupations depends on appearance. Premature wrinkling of skin on the face and eyelids or premature looseness of these tissues can create an insurmountable psychological barrier. In these situations, cosmetic surgery such as rhytidectomy (face lift) or blepharoplasty (the removal of excess tissue around the eyelids) may be performed.

Face lift is the term used for the excision and pulling upward of sagging skin on the face. This cosmetic procedure can smooth wrinkles and provide a more attractive profile, but there are drawbacks: the patient's appearance may be changed too dramatically, and the procedure must be repeated periodically to maintain the desired results.

Surgical face lifting involves making an incision at the hairline and extending it downward; the length of the incision is dependent on the amount of skin sagging that is present. The skin is gently separated from the underlying fascia and is pulled back and tightened until the desired degree of wrinkle elimination is achieved. Excess skin at the posterior (back) margins is removed. The surgeon may also remove fat under the skin and tighten the muscles of the face. When this is complete, the edges of the incision are carefully brought together and secured with fine sutures or adhesive closures. The patient returns to the plastic surgeon in seven to ten days for follow-up evaluation.

Blepharoplasty refers to the surgical alteration of the eyelids. The surgery is similar to that used for a total face lift. An incision is made along the lower margin of the eyebrow. Skin is separated from the fascia. Sometimes, small amounts of fat

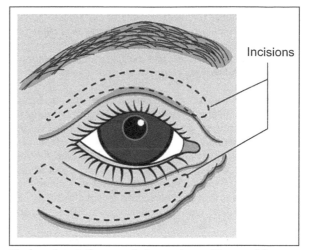

Incisions

Blepharoplasty is the removal of excess, baggy skin around the eyes.

are also removed. The skin of the upper eyelid is tightened. After excess tissue is removed, the free edges are attached with fine sutures. Cosmetic alteration of the lower eyelid can also be accomplished surgically through a similar method. The patient returns to the plastic surgeon in approximately one week for removal of the sutures. Chemical peeling or dermabrasion are additional techniques that can be used to remove fine wrinkles and lines in skin.

Uses and Complications

A face lift is a form of cosmetic surgery and is usually undertaken for aesthetic reasons. Short-term problems include bruising and swelling. Possible long-term complications include infection, scarring, and insufficient removal of unwanted wrinkles. Proper techniques can reduce the first two problems. Realistic expectations can minimize disappointment.

Because of the eyelid's good blood circulation, blepharoplasty performed under sterile conditions seldom results in serious infection. However, the procedure can result in a number of other complications: continued bleeding that requires the reopening of the eyelid wound and either the cauterization of the bleeding vessel or the evacuation of a clot; separation of the edges of the eyelid skin closure, requiring either support tape or sutures; eyelid asymmetry, whereby the eyelids look fine individually but do not match as a pair; and either insufficient or excessive skin removal.

Perspective and Prospects

At birth, human skin contains relatively large amounts of a molecule called collagen. Collagen provides strength to the skin; this is technically called turgor. The function of collagen is similar to that of the fibers in fiberglass or steel reinforcement in concrete: strength. Living on Earth, people are constantly subjected to the effects of gravity and ultraviolet radiation, which over time cause slight damage to the collagen in skin. The turgor is slowly lost, and the skin starts to sag

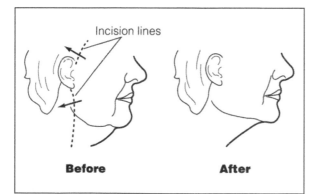

Incision lines

Before   **After**

A "face lift" is the term used for the excision and pulling upward of sagging skin on the face. This cosmetic procedure can smooth wrinkles and provide a more attractive profile, but there are drawbacks: The patient's appearance may be changed too dramatically, and the procedure must be repeated periodically to maintain the desired results.

under the influence of gravity. Excessive exposure to the sun accelerates this process. The use of tanning beds in salons exposes the skin to an increased amount of harmful ultraviolet radiation, which also accelerates the aging process. With sufficient time and exposure, the typical appearance of skin in old age is seen.

There is no way to stop the human body from aging; accepting this inevitable reality can reduce both stress and anxiety. Cosmetic surgical procedures such as blepharoplasty and face lifts are temporary and enable an individual to maintain only an approximation of youthfulness. Over time, the skin will continue to change, necessitating repeat procedures. Each time the procedure is repeated, the result is diminished in comparison to an earlier procedure. Cosmetic surgery can thus only retard the appearance of aging rather than re-create youth.

—*L. Fleming Fallon, Jr., M.D., Ph.D., M.P.H.*

See also Aging; Botox; Collagen; Facial transplantation; Plastic surgery; Skin; Skin disorders.

For Further Information:

A.D.A.M. Medical Encyclopedia. "Facelift." *MedlinePlus*, November 16, 2011.

Aston, Sherrell J., Robert W. Beasley, and Charles H. M. Thorne, eds. *Grabb and Smith's Plastic Surgery*. 6th ed. Philadelphia: Lippincott-Raven, 2007.

"Blepharoplasty." *American Society for Dermatologic Surgery*, 2013.

Bosniak, Stephen L., and Marian Cantisano Zilkha. *Cosmetic Blepharoplasty and Facial Rejuvenation*. 2d ed. Philadelphia: Lippincott-Raven, 1999.

Henry, Kimberly A. *The Face-Lift Sourcebook*. Los Angeles: Lowell House, 2000.

Lewis, Wendy. *The Beauty Battle: The Insider's Guide to Wrinkle Rescue and Cosmetic Perfection from Head to Toe*. Berkeley, Calif.: Laurel Glen Books, 2003.

Loftus, Jean. *The Smart Woman's Guide to Plastic Surgery*. 2d ed. Dubuque, Iowa: McGraw-Hill, 2010.

Marfuggi, Richard A. *Plastic Surgery: What You Need to Know Before, During, and After*. New York: Berkeley, 1998.

McCoy, Krisha. "Blepharoplasty." *Health Library*, January 10, 2013.

Narins, Rhoda, and Paul Jarrod Frank. *Turn Back the Clock Without Losing Time: Everything You Need to Know About Simple Cosmetic Procedures*. New York: Three Rivers Press, 2002.

Turkington, Carol, and Jeffrey S. Dover. *The Encyclopedia of Skin and Skin Disorders*. 3d ed. New York: Facts On File, 2007.

Wyer, E. Bingo. *The Unofficial Guide to Cosmetic Surgery*. New York: Wiley, 1999.

FACIAL PALSY. *See* BELL'S PALSY.

FACIAL TRANSPLANTATION

Procedure

Anatomy or system affected: Blood vessels, bones, circulatory system, ears, eyes, head, immune system, mouth, muscles, neck, nerves, nervous system, nose, skin

Specialties and related fields: Dermatology, ethics, physical therapy, plastic surgery, psychology

Definition: A surgical procedure to transplant all or part of the face from a donor's corpse onto the severely disfigured face of a living person in order to provide a dramatic improvement in the appearance of the recipient.

Key terms:

composite tissue allotransplantation (CTA): the grafting of several structures (such as skin, bones, muscles, and nerves) between two or more individuals

immunosuppressants: medications used to prevent the body from rejecting transplanted tissue and organs

transplant: to transfer organs or tissue from one part or individual to another

Indications and Procedures

Facial transplantation is a procedure that is reserved for people with extensive facial disfigurements who have exhausted all other options, including reconstructive surgery. Accidents such as burns, trauma, maulings, and gunshot wounds; diseases such as cancer and infection; and craniofacial anomalies affect thousands of people each year, causing disfigurement to the face. For most people, surgery can correct all or most of the disfigurement. For the few people who experience a great loss of tissue, however, reconstructive surgery is very limited in returning normal function and appearance.

Facial transplantation is technically easier than other facial reconstruction surgeries, should involve fewer surgeries, and can improve appearance and mobility. In traditional facial reconstruction, tissue is surgically reattached or taken from another part of the person's own body. These reconstructions, however, do not transfer the subtle muscles needed for expression, which creates an expressionless, masklike appearance.

People with severe facial disfigurement may have limited facial movement, which can cause difficulty talking, eating, and even closing the eyes. People with facial disfigurement often have low self-esteem and experience social isolation, depression, anxiety, and poor quality of life. They may have difficulty making friends and finding employment.

The transplantation involves three separate surgeries. The first surgery, which takes ten to twelve hours, degloves the corpse of the donor. An incision is made across the hairline, down the temples, behind or around the ears, and around the jaw line. The face, including the eyebrows, eyelids, nose, mouth, and lips, is then detached, as is underlying fat and connective tissue. Surgeons must be careful not to damage the nerves controlling facial expression, eye movement, and facial sensation. If the donor's face is healthy enough for the transplant, then the surgeons begin the second surgery, in which they deglove the patient's face. This surgery takes longer, since the surgeons must clamp off the veins and arteries and take special care not to damage the nerves. Bone grafts are performed if the patient needs bone replacement. The third surgery involves attaching the new face, including veins, arteries, and nerves, and may take as long as twenty-four hours to complete.

Temporary tubing and drains are installed to remove fluid buildup. After about two months, the patient's face returns to normal size. Depending on the nerve damage before the transplant and the success in nerve reattachment, the patient's

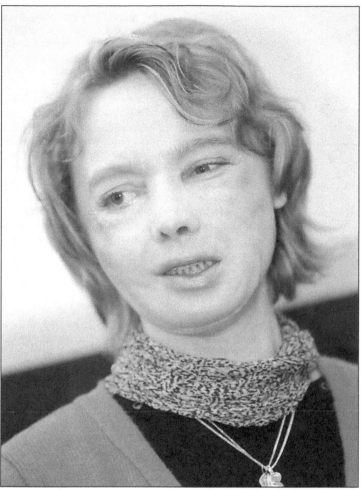

Isabelle Dinoire, the first person to undergo a partial face transplant. (AP/Wide World Photos)

facial movements may not be normal for several months to over a year. The patient must take immunosuppressants for life to prevent the body from rejecting the donated tissue.

Uses and Complications

Few facial transplantations have been performed worldwide, and many of the risks involved remain unknown. In general, skin grafts are more susceptible to rejection than are most organ or other tissue transplants. In addition, skin transplants carry a life-threatening risk, and a rejected facial transplant would leave the patient in worse condition physically, emotionally, and psychologically.

Other risks include tissue damage that occurs because of cell death from the time of removal to reattachment. If the sensory nerves are not properly reconnected, then permanent numbness will occur. Long-term risks, including tissue mutation or psychological impact, are unknown. Short-term risks include infection, additional scarring, potential tissue rejection, and complications in long-term healing. The side effects

of immunosuppressants include infections, metabolic disorders such as diabetes, malignancies, and decreased kidney and lung function.

Perspective and Prospects

With the introduction of immunosuppressive drugs in the 1980s, composite tissue allotransplantation (CTA) became possible. Prior to the introduction of these drugs, hand and face transplants had been considered almost impossible because of the tissue involved and the high risk of rejection.

In 1994, a surgeon successfully reattached the face of a nine-year-old in India whose face and scalp were ripped off by a threshing machine. Two other surgeries, one in Australia and one in the United States in 2002, also reattached entire faces. Facial transplantation was discussed as a serious therapeutic option in a 2002 meeting of the Plastic Surgical Research Council in Boston, Massachusetts, and by early 2006, teams in the United States, France, and Great Britain had been working for years to develop surgical techniques and protocols for immunosuppression, psychological assessment, and informed consent for potential patients.

In France, on November 27, 2005, doctors transplanted a chin, lips, and nose onto Isabelle Dinoire, a woman who had been mauled by her dog while she was unconscious. In April 2006, doctors in China grafted a nose, cheeks, and upper lip onto a man mauled by a bear years before. In December 2008, doctors in the United States performed the first near-total face transplant on a woman who had been shot in the face four years earlier. By 2012, full face transplants had been successfully performed in France, Spain, and the United States.

Despite these successes, the procedure is still very experimental, involves great risks, and raises numerous ethical questions. Patients are participating in research, not receiving traditional medical care. The results are promising, however, and will likely inspire further procedures.

—*Virginia L. Salmon*

See also Bone grafting; Dermatology; Ethics; Grafts and grafting; Immune system; Oral and maxillofacial surgery; Plastic surgery; Skin; Transplantation.

For Further Information:

Baylis, Françoise. "Changing Faces: Ethics, Identity, and Facial Transplantation." In *Cutting to the Core*, edited by David Benatar. New York: Rowman & Littlefield, 2006.

Center for Reconstructive Transplantation. "Face Transplant." *Cleveland Clinic*, 2013.

Comprehensive Transplant Center. "Face Transplant Surgery." *Johns Hopkins Medicine*, 2013.

Concar, David. "The Boldest Cut." *New Scientist* 182 (May 29, 2004): 32–37.

"Crossing New Frontier: Paving the Way to Make Face Transplantation Reality." *Medical Ethics Advisor*, July 1, 2006.

Division of Plastic Surgery. "Face Transplant Surgery." *Brigham and Women's Hospital*, February 14, 2013.

McLaughlin, Sabrina. "Face to Face" *Current Science* 89, no. 2 (September 12, 2003): 8–9.

Wilson, Jim. "Trading Faces." *Popular Mechanics* 180, no. 11 (November, 2003): 76–79.

Factitious disorders

Disease/Disorder

Anatomy or system affected: Psychic-emotional system, most bodily systems

Specialties and related fields: Family medicine, internal medicine, psychiatry, psychology

Definition: Psychophysiological disorders in which individuals intentionally produce their symptoms in order to play the role of patient.

Causes and Symptoms

Although factitious disorders cover a wide array of physical symptoms and are believed to be closely related to a subset of psychophysiological disorders (somatoform disorders), they are unique in all of medicine for two reasons. The first distinguishing factor is that whatever the physical disease for which treatment is sought and regardless of how serious, the patients who seek its treatment have deliberately and intentionally produced the condition. They may have done so in one of three ways, or in any combination of these three ways. First, patients fabricate, invent, lie about, and make up symptoms that they do not have; for example, they claim to have fever and night sweats or severe back pain that they actually do not have. Second, patients have the actual symptoms that they describe, but they intentionally caused them; for example, they might inject human saliva into their own skin to produce an abscess or ingest a known allergic food to cause the predictable reaction. Third, someone with a known condition such as pancreatitis has a pain episode but exaggerates its severity, or someone else with a history of migraines claims his or her headache to be yet another migraine when it is not. Factitious disorders may manifest as complaints about psychological problems, physical problems, or both.

The second element that makes these disorders unique (and at the same time both fascinating to study and frustrating to treat) is that the sole motivation for causing or claiming the symptoms is for these patients to become and remain patients, to assume the sick role wherein little can be expected from them. These patients are not malingerers, individuals who consciously use actual or feigned symptoms for some other gain (such as claiming a fever so one does not have to go to work or school, or insisting that one's post-traumatic stress is worse than it is to enhance the judgment in a lawsuit). In fact, it is the absence of any discernible external benefit that makes these disorders so intriguing.

Technically, psychiatrists and psychologists understand factitious disorders as having three subtypes. In the first, patients claim to have predominantly psychological symptoms such as memory loss, depression, contemplation of suicide, the hearing of voices, or false memory of childhood molestation. Characteristically, the symptoms worsen whenever the patients know themselves to be under observation. In the second, patients have predominantly physical symptoms that at least superficially suggest some general medical condition. In a more extreme form called Münchausen syndrome, individuals will have spent much of their lives getting admitted to medical facilities and, once there, remain as long as possible. While common complaints include vomiting, dizziness, blacking out, generalized rashes, and bleeding, the symptoms can involve any organ and seem limited only to the individuals" medical knowledge and experience with the medical system. The third subtype combines both psychological and physical complaints in such a way that neither predominates.

Regardless of the subtype, factitious disorders are difficult to diagnose. Usually, the diagnosis is considered when the course of treating either a medical or a mental illness becomes atypical and protracted. Often, the person with a factitious disorder will present in a way that seems odd to the experienced clinician. The person may have an unusually extensive history of traveling, much familiarity with medical procedures and terminology, a complex medical and surgical history, few visitors during the hospitalization, behavioral disruptions and disturbances while hospitalized, exacerbation of symptoms while under observation, and/or fluctuating illness with new symptoms and complications arising as the workup proceeds. When present, these traits along with others make suspicion of factitious disorders reasonable.

No one knows how many people suffer with factitious disorders, but the condition is generally regarded as uncommon. It is certainly rarely reported, but this in part may be attributable to the difficulties in determining the diagnosis. While brief episodes of the condition occur, most people who claim a factitious disorder have it chronically, and they usually move on to another physician or facility when they are confronted with the true nature of their illness. It is therefore likely that some individuals are reported more than once by different hospitals and providers.

There is little certainty about what causes factitious disorders. This is true in large measure because those who know the most about the subject—patients with the disorder—are notoriously unreliable in providing information about their psychological state and often seem only dimly aware of what they are doing to themselves. It may be that they are generally incapable of putting their feelings into words. They are unaware of having inner feelings and may not know, for example, that they are sad or angry. It is possible that they experience emotions more physically, behaviorally, and concretely than do most others.

Another view suggests that people learn to distinguish their primitive emotional states through the responsivity of their primary caretaker. A normal, healthy, average mother responds appropriately to her infant's differing affective states, thereby helping the infant, as he or she develops, to distinguish, define, and eventually name what he or she is feeling. When a primary caretaker is, for any of several reasons, incapable of responding in consistently appropriate ways, the infant's emotional awareness remains undifferentiated and the child experiences confusion and emotional chaos.

It is possible, too, that factitious disorder patients are motivated to assume what sociology defines as a sick role wherein people are required to acknowledge that they are ill and are required to relinquish adult responsibilities as they place themselves in the hands of designated caretakers.

Treatment and Therapy

Understanding how to identify individuals with factitious disorders early in their treatment process is crucial to public health for three important reasons. First, early identification will help the individual obtain a more appropriate referral. Second, it will conserve valuable health care resources, so that clients who have pressing medical needs get the treatment that they deserve. Third, the earlier in the process these individuals can be identified, the sooner valuable health care dollars can be saved, lowering the cost of health care as a whole.

Internists, family practitioners, and surgeons are the specialists most likely to encounter patients with factitious disorders, although psychiatrists and psychologists are often consulted in the management of these patients. These patients pose a special challenge because, in a real sense, they do not wish to become well even as they present themselves for treatment. They are not ill in the usual sense, and their indirect communication and manipulation often make them frustrating to treat using standard goals and expectations.

Sometimes mental and medical specialists" joint, supportive confrontation of these patients results in a disappearance of the troubling and troublesome behavior. During these confrontations, the health professionals are acknowledging that such extreme behavior evidences extreme distress in these patients, and as such is its own reason for psychotherapeutic intervention. These patients are not psychologically minded, however; they also have trouble forming relationships that foster genuine self-disclosure, and they rarely accept the recommendation for psychotherapeutic treatment. Because they believe that their problems are physical, not psychological, they often become irate at the suggestion that their problems are not what they believe them to be. Taken from the patient's perspective, this anger makes some sense. For them, they have endured significant time in evaluation and often also a good bit of money, and if they are lacking insight into their condition, such a confrontation may leave them feeling helpless and misunderstood. As such, even in these circumstances, empathy remains an important element in successful intervention.

—Paul Moglia, Ph.D.;
updated by Nancy A. Piotrowski, Ph.D.

See also Hypochondriasis; Münchausen syndrome by proxy; Psychiatric disorders; Psychiatry; Psychiatry, child and adolescent; Psychiatry, geriatric; Psychoanalysis; Psychosomatic disorders.

For Further Information:

American Psychiatric Association. *Diagnostic and Statistical Manual of Mental Disorders: DSM-5.* 5th ed. Arlington, Va.: Author, 2013.

Feldman, Marc D. *Playing Sick? Untangling the Web of Munchausen Syndrome, Munchausen by Proxy, Malingering, and Factitious Disorder.* New York: Brunner-Routledge, 2004.

Mayo Clinic Staff. "Munchausen Syndrome." *Mayo Clinic,* May 13, 2011.

McCoy, Krisha, Rebecca Stahl, and Brian Randall. "Factitious Disorder." *Health Library,* Mar. 15, 2013.

New, Michelle. "Munchausen by Proxy Syndrome." *KidsHealth.* Nemours Foundation, Mar. 2012.

Phillips, Katherine A., ed. *Somatoform and Factitious Disorders.* Washington, D.C.: American Psychiatric Association, 2001.

FAILURE TO THRIVE
Disease/Disorder

Also known as: Growth impairment, stunting, wasting

Anatomy or system affected: Bones, brain, endocrine system, psychic-emotional system

Specialties and related fields: Endocrinology, family medicine, gastroenterology, genetics, neonatology, pediatrics, psychiatry, psychology

Definition: A disorder of early childhood growth that includes disturbances in psychosocial skills and development.

Causes and Symptoms

Failure to thrive may be organic , inorganic; in many children, the etiology is multifactorial. The onset of growth problems may be prenatal as a result of maternal substance abuse, most notably alcohol use, or of maternal infection, particularly with rubella, cytomegalovirus (CMV), or toxoplasmosis. Chromosome problems, such as Down syndrome and Turner syndrome, are also a medical cause of failure to thrive. Other causes include gastrointestinal diasease, endocrine disease, kidney disease, and heart and lung disease, all of which may decrease a child's appetite and how they process food and thus impair growth. Small size in infants secondary to prematurity resolves by two to three years of age unless there are complications.

Many children with failure to thrive are both stunted (linear growth-affected) and wasted (weight-affected). Assessing which of the two conditions predominates can be done using the body mass index (BMI), which is calculated by dividing weight in kilograms by height in meters squared. A low BMI is a sign of malnutrition. Children with environmental failure to thrive fall into this category.

A child who is small but has an appropriate BMI has short stature rather than failure to thrive. The two leading causes of short stature are familial short stature and constitutional delay.

Treatment and Therapy

The main focus of the medical intervention with failure to thrive is to ensure a nurturing environment and adequate nutrition. Nutritional intervention can be achieved in many ways, such as by securing adequate access to food for the

Information on Failure to Thrive

Causes: Maternal substance abuse or infection during prenatal phase, familial short stature, constitutional delay
Symptoms: Stunted growth, weight impairment
Duration: Two to three years
Treatments: Nurturing environment, nutritional intervention, family counseling

family and offering concentrated formulas, nutritional supplementation, and calorie-dense food, depending on the age of the child. Developmental intervention should also be provided if delay is detected. Likewise, family counseling, especially focusing on parenting skills, may be indicated. Other treatment options include treating the underlying medical condition that is contributing to failure to thrive, such as gastrointestinal disease, kidney disease, HIV and other infectious diseases.

Perspective and Prospects

The term "failure to thrive" originated in 1933; it replaced the term "cease to thrive," which appeared in 1889. Initially, the condition was reported in institutionalized children, including those in orphanages. In the 1940s, however, it was recognized as a condition that could also affect children living at home with their biological or adoptive parents.

Although the list of conditions that can cause growth impairment in children is quite extensive, a systematic approach using history and both physical and psychosocial assessment will provide clues to the diagnosis. Intervention ensures an adequate outcome, with improved prospects for physical growth and brain development.

—*Carol D. Berkowitz, M.D.*

See also Bonding; Cognitive development; Cytomegalovirus (CMV); Developmental disorders; Developmental stages; Fetal alcohol syndrome; Growth; Malnutrition; Neonatology; Nutrition; Pediatrics; Rubella; Toxoplasmosis; Weight loss and gain.

For Further Information:

Berk, Laura E. *Child Development.* 8th ed. Boston: Pearson/Allyn & Bacon, 2009.
Carson-DeWitt, Rosalyn. "Failure-to-Thrive." *Health Library*, September 10, 2012.
Geissler, Catherine A., and Hilary J. Powers, eds. *Human Nutrition.* 12th ed. New York: Churchill Livingstone/Elsevier, 2010.
Kreutler, Patricia A., and Dorice M. Czajka-Narins. *Nutrition in Perspective.* 2d ed. Englewood Cliffs: Prentice Hall, 1987.
Nathanson, Laura Walther. *The Portable Pediatrician: A Practicing Pediatrician's Guide to Your Child's Growth, Development, Health, and Behavior from Birth to Age Five.* 2d ed. New York: HarperCollins, 2002.
Navarini, Susanne, et al. "Giant Cardiac Fibroma: An Unusual Cause of Failure to Thrive." *Pediatric Cardiology* 34, no. 5 (2013): 1264–1266.
Reading, Richard. "Weight Faltering and Failure to Thrive in Infancy and Early Childhood." *Child: Care, Health and Development* 39, no. 1 (2013): 151–152.
Shore, Rima. *Rethinking the Brain: New Insights into Early Development.* Rev. ed. New York: Families and Work Institute, 2003.
Whitney, Ellie, and Sharon Rady Rolfes. *Understanding Nutrition.* 12th ed. Belmont: Wadsworth, 2009.
Winick, Myron, et al. *The Columbia Encyclopedia of Nutrition.* New York: Putnam's Sons, 1988.

FAINTING. SEE DIZZINESS AND FAINTING.

FAMILY MEDICINE
Specialty
Also known as: Family practice
Anatomy or system affected: All
Specialties and related fields: Geriatrics and gerontology, internal medicine, obstetrics, osteopathic medicine, pediatrics, preventive medicine, psychiatry, psychology
Definition: The specialty concerned with the primary health maintenance and medical care of an undifferentiated patient population, in the context of family and community.
Key terms:
ambulatory care: health care provided outside the hospital, usually in a clinic or office and sometimes in the patient's home
biopsychosocial model: a model that examines the effects of illness on all spheres in which the patient functions-the biological sphere, the psychological sphere, and the social sphere
general practice: a primary care field with care provided by physicians who usually have completed less than three years of residency training; the organization from which family medicine evolved
generalism: a medical and political movement concerned with primary care, often associated with the medical specialties of family medicine, general internal medicine, general pediatrics, and sometimes obstetrics and gynecology
health maintenance: the practice of anticipating, finding, preventing, and/or dealing with potential or established medical problems at the earliest possible stage to minimize adverse effects on the patient
internship: a synonym for the first year of residency training
patient advocacy: the representation of the patient's interest in medical diagnosis and treatment decisions, in which the physician acts as an information source and counselor for the patient
primary care: first-line or entry-level care; the health care that most people receive for most illnesses
residency training: medical training provided in a specialty after graduation from medical school; similar to an apprenticeship and designed to mimic real-life practice as closely as possible
specialist: any physician who practices in a specialty other than the generalist areas of family medicine, general internal medicine, general pediatrics, and obstetrics and gynecology
undifferentiated patient population: patients seen by family physicians regardless of age, sex, or type of problem

Science and Profession

From cradle to grave, family physicians have the ability to take care of patients from all age groups and manage a great variety of medical problems on a daily basis. As the primary care provider, they are central to a patient's care, either by providing it directly (85 percent of all medical problems) or by consulting specialists and following their management recommendations. They act as the patient's advocate even when healthy by providing preventive care services to find disease earlier in an attempt to eliminate it or slow its progression.

In the United States, there are approximately 80,000 practicing family physicians, accounting for more than 240 million annual office visits. More than a third of all US counties have access to only family physicians to provide medical care to their communities.

Family medicine is the direct descendant of general practice. For many years, most physicians were general practitioners. In the mid-to-late twentieth century, however, the explosion of medical knowledge led to the specialization of medicine. For example, increased knowledge of the function and diseases of the heart seemed to demand creation of the specialty of cardiology. The model of the country doctor or jack-of-all-trades physician taking care of a wide range of medical problems seemed doomed to sink in the sea of subspecialization in medicine. The general practitioner, the venerable physician who hung out his or her shingle after medical school and one or more years of internship or residency training, appeared to be headed for extinction. Indeed, in their then-existent forms, the general practitioner and general practice would not have survived. Several forces came into play which did result in the passing of general practice but which also changed general practice into family medicine.

The primary force pushing for general practice to survive and improve was the desire of the general public to retain the family doctor. The services that these physicians rendered and the relationships developed between physician and patients were held in high esteem. Through such voices as the Citizen Commission on Graduate Medical Education appointed by the American Medical Association (AMA), the public requested the rescue of the family doctor.

Other major players in the movement to revive and reshape general practice included the AMA itself and the American Academy of General Practice. On February 8, 1969, approval was granted for the creation of family medicine as medicine's twentieth official specialty. The American Academy of General Practice became the American Academy of Family Physicians (AAFP), and a certifying board, the American Board of Family Practice (ABFP), was established. The name has since been changed to the American Board of Family Medicine (ABFM). After these steps were completed, three-year training programs (residencies) in family medicine were established in medical universities and larger community hospitals to provide the necessary training for family physicians.

Family physicians are trained to provide comprehensive ongoing medical care and health maintenance for their patients. Those people who choose to become family physicians tend to value relationships over technology and service over high financial rewards. Many family physicians find themselves providing service to underserved populations and in mission work both inside and outside the United States. Family physicians often become advocates, providing counseling and advice to patients who are trying to sort out medical treatment options. They generally enjoy close relationships with their patients, who often hold them in high esteem.

Following graduation from medical school, students interested in a career in family medicine begin a three-year residency in the specialty. During the residency, these physicians train in actual practice settings under the supervision of faculty physicians. Family medicine residency training consists of three years of rotations with other medical specialties, such as internal medicine, pediatrics, surgery, and psychiatry. The unifying thread in family medicine residency training is the continuity clinic. Throughout their training, the residents see their own patients several days a week under the supervision of family medicine faculty physicians. Every effort is made to make this training as close as possible to experiences in the real world. Family medicine residents will deliver their patients" babies, hospitalize their patients, and deal with the emotional issues of death and dying, chronic illness, and disability.

Family medicine residents receive intensive training in behavioral and psychosocial issues, as well as "bedside manner" training. Scientific research has shown that many patients who seek care from family physicians have problems that require the physician to be a good listener and a skilled counselor. Family medicine residency training emphasizes these skills. It also emphasizes the functioning (or malfunctioning) of the family as a system and the effect of major changes (such as the birth of a child or retirement) on the health and functioning of the family members.

The length of training (three years versus one year) and the emphasis on psychosocial and family systems training are two of the major differences in the training of a family physician and the training of a general practitioner. Moreover, family physicians spend up to 30 percent of their training time outside the hospital in a clinic. Family medicine was the first medical specialty to emphasize this type of training, and family physicians spend more time in ambulatory (clinic) training than virtually any other specialist.

Following the successful completion of a residency program, a family physician may take a competency examination devised and administered by the ABFM. Passing this examination allows the physician to assume the title of Diplomate of the American Board of Family Medicine and makes him or her eligible to join the American Academy of Family Physicians, the advocacy and educational organization of family medicine.

There are about 330 fellowships now available to graduating family medicine residents: faculty development, geriatrics, obstetrics, preventive medicine, research, rural medicine, sports medicine, and others such as occupational medicine.

If family physicians wish to retain their diplomate status, they must take at least fifty hours per year of medical education. After a family physician fulfills all educational and other requirements of the ABFM, that physician must then retake the certifying examination every seven years or the certification will lapse. This periodic retesting is required by the ABFM to make sure that family physicians keep up their medical education and maintain their knowledge level and clinical skills. Family medicine was the first specialty to require periodic reexamination of its physicians. In fact, since family medicine has mandated reexaminations, many other medical specialty organizations now require periodic reexamination of their members or are considering such a move. Many former general practitioners who did not have a chance to do a three-year family medicine residency took the ABFM certifying examination and became diplomates based on their years of practice experience and successful completion of the certifying examination. This option was closed to general practitioners in 1988.

A new recertification program, called the Maintenance of Certification Program for Family Physicians (MC-FP), is being required by the ABFM starting with diplomates who recertified in 2003 and all diplomates phased in by 2010. To maintain certification, candidates must perform the following every seven years: submit an online application, maintain a valid medical license, verify completion of three hundred credits of accepted CME credits, and pass the cognitive exam.

Currently, the American Academy of Family Physicians requires new active physician members to be residency-trained in family medicine. Diplomate status reflects only an educational effort by the physician and does not directly affect medical licensure. Medical licensure is based on a different testing mechanism, and license requirements vary from state to state. According to a 2012 report published by the Association of American Medical Colleges, there are more than one-hundred thousand family physicians providing health care in the United States. Family medicine residency programs are approximately 460 in number and usually have about three thousand residents in training.

Diagnostic and Treatment Techniques

Service to patients is the primary concern of family medicine and all those who practice, teach, administer, or foster the specialty. Of all the family physicians in practice, more than 80 percent are involved in direct patient care. While family physicians by no means constitute a majority of physicians, they are among the busiest when measured in terms of ambulatory patient visits. Family physicians see 30 percent of all ambulatory patients in the United States, which is more than the number of ambulatory visits to the next two specialty groups combined. Because of their training, family physicians can successfully care for more than 85 percent of all patient problems they encounter. Consultation with other specialty physicians is sought for the problems that are outside the scope of the family physician's knowledge or abilities.

This level of consultation is not unique to family physicians, as other specialty physicians find it necessary to seek consultation for 10 to 15 percent of their patients as well.

Family physicians can be found in all areas of the United States and in virtually all types of practice situations, providing a wide range of medical services. Family physicians can successfully practice in metropolitan areas or rural communities of one thousand people (or less), and they can be found teaching or doing research in medical colleges. Because of their training and the fact that they see a truly undifferentiated patient population, family physicians deliver a wide range of medical services. Besides seeing many patients in their offices, family physicians care for patients in nursing homes, make house calls, and admit patients to the hospital. Within the hospital, many family physicians care for patients in intensive care and other special care units and assist in surgery when their patients have operations. A small number perform extensive surgical procedures in the hospital setting. A sizable minority of family physicians take care of pregnant women and deliver their children; some of these physicians also perform cesarean sections. Because family physicians see anyone that walks through the door, it is not unheard of for a family physician to deliver a child in the morning, see the siblings in the office in the afternoon, and make a house call to the grandparents in the evening. Over 80 percent of family physicians perform dermatologic procedures, musculoskeletal injections, and electrocardiograms (EKGs) in their own offices.

The thing that makes family physicians different from other physicians is their attention to the physician-patient relationship. The family physician has first contact with the patient and is in a position to bond with the patient. The family physician evaluates the patient's complete health needs and provides personal care in one or more areas of medicine. Such care is not limited to any particular type of problem, be it biological, behavioral, or social, and the patients seen are not screened according to age, sex, or illness. The family physician utilizes knowledge of the patient's functioning in the family and community and maintains continuity of care for the patient in a hospital, clinic, or nursing home or in the patient's own home. Thus, in family medicine, the patient-physician relationship is initiated, established, and nurtured for both sexes, for all ages, and across time for many types of problems.

Because of their training, family physicians are highly sought-after care providers. Small rural communities, insurance companies, and government agencies at all levels actively seek family physicians to care for patients in a wide variety of settings. In this respect, family medicine is the most versatile medical specialty. Family physicians are able to practice and live in communities that are too small to support any other types of physician.

In two reports released by Merritt Hawkins, a national recruiting company, requests for family physicians surged by 55 percent, more than all other specialties. According to data from the Massachussetts Medical Society, community hospitals reported family physicians constituted their "most critical shortage."

While the vast majority of family physicians find themselves providing care for patients, there is a minority of family physicians who serve in other, equally important roles. Roughly 1.5 percent of family physicians serve as administrators and educators. They can be found working in state, federal, and local governments; in the insurance industry; and in residency programs and medical schools. Family physicians in residency programs provide instruction and role modeling for family medicine residents in community-based and university-based residency programs. Family physicians in medical colleges design, implement, administer, and evaluate educational programs for medical students during the four years of medical school. The Society of Teachers of Family Medicine (STFM) is the organization that supports family physicians in their teaching role.

One problem facing the specialty of family medicine is the very small percentage who are dedicated to research: only 0.2 percent of all family physicians. There is a large need for research in family medicine to determine the natural course of illnesses, how best to treat them, and the effects of illness on the functioning of the family unit. The need for research in the ambulatory setting is especially acute because, while most medical research is done in the hospital setting, most medical care in the United States is provided in clinics and offices. This problem will not be easily solved because of the service focus of family medicine training and the small number of family physicians dedicated to research.

Perspective and Prospects

Family medicine developed as a medical specialty because of the demands of the citizens of the United States; it is the only medical specialty with that claim. The ancestor of family medicine was general practice, and there is a direct link from the family physician to the general practitioner. Family medicine has grown and evolved into the specialty best suited to provide for the primary health care needs of most patients. Because of their broad scope of practice, cost-effective methods, and versatility, family physicians are found in virtually every type of medical and administrative setting. Family physicians provide a large portion of all ambulatory health care in the United States, and in some settings they are the sole providers of health care. General practice has been around as long as there have been physicians—Hippocrates was a general practitioner—but family medicine has a definite point of origin. It was created from general practice on February 8, 1969.

In January, 2000, a leadership team consisting of seven national family medicine organizations began the Future of Family Medicine (FMM) Project with its goal being "to develop a strategy to transform and renew the specialty of family medicine to meet the needs of patients in a changing health care environment." Six task forces were created as a result, with each one formed to address specific issues that aid in meeting the core needs of the people receiving care, the family physicians delivering that care, and shaping a quality health care delivery system. The FFM Leadership Committee has focused on improving the American health care system by implementing the following strategies:

taking steps to ensure that every American has a personal medical home, has health care coverage for basic services and protection against extraordinary health care costs, promoting the use and reporting of quality measures to improve performance and service, advancing research that supports the clinical decision making of family physicians, developing reimbursement models to sustain family medicine and primary care offices, and asserting family medicine's leadership to help transform the US health care system.

The present role of the family physician is and will continue to be to seek to improve the health of the people of the United States at all levels. Major problems exist for family medicine, including attrition as older family physicians retire or die, lack of medical student interest in family medicine as a career choice, and the lack of a solid cadre of researchers to advance medical knowledge in family medicine. The major strengths supporting family medicine are its service ethic, attention to the physician-patient relationship, and cost-effectiveness.

After their near demise as a recognizable group in the mid-twentieth century, family physicians have a number of reasons to expect that they will have expanded opportunities to provide for the health care needs of their patients in the future. As the United States, for example, examines its system of health care, which is the most costly and the least effective of any health care system in the developed world, many medical and political leaders look to generalism, and particularly family medicine, to provide answers. Research has shown that, for many medical problems, family physicians can provide outcomes very similar to those provided by specialists. When one couples that fact with the versatility and cost-effectiveness of generalist physicians, it can be argued that to save health care dollars the nation must reverse the 30 percent to 70 percent ratio of generalist to specialist physicians. A ratio of 50 percent to 50 percent generalist to specialist physicians has been proposed at many levels in medicine and government.

As the population ages due to improved mortality statistics and the addition of baby boomers to the geriatric age group, a further shortage of general practitioners such as family physicians is inevitable. This situation will force the United States to deal with its health care issues in order to provide its citizens with cost-effective and adequate coverage. The shortage of family physicians specifically in rural areas has led to approximately 65 million Americans living in federally designated health professions shortage areas (HPSAs), defined as less than 1 primary care physician per 3,500 people. A growing challenge exists for those physicians living in rural areas as a lack of training and preparation for practice in their medical education and residency training has led to a steady decline in their choosing to practice there.

—*Paul M. Paulman, M.D.;*
updated by Kenneth Dill, M.D.

See also African American health; Allergies; American Indian health; Anemia; Asian American health; Athlete's foot; Bacterial infections; Bronchitis; Bruises; Chickenpox; Childhood infectious diseases; Cholesterol; Common cold; Constipation; Coughing; Cytomegalovirus (CMV); Death and dying; Diarrhea and dysentery; Diagnosis; Digestion; Dizziness and fainting; Domestic violence; Ear infections and disorders; Exercise physiology; Eye infections and disorders; Fatigue; Fever; Fungal infections; Geriatrics and gerontology; Grief and guilt; Halitosis; Headaches; Healing; Heartburn; Hypercholesterolemia; Hyperlipidemia; Hypertension; Hypoglycemia; Indigestion; Infection; Inflammation; Influenza; Laryngitis; Measles; Men's health; Mercury poisoning; Mononucleosis; Mumps; Muscle sprains, spasms, and disorders; Nutrition; Obesity; Obesity, childhood; Osteopathic medicine; Over-the-counter medications; Pain; Pediatrics; Pharmacology; Pharmacy; Physical examination; Pneumonia; Poisonous plants; Preventive medicine; Psychology; Puberty and adolescence; Rashes; Rheumatic fever; Rubella; Scabies; Scarlet fever; Sciatica; Shingles; Shock; Signs and symptoms; Sinusitis; Sleep disorders; Sore throat; Strep throat; Stress; Telemedicine; Tetanus; Tonsillitis; Toxicology; Ulcers; Viral infections; Vitamins and minerals; Wheezing; Whooping cough; Women's health; Wounds.

For Further Information:

American Academy of Family Physicians. http://www.aafp.org.

American Board of Family Medicine. http://www .theabfm.org.

Behrman, Richard E., Robert M. Kliegman, and Hal B. Jenson, eds. *Nelson Textbook of Pediatrics.* 18th ed. Philadelphia: Saunders/Elsevier, 2007.

Lippman, Helen. "How Apps are Changing Family Medicine." *Journal of Family Practice* 62, no. 7 (July 2013): 362–367.

Rakel, Robert E., ed. *Essential Family Medicine: Fundamentals and Case Studies.* 3d ed. Philadelphia: Saunders/Elsevier, 2006.

Scherger, Joseph E., et al. "Responses to Questions by Medical Students About Family Practice." *Journal of Family Practice* 26, no. 2 (1988): 169-176.

Sloane, Philip D., et al., eds. *Essentials of Family Medicine.* 5th ed. Philadelphia: Lippincott Williams & Wilkins, 2008.

Tuggy, Michael, et al. "The 'Family' of Family Medicine." *Annals of Family Medicine* 11, no. 4 (July/August 2013): 385–386.

Woolley, Amanda. "Clinical Intuition in Family Medicine: More Than First Impressions." *Annals of Family Medicine* 11, no. 1 (January/February 2013): 60–66.oxy_options track_changes="on"?

FASCIA

Anatomy

Also known as: Connective tissue

Anatomy or system affected: All

Specialties and related fields: Exercise physiology, neurology, orthopedics, osteopathic medicine, physical therapy

Definition: A network of connective tissue that extends throughout the body. It functions as a shock absorber, a structural component of the body, and a medium that permits intracellular communication.

Key terms:

connective tissue: the tissue in the body that binds and supports body parts

parasympathetic nervous system: part of the autonomic nervous system that restores and conserves the body's resources

synovial: related to or producing synovial fluid; many of the body's joints have a sack of synovial fluid that surrounds the joint and provides lubrication

Structure and Functions

There are three layers of fascia: the superficial fascia, the deep fascia, and the visceral fascia. The superficial fascia, also known as the subcutaneous tissue, is a layer of adipose or fatty tissue that lies under the skin. The deep fascia is a layer of dense, fibrous tissue that lies under the superficial fascia, surrounding and penetrating the muscles, bones, nerves, body organs, and blood vessels. The deep fascia has extensions that stretch from the tendons that attach muscles to bone and lie in broad, flat sheets, called an aponeurosis. The deep fascia is so strong that it is rarely damaged, even in traumatic injuries. The visceral fascia surrounds the body organs, suspends them, and wraps them in a protective layer of connective tissue.

The superficial fascia has the capability of stretching to accommodate pregnancy and weight gain. Usually, it slowly reverts to its normal tension level after pregnancy or weight loss. The visceral fascia lacks the elastic properties of the superficial fascia, since its role is to protect the body organs. It provides for limited movement of the organs within their cavities, while not constricting the organs. The deep fascia contains many sensory receptors that are able to report pain and changes in body movement, in pressure and vibration within the body, in the chemicals produced by the body, and in body temperature.

The deep fascia contracts during the response to a threat, known as the "fight or flight" reflex. This increased tension increases the strength of it. The deep fascia relaxes at times when the body is stressed beyond what it can tolerate and when the body is put in a relaxing position. If the tension on the deep fascia persists, then it responds by adding collagen and other proteins, which bind to the existing proteins. While this increases the strength of the body, it can restrict the structures that it is supposed to protect. Hormones produced by the body can relax the deep fascia. For example, parasympathetic nervous system hormones can trigger its relaxation.

Disorders and Diseases

Due to the presence of fascia throughout the body, many conditions can be caused by its disorders. Some examples are adhesions, carpal tunnel syndrome, compartment syndrome, fibromyalgia, hernia, Marfan syndrome, meningitis, mixed connective tissue disease, myofascial pain syndrome, necrotizing fasciitis, pericardial effusion, plantar fasciitis, pleural effusion, polyarteritis nodosa, rheumatoid arthritis, scleroderma, and tendinitis.

Common conditions that affect the fascia are carpal tunnel syndrome, inguinal hernia, plantar fasciitis (heel spur), rheumatoid arthritis, and tendonitis. Carpal tunnel syndrome affects a small opening through the wrist into the hand. The median nerve and the carpal ligament pass through this opening. Narrowing of the opening pinches these structures and causes pain and numbness in the hand. The treatment includes physical therapy, wrist splints, and possibly surgery. An inguinal hernia is the protrusion of part of the bowel through an opening in the fascia. It protrudes through the openings in the abdominal aponeurosis for the two saphenous veins. Inguinal hernias are treated by surgery to support the aponeurosis in the area of these openings.

Plantar fasciitis is caused by chronic inflammation of the fascia that supports the arch of the foot, leading to calcification on the bottom of the heel. This condition is treated with orthotics or surgery. Rheumatoid arthritis is an autoimmune condition that affects symmetric joints in the body and causes chronic inflammation of the synovial membranes in the joints, leading to joint damage. Many medications are available to treat rheumatoid arthritis, but they suppress the immune response of the body and so have risks. Tendinitis is inflammation of a tendon, often as a result of injury or repetitive use, such as tennis elbow. This condition is treated with corticosteroid injections into the joint, the application of ice or heat, and rest.

Perspective and Prospects

The importance of the fascia has been embraced by practitioners other than doctors of traditional medicine. The fascia forms the basis for therapies such as Rolfing, massage, chiropractic, physical therapy, osteopathy, yoga, and Tai Chi Chuan. In the late 1800s, Sweden's Pehr Henrik Ling, with his associates, wrote of the relationship of mind and body. His therapy was aimed at improving the mental status of a person by improving their ability to move their body. In 1984, Raymond Nimmo wrote of the importance of treating the fascia, as well as trigger points in the body.

Ida P. Rolf (1896–1979) was a notable pioneer in the understanding of the importance of the body fascia. Rolf felt that the fascia had been largely ignored by the medical community and developed a technique centered on structural integrity and the importance of gravity. Structural integrity deals with the property of the fascia that causes it to adapt to changes in the body, even when the change puts the body off balance, out of alignment, or causes pain. Rolf devoted much of her life to treating those disabled who had not responded to medical treatment. Her therapy is called Rolfing.

Medical doctors specializing in exercise physiology, neurology, and orthopedics are becoming more cognizant of the role of the fascia in the body. However, chiropractors continue to hold the primary role in dealing with problems of the fascia that do not respond to medical treatment. In 2007, the first International Fascia Research Congress was held in Boston, Massachusetts.

—*Christine M. Carroll, R.N., B.S.N., M.B.A.*

See also Carpal tunnel syndrome; Chiropractic; Connective tissue; Hernia; Rheumatoid arthritis; Stress; Tendinitis; Tendons.

For Further Information:

"Bones, Joints, and Muscles." *MedlinePlus*, December 5, 2011.

"Carpal Tunnel Syndrome." *MedlinePlus*, April 19, 2013.

Chwistek, Marcin. "Rheumatoid Arthritis." *Health Library*, September 30, 2012.

Leach, Robert E., and Teresa Briedwell. "Tendinopathy." *Health Library*, March 18, 2013.

Lindsay, Mark. *Fascia: Clinical Applications for Health and Human Performance*. Clifton Park, N.Y.: Delmar Cengage Learning, 2008.

Paoletti, Serge. *The Fasciae: Anatomy, Dysfunction, and Treatment*. Lisbon, Maine: Eastland Press, 2006.

Scholten, Amy, and Peter Lucas. "Groin Hernia—Adult." *Health Library*, March 18, 2013.

Schultz, R. Louis, and Rosemary Feltis. *The Endless Web: Fascial Anatomy and Physical Reality*. Berkeley, Calif.: North Atlantic Books, 1996.

Vorvick, Linda J., C. Benjamin Ma, and David Zieve. "Plantar Fasciitis." *MedlinePlus*, March 1, 2012.

FATIGUE

Disease/Disorder

Anatomy or system affected: All

Specialties and related fields: Family medicine, geriatrics and gerontology, internal medicine, psychiatry

Definition: A general symptom of tiredness, malaise, depression, and sometimes anxiety associated with many diseases and disorders; in some cases, no specific cause can be found.

Key terms:

physical deconditioning: a condition that results when a person who has previously been exercising (has become conditioned) stops exercising

psychogenic fatigue: fatigue caused by mental factors, such as anxiety, and not attributable to any physical cause

sleep apnea: cessation of breathing during sleep, which may result from either an inhibition of the respiratory center (central apnea) or an obstruction to the flow of air (obstructive apnea)

sleep disorders: conditions resulting in sleep interruption, interfering with the restorative functions of sleep

syndrome: a collection of complaints (symptoms) and signs (abnormal findings on clinical examination) that do not match any specific disease

Causes and Symptoms

Almost all people suffer from fatigue at some point in their lives. It is a nonspecific complaint including tiredness, lack of energy, listlessness, or malaise. Patients often confuse fatigue with weakness, breathlessness, or dizziness, which indicate the existence of other physical disorders. Rest or a change in the daily routine ordinarily alleviates fatigue in healthy individuals. Though normally short in duration, fatigue occasionally lasts for weeks, months, or even years in some individuals. In such cases, it limits the amount of physical and mental activity in which the person can participate.

Long-term fatigue can have serious consequences. Often, patients begin to withdraw from their normal activities. They may withdraw from society in general and may gradually become more apathetic and depressed. As a result of this progression, a patient's physical and mental capabilities may begin to deteriorate. Fatigue may be aggravated further by a reduced appetite and inadequate nutritional intake. Ultimately, these symptoms lead to malnutrition and multiple vitamin deficiencies, which intensify the fatigue state and

---

Information on Fatigue

Causes: Disease, depression, sleep disorders, physical and/or mental overactivity, excessive intake of stimulants, medications

Symptoms: Tiredness, malaise, depression, anxiety, withdrawal

Duration: Typically short-term but can be chronic

Treatments: Rest and relaxation, medications, counseling

---

trigger a vicious circle.

This fatigue cycle ends with a person who lacks interest and energy. Such patients may lose interest in daily events and social contacts. In later stages of fatigue, they may neglect themselves and lose track of their goals in life. The will to live and fight decreases, making them prime targets for accidents and repeated infections. They may also become potential candidates for suicide.

Physical and/or mental overactivity commonly cause recent-onset fatigue. Management of such fatigue is simple: Adequate physical and mental relaxation typically relieve it. Fortunately, many persistent fatigue states can be easily diagnosed and successfully treated. In some cases, however, fatigue does not respond to simple measures.

Fatigue can stem from depression. Depressed individuals often reflect boredom and a lack of interest, and frequently express uncertainty and anxiety about the future. These people usually appear "down." They may walk slowly with their head down, slump their shoulders, and sigh frequently. They often take unusually long to respond to questions or requests. They also show little motivation. Depressed individuals typically relate feelings of dejection, sadness, worthlessness, or helplessness. Often, they complain of feeling tired when they wake up in the morning, and no amount of sleep or rest improves their condition. In fact, they feel weary all day and frequently complain of feeling weak. They often have poor appetites and sometimes lose weight. Once these patients are questioned by a physician, however, it may become apparent that their state of fatigue actually fluctuates. At times they feel exhausted, while at other times (sometimes only minutes later) they feel refreshed and full of energy.

Other manifestations of depression include sleep disorders (particularly early morning waking), reduced appetite, altered bowel habits, and difficulty concentrating. Depressed individuals sometimes fail to recognize their condition. They may channel their depression into physical complaints such as abdominal pain, headaches, joint pain, or vaguely defined aches and pains. In older people, depression sometimes manifests itself as impaired memory.

Anxiety, another major cause of fatigue, interferes with the patient's ability to achieve adequate mental and physical rest. Anxious individuals often appear scared, worried, or fearful. They frequently report multiple physical complaints, including neck muscle tension, headaches, palpitations, difficulty in breathing, chest tightness, intestinal cramping, and trouble

falling asleep. In some cases, both depression and anxiety may be present simultaneously.

Medications also constitute a major cause of fatigue. Most drugs—prescription, over-the-counter, or recreational—can cause fatigue. Medications for sleep, antidepressants, antianxiety medications, muscle relaxants, allergy medications, cold medications, and certain blood pressure medications can lead to problems with fatigue.

An excessive intake of stimulants, paradoxically, sometimes leads to easy fatigability. Stimulants can interfere with proper sleeping habits and relaxation. Common culprits include caffeine and medications (such as some diet pills and nasal decongestants) that can be purchased without a prescription. Recreational drugs can also contribute to chronic fatigue. Depending on their tendencies, they function to cause fatigue in much the same way as the prescription and over-the-counter drugs already discussed. Cocaine and amphetamines, for example, act as stimulants. Narcotics such as heroin and barbiturates (downers) possess strong sedative qualities. Alcohol consumption in an attempt to escape loneliness, depression, or boredom may further exacerbate a sense of fatigue. Alcohol produces fatigue in two ways. It has sedative qualities, and it also intensifies the sedative effects of other medications, if taken with them.

Other drugs that may induce fatigue include diuretics and those that lower blood pressure. These medications increase the excretions of many substances through the kidneys. If inappropriately given or regulated, these drugs may alter the blood concentration of other medications taken concurrently.

Painkillers can lead to fatigue in a different way. In some individuals, they irritate the lining of the stomach and cause it to bleed. Such bleeding usually occurs in small amounts and goes unnoticed by the patient. This slight blood loss can gradually lead to anemia and fatigue.

Medications are particularly likely to cause fatigue in elderly individuals. With many drugs, their elimination from the body through metabolism or excretion may decrease with age. This often leads to higher drug concentrations in the blood than intended, resulting in a state of constant sedation and lethargy. Also, elderly individuals" brains may be more sensitive to sedation than those of younger individuals. Finally, the elderly tend to take more medication for more illnesses than younger adults. The additive side effects of multiple medicines can contribute to fatigue problems.

Sleep deprivation or frequent sleep interruptions lead to fatigue. A change in environment can induce sleep disorders, especially if accompanied by unfamiliar noises, excessive lighting, uncomfortable temperatures, or an excessive degree of humidity or dryness. Total sleep time may be adequate under such conditions, but quality of sleep is usually poor. Nightmares can also interrupt sleep, and if numerous and recurring, they also cause fatigue.

Some sleep interruptions are not so readily apparent. In sleep apnea, a specific and increasingly diagnosed sleep disorder, the patient temporarily stops breathing while sleeping. This results in reduced oxygen levels and increased carbon dioxide levels in the blood. When a critical level is reached, the patient awakens briefly, takes a few deep breaths, and then falls asleep again. Many episodes of sleep apnea may occur during the night, making the sleep interrupted and less refreshing than it should be. The next day, the patient often feels tired and fatigued but may not recognize the source of the problem. Obstructive sleep apnea normally develops in grossly overweight patients or in those with large tonsils or adenoids. Patients with obstructive sleep apnea usually snore while sleeping, and typically they are unaware of their snoring and sleep disturbance.

A number of diseases can lead to easy fatigability. In most illnesses, rest relieves fatigue and individuals awake refreshed after a nap or a good night's sleep. Unfortunately, they also tire quickly. Unlike psychogenic fatigue or fatigue induced by drugs, disease-related fatigue is not usually the patient's main symptom. Other symptoms and signs frequently reveal the underlying diagnosis. Individuals who suffer from severe malnutrition, anemia, endocrine system malfunction, chronic infections, tuberculosis, Lyme disease, bacterial endocarditis (a bacterial infection of the valves of the heart), chronic sinusitis, mononucleosis, hepatitis, parasitic infections, and fungal infections may all experience chronic fatigue.

In early stages of acquired immunodeficiency syndrome (AIDS), fatigue may be the only symptom. Persons at high risk for contracting the human immunodeficiency virus (HIV)—those with multiple sexual partners, those who have unprotected sex, those with a history of blood transfusion, or intravenous drug users—who complain of persistent fatigue should be tested for HIV infection.

Abnormalities of mineral or electrolyte concentrations—potassium, sodium, chloride, and calcium are the most important of these—may also cause fatigue. Such abnormalities may result from medications (diuretics are frequently responsible), diarrhea, vomiting, dietary fads, and endocrine or bone disorders.

Some less common medical causes of chronic fatigue include dysfunction of specific organs such as kidney failure or liver failure. Allergies can also produce chronic fatigue. Cancer can cause fatigue, but other symptoms usually surface and lead to a diagnosis before the patient begins to notice chronic weariness.

Treatment and Therapy

When an individual's fatigue persists in spite of adequate rest, medical help becomes necessary in order to determine the cause. Common diseases known to be associated with fatigue should be considered. Initially, the physician makes detailed inquiries about the severity of the fatigue and how long ago it started. Other important questions include whether it is progressive, whether there are any factors that make it worse or relieve it, or whether it is worse during specific times of the day. An examination of the patient's psychological state may also be necessary.

The physician should ask about the presence of any symptoms that occur along with the general sense of fatigue. For example, breathlessness may indicate a cardiovascular or respiratory disease. Abdominal pain might arouse the suspicion of a gastrointestinal disease. Weakness may point to a neuromuscular collagen disease. Excessive thirst and increased urine output may suggest diabetes mellitus, and weight loss may accompany metabolic or endocrinal abnormalities, chronic infections, or cancer.

Whether they have been prescribed by a physician or purchased over the counter, the medications taken regularly by a patient should be reviewed. The doctor should also inquire about alcohol and tobacco use and dietary fads. A thorough physical examination may be required. During an examination, the doctor sometimes uncovers physical signs of fatigue-inducing diseases. Blood tests and other laboratory investigations may also be needed, especially because a physical examination does not always reveal the cause.

Often, however, despite an extensive workup, no specific cause for the persistent fatigue appears. At this stage, the diagnosis of chronic fatigue syndrome should be considered. To fit this diagnosis, patients must have several of the symptoms associated with this syndrome. They must have complained of fatigue for at least six months, and the fatigue should be of such an extent that it interferes with normal daily activities. Since many of the symptoms associated with chronic fatigue syndrome overlap with other disorders, these other fatigue-inducing conditions must be considered and ruled out.

To fit the diagnosis of chronic fatigue syndrome, patients must have at least six of the classic symptoms. These include a mild fever and sore throat, painful lymph nodes in the neck or axilla, unexplained generalized weakness, and muscle pain or discomfort. Patients may describe marked fatigue lasting for more than twenty-four hours that is induced by levels of exercise that would have been easily tolerated before the onset of fatigue. They may suffer from generalized headaches of a type, severity, or pattern that is different from headaches experienced before the onset of chronic fatigue. Patients may also have joint pain without swelling or redness and neuropsychologic complaints such as a bad memory and excessive irritability. Confusion, difficulty in thinking, inability to concentrate, depression, and sleep disturbances are also on the list of associated symptoms.

No one knows the exact cause of chronic fatigue syndrome. Researchers continue to study the disease and come up with hypotheses, though none have proven entirely satisfactory. One theory argues that since patients with chronic fatigue syndrome appear to have a reduced aerobic work capacity, defects in the muscles may cause the condition. This, however, constitutes only one of many theories concerning the syndrome and its origin.

Many patients with chronic fatigue syndrome relate that they suffered from an infectious illness immediately preceding the onset of fatigue. This pattern causes some scientists to suspect a viral origin. Typically, the illness that precedes the patient's problems with fatigue is not severe, and resembles other upper respiratory tract infections experienced previously. The implicated viruses include the Epstein-Barr virus, Coxsackie B virus, herpes simplex virus, cytomegalovirus, human herpesvirus 6, and the measles virus. It should be mentioned, however, that some patients with long-term fatigue do not have a history of a triggering infectious disease before the onset of fatigue.

Patients with chronic fatigue syndrome sometimes have a number of immune system abnormalities. Laboratory evidence exists of immune dysfunction in many patients with this syndrome, and there have been reports of improvement when immunoglobulin (antibody) therapy was given. The significance of immunological abnormalities in chronic fatigue syndrome, however, remains uncertain. Most of these abnormalities do not occur in all patients with this syndrome. Furthermore, the degree of immunologic abnormality does not always correspond with the severity of the symptoms.

Some researchers believe that the acute infectious disease that often precedes the onset of chronic fatigue syndrome forces the patient to become physically inactive. This inactivity leads to physical deconditioning, and the progression ends in chronic fatigue syndrome. Experiments in which patients with chronic fatigue syndrome were given exercise testing, however, do not support this theory completely. In the case of physical deconditioning, the heart rates of patients with chronic fatigue syndrome should have risen more rapidly with exercise than those without the syndrome. The exact opposite was found. The data were not determined consistent with the suggestion that physical deconditioning causes chronic fatigue syndrome.

A high prevalence of unrecognized psychiatric disorders exists in patients with chronic fatigue, especially depression. Depression affects approximately half of chronic fatigue syndrome patients and precedes other symptoms in about half of them as well. Yet a critical question remains unanswered concerning chronic fatigue syndrome: Are patients with this syndrome fatigued because they have a primary mood disorder, or has the mood disorder developed as a secondary component of the chronic fatigue syndrome?

No completely satisfactory treatment exists for chronic fatigue syndrome. A group of researchers using intravenous immunoglobulin therapy met with varying degrees of success, but other investigators could not reproduce these results. Other therapeutic trials used high doses of medications such as acyclovir, liver extract, folic acid, and cyanocobalamine. A mixture of evening primrose oil and fish oil was also administered with some degree of success. Claims have also been made that patients administered magnesium sulfate improved to a larger extent than those receiving a placebo. Other therapeutic options include cognitive behavioral therapy, programs of gradually increasing physical activity, analgesics, nonsteroidal anti-inflammatory drugs (NSAIDs), and antidepressants. Finally, a number of self-help groups exist for chronic fatigue sufferers.

The prognosis and natural history of chronic fatigue syndrome are still poorly defined. Chronic fatigue syndrome does not kill patients, but it does significantly decrease the quality of life for sufferers. For the physician, management of this syndrome remains challenging. In addition to correcting any physical abnormalities present, the physician should attempt to find an activity that interests the patient and encourage him or her to become involved in it.

Perspective and Prospects

Fatigue is generally considered a normal bodily response, protecting the individual from excessive physical and mental activity. After all, the normal levels of performance for individuals who do not rest usually decline. In the case of overactivity, fatigue should be viewed as a positive warning sign. Using relaxation and rest (both mental and physical), the individual can often alleviate weariness and optimize performance.

In some cases, however, fatigue does not derive from physical or mental overactivity, nor does it respond adequately to relaxation and rest. In these instances, it interferes with an individual's ability to cope with everyday life and enjoy usual activities. The patient begins referring to fatigue as the reason for not participating in normal physical, mental, and social activities.

Unfortunately, physicians, health care professionals, society, and even the patients themselves dismiss fatigue as a trivial complaint. As a result, sufferers seek medical help only after the condition becomes advanced. This dangerous, negative attitude can delay the correct diagnosis of the underlying pathology and threaten the patient's chances for a quick recovery.

The diagnosis and management of chronic fatigue syndrome prove challenging for both physician and patient. It is important to note that chronic fatigue syndrome often stems from nonmedical causes. While the possibility of a serious medical illness should be addressed, illness-related fatigue usually occurs along with other, more prominent symptoms. The causes of chronic fatigue syndrome are numerous and can take time to define. Patients need to answer all questions related to their complaints as thoroughly and accurately as possible, so that their physicians can reach accurate diagnoses using the minimum number of tests. Extensive testing for rare medical causes of fatigue can become extraordinarily expensive and uncomfortable, so doctors select the tests that they are ordering cautiously. They must balance the benefit, the cost, and the risk of each test to the patient. Such decisions should be based on their own experience and on the available data.

Open communication between the patient and doctor is of paramount importance. It ensures a correct diagnosis, followed by the most effective treatment. Follow-up visits and reassurance may be the best therapy in many cases. Professional counselors can offer assistance with fatigue-inducing psychological disorders. Examination of sleep and relaxation habits can reveal potential problems, and steps can be taken to ensure adequate rest.

Persistent fatigue should not be regarded lightly, and serious attempts should be made to determine its underlying causes. In this respect, it may be appropriate to recall one of Hippocrates" aphorisms, "Unprovoked fatigue means disease."

—*Ronald C. Hamdy, M.D., Mark R. Doman, M.D., and*
Katherine Hoffman Doman

See also Aging; Anemia; Anxiety; Apnea; Chronic fatigue syndrome; Depression; Dizziness and fainting; Epstein-Barr virus; Fibromyalgia; Malnutrition; Multiple chemical sensitivity syndrome; Narcolepsy; Overtraining syndrome; Sleep; Sleep disorders; Sleeping sickness; Stress; Stress reduction.

For Further Information:

Archer, James, Jr. *Managing Anxiety and Stress.* 2d ed. New York: Routledge, 1991. Print.

Clever, Linda Hawes, and Dean Omish. *The Fatigue Perscription: Four Steps to Renewing Your Energy, Health, and Life.* Berkeley: Cleis, 2010. Print.

DePaulo, J. Raymond, Jr., and Leslie Ann Horvitz. *Understanding Depression: What We Know and What You Can Do About It.* New York: Wiley, 2003. Print.

Feiden, Karyn. *Hope and Help for Chronic Fatigue Syndrome: The Official Guide of the CFS-CFIDS Network.* New York: Prentice, 1990. Print.

Goroll, Allan H., and Albert G. Mulley, eds. *Primary Care Medicine.* 5th ed. Philadelphia: Wilkins, 2006. Print.

Patarca-Montero, Roberto. *Chronic Fatigue Syndrome and the Body's Immune Defense System.* New York: Haworth, 2002. Print.

Poppe, Carine, et al. "Cognitive Behavior Therapy in patients with Chronic fatigue Syndrome: The Role of Illness Acceptance and Neuroticism." *Journal of Psychosomatic Research* 74.5 (2013): 367–72. Print.

Smith, Howard S. *Handbook of Fatigue in Health and Disease.* New York: Nova, 2011. Print.

Talley, Joseph. *Family Practitioner's Guide to Treating Depressive Illness.* Chicago: Precept, 1987. Print.

Wilson, James L. *Adrenal Fatigue: The Twenty-first Century Stress Syndrome.* Petaluma: Smart, 2004. Print.

Zgourides, George D., and Christie Zgourides. *Stop Feeling Tired! Ten Mind-Body Steps to Fight Fatigue and Feel Your Best.* Oakland: Harbinger, 2003. Print.

FATTY ACID OXIDATION DISORDERS
Disease/Disorder

Anatomy or system affected: Heart, liver, muscles
Specialties and related fields: Biochemistry, biotechnology, nutrition, pediatrics, perinatology
Definition: Inherited metabolic defects that prevent the breakdown of fatty acids in the liver, muscles, and heart.

Causes and Symptoms

Fatty acid oxidation disorders are inherited defects in the enzymes that break down fatty acids to generate metabolic energy. Defects in at least eleven of the twenty enzymes involved with this process have been identified and can be diagnosed by enzymatic analysis of a tissue biopsy. Some generate unique profiles of metabolites in the blood or urine that can be used for diagnosis. These disorders are inherited as autosomal recessive traits, and, in many cases, the causative deoxyribonucleic acid (DNA) mutations have been determined. Fatty acid oxidation disorders can affect the liver, which breaks down fatty acids for its own needs and, by converting them to ketone bodies, for energy generation in other body tissues; they can also affect muscles and the heart, which use fatty acids as a source of energy.

Symptoms appear only under fasting conditions, either overnight or when exacerbated by infection or fever. Under

---

> ## Information on
> ## Fatty Acid Oxidation Disorders
>
> **Causes:** Genetic enzyme deficiency
> **Symptoms:** Only under fasting conditions (overnight or when exacerbated by infection or fever), vomiting, coma, and sometimes death; some disorders largely asymptomatic
> **Duration:** Chronic with acute episodes
> **Treatments:** Minimizing of fasting (snacking before sleep), intravenous glucose for acute episodes

these conditions, as glycogen stores are depleted, the body depends increasingly on fatty acids for energy. If fatty acids cannot be broken down completely, an energy deficit and the accumulation of deleterious intermediates lead to vomiting, coma, and, in severe cases, death. The levels of blood glucose are low because the energy needed for its synthesis is lacking. The first episode may occur in the first two years of life; such an episode can be fatal and may be mistakenly attributed to sudden infant death syndrome (SIDS). Some fatty acid oxidation disorders, however, are largely asymptomatic.

Treatment and Therapy

The general treatment for fatty acid oxidation disorders is to minimize fasting, as by snacking before sleep, and, in acute episodes, to administer intravenous glucose. This treatment restores depleted blood glucose and reduces the demand for fatty acid oxidation. Some defects also benefit from a low intake of dietary fat. Fasting or low carbohydrate diets, for weight loss or other reasons, are contraindicated for individuals with these disorders.

One of these diseases is attributable to the defective cellular uptake of carnitine, which is needed to transport fatty acids into mitochondria, where they are oxidized; this type can be treated with supplemental carnitine. In acute episodes with some other disorders, treatment with carnitine has proven beneficial in increasing the urinary excretion of deleterious intermediates.

Perspective and Prospects

The first observation of a defect in fatty acid oxidation was made in 1972. Although not reported until 1982, one such disorder, medium-chain acyl-coenzyme A dehydrogenase (MCAD) deficiency, is among the most common inborn errors of metabolism, with a frequency of 1 in 9,000 live births. Each disorder of fatty acid oxidation is a candidate for enzyme replacement therapy or gene replacement therapy, although these remain experimental treatments.

—James L. Robinson, Ph.D.

See also Enzyme therapy; Enzymes; Food biochemistry; Glycogen storage diseases; Metabolic disorders; Metabolism.

For Further Information:

Devlin, Thomas M., ed. *Textbook of Biochemistry: With Clinical Correlations.* 7th ed. Hoboken, N.J.: Wiley-Liss, 2011.

Hay, William W., Jr., et al., eds. *Current Diagnosis and Treatment in*

Pediatrics. 21st ed. New York: Lange Medical Books/McGraw-Hill, 2012.

"Medium-Chain Acyl-CoA Dehydrogenase Deficiency." *Genetics Home Reference*, May 13, 2013.

Roe, C. R., and J. Ding. "Mitochondrial Fatty Acid Oxidation Disorders." In *The Metabolic and Molecular Bases of Inherited Disease*, edited by Charles R. Scriver et al. 8th ed. New York: McGraw-Hill, 2001.

Sanders, Lee M. "Disorders of Lipid Metabolism." *Merck Manual Home Health Handbook*, Feb. 2009.

FEET

Anatomy

Anatomy or system affected: Bones, musculoskeletal system

Specialties and related fields: Orthopedics, podiatry

Definition: The lowest extremities, composed of a complex system of muscles and bones, that act as levers to propel the body and that must support the weight of the body in standing, walking, or running.

Key terms:

distal: referring to a particular body part that is farther from the point of attachment or farther from the trunk than another part

extension: movement that increases the angle between the bones, causing them to move farther apart; straightening or extension of the ankle occurs when the toes point away from the shin

flexion: a bending movement that decreases the angle of the joint and brings two bones closer together; flexion of the ankle pulls the foot closer to the shin

hallucis: a term referring to the big toe; the flexor hallucis longus is a muscle that flexes the big toe

inferior: situated below another part; the ankle bones are inferior to the bones of the lower leg

lateral: toward the side with respect to the body's imaginary midline; away from the midline of the body, a limb, or any understood point of reference

medial: closer to an imaginary midline dividing the body into equal right and left halves than another part

plantar: having to do with the sole of the foot (for example, a plantar wart)

podiatry: the branch of medicine that deals with the study, examination, diagnosis, treatment, and prevention of diseases and malfunctions of the foot

proximal: referring to a particular body part that is closer to a point of attachment than another part

superior: above another part or closer to the head; the ankle bones are superior to the bones of the feet

Structure and Functions

The anatomy of the foot is very similar to that of the hand; however, the foot is adapted to perform very different functions. The human hand has the ability to perform fine movements such as grasping and writing, while the foot is involved mainly in support and movement. Therefore, the bones and muscles of the foot tend to be heavier and function without the same dexterity as the hand.

The twenty-six bones of the foot include the tarsals, meta-tarsals, and phalanges. The proximal portion of the foot next to the ankle is composed of seven tarsal bones: the calcaneus, talus, navicular, cuboid, medial cuneiform, intermediate cuneiform, and lateral cuneiform. The bones are rather irregular in shape and form gliding joints; these joints allow only a limited movement when compared to other joints in the body. The calcaneus forms the large heel bone, which serves as a major attachment for the muscles that are located in the back of the lower leg. Just above the calcaneus is another large foot bone called the talus. The talus rests between the tibia and the fibula, the two lower leg bones. Interestingly, the talus is the single bone that receives the entire weight of the body when an individual is standing; it must then transmit this weight to the rest of the foot below. The cuboid and the three cuneiform bones meet the proximal end of the long foot bones, the metatarsals.

The five separate metatarsal bones are relatively long and thin when compared to the tarsal bones. Anatomists distinguish between the five metatarsals by number. If one begins numbering from the medial (or inside) part of the foot, that metatarsal is number one and the lateral (or outside) metatarsal is number five. The distal portion of each metatarsal articulates (meets) with the toe bones, or phalanges.

Humans have toes that are very similar to their fingers. In fact, the numbers and names of the toe and finger bones, phalanges, are identical. The major differences lie in the fact that the finger phalanges are longer than the phalanges that make up toes. Hinge joints are located between each phalanx and allow for flexion and extension movements only. Human toes (or fingers) are made up of fourteen different phalanges. Each toe (or finger) has three phalanges except for the big toe (or thumb), which has only two. The toes are named in a similar way as the metatarsals; that is, the big toe is number one and the little toe is number five. The three phalanges that make up each toe (except for the big toe) are named according to location. The phalanx meeting the metatarsal is referred to as the proximal phalanx. The bone at the tip of the toe is the distal phalanx, and the one in between is the middle phalanx. Since the big toe only has two phalanges, they are called proximal and distal phalanges.

Although it seems that there is only a single arch in each foot, podiatrists and anatomists identify three arches: the medial and lateral longitudinal arches and the transverse, or metatarsal, arch. The medial longitudinal arch, as the name implies, is located on the medial surface of the foot and follows the long axis from the calcaneus to the big toe. Likewise, the lateral longitudinal arch is on the lateral surface and runs from the heel to the little toe. The transverse, or metatarsal, arch crosses the width of the foot near the proximal end of the metatarsals. The bones are only one factor that maintains arches in the feet and prevents them from flattening under the weight of the body. Ligaments (which connect bones), muscles, and tendons (which attach muscles to bones) are primarily responsible for the support of the arches. The arches function to distribute body weight between the calcaneus and the distal end of the metatarsals (the balls of the feet). They also are flexible enough to absorb some of the shock to the feet from walking, running, and jumping.

While the feet seem to be composed of only bones, tendons, and ligaments, the movements of the toes and feet require an extensive system of muscles. Most of the larger muscles that act on the foot and toes are actually located in the lower leg. Anatomists divide these muscles into separate compartments: anterior, posterior, and lateral.

The muscles of the anterior compartment move the foot upward (dorsiflex) and extend the toes. These muscles include the tibialis anterior, extensor digitorum longus, extensor hallucis longus, and peroneus tertius. The tibialis anterior is attached to the top of the first metatarsal and pulls the medial part of the foot upward and slightly lateral. All of the toes except the big toe are pulled up (extended) by the extensor digitorum longus. The extensor hallucis longus moves only the big toe upward, while the peroneus tertius is attached to the fifth metatarsal and moves the foot upward.

The muscles of the lateral compartment act to move the foot in a lateral or outward direction. The peroneus longus and peroneus brevis are attached to the first and fifth metatarsal, respectively. Using these attachments, the muscles can pull the foot laterally.

The muscles of the posterior compartment are the largest group and act to flex the foot and toes. All of these muscles share a common tendon, the calcaneus (or Achilles) tendon. As the name suggests, this large tendon attaches to the calcaneus bone. The larger, more superficial muscles include the gastrocnemius, soleus, and plantaris; these powerful muscles are commonly called the calf muscles. Also in the posterior compartment are four smaller muscles located beneath the calf muscles: the popliteus (located directly behind the knee joint), flexor hallucis longus, flexor digitorum longus, and tibialis posterior. The popliteus rotates the lower leg medially. The flexor hallucis longus flexes the big toe. The remaining toes are flexed by the flexor digitorum longus, while the tibialis posterior acts opposite the tibialis anterior to flex the foot.

Within the foot itself are some muscles known as the intrinsic foot muscles. All but one of these muscles are located on the bottom surface of the foot. This one muscle extends all of the toes except the little toe. The remaining intrinsic muscles are on the plantar (bottom) surface and serve to flex the toes.

The major vessels that provide blood to the foot include branches from the anterior tibial artery. This relatively large artery is located along the anterior surface of the lower leg and branches into the dorsalis pedis artery, which serves the ankle and upper part of the foot. Physicians often check for a pulse in this foot artery to provide information about circulation to the foot and circulation in general, as this is the point farthest from the heart. The bottom parts of the feet are supplied with blood by branches of the peroneal artery. At the ankle, this artery branches into plantar arteries, which supply the structures on the sole of the foot. The human toes receive most of their blood from branches of the plantar arteries called the digital arteries.

Disorders and Diseases

Even though the anatomy of the foot is resistant to the

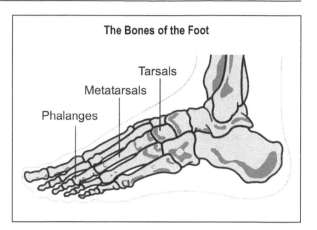

The Bones of the Foot

Phalanges
Metatarsals
Tarsals

tremendous amount of force that the body places on it, it can be injured. Force injuries to the foot commonly result in fractures or breaks of the metatarsals and phalanges. Occasionally, the calcaneus may fracture from a fall on a hard surface. More commonly, patients complain of painful heel syndrome.

Because the shock-absorbing pads of tissue on the heel become thinner with age, repeated pressure on the heel can cause pain. Prolonged standing, walking, or running can add to the pressure, as can being overweight. One cause of pain is plantar fasciitis, an inflammation of the tough band of connective tissue on the sole. The inflammation occurs when the muscles located on the back of the lower leg that are attached to the connective tissue at the calcaneus pull under stress. This may even be associated with small fractures. X-rays may show small spurs of bone near the site of stress; however, these spurs are not believed to be the cause of pain.

Deformities of the foot at birth are fairly common and include clubfoot, flat foot, and clawfoot. The cause of these anomalies is abnormal development. The foot of the fetus normally goes through stages where it is turned outward and inward but gradually assumes a normal position by about the seventh month of gestation. In the case of clubfoot, arrested development in the stage when the foot is turned inward causes the muscles, bones, and joints to develop in this abnormal anatomical position. At the time of birth, the deformity is readily observable and the foot immobile. Treatment includes splints, casting, and surgery. If treatment is begun at birth, the foot may look relatively normal after approximately one year.

Almost everyone is born with feet that are flat because the arches do not begin to develop until the ligaments and muscles function normally. In most people, the arches are fully formed by the age of six. In some individuals, however, the ligaments and muscles remain weak and the feet do not develop a normal arch. Flat feet can also develop in adult life, at which time they are called "fallen arches." Body weight moves along a precise path during walking or running, beginning with the heel touching the ground. Then, as the foot steps, the arch receives the forces pushing down on the foot. Because the bones, muscles, and ligaments form an arch in the foot, the arch can deform slightly and absorb some of the downward force. With further movement, the weight passes to the ball of the foot (the distal metatarsals). A fallen arch has lost this flexibility and shock-absorbing capability. The arch "falls" because of improper weight distribution along the foot, causing the arch to stretch excessively and to weaken with time. Without proper arch support, the foot begins to twist inward, or medially, causing the body weight to be transmitted to the inside of the foot rather than in a straight line toward the toes. This problem often occurs in runners who have improperly fitted shoes or a poor running style (although anyone can suffer from fallen longitudinal arches, regardless of the individual's level of physical activity). As a runner increases distance and speed without correcting his or her shoes or running form, the force applied to the feet increases. Fallen arches appear to occur particularly in runners or joggers who exercise on hard surfaces without proper technique or arch support.

A number of disorders can affect the skin of the foot. Corns are small areas of thickened skin on a toe that are usually caused by tight-fitting shoes. People with high arches are affected most because the arch increases the pressure applied to the toes during walking. If the corn becomes painful, the easiest treatment is for the person to wear better-fitting shoes. If the pain persists, a clinician can pare down the growth with a scalpel.

Plantar warts appear on the skin of the sole and are caused by a papillomavirus. Because of pressure from the weight of the body, the plantar wart is often flattened and forced into the skin of the sole. The wart may disappear without treatment. If it persists, surgery or chemical therapy can be used to relieve the discomfort.

Athlete's foot is a common fungal infection that causes the foot to become itchy, sore, and cracked. It is usually treated with antifungal agents such as miconazole. Preventive measures include keeping the feet dry and disinfecting areas where the fungus may live, such as shower stalls.

Another common deformity is a bunion, which is a bursa (fluid-filled pad) overlying the joint at the base of the big toe. Normal structure of the first metatarsal, first phalange, and their joint is necessary to withstand the force applied to them in everyday activities. A bunion is caused by an abnormal outward projection of the joint and an inward projection of the big toe. Treatment involves correcting the position of the big toe and keeping it in a normal position. Sometimes surgery is necessary if the tissues become too swollen. In fact, some severe cases of bunions have required complete reconstruction of the toe. Unless treated, a bunion will get progressively worse.

Gout is a metabolic disorder, mainly found in men, which causes uric acid crystals to form in joints. Even though any joint can be affected, the big toe joint is likely the major site for gout because it is under chronic stress from walking. The joint is usually red, swollen, and very tender and painful. The first attack usually involves only one joint and lasts a few days. Some patients never experience another attack, but most have a second episode between six months and two years after the first. After the second attack, more joints may become involved. Treatment includes anti-inflammatory drugs and colchicine. These drugs help reduce the pain by decreasing the amount of inflammation around the joint. Physicians may also prescribe allopurinol to reduce the amount of uric acid that the body produces. Drugs are also available that increase the kidneys" ability to excrete uric acid; examples of these agents are probenecid and sulfinpyrazone.

Perspective and Prospects

Even though the feet constitute a relatively small area of the body, ailments of the feet afflict more than half the world's population. For a long time, disorders of the foot were not taken as seriously as those found in other parts of the body. It is now known, however, that poor foot health can have serious effects. For example, in children a painful foot condition not properly diagnosed and treated can result in lost school days and decreased participation in other activities. More important, an uncorrected congenital abnormality, if neglected, could have irreversible consequences. For the elderly, foot problems hinder or prevent normal activities such as taking care of personal needs, exercising, and socializing. Anything that affects the feet affects that individual's overall health and well-being.

Because of the potentially devastating problems of improper foot care, a branch of medicine developed that specifically addresses problems of the feet. Physicians known as podiatrists practice a specialized branch of medicine called podiatry. It is the job of the podiatrist to assess the cause of the foot problem and the patient's general medical condition in determining the need for and the course of treatment. This assessment often calls for contact with the patient's primary care physician for access to the patient's medical records, as many diseases affect the whole body but present signs and symptoms in the feet. The podiatrist or other physician, such as an orthopedist, will evaluate a disorder through physical exams, laboratory tests, and anatomical tests to examine the internal structures; the latter may include X-rays, computed tomography (CT) scans, or magnetic resonance imaging (MRI). The physician will then diagnose and begin treating the disorder using surgery, medical therapy, or physical therapy.

As more individuals become physically active throughout their lives, clinicians who practice sports medicine are paying closer attention to problems of the foot. Many people seek to improve their health by walking, jogging, and bicycling. All these activities have proven to be excellent for maintaining cardiovascular health, but all place additional stress on the foot. Physicians who counsel patients on physical fitness programs attempt to identify individuals who may be injury-prone. Failure to recognize an anatomical anomaly of the feet could lead to an injury or series of injuries that restrict certain activities or even cause permanent damage. Occasionally, individuals are too enthusiastic about their exercise program and experience overuse injuries involving the feet. Such injuries may cause a sudden cessation of the physical activity and may have a significant demoralizing effect on individuals who finally decide to take steps to improve their health and well-being.

People commonly neglect their feet and underemphasize the importance of the normal functional anatomy of the foot. Individuals who experience a foot injury, however, begin to appreciate the absolute importance of this rather complex but often overlooked structure.

—*Matthew Berria, Ph.D.*

See also Anatomy; Athlete's foot; Bones and the skeleton; Bunions; Cysts; Flat feet; Foot disorders; Frostbite; Ganglion removal; Gout; Hammertoe correction; Hammertoes; Heel spur removal; Lower extremities; Nail removal; Nails; Orthopedic surgery; Orthopedics; Orthopedics, pediatric; Podiatry; Sports medicine; Tendon repair; Warts.

For Further Information:

"Bones, Joints, and Muscles." *MedlinePlus*, December 5, 2011.

Currey, John D. *Bones: Structures and Mechanics*. 2d ed. Princeton, N.J.: Princeton University Press, 2006.

Hales, Dianne. *An Invitation to Health Brief*. Updated ed. Belmont, Calif.: Wadsworth/Cengage Learning, 2010.

"Heel Injuries and Disorders." *MedlinePlus*, June 28, 2013.

Lippert, Frederick G., and Sigvard T. Hansen. *Foot and Ankle Disorders: Tricks of the Trade*. New York: Thieme, 2003.

Mader, Sylvia S. *Human Biology*. 13th ed. Dubuque, Iowa: McGraw-Hill, 2014.

Marieb, Elaine N., and Katja Hoehn. *Human Anatomy and Physiology*. 9th ed. San Francisco: Pearson/Benjamin Cummings, 2013.

Shier, David N., Jackie L. Butler, and Ricki Lewis. *Hole's Essentials of Human Anatomy and Physiology*. 11th ed. Boston: McGraw-Hill, 2012.

Van De Graaff, Kent M., and Stuart I. Fox. *Concepts of Human Anatomy and Physiology*. 5th ed. Dubuque, Iowa: Wm. C. Brown, 2000.

FETAL ALCOHOL SYNDROME
Disease/Disorder

Also known as: Fetal alcohol spectrum disorder (FASD), alcohol-related neurodevelopmental disorder (ARND), alcohol-related birth defects (ARBD), fetal alcohol effects (FAE)

Anatomy or system affected: Brain, ears, eyes, hands, head, heart, mouth

Specialties and related fields: All

Definition: Prenatal alcohol exposure of the fetus, resulting in specific facial and central nervous system abnormalities, impairment of physical growth (especially linear growth), and other associated anomalies.

Causes and Symptoms

Fetal alcohol syndrome was first described in 1973 after recognition of a specific pattern of craniofacial, limb, and cardiac defects in unrelated infants born to alcoholic mothers.

Alcohol is a potent teratogen. Ethanol toxicity was initially suspected and has since been proven as the etiology of this syndrome. Fetal alcohol syndrome is not genetically inherited but rather is an acquired syndrome.

Alcohol induces abnormalities in neurogenesis and synaptogenesis and is the leading cause of preventable devel-

---

> ### Information on Fetal Alcohol Syndrome
>
> **Causes:** Alcohol consumption by mother during pregnancy
>
> **Symptoms:** Growth retardation, certain facial anomalies, central nervous system impairment, clumsiness, behavioral problems, brief attention span, poor judgment, impaired memory, diminished capacity to learn from experience
>
> **Duration:** Chronic
>
> **Treatments:** None; preventive measures during pregnancy

opmental disabilities in the United States. These processes result in central nervous system structural anomalies and microcephaly (small head size). Attention deficit, hyperactivity, and behavioral and learning difficulties; planning difficulties; memory problems; receptive language skill deficits; and math and verbal processing difficulties are common with fetal alcohol syndrome. Alcohol also has lifelong negative effects on fine motor coordination and balance. Prenatal and postnatal growth is below the 10th percentile for age and ethnicity.

Additionally, prenatal alcohol exposure results in numerous cardiovascular problems and facial and limb anomalies. Distinguishing features include short palpebral (eyelid) fissures, a thin vermilion (upper edge of the lip), and a long, smooth philtrum (vertical groove in the upper lip). Underdeveloped ears, clinodactyly (curvature of the little fingers), camptodactyly (bent fingers that cannot straighten), "hockey stick" palmar creases, and cardiac defects are common.

Treatment and Therapy

Primary prevention is the optimal treatment. Programs to educate health care providers and the general public regarding the adverse effects of alcohol usage during pregnancy may be effective in reducing the incidence of fetal alcohol syndrome. For individuals with this disorder, lifelong therapy directed toward educational planning, including improving cognitive, motor, behavioral, and psychosocial skills, is warranted. In addition, medical care is required for various associated anomalies such as cardiac defects.

Perspective and Prospects

Alcohol exposure—as a fetus, adolescent, or adult—leads to an increased probability of further alcohol ingestion at other developmental stages. An interruption of this cycle is imperative in order to reduce the incidence of fetal alcohol syndrome. Prevention of alcohol-affected pregnancies depends on developing and implementing evidence-based tools for fetal alcohol syndrome prevention, diagnosis, and treatment. There is no safe dose of alcohol during pregnancy, and current recommendations note that no alcohol should be ingested at conception and throughout gestation.

—*Wanda Todd Bradshaw, M.S.N., N.N.P., P.N.P., C.C.R.N.*

See also Addiction; Alcoholism; Birth defects; Brain disorders;

Childbirth; Childbirth complications; Embryology; Learning disabilities; Mental retardation; Neonatology; Obstetrics; Perinatology; Pregnancy and gestation.

For Further Information:

A.D.A.M. Health Solutions, et al. "Fetal Alcohol Syndrome." *MedlinePlus*, Aug. 8, 2012.

Calhoun, Faye, et al. "National Institute on Alcohol Abuse and Alcoholism and the Study of Fetal Alcohol Spectrum Disorders: The International Consortium." *Annali dell'Istituto superiore di sanitÀ* 42, no. 1 (2006): 4–7.

Chudley, Albert, et al. "Fetal Alcohol Spectrum Disorder: Canadian Guidelines for Diagnosis." *Canadian Medical Association Journal* 172, suppl. 5 (2005): S1–21.

"Fetal Alcohol Spectrum Disorders." *MedlinePlus*, May 2, 2013.

"Fetal Alcohol Syndrome." *KidsHealth*. Nemours Foundation, Nov. 2011.

Gerberding, Julie Louise, Jose Cordero, and R. Louise Floyd. *Fetal Alcohol Syndrome: Guidelines for Referral and Diagnosis*. Atlanta: CDC National Task Force on Fetal Alcohol Syndrome and Fetal Alcohol Effect, 2004.

Hoyme, H. Eugene, et al. "A Practical Clinical Approach to Diagnosis of Fetal Alcohol Spectrum Disorders: Clarification of the 1996 Institute of Medicine Criteria." *Pediatrics* 115, no. 1 (2005): 39–47.

"About FASD." *National Organization on Fetal Alcohol Syndrome* (NOFAS), 2012.

Wattendorf, Daniel, and Maximilian Muenke. "Fetal Alcohol Spectrum Disorders." *American Family Physician* 72 (2005): 279–282, 285.

Wood, Debra, and Rimas Lukas. "Fetal Alcohol Syndrome." *Health Library*, Sept. 10, 2012.

FETAL SURGERY

Procedure

Anatomy or system affected: Bladder, blood, brain, liver, lungs, respiratory system, urinary system

Specialties and related fields: Cardiology, ethics, genetics, neonatology, obstetrics, pediatrics, urology

Definition: Surgical intervention in utero, before birth, if the fetus has a life-threatening condition or congenital abnormality that can be alleviated.

Key terms:

amniocentesis: the drawing of amniotic fluid through the abdominal wall of a pregnant woman in the fifteenth or sixteenth week of pregnancy to test for fetal abnormalities, particularly Down syndrome

diaphragmatic hernia: a protrusion of the stomach into the diaphragm

hiatal hernia: a protrusion of the stomach into the opening normally occupied in the diaphragm by the esophagus

hydronephrosis: swelling (distension) of the kidney

hypotonic: the presence of a low osmotic pressure

in utero: the Latin term for "inside or within the womb"

neonatologist: a physician who specializes in treating newborn infants

osmotic pressure: the pressure between two solutions separated by a membrane

teratoma: a tumor composed of tissue not normally found at that site

thorax: the bone and cartilage cage attached to the sternum; generally referred to as the rib cage

uropathy: any disease of the urinary tract

Indications and Procedures

As early as the 1960s, some unborn infants suffering from progressive anemia caused by antibodies that drew away their strength were saved by receiving blood transfusions in utero. These early procedures marked the beginnings of invasive medical intervention in dealing with fetal problems.

Not until the technical advances of the 1970s and beyond, however, was it possible to observe human fetuses in the uterus. With the development of ultrasound imaging, it became possible to examine in considerable detail the size, growth, and contour of fetuses. The use of ultrasound enabled physicians to assess with considerable accuracy the age of fetuses, their probable date of birth, and a number of congenital abnormalities, such as spina bifida.

Laparoscopes with diameters of less than 0.1 inch make it possible to examine the fetal stomach. The use of lasers and tiny instruments guided by computers has allowed methods of fetal surgery that were inconceivable in the mid-twentieth century. These instruments greatly reduce blood loss in all types of surgery, including fetal surgery, and greatly improve the prognosis in such procedures. They are used to repair ruptured membranes in fetuses, to install shunts to relieve blockages, and, with the laser excision of placental vessels, to equalize osmotic pressure in twin-twin transfusion syndrome.

It has become possible for obstetricians to observe all significant fetal organs. Whereas physicians earlier could barely hear the beat of the fetal heart, they now can monitor all four of its chambers in the unborn to detect defects early, and, in some cases, to repair them surgically. Ultrasound enables physicians to observe fetal movement within the uterus and to monitor fetal breathing and swallowing.

Because physicians can now gather specific information about the fetus and its health, abnormalities and life-threatening physical problems can be detected several months prior to delivery. Whereas neonatologists have regularly encountered such problems as intestinal and urinary tract obstructions, heart defects, protrusions of the wall of the stomach into the thorax (diaphragmatic hernia) or into the esophageal region (hiatal hernia), swelling of the kidney (hydronephrosis), tumors (sacrococcygeal teratomas), hydrocephalus (water on the brain), and defects of the chromosomes shortly after the birth of a child, it is now possible to detect and, in some cases, to treat these defects surgically in utero.

In cases where fetal surgery appears to offer the most reasonable solution to a difficult problem, the mother may be sent to one of the few centers in the United States where this highly specialized and controversial form of surgery is performed regularly. With the development of sophisticated computer-operated instrumentation, surgeons geographically distant from their patients can perform highly specialized surgery on them. Eventually, such surgery will likely be performed without uprooting mothers.

The current success rate of fetal surgery is not encouraging, although some remarkable outcomes have occurred through its use. Fetal surgical procedures often result in miscarriages and sometimes in the death of both the mother and the fetus.

Two conditions that frequently require fetal surgery are obstructions in the urinary tract that, if untreated until birth, may lead to kidney failure, and hydrocephalus, in which cerebral swelling makes it difficult or impossible for brain cerebrospinal fluid to circulate. Both conditions, which occur in 1 of every 5,000 to 10,000 births, require immediate attention to prevent long-term problems or death. Stents can overcome blockages. Instruments have been developed to drain fluid from the brain in instances of hydrocephalus.

When surgery is performed to allow fetal lungs to develop normally, the fetus, attached to the mother through the umbilical cord, exists in the most protective environment it is ever likely to know. If corrections are made in the uterus, then the fetal lungs are in the safest possible environment for becoming stronger before they are forced to function on their own.

In cases of obstructive uropathy (obstruction of the urinary tract), surgery may help injured kidneys to recover and develop. Hypotonic urine found in fetal samples indicates that normal kidney function might be restored and suggests that surgery may permit the affected kidneys to gain strength within the uterus. On the other hand, the presence of isotonic urine in fetal samples indicates kidneys that are too badly compromised to regain normal function. Treatments currently available offer no solution to this problem.

One of the more routine procedures connected with pregnancy is amniocentesis, testing for chromosomal abnormalities through the analysis of amniotic fluid drawn through the abdominal wall of the mother and of blood drawn from the umbilical cord. This procedure is not without risks to mothers and fetuses. It is commonly used, however, because the benefits derived from it are generally thought to outweigh the risks.

Nevertheless, amniocentesis remains a controversial procedure, and major ethical questions surround its use. If the test reveals a chromosomal abnormality, the parents are left with the decision of whether to seek a therapeutic abortion to terminate the pregnancy, which in many jurisdictions would be considered a realistic option. With many such abnormalities, however, the fetus might be delivered alive and, although significantly handicapped, have a life expectancy of many years.

Fetal surgery is indicated when physicians are convinced that a fetus will not survive long enough to be delivered or when it appears certain that the newborn will be unable to survive long after its birth. For example, if it appears through ultrasound that a fetus suffers from a severe kind of congenital diaphragmatic hernia in which the liver is in the chest, then it is obvious that the development of the lungs will be seriously compromised without surgical interven-

tion. Fetal surgery becomes a stopgap measure in such cases to lessen the severity of the problem so that the fetus can grow to term and be delivered, after which corrective surgery outside the uterus can be undertaken. This procedure involves substantial risk, however, because the liver can be destroyed in the process of trying to restore it to its normal position below the diaphragm.

Sometimes ultrasound reveals noncancerous sacrococcygeal tumors. Such tumors, if untreated, can become large enough in a fetus to put a strain on the heart sufficient to cause heart failure. This severely compromises the survival of the fetus. Guided by ultrasound imagery, surgeons can cut off the blood supply to such tumors and starve them before they do irreparable damage to the fetus. When this procedure is used, the destroyed tumor can be removed surgically after birth.

Another growing use of fetal surgery is in cases where spina bifida, usually identified through ultrasound around the sixteenth week of pregnancy, is present. This congenital defect involves a malformation in the vertebral arch, in which the neural tube connected to the brain and the spine is exposed. When this condition is diagnosed and treated early in the development of the fetus, considerable spinal cord function can be preserved. This makes postnatal treatment more effective than it would be were the condition not discovered until after delivery.

There are essentially two major forms of fetal surgery. The more drastic of these involves performing a cesarean section, after which the fetus is carefully removed from the uterus and

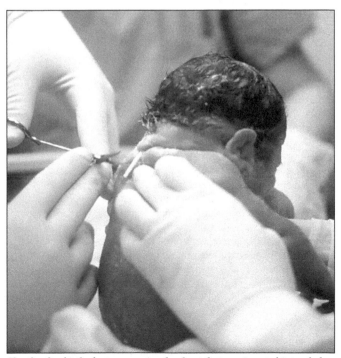

Shortly after birth, doctors examine the shunt that was inserted into a baby two months earlier in an effort to correct his hydrocephalus. (AP/Wide World Photos)

treated. It is then returned to the uterus, which is closed with sutures. The umbilical cord is not cut, so that the fetus is still receiving oxygen and need not breathe on its own before its lungs have developed sufficiently. This procedure is indicated when some congenital defect, possibly a teratoma (tumor), blocks the airway. Clearing the fetal airway enables the baby to breathe independently upon delivery. The other form of fetal surgery is done without removing the fetus from the uterus and is made possible by the use of laparoscopes and other specialized instruments. This is the preferred method if a choice is offered.

Uses and Complications

As fetal surgery becomes more significant and more common in the treatment and elimination of many threatening prenatal conditions, numerous complications, both ethical and physical, necessarily arise. Any surgery involves risk, and in fetal surgery a dual risk exists: risk to the fetus and risk to the mother. Therefore, physicians who perform fetal surgery have simultaneously as patients both prospective mothers and fetuses. Because fetuses cannot speak for themselves or make their own decisions, fetal surgeons often find themselves in an ethical quagmire. Most physicians hesitate to recommend fetal surgery except in such extreme cases that fetal death or severe disability without such surgery seems inevitable.

Sometimes wrenching decisions must be made about whether to save the life of the mother or the life of the fetus. Questions also arise about whether to allow a fetus to come to term if it is obvious that it will suffer from birth defects that will either severely limit the length of its life or adversely compromise its quality of life, which in some cases may involve a normal life span. Many notable people who suffered from severe birth defects have made significant contributions to society and have led productive and rewarding lives.

One of the more significant uses of fetal surgery is in the treatment of twin-twin transfusion syndrome. In the United States, this syndrome occurs in about one thousand pregnancies each year. Twin-twin transfusion syndrome results in a pair of twins being of unequal size in the fetal state because of abnormal circulation of amniotic fluid between them within the placenta that they share. The larger of the two is surrounded by considerably more amniotic fluid than the smaller one. This disproportion can result in the death of one or both of the fetuses. Attempts can be made to equalize the amniotic fluid by inserting a hollow needle through the mother's abdomen and drawing out excess fluid, a procedure that can threaten the viability of one or both of the fetuses.

Another more sophisticated treatment of twin-twin transfusion syndrome involves inserting a fetoscope into the uterus and using heat from a laser to seal off the blood vessels between the fetuses. This treatment is directed toward separating the circulation between the twins, which accounts for the condition. Regardless of which treatment is employed, the mortality rate is currently quite high in such cases, and premature delivery is a virtual certainty in them. Without intervention, however, these fetuses inevitably die in the uterus.

One of the greatest complications of fetal surgery is premature delivery. Fetuses were once thought to be viable only in the seventh month and beyond. Now the means are available to make survival outside the uterus possible earlier than that, although extraordinary care, attention, and equipment are required for extended periods following the delivery of a baby short of seven months and hospitalization in the neonatal intensive care unit (NICU) may continue for many months following such a birth.

When fetal surgery is performed, the mother is routinely medicated with drugs that will both reduce her pain and substantially decrease the possibility of miscarriage or premature delivery. As the field grows and becomes increasingly sophisticated, many of the current problems that it poses will surely be overcome.

Perspective and Prospects

The development of highly specialized instruments, including fiber-optic telescopes and instruments specially designed to enter the uterus through minute incisions, has made possible the field of fetal surgery. Obstetrical surgeons can now correct life-threatening defects and malformations through the smallest, least invasive of openings while the fetus remains within the protection of the mother's body. This procedure, referred to as fetoscopic surgery, is the method preferred whenever it is possible because it reduces substantially the danger of bringing about premature labor at a time when the fetus cannot breathe on its own.

Because fetal surgery is in its infancy, relatively few surgeons specialize in it and the full range of its uses and promises has yet to be explored. The two major centers in the United States that have pioneered development in this field are the Children's Hospital in Philadelphia and the University of California Hospital in San Francisco.

Considerable research in fetal surgery is being conducted at both of these institutions and in laboratories and hospitals throughout the country. It is a matter of time before improved technology will exist to eradicate some of the major barriers to more extensive fetal surgery. Surgery of all kinds is becoming less invasive, which reduces considerably the shock that it delivers to patients" bodies, including blood loss and recovery time. Noninvasive fetal surgery is particularly important to ensure the physical welfare of both the fetus and the mother.

—R. Baird Shuman, Ph.D.;
updated by Alexander Sandra, M.D.

See also Abortion; Amniocentesis; Birth defects; Brain disorders; Cesarean section; Chorionic villus sampling; Down syndrome; Embryology; Ethics; Genetic diseases; Genetics and inheritance; Hernia; Hernia repair; Hydrocephalus; Laparoscopy; Miscarriage; Multiple births; Neonatology; Obstetrics; Perinatology; Pregnancy and gestation; Premature birth; Spina bifida; Stillbirth; Teratogens; Ultrasonography; Umbilical cord.

For Further Information:

Barron, S. L., and D. F. Roberts, eds. *Issues in Fetal Medicine: Proceedings of the Twenty-ninth Annual Symposium of the Galton Institute, London, 1992.* New York: St. Martin's Press, 1995.

Dickens, Bernard M., and Rebecca J. Cook. "Legal and Ethical Issues in Fetal Surgery." *International Journal of Gynecology & Obstetrics* 115, no. 1 (October, 2011): 80–83.

Harrison, Michael, et al. *The Unborn Patient: The Art and Science of Fetal Therapy.* 3d ed. Philadelphia: W. B. Saunders, 2001.

Hartmann, Katherine E., et al. "Evidence to Inform Decisions About Maternal-Fetal Surgery." *Obstetrics & Gynecology* 117, no. 5 (May, 2011): 1191–1204.

O'Neill, J. A., Jr. "The Fetus as a Patient." *Annals of Surgery* 213 (1991): 277-278.

Wise, Barbara, et al., eds. *Nursing Care of the General Pediatric Surgical Patient.* Gaithersburg, Md.: Aspen, 2000.

Vrecenak, Jesse, and Alan Flake. "Fetal Surgical Intervention: Progress and Perspectives." *Pediatric Surgery International* 29, no. 5 (May, 2013): 407–417.

FETAL TISSUE TRANSPLANTATION

Procedure

Anatomy or system affected: Blood, brain, eyes, immune system, nervous system, pancreas, spine

Specialties and related fields: Embryology, ethics, immunology, neurology

Definition: The experimental and controversial use of tissue from aborted human fetuses to replace damaged tissue in patients with diseases in which the patient's own tissue has been destroyed (such as Parkinson's disease or diabetes mellitus).

Key terms:

allograft: a transplanted tissue or organ from a genetically different member of the same species as the recipient

autograft: tissue transplanted from one site to another in the same patient

cannula: a narrow tube used in surgery to drain fluid or to deliver cell suspensions for a transplant

fetal: in humans, a term normally referring to the developmental period following eight weeks of gestation; in fetal tissue transplantation, refers to tissue from earlier developmental stages as well

in utero: a Latin term meaning "in the womb"

isograft: a transplanted tissue or organ from a genetically identical individual (identical twin)

Parkinson's disease: a disease in which the dopamine-secreting cells of the midbrain degenerate, resulting in reduced levels of the neurotransmitter dopamine, tremors, uncontrolled and slow movement, and rigidity

stereotaxic computed tomography (CT): a method of imaging using a series of X rays that are compiled by a computer to give a three-dimensional image of internal structures

xenograft: a transplanted tissue or organ obtained from a member of a species different from that of the recipient

Indications and Procedures

Advances in technology sometimes catapult a society into ethical arenas that are not yet circumscribed by laws and clear moral boundaries. Fetal tissue transplantation is one of these advances. It is a technology that carries the hope of curing a diverse array of severe, often tragic, ailments but one that raises many difficult questions. Tissues from aborted fetuses have been shown in experimental trials to be an excellent source of replacement tissue for patients whose diseases have destroyed their own vital tissues. Parkinson's, Huntington's, and Alzheimer's diseases (in which regions of the brain deteriorate) or juvenile-onset diabetes mellitus (in which insulin-secreting cells of the pancreas degenerate) theoretically could be cured with suitable tissue replacement.

The two sources of tissue used in transplantations, donations from adult cadavers and from aborted fetuses, differ significantly in their suitability. Tissues from cadavers have the severe disadvantage of being immunologically rejected when grafted into anyone who is not an identical twin. The body's surveillance system that protects against infection is designed to attack and destroy any cells that carry molecular markers identifying them as foreign. Patients receiving tissue transplants from other individuals, therefore, will tolerate the tissue graft only if their immune systems are first suppressed with a battery of potent drugs, leaving the patient dangerously unarmed against infection.

Other disadvantages of cadaveric tissues are cell death due to extended postmortem interval (time between individual's death and collection of the tissue) and poor integration into the recipient organ. Porcine xenografts into patients with Parkinson's disease have also been attempted, but they were unsuccessful because of the rejection of the majority of transplanted cells despite aggressive immunosuppression. Taken together, allografts, a transplanted tissue or organ from a genetically different member of the same species, are generally much better tolerated than are xenografts, a transplanted tissue or organ obtained from a member of a species different from that of the recipient. In contrast, isografts, which utilize tissue from a genetically identical twin, are not rejected. Of note is that transplant rejection decreases with the recipient's age, possibly due to immunosenescence and the increased effectiveness of immunosuppressive drugs.

Fetal tissues, however, do not induce a full-scale immune response when transplanted. This is particularly true when cells are transplanted into an organ such as the brain, which is considered an immunologically privileged site along with other locations in the body, such as the anterior chamber of the eye, testis, renal tubule, and uterus. At these sites, the immune response to antigens is reduced and/or not destructive to the transplanted tissue. Nevertheless, transplanted fetal tissues do attract lymphocytes (a type of white blood cell of the immune system) and other immune cells, but the role of this process in graft survival and function is not well understood.

Other properties add to the suitability of fetal tissue for transplantation. Because it is not yet fully differentiated, fetal tissue is said to be very plastic in its abilities to adapt to new locations. Moreover, once placed in a patient, it secretes factors that promote its own growth and those of the new blood vessels at the site. Tissue from an adult source does not have these properties and consequently is slow-growing and poorly vascularized. Though growth factors can be added along with the graft, adult tissue is less responsive to these hormones than is fetal tissue.

It is the source of fetal tissue that has fired such debate over its use for transplantation. Though there has been general acceptance of using tissue from spontaneous abortions or from ectopic pregnancies which, because of their location outside the womb, endanger the life of the mother and must be terminated, these sources are not well suited to transplantation. Spontaneous abortions rarely produce viable tissue, since in most cases the fetus has died two to three weeks before it is expelled. In addition, there are usually major genetic defects in the aborted fetus. In ectopic pregnancies as well, more than 50 percent of the fetuses are genetically abnormal, and most resolve themselves in spontaneous abortion outside a clinic setting. These types of abortions are almost always accompanied by a sense of tragic loss felt by the parents. Many researchers find it unacceptable to request permission from these parents to transplant tissue from the lost fetus.

The alternative source of fetal tissue is elected abortions. One-and-a-half million of these abortions occur in the United States every year. The debate over the ethical correctness of elected abortions has left a cloud of confusion over the issue of using this tissue for transplantation.

When an elective abortion is performed in a clinic, the tissue is removed by suction through a narrow tube. Normally, the tissue would be thrown away. If it is to be used for transplantation, written permission must be obtained from the woman after the abortion is completed. No discussion of transplantation is to take place prior to the abortion, and no alteration in the abortion procedure, except to keep the tissue sterile during collection, is to be made. The donor may not be paid for the tissue, and both the donor and the recipient of the tissue must remain anonymous to each other.

Once collected, the tissue is searched through to locate suitable tissue for transplantation. Although the size of the transplanted tissue varies depending on the type of cell replacement, often only a small block of tissue is used, about eight cubic millimeters (the size of a thin slice of pencil eraser). The tissue is screened for infectious diseases such as hepatitis B and human immunodeficiency virus (HIV). Tissue that is collected is washed a number of times in a sterile solution to ensure that there is no bacterial contamination, and then it is maintained in a sterile, buffered salt solution until it is used. To increase the amount of usable tissue, the tissue may be grown in culture on a nutritive medium under carefully controlled conditions of humidity (95 percent), temperature (37 degrees Celsius), and gas (5 percent carbon dioxide in air) to stimulate normal growing conditions. Preservation of the tissue for long-term storage has been made possible by the highly refined technique of freezing the tissue in liquid nitrogen (cryostorage). Fetal tissue has been kept for as long as ten months in this manner before being used successfully in transplantation. Although the technique should provide methods of maintaining tissue indefinitely, not all types of cells contained in such tissues survive cryopreservation well. For example, despite many attempts to optimize storage conditions, fetal neurons are severely harmed by freezing.

The actual transplantation of the tissue is usually relatively quick and in some cases relatively noninvasive. Often the tissue is injected into the patient as a suspension of individual cells. This permits the use of a small-bore tube called a cannula to deliver the cells to the target organ, thereby avoiding large surgical incisions. Because of modern stereotaxic imaging equipment such as computed tomography (CT) scanning and ultrasound, the physician is able to determine with extreme precision exactly where the cells are to be delivered and can visualize the position of the transplant cannula as the cells are injected. In this way, an entire region of an organ can be seeded with fetal cells. Often the patient is under only a local anesthetic. This aspect of the surgery is especially important when fetal cells are being inserted into the brain, since the physicians can then monitor the patient's ability to speak and move, to ensure that no major damage to the brain is occurring. Usually, antibiotics are given on the day of the transplantation procedure and for two additional days to avoid infection. Although the procedure is relatively safe and recovery is quick—patients often go home in less than three days—transplantation into the central nervous system (CNS) carries risk of hemorrhage (bleeding) and blood clot formation that can damage neurons in the affected area.

Fetal tissue transplantation is still considered an experimental procedure, and further trials are needed to fine-tune the techniques. For example, the precise age of fetal tissue that would be most effective in various cases is uncertain, though it is generally agreed that tissue from a first-trimester fetus is optimal, and six to eight weeks of gestation is most suitable for grafts into brains of Parkinson's sufferers. Often it is not known which patients would respond best to the therapy, but in case of neurotransplantation in Parkinson's disease patients, those with good response to levodopa (L-dopa), a precursor of dopamine, benefit the most. Researchers are also uncertain about whether immunosuppressive drugs should be administered. In animal trials using mice, rats, and monkeys, fetal tissue allografts, but not xenografts, have been well tolerated in the absence of immunosuppression. In humans as well, fetal tissue appears to be readily accepted, with no signs of rejection, and in one study, patients did better without immunosuppression. Some surgeons, however, unwilling to risk tissue rejection, routinely give the transplant patient immunosuppressive drugs, such as cyclosporine and prednisone.

Uses and Complications

The major focus for fetal tissue transplantation has been the treatment of patients with Parkinson's disease, and results have been encouraging. The disease is caused by a deterioration of dopamine-producing regions of the midbrain, the substantia nigra, so named because of the presence of pigmented neurons, which secrete dopamine, in the putamen and caudate nucleus of the basal ganglia. There these neurons send their processes (projecting parts). There is an accompanying loss of motor control causing slowness of movement (bradykinesia), tremors, rigidity, and finally paralysis. Death is most typically a result of accompanying illnesses, such as infections, or caused by the loss of balance and falls. The key drug used to treat the disorder, L-dopa, produces side effects that cause unrelenting and uncontrolled movement of the limbs (dyskinesias) and hallucinations, and the drug loses its effectiveness over time. Advanced patients, who are no longer taking the medication, often remain in a "frozen" state.

A number of patients who have received fetal tissue transplants have shown remarkable improvement and diminished requirements for drug treatment. The first case in the United States to be treated was a man with a twenty-year history of parkinsonian symptoms. He had frequent freezing spells, could not walk without a cane, and suffered from chronic constipation. He also was unable to whistle, a beloved hobby of his. He was operated on by Curt R. Freed and his associates in 1988. Following the operation, initial improvement was slow, but within a year, he was walking without a cane, his speed of movement had considerably improved, and his constipation had resolved itself. He also had regained his ability to whistle. Even after four years, improvements continued. Such results have occurred with many parkinsonian patients receiving fetal tissue transplants.

Beneficial effects of transplants have also been obtained in patients with induced Parkinson-like symptoms. In 1982, some intravenous drug users developed Parkinson-like symptoms after using a homemade preparation of "synthetic heroin" that was contaminated with 1-methyl-4-phenyl-1,2,5,6-tetrahydropyridine (MPTP). MPTP destroys dopamine-secreting cells of the substantia nigra. Two of these patients received fetal tissue transplants in Sweden. Within a year after their operation, they were able to walk with a normal gait, resume chores, and be virtually free of their previously uncontrollable movements.

Because no patient with Parkinson's disease or with Parkinson-like symptoms has yet been cured by a fetal tissue transplant, some have considered the results of such experiments to be disappointing. The expectation of complete cures from a technique that is still in its early experimental phase, however, is overly optimistic. Many patients themselves are encouraged, and many have resumed driving and the other tasks of normal daily life. Altogether, more than two hundred patients with Parkinson's disease have received fetal tissue transplants worldwide. It is important to note that fetal tissue transplants are not stem cell transplants, or grafts of tissue produced from stem cells. Coincidentally, fetal tissue usually contains some stem cells, but the transplant effects are thought to be mostly mediated by the mature or maturing cells in the donor tissue (dopamine neurons or pancreatic beta cells, for example).

That transplanted fetal brain tissue can replace damaged brain tissue to any extent has opened the doors of hope for many diseases. For example, Huntington's disease, a genetic disorder that destroys a different set of neurons but in the same region as that affected by parkinsonism, brings a slow death to those carrying the dominant trait. Its severe dementia and uncontrollable jerking and writhing that steadily progress have had no treatment and no cure. In animal studies in which fetal brain tissue was transplanted into rats with symptoms mimicking Huntington's disease, results have been encouraging enough to warrant human trials, and one human trial, reported by a surgeon in Mexico, has shown limited success. Another

such study is ongoing in France. Researchers are hopeful, though less optimistic, that Alzheimer's disease, a form of dementia that is characterized by neuronal death within the brain, also may be treatable with fetal tissue transplants. Because the destruction is so widespread, however, it is difficult to determine where the transplants should be placed.

Type 1 insulin-dependent diabetes, often called juvenile-onset diabetes, also has been treated with fetal tissue transplants. More than a million people in the United States suffer from this disease caused by the destruction of pancreatic beta cells, the insulin-secreting cells that regulate sugar metabolism. Though the disease can be controlled with regular insulin shots, the long-term effects of diabetes can lead to blindness, premature aging, and renal and circulatory problems. After animal tests showed a complete reversal of the disease when fetal pancreatic tissue was transplanted into diabetic rats, human trials were initiated with great expectations. Though complete success has not been achieved, the sixteen diabetic patients who were given fetal pancreatic tissue transplants by Kevin Lafferty between 1987 and 1992 all showed significant drops in the amount of insulin needed to manage their disease. The transplanted tissue continued to pump out insulin.

An unusual variation of such procedures has been to transplant fetal tissue into fetuses diagnosed with severe metabolic diseases. It is more effective to treat the condition while the fetus is still in the womb than to wait until after birth, when damage from the disease may already be extensive. Fetuses with Hurler's syndrome and similar "storage" diseases have been treated in this way. Hurler's syndrome is a lethal condition in which tissues become clogged with stored mucopolysaccharides, long-chain sugars that the body is unable to break down because it lacks the appropriate enzyme. One of the fetuses to receive this treatment was the child of a couple who had lost two children to the disease. With the transplanted tissue, the child lived and by one year of age was producing therapeutic levels of the enzyme. It has been estimated that there are at least 155 other genetic disorders that could be similarly treated by fetal tissue transplants in utero.

The list of ailments that fetal tissue transplants may alleviate includes some of the major concerns of modern medicine. In addition to those already mentioned are macular degeneration, sickle cell disease, thalassemias, metabolic disorders, immune deficiencies, myelin disorders, and spinal cord injuries. In interpreting the value of these applications, however, it is important to separate the politics of abortion from the medical issue of fetal tissue transplantation.

Perspective and Prospects

Though controversy surrounds the use of fetal tissue for transplantation, such controversy has not included all facets of fetal tissue research. Indeed, fetal cells were used in the 1950s to develop the Salk polio vaccine and later the vaccine against rubella (German measles). With the scourge of acquired immunodeficiency syndrome (AIDS), in the 1990s fetal cells were first used to help design treatments against the AIDS virus. Even the early attempts at fetal tissue transplantation occurred quietly. Reports date as far back as 1928, when Italian surgeons attempted unsuccessfully to cure a patient with diabetes using fetal pancreatic tissue, a procedure repeated, again unsuccessfully, in the United States in 1939. In 1959, American physicians tried to cure leukemia with fetal tissue transplants, but again without success.

The first real indicator that such techniques might work came in 1968, when fetal liver cells were used to treat a patient with DiGeorge syndrome. The success of this procedure resulted in its becoming the accepted treatment for this usually fatal genetic disorder, which results from a deletion of a part of chromosome 22. Because many of the DiGeorge patients are athymic (fail to develop a thymus), they lack T cells, making them immunodeficient. Because the fetal liver supports hematopoiesis (the production of blood cells, including immune cells) during development, fetal liver cells have some value in the treatment of immunodeficiency. However, fetal thymus transplantation can promote more complete immune system reconstitution and is now used as a treatment in athymic patients.

Because suitable fetal tissues are often very difficult to obtain, recently the focus on donor cells for transplantation has shifted toward stem cell-derived cells. Stem cells can be relatively easily expanded in numbers in culture and have the potential to generate a large supply of different cell types for transplantation, thereby averting some of the issues that have decelerated the field of fetal transplantation. Donor cells differentiated from one's own stem cells could be used in an autograft and thereby circumvent both immunological and ethical issues. Studies to explore the potential of such technologies are ongoing. Thus the next chapter in the fetal tissue transplantation story may involve the fast-evolving fields of stem cell research and regenerative medicine.

It was not until 1987 that ethical issues over fetal tissue transplants truly surfaced in the United States. Debate was precipitated when the director of the National Institutes of Health (NIH) submitted a request to the Department of Health and Human Services to transplant fetal tissue into patients with Parkinson's disease. Rather than receiving approval, the request was tabled, pending a thorough study of the issue by an NIH panel on fetal tissue transplantation. The panel made a detailed report on the ethical, legal, and scientific implications of fetal tissue transplantation, concluding that it was acceptable public policy. Despite the report, however, the Secretary of Health and Human Services instituted a ban against the use of government funds for transplanting fetal tissue derived from elective abortions. While in effect, the ban influenced private funding as well. Physicians who performed fetal tissue transplants, unable to obtain grant money, were forced to charge their patients—a bill that could reach as high as forty thousand dollars per transplant. President Bill Clinton's lifting of the ban in 1993, on his third day in office, paved the way for research advances, including isolating and propagating human stem cells. The opposition of Clinton's successor, George W. Bush, to the use of fetal tissue and stem cells for scientific purposes led to several legislative battles and cast some doubts on the future of this field. President Barack Obama restored the use of government funds for stem cell research upon taking office in 2009.

The debates over fetal tissue transplantation are far from over. Though a strict set of guidelines are in place concerning the procurement of fetal tissue, ensuring that the needs never influence decisions concerning abortion, other issues have not been addressed. Some ask whether a fetal tissue bank should be established and, if so, whether it should be government-funded to avoid commercialization. As technology continues to create increasingly complicated ethical issues, society's responsibility increases, as does its need to be scientifically informed.

—Mary S. Tyler, Ph.D.;
updated by W. Michael Zawada, Ph.D.

See also Abortion; Alzheimer's disease; Brain; Brain disorders; Diabetes mellitus; Ethics; Genetic diseases; Genetic engineering; Neurology; Pancreas; Parkinson's disease; Stem cells; Transplantation.

For Further Information:

Barker, Roger A., et al. "The Long-Term Safety and Efficacy of Bilateral Transplantation of Human Fetal Striatal Tissue in Patients with Mild to Moderate Huntington's Disease." *Journal of Neurology* 84, no. 6 (June 2013): 657–665.

Beardsley, Tim. "Aborting Research." *Scientific American* 267, no. 2 (August, 1992): 17–18.

Beauchamp, Tom, and James F. Childress. *Principles of Biomedical Ethics.* 6th ed. New York: Oxford University Press, 2009.

Begley, Sharon. "From Human Embryos, Hope for 'Spare Parts.'" *Newsweek*, November 16, 1998, 73.

Brundin, Patrik, and C. Warren Olanow, eds. *Restorative Therapies in Parkinson's Disease.* New York: Springer, 2006.

Clinical Trials. http://www.clinicaltrials.gov.

"Fetal Cell Study Shows Promise for Parkinson's." *Los Angeles Times*, April 22, 1999, p. 29.

Freed, Curt R., Robert Breeze, and Neil Rosenberg. "Transplantation of Human Fetal Dopamine Cells for Parkinson's Disease." *Archives of Neurology* 47, no. 5 (May 1, 1990): 505–512.

Freed, Curt R., and Simon LeVay. *Healing the Brain: A Doctor's Controversial Quest for a Cell Therapy to Cure Parkinson's Disease.* New York: Times Books/Henry Holt, 2002.

Holland, Suzanne, Karen Lebacqz, and Laurie Zoloth, eds. *The Human Embryonic Stem Cell Debate: Science, Ethics, and Public Policy.* Cambridge, Mass.: MIT Press, 2001.

Lindvall, Olle, Patrik Brundin, and Håkan Widner. "Grafts of Fetal Dopamine Neurons Survive and Improve Motor Function in Parkinson's Disease." *Science* 247 (February 2, 1990): 574–577.

Marshak, Daniel R., Richard L. Gardner, and David Gottlieb, eds. *Stem Cell Biology.* Cold Springs Harbor, N.Y.: Cold Springs Harbor Press, 2002.

Millán-Guerrero, Rebeca. "Role of Neural Stem Cells in Parkinson's Disease." *Current Signal Transduction Therapy* 6, no. 3 (September 2011): 337–340.

Seledtsova, G., et al. "Delayed Results of Transplantation of Fetal Neurogenic Tissue in Patients with Consequences of Spinal Cord Trauma." *Bulletin of Experimental Biology & Medicine* 149, no. 4 (April 2010): 530–533.

Singer, Peter, et al., eds. *Embryo Experimentation.* New York: Cambridge University Press, 1993.

U.S. Congress. Senate. Committee on Labor and Human Resources. *Finding Medical Cures: The Promise of Fetal Tissue Transplantation Research.* 102d Congress, 1st session, 1992. Senate Report 1902.

Wade, Nicholas. "Primordial Cells Fuel Debate on Ethics." *The New York Times*, November 10, 1998, p. 1.

FEVER

Disease/Disorder

Anatomy or system affected: All

Specialties and related fields: Family medicine, internal medicine, pediatrics, virology

Definition: A symptom associated with a variety of diseases and disorders, characterized by body temperature above normal (98.6 degrees Fahrenheit, or 37 degrees centigrade or Celsius); considered very serious at 104 degrees Fahrenheit (40 degrees Celsius) and higher.

Key terms:

antipyretic drugs: drugs that are employed to reduce fevers, such as sodium salicylate, indomethacin, and acetaminophen

ectotherms: organisms that rely on external temperature conditions in order to maintain their internal temperature

endotherms: organisms that control the internal temperature of their bodies by the conversion of calories to heat

febrile response: an upward adjustment of the thermoregulatory set point

metabolic rate: a measurement of the Calories (kilocalories) that are converted into heat energy in order to maintain body temperature and/or for physical exertion

pyrogens: protein substances that appear at the outset of the process that leads to a fever reaction

thermoregulatory set point: the ultimate neural control that maintains the human internal body temperature at 37 degrees Celsius and can either raise or lower it

Causes and Symptoms

Although the symptoms that often accompany a fever are familiar to everyone—shivering, sweating, thirst, hot skin, and a flushed face—what causes fever and its function during illness are not fully clear even among medical specialists. Considerable literature exists on the differences between warm-blooded organisms (endotherms) and cold-blooded organisms (ectotherms) in what is called the normal state, when no symptoms of disease are present. Cold-blooded organisms depend on temperature conditions in their external environment to maintain various levels of temperature within their bodies. These fluctuations correspond to the various levels of activity that they need to sustain at given moments. Thus, reptiles, for example, may "recharge" themselves internally by moving into the warmth of the sun. Warm-blooded organisms, on the other hand, including all mammals, utilize energy released from the digestion of food to maintain a constant level of heat within their bodies. This level—a "normal" temperature—is approximately 37 degrees Celsius (98.6 degrees Fahrenheit) in humans. An internal body temperature that rises above this level is called a febrile temperature, or a fever.

If the temperature in the surrounding environment is low, warm-blooded organisms must raise their metabolic rate (a measurement, in Calories, of converted energy) accordingly to maintain a normal internal body temperature. In humans, this rate of energy expenditure is about 1,800 Calories per day. If insufficient food is taken in to supply the necessary potential energy for this metabolic conversion into heat, the body will draw on its storage resource—fat—to fulfill this vital need. The potentially fatal condition called hypothermia, in which the body is too fatigued to maintain metabolic functions or has exhausted all of its stores of Calories, occurs when the internal temperature falls below normal. Although cold-blooded animals must also protect themselves against the danger that their body heat may fall too low to sustain life functions, they can support adjustments in their own internal temperature down to about 20 degrees Celsius. At the same time, metabolic expenditures, as measured in Calories, are very low in cold-blooded animals; for example, alligators must expend only 60 Calories per day to create the same amount of heat as 1,800 Calories per day in warm-blooded humans.

The question of internal temperature in warm-blooded animals is closely tied to management efficiency in the body. This function becomes critical when one considers abnormally high internal temperature, or fever. Generally speaking, all essential biochemical functions in the human body can be carried out at optimal levels of efficiency at the set point of 37 degrees Celsius. In the simplest of terms, any increase or decrease in temperature creates either more or less kinetic energy and has the potential to affect the chemistry of all body functions.

Endotherms are able to tolerate a certain range of involuntary change in their internal body temperature (brought about by disease or illness), but there is an upper limit of 45 degrees Celsius, which constitutes a high fever. If the self-regulating higher set point associated with fever goes beyond this point, destructive biochemical phenomena will occur in the body—in particular, a breaking down of protein molecules. If these phenomena are not checked, they can bring about death.

Modern scientific approaches to the internal body processes that lead to fever, like a medical discussion of the effects that occur once fever is operating in the body, are much more complicated. They revolve around the concept of a change in the set point monitored in the brain. When this change in the brain's normal (37 degree) thermostatic signal is called for, a process called phagocytosis begins, leading to a higher internal body heat level throughout the organism.

Phagocytosis, the ingestion of a solid substance (especially foreign material such as invading bacteria), involves the appearance in the host's system of large numbers of leukocyte cells. When these cells ingest the bacteria, small quantities of protein called leukocytic pyrogens are produced. According to most modern theories, these protein pyrogens trigger the biochemical reactions in the brain that alter the body's temperature set point. After this point, changes that occur throughout the system and raise the body's internal temperature depend on a component of the bacterial cell wall called endotoxin. By the end of the 1960s, researchers had drawn attention to at least twenty effects that activated endotoxins may have on the host organism. Key effects include enhancement of the production of new white blood cells (leukocytosis), enhancement of various forms of immuno-

Information on Fever

Causes: Infection, various diseases
Symptoms: Shivering, sweating, thirst, hot skin, flushed face
Duration: Acute
Treatments: Medication, comfort measures (e.g., cool compress), rest

logical resistance, reduction of serum iron levels, and lowering of blood pressure.

Most, if not all, of these effects brought about by endotoxins are accompanied by higher levels of heat throughout the body, the definition of fever. Closer biochemical examination of the source of the added heat yielded the suggestion, made by P. B. Beeson in 1948, that the host's endotoxin-affected cells begin to produce a distinct form of protein, now called endogenous pyrogens. Pyrogens are thought to induce the first stage of fever by interacting with cells in tissues very close to the brain, specifically in the brain stem itself. Laboratory experiments in the first half of the twentieth century allowed researchers to produce almost immediate fever reactions when they injected pyrogen protein material into rabbits. Studies of the induced febrile state in laboratory animals, and therefore presumably also in humans, linked fever to immunological (virus-resistant and bacteria-resistant) reactions, not necessarily in the initially affected tissues around the brain but in various places throughout the organism.

Although scientific research has produced many hypotheses concerning the origins of fever in the body, experts admit that the process is not well understood. Matthew J. Kluger, in *Fever: Its Biology, Evolution, and Function* (1979), claims that "the precise mechanism behind endogenous pyrogens" effect on the thermoregulatory set-point is unknown."

Treatment and Therapy

The febrile response has been noted in five of the seven extant classes of vertebrates on earth (Agnatha, such as lampreys, and Chondrichthyes, such as sharks, are excluded). Scientists have determined that its function as a reaction to bacterial infection can be traced back as far as 400 million years in primitive bony fishes. The question of whether the natural phenomenon of fever actually aids in combating disease in the body, however, has not been fully resolved.

In ancient and medieval times, it was believed that fever served to "cook" and separate out one of the four essential body "humors"—blood, phlegm, yellow bile, and black bile—that had become excessively dominant. Throughout the centuries, such beliefs even caused some physicians to try to induce higher internal body temperatures as a means of treating disease. Use of modern antipyretic drugs to reduce fever remained unthinkable until the nineteenth century.

It was the German physician Carl von Liebermeister who, by the end of the nineteenth century, set some of the guidelines that are still generally observed in deciding whether antipyretic drugs should or should not be used to reduce a nat-

urally occurring fever during illness. Liebermeister insisted that the phenomenon of fever was not one of body temperature gone "out of control" but rather a sign that the organism was regulating its own temperature. He also demonstrated that part of the process leading to increased internal temperature could be seen in reactions that actually reduce heat loss at the body's surface, notably decreases in skin blood flow and evaporative cooling through perspiration. Liebermeister determined that one of the positive effects of higher temperatures inside the body was to impede the growth of harmful microorganisms. At the same time, however, other side effects of fever during illness were deemed to be negative, such as loss of appetite, and, in some cases, actual degeneration of key internal organs. Liebermeister's generation of physicians, therefore, tended to rely on antipyretic drugs only when high fevers persisted for long periods of time. Moderate fevers or even high fevers, if they did not continue too long, were deemed to contribute to the overall process of natural body resistance to disease.

In fact, a limited school of physicians followed the teaching of 1927 Nobel laureate Julius Wagner-Jauregg, who claimed that "fever therapy" methods should be adopted for the treatment of certain diseases. Wagner-Jauregg himself had pioneered this theory by inoculating victims of neurosyphilis with fever-producing malaria. Part of his argument in favor of this experimental therapy was that malaria, with its accompanying fever, was a treatable disease (through the use of quinine) and could be controlled at regular intervals during its "service" as a fighter against a disease that still had no known cure. Later use of fever therapy for treatment of other sexually transmitted diseases, specifically gonorrhea, proved to be moderately successful. When typhoid vaccine was used to induce fevers in some patients, however, side effects such as hypotension (low blood pressure) or cardiovascular shock introduced what some considered to be dangerous risk factors. Nevertheless, certain fields of medicine, especially those involved with eye diseases and related eye ailments, have proved that fever-inducing agents (specifically those contained in typhoid and typhoid-paratyphoid vaccines) also induce beneficial secretion of the anti-inflammatory hormone cortisol.

By the second half of the twentieth century, the medical use of antipyretic drugs, containing such components as salicylates and indomethacin, had become widespread. This phenomenon was not caused by any compelling reversal of earlier general assumptions that moderate levels of fever, being a natural body reaction, were not necessarily harmful to patients suffering from a wide variety of diseases. Rather, physicians may have opted to use such drugs as much for their pain-relieving qualities as for their fever-reducing characteristics. Although patients receiving such drug treatment notice a diminishing of severe pains or general aching, the cause of the disease has not been combated merely by the removal of such symptoms as fever and pain.

Modern medical science has tended to support further study of particular circumstances in which induced fevers can actually produce disease-combating reactions. A newly

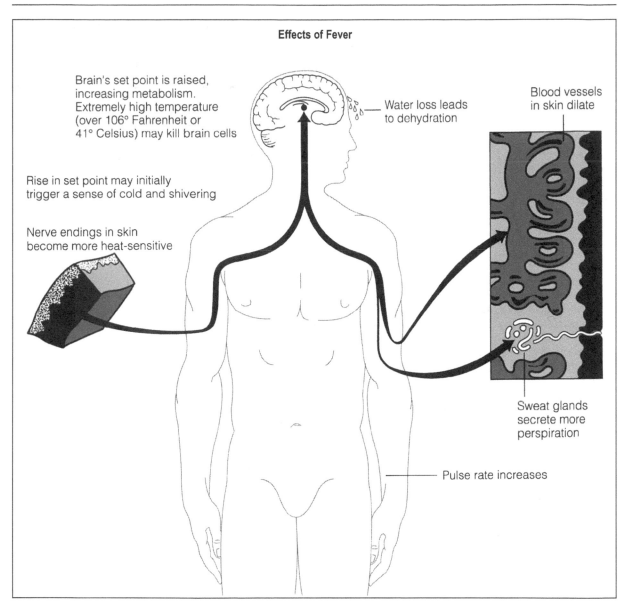

Effects of Fever

Brain's set point is raised, increasing metabolism. Extremely high temperature (over 106° Fahrenheit or 41° Celsius) may kill brain cells

Rise in set point may initially trigger a sense of cold and shivering

Nerve endings in skin become more heat-sensitive

Water loss leads to dehydration

Blood vessels in skin dilate

Sweat glands secrete more perspiration

Pulse rate increases

emerging field by the late 1970s, for example, involved studying the benefits of higher temperatures in newborn infants fighting viral infections. Although specific circumstances and the nature of disease prevent a generalized conclusion in terms of the use of induced fevers as a form of treatment, researchers have shown that an elevated body temperature serves to increase the speed at which white blood cells, the body's natural enemies against disease, move to infected areas.

Perspective and Prospects

Although doctors have been aware of the symptoms of fever since the beginnings of medical history, centuries passed before its importance as an indicator of disease was accepted. A certain degree of sophistication in the study of fevers became possible largely as a result of the development of the common thermometer, in a rudimentary form in the seventeenth century and then with greater technical accuracy in the eighteenth century. Systematic use of the thermometer in the eighteenth century enabled doctors to observe such phenomena as morning remission and evening peaking of fever intensity. Studies involving the recording of temperature in healthy individuals also yielded important discoveries. One such discovery was made in 1774, when use of the thermometer showed that, even in a room heated to the boiling point of water (100 degrees Celsius), healthy subjects maintained an internal body heat that was very close to the normal 37-degree level.

Medical reports as late as the end of the eighteenth century, however, indicate that even internationally recognized pioneers of science were still not close to understanding the causes of fever. The English doctor John Hunter, for example, declared himself opposed to the prevailing view that rising body heat came from the circulation of warmer blood throughout the body. Hunter suspected that the warmth was produced by an entirely different agent that was independent of the circulatory system. He never learned what that agent might be, however, and failed in defense of his theory that the source of added body heat was in the stomach. Even the famous French chemist Antoine-Laurent Lavoisier erred when he tried to explain fever in terms of some form of chemical "combustion" involving hydrogen and carbon. Lavoisier identified the lungs as the possible location for this spontaneous production of internal body heat.

Although these theories were identified as erroneous, the late eighteenth and early nineteenth centuries left one legacy that would develop into the twentieth century and is still practiced by physicians: systematic thermometry. In essence, thermometry involves the tracing of the upward or downward direction of fever during illness in order to judge the course of the disease and the effects brought about by different stages of treatment. In many diseases, for example, clinical records of the full course of previous cases can be studied by doctors responsible for treating an individual patient. With thermometry, the doctor is able to determine how far the body's struggle against a certain disease has progressed. If thermometry shows a marked departure from what clinical records have charted as the normal course of disease under certain forms of treatment, then the physician may look for signs of another disease.

—*Byron D. Cannon, Ph.D.*

See also Avian influenza; Bacterial infections; Common cold; Heat exhaustion and heatstroke; Hyperthermia and hypothermia; Influenza; Kawasaki disease; Reye's syndrome; Rheumatic fever; Scarlet fever; Sweating; Typhoid fever; Typhus; Viral infections; Yellow fever; *other specific diseases.*

For Further Information:

Brassfield, Krista, and Kenneth P. Steckel. *Fevers: Types, Treatments and Health Risks (Human Anatomy and Physiology)*. Hauppauge: Nova Biomedical, 2013.

Kemper, Kathi J. *The Holistic Pediatrician: A Pediatrician's Comprehensive Guide to Safe and Effective Therapies for the Twenty-five Most Common Ailments of Infants, Children, and Adolescents*. Rev. ed. New York: Quill, 2002.

Kluger, Matthew J. *Fever: Its Biology, Evolution, and Function*. Princeton: Princeton University Press, 1979.

Kluger, Matthew J., Tamas Bartfai, and Charles A. Dinarello, eds. *Molecular Mechanisms of Fever*. New York: New York Academy of Sciences, 1998.

Litin, Scott C., ed. *Mayo Clinic Family Health Book*. 4th ed. New York: HarperResource, 2009.

Mackowiak, Philip A., ed. *Fever: Basic Mechanisms and Management*. 2d ed. Philadelphia: Lippincott-Raven, 1997.

Nathanson, Laura Walther. *The Portable Pediatrician: A Practicing Pediatrician's Guide to Your Child's Growth, Development, Health, and Behavior from Birth to Age Five*. 2d ed. New York: HarperCollins, 2002.

Polsdorfer, Ricker. "Fever of Unknown Origin." *Health Library*, July 3, 2013.

Vasey, Christopher. *The Healing Power of Fever: Your Body's Natural Defense Against Disease*. Rochester: Healing Arts, 2011.

Fiber

Biology

Anatomy or system affected: Gastrointestinal system, intestines

Specialties and related fields: Alternative medicine, family practice, gastroenterology, geriatrics and gerontology, internal medicine, nursing, nutrition, preventive medicine, sports medicine

Definition: Plant fiber components include hemicelluloses and pectin and are long, threadlike structures. Animal fiber is composed of protein collagen or segments of loose connective tissue in skin and organ tissue.

Structure and Functions

Dietary fiber helps regulate the passage of food material through the gastrointestinal tract and influences the absorption of various nutrients. It represents the content of substances that cannot be broken down by human digestive enzymes or absorbed by the gastrointestinal tract. Nearly all dietary fiber content is contributed by the insoluble structural matter of plants. Cellulose is an insoluble unbranched glucose polymer that can absorb relatively large volumes of water. Hemicellulose is the name for a wide variety of polymers of five carbon sugars. Pectin is a water-soluble polymer that forms gels and binds water, cations, and bile acids. Gums and mucilages are highly branched polysaccharides that form gels and bind water and other organic material. Increased fiber intake may promote health by promoting the normal elimination of waste products of digestion, by promoting satiety, by helping control serum cholesterol, and by other mechanisms. Greatly increased fiber intake, however, may reduce the absorption of some nutrients.

Disorders and Diseases

The ingestion of too much fiber can result in the formation of an obstructing bolus in a narrowed intestinal or esophageal lumen. The purpose of a low-fiber or fiber-restricted diet is to help prevent this occurrence and to rest the gastrointestinal tract. In acute phases of ulcerative colitis, a fiber-restricted diet lessens the pain and stress of defecation by decreasing the weight and bulk of the stool and delaying intestinal transit time.

A low-fiber diet contains approximately two grams of crude fiber. Foods included are refined bread and cereal products, cooked fruits and vegetables that are low in fiber, and juices. Nuts, legumes, and whole-grain bread and cereal products are restricted. Minimal-fiber diets consist of strained fruit and vegetable juices and white potatoes without skins. Milk is limited to two cups per day, as it indirectly contributes to fecal residue even though it contains no fiber. Continued use of a low-fiber diet in refined carbohydrates, however, is believed to cause diverticular disease of the colon.

Reduced bulk causes the colonic lumen to narrow.

A high-fiber diet contains increased amounts of foods containing cellulose, hemicelluloses, lignin, and pectin, and reduced amounts of refined carbohydrates. Insoluble fibers increase the volume and weight of the residue to maintain the normal size of the colonic lumen and to increase gastrointestinal mobility. Soluble fibers, such as gums and pectins, reduce the rate of intestinal absorption, altering the metabolic effects. High-fiber intake necessitates increased fluids.

Certain individuals should not be encouraged to increase the amount of fiber in their diet. Those who have had gastric surgery, vagotomy, pyloroplasty or Roux-en-Y, and some diabetics with gastroparesis diabeticorum have less acid secretion or decreased gastrointestinal motility and may encounter bezoar formation, a compacted mass that does not pass into the intestine. The high-fiber diet has been recommended, however, in the treatment or prevention of dumping syndrome, hyperlipidemia, gallstones, diabetes, and many other diseases and disorders.

—*Jane C. Norman, Ph.D., R.N., C.N.E.*

See also Carbohydrates; Colitis; Constipation; Diarrhea and dysentery; Dietary reference intakes (DRIs); Digestion; Enzymes; Food biochemistry; Food Guide Pyramid; Gastroenterology; Gastroenterology, pediatric; Gastrointestinal disorders; Gastrointestinal system; Gluten intolerance; Malabsorption; Metabolism; Nutrition; Peristalsis; Phytonutrients; Protein.

For Further Information:
"Dietary Fiber." *MedlinePlus*, May 8, 2013.
"Digestive System." *MedlinePlus*, January 14, 2013.
Dudek, Susan G. *Nutrition Essentials for Nursing Practice.* 6th ed. Philadelphia: Lippincott, Williams and Wilkins, 2010.
Kirschmann, John D. *Nutrition Almanac.* 6th ed. New York: McGraw-Hill, 2007.
Nix, Staci. *Williams" Basic Nutrition and Diet Therapy.* 14th ed. New York: Elsevier Health Sciences, 2013.
Sizer, Frances, and Ellie Whitney. *Nutrition: Concepts and Controversies.* 13th ed. New York: Cengage Learning, 2013.
Whitney, Eleanor Noss, and Sharon Rady Rolfes. *Understanding Nutrition.* Updated 12th ed. New York: Cengage Learning, 2011.

FIBROCYSTIC BREAST CONDITION
Disease/Disorder
Also known as: Fibrocystic breast changes, benign breast disease, benign breast lesions, diffuse cystic mastopathy, mammary dysplasia, nonmalignant breast neoplasms
Anatomy or system affected: Breasts, endocrine system, skin
Specialties and related fields: Gynecology, histopathology, oncology
Definition: The most common type of noncancerous breast condition, affecting approximately 60 percent of all women, the majority of whom are premenopausal. Because of its widespread incidence, the condition is now considered to be a normal physiologic variant. It is characterized by stromal tissue and glandular (lobules and ducts) changes in the breast or breasts that result in lumpiness, thickening, and localized edema (swelling).

Key terms:
collecting duct: a tubular canal that transports milk from the milk duct to the nipple
lobule: a small gland that, when sent appropriate hormonal cues, produces milk
mammary gland: a group of milk-producing cells consisting of lobules and ducts
milk duct: a tubular canal that transports milk from the lobule to the collecting duct
stroma: the deeper layer of breast tissue

Causes and Symptoms
Fibrocystic breast change is the most common type of noncancerous breast condition. Its incidence rate in females is estimated to be more than 60 percent. Therefore, although once classified as a disease, it is now considered to be a normal physiologic variant. It occurs more commonly in females between the ages of thirty and fifty. Its cause is hypothesized to be an excess of circulating estrogen.

Female breast development begins at puberty, triggered by an increase in estrogen level. The four main components of the mature female breast are adipose tissue (fat), ducts (milk ducts and collecting ducts), groups of lobules (referred to as lobes), and connective tissue consisting of a matrix of suspensory ligaments (strong fibrous bands). Each breast contains approximately fifteen to twenty lobes that radiate from the nipple area in a spokelike pattern, with the highest distribution being in the upper outer quadrant of each breast. Breast lobe consistency tends to be firm and slightly nodular, but may vary by breast or by individual, while breast fat is almost always soft. Breasts of younger women primarily consist of glandular tissue. Aging changes result in shrinkage of glandular tissue and replacement with fat, which causes the breast to become softer and less well supported.

Symptoms of fibrocystic breast change result from hormone-induced alterations in the stromal (deeper layer) tissue, glands (lobules) and ducts within the breast. Those changes include possible fibrosis (formation of fibrous tissue like that of scar tissue) and/or formation of cysts, as fluid accumulates inside the glands. Small amounts of accumulated fluid result in microscopic cysts (microcysts); larger amounts of accumulated fluid result in palpable macrocysts that may grow to an inch or more in size. The two major types of breast cysts are type I, characterized by high concentrations of androgen

---

Information on Fibrocystic Breast Condition
Causes: Possibly hormonal variations during the menstrual cycle; excess amount of circulating estrogen
Symptoms: Dense, irregular lumpiness in breast tissue, discomfort and tenderness, dull pain, localized edema (swelling), feeling of fullness, possible nipple discharge
Duration: Varies; usually cyclic
Treatments: Symptom dependent, from breast self-examination and properly fitting support bra to hormone therapy

and estrogen conjugates, epidermal growth factor, and potassium and low concentrations of sodium and chloride; and type II, characterized by high concentrations of sodium and chloride and lower concentrations of androgen and estrogen conjugates, epidermal growth factor, and potassium.

Symptoms of fibrocystic breast change include dense and irregular lumpiness in breast tissue, discomfort, dull pain, localized edema (swelling) and feeling of fullness, tenderness, and possible nipple discharge. Symptoms may vary in intensity throughout the menstrual cycle, peak just prior to menstruation, and range from mild to severe. Symptoms and signs of fibrocystic change may remit after menopause because of decreased amounts of glandular tissue in the breast and decreased levels of estrogen and progesterone.

Treatment and Therapy

Treatment is not for the condition itself but rather for the symptoms. For those women who are asymptomatic, no treatment beyond monitoring via breast self-examination is required. For those women who are symptomatic, treatment options range from use of a properly fitting support bra to use of hormone therapy—via oral contraceptives, androgens, or tamoxifen (a drug that blocks estrogen activity)—which has the potential to cause side effects. Cysts may require fine needle aspiration or ultrasonogrphy to determine whether a biopsy is needed.

Anecdotal evidence suggests that avoidance of methylxanthine-containing items such as coffee, tea, chocolate, and certain sodas; reduction in sodium intake; use of vitamin supplements; and/or use of herbal supplements may ameliorate symptoms caused by fibrocystic changes. However, these findings have not been clinically proven.

Perspective and Prospects

The preferred term for fibrocystic breast disease is now "fibrocystic breast changes" or "fibrocystic breast condition." It may also be referred to as benign breast disease, benign breast lesions, diffuse cystic mastopathy, mammary dysplasia, or nonmalignant breast neoplasms. Cohort studies of risk factors associated with this condition have been conducted for up to thirty years. A family history of fibrocystic breast condition is believed to be the highest risk factor. Consumption of a high-fat diet may be a cofactor. No association has been found between incidence rate of this condition and alcohol consumption or cigarette smoking.

Breast tissue changes as a result of fibrocystic breast condition may make breast examination and mammography interpretation more difficult. However, while presence of type I macrocytes—a fibrocystic change characterized by high concentrations of androgen and estrogen conjugates, epidermal growth factor, and potassium—may be linked to a moderate increase in breast cancer risk, most fibrocystic changes associated with fibrocystic breast condition (fibrosis, microcysts, and type II macrocysts) are not associated with an increased risk of breast cancer.

—*Cynthia L. De Vine*

See also Breast biopsy; Breast disorders; Breasts, female; Cyst removal; Cysts; Hormones; Lesions; Mammography; Menopause; Women's health.

For Further Information:

Ajao, O. G. "Benign Breast Lesions." *Journal of the National Medical Association* 71, no. 9 (1979): 867–868.

Bhimji, Shabir, et al. "Fibrocystic Breast Changes." *MedlinePlus*, Nov. 5, 2012.

"Breast Diseases." *MedlinePlus*, May 3, 2013.

Bruzzi P., L. Dogliotti, and C. Naldoni, et al. "Cohort Study of Association of Risk of Breast Cancer with Cyst Type in Women with Gross Cystic Disease of the Breast." *BMJ* 314 (1997): 925–928.

Dixon, J. M., A. B. Lumsden, and W. R. Miller. "The Relationship of Cyst Type to Risk Factors for Breast Cancer and the Subsequent Development of Breast Cancer in Patients with Breast Cystic Disease." *European Journal of Cancer and Clinical Oncology* 21 (1985): 1047–1050.

"Fibrosis and Simple Cysts." American Cancer Society, Aug. 24, 2012.

Guray, M. Sahin. "Benign Breast Diseases: Classification, Diagnosis, and Management." *Oncologist* 11 (2006): 435–449.

Haagensen, C. D., C. Bodian, and D. E. Haagensen, Jr., eds. *Breast Carcinoma: Risk and Detection*. Philadelphia: W. B. Saunders, 1981.

Hartmann, L. C., T. A. Sellers, M. H. Frost, et al. "Benign Breast Disease and the Risk of Breast Cancer." *New England Journal of Medicine* 353 (2005): 229–237.

Kamel, O. W., R. L. Kempson, and M. R. Hendrickson. "In situ Proliferative Epithelial Lesions of the Breast." *Pathology* 1 (1992): 65–102.

Miller, W. R., et al. "Using Biological Measurements: Can Patients with Benign Breast Disease Who Are at High Risk for Breast Cancer Be Identified?" *Cancer Detection and Prevention* 16 Suppl. (1992): 13–20.

Polsdorfer, Ricker, and Andrea Chisholm. "Fibrocystic Disease." *Health Library*, Sept. 28, 2012.

Santen, R. J., and R. Mansel. "Benign Breast Disorders." *New England Journal of Medicine* 353 (2005): 275–285.

Sauter, Edward R., and Mary B. Daly. *Breast Cancer Risk Reduction and Early Dectection*. New York: Spring, 2010.

Schnitt, S. J., and J. L. Connolly. "Pathology of Benign Breast Disorders." In *Diseases of the Breast*, edited by J. R. Harris et al. 4th ed. Philadelphia: Lippincott Williams & Wilkins, 2010.

"Understanding Breast Changes: A Health Guide for Women." *National Cancer Institute*, Nov. 2, 2012.

Washington C., et al. "Loss of Heterozygosity in Fibrocystic Change of the Breast: Genetic Relationship Between Proliferative Lesions and Associated Carcinomas." *American Journal of Pathology* 157, no. 1 (2000): 323–329.

FIBROMYALGIA

Disease/Disorder

Also known as: Fibromyalgia syndrome

Anatomy or system affected: Brain, head, muscles, musculoskeletal system, nerves, nervous system, psychic-emotional system

Specialties and related fields: Rheumatology

Definition: A connective, soft tissue disease involving chronic, spontaneous, and widespread musculoskeletal pain, as well as recurrent fatigue and sleep disturbance.

Key terms:

connective tissue: the supporting framework of the body, particularly tendons and ligaments *fibrositis:* an earlier, less common term for fibromyalgia

flare-up: an episode of heightened pain and debilitation in fibromyalgia; sometimes flare-ups do not have an immediate, precipitating cause that is identifiable, while other times they are associated with humidity, cold, physical exertion, or psychological stress

functional somatic syndromes: a continuum or spectrum of disorders (such as chronic fatigue syndrome, Epstein-Barr virus, and primary headaches) characterized by complex interactions between symptoms and patients' personal stress

tender points: specific, precise, and localized areas of moderately to severely intense pain

Causes and Symptoms

The cause of fibromyalgia is unknown. Some researchers believe that an injury or trauma to the central nervous system causes the disorder. Other researchers believe that changes in muscle and connective tissue metabolism produce decreased blood flow, beginning a pathological cycle of weakness, fatigue, and decreased strength that eventually results in the full-blown syndrome. Still others believe that an as-yet-undiscovered virus or infectious agent attacks people who are naturally susceptible to the infection, who then develop the syndrome.

The most salient feature of fibromyalgia syndrome is pain. Described by sufferers as "having no boundaries," the pain is characteristically variable. The same sufferer experiences pain ranging from deep muscle aching to throbbing, stabbing, or shooting pains to a burning sensation that has been called "acid running through blood vessels." The pain frequently causes joint and muscle stiffness. Pain and stiffness may be worse in the morning and may be more intense in the joints and muscle groups that are used more often. Patients may have tender points, as in the knee, hips, spine, shoulders, and neck. There are typically eighteen potential tender points, and at least eleven must be painful for a diagnosis of fibromyalgia to be made.

Sufferers also experience fatigue and weakness, ranging from mild to debilitating. Patients liken the fatigue to having their arms and legs tied to concrete, and many feel that they are living in a kind of mental fog, unable to focus or concentrate. Between 40 and 70 percent of patients also have some variation of irritable bowel syndrome (IBS): frequent abdominal cramping, nausea, and chronic constipation or diarrhea. About half of all sufferers also experience concurrent migraine or tension headaches. The condition is often mental as well as physical, as sufferers may also suffer from major depressive disorder and anxiety.

Less common, but readily found, are a constellation of symptoms that, in order of prevalence, include jaw, face, and head pain, which is easily misdiagnosed as temporomandibular joint syndrome (TMJ); hypersensitivities to odors, bright lights, and even fibromyalgia medications; painful menstruation; memory problems; and muscle twitching. Weather (particularly exposure to cold), normal hormonal fluctuation, stress, anxiety, depression, and physi-

---

Information on Fibromyalgia

Causes: Unknown; possibly injury or trauma to central nervous system, changes in muscle and connective tissue metabolism, or infectious agent

Symptoms: Severe muscle pain; joint and muscle stiffness; tender points in knee, hips, spine, shoulders, and neck; fatigue; weakness; sometimes concurrent irritable bowel syndrome (IBS) and migraine or tension headaches

Duration: Chronic with acute episodes

Treatments: Alleviation of symptoms through medications, physical therapy, massage therapy, acupuncture, behavioral therapy

---

cal exertion can aggravate fibromyalgia and produce flare-ups.

Treatment and Therapy

Because the cause of fibromyalgia is unknown, only its symptoms can be addressed. The treatment plan must be individualized and flexible, and it is considered long-term management. Rigid, stereotyped approaches can be worse than no management at all.

Because difficulty sleeping and pain can be both contributors to and outcomes of fibromyalgia, traditional treatment approaches focus on improving quality of sleep and reducing pain. Physicians commonly prescribe medications that increase the neurotransmitters serotonin and norepinephrine, which modulate sleep, pain, and the immune system. These medications may be prescribed in low doses; they benefit one-third to one-half of patients. Alone or in combination, these medicines improve sleep staging, elevate mood, and relax overtense, stiff, and spasm-prone muscle groups. Three other medications, Lyrica (pregabalin), Cymbalta (duloxetine), and Savella (milnacipran), have been specifically approved to treat fibromyalgia.

More comprehensive are approaches that use medications as part of a well-rounded treatment plan. Physical therapy, massage therapy, acupuncture, and behavioral health are other treatment options. Physical therapy and aerobic exercises such as swimming and walking reduce muscle tenderness and pain while improving muscle conditioning and fitness. Because of fibromyalgia sufferers" sensitivity to cold and frequent stiffness, applied heat and therapeutic massage can render short-term relief. Though acupuncture is less well studied, anecdotal accounts claim its effectiveness, making it a sought-after therapy. Psychological counseling, or psychotherapy, can be effective for patients as well.

Perspective and Prospects

Until the 1990s, fibromyalgia syndrome—or fibrositis, as it was then more often called—was not widely accepted by primary care specialists as a legitimate condition. Difficult to diagnose, it was often mistaken as chronic fatigue syndrome (itself a condition not widely recognized in primary care medicine), a sort of chronic pain syndrome, or some condition that was completely psychosomatic (that is, all in the patient's head). Fibromyalgia syndrome was often thought of as a "garbage can diagnosis"—a little bit of everything, but not a real syndrome that could be treated. Sufferers had difficulty finding sympathetic medical help and were often at odds with family, friends, and coworkers who misattributed the causes of this connective, soft tissue disease whose existence could not be proven.

Advances in rheumatological research and the American College of Rheumatology's establishment of diagnostic criteria for fibromyalgia have made it a legitimate medical condition for which treatment can be sought. Previously, those with fibromyalgia often suffered from this painful, fatiguing condition and felt blamed for causing it—or worse, for "making it up." Even today, the Fibromyalgia Network, a grassroots informational clearinghouse, underscores research that proves fibromyalgia syndrome is real.

Despite differing theories about the cause of fibromyalgia, ongoing research has produced some results that all investigators consider reliable. This syndrome seems to involve a relationship among the nervous system, the endocrine system, and sleep. When sleep electroencephalograms (EEGs) for patients known to have fibromyalgia are compared with those for nonpatient subjects, disturbances in the non-rapid eye movement (non-REM) stages become evident. There are five well-known and easily recognized stages of sleep: four non-REM stages and then an REM stage. Most people effortlessly progress through non-REM and REM stages. When they reach stage 4, a non-REM stage, they have reached sleep at its deepest. This is the stage during which tissue repair, antibody production, and possibly neurotransmitter regulation occur. Fibromyalgia EEGs show that these patients revert to stage 2 after stage 3, without having reached stage 4. Specialists refer to this sleep disorder as the alpha-EEG anomaly.

This EEG finding corresponds directly with fibromyalgia patients" anecdotal reports that they frequently do not feel rested or refreshed after a night's sleep. This result also contributes to an understanding of why sufferers are fatigued so often. The disturbance of non-REM sleep helps to produce the symptoms of insufficient sleep: tiredness, reduced mental acuity, irritability, and autoimmune susceptibilities. The various stages of sleep also have corresponding hormonal activity, with different hormones and different levels released during each. Stages 3 and 4 are when growth hormones, including insulin growth factor (IGF), are primarily released. Fibromyalgia patients have low IGF levels.

A few other characteristic findings in these patients are not related to sleep. First, the neurotransmitter cerebrospinal fluid P (CSF P), also called substance P, is found in fibromyalgia patients at three times the normal level. Significantly, CSF P is associated with enhanced pain perception. Second, sufferers have low cortisol levels, suggesting that the hypopituitary-adrenal axis is adversely altered. Among much else, this axis mediates the fight-or-flight response and relaxation. Third, using an office procedure called tilt table testing, fibromyalgia symptoms can be provoked, accompanied by a rapid lowering of blood pressure in those with fibromyalgia

but not in those without the disease. These findings all provide evidence that problems in the autonomic and endocrine systems cause fibromyalgia. What would set these problems into motion in the first place, however, is unknown, although many sufferers have experienced significant physical and/or psychological trauma before any syndrome-specific symptoms began.

—*Paul Moglia, Ph.D.*

See also Anxiety; Chronic fatigue syndrome; Depression; Fatigue; Headaches; Irritable bowel syndrome (IBS); Migraine headaches; Muscle sprains, spasms, and disorders; Muscles; Pain; Pain management; Sleep; Sleep disorders; Stress; Stress reduction.

For Further Information:

"About Fibromyalgia." *National Fibromyalgia Association*, 2009.
Alan, Rick, and Rimas Lukas. "Fibromyalgia." *Health Library*, Sept. 30, 2012.
"Fibro Basics." *Fibromyalgia Network*, 2010.
"Fibromyalgia." *MedlinePlus*, May 13, 2013.
Goldenberg, Don L. *Fibromyalgia: A Leading Expert's Guide to Understanding and Getting Relief from the Pain That Won't Go Away.* Berkeley, Calif.: Berkeley Publishing Group, 2002.
Jones, Kim D., and Janice H. Hoffman. *Fibromyalgia.* Santa Barbara, Calif.: Greenwood Press/ABC-CLIO, 2009.
McCarberg, Bill. H., and Daniel J. Clauw, eds. *Fibromyalgia.* New York: Informa Healthcare, 2009.
Pellegrino, Mark. *Inside Fibromyalgia.* Columbus, Ohio: Anadem, 2001.
"Questions and Answers about Fibromyalgia." *National Institute of Arthritis and Musculoskeletal and Skin Diseases*, Aug. 2012.
Wallace, Daniel J., and Daniel J. Clauw, eds. *Fibromyalgia and Other Central Pain Syndromes.* Philadelphia: Lippincott Williams & Wilkins, 2005.
Wallace, Daniel J., and Janice Brock Wallace. *All About Fibromyalgia: A Guide for Patients and Their Families.* 2d ed. New York: Oxford University Press, 2007.

FIFTH DISEASE

Disease/Disorder

Also known as: Erythema infectiosum

Anatomy or system affected: Nose, skin, throat

Specialties and related fields: Family medicine, pediatrics

Definition: An infectious disease of children characterized by an erythematous (reddish) rash and low-grade fever.

Causes and Symptoms

Fifth disease is caused by infection with the human parvovirus (HPV) B19. The disease is more prevalent during late winter or early spring. Fifth disease is most commonly observed in young children, with the peak attack rate between five and fourteen years of age. Adults may become infected, but they rarely show evidence of disease.

The virus is spread from person to person through nasal secretions or sneezing. Following an incubation period of several days, a rash develops on the face, which has the appearance of slapped cheeks. The bright red color fades as the rash spreads over the rest of the body. An erythematous, pimply eruption may also appear on the trunk or extremities. A mild fever, sore throat, and nasal stuffiness may also be apparent. The rash generally lasts from ten days to two weeks. Often, it

---

Information on Fifth Disease

Causes: Viral infection
Symptoms: "Slapped cheek" rash, fever, sore throat, achiness, malaise
Duration: Ten to fourteen days
Treatments: Alleviation of symptoms through bed rest, administration of liquids

---

will fade only to reappear a short time later. Sunlight may aggravate the skin during this period, also causing a reappearance of the rash.

The diagnosis of fifth disease is primarily clinical, based on the symptoms. Laboratory tests for the virus are generally not performed.

Treatment and Therapy

No antiviral medication is available for fifth disease. Since the disease is rarely serious, treatment is mainly symptomatic, including medications for fever, pain, and itchiness. Bed rest and the administration of liquids, as commonly used in treating mild illness in children, are generally sufficient. Isolation is unnecessary since transmission is unlikely following appearance of the rash.

Perspective and Prospects

Fifth disease was first described during the late nineteenth century as the fifth in the series of erythematous illnesses often encountered by children; the others are measles, mumps, chickenpox, and rubella. HPV B19 was isolated in 1975 and shown to be the etiological agent of the disease in the mid-1980s.

The disease is common and generally benign. HPV B19 has been implicated, however, in certain forms of hemolytic anemias and arthritis in adults, and research continues on the virus.

—*Richard Adler, Ph.D.*

See also Childhood infectious diseases; Fever; Rashes; Sneezing; Sore throat; Viral infections.

For Further Information:

Kliegman, Robert, and Waldo E. Nelson, eds. *Nelson Textbook of Pediatrics*. 19th ed. Philadelphia: Saunders/Elsevier, 2011.
Burg, Fredric D., et al., eds. *Treatment of Infants, Children, and Adolescents*. Philadelphia: W. B. Saunders, 1990.
"Fifth Disease." *MedlinePlus*, May 2, 2013.
Kemper, Kathi J. *The Holistic Pediatrician: A Pediatrician's Comprehensive Guide to Safe and Effective Therapies for the Twenty-five Most Common Ailments of Infants, Children, and Adolescents*. 2d ed. New York: HarperCollins, 2007.
Kumar, Vinay, Abul K. Abbas, and Nelson Fausto, eds. *Robbins and Cotran Pathologic Basis of Disease*. 8th ed. Philadelphia: Saunders/Elsevier, 2010.
McCoy, Krisha, and Michael Woods. "Fifth Disease." *Health Library*, Sept. 26, 2012.
"Parvovirus B19 and Fifth Disease." *Centers for Disease Control and Prevention*, Feb. 14, 2012.
Sompayrac, Lauren. *How Pathogenic Viruses Work*. Boston: Jones and Bartlett, 2002.

FINGERNAIL REMOVAL. *See* **NAIL REMOVAL.**

FIRST AID
Treatment
Also known as: Emergency aid
Anatomy or system affected: All
Specialties and related fields: All
Definition: The National First Aid Science Advisory Board defines "first aid" as "assessments and interventions that can be performed by a bystander (or by the victim) with minimal or no medical equipment."

Introduction

In 2005, the American Red Cross and the American Heart Association created the National First Aid Science Advisory Board (NFASAB) to review scientific literature on first aid. The board's review found few published studies on first-aid practices and concluded that most of them are based on professional experience and expert opinion. The board then published evidence-based first-aid guidelines that can be used to update training programs.

First aid administered at the scene of an accident can be lifesaving. As a general rule, a victim should not be moved if spinal injury is suspected. Advanced first-aid training should include the proper use of immobilization devices for suspected spinal injuries.

Common first-aid breathing emergencies include asthma attacks, allergic anaphylaxis, seizures, and choking. A first-aid responder to an asthma attack can assist a victim in administering his or her prescribed medication, usually an inhaler, while waiting for professional aid. For anaphylaxis due to allergies to insect stings or food, first-aid responders should be trained to administer epinephrine in an emergency, if state law permits, or to assist a victim in self-administering. Seizure treatment should focus on preventing injury and keeping the airway open. Restraining a victim during a seizure is not recommended, as it can cause bruising or injury. Placing an object in the mouth can damage teeth or obstruct airways and is also not recommended. Choking can occur in adults and children when an object gets stuck in the throat and cuts off air. First-aid techniques for choking include using the heel of the hand to administer five firm blows between a person's shoulder blades and, if that fails to dislodge the object, administering the Heimlich maneuver. Both techniques can injure a person if not done correctly. Standard first-aid training should include common breathing emergency techniques.

Common injury-related first aid includes bleeding control and wound management. Excessive bleeding should be controlled by applying pressure over the area until the bleeding stops. Gauze or other clean, soft material can be placed over the wound while applying pressure and should not be removed prematurely. The use of pressure points and the elevation of a limb to help control excessive bleeding are not well studied and should not be used instead of the proven method of applying pressure to the wound. The safety and effective use of tourniquets is also under review.

Cuts, scrapes, and puncture wounds should all be cleaned with cool water. Soap and a soft cloth should be used to clean around the wound, and sterile tweezers should be used to remove any dirt that remains in the wound after rinsing with water. Bleeding can help clean out a shallow wound and usually stops in a few minutes. Deeper cuts may require gentle, firm pressure with gauze or other sterile material. If the wound is on the leg or arm, after bleeding has been controlled, raising it above the patient's head may help, but this should not be used if it interferes with the application of pressure. The wound should be covered if it will get dirty or rub against something; otherwise a shallow wound can remain uncovered to help it dry and heal faster. Large-area scrapes need to be kept moist and covered to avoid scarring. Bandages should be changed at least every day. Antibiotic cream can help prevent infections; triple antibiotic cream is recommended as the most effective.

First-aid training for burns includes how to identify first-, second-, and third-degree burns. Serious burns can result from exposure to fire, heat sources, the sun, electricity, chemicals, or radiation. A serious burn can be any burn more than several inches in diameter or one that turns the skin white or looks charred. Stabilizing treatment includes soaking the burned area in cool water (five minutes for a first-degree burn, fifteen minutes for a second-degree burn), then treating with a skin ointment such as aloe or antibacterial cream and covering the burn area with loose gauze to keep air off and keep the area clean. Over-the-counter pain or anti-inflammatory medicine may help reduce pain and swelling. Direct application of ice cubes to skin is not recommended. Burn blisters should not be popped or removed.

First aid for muscle injuries includes applying a cold pack for no more than twenty minutes to the injury to reduce hemorrhage, edema, pain, and disability. Use of a compression bandage to reduce edema has not been well studied. If an injured extremity is blue or extremely pale, then immediate medical care is needed.

There are many toxic or poisonous substances in the home and workplace. First-aid training includes instruction in emergency procedures for different classes of poisons. Government-sponsored poison-control centers are a good resource. Poisoning can occur by swallowing a poisonous substance, breathing in poisonous air, or contacting a poisonous substance with bare skin. Poison-control centers can provide advice. First-aid training for poison response includes strategies for stabilizing the victim, identifying the poison, and minimizing the responder's exposure to poisonous substances. For ingested poisons, some commonsense approaches or older methods are no longer recommended. Inducing vomiting with syrup of ipecac is not recommended, nor is administering charcoal. If poisons have been inhaled, then removing the person to a place with fresh air as fast as possible is essential.

Standard first aid includes recognition and treatment of insect, snake, and animal bites. Some insect bites or stings, such as from bees, wasps, yellow jackets, and fire ants, can cause localized pain and swelling; if a person is allergic, they can cause more serious reactions, including life-threatening swelling of airway passages (anaphylaxis). Only a small number of spiders cause serious reactions in nonallergic people; chief among these are the black widow and the brown recluse. First-aid training should cover treatment for insect bites or stings, including tick bites, as well as animal bites. The latter should also feature assessment of the possibility of rabies infection. Poisonous snakebites are a medical emergency. First-aid recommendations focus on limiting the spread of venom in the bloodstream by not moving the affected area. It is not advised to try to suck out the venom or cut out the bitten area.

Wilderness first aid requires some additional skills and supplies. Stabilizing an injured person and assisting them in evacuating a remote area are critical skills. Components of wilderness first-aid training can include how to treat hyperthermia, hypothermia, frostbite, and altitude sickness; specific knowledge of marine hazards, such as stinging jellyfish; emergency treatment for diarrhea and dehydration; and how to make splints and other supports from available materials. Hikers and explorers should learn specifics about first aid for the area where they will be traveling.

Discussion

First-aid training is often available through local Red Cross chapters or local community or health centers. Key components of first-aid training should include knowing how to get help, knowing how to position a victim, and knowing how to handle medical emergencies. Key medical emergencies include breathing difficulties, anaphylaxis, and seizures. Key injury emergencies include bleeding; wounds and abrasions; burns; spine injuries; musculoskeletal injuries such as sprains, strains, and fractures; and dental injuries. Key environmental emergencies include hypothermia, drowning, poisoning, and snakebites. More complex first-aid training may include safe handling of blood-borne pathogens and administration of oxygen and cardiopulmonary resuscitation (CPR). Specific first-aid training, such as wilderness first aid and travel first aid, are offered by a number of organizations.

The most common first-aid courses offer home first-aid training for parents and other caregivers. Basic first-aid training for the home includes how to respond to common illnesses and conditions such as croup, stroke, angina, asthma, diabetes, epilepsy, meningitis, anaphylaxis, heart attack, and febrile convulsions. It can also include how to identify and respond to common household poisonings, eye injury, head injury, crush injury, spinal injury, and the effects of temperature extremes. Other topics include how to respond to minor injuries and illness such as fever, cramps, blisters, fainting, earache, vomiting, headache, diarrhea, toothache, sore throat, abdominal pain, crushed fingers, burns and scalds, allergic reactions, stings, splinters, and small wounds and grazes.

First-aid kits are a key component of any first-aid effort. First-aid kits should be available in every home, school, work site, and vehicle. A standard kit should include a first-aid manual; bandages, including elastic bandages and sterile gauze; adhesive tape; disinfectants, such as antiseptic wipes or solutions; antibiotic ointment; over-the-counter pain and anti-inflammatory medicine, such as acetaminophen and ibuprofen; various tools, such as tweezers, sharp scissors, and safety pins; a thermometer; and plastic gloves.

Perspective and Prospects

First aid has been a part of organized Western medicine since the mid-nineteenth century, when it was expanded from efforts to tend to wounded soldiers. It began as basic training for soldiers to tend war casualties. The term "first aid" was coined from the terms "first response" and "National Aid" (the precursor to the British Red Cross) in 1878 by British Army officer and doctor Peter Shepherd, who, together with fellow officer Francis Duncan, introduced the concept of training civilians in first aid. Participants in these training courses received a certificate and volunteered to help care for wounded soldiers.

First aid became an established form of emergency care in the late nineteenth century. In Great Britain, the St. John Ambulance Brigade was established in 1873 to provide first aid to the public, and the St. John Ambulance Association was established in 1877 to train civilians in first-aid care. The primary focus was on providing aid to industrial workers. As part of the St. John Ambulance Association program, first-aid volunteers also helped in public disaster response. Both these groups have their roots in the Order of St. John, a religious order that provided medical services to soldiers as early as the twelfth century. St. John Ambulance remains one of the largest providers of first aid worldwide, operating in thirty-nine countries.

At about the same time that the Order of St. John was establishing first-aid classes, the International Red Cross committee was working to provide humanitarian aid to soldiers worldwide. In 1863, Henry Dunant founded the International Committee of the Red Cross as a reaction to the mass war casualties that he witnessed during a business trip to Italy and the lack of medical and humanitarian care available to wounded soldiers. This was the beginning of international efforts to establish Red Cross societies around the world. In the United States, Clara Barton, a nurse and teacher, became president of the American Red Cross in 1881. She expanded basic first-aid training for soldiers to include training for industrial accidents and disaster relief. Today, national Red Cross societies exist in most countries.

—Sandra Ripley Distelhorst

See also Accidents; Bites and stings; Bleeding; Burns and scalds; Cardiopulmonary resuscitation (CPR); Choking; Concussion; Critical care; Critical care, pediatric; Drowning; Electrical shock; Emergency medicine; Emergency medicine, pediatric; Fracture and dislocation; Fracture repair; Frostbite; Heart attack; Heat exhaustion and heatstroke; Hyperthermia and hypothermia; Laceration repair; Paramedics; Poisoning; Resuscitation; Shock; Snakebites; Sports medicine; Unconsciousness; Wounds.

For Further Information:

American Red Cross and Kathleen A. Handal. *The American Red Cross First Aid and Safety Handbook.* Boston: Little, Brown, 1992.
"First Aid." *MedlinePlus*, May 28, 2013.
Krohmer, Jon R., ed. *American College of Emergency Physicians First Aid Manual.* 2d ed. New York: DK, 2004.
Subbarao, Italo, Jim Lyznicki, and James J. James, eds. *The American Medical Association Handbook of First Aid and Emergency Care.* Rev. ed. New York: Random House Reference, 2009.
Weiss, Eric A. *Wilderness and Travel Medicine: A Comprehensive Guide.* 4th ed. Seattle: Mountaineers, 2012.

FIRST RESPONDER

Anatomy or system affected: All

Specialties and related fields: Firefighter, law enforcement officer, emergency medical technician (EMT), community emergency response teams (CERT), medical/paramedical personnel, community nurses, Hazardous materials and items (HAZMAT) team

Definition: The initial person(s) to arrive on the scene who has received training in the rescue and prehospital care of individuals involved in or affected by an emergency situation.

History of the Role

The history of the First Responder role has evolved simultaneously over the years as the level of emergency response has matured. In 1979, an effort was made to improve the then Emergency Crash Response Program to include more comprehensive and structured prehospital care. The program to train First Responders expanded from an eight-hour program, first proposed by the American Red Cross, to a more comprehensive program. Subsequently, as the need for First Responders increased, in 1995, the U.S. Department of Transportation (DOT) took a closer look at the role and developed guidelines for the certification of the First Responder in America. This program matured to a 40-60 hour instructional program to recruit individuals to respond to their community emergency needs. The emergency crises that resulted from the collapse of the World Trade Center provided even more dimension to the maturing role of the First Responder. For the first time in American history, legislation was signed into law providing financial support for those First Responders affected by the 9/11 tragedy (The James L. Zadroga 9/11 Health and Compensation Act).

Science and Profession

First Responders provide rescue and prehospital care to individuals acutely ill/injured or in need of emergency transport from an emergency situation or catastrophic event in the community they serve. Those First Responders who have been previously trained can provide emergency care to individuals in need of immediate response/help. However, First Responders are usually trained to elicit the help of more emergency/medically trained personnel as soon as feasibly possible. This may include the help of the fire department, law enforcement, emergency medical technicians and other medical services. First Responders are trained to recognize the emergency, medical situation, or emergent environment of a circumstance and coordinate or manage the emergency care or safe evacuation of the person in need. This is why so many facets of emergency services may be utilized/employed.

Perspective and Prospects

First Responder is a dynamic and exciting field of study. It is a field that is open to many individuals regardless of academic preparation. Few areas offer more opportunity to serve the community they live in, in a way that uniquely fits the individual's ability and skills. There is an opportunity to become certified in this area through local community groups. These programs may be organized and provided by the local fire department/police department or, as in New York City, the Office of Emergency Management (OEM). The need for the services of First Responders continues to grow with the threat of ongoing climate change, catastrophic emergencies, and terrorist activities. Recruitment continues to be a challenge for all communities as well as developing agencies that can address the responsibility to oversee the dynamics of these ongoing programs.

—*Mary Frances McGibbon, DNP, RN, MSN, FNP-BC*

For Further Information:

Hamilton, Glenn C., et al. *Emergency Medicine: An Approach to the Clinical-Problem Solving.* 2nd ed. New York: W.B. Saunders, 2003. Provides an understanding of the emergency scene and response examples.

McGibbon, M.F. *Support for First Responders Health Care: In the Aftermath of the World Trade Center Disaster, An Historical Overview.* Washington, D.C.: National Archives: 2011. Provides background information on the First Responders and the effects of 9/11 exposure and legislation in this area.

National Training and Education Division (NTED): https://www.firstrespondertraining.gov/content.do. Guidelines and training for First Responders from the U.S. government agency that serves them.

North Shore/Long Island Jewish Hospital's Certifies First Responder Course: http://www.northshorelij.com/hospitals/location/certified-first-responder-course. Information on a 70-hour course designed to address the needs of the new First Responder.

FISTULA REPAIR

Procedure

Anatomy or system affected: Abdomen, anus, bladder, blood, gallbladder, gastrointestinal system, intestines, reproductive system, urinary system, uterus

Specialties and related fields: Gastroenterology, general surgery, pediatrics, proctology

Definition: The removal of any abnormal passage associated with body sites or tissues.

Key terms:

anorectal: associated with the anal portion of the large intestine

arteriovenous: associated with arteries and/or veins

Crohn's disease: a chronic inflammation of the bowel, often as a result of an autoimmune disease

crypt: a pit or depression in the body

fistulectomy: the surgical elimination of a fistula

Indications and Procedures

A fistula is any abnormal opening or passage between internal organs or between an internal organ and the surface of the body. Fistulas can occur nearly anywhere in the body, but they are most commonly associated with the anorectal portion of the anatomy. Some fistulas may result from congenital defects, while others may be created surgically in association with specific procedures. For example, an arteriovenous fistula may be created to allow the insertion of a cannula (tube) for hemodialysis.

Common Sites of Fistulas

Fistulas are abnormal passages between organs or an organ and the outside of the body. They are more common in the rectal and genital regions of women, such as between the intestines and vagina (enterovaginal), the bladder and uterus (vesicouterine), the bladder and vagina (vesicovaginal), the urethra and vagina (urethrovaginal), and the rectum and vagina (rectovaginal).

Anorectal fistulas usually begin as an abscess within the anal region or internal crypt that then spreads to adjacent tissue or to the surface of the body. Pain, itching, or tenderness in the region is often the first sign of a problem. The discomfort may be aggravated by bowel movements. Since infection is common, the opening may become purulent (pus producing).

Treatment of anorectal fistulas usually requires surgery. A crypt hook may be used if the site of the original crypt must be located, though this is often unnecessary. The crypt may also be observed through an anoscope or as part of a proctoscopic examination. Often, digital examination of the anal canal may detect a nodule, representing the abscess itself.

Any abscess must first be drained and treated. If the fistula is small, it may heal itself. The surgical procedure, commonly referred to as a fistulectomy, is a relatively simple operation carried out under general anesthesia. The fistula must be reduced or removed. Surgical repair begins at the primary opening. Generally the entire tract is opened, both to allow for proper drainage of infectious material and to promote healing. If the surgery is carried out properly, the incision should heal relatively quickly.

Difficult labor in women may create a variety of fistulas. A vesicovaginal fistula, created between the urinary bladder and the vagina, may be indicated by the presence of urine in the vaginal tract. As with any opening to the surface of the body, infection may develop. Likewise, a rectovaginal fistula, between the rectum and vagina, was formerly a possible serious complication of difficult childbirth. Such openings, like any fistulas, must be opened, drained, and sutured for healing.

Fistula formation may also be internal, as in biliary fistulas between the gallbladder and intestine. Such connections can occur as a consequence of gallstones, ulcers, or tumor formation. Often, the major symptom may be an intestinal blockage resulting from the stone or tumor itself. Bile may leak from the gallbladder into the peritoneum or body cavities, resulting in infection. Therapy for such fistula formation first requires an analysis of the channel itself. If the fistula is external, con-

Common Sites of Fistulas

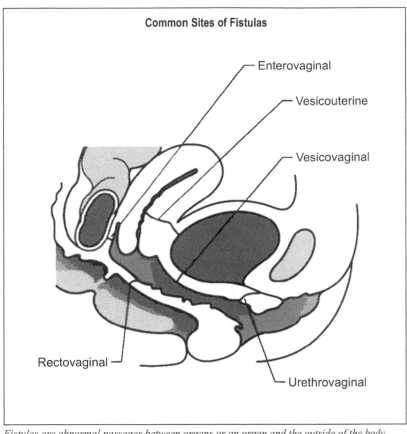

- Enterovaginal
- Vesicouterine
- Vesicovaginal
- Urethrovaginal
- Rectovaginal

Fistulas are abnormal passages between organs or an organ and the outside of the body. They are more common in the rectal and genital regions of women, such as between the intestines and vagina (enterovaginal), the bladder and uterus (vesicouterine), the bladder and vagina (vesicovaginal), the urethra and vagina (urethrovaginal), and the rectum and vagina (rectovaginal).

trast material may be injected into the site to analyze the tract. If it is internal, the extent of the tract may require cholangiography, the injection of a radiopaque material to outline the bile duct. General surgery is required for the proper correction of any underlying problem.

Uses and Complications

Surgical repair of a fistula has a number of functions, in addition to the elimination of the fistula itself. The goal of repair is to support the healing process, while at the same time attempting to maintain the normal function (and appearance, when applicable) of the tissue.

The anal fistula represents one of the more common types. Frequently, it begins as an abscess or break in the anal or rectal wall. The underlying cause is often inflammation of the colon as a result of ulcerative colitis or Crohn's disease, an autoimmune disease that can cause ulceration of the intestinal wall. The fistula itself may become chronically infected, resulting in pain and discomfort. Cancer development in the area of the fistula, while uncommon, has been known to occur.

The major complication of anorectal surgery to repair the fistula is delayed healing. If not completely drained or covered, the area may continue to become infected. If the fistula is deep, damage to muscles during surgical repair may result in incontinence. Assuming that the fistula does not recur and postoperative care is properly provided, however, the prognosis is generally excellent.

Surgical procedures can also be used in the intentional formation of a fistula. For example, a site must be prepared for insertion of a cannula to carry out hemodialysis, the removal of waste from the blood under conditions of renal insufficiency. Generally, such a fistula between an artery and a vein is prepared one to two months prior to insertion of the cannula. The fistula is created either by grafting a section of bovine carotid artery into the site or by using a graft prepared from synthetic material. Proper circulation through the fistula must be monitored to ensure that infection does not develop.

Perspective and Prospects

The development and widespread use of antibiotics in the mid-twentieth century provided a means for the effective treatment of infection, which is the major complication associated with fistula development. Fistulas may result in abscess formation or may be secondary to problems elsewhere, as with Crohn's disease. Better treatment of those infections associated with fistula formation, such as tuberculosis, has reduced their incidence. Likewise, proper prenatal care has largely controlled fistula development secondary to difficult labor in women.

—*Richard Adler, Ph.D.*

See also Abscess drainage; Abscesses; Anus; Childbirth complications; Colon; Colorectal surgery; Crohn's disease; Gallbladder; Gastroenterology; Gastroenterology, pediatric; Gastrointestinal disorders; Gastrointestinal system; Grafts and grafting; Gynecology; Infection; Intestines; Proctology; Rectum; Reproductive system; Stone removal; Stones; Tumor removal; Tumors; Ulcer surgery; Ulcers; Urinary system; Urology; Urology, pediatric.

For Further Information:

American Medical Association. *American Medical Association Family Medical Guide.* 4th rev. ed. Hoboken, N.J.: John Wiley & Sons, 2004.

Cameron, John L., and Andrew M. Cameron, eds. *Current Surgical Therapy.* 10th ed. Philadelphia: Elsevier/Saunders, 2011.

Doherty, Gerard M., and Lawrence W. Way, eds. *Current Surgical*

Diagnosis and Treatment. 13th ed. New York: Lange Medical Books/McGraw-Hill, 2010.

"Fistulas." *MedlinePlus*, October 31, 2012.

Papadakis, Maxine A., and Stephen J. McPhee, eds. *Current Medical Diagnosis and Treatment 2013*. New York: McGraw-Hill, 2013.

Peikin, Steven R. *Gastrointestinal Health: The Proven Nutritional Program to Prevent, Cure, or Alleviate Irritable Bowel Syndrome (IBS), Ulcers, Gas, Constipation, Heartburn, and Many Other Digestive Disorders*. 3d ed. New York: Perennial Currents, 2004.

Saibil, Fred. *Crohn's Disease and Ulcerative Colitis: Everything You Need to Know*. 3d ed. Richmond Hill, Ont.: Firefly Books, 2011.

FLAT FEET
Disease/Disorder

Also known as: Pes planus, talipes planus

Anatomy or system affected: Feet, ligaments, muscles, musculoskeletal system

Specialties and related fields: Orthopedics, podiatry

Definition: A congenital or acquired flatness of the longitudinal arch of the foot.

Causes and Symptoms

Congenital flat feet are considered to be hereditary. Acquired flat feet can be caused by stretching of the arch ligaments and a weakness of the muscles found in the arches; this produces flexible flat feet. Rigid flat feet are caused by changes in the shape of the foot bones or a short Achilles tendon. Other causes of flat feet include injury and a lack of muscle tone or weak foot muscles that cannot sustain the body's weight.

All infants appear to be flat-footed because of a pad of fat under each instep. Arch formation in the feet takes place once they begin walking. Flat feet are often detected by parents when an infant experiences delays in learning how to walk.

Flat feet usually are painless and do not contribute to changes in posture or the ability to walk. Adolescents and adults are occasionally prone to fallen arches, or temporary foot strain caused by an activity that overstretches the ligaments in the arch; this condition is accompanied by pain. Rigid flat feet caused by a short Achilles tendon and spastic flat feet caused by a deformity of the heel result in pain and clumsiness in walking.

Treatment and Therapy

Flexible, pain-free flat feet require no treatment. Special orthopedic shoes with arch supports do not change the shape of the feet over time, while foot exercises and prescribed

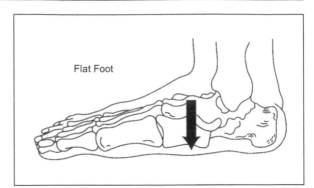

Flat feet, or abnormally flat arches, can arise from muscle weakness, improper walking, or developmental defects.

changes in gait are hard to enforce in children.

In cases of fallen arches accompanied by fatigue or pain, however, rest, foot exercises, and the use of arch supports are recommended. If the Achilles tendon is too short or tight, it can be stretched by placing the foot in a cast. Severe cases of flat feet require surgery that removes excess bone or reconstructs the soft tissue of the foot.

—Rose Secrest

See also Arthritis; Bone disorders; Bones and the skeleton; Feet; Foot disorders; Lower extremities; Orthopedics; Orthopedics, pediatric; Podiatry.

For Further Information:

Copeland, Glenn, and Stan Solomon. *The Foot Doctor: Lifetime Relief for Your Aching Feet*. Rev. ed. Toronto, Ont.: Macmillan Canada, 1996.

Currey, John D. *Bones: Structure and Mechanics*. 2d ed. Princeton, N.J.: Princeton University Press, 2006.

"Flat Feet and Fallen Arches." *HealthyChildren.org*. American Academy of Pediatrics, Oct. 12, 2012.

"Flexible Flatfoot." *Foot Health Facts*. American College of Foot and Ankle Surgeons, Dec. 18, 2009.

Frowen, Paul, et al., eds. *Neale's Disorders of the Foot*. 8th ed. Edinburgh: Churchill Livingstone, 2010.

Lippert, Frederick G., and Sigvard T. Hansen. *Foot and Ankle Disorders: Tricks of the Trade*. New York: Thieme, 2003.

Ma, C. Benjamin, et al. "Flat Feet." *MedlinePlus*, Jan. 17, 2013.

"Pediatric Flatfoot." *Foot Health Facts*. American College of Foot and Ankle Surgeons, Mar. 31, 2010.

Polsdorfer, Ricker, and Michael Woods. "Flat Foot." *Health Library*, May 2, 2013.

Van De Graaff, Kent M. *Human Anatomy*. 6th ed. New York: McGraw-Hill, 2002.

FLUIDS AND ELECTROLYTES
Biology

Anatomy or system affected: Blood, cells, respiratory system

Specialties and related fields: Biochemistry, cytology, hematology, histology, pharmacology, pulmonary medicine, serology, urology

Definition: Body fluids are intracellular or extracellular solutions of water and other substances, the concentrations of which must be regulated to achieve proper physiological

---

Information on Flat Feet

Causes: Congenital weakness of muscles in arches, changes in shape of foot bones, short Achilles tendon, injury

Symptoms: Delays in learning how to walk, pain, clumsiness in walking

Duration: Typically short-term

Treatments: Depends on severity; ranges from orthopedic shoes with arch supports, foot exercises, and rest to casts or surgery

functioning; electrolytes are chemicals that become electrically charged particles when they dissolve in water.

Key terms:

adenosine triphosphate: a chemical that, when it reacts to lose a phosphate group, gives off free energy that is available for bodily processes

edema: the abnormal accumulation of fluid in tissues or cavities of the body

electrolyte: a chemical that, when it dissolves in water, dissociates to form positive and negative ions so that the resulting solution is an electrical conductor

homeostasis: the tendency of the body to maintain a beneficial balance among its parts

physiology: the study of the processes and mechanisms by which living organisms function

resorption: the process in which bones dissolve and return their components to the body fluids

semipermeable membrane: a barrier that allows some materials to pass but blocks others

solute: a material that has gone into solution and in so doing has changed its phase

Structure and Functions

Humans live in a wide variety of environmental conditions. Some days are hot and wet, others are cold and dry, and most are somewhere between. At the same time, as foods and liquid are taken in, the body is exposed to a variety of chemical substances over a wide range of concentrations. Amid these widely changing circumstances, the internal environment, to which the body's cells are exposed, remains essentially unchanged. This regulation of the internal environment, which is called homeostasis, is necessary for the correct functioning of the body. Essentially, all the organs and tissues of the body play roles in the homeostatic processes, and the main control mechanism operates through the movement of body fluids.

There are several different body fluids, but they are all solutions of solutes in water. The identity of the solutes and their concentrations differentiates one body fluid from another. Among the solutes, two categories exist. Some solutes dissociate into electrically charged particles when they dissolve and are thus called electrolytes. Others remain as neutral particles dissolved in the water and are nonelectrolytes. Both types of solutes play important roles in the correct physiological functioning of the body, but it is the electrolytes that draw the most attention. This is the case because the fluids and the electrolytes are interdependent and because imbalances of these factors are associated with a vast array of illnesses.

Although subject to some variation with age, gender, and physical condition, the body is composed of about 60 percent water by weight. For purposes of classification, this water is considered to be present in compartments. It is important to recognize that this terminology is conceptual only and does not refer to the existence of any real, separate, water-containing compartments in the body. Approximately twenty-five cubic decimeters of water are contained within the body's cells; this is the intracellular fluid. Most of the remaining fluid, about twelve cubic decimeters, is termed extracellular

and exists in the regions exterior to cells. The extracellular fluid is further subdivided into the categories of interstitial fluid, which surrounds the cells; intravascular fluid, which is located within the blood vessels; and transcellular fluid, which includes the fluid found in the spinal column, the region of the lungs, the area surrounding the heart, the sinuses, and the eyes, along with sweat and digestive secretions. These subcategories are listed in order of the amount of fluid present. Of all these types, only the intravascular fluid is directly affected when a person drinks or eliminates fluid. Alterations in the other regions occur in response to that change, however, and there is a continual dynamic exchange of fluid among all compartments. The balance of conditions created by this exchange determines the state of health of the individual.

The solutes that are electrolytes generate positively charged ions called cations and negatively charged ions called anions. The amount of positive charge present in a solution is always equal to the amount of negative charge. The major cations present are hydrogen, sodium, potassium, calcium, and magnesium. The most important anions are chloride, hydrogen carbonate, hydrogen phosphate, sulfate, and those derived from organic acids such as acetic acid. Several other ions of both types are present at very low levels. The nonelectrolytes present include urea, creatinine, bilirubin, and glucose. All these solutes are involved with particular biological changes in the body, so their presence at the correct concentration is vital.

The fluid and its solutes move within the body by means of several transport mechanisms, some of which move solutes through the fluid and some of which move either water or the solutes from one side of a cell membrane to the other. The mechanisms available are diffusion, active transport, filtration, and osmosis. Diffusion is the movement of particles through a solution from a region in which the concentration of the particles is high to a region in which it is lower. The energy that drives this motion is thermal energy, and the transport rate is increased by increasing the temperature, which increases the concentration difference from point to point and is faster for smaller particles. Cell walls are a barrier to this type of transport unless the solute particles are small enough to pass through pores in the wall or are soluble in the cell wall itself. Active transport provides another means of moving solutes across cell walls. The energy for such movement is provided by a series of chemical reactions involving adenosine triphosphate. The movement of sodium out of and potassium into cells, as well as the transport of amino acids into cells, occurs in this manner. Filtration is a means by which both water and some solutes are transported through a porous membrane. The solutes transported are those that are small enough to pass through the pores in the membrane. The driving force for filtration is provided by a difference in pressure on the two sides of the membrane, and the motion occurs from the high-pressure side to the low-pressure side. The pressure in this case results from gravity and from the pumping action of the heart. Osmosis is a process by which water is moved across a semipermeable membrane as the result of the influence of a different type of pressure. When two solutions of different concentrations of solute particles are separated by a semipermeable membrane, an osmotic pressure develops that acts as the driving force to move water from the side of the membrane where the concentration of solute particles is lower to the side where the solute particle concentration is higher.

A solute's concentration in the body fluid has a great effect on the transport of materials and thus on the body's health. Concentrations in body fluids are expressed in several ways. Electrolyte concentration is often expressed in terms of milliequivalents of solute per cubic decimeter of solution. This is a measure of the amount of change, positive or negative, provided by that solute. A solution with twice the number of milliequivalents per cubic decimeter will have twice the concentration of change. This also measures the solute's combining power, because one milliequivalent of cations will chemically combine with one milliequivalent of anions. Osmolality, osmolarity, and tonicity refer to a solution's ability to provide an osmotic pressure. Osmolality and osmolarity are proportional to the number of particles of solute present in the solution. When solutions of different osmolalities or osmolarities are separated by a semipermeable membrane, there will be a flow of solvent across the membrane. Isotonic solutions have equal osmotic effects. Tonicity is a way of comparing the osmotic potential of solutions by referring to one as being hypotonic, isotonic, or hypertonic to the other.

Disorders and Diseases

There are two ways to approach thinking about the health role of body fluids and electrolytes. One is to consider one particular fluid component, such as sodium, that is out of balance and proceed to trace possible causes of the imbalance and appropriate treatment modes. It must be noted, however, that there are many possible illnesses that could cause any particular imbalance. The second approach is to consider a representative number of specific diseases and to look at their effect on the fluid and electrolyte balance and how such effects may be treated.

The first of these two approaches is adopted here because it highlights the fluids and electrolytes themselves rather than the diseases. Two imbalances will be considered as examples of the types of effects seen. First to be considered is the volume of fluid itself. Second, the balance of calcium will be given attention because of the connection of calcium deficiency with the bone brittleness that often occurs during aging.

Volume imbalance that is larger than the system's normal regulatory ability to control may occur in either the intracellular or extracellular fluid or both and may be in the direction of too little fluid (dehydration) or too much (overhydration). Both of these effects may result from a number of underlying illnesses, but each is, by itself, life-threatening and requires direct treatment. Often, this treatment precedes the diagnosis of the root cause.

The body apparently senses fluid volume imbalance with receptors near the heart, and several coping responses are triggered. Dehydration can be the result of vomiting, diarrhea, excessive perspiration, or blood loss. In such cases, the body's responses are in the direction of maintaining the flow of blood to vital organs. Vessels at the extremities are constricted, and those in the regions of the vital organs are dilated. Kidney function is greatly slowed, the reabsorption of sodium is increased, and the production of urine is markedly decreased, ensuring water retention. Centers in the hypothalamus respond and cause the individual to become thirsty. Thus, the body acts to protect its most important functions while at the same time stimulating actions from the individual that will bring additional fluid volume into the system. The manner in which the individual responds to being thirsty will determine other bodily changes. If plain water is used to quench the thirst, the extracellular fluid becomes less concentrated in electrolytes than is the intracellular fluid, causing an osmotic pressure imbalance that the body regulates by transporting more water into the cells, producing overhydration there and aggravating the original dehydration in the extracellular fluid. Notice that this means that drinking large amounts of water can, strange though it may seem, cause dehydration. If saltwater is ingested, the reverse occurs, with a resulting dehydration of the cells that in turn triggers extreme thirst but few cardiovascular problems. Proper volume replacement thus requires that the water brought into the system be of the same electrolyte concentration as the cellular fluids—that is, that they be isotonic. In that case, the osmotic pressure remains balanced and the fluid volumes in both of the major compartments can be built up.

Overhydration is a less common occurrence that is usually associated with cardiovascular disease, severe malnutrition and kidney disease, or surgical stress. When the heart is not able to act as an effective pump, a back pressure builds in the circulatory system that causes fluid to be filtered through the walls of the vessels and that results in the accumulation of fluid in the interstitial regions around the heart and lungs. A decrease in proteins in the bloodstream, resulting from either malnutrition or kidney malfunction, lowers the osmotic pressure in the blood and causes water retention in the interstitial spaces. Accumulation of excess fluid in the interstitial spaces is called edema. This same end condition also arises when the kidney excessively filters fluid from the bloodstream into the interstitial spaces. The treatment of overhydration takes the form of fluid intake restriction, restriction of dietary sodium, and the use of diuretic therapy to stimulate urine production.

Calcium, much of which comes from milk and milk products, is the fifth most abundant ion in the body and is involved with the formation of the mineral component of teeth and bones, the contraction of muscles, proper blood clotting, and the maintenance of cell wall permeability. Calcium is added to extracellular fluid as a result of the intestinal absorption of dietary calcium and bone resorption. It is lost from the extracellular fluid via secretion into the intestinal tract, urinary excretion, and deposition in bone. The maintenance of a proper calcium level mainly depends on processes occurring in the intestinal tract. Only a very small part of the body's total calcium is in fluids. Both hypocalcemia and hypercalcemia, the shortage and the overabundance of calcium in the fluids, may occur. Unlike the case of water shortage or excess, however, there are few direct visual consequences of a calcium imbalance; one must rely on laboratory testing of the fluid and on indirect physical assessment.

Hypocalcemia in the blood is associated with reduced intake, increased loss, or altered regulation, as in hypoparathyroidism. Bone, a living material, continually absorbs and desorbs calcium. The parathyroid gland secretes a hormone that regulates bone resorption and thus can raise the calcium level in the extracellular fluid at the expense of decreasing the amount of bone. Obviously, this cannot be a long-term mechanism to provide calcium. The same hormone also regulates the absorption of calcium from the intestines and the kidneys. Vitamin D is an essential, although indirect, factor in permitting the absorption of calcium from the intestine. A deficiency of this vitamin is a major cause of hypocalcemia. When the calcium level in the extracellular fluid falls below normal, the nervous system becomes increasingly excited. If the level continues to fall, the nerve fibers begin to discharge spontaneously, passing impulses to the peripheral skeletal muscles, where they cause a contractive spasm. Often, this is first seen in a contracting of the fingers. Generalized muscular spasming can be lethal if the calcium imbalance is not corrected quickly. Immediate calcium deficiency is treated with the administration of either oral or intravenous calcium compounds, with vitamin D therapy, and with the inclusion of foods of high calcium content in the diet. In the longer term, treatment of the underlying illness is necessary.

The opposite imbalance, hypercalcemia, can occur as a result of an excessive intake of calcium supplements and vitamin D, in conjunction with a high-calcium diet. Calcium excess is also associated with some tumors and with kidney or glandular diseases. It has also been found to be caused by prolonged immobility, in which case the bones resorb because of the lack of bone stress. This latter effect has been of major concern in the space program. Too high a level of calcium in the intercellular fluid causes a depression of the nervous system and a slowing of reflexes. Lack of appetite and constipation are also common results. At very high levels, calcium salts may precipitate in the blood system, an effect that can be rapidly lethal. Again, in the long term, the underlying cause of the imbalance must be corrected, but treatments do exist for more immediate alleviation. As long as the kidneys are functioning correctly, intravenous treatment with saline serves as a means of flushing out excess calcium. Calcium also can be bound to phosphate that is delivered intravenously, but there is a risk of causing soft tissue precipitation of the calcium phosphate compound. Dietary control is used, at times in concert with steroid therapy, to counter high calcium levels. If resorption is the cause of the excess, there are therapies, both chemical and physical, that are effective in increasing bone deposition.

Perspective and Prospects

From the earliest times, those concerned with the treatment of illnesses have had their attention drawn to the fluids present in or exuded by the human body. The color, smell, and texture of fluids being given off by a sick or injured person provided clues to the nature of the illness or injury. Bleeding was commonly practiced as a means of venting the illness so that health could be restored. Lancing of ulcerative conditions was also practiced by early healers. These early attempts at understanding and of treatment have been greatly refined, and the search for better understanding and improved treatment modes continues.

This concern with fluids and electrolytes is easy to understand. The fluids and their components constitute both the external and the internal environment for all the body's tissues and cells. Any abnormality in the cells or tissues is reflected in a variation from normal conditions in the fluids. All major illnesses and many minor ones have associated with them a fluid and electrolyte disorder. Fluids are more readily accessible for study than are tissues from deep within the body; hence, a considerable effort has been directed at measuring fluid constituents and interpreting the findings. The testing of fluids has evolved from highly labor intensive measurements of a few components to highly automated testing procedures applied to dozens of components. The reliability and precision of the measurements continue to increase, and the scope of measurements continues to expand.

Not all that is to be known about fluids and electrolytes, however, depends on laboratory testing. Some knowledge can be collected from close observation of the patient. Although the resulting measurements are not precise, they are nevertheless important because they are much more immediately available. Physical symptoms that carry information about fluids and electrolytes include the following: sudden weight gain or loss; changes in abdominal girth; changes in either the intake or output of fluids; body temperature; depth of respiration; heart rate; blood pressure; skin moisture, color, and temperature; the skin's ability to relax to normal after being pinched; the swelling of tissue; the condition of the tongue; the appearance of visible veins; reflexive responses; apparent mental state; and thirst. Each of these observations, and more, is readily available to one who is monitoring the health of an individual.

As is the case with most testing and data-gathering situations, interpreting the test and observation results is the critical step. Any one measure, by itself, points to a vast array of possible illnesses. Only by considering the whole and recognizing the existence of patterns in the information can a health professional narrow the possibilities. It is this recognition of patterns that develops with education and experience, and it is this step that relies on judgment that makes medicine an art as well as a science.

—Kenneth H. Brown, Ph.D.

See also Acid-base chemistry; Bile; Blood and blood disorders; Cells; Chyme; Circulation; Cytology; Dehydration; Edema; Fever; Hyperhidrosis; Hypertension; Hypotension; Lipids; Lymph; Physiology; Semen; Sweating; Tears and tear ducts; Vascular system; Weight loss and gain.

For Further Information:

Campbell, Neil A., et al. *Biology: Concepts and Connections*. 6th ed. San Francisco: Pearson/Benjamin Cummings, 2009.

Centers for Disease Control and Prevention. "Water: Meeting Your Daily Fluid Needs." *Centers for Disease Control and Prevention*, October 10, 2012.

Chambers, Jeanette K., Marilyn J. Rantz, and Meridean Maas, eds. *Common Fluid and Electrolyte Disorders, Nursing Diagnoses: Implementation*. Philadelphia: W. B. Saunders, 1987.

Dugdale, David C., III. "Electrolytes." *MedlinePlus*, September 20, 2011.

Guyton, Arthur C., and John E. Hall. *Human Physiology and Mechanisms of Disease*. 6th ed. Philadelphia: W. B. Saunders, 1997.

Horne, Mima M., Ursula Easterday Heitz, and Pamela L. Swearingen. *Fluid, Electrolyte, and Acid-Base Balance: A Case Study Approach*. St. Louis, Mo.: Mosby Year Book, 1991.

Kee, Joyce LeFever, Betty J. Paulanka, and Larry D. Purnell. *Fluids and Electrolytes with Clinical Applications: A Programmed Approach*. 8th ed. Clifton Park, N.Y.: Thomson/Delmar Learning, 2010.

Lee, Carla A. Bouska, C. Ann Barrett, and Donna D. Ignatavicius. *Fluids and Electrolytes: A Practical Approach*. 4th ed. Philadelphia: F. A. Davis, 1996.

MedlinePlus. "Fluid and Electrolyte Balance." *MedlinePlus*, July 4, 2013.

Speakman, Elizabeth, and Norma Jean Weldy. *Body Fluids and Electrolytes*. 8th ed. New York: Elsevier, 2002.

FLUORIDE TREATMENTS

Procedure

Anatomy or system affected: Gums, mouth, teeth

Specialties and related fields: Bacteriology, biochemistry, dentistry, microbiology

Definition: Treatment of the teeth with a fluoride-releasing substance to help the enamel resist tooth decay.

Indications and Procedures

Tooth decay involves the solubility of food during eating. Consumed carbohydrates are oxidized to organic acids, such as lactic acid, by the action of specific bacteria that adhere to the teeth. These acids dissolve tooth enamel, which mainly consists of a mineral called "hydroxyapatite" and is considered the hardest substance in the body. The protection of the enamel, and thus the inner part of the tooth, from decomposition can be achieved through fluoride treatments.

Fluoride treatment involves the ingestion of fluoride ions in drinking water, toothpaste, and other sources to change the nature and composition of hydroxyapatite by producing a new compound called "fluorapatite." Because it is less alkaline than hydroxyapatite, fluorapatite forms a more resistant enamel. Because of its effectiveness in preventing cavities, fluoride is added in the form of sodium fluoride or sodium hexafluorosilicate to the public water supply of many US municipalities in concentrations of 0.7 milligram per milliliter, or just under 1 part per million.

Uses and Complications

As a result of this fluoridation process, a drastic reduction in dental decay has been observed. In addition, most commercially available toothpastes and gels contain fluoride, in the

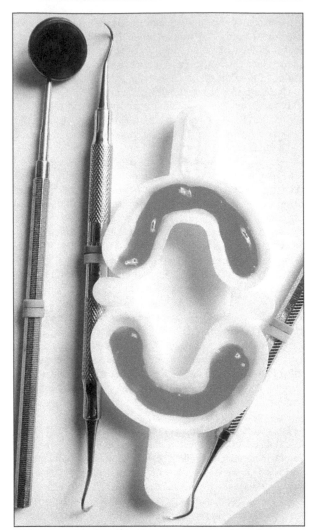

Children may be given fluoride treatments as a gel in a foam mouthpiece in order to protect against the formation of cavities. (AP/Wide World Photos)

form of sodium monofluorophosphate or sodium fluoride in concentrations of about 0.1 percent fluoride by weight. Stannous fluoride, introduced in the 1950s, has been less commonly used since the 1990s.

The recommended annual or semiannual dental cleaning by a dentist or oral hygienist removes accumulated plaque and may include further application with a fluoride substance in the form of a gel, foam, or varnish. Generally, only children and teenagers receive such a fluoride treatment, although some adults may also have it.

It must be noted that fluoride ions are toxic in large quantities. As a result, when the fluoride concentration in water is about 2–4 parts per million, discoloration (mottling) or damage of the teeth may occur. Study data conflict regarding whether fluoridation is associated with increased risk of osteoporosis and bone fractures in older adults. Fluoride toxicity is weight- and age-dependent, so the risks are greatest in young children.

—*Soraya Ghayourmanesh, Ph.D.*

See also Cavities; Dental diseases; Dentistry; Dentistry, pediatric; Plaque, dental; Teeth; Wisdom teeth.

For Further Information:

A.D.A.M. Medical Encyclopedia. "Fluoride in Diet." *MedlinePlus*, June 14, 2011.

Ash, Major M., Jr., and Stanley J. Nelson. *Wheeler's Dental Anatomy, Physiology, and Occlusion*. 9th ed. St. Louis, Mo.: Saunders/Elsevier, 2010.

"Fact Sheets: Oral Health." *World Health Organization*, April 2012.

Foster, Malcolm S. *Protecting Our Children's Teeth: A Guide to Quality Dental Care from Infancy Through Age Twelve*. New York: Insight Books, 1992.

National Center for Chronic Disease Prevention and Health Promotion, Division of Oral Health. "Community Water Fluoridation: Fluoridation Basics." *Centers for Disease Control and Prevention*, April 27, 2012.

Smith, Rebecca W. *The Columbia University School of Dental and Oral Surgery's Guide to Family Dental Care*. New York: W. W. Norton, 1997.

Wood, Debra, and Brian Randall. "Fluoride and Your Bones: A Mixed Bag." *Health Library*, June 13, 2012.

Woodall, Irene R., ed. *Comprehensive Dental Hygiene Care*. 4th ed. St. Louis, Mo.: Mosby, 1993.

FLUOROSCOPY. *See* IMAGING AND RADIOLOGY.

FOOD ALLERGIES
Disease/Disorder

Anatomy or system affected: Circulatory system, gastrointestinal system, immune system, respiratory system, skin

Specialties and related fields: Gastroenterology, immunology, nutrition

Definition: An abnormal response by the immune system to some foods, causing mild to severe symptoms that may become life threatening.

Key terms:

allergen: any substance that causes an allergic reaction

anaphylaxis: a severe allergic reaction involving the circulatory and respiratory systems; often fatal without immediate treatment

biphasic reaction: delayed allergic reaction to an allergen, between one to four hours after the initial reaction

Epi-Pen: a device that administers a prescribed dose of injectable epinephrine

epinephrine: a hormone that acts as a vasoconstrictor and cardiac stimulant

food allergy action plan: a care plan outlining lifesaving strategies when experiencing a food allergy reaction

immunoglobulin antibody: a protein activated during allergic reactions by the immune system

RAST: the most accurate blood test available to diagnose allergies

Causes and Symptoms

Allergic reactions occur when the immune system is stimulated to protect the body from foreign organisms known as allergens. Allergens, usually proteins, are perceived by the body as potentially harmful. When the immune system is activated, two types of white blood cells respond: phagocytes and lymphocytes. Phagocytes destroy bacteria, viruses, and parasites. Lymphocytes destroy other types of harmful organisms, and it is these white blood cells that respond when a food is perceived as harmful. Therefore, when an allergen is encountered, white blood cells respond and attach an immunoglobulin (Ig) antibody to it. Five different immunoglobulin antibodies can be activated, and each has a different responsibility. Immunoglobulin E (IgE) is the antibody that responds during a food allergy reaction. Marking an allergen with an Ig antibody distinguishes it from healthy tissue and cells. This in turn allows white blood cells to release a chemical spray, usually histamine, which targets and destroys only the harmful allergen.

Food is essential for life and good health, and the exact reason why a food substance is identified as harmful is still inconclusive. Genetics provide the strongest link to food allergy incidence. Research studies show that a family history of allergies increases the chance of developing all allergies, including those to food. If both parents have an allergy, there is a 70 to 80 percent chance that their children will also develop an allergy. Even those who have no family history of allergies can still develop them, however, indicating that other factors play a role. Many theories have been proposed. The hygiene hypothesis suggests that the Western world's habit of cleanliness causes the immune system to become bored and attack itself. Introducing foods at too early of an age may overstimulate an immature gastrointestinal tract and trigger an allergic reaction. The leaky gut theory, in which an unhealthy gastrointestinal tract leaks allergens into the bloodstream, is also theorized to promote allergies. Many foods also contain proteins, and it is thought the body confuses food proteins with an allergenic protein from another source. Frequent use of antacids, food additives, and vaccines, genetic manipulations of food crops, and exposure to environmental toxins are also linked to an abnormal immune system response to foods.

More than two hundred foods, some food additives, and foods naturally high in histamine have been reported to cause adverse food reactions. However, not all adverse food reactions are diagnosed as a food allergy. An estimated 3 to 4 percent of adults and 6 to 8 percent of children worldwide are diagnosed with a food allergy. Approximately 90 percent of food allergies are to cow's milk, eggs, fish, peanuts, shellfish, soybeans, tree nuts, and wheat. Frequently, food allergy symptoms mimic food intolerances, sensitivities, and other medical disorders, making diagnosis difficult. In general, a true food allergy reaction occurs anywhere from minutes to two hours after eating a specific food. Symptoms range from mild to a severe, life-threatening anaphylaxis. Severity of reactions is unpredictable, no matter how mild or severe the previous reaction was. Most symptoms involve the circula-

Information on Food Allergies

Causes: Substance found in food (usually a protein), histamine, some food additives; often cow's milk, eggs, fish, peanuts, shellfish, soybeans, tree nuts, or wheat

Symptoms: Anaphylaxis, angioedema, asthma, abdominal pain, low blood pressure, difficulty breathing, diarrhea, gastrointestinal bloating, difficulty swallowing, dizziness, faintness, headache, hives, itchy mouth, metallic taste in mouth, tightness in chest, vomiting, wheezing

Duration: Minutes to hours; may be fatal without immediate treatment

Treatments: Epinephrine injection and/or oral antihistamine medications, intravenous or oral steroids, topical hydrocortisone ointments; often immediate emergency medical care

tory and respiratory systems, and common symptoms include difficulty breathing, facial swelling, heart arrhythmias, runny or stuffy nose, and fainting. Mild symptoms often affect the skin, causing angioedema, eczema, and hives. The gastrointestinal system may be affected, causing abdominal pain, bloating, diarrhea, metallic taste in the mouth, difficulty swallowing, and vomiting. Children may experience weight loss or poor growth. Malnutrition and eating disorders may also occur over time when one or more food groups must be eliminated from the diet or there is fear of experiencing a reaction.

Many individuals assume, without a medical evaluation, that they have a food allergy. If a food allergy is suspected, then a food allergist, as well as a gastroenterologist when indicated, should be consulted. A combination of medical and family history, blood and skin tests, and an elimination diet are the tools used to make a firm diagnosis of food allergies. Blood tests include checking serum IgE antibody concentrations and the radioallergosorbent test (RAST), which tests if a reaction to a specific food allergen occurs. The RAST is considered to be one of the most reliable tests in use to diagnose food allergies. However, between 50 and 60 percent of positive RAST scores are false positives and 10 to 30 percent are false negatives. Skin tests involve scratching the skin with food extracts and monitoring for allergic reactions, such as hives, but these tests also have a large percentage of false positives. Therefore, an elimination diet, in which suspected food allergens are eliminated from the diet for two to four weeks, is often prescribed and symptom changes evaluated.

Treatment and Therapy

Allergic reactions to foods must always be taken seriously since symptoms can escalate from minor to life-threatening in a matter of minutes. Individuals with asthma are at the highest risk for severe food reactions. When a severe food reaction occurs, an injection of epinephrine and emergency medical treatment must be administered as quickly as possible. Mild reactions may require an oral/intravenous antihistamine or steroid medication or topical hydrocortisone ointment. Even when symptoms seem to be over or under control, the individual must still be continually monitored for four to six hours after the initial reaction because symptoms can progress rapidly to life-threatening as a result of a delayed reaction known as a biphasic reaction.

The only way to prevent a food allergy reaction is by strictly avoiding the food. Allergic individuals must be careful at all times about every food that they eat because food allergens can go airborne or be used in the processing or cooking of a food. Reading food ingredient labels (disclosures by food processing manufacturers are required by law) and questioning food preparers about prepared foods are critical prevention steps that anyone living with a food allergy must take. However, accidental exposures can still occur no matter how careful an individual is. Therefore, it is essential that an EpiPen or similar device and a food allergy action plan be carried at all times.

An EpiPen is a device that administers a prescribed dose of injectable epinephrine during severe allergic reactions; quick treatment with it can mean the difference between life and death. Food allergy action plans are also important because they identify the problem and outline a quick and appropriate lifesaving plan of care when an individual is unconscious. A food allergy action plan lists allergenic foods, symptoms, medications and dose prescribed, sequence of steps to follow during an emergency, emergency contact information, and the name and phone number of the treating physician. Wearing medical alert jewelry is also advised.

While adults can develop food allergies as they age, young children frequently outgrow them, although this is not always true for fish, peanut, shellfish, and tree nut allergies. Therefore, it may be recommended that children undergo food challenges periodically to evaluate if they remain allergic to a specific food. Food challenges reintroduce an allergenic food into the diet under strict medical supervision only, since the potential for a severe and fatal allergic reaction is high.

Perspective and Prospects

It has long been recognized that surviving an illness often provides protection against that illness in the future. This connection between immunity and disease was particularly apparent during the ancient plagues of smallpox. Smallpox, an infectious virus, is estimated to have killed three hundred to five hundred million people worldwide in just the twentieth century. Ancient Egyptian mummies show the ravages of this disease and Greek historians record the decimated population during the Athenian plague (430–426 BCE). Historians have recorded efforts to increase population survival rates, namely the inhaling of crushed smallpox scabs (early immunization technique) and inoculations using pus from smallpox lesions (early vaccination technique) to prevent the disease.

During the eighteenth and nineteenth centuries, many lifesaving advances were made in the fields of science and medicine. The body's defense mechanisms, the immune system, were explored and many diseases were successfully eradicated over time. Preventative vaccines to protect and increase life span were developed and are now accepted medical practice. However, understanding the mechanism of food allergies has taken much longer. In the twentieth century, Carl Prausnitz-Giles, a bacteriologist-immunologist, was the first to discover that food allergies are intimately tied to the immune system. Scientists Kimishige Ishizaka and Terako Ishizaka discovered that IgE is the principal agent for food allergy reactions.

Research in the area of food allergies has greatly expanded in recent years, since many countries are experiencing an increase in food allergy incidence. In 2008, the United States implemented the Exploratory Investigations in Food Allergy program to focus on research into the origin and epidemiology of food allergies and the discovery of more reliable testing methods and effective treatments. The EuroPrevall Project includes European countries as well as Australia, China, Ghana, India, and New Zealand. The program was initiated in 2005 to improve the quality of life for those who live and struggle with food allergies as well as to discover breakthroughs in clinical research.

Progress is being made in developing more reliable diagnostic methods and treatment options. Promising areas include using pure allergens rather than extracts for skin and blood tests and improved technologies to measure IgE antibodies and the immune response to foods. Also promising are the development of safe injectable and sublingual immunotherapies as preventive treatments, along with anti-IgE medicines that may block allergic reactions.

—*Alice C. Richer, R.D., M.B.A., L.D.*

See also Allergies; Antihistamines; Asthma; Autoimmune disorders; Celiac sprue; Food biochemistry; Food poisoning; Gastroenterology; Gastroenterology, pediatric; Gastrointestinal disorders; Gastrointestinal system; Gluten intolerance; Hives; Host-defense mechanisms; Immune system; Immunization and vaccination; Immunology; Lactose intolerance; Poisonous plants; Pulmonary medicine; Pulmonary medicine, pediatric; Rashes; Shock.

For Further Information:

American Academy of Allergy Asthma & Immunology, 26 July 2013.
"Food Allergy." *MedlinePlus*, 22 July 2013.
"Food Allergy." *National Institute of Allergy and Infectious Diseases*, 29 Feb. 2012.
FARE. Food Allergy Research & Education, 1 Aug. 2013.
Melina, Vesanto, Jo Stepaniak, and Dina Aronson. *Food Allergy Survival Guide*. Summertown, Tenn.: Healthy Living, 2004.
Richer, Alice C. *Food Allergies*. Westport, Conn.: Greenwood Press, 2009.
Sicherer, Scott H. *Understanding and Managing Your Child's Food Allergies*. Baltimore: Johns Hopkins University Press, 2006.
Wood, Robert A. *Food Allergies for Dummies*. Hoboken, N.J.: Wiley, 2007.

FOOD AND DRUG ADMINISTRATION (FDA)
Organization

Also known as: Bureau of Chemistry (1906-1927); Food, Drug, and Insecticide Administration (1927-1931)

Definition: An agency in the United States Department of Health and Human Services whose responsibilities include protecting citizens against harmful or falsely labeled foods, food additives, drugs, cosmetics, or medical devices.

Key terms:

Generally Recognized as Safe (GRAS) list: food ingredients or chemicals designated by the FDA as harmless to human beings when used as intended

generic drugs: copycat versions of brand-name originals that are no longer protected by patents

orphan drug: a drug developed for a very rare disease (legally, drugs for two hundred thousand or fewer potential users)

thalidomide: a sedative and sleep-inducing drug that was found to produce phocomelia (a birth defect in which hands or feet are attached to the body by short, flipperlike stumps) in developing fetuses and newborns

Structure and Function

The mission of the Food and Drug Administration (FDA) is to protect the nation's health. Consequently, the US Congress empowered this agency to prevent the sale of harmful products. The FDA's specific duty is to enforce the numerous federal laws that have been passed to ensure that foods and drugs are pure and safe and that all such products are correctly labeled. With the multiplication of its responsibilities over time came a concomitant growth in the FDA's administrative, technical, and service staffs both in Washington, DC, and in ten regions around the country. Officials in each region are responsible for enforcing the relevant laws in their jurisdictions, and they are helped in this by inspectors and scientists.

The activities of FDA personnel include research, inspection, and legal action. In FDA laboratories, scientists verify manufacturers" claims of the safety and effectiveness of food additives, drugs, and cosmetics before they are put onto the market. In addition to studying the long-term effects of various products, FDA workers also study how foods are processed, preserved, packaged, and stored. Using their field staffs, FDA officials send their inspectors to monitor manufacturing facilities and assist industrial employees in setting up procedures to prevent violations of the law. The FDA also has the duty of enforcing laws against illegal sales of prescription drugs, and FDA employees periodically examine imports of foods, drugs, cosmetics, and therapeutic devices to make sure that they comply with federal laws.

Even though the FDA has the responsibility of protecting consumers from various lawbreakers, its enforcement of relevant laws is limited by the courts. In fact, the agency must have the cooperation of attorneys and judges to prosecute persons or firms, impose fines, or seize products. FDA inspectors collect evidence of violations, and administrators review this evidence before deciding which cases will be presented to the federal courts for action. As a federal agency, the FDA is restricted to products involved in interstate commerce.

Because of physicians" professional concerns with nutrition, prescription and nonprescription drugs, and medical technologies, they have a vested interest in the FDA and its activities. According to several studies, physicians are protective of their independence and the integrity of the doctor-patient relationship, and many doctors are wary of governmental involvement in how they practice medicine. On the other hand, critics have pointed out the dangers of the close relationship that has developed between doctors and drug companies.

The FDA supervises the development and marketing of all drugs sold in the United States. New drugs originate in pharmaceutical or chemical companies, government laboratories, medical schools, or universities. An inventor or discoverer of a new drug can be granted a patent for the drug itself or for how it is made or used. Patents give the developer exclusive rights to a drug for seventeen years. After a patent has expired, other companies may sell a generic version of the drug, usually at a much lower price. The FDA's approval of a generic drug is based on laboratory studies to guarantee that the copy has the safety and effectiveness of the original. Since the generic drug manufacturer who is first to market a new generic drug reaps huge financial rewards, great pressures exist on the FDA to facilitate this process.

In 1988, generic drugs became the focus of a congressional subcommittee. It discovered that three generic drug companies were receiving accelerated approval of their applications in exchange for payoffs to FDA employees. When this generic drug scandal was over, federal courts had convicted ten companies and forty-two people of corruption. This scandal also revealed a potentially corrupting collusion between FDA workers and pharmaceutical companies, since FDA employees often leave their government jobs for highly paid positions at the companies they had formerly regulated.

Controversies and Ethical Debates

As the federal agency charged with protecting the health of Americans, the FDA is often entangled in controversial and ethical issues. For example, it is responsible for the regulation of investigational new drugs (INDs)—drugs approved for testing but not for sale. For a drug to become an IND, it must first be given to animals, since a correlation often exists between a drug's adverse effect on animals and its similar effect on humans. The FDA's procedure for testing INDs includes three phases: In Phase I, small groups of healthy volunteers are given the IND to help researchers study its effectiveness, dosage, and metabolism; in Phase II, one to two hundred patients with the drug-targeted disease are monitored for the drug's safety, efficacy, and side effects; in Phase III, even larger numbers of patients take the drug to refine optimum dosages and, with the use of placebos, to make sure that the IND's effects are not due to chance or the developer's optimism.

In the 1970s, the FDA's handling of INDs came under attack. The General Accounting Office (GAO) studied ten of the more than six thousand drugs then classified as INDs, concluding that in eight cases the FDA failed to halt human tests after receiving indications that the new drugs were unsafe. Furthermore, the GAO found that drug companies delayed reporting adverse drug effects to the FDA. Others pointed out that the FDA tested INDs singly, whereas some drugs have the potential of causing great harm when they interact with other drugs (the so-called synergistic effect). Some criticized the FDA for approving too many drugs too quickly, thereby increasing risks, while others blamed the FDA for increasing risks by approving too few drugs too slowly. Defenders of the FDA responded by saying that it is impossible to eliminate all risks from the use of medicines.

A specific example of what some see as the FDA's excessive regulation of foods and drugs is the controversy over dietary supplements. Initially, the FDA tried to restrict the public's right to choose these supplements. Some scientists thought that the FDA's vitamin regulations were reasonable, but public discontent forced Congress to pass a law guaranteeing consumers freedom to choose nutritional supplements. In the 1970s, this debate centered on laetrile (also known as vitamin B_{17}), a substance found naturally in apricot pits. Many countries permitted the sale of laetrile as a supplement, but the FDA banned it, pointing out that it causes the release of cyanide in the body. Advocates believed that laetrile relieved the symptoms and slowed the growth of cancers, and some states legalized laetrile, challenging the FDA ban. However, in 1979, the Supreme Court ruled unanimously that the FDA had the power to ban the interstate sale and distribution of laetrile. This and such controversies as disputes over artificial hearts, cigarettes as "drug-delivery devices," and various acquired immunodeficiency syndrome (AIDS) drugs helped define the FDA's role in American society, just as similar controversies have throughout the history of the agency.

Perspective and Prospects

Most scholars trace the history of the FDA to the Pure Food and Drug Act of 1906. This law, like many that would follow it, originated from public outrage over tragedies caused by impure foods and drugs. More than a century ago, food producers commonly added water to milk and adulterated coffee with charcoal. They colored foods and drinks with harmful dyes, and they used such injurious preservatives as formaldehyde, sodium benzoate, and borax. Consumers had to choose drugs based on false or misleading labels. This intolerable situation inspired the crusade of Harvey Wiley, who, because of his attacks on adulterated or pernicious foods and drugs, became known as the founder of the pure food and drug law. In his position as chief of the Bureau of Chemistry of the Department of Agriculture, Wiley gathered a group of idealistic young chemists, nicknamed the Poison Squad, to study the physiological effects of various chemical additives in foods. Their studies aroused public concern over food additives, but "Wiley's Law" would never have become a reality were it not for Upton Sinclair, whose novel *The Jungle* (1906) dramatizes unsanitary practices in the meatpacking industry, and for US president Theodore Roosevelt, who, disgusted by scandals in the drug trade, prodded members of Congress to pass the law. The Food and Drug Act of 1906 prohibited the "manufacture, sale, or transportation of adulterated or misbranded or poisonous or deleterious foods, drugs,

In the News:
Creation of Drug Safety Oversight Board

On February 15, 2005, the Food and Drug Administration (FDA) announced the creation of the Drug Safety Oversight Board, independent of the existing Office of Drug Safety. The board would be responsible for overseeing drug safety policies and resolving disputes involving drug risks.

The board was the result of several scientific controversies regarding the safety of drugs that the FDA had approved for public sale. Recall of the popular and widely advertised painkiller Vioxx by Merck, amid revelations that continued use increased the risk of heart attack or stroke, as well as disclosure that frequently prescribed antidepressants increased suicidal thoughts among children, shook the agency. In each case, the FDA was accused of being slow to act, of ignoring warnings from its own Office of Drug Safety, and of being reluctant to inform the public about problems with drugs already on the market.

The board has fifteen voting members appointed by the FDA commissioner; thirteen are senior scientific managers at the FDA and the other two are staff physicians at the National Institutes of Health and the U.S. Department of Veterans Affairs. In its first year, the board held five private meetings and issued safety alerts on forty-four drugs, of which three were suspended and two withdrawn.

Criticism of the board's composition and methods of operation came quickly and continued. Lawmakers and consumer groups argued that since all members came from within the FDA, the board lacked true independence, which was not possible as long as the same agency approved drugs and evaluated their postmarket safety. The FDA defended holding closed meetings on the grounds that the board considered proprietary information of drug companies, but lawmakers complained that the lack of transparency meant they did not know what the board actually did. The original FDA announcement said that medical experts and patient and consumer groups would act as consultants to the board, but no consultations were held during the first year. Although the FDA promised to set up a Web site to post actions of the board, it did not do so.

—Milton Berman, Ph.D.

medicines, and liquors." The Bureau of Chemistry administered the new law, and Wiley and his successors developed an organization that won many victories for pure foods and drugs in the courts.

In 1928, Congress authorized the creation of the Food, Drug, and Insecticide Administration as the executor of the Pure Food and Drug Act. The Agricultural Appropriation Act of 1931 changed the agency's name to the Food and Drug Administration. When Franklin D. Roosevelt became president in 1933, he and his team of "New Dealers" tried to get through Congress a number of fiscal and social reforms, including an expansion of the FDA's mission, since companies were continuing to make dangerous medicines. Little was accomplished until 1937, when the Massengill Company shipped its Elixir Sulfanilamide to pharmacists. This drug, which was intended to cure infections, eventually caused the deaths of 107 people. Within months of this tragedy, Congress finally passed the Federal Food, Drug, and Cosmetic Act of 1938. This law required drug manufacturers to provide scientific proof, through tests on animals and humans, that all their new drugs were safe before they were put on the market.

To isolate the FDA from advocacy groups, it became part of the Federal Security Agency in 1940. World War II expanded the FDA's workload, especially with the discovery of new "wonder drugs" that had to be tested. After the war, the number, variety, and power of new drugs increased dramatically. With the FDA's emphasis on prescription drugs, new

industries emerged and, because of high profits, these companies grew in size and influence. The profitability of the postwar food and drug industries brought both abuses and legislative remedies.

During the 1950s and 1960s, the 1938 act was periodically amended, including the Humphrey-Durham Drug Prescription Act (1951), the Food Additives Amendment (1958), the Color Additives Amendment (1961), and the Kefauver-Harris Drug Amendment (1962). After the FDA became part of the Department of Health, Education, and Welfare in 1953, it used these new laws to concentrate control of powerful new drugs in the hands of FDA officials and doctors. Some of these new laws gave the FDA responsibility for determining the safety of food ingredients, even those on the Generally Recognized as Safe (GRAS) list that had previously been used with no apparent ill effects. For example, sodium cyclamate, an additive used as an artificial sweetener, had originally been classified as GRAS but was later banned as being possibly carcinogenic. The Delaney Clause (1958) prohibited the use of substances in food if they caused cancer in laboratory animals. This law led to a controversial ban of another artificial sweetener, saccharin, a weak carcinogen (the Delaney Clause was replaced, in 1996, by a less stringent standard).

In the late 1950s, the thalidomide tragedy in Europe, during which thousands of deformed infants were born, helped to enhance public support for legislation strengthening the Food, Drug, and Cosmetic Act. Widespread use of thalidomide in America was prevented by Frances Kelsey, an FDA examiner, who used the pretext of insufficient information to turn down a company's repeated applications to market this drug in the United States. Congress responded to the thalidomide tragedy by passing the Kefauver-Harris Amendment in 1962. This law changed the ways in which drugs were created, tested, developed, prescribed, and sold. The burden was now on the companies sponsoring a new drug to show that it was safe and effective. The FDA also issued new regulations that made the drug review process extremely stringent; some said too stringent, because FDA officials, fearful of another thalidomide-like tragedy, delayed new drug approval by asking for study after study.

During the 1970s, 1980s, and 1990s, the Food, Drug, and Cosmetic Act of 1938 was constantly revised and amended. For example, an amendment in 1976 strengthened the FDA's authority to regulate medical devices, and in 1980, serious illnesses in babies caused Congress to pass an Infant Formula

Act requiring strict controls over the nutritional content and safety of commercial baby foods. In 1982, seven deaths from cyanide poisoning later traced to Tylenol capsules caused the FDA to issue regulations requiring tamper-resistant packaging. The Orphan Drug Act of 1983 offered economic inducement to encourage pharmaceutical companies to develop drugs for rare diseases affecting small populations. However, the multiplication of regulations did not prevent the generic drug scandals of the late 1980s. In fact, for many critics, the FDA had become an inefficient agency, under constant attack from congressional subcommittees, newspaper reporters, public interest groups, and industry executives.

In the 1990s, the FDA struggled to retrieve its credibility and authority by becoming once again the guardian of the nation's health. In 1992, the Prescription Drug User Fee Act required $100,000 for each new drug application, rising to $233,000 per application in five years. In return, the FDA hired six hundred new examiners to cut the review time for important new drugs. The FDA also improved standards of risk assessment for food additives, drugs, and medical devices, and it increased inspections of food and drug factories. By the end of the twentieth century, the FDA was an agency trying to keep up with the revolutionary advances in the chemical, biological, and medical sciences.

The beginning of the twenty-first century introduced an interesting era for the FDA. Because of a slowdown in the creation of innovative drugs and medical devices, the FDA rolled out new guidelines to help pharmaceutical companies better prove how a drug works in efforts to streamline the process of approval and get new treatments to the consumer market faster. Noting that drug companies went from sending a high of sixty never-before-seen drugs in 1995 for FDA approval down to just seventeen in 2002, the agency decided to make their requirements for approval more clear so that companies could do better research faster and be more willing to take chances on truly novel treatments instead of safer "copycat" medications. Some of these requirements included helping companies avoid incomplete applications, developing special guidelines for brand-new technology so that companies can design the right studies from the beginning, and providing more training of FDA reviewers.

The terrorist attacks on the World Trade Center in New York City and the Pentagon on September 11, 2001, also introduced a change in the FDA's approval process. To help in the development of bioterrorism antidotes, the agency announced that it would approve certain drugs based only on animal studies if human drug testing would be impossible. The new approach to the evaluation process includes only those drugs that would treat or prevent the potentially lethal or disabling toxicity of chemical, biological, or nuclear substances.

—*Robert J. Paradowski, Ph.D.*

See also Animal rights vs. research; Antibiotics; Anti-inflammatory drugs; Clinical trials; Creutzfeldt-Jakob disease (CJD); Food biochemistry; Food poisoning; Iatrogenic disorders; Over-the-counter medications; Pharmacology; Pharmacy; Screening.

For Further Information:
Hickmann, Meredith A., ed. *The Food and Drug Administration (FDA)*. Hauppauge, N.Y.: Nova Science, 2003.
Hilts, Philip J. *Protecting America's Health: The FDA, Business, and One Hundred Years of Regulation*. New York: Alfred Knopf, 2003.
Jackson, Charles O. *Food and Drug Legislation in the New Deal*. Princeton, N.J.: Princeton University Press, 1970.
Liska, Ken. *Drugs and the Human Body, with Implications for Society*. 8th ed. Upper Saddle River, N.J.: Pearson/Prentice Hall, 2009. Print.
Lofstedt, Ragnar, et al. "Transparency and the Food and Drug Administration—A Quantitative Study." *Journal of Health Communication* 18, no. 4 (April 2013): 391–296.
Mahajan, Rajiv. "Food and Drug Administration's Critical Path Initiative and Innovations in Drug Development Paradigm: Challenges, Progress, and Controversies." *Journal of Pharmacy & Bioallied Sciences* 2, no. 4 (October–December 2010): 307–313.
O'Reilly, James T. *Food and Drug Administration*. 3d ed. St. Paul, Minn.: Thomson/West, 2007.
Parrish, Richard. *Defining Drugs: How Government Became the Arbiter of Pharmaceutical Fact*. Somerset, N.J.: Transaction, 2003. Print.
Pisano, Douglas. *Essentials of Pharmacy Law*. Boca Raton, Fla.: CRC Press, 2003.
Schweitzer, Stuart O. "How the US Food and Drug Administration Can Solve the Prescription Drug Shortage Problem." *American Journal of Public Health* 103, no. 5 (May, 2013): 10–14.
Young, James Harvey. *Pure Food: Securing the Federal Food and Drugs Act of 1906*. Princeton, N.J.: Princeton University Press, 1989. oxy_options track_changes="on"?

FOOD BIOCHEMISTRY
Biology

Anatomy or system affected: Cells, gastrointestinal system, pancreas, stomach

Specialties and related fields: Biochemistry, cytology, gastroenterology, nutrition, pharmacology

Definition: The breakdown of food by cells, a process in which nutrients are converted to energy and other components needed by the body.

Key terms:

amino acids: the organic compounds that make up proteins; twenty are necessary for growth, nine of which must be obtained in the diet

Calorie: the basic unit of energy; the amount of heat needed to change the temperature of one liter of water from 14.5 degrees Celsius to 15.5 degrees Celsius

carbohydrates: a group of organic compounds that includes the sugars and the starches; one of three classes of nutrients and a basic source of energy

fats: a group of organic compounds, also called lipids, that store energy; one of three classes of nutrients

glycolysis: a metabolic pathway that converts the sugar glucose to pyruvate for energy without the use of oxygen

metabolism: the totality of a cell's biochemical processes; the process by which food molecules release their stored energy

minerals: inorganic compounds that are essential for human life; seventeen are required in the diet

proteins: organic compounds that are composed of amino acids and function as enzymes, speeding up metabolic reactions; one of three classes of nutrients

vitamins: organic compounds, essential for life but required in very minute quantities, that participate in biochemical reactions and help to release energy from the three classes of nutrients

Structure and Functions

Food biochemistry is concerned with the breakdown of food in the cell as a source of energy. Each cell is a factory that converts the nutrients of the food one eats to energy and other structural components of the body. The amount of energy that these nutrients supply is expressed in Calories (kilocalories). The number of Calories consumed will determine the energy balance of the individual and whether one loses or gains weight. The nutrients come in a variety of forms, but they can be divided into three major categories: carbohydrates, lipids (fats), and proteins. These nutrients are broken down by the cell metabolically to produce energy for cellular processes. Other components are used by the cell and the entire body for structure and transport. Each of these nutrients is essential to a well-balanced diet and good health. Two other components of a successful diet are vitamins and minerals.

Carbohydrates are molecules composed of carbon, hydrogen, and oxygen. They range from the simple sugars all the way to the complex carbohydrates. The simplest carbohydrates are the monosaccharides (one-sugar molecules), primarily glucose and fructose. The simple monosaccharides are usually joined to form disaccharides (two-sugar molecules), such as sucrose (glucose and fructose, or cane sugar), lactose (glucose and galactose, or milk sugar), and maltose (two glucoses, which is found in grains). The complex carbohydrates are the polysaccharides (multiple sugar molecules), which are composed of many monosaccharides, usually glucose. There are two main types: starch, which is found in plants such as potatoes, and glycogen, in which form humans store carbohydrate energy for the short term (up to twelve hours) in the liver.

The next major group of molecules is the lipids, which are made up of the solid fats and liquid oils. These molecules are primarily composed of carbon and hydrogen. They form three major groups: the triglycerides, phospholipids, and sterols. The triglycerides are composed of three fatty acids attached to a glycerol (a three-carbon molecule); this is the group that makes up the fats and oils. Fats, which are primarily of animal origin, are triglycerides that are solid at room temperature; such triglycerides are saturated, which means that there are no double bonds between their carbon molecules. Oils are liquid at room temperature, primarily of plant origin, and either monounsaturated or polyunsaturated (there are one or more double bonds between the carbon molecules in the chain). This group provides long-term energy in humans and is stored as adipose (fat) tissue. Each gram of fat stores approximately nine Calories of energy per gram, which is about twice that of carbohydrates and proteins (four Calories per gram). The adipose tissue also provides impor-

tant insulation in maintaining body temperature. Phospholipids are similar to triglycerides in structure, but they have two fatty acids and a phosphate attached to the glycerol molecule. Phospholipids are the building blocks of the cell membranes that form the barrier between the inside and the outside of the cell. Sterols are considered lipids, but they have a completely different structure. This group includes cholesterol, vitamin D, estrogen, and testosterone. The sterols function in the structure of the cell membrane (as cholesterol does) or as hormones (as do testosterone and estrogen).

The last major group of molecules is that of the proteins, which are composed of carbon, hydrogen, oxygen, and nitrogen. Proteins are long chains of amino acids; each protein is composed of varying amounts of the twenty different amino acids. Proteins are used in the body as enzymes, substances that catalyze (generally, speed up) the biochemical reactions that take place in cells. They also function as transport molecules (such as hemoglobin, which transports oxygen) and provide structure (as does keratin, the protein in hair and nails). The human body can synthesize eleven of the twenty amino acids; the other nine are considered essential amino acids because they cannot be synthesized and are required in the diet.

Two other groups of essential compounds are necessary in the diet for the body's metabolism: vitamins and minerals. The vitamins are organic compounds (made up of carbon) that are required in only milligram or microgram quantities per day. The vitamins are classified into two groups: the water-soluble vitamins (the B vitamins and vitamin C) and the fat-soluble vitamins (vitamins A, D, E, and K). Vitamins are vital components of enzymes.

The minerals are inorganic nutrients that can be divided into two classes, depending on the amounts needed by the body. The major minerals are required in amounts greater than one hundred milligrams per day; these minerals are calcium, phosphorus, magnesium, sodium, chloride, sulfur, and potassium. The trace elements, those needed in amounts of only a few milligrams per day, are iron, zinc, iodine, fluoride, copper, selenium, chromium, manganese, and molybdenum. Although they are required in small quantities, the minerals play an important role in the human body. Calcium is involved in bone and teeth formation and muscle contractions. Iron is found in hemoglobin and aids in the transportation of oxygen throughout the body. Potassium helps nerves send electrical impulses. Sodium and chloride maintain water balance in tissues and vascular fluid.

An adequate diet is one that supplies the body and cells with sources of energy and building blocks. The first priority of the diet is to supply the bulk nutrients—carbohydrates, fats, and proteins. An average young adult requires between 2,100 and 2,900 Calories per day, taking into account the amount of energy required for rest and work. Carbohydrates, fats, and proteins are taken in during a meal and digested—that is, broken into smaller components. Starch is broken down to glucose, and sucrose is broken down to fructose and glucose and absorbed by the bloodstream. Fats are broken down to triglycerides, and proteins are divided into their separate amino acids, to be absorbed by the bloodstream and transported throughout the body. Each cell then takes up essential nutrients for energy and to use as building parts of the cell.

Once the nutrients enter the cell, they are broken down into energy through a series of metabolic reactions. The first step in the metabolic process is called glycolysis. Glucose is broken down through a series of reactions to produce adenosine triphosphate (ATP), a molecule used to fuel other biochemical pathways in the cell. Glycolysis gives off a small amount of energy and does not require oxygen. This process can provide the energy for a short sprint; lactic acid buildup in the muscles will lead to fatigue, however, if there is insufficient oxygen.

Long-term energy requires oxygen. Aerobic respiration can metabolize not only the sugars produced by glycolysis but triglycerides and amino acids as well. The molecules enter what is called the Krebs cycle, an aerobic pathway that provides eighteen times more energy than glycolysis. The waste products of this pathway are carbon dioxide and water, which are exhaled.

Disorders and Diseases

Diet plays a major role in the metabolism of the cells. One major problem in diet is the overconsumption of Calories, which can lead to weight gain and eventual obesity. Obesity is defined as being 20 percent over one's ideal weight for one's body size. A number of problems are associated with obesity, such as high blood pressure, high levels of cholesterol, increased risk of cancer, heart disease, and early death.

At the other end of the scale is malnutrition. Carbohydrates are the preferred energy source in the form of either blood glucose or glycogen, which is found in the liver and muscles. This source gives a person approximately four to twelve hours of energy. Long-term storage of energy occurs as fat, which constitutes anywhere from 15 percent to 25 percent of body composition. During times of starvation, when the carbohydrate reserve is almost zero, fat will be mobilized for energy. Fat will also be used to make glucose for the blood because the brain requires glucose as its energy source. In extreme starvation, the body will begin to degrade the protein in muscles down to its constituent amino acids in order to produce energy.

Malnutrition can also occur if essential vitamins and minerals are excluded from the diet. Vitamin deficiencies affect the metabolism of the cell since these compounds are often required to aid the enzymes in producing energy. A number of medical problems are associated with vitamin deficiencies. A deficiency in thiamine will result in the metabolic disorder called beriberi. A loss of the thiamine found in wheat and rice can occur in the refinement process, making it more difficult to obtain enough of this vitamin from the diet. Alcoholics have an increased thiamine requirement, to help in the metabolism of alcohol, and usually have a low level of food consumption; thus, they are at risk for developing beriberi. Lack of vitamin A results in night blindness, and lack of vitamin D results in rickets, in which the bones are weakened as a result of poor calcium uptake.

One interesting feature about diet and the metabolic pathways concerns how different molecules are treated. Some people mistakenly believe that it is better to eat fruit sugar than other sugars. Fruit sugar, the simple sugar fructose, is chemically related to glucose. Because glucose and fructose are converted to each other during glycolysis, it does not matter which sugar is eaten. Far more important to proper nutrition is what accompanies the sugar. Table sugar provides only calories, while a piece of fruit contains both fruit sugar and vitamins, minerals, and fiber for a more complete diet.

Many errors in metabolism occur because genes do not carry the proper information. The result may be an enzyme that, although critical to a biochemical pathway, does not function properly or is missing altogether. One disorder of carbohydrate metabolism is called galactosemia. Mother's milk contains lactose, which is normally broken down into galactose and glucose. With galactosemia, the cells take in the galactose but are unable to convert it to glucose because of the lack of an enzyme. Thus, galactose levels build up in the blood, liver, and other organs, impairing their function. This condition can lead to death in an infant, but the effects of galactosemia are usually detected and the diet modified by use of a milk substitute.

Amino acid metabolism can also be defective, leading to the accumulation of toxic by-products. One of the best-known examples involves the amino acid phenylalanine. About one in ten thousand infants is born with a defective pathway, a disorder called phenylketonuria (PKU). If PKU is not discovered in time, by-products can accumulate, causing poor brain development and severe mental retardation. PKU must be diagnosed early in life, and a special, controlled diet must be given to the infant. Because phenylalanine is an essential amino acid, limited amounts are included in the diet for proper growth, but large amounts need to be excluded. The artificial sweetener aspartame (NutraSweet) poses a problem for those with PKU. Aspartame is composed of two amino acids, phenylalanine and aspartic acid. When aspartame is broken down during digestion, phenylalanine enters the bloodstream. Individuals with PKU should not ingest aspartame; there is a warning to that effect on products containing this chemical.

Other errors of metabolism are noted later in life. One example is lactose intolerance, in which lactose is cleaved by the enzyme lactase into glucose and galactose. The enzyme lactase, found in the digestive tract, is very active in suckling infants, but only northern Europeans and members of some African tribes retain lactase activity into adulthood. Other groups, such as Asian, Arab, Jewish, Indian, and Mediterranean peoples, show little lactase activity as adults. These people cannot digest the lactose in milk products, which then cannot be absorbed in the intestinal tract. A buildup of lactose can lead to diarrhea and colic. Usually in those parts of the world milk is not used by adults as food. In the United States, one can purchase milk that contains lactose which has been partially broken down into galactose and glucose. One can also purchase the lactase enzyme itself and add it to milk.

Another error of metabolism results in diabetes mellitus, which means "excessive excretion of sweet urine." A telltale sign of this condition is sugar, specifically glucose, in the urine. In normal people, blood glucose levels remain relatively stable. After a meal, when the blood glucose levels rise, the pancreas starts to secrete the hormone insulin. Insulin causes the cells to take in the extra blood glucose and convert it to glycogen or fat, thus storing the extra energy. In diabetics, there is little or no insulin production or release, or the target cells may have faulty receptors. As a result, the blood glucose level remains high. The excess glucose is then excreted in the urine, leading to the symptom of excess thirst. The body is forced to rely much more heavily on fats as an energy source, leading to high levels of circulating fats and cholesterol in the blood. These substances can be deposited in the blood vessels, causing high blood pressure and heart disease. Excess fats, in levels that exceed the body's ability to metabolize and burn them, may produce acetone, which gives the breath of diabetics a sweet odor. A buildup of acetone can lead to ketoacidosis, a pathologic condition in which the blood pH drops from 7.4 to 6.8. Complications arising from diabetes also include blindness, kidney disease, and nerve damage. Furthermore, resulting peripheral vascular disease, in which the body's extremities do not get enough blood, leads to tissue death and gangrene.

Perspective and Prospects

The study of food biochemistry has evolved over the years from a strictly biochemical approach to one in which diet and nutrition play a major role. An understanding of diet and nutrition required vital information about the metabolic processes occurring in the cell, supplied by the field of biochemistry.

This information started to become available in 1898 when Eduard Buchner discovered that the fermentation of glucose to alcohol and carbon dioxide could occur in a cell-free extract. The early twentieth century led to the complete discovery of the glycolytic pathway and the enzymes that were involved in the process. In the 1930s, other pathways of metabolism were elucidated.

In conjunction with Buchner's discovery, British physician Archibald Garrod in 1909 hypothesized that genes control a person's appearance through enzymes that catalyze certain metabolic processes in the cell. Garrod thought that some inherited diseases resulted from a patient's inability to make a particular enzyme, and he called them "inborn errors of metabolism." One example he gave was a condition called alkaptonuria, in which the urine turns black upon exposure to the air.

Some of the earliest nutritional studies date back to the time of Aristotle, who knew that raw liver contained an ingredient that could cure night blindness. Christiaan Eijkman studied beriberi in the Dutch East Indies and traced the problem to diet. Sir Frederick Hopkins was an English biochemist who conducted pioneering work on vitamins and the essentiality of amino acids in the early twentieth century.

Hopkins realized that the type of protein is important in the diet as well as the quantity. Hopkins hypothesized that some trace substance in addition to proteins, fats, and carbohydrates may be required in the diet for growth; this substance was later identified as the vitamin. Hopkins was the first biochemist to explore diet and metabolic function.

Working with this broad base, scientists have made tremendous advances in the study of diet and nutrition based on the biochemistry of the cell. In 1943, the first recommended daily (or dietary) allowances (RDAs) were published to provide standards for diet and good nutrition; the term now used is dietary reference intake (DRI). The DRIs suggest the amounts of protein, fats, carbohydrates, vitamins, and minerals required for adequate nutrient uptake. The major uses of the DRIs are for schools and other institutions in planning menus, obtaining food supplies, and preparing food labels.

Since the 1970s, research has consistently associated nutritional factors with six of the ten leading causes of death in the United States: high blood pressure, heart disease, cancer, cardiovascular disease, chronic liver disease, and non-insulin-dependent diabetes mellitus. This research has led to improvements in the American diet.

—*Lonnie J. Guralnick, Ph.D.*

See also Antioxidants; Appetite loss; Caffeine; Carbohydrates; Cholesterol; Cytology; Diabetes mellitus; Dietary reference intakes (DRIs); Digestion; Enzymes; Fatty acid oxidation disorders; Fiber; Food Guide Pyramid; Glycogen storage diseases; Glycolysis; Lactose intolerance; Macronutrients; Malnutrition; Metabolism; Nutrition; Phenylketonuria (PKU); Phytochemicals; Protein; Supplements; Vitamins and minerals.

For Further Information:

Bonci, Leslie. *American Dietetic Association Guide to Better Digestion*. New York: Wiley, 2003.

Campbell, Neil A., et al. *Biology: Concepts and Connections*. 6th ed. San Francisco: Pearson/Benjamin Cummings, 2008.

Clark, Nancy. *Nancy Clark's Sports Nutrition Guidebook*. 4th ed. Champaign, Ill.: Human Kinetics, 2008.

Duyff, Roberta Larson. *American Dietetic Association Complete Food and Nutrition Guide*. 3d ed. Hoboken, N.J.: John Wiley & Sons, 2007.

"Malnutrition." *MedlinePlus*, June 14, 2011.

Margen, Sheldon. *Wellness Foods A to Z: An Indispensable Guide for Health-Conscious Food Lovers*. New York: Rebus, 2002.

Marlow, Amy. "Phenylketonuria." *Health Library*, November 26, 2012.

Nasset, Edmund S. *Nutrition Handbook*. 3d ed. New York: Harper & Row, 1982.

Nelson, David L., and Michael M. Cox. *Lehninger Principles of Biochemistry*. 5th ed. New York: W. H. Freeman, 2009.

Nieman, David C., Diane E. Butterworth, and Catherine N. Nieman. *Nutrition*. Rev. ed. Dubuque, Iowa: Wm. C. Brown, 1992.

Wood, Debra. "Lactose Intolerance." *Health Library*, May 11, 2013.

FOOD GUIDE PLATE

Also known as: MyPlate

Anatomy or system affected: All

Specialties and related fields: Biochemistry, nutrition, preventive medicine, public health

Definition: An icon designed to remind consumers to make better food choices based on recommendations from Dietary Guidelines for Americans 2010. Along with supporting information from the website ChooseMyPlate.gov, people can learn new eating and activity behaviors to enhance their overall health.

Key terms:

body mass index: A calculation based on the weight and height of adults or weight, height, and age of children that is generally an indicator of body fatness and is used to screen for weight categories that may lead to future health problems

nutrients: substances in food that provide energy and are required by the body to support growth and maintenance of life

overweight: weighing more than is generally considered healthy

obese: the Centers for Disease Control and Prevention (CDC) defines obese as adults with a Body Mass Index (BMI) of thirty or more, or children with a BMI above the ninety-fifth percentile for age

sedentary: spending a great deal of time seated, engaging in little physical activity

Introduction

Eating habits that provide excess energy but are lacking in certain nutrients and a sedentary lifestyle are associated with the major causes of chronic disease and death in adults, such as heart disease, stroke, cancer, and diabetes. Poor eating habits and insufficient physical activity have also contributed to the current epidemic of overweight and obesity among young Americans. According to the CDC more than one-third of children and adolescents in the United States were overweight or obese in 2010, leading to concerns about immediate and long-term health effects in this population. Nutrition-related health concerns were addressed by the Dietary Guidelines Advisory Committee (DGAC) in their systemic review of nutrition research, which was used, in combination with other scientific reports, to create the *Dietary Guidelines for Americans 2010 (DGA 2010)*. These guidelines are used to set federal nutrition policy and coordinate nutrition education for the American public.

In June 2011, the United States Department of Agriculture (USDA) Center for Nutrition Policy and Promotion issued updated food patterns based on the *DGA 2010* and released the MyPlate icon and ChooseMyPlate.gov website. MyPlate replaced the previous Food Guide Pyramid. Critics of the Food Guide Pyramid claimed that it was confusing and difficult for people to use. The MyPlate food guide was developed with input from consumer focus groups and designed to be a visual cue linked to a more familiar mealtime symbol, the plate.

The Food Guide Plate is a simple illustration to remind people to eat healthfully. Five food groups are represented in the picture. The MyPlate icon consists of a plate divided into four parts, and a smaller circle at the top right of the plate, representing a beverage. The left half of the plate contains a red wedge labeled "Fruits" and below that, a slightly larger green wedge labeled "Vegetables." The right half of the plate contains a purple wedge labeled "Protein" and above that a slightly larger brown wedge labeled "Grains". The small blue circle is labeled "Dairy." At the bottom of the icon is the web address "ChooseMyPlate.gov."

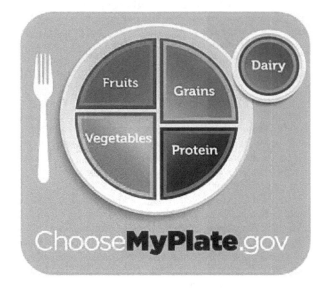

The Food Guide Plate icon directs attention to the proportions of various types of food in meal planning, represented by the size of the divisions on the plate, and to variety by showing five basic food groups. It does not address other foods such as sweets and fats, nor directly teaches people to avoid excess energy intake. These topics and more details about the best food choices are addressed at the ChooseMyPlate.gov website.

Visitors to this website are guided through key messages to adopt eating patterns that meet nutrient needs without promoting overweight/obesity and to understand how foods and beverages can fit within a healthy eating pattern. Messages to "focus on fruits," "vary your veggies," "make at least half your grains whole," "go lean with protein," and, "get your calcium-rich foods" are supported with more detailed information. The website also contains recommendations concerning weight management and physical activity, and the Supertracker (a tool to plan, analyze, and track personal diet and exercise).

Perspective and Prospects

The goal in early nutrition research was to identify essential nutrients in foods, aiming to eliminate nutritional deficiency diseases. In 1916, the USDA issued its first food guide, *Food for Young Children,* followed in 1917 by *How to Select Food.* Nutrition messages in that era focused on the selection of "protective food."

By the 1940s, the USDA food guide had evolved into *A Guide to Good Eating* and included seven food groups with a recommended number of servings each day, although serving sizes were not specified. Various food guides developed over the next three decades, and they emphasized planning meals for nutritional adequacy.

By the late 1970s cardiovascular disease mortality rates were at an all-time high. The American diet, high in total and saturated fat, contributed to this epidemic. Therefore, in 1977, the U.S. Senate Select Committee on Nutrition and Human Needs recommended that dietary goals for Americans be established. The first *Dietary Guidelines for Americans* was issued in 1980 as a nineteen-page brochure containing seven guidelines for healthy people. Since then, food guides have taken a total diet approach, addressing both nutrient adequacy and moderation.

Though much of the dietary advice has not changed dramatically since 1980, the underlying scientific research has expanded extensively, and is being incorporated in the every-five-year updates of the *DGA*. The 2010 report was the first entirely evidence-based DGAC Report, and it included a systematic, detailed review of information from the USDA Nutrition Evidence Library and a ranking system that qualifies the amount and type of evidence available. It also addressed the epidemic of overweight and obesity in America and emphasized primary prevention of obesity before birth and during infancy and childhood as the most potentially effective method for reversing this problem.

As of 2013, the USDA had launched specific initiatives to teach healthy diet and activity behaviors to children (the MyPlate Kid's Place) and to college students (MyPlate on Campus). Also, initiatives for older adults and children under age two are under development.

—*Carol A. Selden, R.D.*

See also Exercise physiology; Malnutrition; Obesity; Obesity, childhood

For Further Information:

Blake, Joan Salge. *Nutrition and You, My Plate Edition.* 2nd ed. San Francisco: Pearson Benjamin Cummings, 2012.

Duyff, Roberta Larson. *American Dietetic Association Complete Food and Nutrition Guide.* 4th ed. Hoboken, NJ: John Wiley and Sons, 2012.

Suitor, Carol West, and Suzanne P. Murphy. "Chapter 13-Nutrition Guidelines to Maintain Health." *Nutrition in the Prevention and Treatment of Disease.* 3rd ed., edited by Ann M. Coulston, Carol J. Boushey, and Mario Ferruzzi. Amsterdam: Elsevier/Academic Press, 2012.

10 June. 2011.

FOOD POISONING
Disease/Disorder

Anatomy or system affected: Gastrointestinal system, intestines, stomach

Specialties and related fields: Environmental health, epidemiology, gastroenterology, public health, toxicology

Definition: Food-borne illness caused by bacteria, viruses, or parasites consumed in food and resulting in acute gastrointestinal disturbance that may include diarrhea, nausea, vomiting, and abdominal discomfort.

Key terms:

contamination: infection of a food item by a pathogen

food-borne infection: disease caused by eating foods contaminated by infectious microorganisms, with onset occurring within twenty-four hours (for example, salmonellosis)

food-borne intoxication: disease caused by eating foods containing microorganisms that produce toxins, with onset occurring within six hours (for example, botulism)

microorganism: an organism that is too small to be seen with the naked eye

parasite: an organism that lives on another organism (the host) and causes harm to the host while it benefits

pathogen: a disease-causing organism

thermal death point: the lowest temperature that can destroy a food-borne organism

Causes and Symptoms

Often a person feeling the symptoms of nausea, vomiting, diarrhea, and abdominal discomfort assumes that he or she has contracted influenza. The presence of a true influenza virus, however, is uncommon. More likely, these symptoms are caused by eating food that contains undesirable bacteria, viruses, or parasites. This is called food-borne illness, or food poisoning. Most food-borne pathogens are colorless, odorless, and tasteless. Fortunately, there are recommendations based on scientific principles to help prevent food-borne illness.

Food poisoning is a worldwide problem. In developing countries, diarrhea is a factor in child malnutrition and is estimated to cause millions deaths per year. According to the Center for Disease Control and Prevention (CDC), approximately 49 million Americans are affected by food-borne illnesses every year, resting in 3,000 deaths and 128,000 hospitalizations. Despite advances in modern technology, food-borne illness is a major problem in developed countries as well.

Certain foods, particularly foods with a high protein and moisture content, provide an ideal environment for the multiplication of pathogens. The foods with high risk in the United States are raw shellfish (especially mollusks), underdone poultry, raw eggs, rare meats, raw milk, and cooked food that another person handled before it was packaged and chilled. In addition to those foods listed, some developing countries could add raw vegetables, raw fruits that cannot be peeled, foods from sidewalk vendors, and tap water or water from unknown and contaminated sources.

Most of the documented cases of food-borne illness are caused by only a few bacteria, viruses, and parasites. Bacteria known as *Salmonella* are ingested by humans in contaminated foods such as beef, poultry, and eggs; they may also be transmitted by kitchen utensils and the hands of people who have handled infected food or utensils. Once the bacteria are inside the body, the incubation time is from eight to twenty-four hours. Since the bacteria multiply inside the body and attack the gastrointestinal tract, this disease is known as a true food infection. The main symptoms are diarrhea, abdominal cramps, and vomiting. The bacteria are killed by cooking

---

Information on Food Poisoning

Causes: Bacteria, viruses, or parasites consumed in food

Symptoms: Diarrhea, nausea, vomiting, fever, abdominal discomfort

Duration: One to three days

Treatments: Rest, avoidance of food, extra fluid intake

---

foods to the well-done stage.

The major food-borne intoxication in the United States is caused by eating food contaminated with the toxin of *Staphylococcus* bacteria. Because the toxin or poison has already been produced in the food item that is ingested, the onset of symptoms is usually very rapid (between one-half hour and six hours). Improperly stored or cooked foods (particularly meats, tuna, and potato salad) are the main carriers of these bacteria. Since this toxin cannot be killed by reheating the food items to a high temperature, it is important that foods are properly stored.

Botulism is a rare food poisoning caused by the toxin of *Clostridium botulinum*. It is anaerobic, meaning that it multiplies in environments without oxygen, and is mainly found in improperly home-canned food items. Originally one of the sources of the disease was from eating sausages (the Latin word for which is *botulus*)—hence, the term "botulism." A very small amount of toxin, the size of a grain of salt, could kill hundreds of people within an hour. Danger signs include double vision and difficulty swallowing and breathing.

Though everyone is at risk for food-borne illness, certain groups of people develop more severe symptoms and are at a greater risk for serious illness and death. Higher-risk groups include pregnant women, very young children, the elderly, and immunocompromised individuals, such as patients with acquired immunodeficiency syndrome (AIDS) and cancer.

Bacteria known as *Listeria* were first documented in 1981 as being transmitted by food. Most people are at low risk of becoming ill after ingesting these bacteria; however, pregnant women are at high risk. *Listeria* infection is rare in the United States, but it does cause serious illness. It is associated with consumption of raw (unpasteurized) milk, nonreheated hot dogs, undercooked chicken, various soft cheeses (Mexican style, feta, Brie, Camembert, and blue-veined cheese), and food purchased from delicatessen counters. *Listeria* cause a short-term illness in pregnant women; however, this bacteria can cause stillbirths and spontaneous abortions. A parasite called *Toxoplasma gondii* is also of particular risk for pregnant women. For this reason, raw or very rare meat should not be eaten. (In addition, since cats may shed these parasites in their feces, it is recommended that pregnant women avoid cleaning cat litter boxes.)

As the protective antibodies from the mother are lost, infants become more susceptible to food poisoning. Botulism generally occurs by ingesting the toxin or poison; however, in infant botulism it is the spores that germinate and produce the toxin within the intestinal tract of the infant. Since honey and corn syrup have been found to contain spores, it is recommended that they not be fed to infants under one year of age, especially those under six months.

Determining whether a disease is caused by a food-borne organism is highly skilled work. The Centers for Disease Control and Prevention (CDC) in Atlanta investigate diseases and their causes. It has been estimated that the true incidence of food-borne illness in the United States is ten to one hundred times greater than that reported to the CDC. The CDC report some of the more interesting cases and outbreaks in narrative form in the *Morbidity and Mortality Weekly Report*.

Treatment and Therapy

In cases of severe food poisoning marked by vomiting, diarrhea, or collapse—especially in cases of botulism and ingestion of poisonous plant material such as suspicious mushrooms—emergency medical attention should be sought immediately, and, if possible, specimens of the suspected food should be submitted for analysis. Identifying the source of the food is especially important if that source is a public venue such as a restaurant, because stemming a widespread outbreak of food poisoning may thereby be possible. In less severe cases of food poisoning, the victim should rest, eat nothing, but drink fluids that contain some salt and sugar; the person should begin to recover after several hours or one or two days and should see a doctor if not well after two or three days.

Some types of food poisoning can be treated with antibiotics, and there is an antitoxin available for cases of botulism. However, the best "treatment" for food poisoning is prevention. While there is ample information regarding the prevention of food poisoning, many outbreaks still occur as a result of carelessness in the kitchen. Good food safety is basically good common sense, yet it can make sense only when one has acquired some knowledge of how food-borne pathogens spread and how to apply food safety steps to prevent food-borne illness. Based on the research literature, as well as on the suggestions made by the World Health Organization (WHO) and other groups, the recommendations are to cook foods well, to prevent cross-contamination, and to keep hot foods hot and cold foods cold.

Cooking foods well means cooking them to a high enough temperature in the slowest-to-heat part and for a long enough time to destroy pathogens that have already gained access to foods. Cooking foods well is only a concern when they have become previously contaminated from other sources or are naturally contaminated. There are a number of possible sources of contamination of food products.

Coastal water may contaminate seafood. Filter-feeding marine animals (such as clams, scallops, oysters, cockles, and mussels) and some fish (such as anchovies, sardines, and herring) live by pumping in seawater and sifting out organisms that they need for food. Therefore, they have the ability to concentrate suspended material by many orders of magnitude. Shellfish grown in contaminated coastal waters are the most frequent carriers of a virus called hepatitis A.

Contaminated eggs can be another vehicle of food-borne

illness. Contamination of eggs can occur from external as well as internal sources. If moist conditions are present and there is a crack in the shell, the fecal material of hens carrying the microorganism can penetrate the shell and membrane of the egg and can multiply. In the early 1990s, *Salmonella enteritidis* began to appear in the intact egg, particularly in the northeastern part of the United States. It is hypothesized that contamination occurs in the oviduct of the hen before the egg is laid. Food vehicles in which *Salmonella enteritidis* has been reported include sandwiches dipped in eggs and cooked, hollandaise sauce, eggs Benedict, commercial frozen pasta with raw egg and cheese stuffing, Caesar salad dressing, and blended food in which cross-contamination had occurred. Foods such as cookie or cake dough or homemade ice cream made with raw eggs are other possible vehicles of food-borne illness.

Milk, especially raw milk, can be contaminated. Sources of milk contaminants could be an unhealthy cow (such as from mastitis, a major infection of the mammary gland of the dairy cow) or unclean methods of milking, such as not cleaning the teats well before attaching them to the milker or unclean utensils (milking tanks). If milk is not cooled fast enough, contaminants can multiply.

Modern mechanized milking procedures have reduced but not eliminated food-borne pathogens. Postpasteurization contamination may occur, especially if bulk tanks or equipment have not been properly cleaned and sanitized. In 1985 in Chicago, one of the largest salmonellosis outbreaks occurred, with the causal food being pasteurized milk. More than sixteen thousand people were infected, and ten died. A small connecting piece in the milk tank which allowed milk and microorganisms to collect was determined to be the source of the contamination. Bulk tanks should be properly maintained and piping should be inspected regularly for opportunities for raw milk to contaminate the pasteurized product.

Recommendations for cooking temperatures are based not only on the temperature required to kill food-borne pathogens but also on aesthetics and palatability. Generally, a margin of safety is built into the cooking temperature because of the possibility of nonuniform heating. Based on generally accepted temperature requirements, cooking red meat until 71 degrees Celsius (160 degrees Fahrenheit) will reach the thermal death point. Hamburger should be well cooked so that it is medium-brown inside. If pressed, it should feel firm and the juices that run out should be clear. Cooking poultry to the well-done stage is done for palatability. Tenderness is indicated when there is a flexible hip joint, and juices should run clear and not pink when the meat is pierced with a fork. Fish should be cooked until it loses its translucent appearance and flakes when pierced with a fork. Eggs should be thoroughly cooked until the yolk is thickened and the white is firm, not runny. Cooked or chilled foods that are served hot (that is, leftovers) should be reheated so that they come to a rolling boil.

Cross-contamination occurs when microorganisms are transmitted from humans, cutting boards, and utensils to food. Contamination between foods, especially from raw meat and poultry to fresh vegetables or other ready-to-eat foods, is a major problem.

One of the best ways to prevent cross-contamination is simply washing one's hands with soap and water. Twenty seconds is the minimum time span that should be spent washing one's hands. To prevent the spread of disease, it is also recommended that the hands be dried with a paper towel, which is then thrown away. Thoroughly washed hands can still be a source of bacteria, however, so one should use tongs and spoons when cooking to prevent contamination.

It is especially important to wash one's hands after certain activities, such as blowing the nose or sneezing, using the lavatory, diapering a baby, smoking, petting animals or pets, and before cooking or handling food.

Other sources of cross-contamination include utensils and cutting surfaces. If people use the same knife and cutting board to cut up raw chicken for a stir-fry and peaches for a fruit salad, they are putting themselves at great risk for food-borne illness. The bacteria on the cutting board and the knife could cross-contaminate the peaches. While the chicken will be cooked until it is well done, the peaches in the salad will not be. In this situation, one could cut the fruit first and then the chicken, and then wash and sanitize the knife and cutting board.

Cleaning and sanitizing is actually a two-step process. Cleaning involves using soap and water and a scrubber or dishcloth to remove the major debris from the surface. The second step, sanitizing, involves using a diluted chloride solution to kill bacteria and viruses.

Wooden cutting boards are one of the worst offenders in terms of causing cross-contamination. Since bacteria and viruses are microscopic, they can adhere to and grow in the grooves of a wooden cutting board and spread to other foods when the cutting board is used again. Use of a plastic or acrylic cutting board prevents this problem.

The danger zone in which bacteria can multiply is a range of 4.4 degrees Celsius (40 degrees Fahrenheit) to 60 degrees Celsius (140 degrees Fahrenheit). Room temperature is generally right in the middle of this danger zone. The danger zone is critical because, even though they cannot be seen, bacteria are increasing in number. They can double and even quadruple in fifteen to thirty minutes. Consequently, perishable foods such as meats, poultry, fish, milk, cooked rice, leftover pizza, hard-cooked eggs, leftover refried beans, and potato salad should not be left in the danger zone for more than two hours. Keeping hot foods hot means keeping them at a temperature higher than 60 degrees Celsius. Keeping cold foods cold means keeping them at a temperature lower than 4 degrees Celsius (40 degrees Fahrenheit).

Other rules are helpful for preventing contamination. When shopping, the grocery store should be the last stop so that foods are not stored in a hot car. When meal time is over, leftovers should be placed in the refrigerator or freezer as soon as possible. When packing for a picnic, food items should be kept in an ice chest to keep them cold or brought slightly frozen. Many instances of food-born illnesses and death could be prevented if such food safety rules were followed.

Perspective and Prospects

When the lifestyle of people changed from a hunting-and-gathering society to a more agrarian one, the need to preserve food from spoilage was necessary for survival. As early as 3000 BCE, salt was used as a meat preservative and the production of cheese had begun in the Near East. The production of wine and the preservation of fish by smoking were also introduced at that time. Even though throughout history people had tried many methods to preserve foods and keep them from spoiling, the relationship between illness and pathogens or toxins in food was not recognized and documented until 1857. It was then that the French chemist Louis Pasteur demonstrated that the microorganisms in raw milk caused spoilage.

Stories from the American Civil War (1860–1865) demonstrate the problems of institutional feeding of many people for long periods of time. Gastrointestinal diseases were rampant during that time period. During the first year of the war, of the people who had diarrhea and dysentery, the morbidity rate was 640 per 1,000 and increased to 995 per 1,000 in 1862. More men died of disease and illness than were killed in battle.

Food can be contaminated by disease-causing organisms at any step of the food-handling chain, from the farm to the table. An important role of government and industry is to ensure a safe food supply. In the United States, setting and monitoring of food safety standards are the responsibility of the Food and Drug Administration (FDA) under the auspices of the US Department of Health and Human Services and the Food Safety and Inspection Service (FSIS) under the auspices of the US Department of Agriculture (USDA). The FDA is responsible for the wholesomeness of all food sold in interstate commerce, except meat and poultry, while the USDA is responsible for the inspection of meat and poultry sold in interstate commerce and internationally. Some major food safety laws and policies that have guided the provision of safe food are the Federal Food and Drugs Act in 1906; the Federal Meat Inspection Act in 1906–1907; the Food, Drug, and Cosmetic Act in 1938; and the Poultry Products Inspection Act in 1957.

Historically, the diseases of tuberculosis, scarlet fever, strep throat, typhoid fever, and diphtheria have been associated with raw or unpasteurized milk. The reporting of foodborne illness was initiated in the 1920s by the US Public Health Service (USPHS) when annual summaries of outbreaks of milk-borne disease were recorded and reported. Later, reports of waterborne and food-borne diseases were added.

The public attitude about what is hazardous in the food supply and that of the FDA have often differed. The public generally believes that the safety of additives and chemical contaminants in food is of a higher priority than that of the microbiological and nutritional hazards—the exact opposite of the FDA's priorities. (For example, in the mid-1980s, the story about Alar, a chemical used to slow the ripening of apples, represented a very emotional topic. There was particular concern about the risks that this chemical might pose to children who ate large amounts of apple products.) As more reliable information is available about both areas of concern, the situation regarding priorities is likely to change.

—*Martha M. Henze, M.S., R.D.;*
updated by Maria Pacheco, Ph.D.

See also Bacterial infections; Biological and chemical weapons; Botulism; *Campylobacter* infections; Diarrhea and dysentery; *E. coli* infection; Enterocolitis; Gangrene; Gastroenteritis; Gastroenterology; Gastroenterology, pediatric; Gastrointestinal disorders; Gastrointestinal system; Indigestion; Intestinal disorders; Intestines; Lead poisoning; *Listeria* infections; Mercury poisoning; Nausea and vomiting; Noroviruses; Parasitic diseases; Poisoning; Rotavirus; Salmonella infection; Shigellosis; Trichinosis; Tularemia; Ulcers; Viral infections.

For Further Information:

Carson-DeWitt, Roasalyn. "Food Poisoning." *Health Library*, March 22, 2013.

Cliver, Dean O., and Hans P. Riemann, eds. *Foodborne Diseases*. 2d ed. San Diego: Academic Press, 2002.

Gaman, P. M., and K. B. Sherrington. *The Science of Food: An Introduction to Food Science, Nutrition, and Microbiology*. 4th ed. Boston: Butterworth-Heinemann/Elsevier, 2008.

Griffith, C. J. "Do Businesses Get the Food Poisoning They Deserve? The Importance of Food Safety Culture." *British Food Journal* 112, no. 4 (2010): 416–425.

Hobbs, Betty C., Jim McLauchlin, and Christina Louis Little. *Hobbs" Food Poisoning and Food Hygiene*. 7th ed. London: Hodder Arnold, 2007.

Jay, James M., Martin J. Loessner, and David A. Golden. *Modern Food Microbiology*. 7th ed. New York: Springer, 2005.

Leon, Warren, and Caroline Smith DeWaal. *Is Our Food Safe? A Consumer's Guide to Protecting Your Health and the Environment*. New York: Crown, 2002.

Lew, Kristi. *Food Poisoning: E. Coli and the Food Supply*. New York: Rosen Publishers, 2011.

Longrée, Karla, and Gertrude Armbruster. *Quantity Food Sanitation*. 5th ed. New York: John Wiley & Sons, 1996.

Marriot, Norman G., and Robert B. Gravani. *Principles of Food Sanitation*. 5th ed. New York: Springer, 2006.

Nestle, Marion. *Safe Food: The Politics of Food Safety*. Updated ed. Berkeley: University of California Press, 2010.

Ray, Bibek. *Fundamental Food Microbiology*. 4th ed. Boca Raton: Taylor & Francis, 2008.

Troncoso, Alcides, Cecilia Ramos Clausen, and Jessica Rivas. *Where Can You Catch Botulism Food Poisoning?: Foodborne Botulism*. Saarbrücken: Lambert Academic Publishing, 2012.

Wilson, Michael, Brian Henderson, and Rod McNab. *Bacterial Disease Mechanisms: An Introduction to Cellular Microbiology*. New York: Cambridge University Press, 2002.

FOOT DISORDERS

Disease/Disorder

Anatomy or system affected: Bones, feet, muscles, musculoskeletal system

Specialties and related fields: Orthopedics, podiatry

Definition: Disorders involving the muscles, bones, nerves, or skin of the feet.

Because of the constant and heavy use of feet by humans as bipeds, they are prone to many problems. In spite of what is commonly believed, most cases of foot bone and joint abnormalities are developmental in origin instead of being caused

Information on Foot Disorders

Causes: Congenital and developmental factors, improper footwear, muscle weakness, incorrect weight-bearing, short Achilles tendon, nerve disorders, dermatologic disorders

Symptoms: Pain, swelling, limping, numbness, tingling

Duration: Short-term or chronic

Treatments: Medication, ointments, surgery, orthopedic footwear

by poorly fitting footwear.

Developmental, muscle, and bone disorders of the feet. Clubfoot, also called talipes, is one of the developmental, or congenital, disorders affecting the feet. It occurs in approximately one of every one thousand live human births and is characterized by deformities such as the foot turning down and under, such that a child will walk on the top of his or her foot. Over time, tendon and ligament contraction reinforces the deformity; thus, either casting or surgery is needed for realignment.

Flat foot, or pes planus, is an abnormally flat arch in the foot, accompanied by a characteristic gait, both of which can occur in varying degrees. Muscle weakness, incorrect weight-bearing, a short Achilles tendon, and developmental defects may all contribute to this deformity. Flat foot may or may not produce a pathologic condition such as arthritis.

A bunion is the relocation of bone from the first metatarsal to the inner portion of the joint connecting it to the big toe. This prominence at the base of the big toe makes the soft tissue in the area subject to pressure from shoes, causing swelling and pain in the protective sac above the metatarsophalangeal joint in a condition called bursitis. Cortisone injections may relieve symptoms, but surgery is required in extreme cases to realign the first metatarsal. Flat foot usually accompanies bunions and is a factor in their development.

Muscular imbalances inherent in the foot are the reason for the curvature of the individual bones of the toes. Abnormally curved bones produce hammertoe, or claw toe, which usually requires little treatment other than a padding of the shoes to avoid corn or callus development. Excessive muscle tension at the heel can produce bony growths called heel spurs or calcaneal exostoses. Inflammation may develop in a neighboring joint's bursa, causing a throbbing pain.

Inflammation of the calcaneus or heel bone can occur in childhood while the heel is still fusing from the two bones that constitute the heel. When a piece of separated bone, called an apophysis, becomes inflamed, apophysitis occurs. This condition can injure the connecting, softer cartilage between the two, not-yet-connected, bones. Apophysitis usually disappears as children grow and the heel fuses whole.

Nerve and skin disorders of the feet. Factors including footwear, the structures of the foot itself, and harmful external forces acting on the foot may all contribute to irritation and/or damage to the nerves of the foot. Morton's neuroma is the thickening of the nerve located between the metatarsals of the third and fourth toes, followed by the formation of a small benign tumor. Painful burning, numbness, or tingling sensations may be alleviated by wearing more comfortable footwear or by the surgical removal of the tumor. Tarsal tunnel syndrome occurs when a nerve traveling along the bottom of the foot through a channel called the tarsal canal becomes compressed and damaged. Cortisone injections into this canal can relieve pressure on the nerve, and surgery can be used to treat severe cases.

The skin of the foot is subject to much pressure and rubbing; thus, it responds by producing changes, termed dermatologic disorders, which themselves cause pain. A corn, or heloma, is a small, sharply defined, raised area of thickened skin containing much of the fibrous protein called keratin. Calluses are also composed of keratin but are flatter and do not possess the defined borders of corns. Both types of

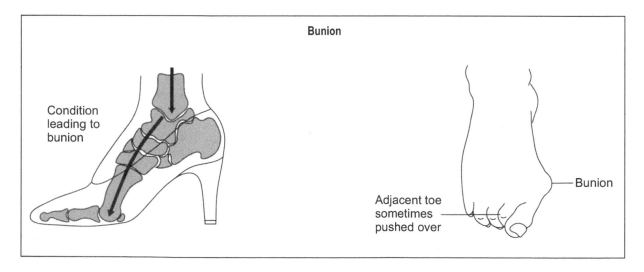

Bunion

Condition leading to bunion

Adjacent toe sometimes pushed over

Bunion

thickened keratinized skin are usually attributed to incorrect positioning of the underlying bone.

Warts, or verrucae, are actually skin tumors caused by the human papillomavirus. They occur most commonly on the sole of the foot, where they are named plantar warts. Warts can be transmitted from person to person, and the lymphatic communication between warts within an individual explains their ability to spread. Warts on the foot are invariably benign, however, and should not be treated with x-ray or radium therapy lest the surrounding areas undergo change themselves and eventually produce tumors.

Dermatitis venenata is often caused by chemicals used in the binding or dyeing of shoes. Angiokeratoma is a lesion on the bottom of the foot commonly mistaken for a wart. Fibroma is the name of the benign growth that may spread under the toenails as a result of insect bites in the vicinity or manifestations of other skin diseases.

Ingrown toenails, or onychocryptoses, occur when the free end of the toenail penetrates the surrounding soft tissue. Reasons for this painful disorder are commonly badly fitted footwear, nail disease, and foot or nail structural abnormalities.

Systemic diseases affecting the feet. Rheumatoid arthritis is a condition involving connective tissue, unknown in origin, in which the synovial membrane of joints proliferates while invading and even destroying cartilage and bone. Women acquire this disease three times more often than do men. Steroid hormones are sometimes applied to aid in the treatment of rheumatoid arthritis, but gold salt injection is the only therapy resulting in a permanent cure. The chances of a cure are greater when this disease occurs in children. The condition is then known as juvenile rheumatoid arthritis, or Still's disease.

Several normally fatal diseases may accompany rheumatoid arthritis. Systemic lupus erythematosus can be masked by the arthritic condition until inflammation spreads to small arteries of the body's organs. Polyarteritis nodosa also involves arteries throughout the body, and its true diagnosis may be prevented by the misleading arthritic condition. Scleroderma involves the thickening of the skin on the face, hands, and feet; depigmentation; loss of hair; and lesions. Sarcoidosis manifests itself in the hands and feet and causes microscopic lesions in the bone that eventually become visible by x-ray examination. Henoch-Schönlein syndrome is an allergic reaction that can resemble the synovitis of rheumatic fever.

Rheumatic fever affects fibrous tissues in a widespread fashion involving the joints and later the heart. It is related to streptococcal infections and occurs as a migrating arthritis producing no lasting joint damage in the feet, but it can cause permanent damage to the cardiac valve. Osteoarthritis causes the degeneration of cartilage and the overgrowth of bone surfaces. The effects of this condition are limited to the joints, unlike rheumatoid arthritis, which can spread to nearby cartilage and bone. Staphylococci, streptococci, and coliform bacteria are the infective agents involved in pyogenic arthritis. In this condition, the organism is carried by the blood to the joint interior. Ulcers of the feet may be caused by a variety of conditions, including diabetes mellitus, syphilis, anemia, and leprosy.

If there is sustained pain in the foot or ankle with no known cause such as injury, a continuously low leukocyte count, and negative laboratory tests for the presence of bacteria, then a viral infection is likely present. An elevated leukocyte count is often indicative of a bacterial infection.

—Ryan C. Horst and Roman J. Miller, Ph.D.

See also Athlete's foot; Birth defects; Bones and the skeleton; Bunions; Feet; Flat feet; Fracture and dislocation; Frostbite; Fungal infections; Ganglion removal; Gout; Hammertoe correction; Hammertoes; Heel spur removal; Lower extremities; Nail removal; Nails; Orthopedic surgery; Orthopedics; Orthopedics, pediatric; Osteonecrosis; Podiatry; Tendon repair; Warts.

For Further Information:

American Podiatric Medical Association. http://www .apma.org.

Copeland, Glenn, and Stan Solomon. *The Foot Doctor: Lifetime Relief for Your Aching Feet.* Rev. ed. Toronto, Ont.: Macmillan Canada, 1996.

Lippert, Frederick G., and Sigvard T. Hansen. *Foot and Ankle Disorders: Tricks of the Trade.* New York: Thieme, 2003.

Lorimer, Donald L., et al., eds. *Neale's Disorders of the Foot.* 7th ed. New York: Churchill Livingstone/Elsevier, 2006.

Mooney, Jean. *Illustrated Dictionary of Podiatry and Foot Science.* New York: Churchill Livingstone, 2009.

Rose, Jonathan D., Vincent J. Martorana. *The Foot Book: A Complete Guide to Healthy Feet.* Baltimore: Johns Hopkins University Press, 2011.

Thordarson, David B. *Foot and Ankle.* 2nd ed. Philadelphia: Wolters Kluwer/Lippincott, Williams, & Wilkins, 2013.

Van De Graaff, Kent M. *Human Anatomy.* 6th ed. New York: McGraw-Hill, 2002.

FORENSIC PATHOLOGY

Specialty

Anatomy or system affected: All

Specialties and related fields: Dentistry, epidemiology, hematology, histology, pathology, psychology, public health, pulmonary medicine, serology, toxicology

Definition: A science that brings medical knowledge to bear in order to resolve legal issues, usually through the performance of an autopsy.

Key terms:

anthropology: the study of human remains, especially skeletal ones

autopsy: the examination of a body to determine the cause and circumstances of death

forensic: having to do or in connection with the operation of the law, usually criminal law

histology: the microscopic study of plant and animal tissue

odontology: the study of teeth

pathology: the study of disease and the deviations from normalcy that it causes

psychiatry: the medical discipline concerned with mental, emotional, and behavioral disorders

serology: the study of body fluids

toxicology: the study of poisons and their effects

trace evidence: minute, often microscopic, signs or indications of an event or a presence

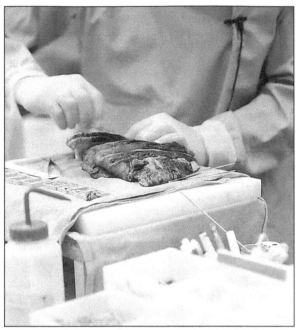

A pathologist studies a tissue sample. (PhotoDisc)

Science and Profession

Forensic medicine probably is best known to most people because of the work of forensic pathologists, principally for the autopsies that they perform as coroners and medical examiners. Other experts, however, also are key participants in the field. They include anthropologists, histologists, odontologists, psychiatrists, serologists, toxicologists, police officers, and specialists in trace evidence. Except for the forensic psychiatrist, who is called on to determine the sanity of an accused individual and thus that person's fitness to stand trial, the above-listed specialists generally do not become involved in the work of forensic medicine until a death has occurred that obviously is other than from natural causes.

In the United States, a forensic pathologist is a medical doctor who typically will spend three to four years preparing in that field after being graduated from medical school and two or so years beyond that before being certified by the American Society of Clinical Pathologists. Other forensic specialties generally require a four-year college degree as well as specialized training after that.

Forensic medicine is not a crowded field. Indeed, there is a shortage of trained and qualified people because most such jobs are in the public sector, where salaries are good but not as high as similar skills and knowledge will command in the private sector. Those who choose careers in forensic medicine, however, find the fascinating and exciting work, intellectual challenge, and personal satisfaction that private-sector jobs seldom offer.

Duties and Investigative Techniques

As a general rule, the coroner, supported to a greater or lesser extent by one or more of the specialists listed above, will become involved in a death when a person dies of criminal or other violent means, by suicide, suddenly when in apparent good health, or in any suspicious or unusual manner. In such a case, the coroner typically is charged by law with determining the cause, mode, and manner of death, with each of those terms having a specific meaning. The physical cause of death is a purely medical determination. Legal considerations, on the other hand, are broader and more inclusive.

Both medical and legal aspects, however, are so interrelated that they cannot be separated. For example, to determine the physical cause of death, it would be sufficient to show a penetrating wound to the heart. To determine the mode of death, however, it would be necessary to establish whether the wound was caused by a bullet or a sharp instrument. An autopsy would reveal the mode of death. The next question is legal: What was the manner of death? In other words, how was the wound inflicted? Was it self-inflicted? If it was, was it intentional (suicide) or accidental? If it was inflicted by another person, was it an accident or was it homicide? Investigation of the scene where the injury was sustained, examination of the evidence found there, and statements of witnesses would furnish information as to the circumstances of the incident.

The actual autopsy involves the dissection and examination of a dead body—surgery performed postmortem. It begins with what is called a gross examination—that is, a visual examination with the naked eye, first externally and then internally. For the internal examination, a Y-shaped incision is made beginning at each shoulder, running down to and meeting just below the sternum or breastbone and continuing as a single cut down to the lower portion of the abdomen just above the genital area. Rib cutters are used to expose the thoracic area. The internal organs are removed and examined. Fluids are drawn for laboratory tests, and tissue samples are taken for microscopic examination. Access to the brain is gained by using a small powersaw to remove the top part of the skull. The third portion of the autopsy involves the toxicological examination of body fluids, including blood, urine, and the vitreous humor of the eye. After examination, the body is restored, and the incisions are carefully sewn.

Perspective and Prospects

Probably the first well-known person to be the subject of a postmortem examination was Julius Caesar. A physician named Antisius determined that of the twenty-three wounds that Caesar sustained, the one that perforated the thorax was the cause of death. The Justinian Code of the sixth century required the opinion of a physician in certain circumstances and often is credited as the first recognition of the correlation of law and medicine in effecting legal justice. By the sixteenth century in England, investigations were being made by a representative of the king, who had the title of Custos Placitorum Coronae (guardian of the decrees of the crown), from which comes the word "coroner." It is believed that William Penn appointed the first coroner in the American colonies. In the nineteenth century, forensic medicine became established as a distinct specialty and has continued to mature into the advanced and sophisticated field that it is today.

The capabilities of and advances in forensic medicine traditionally are tied to those of science in general and applicable medical specialties. They set the pace for the development of forensic medicine. The future should prove no different. The advances in overall knowledge of deoxyribonucleic acid (DNA), the development of scanning electron microscopy, improvements in spectrographic analysis, and advances in computer graphics capabilities, for example, occurred outside the field of forensic medicine and subsequently were adopted by it.

—John M. Shaw;
updated by Karen E. Kalumuck, Ph.D.

See also Anatomy; Autopsy; Death and dying; Diagnosis; DNA and RNA; Histology; Laboratory tests; Law and medicine; Pathology; Suicide; Toxicology.

For Further Information:

Browning, Michael, and William R. Maples. *Dead Men Do Tell Tales: The Strange and Fascinating Cases of a Forensic Anthropologist.* New York: Main Street Books, 1995.

Camenson, Blythe. *Opportunities in Forensic Science Careers.* Rev. ed. New York: McGraw-Hill, 2009.

Evans, Colin. *The Casebook of Forensic Detection: How Science Solved One Hundred of the World's Most Baffling Crimes.* New York: John Wiley & Sons, 1996.

Genge, N. E. *The Forensic Casebook: The Science of Crime Scene Investigation.* New York: Random House, 2002.

James, Stuart H., and Jon J. Nordby. *Forensic Science: An Introduction to Scientific and Investigative Techniques.* 2d ed. Boca Raton: CRC Press, 2005.

Joyce, Christopher, and Eric Stover. *Witnesses from the Grave: The Stories Bones Tell.* Boston: Little, Brown, 1991.

Klawans, Harold L. *Trials of an Expert Witness: Tales of Clinical Neurology and the Law.* Boston: Little, Brown, 1998.

Maeda, Hitoshi, et al. "Forensic Molecular Pathology of Violent Deaths." *Forensic Science International* 203, no. 1–3 (December 2010): 83–92.

Miller, Hugh. *What the Corpse Revealed: Murder and the Science of Forensic Detection.* New York: St. Martin's Press, 1999.

Pollanen, Michael. "Forensic Pathology and the Miscarriage of Justice." *Forensic Science, Medicine & Pathology* 8, no. 3 (September 2012): 285–289.

Schuliar, Yves, and Peter Knudsen. "Role of Forensic Pathologists in Mass Disasters." *Forensic Science, Medicine & Pathology* 8, no. 2 (June 2012): 164–173.

Ubelaker, Douglas H., and Henry Scammel. *Bones: A Forensic Detective's Casebook.* New York: M. Evans, 2000.oxy_options track_changes="on"?

FRACTURE AND DISLOCATION
Disease/Disorder

Anatomy or system affected: Arms, bones, hands, hips, joints, knees, legs, musculoskeletal system

Specialties and related fields: Emergency medicine, orthopedics, sports medicine

Definition: A fracture is a break in a bone, which may be partial or complete; a dislocation is the forceful separation of bones in a joint.

Key terms:

anesthesia: a state characterized by loss of sensation, caused by or resulting from the pharmacological depression of normal nerve function

callus: a hard, bone-like substance made by osteocytes that is found in and around the ends of a fractured bone; it temporarily maintains bony alignment and is resorbed after complete healing or union of a fracture occurs

ecchymosis: a purplish patch on the skin caused by bleeding; the spots are easily visible to the naked eye

embolus: an obstruction or occlusion of a vessel (most commonly, an artery or vein) caused by a transported blood clot, vegetation, mass of bacteria, or other foreign material

epiphysis: the part of a long bone from which growth or elongation occurs

instability: excessive mobility of two or more bones caused by damage to ligaments, the joint capsule, or fracture of one or more bones

ischemia: a local anemia or area of diminished or insufficient blood supply due to mechanical obstruction, commonly narrowing of an artery

kyphoplasty: similar to vertebroplasty (see below), but uses a special balloon in order to restore vertebral height and lessen spinal deformity

osteoblast: a bone-forming cell

osteocyte: a bone cell

paralysis: the loss of power of voluntary movement or other function of a muscle as a result of disease or injury to its nerve supply

petechiae: minute spots caused by hemorrhage or bleeding into the skin; the spots are the size of pinheads

prone: the position of the body when face downward, on one's stomach and abdomen

pulse: the rhythmical dilation of an artery, produced by the increased volume of blood forced into the vessel by the contraction of the heart

transection: a partial or complete severance of the spinal cord

vertebroplasty: medical procedure where acrylic cement is injected into the body of the vertebra for stabilization

Causes and Symptoms

A fracture is a linear deformation or discontinuity of a bone produced by the application of a force that exceeds the modulus of elasticity (ability to bend) of a bone. Normal bones require excessive force to fracture. Disease, tumor-related diseases, or tumors themselves weaken the physical structure of bones, which reduces their ability to withstand an impact. Bones respond to stresses placed upon them and can thus be strengthened through physical conditioning and made more resistant to fracture. This is a normal part of training in many athletic activities.

Fractures are classified according to the type of break or, more correctly, by the plane or surface that is fractured. A break that is at a right angle to the axis of the bone is called transverse. An oblique fracture is similar, but is found at any angle, other than perpendicular to the main axis of the bone. If a twisting force is applied, the break may be spiral, or twisted. A comminuted fracture is a break that results in two or more fragments of bone. If the pieces of bone remain in their origi-

Information on Fracture and Dislocation

Causes: Usually injury, sometimes disease or infection
Symptoms: Varies widely; typically inflammation, pain, swelling, deformity, bruising
Duration: Acute or chronic depending on severity
Treatments: Reduction (return of fractured bone to normal position), immobilization, surgery, orthopedic appliances

nal positions, the fracture is undisplaced. In a displaced fracture, the portions of bone are not properly aligned.

If bones do not penetrate the skin, the fracture is called closed, or simple. When bones protrude through the skin, the result is an open, or compound, fracture. Other types of fractures are associated with pathologic or disease processes. A stress fracture results from repeated stress or trauma to the same site of a bone. None of the individual stresses is sufficient to cause a break. If these stresses cause a callus to form, the bone will be strengthened and actual separation of fragments will not occur. A pathologic fracture occurs at the site of a tumor, infection, or other bone disease. A compression fracture results when bone is crushed; the force applied is greater than the ability of the bone to withstand it. A greenstick fracture is an incomplete separation of bone.

The diagnosis of a fracture is based on several criteria: instability, pain, swelling, deformity, and ecchymosis. The most reliable diagnostic criterion is instability. Pain is not universally present at a fracture site. Swelling may be delayed and occur at some time after a fracture is sustained. Deformity is obvious with open fractures but may not be apparent with other, undisplaced breaks.

Ecchymosis is a purplish patch caused by bleeding into skin; it will not be present if blood vessels are not broken. A definitive diagnosis is made with two-plane film X-rays taken at the site of a fracture at right angles to one another. If the fracture site is visually examined and palpated shortly after the injury occurs, an accurate tentative diagnosis may be made; this should be confirmed with X-rays as soon as it is convenient. Occasionally, an X-ray will not show undisplaced or chip fracture. If a patient experiences symptoms of pain, swelling, or ecchymosis but has a negative X-ray for a fracture, the site should be immobilized and X-rayed again in two to three weeks.

Fractures occur most commonly in the extremities: arms or legs. Such fractures must be evaluated to determine if injuries have occurred to other tissues such as nerves or blood vessels. The presence of bruising or ecchymosis indicates blood vessel damage. The absence of peripheral pulses with severe bruising indicates that the major arteries are injured. Venous flow is more difficult to evaluate. The venous circulation is a lower pressure system than arterial, so venous bleeding can be considered of lesser importance and therefore temporarily tolerated.

Neurologic functioning may be assessed by the ability of the patient to contract muscles or sense skin touches or pinpricks. Temporary immobilization may be necessary before nerve status can be evaluated accurately.

An open fracture creates a direct pathway between the skin surface and underlying tissues. If bacteria contaminate the site, an opportunity for osteomyelitis (infection of the bone) to form is created. Inadequate treatment by the initial surgeon may result in skin loss, delayed union, loss of joint mobility, osteomyelitis, and even amputation.

Skin damage may or may not be related to a fracture. When skin integrity is broken over or near a fracture site, bone involvement must be assumed. If there is infection of the fracture site; appropriate antibiotics are normally administered. If skin damage is extensive, final surgical reduction of the underlying fracture may have to be delayed until the skin is healed.

Delayed union refers to the inability of a fractured bone to heal. This is a potentially serious problem, as normal stability is not possible as long as a fracture exists. Joints may not function normally in the presence of a fracture. If a fracture heals improperly, bones may be misaligned and cause pain with movement, leading to limitations of motion. If the bones are affected by osteomyelitis, the infection may spread to the joint capsule and reduce the normal range of motion for the bones or the joint. Amputation may become necessary if infection becomes extensive in the area of a fracture. An infection, which becomes firmly established in bones or spreads widely into adjacent muscle tissue, may lead to cellulitis or gangrene and may compromise a portion of an extremity. Amputation may be performed if the pathologic process cannot be treated with antibiotics and/or surgery.

Adequate blood supply to tissues is critical for survival. In an extremity, the maximum time limit for complete ischemia (lack of blood flow) is six to eight hours; after that time, the likelihood of later amputation increases. Pain, pallor, pulselessness, and paralysis are indicators of impaired circulation. When two of these signs are present, the possibility of vascular damage must be thoroughly explored.

Dislocations occur at joints and are caused by an applied force that is greater than the strength of the ligaments and muscles that keep a joint intact. The result is a stretching deformity or injury to a joint and an abnormal movement of a bone out of the joint. Accidental trauma, commonly the result of an athletic injury or automobile accident, is the most common cause of a dislocation. Joints that are frequently dislocated include the shoulder and digits (fingers and toes). Dislocations of the ankle and hip are infrequent but serious; they require immediate management. Dislocations may accompany fractures, but the two injuries need not occur together.

When dislocations are reduced, the bones of the joint are returned to normal position. Reduction of a dislocation is accomplished by relaxing adjacent muscles and applying traction (pulling force) to the bone until it returns to its normal position within the joint. For most dislocations of the shoulder, the victim lies in a prone position and the dislocated arm hangs down freely. Gradual traction is applied until reduction occurs. This can be accomplished by bandaging a pail to the

Types of Fracture

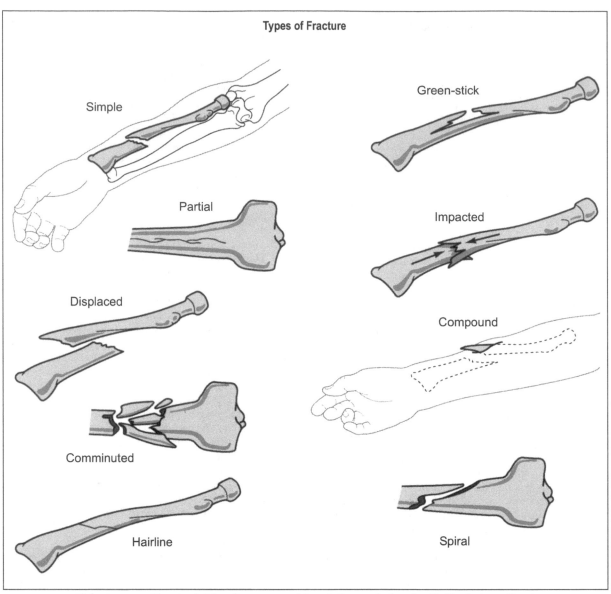

Simple

Partial

Displaced

Comminuted

Hairline

Green-stick

Impacted

Compound

Spiral

All fractures are either simple (closed) or compound (open); they are further classified by the type of break.

arm and slowly filling it with water. Alternatively, the victim can hold a heavy book while the muscles of the arm are allowed to relax until the dislocation is reduced. Such treatments are usually reserved for situations in which medical assistance is unavailable. Digits are reduced in a similar manner, by gentle pulling of the end of the finger or toe. Ankle and hip dislocations are potentially more serious because these joints are more complex and have extensive blood supplies. Reduction of dislocated ankles and hips should be undertaken by qualified medical personnel in an expedited manner.

After reduction, competent medical personnel should evaluate all dislocations. With dislocated digits, long-term damage is relatively unlikely but can occur because of ligament damage sustained in the initial injury. Dislocations of the shoulder may be accompanied by a fracture of the clavicle or collarbone and may involve nerve damage in the shoulder joint. Dislocations of the ankle and hip may lead to avascular necrosis (damage to the bone as a result of inadequate blood supply) if not evaluated and reduced promptly.

Treatment and Therapy

Fractures are usually treated by reduction and immobilization. Reduction, which refers to the process of returning the fractured bones to the normal position, may be either closed or open. Closed reduction is accomplished without surgery

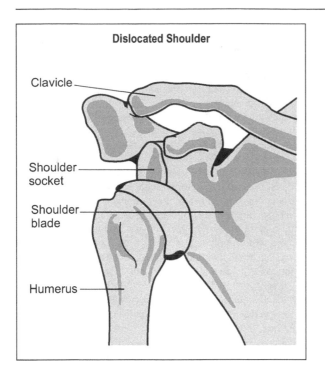

Dislocated Shoulder

Clavicle

Shoulder socket

Shoulder blade

Humerus

by manipulating the broken bone through overlying skin and muscles. Open reduction requires surgical intervention in which the broken pieces are exposed and returned to the normal position. Orthopedic appliances may be used to hold the bones in the correct position. The most common of these appliances are pins and screws, but metal plates and wires may also be employed. Orthopedic appliances are usually made of stainless steel. These may be left in the body indefinitely or may be surgically removed after healing is complete. Local anesthesia is usually used with closed reductions; open reductions are performed in an operating room, under sterile conditions using general anesthesia.

Immobilization is generally accomplished by the use of a cast. Casts are often made of plaster, but they may be constructed of inflatable plastic. It is important to hold bones in a rigid, fixed position for a sufficient length of time for the broken ends to unite and heal. The cast must be loose enough, however, to allow blood to circulate. Padding is usually put in place before plaster is applied to form a cast. Whenever possible, the newly immobilized body part is elevated to reduce the chance of swelling in the cast, which would compromise the blood supply to the fracture site and the portion of the body beyond the cast. Casts should be checked periodically to ensure that they do not impair circulation.

The broken bone and accompanying body part must be placed in an anatomically neutral position. This is done to minimize postfracture disability and improve the prospect for rehabilitation. The length of time that a fractured bone is immobilized is highly variable and dependent on a number of factors.

Traction may also be used to immobilize a fracture. Trac-

tion is the external application of force to overcome muscular resistance and hold bones in a desired position. Commonly, holes are drilled through bones and pins are inserted; the ends of these pins extend through the surface of the skin. Part of the body is fixed in position through the use of a strap or weights, and wires are attached to the pins in the body part to be stretched. Weights or tension is applied to the wires until the broken bone parts move into the desired position. Traction is maintained until healing has occurred.

Individual ends of a single fractured bone are sometimes held in position by external pins and screws. Holes are drilled through the bone, and pins are inserted. The pins on opposite sides of the fracture site are then attached to each other with threaded rods and locked in position by nuts. This process allows a fractured bone to be immobilized without using a cast.

Different bones require different amounts of time to heal. Furthermore, age is a factor in fracture healing. Fractures in young children heal more quickly than do broken bones in adults. The elderly typically require even more time for healing. The availability of nutrients like calcium and vitamin D also affects the speed with which a fracture heals.

Delayed union of fractures is a term applied to fractures that either do not heal or take longer than normal to heal; there is no precise time frame associated with delayed union. Nonunion refers to fractures in which healing is not observed and cannot be expected even with prolonged immobilization. X-ray analysis of a nonunion will show that the bone ends have sclerosed (hardened), that the ends of the marrow canal have become plugged, and that a gap persists between the ends of a fractured bone. Nonunion may be caused by inadequate blood supply to the fracture site, which leads to the formation of cartilage instead of new bone between the broken pieces of bone. Nonunion may also be caused by injury to the soft tissues that surround a fracture site. This damage impairs the formation of a callus and the reestablishment of an adequate blood supply to the fracture site; it is frequently seen in young children. Inadequate immobilization may also allow soft tissue to enter the fracture site by slipping between the bone fragments, and may lead to nonunion. Respect for tissue and minimizing damage in the vicinity of a fracture, especially with open reduction, will minimize problems of nonunion. Subjecting the nonuniting fracture site to a low-level electromagnetic field will usually stimulate osteoblastic (bone-forming cell) activity and lead to healing.

The epiphyseal plate is the portion of bone where growth occurs. Bony epiphyses are active in children until they attain their adult height, at which time the epiphyses become inactive and close. Once an epiphysis ceases to function, further growth does not occur. In children, a fracture involving the epiphyseal plate is potentially dangerous because bone growth may be interrupted or halted. This situation can lead to inequalities in the length of extremities or impaired range of movement in joints. Accurate reduction of injuries involving an epiphyseal plate is necessary to minimize subsequent deformity. A key factor is blood supply to the injured area: If adequate blood supply is maintained, epiphyseal plate damage is minimized.

Fractures of the spinal vertebrae are potentially very dangerous because they can cause injury to the nerves and tracts of the spinal cord. Fractures of the vertebrae are commonly sustained in automobile accidents, athletic injuries, falls from heights, and other situations involving rapid deceleration. When vertebrae are fractured, the spinal cord can be compromised. Spinal cord injury can be direct and cut all or a portion of the spinal nerves at the site of the fracture. The extent of the damage is dependent on the level of the injury. An accident that completely severs the spinal cord will lead to a complete loss of function for all structures below the level of injury. Since spinal nerves are arranged segmentally, cord damage at a lower level involves compromise of fewer structures. As the level of injury becomes higher in the spinal cord, more vital structures are involved. Transection of the spinal cord in the neck usually leads to complete paralysis of the entire body; it can cause death if high enough to cut the nerves controlling the lungs. Individuals in whom vertebral fractures and thus spinal cord injuries are suspected must have the spinal column immobilized before they are moved. Only a highly skilled professional should undertake reduction of spinal cord fractures.

When bones having large marrow cavities such as the femur (thighbone) are fractured, fat globules may escape from the marrow and enter the bloodstream. Such a fat globule is then called an embolus (plural is emboli). Fat emboli are potentially dangerous in that they can become lodged in the capillaries of the lungs. This causes pain and can lead to impaired oxygenation of blood, a condition called hypoxemia. About 10 to 20 percent of individuals sustaining a fractured femur also have central nervous system depression and skin petechiae (minute spots caused by hemorrhage or bleeding into the skin) in addition to hypoxemia in the two to three days after the injury. This triad of signs is called fat embolism syndrome. It is treated medically with oxygen, steroids, and anticoagulant drugs.

Perspective and Prospects

Fractures rarely threaten a patient's life directly, and injuries to the brain, heart, circulatory system, and abdominal cavity must receive priority of treatment. It is imperative, however, not to move a patient in whom a fracture is suspected without first immobilizing the potential fracture site. This is especially true with suspected fractures of the spine. Instability may not be apparent when a patient is lying down but can become catastrophic if the person is moved without proper preparation and immobilization.

Crush injuries of the spinal cord are relatively common among victims of osteoporosis. Osteoporosis is a pathological syndrome defined by a decrease in the density of a bone below the level required for mechanical support and is frequently associated with a deficiency of calcium, problems related to calcium in the body, or a rate of bone cell breakdown that is greater than the rate of bone cell remodeling. Crush fractures occur when the bones become so weak that the weight of the upper portion of the body is greater than the ability of the vertebrae to support it. These crush injuries may

occur slowly over time and cause no serious injury to the underlying spinal cord. The resulting deformity of the spine, however, impairs movement. There are limited treatments for osteoporotic crush fractures of the vertebrae. Most of the treatments aim to strengthen nearby muscles and aid in nutritional deficiencies causing the osteoporosis. However surgeries such as vertebroplasty, balloon kyphoplasty, and spinal fusion are available as last-line treatments for reoccurring or nonhealing (painful) vertebral fractures.

Occupational exposures may lead to fractures and dislocations. Professional athletes are clearly at increased risk for skeletal injuries. These individuals are also usually well conditioned, however, and so can withstand increased impacts and blows to the body. Many are also trained in methods that minimize the force of impact; they know how to fall properly.

The vast proportions of workers are not conditioned and are given minimal training to avoid situations that lead to fractures. Accident analysis reveals that carelessness is the most common predisposing factor. Workers operating without safety equipment such as belaying lines or belts may become overconfident. In such a situation, slips or falls can occur, and fractures result. Unsafe equipment can lead to hazardous situations and cause fractures or dislocations. Machinery that is not properly maintained can fail; parts may become detached, hit nearby workers, and cause fractures.

Recreational activities also result in fractures. Individuals who once were well conditioned may engage in sports without proper equipment and sustain fractures or dislocations. Contact sports such as hockey, football, and basketball are primary examples of such activities. Riding bicycles and motorized recreational vehicles without proper safety equipment can lead to serious skeletal injuries. Activities such as rock climbing are inherently dangerous. With proper training and use of safety equipment, accidents can be reduced or their severity minimized. The keys to avoiding fractures and dislocations when participating in recreational activities are receiving proper instruction and training, employing adequate safety equipment, and using common sense by avoiding difficult or hazardous situations that are beyond one's physical abilities or skill level.

—*L. Fleming Fallon, Jr., M.D., Ph.D., M.P.H.;*
updated by Mikhail Varshavski, OMS-IV

See also Bone disorders; Bone grafting; Bones and the skeleton; Casts and splints; Fracture repair; Head and neck disorders; Hip fracture repair; Joints; Orthopedic surgery; Orthopedics; Orthopedics, pediatric; Osteonecrosis; Osteoporosis; Physical rehabilitation; Spinal cord disorders; Spine, vertebrae, and disks; Wounds

For Further Information:

Brunicardi, F. Charles, et al., eds. *Schwartz's Principles of Surgery.* 9th ed. New York: McGraw-Hill, 2010. A standard textbook of surgery containing sections on fractures and dislocations. Its intended audience is practicing surgeons, and thus the language is sometimes technical. Nevertheless, the serious reader can obtain much useful detail from this work.

Currey, John D. *Bones: Structures and Mechanics.* Princeton, NJ: Princeton University Press, 2006. Very accessible overview of a range of information related to whole bones, bone tissue, and dentin and enamel. Topics include stiffness, strength, viscoelasticity, fatigue, fracture mechanics properties, buckling, impact fracture, and properties of cancellous bone.

Doherty, Gerard M., and Lawrence W. Way, eds. *Current Surgical Diagnosis and Treatment.* 13th ed. New York: Lange Medical Books/McGraw-Hill, 2009. The diagnosis and treatment of fractures and dislocations is discussed in a brief and concise format emphasizing treatment modalities. The different section authors are recognized experts in their fields. The material is accessible to the general reader and the sections are brief.

Egol, Kenneth, Kovai, Kenneth J, et al., eds. *Handbook of Fractures.* 4th ed. Philadelphia: Lippincott Williams and Wilkins, 2010. Handbook of different types of fractures published for residents, but material is understandable by general reader. Easy access to charts, pictures, and tables in order to understand more about all types of fractures. Provides great visuals along with step-by-step explanations for treatment.

Marieb, Elaine N., and Katja Hoehn. *Human Anatomy and Physiology.* 9th ed. San Francisco: Pearson/ Benjamin Cummings, 2012. Nonscientists at the advanced high school level or above will be able to understand this fine textbook. The chapters "Bones and Bone Tissue," "The Skeleton," and "Joints" are very well illustrated.

Townsend, Courtney M., Jr., et al., eds. *Sabiston Textbook of Surgery.* 19th ed. Philadelphia: Saunders/Elsevier, 2012. A standard textbook of surgery that contains an extensive discussion of different types of fractures and dislocations and how they are treated. Intended for practicing professionals but can be generally understood by the layperson.

FRACTURE REPAIR

Procedure

Anatomy or system affected: Arms, bones, hips, legs, musculoskeletal system, teeth

Specialties and related fields: Dentistry, orthopedics

Definition: The placement and fixation of broken portions of bones in their correct positions until they have grown together.

Indications and Procedures

A fracture is a break in a bone, either partial or complete, resulting from an applied force that is greater than the bone's internal strength. The most common causes of fractures are accidents and trauma.

Types of Fracture Repair

Severe leg fractures can be immobilized through external or internal fixation. External fixation involves the use of long pins that are inserted through the bone and held in place with a steel rod on the outside of the body. Internal fixation involves the use of screws, pins, and plates that are attached directly to the bones and often left there permanently.

Fractures are usually treated by reduction and immobilization. Reduction, which may be either closed or open, refers to the process of returning the fractured bones to their normal position. Closed reduction is accomplished without surgery by manipulating the broken bone through overlying skin and muscles. Open reduction requires surgical intervention. The broken pieces are exposed and returned to their normal positions. Orthopedic appliances may be used to hold the bones in the proper position (internal fixation); the most common appliances are stainless-steel pins and screws, but metal plates and wires may also be employed. These devices can be left in the body indefinitely or may be surgically removed after healing is complete. Local anesthesia is usually used with closed reductions; open reductions are performed in an operating room under sterile conditions, using general anesthesia.

After reduction, the broken bone and accompanying body part must be placed in an anatomically neutral position. Immobilization is generally accomplished by the use of a cast. Casts are usually made of plaster, but they may be constructed of inflatable plastic.

Individual ends of a single fractured bone are sometimes held in position by external pins and screws (external fixation). Holes are drilled through the bone, and pins are inserted as described above. The pins on opposite sides of the fracture site are then attached to each other with threaded rods and locked in position by nuts. This process allows a fractured bone to be immobilized without using a cast.

Traction, the external application of force to overcome muscular resistance and hold bones in a desired position, may also be used to immobilize a fracture. Commonly, holes are drilled through bones and pins are inserted; the ends of these pins extend through the surface of the skin. Part of the body is fixed in position through the use of a strap or weights. Wires are attached to the pins in the body part to be stretched. Force is applied to the wires via weights or tension until the broken bone parts are in the desired position. Traction is maintained until complete healing has occurred.

Uses and Complications

All broken bones must be held in position until healing takes place. The complications associated with repairing fractures include infection, which is rare, and loss of function. The potential for loss of function is minimized by placing the limb in an anatomically neutral position prior to the application of a cast.

The techniques of fracture repair have not changed radically in decades. New methods, however, are being tried. For example, electromagnetic fields are used with fractures that do not heal spontaneously. Such fields induce the growth of osteoblasts, which are bone-forming cells.

—*L. Fleming Fallon, Jr., M.D., Ph.D., M.P.H.*

See also Bone grafting; Bones and the skeleton; Casts and splints; Dentistry; Emergency medicine; Fracture and dislocation; Hip fracture repair; Jaw wiring; Orthopedic surgery; Orthopedics; Orthopedics, pediatric; Osteoporosis; Teeth.

For Further Information:

Browner, Bruce D., et al. *Skeletal Trauma: Basic Science, Management, and Reconstruction.* 4th ed. Philadelphia: Saunders/Elsevier, 2009.

Eiff, M. Patrice, and Robert L. Hatch. *Fracture Management for Primary Care.* 3d ed. Philadelphia: Saunders/Elsevier, 2012.

"Fractures." *MedlinePlus*, May 15, 2013.

Gregg, Paul J., Jack Stevens, and Peter H. Worlock. *Fractures and Dislocations: Principles of Management.* Cambridge, Mass.: Blackwell Science, 1996.

Types of Fracture Repair

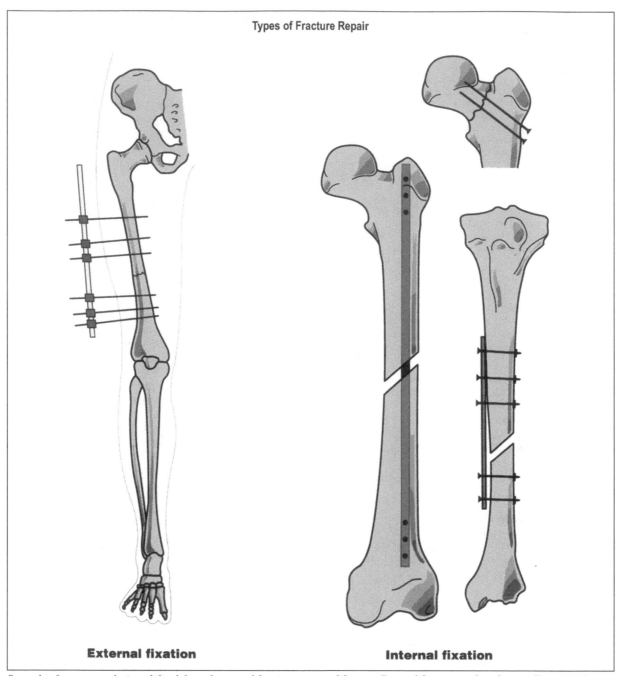

External fixation

Internal fixation

Severe leg fractures can be immobilized through external fixation or internal fixation. External fixation involves the use of long pins that are inserted through the bone and held in place with a steel rod on the outside of the body. Internal fixation involves the use of screws, pins, and plates that are attached directly to the bones and often left there permanently.

Gustilo, Ramon B., Richard F. Kyle, and David C. Templeman, eds. *Fractures and Dislocations.* St. Louis, Mo.: Mosby, 1993.

"Helping Fractures Heal (Orthobiologics)." *OrthoInfo*, January 2010.

Hodgson, Stephen F., ed. *Mayo Clinic on Osteoporosis: Keeping Bones Healthy and Strong and Reducing the Risk of Fractures.* Rochester, Minn.: Mayo Clinic, 2003.

Magee, David J. *Orthopedic Physical Assessment.* 5th ed. St. Louis, Mo.: Saunders/Elsevier, 2008.

Ruiz, Ernest, and James J. Cicero, eds. *Emergency Management of Skeletal Injuries.* St. Louis, Mo.: Mosby, 1995.

Salter, Robert Bruce. *Textbook of Disorders and Injuries of the Musculoskeletal System.* 3d ed. Baltimore: Williams & Wilkins, 1999.

FRAGILE X SYNDROME
Disease/Disorder
Also known as: Martin-Bell syndrome
Anatomy or system affected: Brain, ears, feet, genitals, hands, joints
Specialties and related fields: Genetics
Definition: A genetic disorder of variable expression, with mental retardation being the most common feature.

Causes and Symptoms
Fragile X syndrome is caused by a change in a gene located on the long arm of the X chromosome. It is a sex-linked inherited disease, transmitted from parent to child, with boys being affected much more often and more severely than girls. The prevalence of the disorder is estimated to be 1 in 4,000 males and 1 in 6 to 8,000 females worldwide.

While symptoms and their severity vary widely, common physical features of fragile X syndrome include a long, thin face, a prominent jaw and ears, a broad nose, a high palate, large testicles (macroorchidism) in males, and large hands with loose finger joints. Physical features are more subtle in females. Nonphysical features include a range of intellectual and learning disabilities, with the majority of affected males demonstrating a range from low-normal intelligence to severe intellectual disability. More recent research has found that the intelligence quotients (IQs) of males with fragile X syndrome appear to decline throughout childhood. Associated behavioral symptoms include unusual speech patterns, problems with attention span, hyperactivity, motor delays, and occasional autistic-type behaviors, such as poor eye contact, hand-biting, or hand-flapping.

Treatment and Therapy
While there is no cure for fragile X syndrome, a number of possible interventions can address various symptoms. Medications can be administered to assist with attention span and hyperactivity, as well as with aggressive behavior. Schools can provide children with assistance in speech, physical therapy, and vocational planning. Early childhood special education services for children prior to school age can provide necessary early intervention that may prove most helpful if indeed the rate of learning for children with fragile X syndrome slows with age. Genetic counseling is advised for families who carry the gene.

Information on Fragile X Syndrome

Causes: Genetic
Symptoms: Thin face, prominent jaw and ears, broad nose, large testicles in males, large hands with loose finger joints, mental impairment ranging from severe retardation to learning disabilities, unusual speech patterns, problems with attention span and hyperactivity, motor delays, occasional autistic-type behaviors
Duration: Chronic
Treatments: None; alleviation of symptoms

Perspective and Prospects
In 1969, the discovery was made of a break or fragile site on the long arm of the X chromosome. It was not until the 1980s, however, that consistent diagnoses of fragile X syndrome were made. In 1991, the responsible gene was sequenced and named the FMR-1 gene. Cytogenetic and deoxyribonucleic acid (DNA) testing are now available to identify affected persons.

—*Robin Hasslen, Ph.D.*

See also Autism; Developmental disorders; Genetic diseases; Genetics and inheritance; Learning disabilities; Mental retardation; Motor skill development; Speech disorders.

For Further Information:
Alan, Rick, and Rimas Lukas. "Fragile X Syndrome." *Health Library*, Oct. 11, 2012.
"Facts about Fragile X Syndrome." *Centers for Disease Control and Prevention*, Apr. 15, 2013.
"Fragile X Syndrome." *MedlinePlus*, May 13, 2013.
Hagerman, Randi Jensen, and Paul J. Henssen. *Fragile X Syndrome: Diagnosis, Treatment, and Research.* 3d ed. Baltimore: Johns Hopkins University Press, 2002.
Maxson, Linda, and Charles Daugherty. 3d ed. *Genetics: A Human Perspective.* Dubuque, Iowa: Wm. C. Brown, 1992.
Moore, Keith L., and T. V. N. Persaud. *The Developing Human: Clinically Oriented Embryology.* 9th ed. Philadelphia: Saunders/Elsevier, 2013.
National Fragile X Foundation. *Fragile X–Associated Disorders (FXD).* 3d ed. Walnut Creek, Calif.: National Fragile X Foundation, Sept. 2009.
Parker, James N., and Philip M. Parker, eds. *The Official Parent's Sourcebook on Fragile X Syndrome.* Rev. ed. San Diego, Calif.: Icon Health, 2005.
Sherwood, Lauralee. *Human Physiology: From Cells to Systems.* 8th ed. Pacific Grove, Calif.: Brooks/Cole/Cengage Learning, 2013.
Webb, Jayne Dixon, ed. *Children with Fragile X Syndrome: A Parents" Guide.* Bethesda, Md.: Woodbine House, 2000.
"What is Fragile X?" *FRAXA Research Foundation*, 2013.

FRONTAL LOBE SYNDROME
Disease/Disorder

Anatomy or system affected: Frontal lobe of the brain, disinhibition, impulsivity, personality, regulation of emotion, attention, awareness, execution of sequential tasks
Specialties and related fields: Geropsychology, neurology, neuropsychology, neuroscience, psychology
Definition: An organic disorder of the brain affecting cognitive ability, personality, and behavior.
Key terms:
aneurysm: an expansion of a segment of blood vessel that causes damage to the surrounding areas, sometimes causing additional damage when the weak area bursts, resulting in internal bleeding; brain injury is sustained from both the pressured displacement of brain structures and deterioration of brain tissue caused by blood contact with the brain
anterior: a term of location meaning towards the front
Broca's area: part of the motor cortex that controls speech; it is typically located in the left hemisphere, just anterior to the ear; lesions to this are associated with speech dysfunction

embolism: a blockage of a blood vessel interrupting blood flow; a cerebral embolism is likely to cause a stroke

frontal lobe: the cerebral cortex of the brain is divided into two sections called hemispheres: the left hemisphere and right hemisphere; each hemisphere is further divided into quadrants called lobes: the frontal lobe is the most anterior lobe, located just behind the eyes; the other lobes are the parietal, occipital, and temporal; the frontal lobe is associated with executive function, thought process, personality, and execution of intentional voluntary physical movement

lesion: a term used to described injury or abnormal change in an area of the brain

motor cortex: the primary, secondary and tertiary motor cortex is part of the frontal lobe that controls movement; this includes speech

Causes and Symptoms

The causes are from traumatic brain injury (TBI), such as a car accident involving a blow to the head or repeated exposure to intense blasts from explosives at a close range; transient ischemic attack (TIA); cerebrovascular accident (CVA), such as an embolism or aneurism; dementia; alcohol abuse (Korsakoff's Syndrome) and drug abuse.

Symptoms may include changes in mood such as depression, affect, hypomania, personality traits, ability to make decisions, memory recall, ability to think sequentially, disinhibition, social inappropriateness, apathy, and the ability to communicate ideas.

Treatment and Therapy

Pharmacological treatment can be combined with neuropsychotherapy and behavioral therapy. The neuropsychological approach often addresses the patient's impairment by developing strategies of working around deficits in function to facilitate an improved quality of life. In addition, the treatment often emphasizes psychoeducation for people who interact with the patient to help them contextualize the patient's functioning level, behavior, and personality changes. Behavioral therapy may also be helpful depending on the level of impairment. Other treatments address the psychological symptoms associated with each particular case and implementing the appropriate corresponding treatment.

Perspective and Prospects

One of the first documented cases of frontal lobe syndrome was in 1848. The patient was Phineas Gage, a railway worker who survived having an iron pole driven through his skull from an explosion. The primary area of brain damaged was the left frontal lobe, just behind the left eye. He survived, but those who were familiar with him reported his behavior and personality as uncharacteristic of the person they once knew.

In recent texts, the term is used to indicate a group of syndromes or diagnoses, frontal lobe syndromes, with symptoms indicative of damage to the frontal lobe. Damage is frequently associated with drug and alcohol abuse, chemical exposure, infection, physical trauma, and aging. Practitioners and researchers have pointed out the inherent problems with having an anatomical structure also be the name of a disorder. Some research suggests the symptoms associated with frontal lobe syndrome may not correlate with lesions to the frontal lobe alone, thus pointing out the difficulty of having an anatomical structure as a diagnosis. The diagnosis code for frontal lobe syndrome in the International Code Diagnosis version 9 (ICD-9) has been removed. The ICD-10, scheduled to be released in October, 2014, maps the old diagnosis of frontal lobe syndrome to a diagnosis of personality change due to a known physiological condition. The new edition of the Diagnostic and Statistical Manual for Mental Disorders, version 5, defines neurocognitive disorders (NCDs) as a group of disorders with causes and symptoms of what was termed frontal lobe syndrome. NCDs can present with symptoms of other mental disorders such as mania, hypomania, paranoia, hallucinations, and depression.

Since the behavior of communicating ideas or recalling memories is hindered, it is unclear in each individual case if the person suffers from memory deficits or just the inability or lack of motivation to communicate ideas and memories. Typically, the frontal lobe syndrome would cause a deficit in the organization and execution of sequential tasks, abstract thought, and making meaning, whether it be as simple as the communication of commonalities in apples and bananas, or the complexities of hypothesizing on a construct for the meaning of life.

—*Gregory A. Benitz, Psy.D.*

See also Concussion; Glasgow coma scale; Neurology; Neuropsychology; Neuroscience; Traumatic brain injury

For Further Information:

Buck, Carol J. *2013 ICD-9-CM for Physicians, Volumes 1 and 2 Professional Edition.* 1st ed. St. Louis: Elsevier/Saunders, 2012.

Canavan, A.G., I. Janota, and P.H. Schurr. "Luria's Frontal Lobe Syndrome: Psychological and Anatomical Considerations." *Journal of Neurology, Neurosurgery, & Psychiatry,* 48, no. 10 (October, 1985) 1049-1053.

Cummings, Jeffrey. *Clinical Neuropsychology.* Orlando, FL: Grune & Stratton, Inc., 1985.

Diagnostic and Statistical Manual of Mental Disorders, 5th Edition: DSM-5. Arlington, VA: American Psychiatric Publishing, 2013.

Kolb, Bryan, and Ian Q. Whishaw. *Fundamentals of Human Neuropsychology.* 6th ed. New York: Worth Publishers, 2008.

Levin, Harvey S., Howard M. Eisenberg, and Arthur L. Benton. *Frontal Lobe Function and Dysfunction.* New York: Oxford University Press, 1991.

Lezak, Muriel D. *Neuropsychological Assessment.* 3rd ed. New York: Oxford University Press, 1995.

Parind, Shah. *Frontal Lobe Syndrome-Affective and Personality Changes with Traumatic Brain Injury.* Self-published slideshow: http://www.slideshare.net/shahparind/frontal-lobe-syndrome, 2008.

Purves, Dale, George J. Augustine, David Fitzpatrick, et. al. *Neuroscience.* 5th ed. Sunderland, MA: Sinauer, 2012.

Snyder, Peter J., Paul D. Nussbaum, and Diana L. Robins, eds. *Clinical Neuropsychology: A Pocket Handbook for Assessment.* Washington, D.C.: American Psychological Association, 2006.

Ziauddeen, H., C. Dibben, C. Kipps, J.R. Hodges, and P.J. McKema. "Negative Schizophrenic Symptoms and the Frontal Lobe Syndrome: One and the Same?" *European Archives of Psychiatry and Clinical Neuroscience* 261, no. 1 (February, 2011): 59-67.

FRONTOTEMPORAL DEMENTIA (FTD)
Disease/Disorder

Anatomy or system affected: Brain, nervous system, psychic-emotional system

Specialties and related fields: Neurology, pathology, psychiatry

Definition: Frontotemporal dementia is a descriptive term for a group of neurodegenerative disorders that affect the frontal and temporal lobes of the brain.

Key terms:

aphasia: language difficulty due to understanding, speaking, or writing

dementia: impairment and loss of intellect and personality due to loss or damage of neurons in the brain

frontal lobe: the area of the brain in the front of the skull, responsible for executive functions; each cerebral hemisphere has one frontal lobe

Pick bodies: abnormal clumps of proteins seen in brain tissue of individuals with FTD

temporal lobe: the area of the brain on each lower side of the skull, responsible for language, memory, and emotion

Causes and Symptoms

Frontotemporal dementias (FTDs) are a group of disorders characterized by degeneration of the frontal and temporal lobes of the brain. These areas in the brain are responsible for language, behavior, and personality. Magnetic resonance imaging (MRI) of the brain can show shrinkage of the brain in these areas (frontal and/or temporal lobes). FTDs can show variable symptoms depending on which parts of the brain may be affected. Most individuals have either behavior changes or language disturbances as their main feature.

Behavior changes associated with FTDs include dramatic personality changes, toward either impulsive and disinhibited or apathetic and listless. Frequently, verbal and facial social cues are unrecognizable to affected individuals. Additional behaviors can include isolation, lack of empathy and sympathy, distractibility, loss of insight, dietary changes (sweet food preferences), neglect of personal hygiene, repetitive behaviors, and decreased motivation. Language changes in FTDs are of two main types: loss of ability to speak as a result of difficulty with word recall (primary progressive aphasia) or loss of ability to understand language (semantic dementia).

Frequently, family members bring affected individuals to medical attention because of these behavioral changes, which go unrecognized to the individual. The onset of FTD can be from age forty to seventy; therefore, individuals can be living with the disease many years before family members notice personality and behavior changes or behaviors begin to interfere with activities of daily living.

There are a few rare types of FTDs that involve movement disorders in addition to dementia. One type is FTD with motor neuron disease (MND). Classical MND is also called amyotrophic lateral sclerosis (ALS) or Lou Gehrig's disease. FTD can also be seen with symptoms of Parkinson's disease.

Information on
Frontotemporal Dementia (FTD)

Causes: About half with family history, several genes identified

Symptoms: Behavior changes (apathy, lack of inhibition, repetitiveness), speech and language changes (primary progressive aphasia and semantic dementia), motor neuron disease, Parkinson's disease

Duration: Eight to ten years until death; if with motor neuron disease, three to five years until death

Treatments: None; therapy to manage symptoms

Movement disorder-related symptoms can include tremor, weakness, difficulty swallowing, and poor coordination.

People can be misdiagnosed with psychiatric problems, especially with the young age of onset seen in FTDs. Others can be misdiagnosed with Alzheimer's disease because of the fact that it is much more commonly seen by physicians.

Men and women are affected equally by FTD. Family history is the greatest risk factor for FTDs, with approximately 50 percent of all FTD cases showing familial inheritance. Mutations in several genes have been shown to cause several types of FTDs. Genetic testing may be offered. Individuals with FTD symptoms will undergo a variety of tests to try to rule out other illnesses that may mimic the symptoms of FTD. These tests may include blood count, electrolytes, liver function, thyroid function, and kidney function. Also, images of the brain via magnetic resonance imaging (MRI) and computed tomography (CT) scanning may be obtained to rule out bleeding or tumors that can cause similar symptoms. Finally, neuropsychological testing may be used to help determine if there are language, memory, and/or reasoning deficits to aid in the diagnosis of FTD.

Treatment and Therapy

FTD is a degenerative disorder. There are no treatments to cure or slow the progression of the brain degeneration. The median duration of illness is six to eight years from onset to death, although the length of time can range from less than two years to more than ten years. Individuals with FTD-MND have a shorter survival time, with a median survival of only three years. Most therapy for individuals with FTDs focuses on managing the symptoms and behaviors seen in the disorder. Speech therapy can be helpful to learn new strategies to aid in verbal and written communication. Caregivers can help reduce behavior problems by avoiding behavior triggers (events or activities), anticipating needs, and maintaining a calm environment. Caregivers should focus on building a support network that includes social services, psychiatric care, support groups, respite care in adult care centers, and/or home health aids. Ultimately, individuals with FTDs will progress to require twenty-four-hour care, and nursing home care may be required. Many patients, if able, may wish to help family members with this planning ahead of time, making the transition for caregivers and family members easier knowing that the affected individual was part of the decision-making process.

Medications currently used to treat the behavioral symptoms of FTD include antidepressants and antipsychotics. These drugs have not shown great success. Therapeutic research related to the genetic causes of FTDs, however, has shown promise. For example, the microtubule-associated protein tau (MAPT) gene can be altered to cause toxic clumps and tangles of MAPT protein. These MAPT tangles are seen in several forms of FTDs. Therapies and drugs designed to prevent or fix the MAPT tangles are currently being designed and tested in animal models. Additional testing and validation will be needed before clinical trials begin in humans.

Perspective and Prospects

FTD was originally described by Arnold Pick in the 1890s. He published a case series of patients in which he described the behavioral and language variants now part of the clinical criteria of FTD. In 1926, two neuropathologists, K. Onari and Hugo Spatz, described the brain findings commonly seen in FTD, including shrinkage of the frontal and temporal lobes and Pick bodies. In the 1980s, the term "frontolobe dementia" and "frontotemporal dementia" were derived in a group of papers trying to define the clinical criteria of FTD and help differentiate the disorder from Alzheimer's disease. The recent discovery of several mutated genes that can cause FTD symptoms has helped physicians and scientists define the disorder and will only lead to improved diagnosis and treatments for the future.

—*Elicia Estrella, M.S., C.G.C., L.G.C.*

See also Alzheimer's disease; Amyotrophic lateral sclerosis; Brain; Brain disorders; Dementias; Parkinson's disease; Pick's disease; Psychiatric disorders; Psychiatry; Psychiatry, geriatric.

For Further Information:

Bradley, Walter, et al., eds. *Neurology in Clinical Practice*. 6th ed. Boston: Butterworth Heinemann, 2012.

Cairns, Nigel J., et al. "Neuropathologic Diagnostic and Nosologic Criteria for Frontotemporal Lobar Degeneration: Consensus for the Consortium for Frontotemporal Lobar Degeneration." *Acta Neuropathologica* 114 (2007): 5–22.

Carson-DeWitt, Rosalyn, and Rimas Lukas. "Dementia." *Health Library*, Sept. 27, 2012.

"Dementia." *MedlinePlus*, May 7, 2013.

"Frontotemporal Disorders: Information for Patients, Families, and Caregivers." *National Institute on Aging*, Mar. 13, 2013.

Kertesz, Andrew. "Frontotemporal Dementia/Pick's Disease." *Archives of Neurology* 61 (2004): 969–971.

"MAPT." *Genetics Home Reference*, May 13, 2013.

Neary, David, Julie Snowden, and David Mann. "Frontotemporal Dementia." *The Lancet Neurology* 4 (2005): 771–780.

"NINDS Frontotemporal Dementia Information Page." *National Institute of Neurological Disorders and Stroke*, Mar. 20, 2013.

FROSTBITE
Disease/Disorder

Anatomy or system affected: Feet, hands, skin and adjacent tissues

Specialties and related fields: Emergency medicine, environmental health

Definition: Frostbite is localized freezing of tissue, usually of extremities exposed to low temperatures, that results in ice crystals forming within cells, thereby killing them.

Key terms:

anticoagulant: a drug that reduces the clotting of the blood

basal metabolic rate: the rate at which the body burns calories and produces heat energy while the body is at rest or not active

gangrene: the death of part of the body (such as an arm or leg) caused by the death of the cells in that structure

hypothermia: the process by which the body core temperature falls below that needed for the body to function normally

hypoxia: a lack of an adequate amount of oxygen to the tissues; results in a reduction of mental and physical capabilities

maceration: the process of breaking down tissue to a soft mass, either by soaking it or through infection or gangrene

necrosis: the death of body tissue cells

sludging: an increase in red blood cell structures, known as platelets, which slows down the blood flow through vessels and promotes clotting of the blood

sympathectomy: the surgical process of removing or destroying nerves that may be afflicted by frostbite or other injury

vasoconstriction: a decrease in the diameter of vessels transporting blood throughout the body, reducing blood flow and oxygen transport

windchill: the effect of wind blowing across exposed flesh; increased heat is lost from the skin's surface, as if the air were much colder than the actual temperature indicates

Causes and Symptoms

The effect of cold on the human body is to reduce the circulation of blood to surface areas, such as the feet, hands, and face. This reduction restricts the amount of heat lost by the body and helps to prevent the development of hypothermia. Blood constriction may become so severe in severely chilled areas of the body, however, that circulation almost totally ceases. People with poorer circulation, such as the elderly and the exhausted, are not as resistant to low temperatures as are fitter or younger people.

If the skin's temperature falls below -0.53 degrees Celsius, the tissue freezes and frostbite occurs. Rapid freezing causes ice crystals to form within a cell. These crystals rupture the cell wall and destroy structures within the cell, effectively killing it. If freezing is slow, ice crystals form between the cells and grow by extracting water from the cells. The tissue may be injured physically by the ice crystals or by dehydration and the resulting disruption of osmotic and chemical balance within the cells; however, tissue death following frostbite is more likely to be attributable to interruption of the blood supply to the tissue than to the direct action of freezing. Cold also damages the capillaries in the affected areas, causing blood plasma to leak through their walls, thus adding to tissue injury and further impairing circulation by allowing the blood to sludge (that is, clot because of an increase in red blood cells) inside the vessels. All sensation of cold or pain is lost as circulation becomes seriously impaired. Unless the tissue is warmed quickly, the skin and superficial tissues begin to freeze. With continual chilling, the frozen area enlarges and extends to deeper areas. This condition is known as frostbite.

Frostbite was common among soldiers during Napoleon's campaign in Russia in the early nineteenth century, during World War II in Northern Europe, in the Korean War, and in fighting between Indian and Chinese troops in the Himalayas. Air crews, especially waist gunners in the US Air Force in World War II, were particularly prone to frostbite. In 1943, frostbite injuries among these bomber crews were more numerous than all other casualties combined.

Polar travelers before the 1920s suffered severely from frostbite. Mountain climbers are at risk from frostbite at higher elevations. Lower oxygen availability increases the danger of frostbite because the body cannot take in sufficient oxygen in this thinner air. The resulting condition, called hypoxia, reduces mental abilities, which may cause a person to either take inadequate precautions against the cold or neglect such precautions altogether. High winds, often experienced in the mountains, speed heat loss from exposed skin surfaces. This wind chill can be deadly to mountaineers and often leads to hypothermia, which increases the risk of frostbite, as heat is drawn away from extremities to protect the body's core temperature. In addition, the insulating layer of subcutaneous fat decreases with longer periods of time spent at higher elevations, which in turn decreases the insulation of the surface areas of the body against freezing. Inadequate food intake while mountain climbing, often caused by poor appetite at high elevations, also increases the danger of frostbite, as the body does not have enough calories to keep its temperature constant. At higher elevations, most humans function at only about 60 percent of the physiological efficiency that they have at sea level. Women have more resistance to cold and may be less likely to experience frostbite than men.

Frostbite at high altitudes seems to be more common than at the same temperature at lower altitudes. More red blood cells are found in the blood of persons working at higher elevations, thickening the blood and reducing circulation to the extremities, thus lowering the temperature of these extremities. The basal metabolic rate and cardiac output of the body also decrease as one goes higher; both of these actions reduce the body's ability to keep its feet, hands, and face warm.

Blood vessels move heat from the central body core to the skin, after which it radiates into the air from exposed surfaces. This heat loss is greatest in the hands, feet, and head, where the vessels are close to the skin's surface. Respiration causes loss of body heat when cold air is inhaled into the lungs, body heat warms it, and the air is then exhaled. Evaporation, moisture leaving the skin's surface, also draws heat from the body. In low temperatures, spilling gasoline on exposed skin will create frostbite because the fuel evaporates much faster than water, drawing heat away from the body quickly. Convection carries body heat away by wind currents. This wind-chill factor, calculated for Fahrenheit tem-

---

Information on Frostbite

Causes: Exposure to freezing temperatures, causing impaired circulation to nearly cease

Symptoms: Tingling and pain in afflicted tissues, slightly flushed skin before freezing begins followed by white or blotchy blue color, skin that is firm and insensitive to the touch

Duration: Acute

Treatments: Manual or medical rewarming, antibiotics, hyperbaric oxygen, occasionally surgery

---

peratures by subtracting two times the wind speed from the air temperature, determines the amount of heat energy lost from the body's surface. Conduction transfers heat from one substance to another; for example, contact between the body and snow or metal will cause the skin to lose heat.

Although many people work and live in subzero temperatures, frostbite is uncommon. Nevertheless, an accident that prevents one from moving, loss of the ability to shiver in order to generate heat, or inactivity may increase one's chances of developing frostbite. Frostbite can occur in any cold environment. Initial warning symptoms of frostbite include tingling and pain in the afflicted tissues. The skin may be slightly flushed before freezing. It then turns white or a blotchy blue in color and is firm and insensitive to the touch. Tissue that is first painful and then becomes numb and insensitive is frozen.

Treatment and Therapy

Slight cases of frostbite, often termed frostnip or superficial frostbite, can be treated outdoors or in the field with little or no medical help. Such cases are usually reversible, with no permanent damage, as only skin and subcutaneous tissues are involved. In cases of frostnip, also called first-degree frostbite, the frozen part, although white and frozen on the surface, is soft and pliable when pressed gently before thawing. The area is often a cheek or the tip of the nose or the fingers. The frozen area, usually small, can be warmed manually. A hand is placed over the frostnipped area if it is a cheek or nose, while frozen fingers can be placed under the armpit or on a partner's bare stomach for warming. Tissue that has had only a minor amount of frostnip soon returns to normal color. A tingling sensation is felt when frostnipped tissue is thawed.

After thawing, areas that have had more serious superficial frostbite, also called second-degree frostbite, become numb, mottled, or blue or purple in color and then will sting, burn, or swell for a period of time. Small blisters, called blebs, may occur within twenty-four to forty-eight hours. Blistering is more common where the skin is loose. Blister fluid is absorbed slowly; the skin may harden and be insensitive to touch. Throbbing or aching may persist for weeks, and superficial gangrene may develop. With immediate treatment, second-degree frostbite will be mostly healed in two or three months and will not progress to the much more serious injury of deep frostbite.

Tissues vary in their resistance to frostbite. Skin freezes at

-0.53 Celsius, and muscles, blood vessels, and nerves are also highly subject to freezing. Connective tissue, tendons, and bones are relatively resistant to freezing, however, which explains why the blackened extremities of a frostbitten hand or foot can be moved: the tendons under the gangrenous skin remain intact and functional.

Deep frostbite, also called third- or fourth-degree frostbite depending on severity, includes not only skin and subcutaneous tissue but also deeper structures, including muscle, bone, and tendons. The affected area becomes cold, mottled, and blue or gray in color and may remain swollen for months. With deep frostbite, the tissues become quite hard to the touch. The frozen part may be painless at first, but one to three days after thawing, the affected area becomes quite painful, and shooting and throbbing pains may continue for several months after. Blisters, initially small blebs and then large, coalescing ones, may take weeks to develop. Permanent loss of tissue is almost inevitable with deep frostbite. The affected extremity has a severely shriveled look. A limb may return to almost normal over some months, however, and amputation should never be carried out until a considerable period, probably at least six to nine months, has elapsed.

In cases of frostbite, surgical intervention must be minimal. Blackened frostbitten tissue will gradually separate itself from healthy, unfrozen tissue without interference; no efforts should be taken to hasten separation. Most cases of deep frostbite seem to heal in six to twelve months, and the gangrenous tissue, if it has not become infected with bacteria, is essentially superficial and should be able to be removed without amputation. Many unnecessary amputations have been carried out because of impatience at the slow recovery rate of tissue that has suffered deep frostbite; amputation is only necessary when infection has set in and cannot be controlled with antibiotics.

If possible, deep frostbite should be treated under hospital care, not in the field or outdoors. The deep frozen tissue should remain frozen until hospital care is available. If frozen tissues are thawed, the patient will most likely be unable to move as the pain will be severe with any movement. Walking on feet that have been thawed after being frozen will cause permanent damage; however, walking on a frozen foot for twelve to eighteen hours or even longer produces less damage than inadequate warming. As frozen tissue thaws, cells exude fluid. If this tissue is refrozen, ice crystals form and cause more extensive, irreparable damage.

Rapid rewarming is the recommended treatment for deep frostbite and is a proven method of reducing tissue loss. Rubbing the frostbitten area with the hand or snow—akin to rubbing the area with broken glass—should never be done. This treatment does not melt the intracellular ice crystals or increase circulation to the frozen area, but it does break the skin and allow infection to enter into the system. Vasodilator agents do not improve tissue survival. Local antibiotics in aerosol form can be used, but it is unwise to rely on this method alone for combating infection. Sympathectomy, the removal or destruction of affected nerves, does not improve cell survival. The early use of the drug dextran to prevent

sludging has limited benefit and may have dangerous side effects. The use of hyperbaric oxygen or supplementary oxygen may increase the tissue tension of oxygen and save some cells partially damaged by cold injury.

Rewarming should be carried out in a water bath with water temperatures ranging from 37.7 to 42.2 degrees Celsius (100 to 108 degrees Fahrenheit). Higher temperatures will further damage already-injured tissues. Rewarming in a large bathtub warms the frozen extremity more rapidly, resulting in less tissue loss in many cases, particularly where frostbite has been deep and extensive. A large container also permits more accurate control of the water temperature. If a bathtub is not available, a bucket, large wastebasket, dishpan, or other similar container can be used. During rewarming, hot water usually must be added to the bath occasionally to keep the temperature correct; in such cases, the injured extremity should be removed from the bath and not returned to it until the water has been thoroughly mixed and its temperature measured. An open flame must not come into contact with the area to which

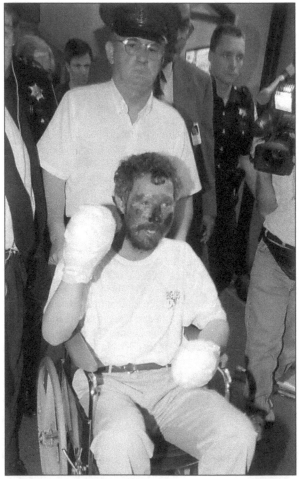

Dr. Seaborn Beck Weathers suffered frostbite to his face and hands when caught in a deadly blizzard on Mount Everest in 1996. (AP/ Wide World Photos)

heat is applied, since sensation is lost as a result of the frostbite and the tissue could be seriously burned without the patient noticing.

For rewarming, the frostbitten extremity should be stripped of all clothing, and any constricting bands, straps, or other objects that might stop circulation should be removed. The injured area should be suspended in the center of the water and not permitted to rest against the side or bottom. Warming should continue for thirty to forty minutes. The frostbitten tissues may become quite painful during this process, so it may be necessary to give painkillers to the patient in order to reduce discomfort during or after thawing. Aspirin (as well as codeine, morphine, or meperidine, if needed) may be given for pain. Aspirin or an anticoagulant increases blood circulation by reducing red blood cell platelet formation and thus reducing sludging. Phenoxybenzamine reduces vasoconstriction.

Following rewarming, the patient must be kept warm and the injured tissue elevated and protected from any kind of trauma. One should avoid rupturing blisters that have formed. Blankets or bedclothes should be supported by a framework to avoid pressure on or rubbing of the injured area.

Subsequent care is directed primarily toward preventing infection. Cleanliness of the frostbitten area is extremely important. It should be soaked daily in a body-temperature water bath to which a germicidal soap has been added. If contamination of the water supply is a possibility, the bath water should be boiled and cooled before use. Dead tissue should not be cut or pulled away; the water baths remove such tissue more efficiently.

The afflicted area should be immobilized and kept sterile. Even contact with sheets can be damaging to a frostbitten limb. Sterile, dry cotton may be placed between the fingers or toes to avoid maceration. If infection appears present, as indicated by the area between the frostbitten tissue and healthy tissue becoming inflamed and feeling tender or throbbing, antibiotics such as ampicillin or cloxicillin should be given every six hours. Wet, antiseptic dressings should be applied if gangrene occurs in the damaged tissue. A tetanus toxoid booster shot, or human antitoxin if the patient has not been previously immunized against tetanus, should be given. Complete rest and a diet high in protein will help healing. Moderate movement of the afflicted area should be encouraged but should be limited to that done by a physical therapist, without assistance by the patient. Considerable reassurance and emotional support may be required by the patient, as the appearance of the frostbitten area can be alarming.

Amputation in response to infected, spreading gangrene may be needed eventually, but it should be delayed until the natural separation of dead from living tissue and bone has taken place. Radionucleotide scanning helps save frostbitten limbs by accurately demonstrating blood flow in frostbitten extremities, thus predicting what tissue will survive.

Perspective and Prospects

Frostbite is an injury that can affect anyone who works or plays in cold conditions. Increased knowledge about what causes this injury, better equipment, and techniques that minimize its effect have reduced its occurrence. Advances in medical knowledge regarding how the injury occurs within the afflicted tissues have produced treatment protocols that reduce the extent of permanent injury from frostbite.

Prevention is the most effective treatment for frostbite, which can occur only when the body lacks enough heat to keep the extremities above freezing. The overall body-heat deficit results from inadequate clothing or equipment, reduced food consumption, exhaustion, injury or inactivity causing a lack of body movement, or some combination of these factors. Those playing or working in a cold environment should know the conditions under which frostbite may develop. For frostnip to occur, the windchill index must exceed 1,400 and the air temperature must be below the freezing point of exposed skin (-0.53 degrees Celsius). An ambient temperature of -10 to -15 degrees Celsius is usually necessary for deep frostbite to develop.

Adequate clothing—especially boots that allow circulation to occur freely, mittens (not gloves) that cover the hands, and a head covering that protects the face, ears, and neck—must be worn. Boots should be well broken in and large enough to fit comfortably with several pairs of socks. The laces at the top of the boots should not be tight. Gaiters or overboots should be worn if deep or wet snow is anticipated. Windproof or insulated pants should be worn to protect the legs from cold and help keep the feet warm. Dry socks and mitten liners should be carried. Moisture greatly reduces the insulative value of clothing, so it is necessary to stay dry; if clothing becomes wet or damp, one should change into dry items. Plastic bags, worn over bare feet, provide a vapor barrier liner that is effective in helping keep one's feet dry and warm under cold conditions. Adequate ventilation avoids dampness from excessive perspiration. Dressing in layers—having several light shirts, jackets, or a windbreaker—is better than wearing only one heavy jacket.

Heat production, resulting from exercise or the protective mechanism of shivering, is just as important as clothing in maintaining body temperature. Injuries that cause the victim to go into shock or lie immobilized predispose the victim to frostbite, even when adequate clothing is worn.

Eating high-energy foods and taking in 6,000 or more kilocalories (Calories) a day may be necessary to keep body temperatures constant under very cold or physically demanding conditions. Adequate rest, including eight or more hours of sleep, helps to reduce fatigue, which in turn increases the body's ability to produce heat. Alcohol and tobacco should be strictly avoided. Alcohol dilates the blood vessels and, although this action temporarily warms the skin, results in increased loss of total body heat. Smoking constricts the blood vessels in the skin and so reduces heat flow to surface areas; this may be sufficient to initiate frostbite in exposed tissue. A person who has sustained frostbite in the past is usually more susceptible to more cold injury. Problems with arthritis may develop in extremities that have been frostbitten.

—David L. Chesemore, Ph.D.

See also Amputation; Cyanosis; Gangrene; Hyperbaric oxygen therapy; Hyperthermia and hypothermia; Skin; Necrosis; Skin disorders.

For Further Information:

Calvert, John H., Jr. "Frostbite." *Flying Safety* 54, no. 10 (October 1998): 24–25.

Carson-DeWitt, Rosalyn, and Peter Lucas. "Frostbite." *Health Library*, September 30, 2012.

"Frostbite." *MedlinePlus*, August 6, 2013.

Phillips, David. "How Frostbite Performs Its Misery." *Canadian Geographic* 115, no. 1 (January/February 1995): 20–21.

Tilton, Buck. *Backcountry First Aid and Extended Care*. 5th ed. Guilford, Conn.: Falcon, 2007.

Tilton, Buck. "The Chill That Bites." *Backpacker* 28, no. 7 (September 2000): 27.

Tredget, Edward E., ed. *Thermal Injuries*. Philadelphia: W. B. Saunders, 2000.

Wilkerson, James A., ed. *Medicine for Mountaineering and Other Wilderness Activities*. 6th ed. Seattle: The Mountaineers Books, 2010.

Zafren, Ken. "Frostbite: Prevention and Initial Management." *High Altitude Medicine and Biology* 14, no. 1 (March 2013): 9–12.

FRUCTOSEMIA

Disease/Disorder

Anatomy or system affected: Gastrointestinal system, intestines, kidneys, liver

Specialties and related fields: Biochemistry, genetics, nutrition, pediatrics

Definition: An inborn error of metabolism in which eating foods containing fructose or sucrose will result in high blood fructose levels.

Causes and Symptoms

Fructosemia may also be called hereditary fructose intolerance; it literally means "fructose in the blood." Fructosemia occurs as a result of a hereditary lack of an enzyme called fructose-1-phosphate aldolase B. This autosomal recessive disease is rare, although some researchers suspect that more people have the disorder than are diagnosed. These individuals may naturally avoid fructose after becoming ill following the consumption of fructose-containing foods. The infant, child, or adult with undiagnosed fructosemia will be normal unless foods containing fructose, sucrose, or sorbitol are eaten. If foods containing these carbohydrates are eaten, then fructose levels will increase in the patient's blood and urine and the person will become ill. Symptoms include vomiting and low blood glucose and may progress to failure to thrive and/or coma. The severity of the disease appears to be variable, being rather mild in some individuals and causing death in others. In severe cases, the liver, kidneys, and intestines may be affected, although this damage usually reverses with the elimination of dietary fructose.

Treatment and Therapy

Treatment for this disorder is entirely dietary. Foods containing fructose, sucrose, or sorbitol must be eliminated from the diet. Fructose is often thought of as "fruit sugar," but far more foods than fruits and juices must be eliminated. Honey

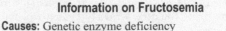

Information on Fructosemia

Causes: Genetic enzyme deficiency

Symptoms: Variable; may include vomiting, low blood glucose, failure to thrive, and coma if foods containing fructose, sucrose, or sorbitol are eaten

Duration: Chronic

Treatments: Avoidance of foods containing fructose, sucrose, or sorbitol

contains fructose, for example. Because half of sucrose becomes fructose when sucrose is metabolized, all foods containing sucrose (sugar) must be eliminated as well. This includes all sugar, whether from cane, beets, or sorghum. Sucrose is also part of maple syrup. Sorbitol metabolism also produces fructose, and so this sugar substitute must be avoided as well. Some infant formulas and baby foods may contain fructose, and many sweetened fruit beverages do. Reading food labels and being familiar with the ingredients of restaurant food is imperative for those with fructosemia.

Perspective and Prospects

Cases of fructosemia were first described in the mid-1950s. Soon after, the biochemical pathway defect was discovered. Today, genetic counseling may be of benefit to those who have fructosemia and want to have children, although strict avoidance of the three carbohydrates fructose, sucrose, and sorbitol will prevent symptoms.

—*Karen Chapman-Novakofski, R.D., L.D.N., Ph.D.*

See also Endocrine disorders; Endocrinology; Endocrinology, pediatric; Enzyme therapy; Enzymes; Galactosemia; Genetic diseases; Lactose intolerance; Metabolic disorders; Metabolism; Nutrition.

For Further Information:

Ali, M., et al. "Hereditary Fructose Intolerance." *Journal of Medical Genetics* 35, no. 5 (May, 1998): 353–365.

Cox, T. M. "Aldolase B and Fructose Intolerance." *FASEB Journal* 8, no. 1 (January, 1994): 62–71.

Haldeman-Englert, Chad, and David Zieve. "Hereditary Fructose Intolerance." *MedlinePlus*, May 15, 2011.

"Hereditary Fructose Intolerance." *Genetics Home Reference*, May 13, 2013.

Sanders, Lee M. "Disorders of Carbohydrate Metabolism." *Merck Manual Home Health Handbook*, Feb. 2009.

Steinmann, Beat, René Santer, and Georges van den Berghe. "Disorders of Fructose Metabolism." In *Inborn Metabolic Diseases: Diagnosis and Treatment*, edited by Jean-Marie Saudubray, et al. 5th ed. New York: Springer, 2012.

FUNGAL INFECTIONS

Disease/Disorder

Anatomy or system affected: Immune system, nails, respiratory system, skin

Specialties and related fields: Dermatology, family medicine, immunology, internal medicine, microbiology, pulmonary medicine

Definition: Infections caused by fungi-simple, plantlike organisms-that range from minor skin diseases to serious, disseminated diseases of the lungs and other organs; patients whose immune systems are impaired are at greater risk of serious fungal infections.

Key terms:

asexual reproduction: the production of new individuals without the mating of two parents of unlike genotype, such as by budding

mycelium: a collection of threadlike fungal strands (hyphae) making up the thallus, or nonreproductive portion, of a fungus

mycosis: a disease of humans, plants, or animals caused by a fungus; the prefix myco- means "fungus," hence mycology (the study of fungi)

pleomorphic fungus: a fungus whose morphology changes markedly from one phase of its life cycle to another, or according to changes in environmental conditions

tinea: a medical term for fungal skin diseases, such as ringworm and athlete's foot, caused by a variety of fungi

yeast: a unicellular fungus which reproduces by budding off smaller cells from the parent cell; yeasts belong to several different groups of fungi, and some fungi are capable of growing either as a yeast or as a filamentous fungus

Types of Fungus

The term "fungus" is a general one for plantlike organisms that do not produce their own food through photosynthesis but live as heterotrophs, absorbing complex carbon compounds from other living or dead organisms. Fungi were formerly classified in the plant kingdom (together with bacteria, all algae, mosses, and green plants); more recently, biologists have realized that there are fundamental differences in cell structure and organization separating the lower plants into a number of groups that merit recognition as kingdoms. Fungi differ from bacteria and actinomycetes in being eukaryotic, that is, in having an organized nucleus with chromosomes within the cell. One division of fungi, which is believed to be distantly related to certain aquatic algae, has spores that swim by means of flagella. These water molds include pathogens of fish and aquatic insect larvae and a few economically important plant pathogens, but none have yet been recorded as causing a defined, nonopportunistic human disease. The other division of fungi lacks flagellated spores at any stage in its life cycle. It encompasses most familiar fungi, including molds, mushrooms, yeasts, wood-rotting fungi, leaf spots, and all fungi reliably reported to cause disease in humans.

Fungi that lack flagellated stages in their life cycles are further divided into three classes and one form-class according to the manner in which the spores are produced. The first of these, the Zygomycetes (for example *Rhizopus*, the black bread mold), produce thick-walled, solitary sexual spores as a result of hyphal fusion; they are a diverse assemblage including many parasites of insects. Species in the genus *Mucor* cause a rare, fulminating, rapidly fatal systemic disease called mucormycosis, generally in acidotic diabetic patients. The Basidiomycetes, characterized by the production of sexual spores externally on a club-shaped structure called a basidium, include mushrooms, plant rusts (such as stem rust

---

Information on Fungal Infections

Causes: Invasion of body tissues or organs by fungi

Symptoms: Varies; can include vascular constriction leading to gangrene of limbs, hallucinations, discolored patches on skin, localized inflammation, thrush, chronic localized tumors, pulmonary infection, miscarriage

Duration: Acute or chronic with recurring episodes

Treatments: Antifungal agents, antibiotics, chemotherapy

---

of wheat), and most wood-rotting fungi. There is one important basidiomycetous human pathogen (*Filobasidiella neoformans*) and a few confirmed opportunists. The Ascomycetes, including most yeasts and lichens, many plant pathogens (such as Dutch elm disease and chestnut blight), and a great diversity of saprophytes growing on wood and herbaceous material, produce sexual spores in a saclike structure called an ascus. One ascomycete, *Piedraia nigra*, regularly produces its characteristic fruiting bodies on its human host; others do so in culture. In addition, there is a form-class Deuteromycetes consisting of fungi that produce only asexual spores. Most are suspected of being stages in the life cycle of Ascomycetes, but some are Basidiomycetes or are of uncertain affinity. Human pathogens, at least as they occur on the host or in typical laboratory culture, are mostly Deuteromycetes.

Medical mycology (the study of fungi) would occupy only a single chapter in a book on the relationship of fungi to human affairs. Relatively few fungi have become adapted to living as parasites of human (or even mammalian) hosts, and of these, the most common ones cause superficial and cutaneous mycoses (fungal infections) with annoying but scarcely life-threatening effects. Serious fungal diseases are mercifully rare among people with normally functioning immune systems.

The majority of fungi are directly dependent on green plants as parasites, as symbionts living in a mutually beneficial association with a plant, or as saprophytes on dead plant material. One large, successful group of Ascomycetes lives in symbiotic association with algae, forming lichens. Fungi play a critical ecological role in maintaining stable plant communities. As plant pathogens, they cause serious economic loss, leading in extreme cases to famine. The ability of saprophytic fungi to transform chemically the substrate on which they are growing has been exploited by the brewing industry since antiquity and has been expanded to other industrial processes. Penicillin, other antibiotics, and some vitamins are extracted from fungi, which produce a vast array of complex organic compounds whose potential is only beginning to be explored and which constitutes a fertile field for those interested in genetic engineering.

This same chemical diversity and complexity also enable fungi to produce mycotoxins—chemicals that have an adverse effect on humans and animals. Saprophytic fungi growing on improperly stored food are a troublesome source of toxic compounds, some of which are carcinogenic. The old adage that "a little mold won't hurt you" is true in the sense that common molds do not cause acute illness when ingested, but it is poor advice in terms of long-term health.

A mycotoxicity problem of considerable medical and veterinary interest is posed by Ascomycetes of the order *Clavicipitaceae*, which are widespread on grasses. Some species of grasses routinely harbor systemic, asymptomatic infections by these fungi, which produce compounds toxic to animals that graze on them. From the point of view of the grass, the relationship is symbiotic, since it discourages grazing; from the point of view of range management, the relationship is deleterious to stock. *Claviceps purpurea*, a pathogen of rye, causes a condition known as ergotism in humans, with symptoms including miscarriage, vascular constriction leading to gangrene of the limbs, and hallucinations. Outbreaks of hallucinatory ergotism are thought by some authors to be responsible for some of the more spectacular perceptions of witchcraft in premodern times. Better control of plant disease and a decreased reliance on rye as a staple grain have virtually eliminated ergotism as a human disease in the twentieth century.

Fungi exhibit a bewildering variety of forms and life cycles; nevertheless, certain generalizations can be made. A fungus starts life as a spore, which may be a single cell or a cluster of cells and is usually microscopic. Under proper conditions, the spore germinates, producing a filament of fungal cells oriented end to end, called a hypha. Hyphae grow into the substrate, secreting enzymes that dissolve structures to provide food for the growing fungus and to provide holes through which the fungus can grow. In an asexually reproducing fungus, some of the hyphae become differentiated, producing specialized cells (spores) that differ from the parent hypha in size and pigmentation and are adapted for dispersal, but that are genetically identical to the parent. In a sexually reproducing fungus, two hyphae (or a hypha and a spore from different individuals) fuse, their nuclei fuse, and meiosis takes place before spores are formed. Spores are often produced in a specialized fruiting body, such as a mushroom.

Fungus spores are ubiquitous. Common saprophytic fungi produce airborne spores in enormous quantities; thus it is difficult to avoid contact with them in all but the most hypersterile environments. In culture, fungi (including pathogenic species) produce large numbers of dry spores that can be transmitted in the air from host to host, making working with fungi in a medical laboratory potentially hazardous.

Fungal Diseases and Treatments

Human fungal diseases are generally placed in four broad categories according to the tissues they attack, and they are further subdivided according to specific pathologies and the organisms involved. The categories of disease are superficial mycoses, cutaneous mycoses, subcutaneous mycoses, and systemic mycoses.

Superficial mycoses affect hair and the outermost layer of the epidermis and do not evoke a cellular response. They include tinea versicolor and tinea nigra, deutermycete infec-

tions that cause discolored patches on skin, and black piedra, caused by an ascomycete growing on hair shafts. They can be treated with a topical fungicide, such as nystatin, or, in the case of piedra, by shaving off the affected hair.

Cutaneous mycoses involve living cells of the skin or mucous membrane and evoke a cellular response, generally localized inflammation. Dermatomycoses (dermatophytes), which affect skin and hair, include tinea capitis (ringworm of the scalp), tinea pedis (athlete's foot), and favus, a scaly infection of the scalp. Domestic animals serve as a reservoir for some cutaneous mycoses. The organisms responsible are generally fungi imperfecti in the genera *Microsporum* and *Trichophyton*. Cutaneous mycoses can be successfully treated with topical nystatin or oral griseofulvin.

Candida albicans, a ubiquitous pleomorphic fungus with both a yeast and a mycelial form, causes a variety of cutaneous mycoses as well as systemic infections collectively named candidiasis. Thrush is a *Candida* yeast infection of the mouth that is most common in infants, especially in infants born to mothers with vaginal candidiasis. Vaginal yeast infections periodically affect 18 to 20 percent of the adult female population and more than 30 percent of pregnant women. *Candida* also causes paronychia, a nailbed infection. Small populations of *Candida* are normally present in the alimentary tract and genital tract of healthy individuals; candidiasis of the mucous membranes tends to develop in response to antibiotic treatment, which disturbs the normal bacterial flora of the body, or in response to metabolic changes or decreasing immune function.

None of the organisms causing cutaneous mycoses elicits a lasting immune response, so recurring infections by these agents is the rule rather than the exception. Even in temperate climates, under modern standards of hygiene, cutaneous mycoses are extremely common.

Subcutaneous mycoses, affecting skin and muscle tissue, are predominantly tropical in distribution and not particularly common. Chromomycosis and maduromycosis are caused by soil fungi that enter the skin through wounds, causing chronic localized tumors, usually on the feet. Sporotrichosis enters through wounds and spreads through the lymphatic system, causing skin ulcers associated with lymph nodes. Amphotericin B, a highly toxic systemic antifungal agent, has been used to treat all three conditions; potassium iodide is used to treat sporotrichosis, and localized chromomycosis and maduromycosis lesions can be surgically removed.

Systemic mycoses, the most serious of fungal infections, have the ability to become generally disseminated in the body. The main nonopportunistic systemic mycoses known in North America are histoplasmosis, caused by *Histoplasma capsulatum*; coccidiomycosis, caused by *Coccidiodes immitis*; blastomycosis, caused by *Ajellomyces* (or *Blastomyces*) *dermatidis*; and cryptococcosis, caused by *Cryptococcus* (or *Filobasidiella*) *neoformans*. Similar infections, caused by related species, occur in other parts of the world.

Coccidiomycosis, also called San Joaquin Valley fever or valley fever, will serve as an example of the etiology of systemic mycoses. The causative organism lives in arid soils in the American southwest; its spores are wind-disseminated. When inhaled, the fungus grows in the lungs, producing a mild respiratory infection that is self-limiting in perhaps 95 percent of the cases. The mild form of the disease is common in rural areas. In a minority of cases, a chronic lung disease whose symptoms resemble tuberculosis develops. There is also a disseminated form of the disease producing meningitis; chronic cutaneous disease, with the production of ulcers and granulomas; and attack of the bones, internal organs, and lymphatic system. A chronic pulmonary infection may become systemic in response to factors that undermine the body's immune system. Factors involved in individual susceptibility among individuals with intact immune systems are poorly understood.

Histoplasmosis (also known as summer fever, cave fever, cave disease, Mississippi Valley fever, or Ohio Valley disease) is even more common; 90 percent of people tested in the southern Mississippi Valley show a positive reaction to this fungus, indicating prior, self-limiting lung infection. The fungus is associated with bird and bat droppings, and severe cases sometimes occur when previously unexposed individuals are exposed to high levels of inoculum in caves where bats roost. A related organism, *Histoplasma duboisii*, occurs in central Africa. Blastomycosis causes chronic pulmonary disease, chronic cutaneous disease, and systemic disease, all of which were usually fatal until the advent of chemotherapy with amphotericin B. The natural habitat of the fungus is unclear. *Cryptococcus neoformans* occurs in pigeon droppings and is worldwide in distribution. The subclinical pulmonary form of the disease is probably common; invasive disease occurs in patients with collagen diseases, such as lupus, and in patients with weakened immune systems. It is the leading cause of invasive fungal disease in patients with acquired immunodeficiency syndrome (AIDS).

Systemic fungal diseases are notoriously difficult to treat. Chemotherapy of systemic, organismally caused diseases depends on finding a chemical compound that will selectively kill or inhibit the invading organism without damaging the host. Therefore, the more closely the parasite species is related biologically to the host species, the more difficult it is to find a compound that will act in such a selective manner. Fungi are, from a biological standpoint, more like humans than they are like bacteria, and antibacterial antibiotics are ineffective against them. If a fungus has invaded the skin or the digestive tract, it can be attacked with toxic substances that are not readily absorbed into the bloodstream, but this approach is not appropriate for a systemic infection. Amphotericin, itraconazole, and fluconazole, the drugs of choice for systemic fungal infections, are highly toxic to humans. Thus, dosage is critical, close clinical supervision is necessary, and long-term therapy may not be feasible.

Perspective and Prospects

Medical mycology textbooks written before 1980 tended to focus on two categories of fungal infection: the common, ubiquitous, and comparatively benign superficial and cutaneous mycoses, frequently seen in clinical practice in the industrialized world, and the subcutaneous and deep mycoses, treated as a rare and/or predominantly tropical problem. Opportunistic systemic infections, if mentioned at all, were regarded as a rare curiosity.

The rising population of patients with compromised immune systems, including cancer patients undergoing chemotherapy, people being treated with steroids for various conditions, transplant patients, and people with AIDS, has dramatically changed this clinical picture. Between 1980 and 1986, more than a hundred fungi, a few previously unknown and the majority common inhabitants of crop plants, rotting vegetable debris, and soil, were identified as causing human disease. The number continues to increase steadily. Compared to organisms routinely isolated from soil and plants, these opportunistic fungi do not seem to have any special characteristics other than the ability to grow at human body temperature; however, the possibility that an opportunistic pathogen might mutate into a form capable of attacking healthy humans is worrisome.

Systemic opportunistic human infections have been attributed to *Alternaria alternata* and *Fusarium oxysporum*, common plant pathogens that cause diseases of tomatoes and strawberries, respectively. Several species of *Aspergillus*, saprophytic molds (many of them thermophilic), have long been implicated in human disease. Colonizing aspergillosis, involving localized growth in the lungs of people exposed to high levels of aspergillus spores (notably agricultural workers working with silage), is not particularly rare among people with normal immune systems, but the more severe invasive form of the disease, in which massive lung lesions form, and disseminated aspergillosis, in which other organs are attacked, almost always involve immunocompromised patients. *Ramichloridium schulzeri*, described originally from wheat roots, causes "golden tongue" in leukemia patients; fortunately this infection responds to amphotericin B. *Scelidosporium inflatum*, first isolated from a serious bone infection in an immunocompromised patient in 1984, is being isolated with increasing frequency in cases of disseminated mycosis; it resists standard drug treatment.

Oral colonization by strains of *Candida* is often the first sign of AIDS-related complex or full-blown AIDS in an individual harboring the human immunodeficiency virus (HIV). Drug therapy with fluconazole is effective against oral candidiasis, but relapse rates of up to 50 percent within a month of the cessation of drug therapy are reported. Reported rates of disseminated candidiasis in AIDS patients range from 1 to 10 percent. Invasive procedures such as intravenous catheters represent a significant risk of introducing *Candida* and other common fungi into the bloodstream of patients.

Pneumocystis jiroveci (formely called *Pneumocystis carinii*), the organism causing a form of pneumonia that is the single most important cause of death in patients with AIDS, was originally classified as a sporozoan—that is, as a parasitic protozoan—but detailed investigations of the life cycle, metabolism, and genetic material of *Pneumocystis* have convinced some biologists that it is actually an ascomycete, although an anomalous one that lacks a cell wall. Unfortunately, while antibiotics and corticosteroids are used to treat the illness, it does not respond to therapy with the antifungal drugs currently in use.

In general, antifungal drug therapy for mycoses in AIDS patients is not very successful. In the absence of significant patient immunity, it is difficult to eradicate a disseminated infection from the body entirely, making a resurgence likely once drug therapy is discontinued. Reinfection is also likely if the organism is a common component of the patient's environment.

Given the increasing number of lethal systemic fungal infections seen in clinical practice, there is substantial impetus for a search for more effective, less toxic antifungal drugs. A number of compounds, produced by bacteria and chemically dissimilar to both antibacterial antibiotics and the most widely used antifungal compounds, have been identified and are being tested. It is also possible that the plant kingdom, which has been under assault by fungi for all its long geologic history, may prove a source for medically useful antifungal compounds.

—Martha Sherwood-Pike, Ph.D.

See also Acquired immunodeficiency syndrome (AIDS); Aspergillosis; Athlete's foot; Candidiasis; Coccidioidomycosis; Diaper rash; Food poisoning; Immune system; Immunodeficiency disorders; Immunology; Immunopathology; Microbiology; Mold and mildew; Nail removal; Nails; Opportunistic infections; Pneumonia; Poisonous plants; Ringworm; Skin; Skin disorders.

For Further Information:

Alcamo, I. Edward. *Microbes and Society: An Introduction to Microbiology.* 2d ed. Sudbury, Mass.: Jones and Bartlett, 2008.

Biddle, Wayne. *A Field Guide to Germs.* 3d ed. New York: Anchor Books, 2010.

Carlile, Michael J., Sarah Watkinson, and Graham W. Gooday. *The Fungi.* 2d ed. San Diego, Calif.: Academic Press, 2008.

Crissey, John Thorne, Heidi Lang, and Lawrence Charles Parish. *Manual of Medical Mycology.* Cambridge, Mass.: Blackwell Scientific, 1995.

"Fungal Diseases." *Centers for Disease Control and Prevention,* Nov. 19, 2012.

"Fungal Infections." *MedlinePlus,* Jan. 31, 2013.

"Fungal Infections." *National Institute of Allergy and Infectious Diseases,* Apr. 16, 2006.

Kumar, Vinay, Abul K. Abbas, and Nelson Fausto, eds. *Robbins and Cotran Pathologic Basis of Disease.* 8th ed. Philadelphia: Saunders/Elsevier, 2010.

Mandell, Gerald L., John E. Bennett, and Raphael Dolin, eds. *Mandell, Douglas, and Bennett's Principles and Practice of Infectious Diseases.* 7th ed. New York: Churchill Livingstone/Elsevier, 2010.

Murray, Patrick R., Ken S. Rosenthal, and Michael A. Pfaller. *Medical Microbiology.* 7th ed. Philadelphia: Mosby/Elsevier, 2013.

Richardson, Malcolm D., and David W. Warnock. *Fungal Infection: Diagnosis and Management.* 4th ed. Hoboken, NJ: Wiley-Blackwell, 2012.

Rippon, John Willard. *Medical Mycology: The Pathogenic Fungi and Pathogenic Actinomycetes.* 3d ed. Philadelphia: W. B. Saunders, 1988.

Shaw, Michael, ed. *Everything You Need to Know About Diseases.* Springhouse, Pa.: Springhouse Press, 1996.

Weedon, David. *Skin Pathology.* 3d ed. New York: Churchill Livingstone/Elsevier, 2010.

GALACTOSEMIA

Disease/Disorder

Anatomy or system affected: Eyes, liver

Specialties and related fields: Biochemistry, genetics, nutrition, pediatrics

Definition: An inherited disorder of carbohydrate metabolism in which an infant is unable to utilize galactose from food.

Causes and Symptoms

In classic I galactosemia, a congenital deficiency of the enzyme galactose-1-phosphate uridyl transferase (GALT) causes galactose to accumulate instead of being converted to glucose for energy production. As galactose accumulates in the child's tissues and organs, it will have a toxic effect and cause various signs and symptoms. Galactosemia means "galactose in the blood." Galactose is a sugar that may be found alone in foods but is usually associated with lactose, a milk sugar.

A gene mutation on the short arm of chromosome 9 has been identified in babies with galactosemia. About one in forty thousand newborns is affected with this autosomal recessive disorder. Both parents serve as carriers; they are not themselves affected, but each conception carries a one in four chance that the child will be born with galactosemia. Prenatal diagnosis is possible in cultured fibroblasts from amniotic fluid. Mandatory screening programs in many states test all newborns for galactosemia during the first week of life.

Galactosemia is an example of a multiple-allele system. In addition to the normal allele (G) and the recessive allele (g), a third allele, known as G^D, has been found. The D allele is named after Duarte, California, where it was discovered. The existence of three alleles produces six possible genotypic combinations in the deoxyribonucleic acid (DNA). These enzymatic activities may range from 0 to 100 percent. Consequently, it is very important to monitor each patient with biochemical studies.

Homozygous recessive infants (gg) are unaffected at birth but develop symptoms a few days later, including jaundice, vomiting, an enlarged liver from extensive fatty deposits, cataracts, and failure to thrive. Mental retardation and death may also occur if dietary treatment has not been started.

Treatment and Therapy

Galactosemia is treated by removing foods that contain galactose from the diet. Since milk and milk products are the most common source of galactose, infants with galactosemia

should not be given these foods. Serious problems can be prevented through this early exclusion of galactose.

While it is not possible for a child with galactosemia to have an entirely galactose-free diet, all persons with galactosemia should limit galactose intake from foods to a very low level. The galactose-1-phosphate levels determine the degree of dietary restriction for each individual. Advice from a dietician is needed.

—Phillip A. Farber, Ph.D.

See also Endocrine system; Endocrinology; Endocrinology, pediatric; Enzyme therapy; Enzymes; Fructosemia; Gaucher's disease; Genetic diseases; Glycogen storage diseases; Lactose intolerance; Mental retardation; Metabolic disorders; Metabolism; Nutrition.

For Further Information:

Badash, Michelle. "Galactosemia." *Health Library*, November 26, 2012.
Berry, Gerard T. "Galactosemia: When is it a Newborn Screening Emergency?" *Molecular Genetics & Metabolism* 106, no. 1: 7–11.
Cummings, Michael R. *Human Heredity: Principles and Issues.* 8th ed. Pacific Grove, Calif.: Brooks/Cole, 2009.
"Galactosemia." *MedlinePlus*, May 1, 2011.
Icon Health. *Galactosemia: A Medical Dictionary, Bibliography, and Annotated Research Guide to Internet References.* San Diego, Calif.: Author, 2004.
Kasper, Dennis L., et al., eds. *Harrison's Principles of Internal Medicine.* 16th ed. New York: McGraw-Hill, 2005.
Rudolph, Colin D., et al., eds. *Rudolph's Pediatrics.* 21st ed. New York: McGraw-Hill, 2003.

GALLBLADDER

Anatomy

Anatomy or system affected: Abdomen, gastrointestinal system

Specialties and related fields: Gastroenterology, internal medicine

Definition: A small, pear-shaped sac located under the liver that stores and concentrates bile.

Key terms:

bile: a fluid made by the liver to help digest fat

bilirubin: a yellow-brown component of bile created when the liver breaks down old red blood cells

cholesterol: a waxy essential substance present in all cells and transported in the blood

gallstones: solid particles that form from substances in the bile

Structure and Functions

The gallbladder is part of the digestive system. Bile originates in the liver then flows into the gallbladder through a system of ducts. Some bile flows directly into the small intestine, but the gallbladder collects and concentrates much of the bile. It then contracts and releases more bile into the small intestine as food is eaten. Bile helps break down the fats and neutralize the acids in the food. The organs and ducts that transport bile are collectively called the biliary system and include the gallbladder, liver, pancreas, stomach, small intestine, and the ducts connecting these organs.

Information on Galactosemia

Causes: Genetic enzyme deficiency

Symptoms: Varies; may include jaundice, vomiting, liver enlargement, cataracts, failure to thrive, and mental retardation if foods containing galactose (milk sugar) are eaten

Duration: Chronic

Treatments: Avoidance of foods containing galactose

Disorders and Diseases

Gallstones are a very common gallbladder problem. Two types of stones may form. Cholesterol stones are the most common type of gallstone, and they form when there is too much cholesterol in the bile. Pigment stones are less common, occurring only about 20 percent of the time; they are formed when there is too much bilirubin in the bile. Gallstones may be any size, ranging from stones that are tiny, like grains of sand, up to the size of a golf ball. When stones are small, they may form a type of "sludge" that affects the functioning of the gallbladder. If they are large, then they may move about and cause blockage of the ducts that drain the bile from the gallbladder into the digestive system, causing pain or a "gallbladder attack." Stones may exit the gallbladder and block other areas of the digestive system, causing pain, infection, or organ damage. However, it is possible to have gallstones that cause no pain or problem at all.

Some risk factors for gallstones include being female (especially females who have been pregnant or have taken hormones), being overweight, losing weight quickly (such as with "crash" dieting), or having high blood cholesterol levels.

Common symptoms of gallstones include pain in the upper right abdomen (especially within thirty minutes after a fatty meal), nausea, vomiting, fever, indigestion, gas, constipation, diarrhea, or bloating. Stones blocking the common bile duct are likely to cause symptoms such as jaundice, dark urine, and rapid drop in blood pressure. Some relief may be found by following a low-fat diet, and some patients find relief through nontraditional methods, such as acupuncture or herbal medicine. More conventional treatments may involve dissolving the gallstones by various methods; however, once gallstones begin to form, they are very likely to return, so this option may not be a long-lasting one. Another possibility is to perform a therapeutic endoscopic retrograde cholangiopancreatography (ERCP), which allows stones to be removed or ducts to be opened. In complicated or recurring cases, the treatment for gallstones involves removing the gallbladder (cholecystectomy). Without the gallbladder, all bile flows directly from the liver into the small intestine. In most people, gallbladder removal has almost no side effects; in a very small percentage (approximately 1 percent), bile traveling directly into the small intestine can cause diarrhea.

Untreated gallstones can become life-threatening due to infection or organ damage because of blockages, and complications including gangrene and perforation of the gallbladder can occur. People with diabetes are, for unknown reasons, more likely to have serious complications from gallstones.

Gallbladder cancer is quite rare, with new cases of less than ten thousand per year in the United States. It is seen most often in people aged seventy and older and is more common in women than in men. The cause of gallbladder cancer is unknown, but risk factors include a history of gallstones, porcelain gallbladder (a rare condition where calcium lines the walls of the gallbladder), smoking, family history of gallbladder cancer, and obesity. There are usually no symptoms of gallbladder cancer; most cancers are found incidentally during surgery to remove gallstones. Surgery to remove the gallbladder, radiation therapy, and/or chemotherapy are all possible treatments for gallbladder cancer.

Perspective and Prospects

The gallbladder has been recognized throughout history as an important organ in the digestive process. It is one of the organs in the "four humors" system of medicine, which may have originated in Mesopotamia or Egypt but reached its height in the Greek system of medicine. In that system, the gallbladder was linked to the season of summer and the element of fire, and an overabundance of bile was thought to cause one to be bad-tempered or "choleric." In traditional Chinese medicine, the gallbladder is thought to affect the quality and length of sleep.

—*Marianne M. Madsen, M.S.*

See also Abdomen; Abdominal disorders; Bile; Cholecystectomy; Cholecystitis; Gallbladder cancer; Gallbladder diseases; Gastroenterology; Gastroenterology, pediatric; Gastrointestinal dis-

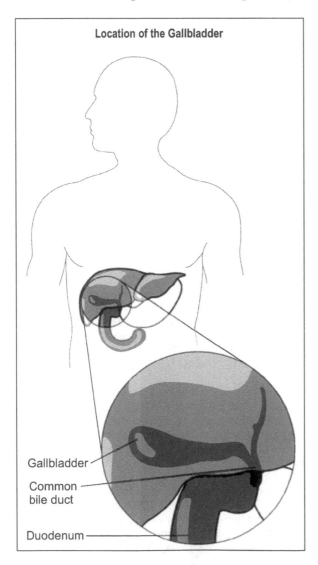

Location of the Gallbladder

Gallbladder
Common bile duct
Duodenum

orders; Internal medicine; Jaundice; Kidney stones; Laparoscopy; Obesity; Stone removal; Stones.

For Further Information:

Andrén-Sandberg, Å...ke. "Diagnosis and Management of Gallbladder Cancer." *North American Journal of Medical Sciences* 4, no. 7 (July, 2012): 293–99.

Clavien, Pierre-Alain, ed. *Diseases of the Gallbladder and Bile Ducts: Diagnosis and Treatment.* 2d ed. Wiley-Blackwell, 2006.

"Gallbadder Removal—Laparoscopic." *MedlinePlus*, August 1, 2011.

Kraus, J. *The Etiology, Symptoms, and Treatment of Gall-Stones.* BiblioLife, 2009.

Lack, Ernest E. *Pathology of the Pancreas, Gallbladder, Extrahepatic Biliary Tract, and Ampullary Region.* New York: Oxford University Press, 2001.

Mitchell, George. *Learn About Your Liver and Gallbladder.* Dupage Digital, 2008.

PM Medical Health. *Twenty-first Century Ultimate Medical Guide to Gallbladder and Bile Duct Disorders: Authoritative Clinical Information for Physicians and Patients.* Progressive Management, 2009.

Savitsky, Diane. "Gallstones." *Health Library*, September 30, 2012.

Thomas, Charles, and Clifton Fuller, eds. *Biliary Tract and Gallbladder Cancer: Diagnosis and Therapy.* Demos, 2008.

Thudichum, John Louis William. *A Treatise on Gall-stones: Their Chemistry, Pathology, and Treatment.* BiblioLife, 2009.

GALLBLADDER CANCER
Disease/Disorder

Also known as: Biliary cancer, biliary tract cancer

Anatomy or system affected: Gallbladder, gastrointestinal system

Specialties and related fields: Gastroenterology, general surgery, oncology, radiology

Definition: A rare type of cancer affecting the gallbladder (a muscular, membranous sac containing bile) and its surrounding organs.

Key terms:

adenocarcinoma: a malignant tumor originating in glandular epithelium

bile: a yellowish-green, viscous fluid secreted by the liver and passed into the duodenum to aid in the breakdown and absorption of fats

cholecystectomy: surgical removal of the gallbladder

gallstones: crystalline accumulations of bile salts within the gallbladder

jaundice: yellowing of the skin, eyes, and other tissues that occurs when bile salts are deposited in these areas of the body

resectable: able to be surgically removed and/or repaired

Causes and Symptoms

The gallbladder is an accessory organ of digestion that stores bile, a yellowish-green, thick fluid produced by the liver. Bile aids in the breakdown and absorption of fats, and it also helps to eliminate waste metabolic products, excess cholesterol, and drugs. Food intake, especially the ingestion of fatty foods, stimulates the release of a hormone, cholecystokinin (CCK), from the small intestine. CCK then stimulates the

---

Information on Gallbladder Cancer

Causes: Possibly gallstones, high alcohol intake, smoking, obesity, high levels of estrogen, inflammatory bowel disease (IBD), carcinogens

Symptoms: Jaundice, extreme itching, nausea, weight loss, abdominal pain

Duration: Depends on stage, from five or more years to between two and four months; often fatal

Treatments: Surgery

---

gallbladder to contract and send bile through the common bile duct and into the duodenum, where fat emulsification and absorption continues.

A rare disease, gallbladder cancer usually occurs in patients who have gallstones. Gallstones form within the gallbladder when bile salts crystallize into hard, rocklike accumulations. These stones may then block the common bile duct, resulting in intense gastrointestinal pain when the gallbladder contracts and tries to squeeze bile into this duct during the process of digestion.

Besides the presence of gallstones, gallbladder cancer has also been associated with high alcohol intake, smoking, obesity, high levels of estrogen, and inflammatory bowel disease (IBD). Patients who have taken certain medications, such as oral contraceptives and methyldopa, may have a higher incidence of this type of cancer. Recent research also indicates that exposure to carcinogens such as asbestos, dioxin, polychlorinated biphenyls (PCBs), and azotoluene may cause gallbladder cancer. The presence in the body of *Salmonella typhi*, a bacterium, may cause chronic gallbladder infections that can lead to cancer.

Patients with gallbladder cancer often suffer from jaundice, extreme itching, nausea, unexplained weight loss, and pain in the upper right abdomen or more generalized abdominal pain. Diagnosis of this cancer may sometimes be made with simple tests, such as a complete blood count, liver function test, or chest X-ray. More bloodwork may be ordered by a physician to search for a specific tumor marker, CA 19-9, which detects the adenocarcinomas of gallbladder cancer. Usually, however, more extensive testing with ultrasound, computed tomography (CT) scans, and magnetic resonance imaging (MRI) is required. Ultrasonography is useful for detecting gallstones and a "porcelain" (highly calcified) gallbladder. CT scans may show invasion of the cancer into the liver, while MRI can also reveal extension into other tissues. A very specific test for biliary tract cancers called endoscopic retrograde cholangiopancreatography (ERCP) is used to check for blockages in the bile ducts. If a tumor is found to be blocking ducts, then a fine tube may be inserted into the area in an attempt to clear the blockage.

In the United States, most patients are female and of American Indian or Mexican American descent. American Indians are five times more likely than the general population to develop gallstones and gallbladder cancer. Women are twice as likely to develop the disease than are men because estrogen, the female sex hormone, causes more cholesterol to be excreted into the bile. High rates of this cancer also occur in Mexico, South America, and Israel. This cancer is usually diagnosed in patients who are in their mid-sixties.

Treatment and Therapy

Surgical removal of the gallbladder, known as cholecystectomy, is the only cure for gallbladder cancer, assuming that the surgeon is able to remove all of the cancer. Unfortunately, only about 25 percent of patients are able to have successful surgery. Because the symptoms of gallbladder cancer mimic those of many other diseases, a majority of patients come to their doctors with a well-advanced stage of cancer. Of the patients diagnosed with this condition, 40 percent to 60 percent have cancer that has already spread to surrounding tissues. For these patients, surgical removal of the gallbladder is essential, and removal of parts of the liver, small intestine, colon, and nearby lymph nodes may also be required. Approximately 30 percent of patients who are diagnosed already have metastatic disease.

As with other cancers, gallbladder cancer is "staged" (the degree of progression of the disease is categorized) according to the tumor, node, metastases (TNM) system of the American Joint Committee on Cancer (AJCC). Stage I and II cancers are localized within the gallbladder and surgically resectable. Stage III cancers have spread to surrounding tissues and are not generally cured by surgery. Stage IV cancers have metastasized.

Radiation therapy is often used as a follow-up to surgery and may help to kill remaining cancer cells. Chemotherapy may also be used after surgery, but oncologists report that it does not work very well for this type of cancer.

Perspective and Prospects

Gallbladder cancer was first diagnosed in 1777. More than two hundred years later, the prognosis for patients with this disease is still generally poor, depending upon the stage of the disease when the patient is first diagnosed. Of patients with stage I and II cancers, 80 percent survive five years or longer. For those with stage III cancer, the five-year survival rate drops to 8 percent, and for those with stage IV, only 2 to 4 percent survive. In the advanced stages of gallbladder cancer, the survival period is usually very short, about two to four months. Hospice referral is considered essential for these patients.

—*Lenela Glass-Godwin, M.W.S.*

See also Abdomen; Abdominal disorders; American Indian health; Cancer; Chemotherapy; Cholecystectomy; Cholecystitis; Gallbladder; Gallbladder diseases; Gastroenterology; Gastrointestinal diseases; Internal medicine; Jaundice; Radiation therapy; Stone removal; Stones.

For Further Information:

Alan, Rick, and Mohei Abouzied. "Gallbladder Cancer." *Health Library*, Nov. 26, 2012.

Clavien, Pierre-Alain, and John Baillie, eds. *Diseases of the Gallbladder and Bile Ducts: Diagnosis and Treatment*. 2d ed. Hoboken, N.J.: Wiley-Blackwell, 2006.

"Gallbladder Cancer." *American Cancer Society*, Jan. 18, 2013.

"Gallbladder Cancer." *MedlinePlus*, Apr. 10, 2013.

"General Information about Gallbladder Cancer." *National Cancer Institute*, Mar. 14, 2013.

Gunderson, L. L., and C. G. Willett. "Pancreas and Hepatobiliary Tract." In *Principles and Practice of Radiation Oncology*, edited by Carlos A. Perez et al. 4th ed. Philadelphia: Lippincott Williams & Wilkins, 2004.

Laczano-Ponce, E. C., et al. "Epidemiology and Molecular Pathology of Gallbladder Cancer." *CA: A Cancer Journal for Clinicians* 51 (2001): 349–364.

Toner, C. B., et al. "Surgical Treatment of Gallbladder Cancer." *Journal of Gastrointestinal Surgery* 8, no. 1 (January, 2004): 83–89.

GALLBLADDER DISEASES
Disease/Disorder

Anatomy or system affected: Abdomen, gallbladder, gastrointestinal system

Specialties and related fields: Gastroenterology, internal medicine

Definition: A family of disorders affecting the gallbladder, usually causing abdominal pain but occasionally symptomless.

Key terms:

bile: a complex solution formed by liver cells which is composed mainly of bile salts, fats, and cholesterol, which aids in fat digestion; it is secreted by the liver into a system of ducts connecting the liver, gallbladder, and intestinal tract

biliary colic: a distinct pain syndrome characterized by severe intermittent waves of right-sided, upper abdominal pain, often brought on by the ingestion of fatty foods; pain occurs when a gallstone obstructs the outflow of bile and usually resolves when the gallstone moves away from the outflow area

cholecystectomy: the surgical procedure that results in the removal of the gallbladder in its entirety; the two main techniques are the traditional open method and the laparoscopically aided method

cholecystitis: the disease that occurs when the gallbladder becomes inflamed or infected, which produces severe right-sided, upper abdominal pain, fever, and other signs of infection; a frequent indication for removal of the gallbladder

cholelithiasis: the presence of gallstones in the gallbladder

gallbladder: a muscular, walled sac located on the undersurface of the liver which stores and concentrates bile; under stimulus from the intestine in response to a meal, the gallbladder contracts and expels bile into the digestive tract to aid in fat digestion

gallstones: particles that form in the gallbladder when the solubility of the components of bile is somehow altered, also resulting in the precipitation of cholesterol; the gallstones, which can grow very large, are made up mostly of cholesterol but can be pigmented or contain other substances

laparoscopic cholecystectomy: a procedure in which the gallbladder is removed with the help of a telescopic eyepiece which is attached to a tube inserted into the patient's body; the surgery is done using four small incisions and allows the patient to recover much faster than the traditional method of open surgery

Causes and Symptoms

Gallbladder diseases affect a large number of people and are among the most common causes of abdominal pain. Most gallbladder problems stem from the presence of gallstones, which may be present in as many as one of every ten adults. In the past, anyone with gallstones was advised to have the gallbladder taken out, but this is no longer the case. It is now known that many people with gallstones never experience difficulty because of them.

A common gallbladder disease is biliary colic. This is usually manifested by severe right-sided, upper abdominal pain that is fairly repetitive. The pain may literally take the patient's breath away, but an episode usually lasts less than thirty minutes. The patient may also complain of right-sided shoulder or back pain, often caused by irritation of the diaphragmatic nerves, which are located just above the liver on the right side. Many people may confuse the pain of biliary colic with indigestion, because in some patients it may be experienced in the middle of the upper abdomen. This pain is almost always brought on by eating, since the gallbladder contracts in response to food in the intestinal tract. The meal triggering such an episode often is described as rich and fatty, and many patients soon learn what types of food to avoid. Biliary colic does not occur unless gallstones are present, because they tend to obstruct the outflow of bile from the gallbladder. The initial treatment for biliary colic usually consists of dietary manipulation, that is, the avoidance of fatty foods or other foods known to trigger the pain, but eventual recurrence and complications are likely, and elective removal of the gallbladder (cholecystectomy) is usually recommended.

When a diagnosis of gallstones is suspected, the physician will take down the patient's medical history and perform a physical examination. In most cases, however, such actions will yield no physical findings that are indicative of gallstone disease. Thus the diagnosis is usually confirmed by an imaging study of the gallbladder, in which the gallstones are either directly or indirectly visualized. The most commonly used imaging modality is the ultrasound test, which can be easily and rapidly performed with very reliable results. While the gallstones cannot actually be seen, they have a density that reflects, rather than transmits, sound waves. As a result, they create specific echoes and shadows that can be interpreted by the radiologists as gallstones. No patient should be treated for gallstone disease without such imaging to confirm the presence of gallstones.

A potentially serious type of gallbladder disease caused by gallstones is acute cholecystitis. In this condition, the outflow of bile is obstructed, usually by a gallstone that is stuck in the outflow tract, and severe inflammation and infection may develop. A patient with acute cholecystitis often complains of pain that does not go away promptly, may have chills or fever, and is usually found to have a very tender abdomen on the upper right side. The treatment of this condition is not controversial, and most physicians would probably recommend removing the gallbladder surgically. The only question remaining is whether the gallbladder should be removed immediately or electively, at a later date, if the patient recovers

---

Information on Gallbladder Diseases

Causes: Presence of gallstones
Symptoms: Varies; often includes severe and repetitive right-sided, upper abdominal pain; inflammation and infection; chills or fever
Duration: Acute
Treatments: Surgery, dietary management

---

from acute cholecystitis with conservative management, including the use of antibiotics and the avoidance of eating until the inflammation subsides.

Inflammation and infection can also occur, although rarely, in gallbladders that do not produce gallstones. This happens in very select circumstances and is called acute acalculous cholecystitis. It usually afflicts very ill patients who have been in an intensive care unit for a long time, patients who have needed a heart-lung machine as a result of open heart surgery, or patients who are unable to eat for an extended period of time because of other problems. These patients are often fed only intravenously, which can lead to severe gallbladder problems. The exact mechanisms are not entirely known, but alterations in blood flow and an impaired ability to fight infection may play a role. Whatever the cause, the treatment often remains the same: removal of the gallbladder that does not respond to conservative therapy.

Gallstones can also move out of the gallbladder and cause serious problems. The main outflow tract of bile from the gallbladder and liver is the common bile duct, and this is a place gallstones frequently lodge. The end of this duct is surrounded by a small muscle called the sphincter of Oddi, which may not allow the passage of gallstones. If they become stuck there, they can completely obstruct the biliary system, and the patient will appear jaundiced. Removal of the gallstones will cure the problem. The presence of gallstones in the common bile duct is also associated with the development of pancreatitis, an inflammation of the pancreas that can be severe and life-threatening. Removal of the gallbladder at an appropriate time will prevent future bouts of pancreatitis.

The gallbladder can also be a source of cancer. Although cancer of the gallbladder is not common, it is estimated that one of every one hundred gallbladders removed will contain cancer. Therefore, all specimens removed must be examined by a qualified pathologist and all reports must be reviewed in their entirety by the surgeon. If the disease is limited to a minor thickness of the gallbladder, no further therapy is needed, but if the tumor is larger, further surgery—including removal of part of the liver may be necessary. Gallbladder cancer grows silently in many patients, and it is often not detected until late in its course.

Treatment and Therapy

Because there is no simple way to prevent gallbladder problems, surgery plays a large role in their management. Removing the gallbladder, a relatively routine operation, results in a complete cure, with acceptably low complication rates and few long-term problems. While several exciting new ways of treating gallbladder and gallstone problems have been developed, the classic and standard method of therapy for gallbladder disease has been open cholecystectomy. This procedure entails making an incision across the upper right side of the abdomen a few inches below and parallel to the bottom of the rib cage. The muscles of the abdominal wall are cut, and the abdominal cavity is opened. The gallbladder, which is usually located right under this incision, is then removed and the incision closed in layers. This method of gallbladder removal has acceptable complication rates and is relatively safe and extremely effective. It allows the surgeon to inspect the entire abdomen and rule out other problems. One must consider, however, that this procedure constitutes major surgery. Most patients need to be in the hospital for a minimum of three to five days, and there is a considerable amount of pain with this incision. These problems have prompted surgeons to find a less invasive way of removing the gallbladder, thereby achieving better pain control and reducing the length of the hospital stay and the time lost from work and other activities.

A laparoscope is an optical instrument, composed of a tube connected to a telescopic eyepiece, that allows the surgeon to perform a procedure inside the patient's body. It has been employed in surgeries for many years, mainly in gynecological procedures, and has been widely adapted for removal of the gallbladder and for other types of surgeries. Laparoscopic cholecystectomy has become a procedure that all surgeons must know to stay current with the profession. The laparoscope and other surgical instruments are inserted directly into the abdomen through several small incisions, and the gallbladder is removed without a large incision having been made. The patients are often discharged the same day of

the surgery, and they return to work much faster than with the open technique.

Despite its advantages, there are some pitfalls with laparoscopic cholecystectomy, and it cannot be used for all patients. There is an increased incidence of certain injuries to other organs and bile ducts at the time of the operation because less of the area can be seen than with an open operation. In addition, patients who have had previous upper abdominal surgery are not candidates for this procedure, and for those with acute cholecystitis, severe inflammation may make this technique unsafe. For most patients, however, laparoscopic cholecystectomy can be performed easily and safely with minimal complications and excellent results. It is becoming the standard of care and will continue to change the way gallbladder surgery is performed. The laparoscope is also being used to perform appendectomies, ulcer surgeries, cancer surveillance, and all types of intra-abdominal surgery.

Radiologists and internists may play an important role in the management of gallbladder disease. In certain circumstances, the techniques performed by these specialists may be indicated for extremely ill patients who might not be able to tolerate an operation, or for whom the anesthesia might be too hazardous. Invasive radiologists can actually place a tube into the gallbladder with help from their imaging equipment and remove infection or troublesome gallstones from the gallbladder. This procedure can alleviate symptoms in some patients, who may not even require any additional intervention. These practices are not common, however, and they are usually reserved for the very ill patient who might not survive an open operation or is at extremely high risk to develop a certain complication.

Gallstones can migrate out of the gallbladder and cause problems if they lodge in and obstruct the common bile duct. This places the patient at high risk for developing jaundice and infection in the biliary system. The standard method for dealing with this problem continues to be open surgery. In this procedure, the gallbladder is removed through an incision and the common bile duct is also opened. The gallstones are removed through a variety of techniques, and the duct is then closed. A tube is placed in the duct to keep it open, because otherwise it could scar and become narrowed. Many of these patients must be hospitalized for a number of days, making this surgery an expensive one.

Internists who specialize in the diseases of the abdomen have become proficient at performing endoscopic techniques. These techniques came about after the development of fiber optics, which allow one to see through a tube, even if it is bent at a variety of angles. An endoscope, composed of surgical instruments, a light source, and fiber-optic cables, can be used to examine the lining of the stomach and intestines, allowing the diagnosis of many conditions.

Endoscopy is performed by inserting the endoscope through the mouth and into the patient's stomach and the first part of the intestines. From this location, the area where the common bile duct opens into the intestines can be seen, and this is often where gallstones become lodged. The gallstones can be removed with instruments attached to the scope, thus

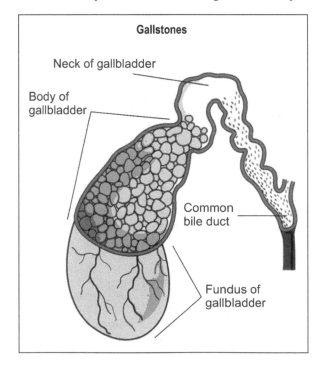

Gallstones

Neck of gallbladder

Body of gallbladder

Common bile duct

Fundus of gallbladder

solving the patient's problem. Unfortunately, this technique does not remove the gallbladder, the source of the gallstones, and the patient is at some risk for a recurrence. This risk can be minimized by enlarging the opening where the duct enters the intestinal tract. This technique, too, is advantageous for patients who are elderly or ill and cannot withstand the trauma of surgery and anesthesia.

There are other options besides surgery or dietary changes for the treatment of patients with gallstones. Medicines are available that can dissolve the gallstones by changing the chemical nature and solubility of bile. Such drugs, however, are not ideal: They work only for certain types of gallstones, are expensive, and may produce side effects. In addition, there may be a recurrence of the gallstones when a patient stops taking these medicines. Such a result indicates that the bile-concentrating action of the gallbladder combines with a given patient's bile composition to create a gallstone-forming environment. Thus, gallstones will continue to form unless the gallbladder is removed or the bile is again altered when the taking of such medicines is resumed. Patients can also have the gallstones broken up into very small pieces, as is often done with kidney stones, by high-frequency sound waves aimed at the gallstones. This procedure, however, known as lithotripsy, has drawbacks: It works in only a small percentage of patients (those with a limited number of small gallstones), and the results have not been uniformly consistent or satisfactory.

Perspective and Prospects

Diseases of the gallbladder and biliary system are common in modern industrialized societies. The exact etiologies are not entirely clear, but they may involve dietary mechanisms or other customs of the Western lifestyle. There is also evidence that genetic factors are important, as gallbladder disease often runs in families. Traditionally, the treatment of non-life-threatening gallbladder disease has been conservative, with dietary discretion being the most important factor. When that failed, or if the condition was more serious, the gallbladder was removed.

Open cholecystectomy was long considered the best method for dealing with these problems. This operation has been recently challenged by endoscopic and laparoscopic techniques, which have become widely available and enjoyed great success. These new treatment options will become more important as increasing medical costs promote the refinement of less invasive and better techniques. Nevertheless, open cholecystectomy is sometimes the only option for a patient, and less invasive techniques can have limitations as well as complications.

Basic scientific research is also important in this field. Investigations into the mechanisms of gallstone formation are critical to the understanding of gallbladder diseases, as gallstones are the cause of many of these problems. As with many other diseases, prevention might be the key to eliminating many gallbladder diseases, making biliary colic, cholecystitis, and common bile duct diseases rare.

—*Mark Wengrovitz, M.D.*

See also Abdomen; Abdominal disorders; Bile; Cholecystectomy; Cholecystitis; Gallbladder; Gallbladder cancer; Gastroenterology; Gastroenterology, pediatric; Gastrointestinal disorders; Internal medicine; Jaundice; Kidney stones; Laparoscopy; Liver; Liver cancer; Liver disorders; Liver transplantation; Obesity; Pain; Pancreatitis; Stone removal; Stones; Ultrasonography.

For Further Information:
Blumgart, L. H., and Y. Fong, eds. *Surgery of the Liver and Biliary Tract.* 3d ed. 2 vols. New York: W. B. Saunders, 2000.
Cameron, John L., and Andrew M. Cameron, eds. *Current Surgical Therapy.* 10th ed. Philadelphia: Mosby/Elsevier, 2011.
Choi, Young, and William B. Silverman. "Biliary Tract Disorders, Gallbladder Disorders, and Gallstone Pancreatitis." *American College of Gastroenterology*, Nov. 2008.
"Gallbladder Diseases." *MedlinePlus*, Apr. 8, 2013.
Krames Communications. *The Gallbladder Surgery Book.* San Bruno, Calif.: Author, 1991.
Krames Communications. *Laparoscopic Gallbladder Surgery.* San Bruno, Calif.: Author, 1991.
Porter, Robert S., et al., eds. *The Merck Manual Home Health Handbook.* 3d ed. Whitehouse Station, N.J.: Merck Research Laboratories, 2011.
Savitsky, Diane, and Marcin Chwistek. "Gallstones." *Health Library*, Sept. 30, 2012.
Zinner, Michael J., et al., eds. *Maingot's Abdominal Operations.* 12th ed. New York: McGraw-Hill, 2013.

GALLBLADDER REMOVAL. *See* CHOLECYSTECTOMY.

GALLSTONES. *See* GALLBLADDER DISEASES; STONE REMOVAL; STONES.

GAMETE INTRAFALLOPIAN TRANSFER (GIFT)
Procedure

Also known as: Assisted reproductive technology

Anatomy or system affected: Reproductive system

Specialties and related fields: Embryology, endocrinology, obstetrics

Definition: A treatment for infertility in which sperm and eggs are introduced surgically into a Fallopian tube, where fertilization (and subsequent implantation in the uterus) are expected to occur naturally.

Key terms:

assisted reproductive technology: any treatment or procedure involving the manipulation of sperm or eggs outside the body in order to achieve pregnancy

Fallopian tube: one of the pair of open-ended ducts branching from the top of the uterus, which collects eggs released from the ovary and in which fertilization usually occurs

fertilization: the union of egg and sperm

gamete: any reproductive cell, either egg or sperm

in vitro fertilization (IVF): the fertilization of eggs outside the body with subsequent implantation of embryos in the uterus

laparoscope: a thin, needlelike medical instrument containing a fiber-optic light source that is inserted through the skin and used both to visualize internal organs and to perform certain surgical procedures

ovulation: the release of a mature egg from an ovary

uterus: the female organ in which the embryo/fetus develops

zygote: a fertilized egg before cell division occurs; after the first division, it is called an embryo

Indications and Procedures

Couples who have sexual intercourse for a year without contraception and do not achieve pregnancy are defined as infertile. So too are couples who conceive but, because of repeated miscarriages, have not had a child. There are many possible causes of infertility. In women, they include abnormal or irregular ovulation, blocked or constricted fallopian tubes, and growths, scarring, or abnormalities of the uterus. In men, infertility may result from failure to ejaculate, low sperm count, abnormalities in sperm cells, or a blocked sperm tube. In many cases, no cause of infertility can be determined.

To have a child, some infertile couples turn to clinics offering assisted reproductive technology (ART) services. The most common form of ART is in vitro fertilization (IVF). Gamete intrafallopian transfer (GIFT) is similar to IVF, but it does not involve fertilization outside the body. Gametes (sperm and egg) are collected and then surgically introduced into a fallopian tube, where fertilization is expected to occur naturally.

Women who have at least one fallopian tube open are considered candidates for any of the ARTs, if sufficient numbers of healthy sperm can be collected from the male partner. GIFT may be the ART of choice for young women who have never undergone laparoscopy and for men with weak or few sperm. GIFT is sometimes employed in cases of unexplained infertility.

Prior to the procedure, egg maturation in the ovaries is stimulated with fertility drugs. With ultrasound guiding the probe, the physician retrieves eggs using a laparoscope. Sperm are collected several hours before the procedure. A laparoscope is also used to inject eggs and sperm into a fallopian tube. The patient may be awake or under general anesthesia for GIFT, which is typically done as a same-day, outpatient procedure. The American Society for Reproductive Medicine recommends that GIFT be performed only in a facility capable of performing IVF, in case GIFT fails or excess eggs are recovered.

Uses and Complications

All ART procedures involve risks, including general surgical risks and pregnancy complications such as multiple fetuses, low birth weight, and possibly certain birth defects. The rate of ectopic pregnancy (implantation outside the uterus) is also slightly higher. Multiple fetuses, which are present in nearly one-third of ART pregnancies, are associated with increased risk of prematurity, low birth weight, and neonatal death in the infant and of cesarean section and hemorrhage in the mother. Although ARTs are emotionally taxing, physically demanding, and expensive, thousands of infertile couples seek them annually.

The possible side effects of the hormonal drugs used to induce ovulation include hot flashes, changes in vision, ovarian cysts (sacs of fluid forming in the ovary), ovarian enlargement, and leakage of fluid into the abdominal cavity, which can trigger kidney failure, strokes, and heart attacks if not treated. IVF entails a slightly increased risk of chromosomal birth defects; whether GIFT carries a similar risk is unknown. ARTs do not appear to increase the overall risk of birth defects, although specific defects, such as vision problems, have been uncovered in some studies.

Some couples choose GIFT because they consider it more natural than IVF. However, GIFT is a riskier procedure than IVF, because laparoscopic surgery is required. Also, because fertilization is not confirmed before the injection of gametes, there is no way of knowing whether it occurred unless pregnancy is achieved. The mother's age is an important factor: the younger the mother, the better the chance of success.

Perspective and Prospects

Before the 1970s, infertility treatment was limited mostly to the surgical repair of blocked Fallopian tubes and the insertion of sperm into the uterus (artificial insemination). In the early 1960s, Min Chang, a scientist at the Worcester Foundation in Shrewsbury, Massachusetts, performed the first IVF. He used sperm and eggs from black rabbits to grow embryos in vitro (meaning literally "in glass," or in a laboratory dish). He then placed the embryos in the uterus of a white rabbit. A litter of black pups was born.

In 1969, English physician Robert G. Edwards successfully fertilized human eggs in vitro. Cell division was achieved a year later. He next collaborated with English physician Patrick Steptoe, who specialized in laparoscopic surgery. Together, they developed reliable techniques for retrieving eggs and maintaining embryos. The result was Louise Brown, the first "test tube baby." She was born in England in 1978. In 1981, the breakthrough was replicated in the United States. During the following twenty years, more than one million IVF babies were born.

After that, the field of reproductive endocrinology flourished, as did the development of ART techniques. Ricardo H. Asch of the University of Texas at San Antonio performed the first successful GIFT in 1984. Another, similar development was zygote intrafallopian transfer (ZIFT), first successfully performed in 1986. ZIFT involves mixing sperm and eggs together outside the body and then confirming fertilization before the zygote is surgically placed in a fallopian tube. Another ART, intracytoplasmic sperm injection (ICSI), was introduced in 1992. It involves injecting a single sperm directly into an egg. It is often used in conjunction with IVF to fertilize eggs before embryo transplantation.

Research and development activities continue to improve ART methods and techniques. Certain conditions within the fallopian tube that interfere with ART can now be treated, and better culture media have been developed for growing and maintaining embryos. The selection of smaller numbers of higher-quality embryos may cut the rate of multiple pregnancies, and improved methods for identifying those couples most likely to benefit from ART are being perfected. Researchers hope that implanting smaller numbers of more mature embryos will reduce the number of multiple births and diminish the risks that they entail.

ARTs raise ethical and social issues. Some churches and religious leaders oppose ARTs because they believe them to be unnatural or because some of the embryos produced in vitro are subsequently destroyed. Other controversies include pregnancies achieved in women past their natural reproductive age and legal issues surrounding the ownership of reproductive cells and frozen embryos.

—*Faith Hickman Brynie, Ph.D.*

See also Assisted reproductive technologies; Conception; Embryology; Ethics; Genetic engineering; Gynecology; In vitro fertilization; Infertility, female; Infertility, male; Multiple births; Obstetrics; Ovaries; Pregnancy and gestation; Reproductive system; Uterus; Women's health.

For Further Information:

A.D.A.M. Health Encyclopedia. "Infertility." *MedlinePlus*, February 26, 2012.

American Society for Reproductive Medicine. "Assisted Reproductive Technologies." *American Society for Reproductive Medicine*, 2013.

Johns Hopkins Medicine Fertility Center. "Gamete Intrafallopian Transfer (GIFT)." *Johns Hopkins Medicine*, 2013.

Meniru, Godwin I. *Cambridge Guide to Infertility Management and Assisted Reproduction*. New York: Cambridge University Press, 2001.

Peoples, Debby, and Harriette Rovner Ferguson. *Experiencing Infertility: An Essential Resource*. New York: W. W. Norton, 2000.

US Department of Health and Human Services. *2002 Assisted Reproductive Technology Success Rates: National Summary and Fertility Clinic Reports*. Atlanta: Author, 2004.

GANGLION REMOVAL
Procedure
Anatomy or system affected: Feet, hands, tendons

Specialties and related fields: Dermatology, family medicine, general surgery

Definition: The removal of fluid-filled sacs which usually develop on the tendons of the wrists, fingers, or feet.

Indications and Procedures

Sacs containing synovial fluid surround tendons to reduce the friction on adjacent tissues during movement. These sacs can form cysts, known as ganglions, that range from the size of a pea to the size of a golf ball. Ganglion formation typically occurs around the tendons of the wrist but may also occur on the foot. Smaller ganglions are more common and often spontaneously disappear. Ganglions are not harmful and typically are not treated unless they cause pain or the patient desires treatment for cosmetic reasons.

To remove a ganglion, the physician will disinfect the skin overlying the cyst and insert a needle attached to a syringe in order to aspirate the fluid from the ganglion. This procedure usually reduces the ganglion's size only temporarily. Some physicians will make an incision into the skin and remove the whole ganglion. This procedure requires thorough disinfection of the skin using alcohol or povidone-iodine and may re-

quire a local anesthetic such as lidocaine to be injected under the skin. Surgical instruments are used to dissect the cyst wall from the tendon and surrounding tissues. The total removal of the ganglion usually prevents recurrence, although ganglions may recur even after surgery in some cases.

Uses and Complications

As in any invasive procedure, the physician performing the surgical removal of a ganglion must be cautious so as to prevent infections or damage to surrounding healthy tissues.

The larger the ganglion, the greater are the potential complications. A longer incision must be made, which allows a large site for potential bacterial invasion and infection. The larger ganglion also requires more extensive dissection from surrounding tissues, which increases the possibility of injury to these structures. Although it is rare, tendons, ligaments, and nerves can be permanently damaged in ganglion removal. For example, if a ganglion was located in the wrist and the underlying tendons and nerves were severely damaged, the result may be a limited use or loss of use of the hand.

—*Matthew Berria, Ph.D.,*
and Douglas Reinhart, M.D.

See also Abscess removal; Abscesses; Cyst removal; Cysts; Nervous system; Neurology; Tendon disorders; Tendon repair.

For Further Information:

American Society for Surgery of the Hand. "Ganglion Cysts." *American Society for Surgery of the Hand*, 2012.

Carson-DeWitt, Rosalyn. "Ganglion Cyst." *Health Library*, June 6, 2013.

Foot Health Facts. "Ganglion Cyst." *American College of Foot and Ankle Surgeons*, 2013.

Icon Health. *Ganglions: A Medical Dictionary, Bibliography, and Annotated Research Guide to Internet References*. San Diego, Calif.: Author, 2004.

Kikuchi, Kenji, and Masahiro Saito. "Ganglion-Cell Tumor of the Filum Terminale: Immunohistochemical Characterization." *Tohoku Journal of Experimental Medicine* 188, no. 3 (July, 1999): 245–56.

Lenfant, C., R. Paoletti, and A. Albertini, eds. *Growth Factors of the Vascular and Nervous Systems: Functional Characterization and Biotechnology*. New York: S. Karger, 1992.

McLendon, Roger E., et al. *Pathology of Tumors of the Central Nervous System: A Guide to Histological Diagnosis*. New York: Oxford University Press, 2000.

GANGLIONS. *See* CYSTS; GANGLION REMOVAL.

GANGRENE
Disease/Disorder
Also known as: Gas gangrene

Anatomy or system affected: Heart, muscles, skin

Specialties and related fields: Bacteriology, dermatology, emergency medicine

Definition: Gas gangrene is an infectious disease usually caused by *Clostridium perfringens*, a spore-producing bacterium that is usually found in soil and the gastrointestinal tract of humans and other animals.

Key terms:

aerobic: living or growing only in the presence of air

anaerobic: living without air

exotoxin: a poisonous substance that is secreted by a microorganism and released into the surrounding environment

myo-: a prefix that refers to muscle

necrosis: death of a cell or tissue as a result of injury or trauma

organism: a form of life that contains mutually independent components

sepsis: local or generalized invasion of the body by an organism or its toxins, which can cause death

spontaneous: growing naturally without cultivation

spore: a walled-off cell that can reproduce directly or indirectly

Causes and Symptoms

Gangrene involves tissue death (necrosis) due to lack of blood flow or bacterial infection. There are three main types of gangrene: dry gangrene, wet gangrene, and gas gangrene. Dry gangrene refers to necrosis caused by blood flow interruption without bacterial infection, as from diseases such as diabetes and atherosclerosis that impair the circulatory system. Dry gangrene affects the extremities, most commonly the toes and feet, and presents as dry, shriveled, purplish or blackened skin that looks like it has been mummified. Wet gangrene and gas gangrene, on the other hand, are both caused by bacterial infections. Wet gangrene can be caused by a variety of bacteria that infect damaged tissue following an injury or trauma, such as bedsores or frostbite. The infected tissue can blister or swell and emit a foul-smelling discharge. Wet gangrene is more dangerous than dry gangrene because of the risk of sepsis, or infection spreading to the whole rest of the body, often resulting in death. Gas gangrene is a specific kind of bacterial infection, usually *Clostridium perfringens* but sometimes *Clostridium septicum*, that affects deep muscle tissue. It is generally the result of trauma or surgery, although it can occur spontaneously. The infection begins deep beneath the skin, but eventually large patches of skin can turn dark purple and develop large dark blisters. The disease is known for its quick progression, muscle and tissue death, gas production, and, ultimately, sepsis. Not every infected wound will progress to wet or gas gangrene; they occur only if there is sufficient tissue death, as the dead tissue provides an excellent environment for the bacteria to grow and flourish.

With gas gangrene that is the result of surgery or trauma, bacteria enter the body through an opening in the skin. When the involved tissue becomes compromised because of a lack of blood, infection occurs and the process of necrosis begins. Spontaneous gas gangrene occurs when the bacteria spread from the gastrointestinal tract (stomach and intestines) in people with colon cancer. When there is a small tear in the gastrointestinal tract, the bacteria enter the bloodstream and spread to the muscles. Spontaneous gas gangrene is caused by *Clostridium septicum*. *C. septicum* is different from *C. perfringens* because it can survive and grow in conditions that are aerobic. In both types of gas gangrene, the real cause

Information on Gangrene
Causes: Trauma, bacterial infection
Symptoms: Pain, fever, blisters, sweating, rapid heart rate
Duration: Acute
Treatments: Antibiotics, surgery, amputation

of the associated problems are the exotoxins that are released. These exotoxins destroy cells, resulting in tissue death that can also affect the heart muscle.

Treatment and Therapy

The usual treatment for gangrene is the removal of dead and dying tissue (a procedure called abridgement), usually surgically, to improve the healing of surrounding tissue. Sometimes skin grafts may be used to repair the damaged area. However, if the damage is too extensive, amputation of the affected digits or limb may be required. In the case of gangrene caused by bacterial infection, an immediate course of intravenous antibiotics is also pursued. Blood thinners may also be administered to prevent blood clots. Gas gangrene is an infectious disease emergency, and the patient should be evaluated immediately. An additional treatment for gas gangrene is a procedure called hyperbaric oxygen therapy, in which the patient is placed in a small chamber that is filled with oxygen at greater than normal atmospheric pressure. This forces more oxygen into the blood, which is detrimental to the growth of *Clostridium septicum*, because it is an anaerobic bacterium, meaning it thrives in the absence of oxygen.

To prevent gangrene, early wound care is mandatory. The use of antibiotics to prevent infection is also important in the care of a patient who has sustained trauma. Once the diagnosis of gangrene has been made, aggressive management that includes cutting away the dead tissue, managing the basic life support parameters, antibiotics, and surgery if needed, will improve the prognosis. Therefore, the mainstay of treatment is early identification and aggressive treatment.

—Rosslynn S. Byous, D.P.A., PA-C

See also Amputation; Bacterial infections; Embolism; Food poisoning; Frostbite; Hernia; Hernia repair; Hyperbaric oxygen therapy; Infection; Necrosis; Poisoning; Thrombosis and thrombus; Wounds.

For Further Information:

Carson-DeWitt, Rosalyn. "Gangrene." *Health Library*, September 30, 2012.

Folstad, Steven G. "Soft Tissue Infections." In *Emergency Medicine: A Comprehensive Study Guide*, edited by Judith E. Tintinalli. 6th ed. New York: McGraw-Hill, 2004.

"Gangrene." *Mayo Clinic*, August 10, 2011.

"Gangrene." *MedlinePlus*, August 24, 2011.

Urschel, John D. "Necrotizing Soft Tissue Infections." *Postgraduate Medical Journal* 75 (November, 1999): 645–649.

Wong, Jason K., et al. "Gas Gangrene." http://www .emedicine.com/ emerg/topic211.htm.

GASTRECTOMY

Procedure

Anatomy or system affected: Abdomen, gastrointestinal system, stomach

Specialties and related fields: Gastroenterology, general surgery, oncology

Definition: The surgical removal of all or part of the stomach.

Key terms:

anesthesia: the use of drugs to inhibit pain and alter consciousness

duodenum: the first part of the small intestine, located just after the stomach and before the jejunum

hemostasis: the control of bleeding

incision: a cut made with a scalpel

jejunum: a region of the small intestine located after the duodenum

suture: a thread used to unite parts of the body

Indications and Procedures

The stomach is an important organ in the gastrointestinal system. It receives the food that has been swallowed from the esophagus and immediately begins to process it. The stomach produces and secretes gastric juices, which include hydrochloric acid and an enzyme called pepsin for digestion. As the stomach collects it, food is churned and mixed with the gastric fluid before it is passed to the first region of the small intestine, the duodenum. Occasionally, the stomach becomes cancerous or has an ulcer that will not heal and thus must be surgically removed.

Complete removal of the stomach, a total gastrectomy, is a relatively rare operation usually performed to treat stomach cancer. Partial gastrectomy, however, in which only the diseased portion of the stomach is removed surgically, is fairly common. A partial gastrectomy is often performed to treat a peptic ulcer that fails to heal after medical treatment. Peptic ulcers, which include gastric and more commonly duodenal ulcers, may not respond to drug therapy and can place the patient at risk for bleeding into the gastrointestinal tract or even complete perforation of the stomach or duodenal wall. Therefore, the indications for gastrectomy include perforation, obstruction, massive bleeding, and severe abdominal pain.

Gastrectomy requires hospitalization, general anesthesia, and postoperative care. An anesthesiologist will administer a general anesthetic, rendering the patient unconscious and insensible to pain during the operation. A nasogastric tube is passed into the stomach via the nose and nasal cavity so that any stomach contents can be removed using suction before an incision is made into the stomach.

During total gastrectomy, the whole stomach is removed and the esophagus is attached to the jejunum. The two most common types of partial gastrectomy surgeries are the Billroth I and Billroth II. A surgeon performing a Billroth I will remove the diseased part of the stomach and attach the remaining healthy stomach to the duodenum. The Billroth I is also known as gastroduodenostomy. This operation preserves most of the digestive functions. Billroth II gastrectomy requires the surgeon to perform a gastrojejunostomy in which the remaining stomach is joined with the jejunum and bypasses the duodenum. Thus the opening of the duodenum must be closed to prevent the digestive contents from escaping into the abdominal cavity.

During the recovery period, the nasogastric tube is left in

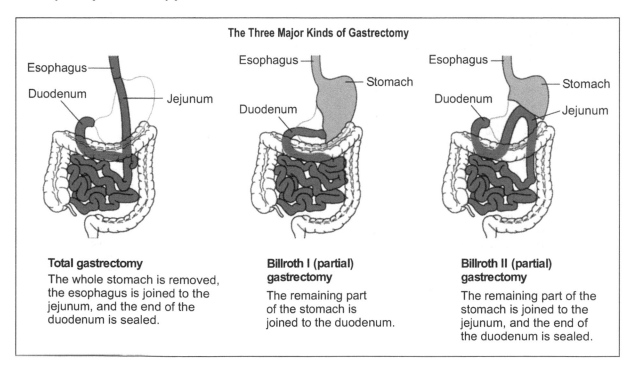

The Three Major Kinds of Gastrectomy

Esophagus — Duodenum — Jejunum

Esophagus — Stomach — Duodenum

Esophagus — Stomach — Duodenum — Jejunum

Total gastrectomy
The whole stomach is removed, the esophagus is joined to the jejunum, and the end of the duodenum is sealed.

Billroth I (partial) gastrectomy
The remaining part of the stomach is joined to the duodenum.

Billroth II (partial) gastrectomy
The remaining part of the stomach is joined to the jejunum, and the end of the duodenum is sealed.

place to help drain the secretions from the gastrointestinal system until the body is recovered enough to eliminate these secretions normally. Once the normal movement of the digestive tract (peristalsis) is detected, the patient is given very small amounts of fluid. If the intestines can process the ingested fluids, then the nasogastric tube is removed and the amount of fluid ingested is gradually increased. Typically, if there is no pain or nausea and vomiting, the patient can be started on a diet containing small amounts of solid food.

Uses and Complications

The risk of complications is relatively high in a total gastrectomy and lessens if smaller portions of the stomach are removed. The overall rate of complications is approximately 10 percent.

Since the stomach has such an important role in the process of digestion, it is not surprising that complications and adverse effects occur postsurgically. Some of the most common symptoms noted after gastrectomy include a feeling of discomfort and fullness after ingesting a relatively small meal. This feeling is attributable to the fact that the stomach volume has been reduced in a partial gastrectomy or eliminated in a total gastrectomy. New ulcers may also form and necessitate further drug treatment. Gastritis (inflammation of the stomach lining) may also occur after surgery, as well as a condition called dumping syndrome. Patients with dumping syndrome feel weak, nauseated, and light-headed after a meal because the food moves too rapidly out of the stomach. Most of these side effects can be treated with medications and dietary changes.

Long-term complications include malabsorption problems. Occasionally after gastrectomy, the digestive system cannot compensate adequately for the loss of the stomach, leading to poor digestion and absorption of nutrients. The most common malabsorptive disorder following gastrectomy is the inability to absorb vitamin B_{12}. The stomach produces a substance called intrinsic factor which is required for the absorption of this essential vitamin. Without intrinsic factor and the ability to absorb vitamin B_{12}, the patient must receive monthly injections of the vitamin for the rest of his or her life.

Perspective and Prospects

Early detection of stomach cancers and ulcers may help reduce the need for gastrectomies. Endoscopic examinations in which the physician can observe the lining of the stomach through a surgical tube passed into the patient's mouth and down the esophagus may aid in the early detection of stomach problems such as cancer and ulcers that are failing to heal.

Aggressive medical management of gastrointestinal ulcers will likely reduce the chance that an ulcer will perforate and require gastrectomy. Antiulcer medications are available to reduce the amount of stomach acid released, to add to the protective barrier of the stomach, and to eradicate the bacteria known to cause many ulcers. Destroying the bacteria, *Helicobacter pylori*, increases the likelihood of curing the patient of ulcer formation.

—Matthew Berria, Ph.D.,
and Douglas Reinhart, M.D.

See also Bariatric surgery; Cancer; Digestion; Gastroenterology; Gastrointestinal disorders; Gastrointestinal system; Ileostomy and colostomy; Oncology; Stomach, intestinal, and pancreatic cancers; Ulcer surgery; Ulcers; Vitamins and minerals.

For Further Information:

Brunicardi, F. Charles, et al., eds. *Schwartz's Principles of Surgery.* 9th ed. New York: McGraw-Hill, 2010.
"Gastrectomy." *MedlinePlus*, December 10, 2012.
Leikin, Jerrold B., and Martin S. Lipsky, eds. *American Medical Association Complete Medical Encyclopedia*. New York: Random House Reference, 2003.
Mohamed, Habeeb. "Laparoscopic Sleeve Gastrectomy: An Ideal Procedure for Control of Morbid Obesity." *World Journal of Laparoscopic Surgery* 5, no. 2 (May–August, 2012): 89–101.
McCoy, Krisha. "Gastrectomy." *Health Library*, November 26, 2012.

GASTRIC BYPASS. *See* BARIATRIC SURGERY.

GASTRITIS. *See* ABDOMINAL DISORDERS; GASTROENTERITIS; GASTROINTESTINAL DISORDERS.

GASTROENTERITIS
Disease/Disorder
Also known as: Stomach flu
Anatomy or system affected: Abdomen, gastrointestinal system, intestines, stomach
Specialties and related fields: Bacteriology, environmental health, gastroenterology, internal medicine, microbiology, virology
Definition: An acute infectious process affecting the gastrointestinal system, usually leading to abdominal discomfort and diarrhea.
Key terms:
colitis: inflammation of the large intestine (colon), which usually is associated with bloody diarrhea and fever
diarrhea: loose or watery stools, usually a decrease in consistency or increase in frequency from an individual baseline
incubation period: the time between first exposure to an organism and onset of symptoms
transmission: the mode of acquiring a disease

Causes and Symptoms

Gastroenteritis refers to the infection of the intestinal tract and is most commonly due to viruses, although bacteria and parasites also contribute to a lesser degree. The most common viruses involved are rotavirus and norovirus, which together cause more than 90 percent of viral gastroenteritis cases. Less common viral etiologies include adenovirus and astrovirus.

Rotavirus is most likely to cause gastroenteritis in infants and young children and can lead to significant dehydration. Infection in adults is less common and is usually without symptoms. Transmission is by the fecal-oral route, and viral shedding from stools can last up to ten days. The incubation period is about forty-eight hours.

Norovirus affects all age groups, usually in settings such as

Information on Gastroenteritis

Causes: Viruses, bacteria, parasites
Symptoms: Fever, abdominal discomfort, diarrhea, nausea, vomiting, rectal urgency, loss of appetite, generalized weakness
Duration: Acute; can be chronic
Treatments: Hydration, antidiarrheals, antibiotics, antiparasitics

restaurants with catered meals, hospitals, nursing centers, schools, day cares, and cruise ships. Transmission is by the fecal-oral route, with an incubation period of twenty-four to forty-eight hours. Norovirus is one of the top contributors of food-borne illnesses and is highly resistant to heating and chlorine disinfectants.

Gastroenteritis due to viruses usually affects the small bowel, leading to symptoms such as large-volume watery diarrhea, abdominal cramping, bloating, and gas. Fever and bloody stools are typically absent, although a low-grade fever can occur.

Bacterial causes of gastroenteritis are commonly due to *Campylobacter, Salmonella, Shigella,* and *E. coli.* Bacterial gastroenteritis is commonly transmitted through either ingestion of improperly cooked or handled food products or person-to-person contact. *Campylobacter jejuni* is the most common cause of *Campylobacter* infections and is often found in the gastrointestinal tract of food animals. Infection is usually caused by the ingestion of contaminated poultry. Most cases of *Salmonella* infections are due to *S. typhimurium* or *S. enteritidis* and are typically acquired from contaminated food products such as eggs, poultry, under-cooked meats, unpasteurized dairy products, seafood, and fresh produce. *Shigella* is most commonly transmitted via person-to-person contact and is commonly due to *S. dysenteriae, S. flexneri, S. boydii,* and *S. sonnei.* There are different strains of *E. coli* that cause gastroenteritis, such as hemorrhagic versus toxigenic strains, the former of which produces more severe symptoms and is usually due to ingestion of undercooked beef. Less common bacterial causes of gastroenteritis include *Vibrio cholera, Yersinia enterocolitica, Clostridium difficile, Staphylococcus aureus,* and *Bacillus cereus.*

Gastroenteritis resulting from bacteria usually affects the large intestine and produces symptoms of colitis, such as fever, small-volume bloody diarrhea, and rectal urgency. The small intestine can also be affected by certain bacteria, and the symptoms are similar to those caused by viruses.

Parasitic causes of gastroenteritis primarily include *Giardia lamblia, Cyclospora, Cryptosporidium,* and *Entamoeba histolytica.* They predominantly lead to persistent watery diarrhea (which can in turn lead to bloody diarrhea), sometimes for weeks; this is contrary to the duration of most cases of viral and bacterial gastroenteritis, which are self-limited and usually resolve in three to five days. The most common mode of transmission is ingestion of contaminated food or water.

Treatment and Therapy

Because most forms of gastroenteritis are self-limited, the mainstay of therapy is symptomatic treatment, focusing on rehydration and replacing important fluids and electrolytes lost through the diarrhea. Typical rehydration fluids consist of water, salt, sugar, and baking soda. During the acute illness, it is also advisable to temporarily avoid lactose products and caffeine.

Antidiarrheal agents are often used in gastroenteritis for symptomatic treatment of diarrhea. Commonly used agents include loperamide, bismuth subsalicylate, and diphenoxylate-atropine. These medications are usually used in viral gastroenteritis or in cases where bloody diarrhea or high fevers are absent, because in the latter cases the use of these agents may worsen the illness.

Antibiotics are typically not warranted unless the illness is severe, as indicated by the presence of persistent high fevers, bloody diarrhea, and frequent bowel movements. Antiparasitics are used if stool tests reveal the presence of these organisms.

Perspective and Prospects

Gastroenteritis is a very common illness that produces significant health issues in developing countries, where the medical care may not be adequate in cases of severe illnesses. This is especially true for malnourished infants and young children, who are more susceptible to the effects of severe dehydration. In developed countries, medical advancements have led to the production of antibiotics, antidiarrheals, and rehydration solutions. Intravenous hydration is also possible in severe cases.

Because infectious gastroenteritis is so common, it is imperative to take standard precautions to prevent transmission of the disease. This includes hand washing after handling suspected sources of infection, such as fecal content or raw meat, as well as ensuring that ingested food and water are properly cooked and processed.

The frequency of rotavirus infections in children has led to the development of a rotavirus vaccine, which was approved in 2006 by the Food and Drug Administration (FDA) and is now universally recommended for infants. A study published in 2013 in the *New England Journal of Medicine* showed that norovirus has become the most common cause of acute gastroenteritis in US children under five, perhaps due to the widespread use of the rotavirus vaccine. Efforts are under way to develop a norovirus vaccine as well.

—*Andrew Ren, M.D.*

See also Bacterial infections; Botulism; *Campylobacter* infections; *Clostridium difficile* infections; Diarrhea and dysentery; *E. coli* infection; Enterocolitis; Food poisoning; Gastroenterology; Gastroenterology, pediatric; Gastrointestinal disorders; Gastrointestinal system; Giardiasis; Intestinal disorders; Intestines; Nausea and vomiting; Noroviruses; Parasitic diseases; Poisoning; Rotavirus; Salmonella infection; Shigellosis; Trichinosis; Tularemia; Viral infections.

For Further Information:

Blaser, Martin, eds. *Infections of the Gastrointestinal Tract.* 2d ed.

Philadelphia: Lippincott Williams & Wilkins, 2002.

Butterton, Joan. "Infectious Diarrheal Diseases and Bacterial Food Poisoning." In *Harrison Principles of Internal Medicine*, edited by Anthony Fauci. 17th ed. New York: McGraw-Hill, 2008.

"Gastroenteritis." *MedlinePlus*, Apr. 19, 2013.

Mandell, Gerald, eds. *Mandell, Douglas, and Bennett Principles and Practice of Infectious Diseases*. 5th ed. Philadelphia: Churchill Livingstone, 2000.

"Norovirus Is Now the Leading Cause of Severe Gastroenteritis in US Children." *Centers for Disease Control and Prevention*, Mar. 21, 2013.

Gastroenterology

Specialty

Anatomy or system affected: Abdomen, gallbladder, gastrointestinal system, intestines, liver, pancreas, stomach, throat

Specialties and related fields: Internal medicine, microbiology, nutrition, oncology

Definition: The subspecialty of internal medicine devoted to the digestive tract and the organs aiding digestion.

Key terms:

biopsy: the use of special needles, forceps, and suction capsules to remove tissue samples for examination

endoscope: a long, maneuverable tube containing fiber optics through which physicians can view the gastrointestinal tract directly

enzyme: any of a large group of cell-produced proteins that act as catalysts for the chemical reactions necessary for digestion

motility: the spontaneous motion of the gastrointestinal tract's organs

peristalsis: the rhythmic waves of muscle contraction that move food through the esophagus, stomach, and intestines

procedure: any medical treatment that involves physical manipulation or invasion of the body

sphincter: a ringlike muscle that acts as a one-way valve to control the flow of fluids and waste

stool: the food wastes, mixed with bile and bacteria, that are eliminated through the anus

stricture: the narrowing of a passageway

Science and Profession

The gastrointestinal (GI), or digestive or alimentary, tract is a hose of layered membranes, about seven to nine meters long, that runs from the throat to the anus, allowing matter from the external world to pass through the human body. Along with its allied organs, glands, and nerve networks, the GI passage extracts the nutrients from food that are needed to fuel the body and excretes any substances that are left over. Physicians specializing in the GI system, gastroenterologists, care for everything from the upper esophageal sphincter to the anus; other specialists care for the mouth.

The GI tract has five major sections, each performing a different service: the esophagus, the stomach, the small intestine, the colon, and the anorectum. The esophagus begins where the throat ends, just below the vocal cords. It is a straight tube, about twenty to twenty-two centimeters long, with a valve at the top (upper esophageal sphincter). When food, formed into a ball and softened by chewing, enters from the mouth, rhythmic waves of muscle contractions (peristalsis) squeeze it smoothly toward the stomach, a trip that lasts about seven seconds. Peristaltic pressure triggers the lower esophageal sphincter to open, dropping the ball of food into the stomach; the sphincter immediately closes so that no stomach acids wash up into the esophagus.

The stomach, an ear-shaped bag that holds one to two liters of material, has three adjoining sections. First, the fundus, just below the lower esophageal sphincter, stores food. Second, the body mixes hydrochloric acid into the food, which breaks down proteins and kills bacteria, as well as a variety of enzymes, most of which also attack protein; a chemical is also introduced that prepares vitamin B_{12} for absorption in the small intestine. Third, the antrum grinds the food and pumps it through a sphincter (the pylorus) into the small intestine. Food usually takes from one to six hours to pass through the stomach.

The small intestine, about three meters long, loops and coils in the region from the rib cage to the pelvis. The first major loop, a squared U-shape, is the duodenum. Here bile from the liver and the gallbladder breaks down fats; water may come in from the blood if the food is salty, and enzymes from the pancreas and intestinal membrane glands continue digestion. The next section, the jejunum, absorbs most of the juices mixed with the food during digestion—up to eight liters—as well as minerals and nutrients. The last section, the ileum, takes out bile salts and vitamin B_{12}. After about three to five hours, the remnants of food, moved by peristalsis, reach another sphincter, the ileocecal valve.

The ileocecal valve admits the remaining contents into the colon, which is wider and has segments like a caterpillar. Also called the large intestine, it rises along the right side of the body in the ascending colon; turns ninety degrees into the transverse colon, which crosses to the left side of the body; and turns another ninety degrees into the descending colon, which drops to the sigmoid (S-shaped) colon—altogether a passage of more than a meter. The colon receives watery matter from the small intestine each day, and colon bacteria, of which there is a great variety, mix with the solids and complete digestion. The colon absorbs most of this remaining water.

The anorectum is the last stop. The rectum stores fecal matter, the waste products of digestion: bile, bacteria, undigested fiber, cells sloughed from intestinal linings, and mucus. When a sufficient mass has built up, about 100 to 200 grams, pressure signals the time for defecation. The puborectalis muscle, which is under conscious control after toilet training, relaxes, tilting the feces into a vertical position. The anal sphincter opens, and the feces exit the body as stool. It normally takes from four to seventy-two hours for wastes to pass through the colon.

Three organs attached to the GI tract participate in digestion: the liver, the gallbladder, and the pancreas. The liver makes bile, an oily green liquid that aids the absorption of fats and fat-soluble vitamins and which stores and processes absorbed nutrients, as well as removing toxic substances from food. Bile travels from the liver through the common bile duct into the duodenum; along the way, the gallbladder, a small pouch, stores the bile until it is needed. In addition to making insulin, the pancreas secretes various enzymes for digestion into the duodenum via the pancreatic duct.

The enteric nervous system (ENS), or "gut brain," regulates peristalsis, secretions, and some immune responses throughout the digestive tract, although its mechanisms are not completely understood. The ENS comprises an intricate network of nerves and ganglia laced through the linings of the gut membranes and muscles, and it senses the presence of food through various hormones and neurotransmitters. The vagus nerve connects the esophagus and stomach to the base of the brain; sacral nerves do the same job for the colon. Other nerves reach from the GI tract to the spinal cord.

Mark Twain advised people to eat whatever they liked and then let the foods fight it out in the stomach. When the GI tract reacts to disagreeable foods, however, the result can be pain; in fact, because of the great number of possible malfunctions (deadly or not), the GI tract is responsible for more discomfort and misery than any other major system.

Gastroenterologists spend the largest percentage of their time treating maladies that cause pain but do no lasting harm. For example, gas, a perennial problem for people of all ages, causes bloating, and its pain is sometimes so severe that it is mistaken for a heart attack. An array of poorly understood functional disorders of the colon, called irritable bowel syndrome (IBS), affects 15 to 20 percent of Americans. Affected individuals have nausea, diarrhea or constipation, and abdominal distress; this condition is popularly known as nervous stomach. Although not dangerous, it produces a bewildering variety of stomachaches. Likewise, chronic stomach and motility irregularities in the esophagus can affect digestion. Proctalgia fugax is intermittent, intense pain in the rectum.

Many GI diseases, however, can be deadly. Various cancers grow in the stomach, esophagus, and, most commonly among Americans, colon. (Cancers rarely begin in the small intestine.) Gastroesophageal reflux disease (GERD) occurs when stomach juices repeatedly sluice into the esophagus, where they irritate and inflame the membrane. Aside from causing a burning sensation, the juices can erode through the membrane, creating ulcers. If the membrane is eaten through entirely, a hole opens into the body cavity around the gut, spilling food, blood, and digestive juices. Emergency surgery is then needed. Although conventional wisdom has long attributed ulcers to emotional stress or bad habits, such as too much alcohol, recent research has determined that virtually all people with stomach or duodenum ulcers have a bacterium known as *Helicobacter pylori* in their gut. Most scientists now believe that *H. pylori* may be necessary for ulcers to form, although there is still some question about whether high levels of acid or long-term use of aspirin can produce ulcers independently of the bacteria. *H. pylori* may also play a role in the development of gastroenterological cancers. Patients with symptoms of ulcers or with cancers of the gastrointestinal tract should be tested for this bacteria and treated with an-

tibiotics. Ulcers can also occur in the stomach and duodenum as a result of motility disorders, excess acid, or drugs, especially alcohol and aspirin, that irritate the membrane. Regardless of cause, symptoms of ulcers are exacerbated by motility disorders, excess acid, or drugs, especially alcohol and aspirin, that irritate the membrane.

Colitis and Crohn's disease are serious inflammations of the gut lining, especially in the colon; except for some forms of colitis that are caused by bacteria, the mechanism behind such inflammation remains unknown, but the disorders frequently require surgery to remove damaged and inflamed areas.

Similarly, tears in the gut lining, strictures, passages blocked by chunks of food, exposed veins (varices), infected sacs in the colon (diverticula), and communicable diseases such as dysentery and hepatitis produce potentially deadly symptoms.

Diagnostic and Treatment Techniques

An extensive battery of tests, procedures, and medications enable gastroenterologists to cure or palliate many GI diseases. In addition to the traditional physician's tools of the physical examination and the patient's medical history, high-tech instruments let gastroenterologists see inside parts of the gut, produce images of it, remove tissue and stones, stop bleeding, and destroy tumors. Medicines kill bacteria, help regulate motility, speed the healing of damaged tissue, and control diarrhea and constipation. Yet the GI tract is a very intricate system, and at times, the gastroenterologist's most effective remedy is sympathy and advice about changing behavior or diet so that patients learn to live with their diseases.

Before treatment can begin, the disease must be identified. An interview with the patient and a medical examination constitute the first step in narrowing the range of possible causes of distressing symptoms. Symptoms described by the patient or discovered by the physician are clues to the underlying causes and suggest the kinds of tests that will most likely isolate the actions of a specific disease. Blood tests can reveal abnormal levels of white cells or chemicals and the presence of infection. Samples of digestive juices likewise can show chemical imbalances, infections, and bleeding, as can stool samples. Biopsies of the gut membrane, liver, and tumors allow pathologists to inspect tissue damage and look for viruses or bacteria. For example, a patient with yellowish skin (jaundice) and a tender liver who complains of nausea and chills may lead a physician to suspect hepatitis. The physician will then order a blood serum test, looking for specific proteins typical of hepatitis infection, and a liver biopsy to learn the type of hepatitis.

Some diseases, especially those destroying or inflaming tissue or involving motility problems, require imaging to identify, as do blockages and strictures. To obtain pictures of the gut, physicians use ultrasonography, X rays, magnetic resonance imaging (MRI), and computed tomography (CT) scans. Ultrasonographs transmit sound waves through the body and judge the density of tissues by the intensity and pattern of reflection; they are particularly useful for spotting gallstones. X rays, MRIs, and CT scans pass radiation through the body and record it on film or by sensors that feed data to a computer to construct an image. Plain X rays show the pattern of air and gas distribution in the digestive tract and can detect obstructions; X rays may also be taken after barium, a radioopaque element, has been swallowed or inserted in the colon so that it coats the GI tract's walls and makes them easier to see. Such imaging helps the physician to locate strictures, perforations, cancers, diverticula, blockages, and distended areas.

Few tests are more revealing, however, than a direct look inside the GI tract. Until the 1960s, this could not be done without exploratory surgery. At that time, the endoscope became widely available. Developed by British, American, and Japanese scientists, the endoscope is a long, flexible, maneuverable tube filled with fiber optic strands and a central channel for inserting various instruments. A light source at its tip illuminates the area ahead of the scope; the fiber optics collect the reflected light and pass it directly to the eye of the examining physician at the scope's opposite end, to a television monitor, or to a camera. There are many types of endoscopes, of which three are most common: The meter-long upper gastrointestinal panendoscope (or gastroscope), inserted through the mouth, can be used for seeing well into the duodenum; the 60-centimeter flexible sigmoidoscope is used in the rectum and sigmoid colon; and the lower panendoscope (or colonoscope)—180, 140, 100, or 70 centimeters long—inserted through the anus, can be worked through the entire colon and as much as 30 centimeters into the ileum. Most of the small intestine cannot be seen by endoscopy.

With endoscopy, gastroenterologists can spot and examine a diseased or damaged area of the gut and perform a biopsy so that tissue can be examined under a microscope. Yet endoscopes can do even more than that. They can push a wad of food obstructing the esophagus into the stomach, stretch open a stricture, or clear a clogged duct with wires inserted through the scope's channel; small balloons can be inflated inside the gut to widen constricted passages. Similarly, endoscopes with wire attachments can open a passage between the surface skin and the stomach, allowing food to be put directly in the stomach for patients incapable of swallowing, a procedure called percutaneous endoscopic gastrostomy (PEG). With looped and electrified wires, they can remove polyps, cut away tissue, and cauterize bleeding vessels and ulcers. One such procedure, endoscopic retrograde-cholangiopancreatography (ERCP), can image the biliary and pancreatic ducts and allow removal of gallstones without surgery. Drugs may also be injected through the endoscope to control bleeding from varicose veins (sclerotherapy), and fiber optics permit the use of lasers to vaporize cancerous tissue. Endoscopic treatments exist for chronic heartburn, including EndoCinch, a procedure that strengthens the lower esophageal sphincter (LES) by putting in stitches that pleat the tissue, and the Stretta procedure, which increases the thickness of the LES using radiofrequency energy. Endoscopy can also be used to treat GERD.

Gastroenterologists use drugs to sedate patients during procedures and to treat dysfunctions and diseases. Other medications available are too numerous and their administration too complex to describe in detail, but basically they ease pain, check diarrhea and vomiting, decrease acid production to permit ulcers to heal, soften the stool of constipated patients, control motility problems (such as spasms), regulate secretions, speed coagulation at bleeding sites, or kill harmful bacteria and parasites. GI pain, especially from irritable bowel syndrome, is notoriously difficult to treat because of the diversity of contributing causes, including emotional problems. Researchers turn out a steady supply of new drugs each year, but improvements are slow, and new drugs require extensive clinical trials to determine proper dosage and detect harmful side effects. Sometimes, a placebo—that is, a pill with no active ingredient, a "sugar pill"—is enough to make a patient feel better. The interaction between a patient's gut, nervous system, and personality is intricate and sometimes highly idiosyncratic.

Gastroenterologists do not simply react to disease and trauma with treatments; they also try to prevent trouble from starting in the first place. A large part of their job involves educating patients. They discuss diets that can reduce GI pain and warn against the abuse of drugs, especially alcohol and tobacco, that are known to contribute to heartburn and ulcers. They routinely screen patients over the age of fifty for cancer, sometimes by endoscopic examination, especially if there is a family history of cancer.

Perspective and Prospects

Jan Baptista van Helmont, a seventeenth century medical chemist, was the first to describe the diseases and digestive juices of the GI tract scientifically. Gastroenterology can be said to have started with his studies (he also coined the word "gas"). Yet no one directly observed the operations of digestion until 1833, when US Army surgeon William Beaumont cared for a French Canadian with a bullet wound to the stomach. The wound remained open, and Beaumont could watch the action of gastric juices and the stomach's mixing and grinding action. Throughout the nineteenth century, there were advances in the understanding and treatment of the GI tract, including the introduction of enemas and gastric lavage (washing out), X rays, and an early form of endoscopy.

As it did for most branches of medicine, twentieth century technology greatly expanded the role of gastroenterology in diagnosing, preventing, and treating disease. Imaging and endoscopy especially have revolutionized the field. In 1932, Rudolph Schindler developed a flexible gastroscope, and in 1943, Lester Dragstedt performed the first vagotomy (surgically cutting the vagus nerve) to reduce stomach acid secretions. Advances were also made to heal peptic ulcers with a special diet. The second half of the twentieth century saw an escalating number of refinements and innovations in procedures but was most remarkable for the development of drugs.

This progress has meant that far fewer surgical procedures are needed for common GI diseases. Because of new medicines, ulcer disease rarely requires surgery. Gallstones in the common bile duct that once necessitated surgical removal now may be taken out during an ERCP; a stent (perforated tube) can be inserted into a blocked bile duct under a gastroenterologist's guidance to keep bile flowing from the liver. Screenings for colon cancer and the removal of polyps, which can become cancerous, often identify cancerous or precancerous areas early and permit surgeons to remove tumors before the cancer spreads, sometimes making surgery unnecessary. Patients who once might have died because of a blocked or strictured esophagus can now be relieved and quickly released from the hospital. The overall trend has been shorter hospital stays and lower medical costs for common ailments. The sophistication of equipment and the training needed to treat difficult problems, however, have correspondingly inflated costs, as has the tendency to medicate painful ailments that sufferers once had to steel themselves to endure, such as irritable bowel syndrome.

Despite the expansion of gastroenterology's procedures and knowledge, it is far from an independent field. Gastroenterologists typically act as consultants, caring for patients only after they have been screened by family practitioners, emergency room doctors, and internists. Moreover, gastroenterologists rely on pathologists to decipher the information in biopsied tissue samples, radiologists to interpret imaging, neurologists to trace nervous system problems, and surgeons to repair perforated gut walls and remove diseased organs or transplant new ones. Finally, specially trained nurses and technicians must help them with many procedures and ensure that patients follow prescribed dietary and drug regimens.

—Roger Smith, Ph.D.;
updated by Caroline M. Small

See also Abdomen; Abdominal disorders; Acid reflux disease; Anus; Appendectomy; Appendicitis; Appetite loss; Bariatric surgery; Bile; Bulimia; Bypass surgery; Celiac sprue; Cholecystectomy; Cholecystitis; Cholera; Chyme; Colic; Colitis; Colon; Colonoscopy and sigmoidoscopy; Colorectal cancer; Colorectal polyp removal; Colorectal surgery; Constipation; Crohn's disease; Diarrhea and dysentery; Digestion; Diverticulitis and diverticulosis; *E. coli* infection; Emergency medicine; Endoscopic retrograde cholangiopancreatography (ERCP); Endoscopy; Enemas; Enzymes; Fistula repair; Food biochemistry; Food poisoning; Gallbladder cancer; Gallbladder diseases; Gastrectomy; Gastroenterology, pediatric; Gastrointestinal disorders; Gastrointestinal system; Gastrostomy; Glands; Heartburn; Hemorrhoid banding and removal; Hemorrhoids; Hernia; Hernia repair; Hirschsprung's disease; Ileostomy and colostomy; Indigestion; Internal medicine; Intestinal disorders; Intestines; Irritable bowel syndrome (IBS); Lactose intolerance; Liver; Liver cancer; Liver disorders; Liver transplantation; Malabsorption; Malnutrition; Metabolism; Nausea and vomiting; Noroviruses; Nutrition; Obstruction; Pancreas; Pancreatitis; Peristalsis; Pinworms; Poisonous plants; Proctology; Pyloric stenosis; Rectum; Rotavirus; Roundworms; Salmonella infection; Shigellosis; Small intestine; Soiling; Stomach, intestinal, and pancreatic cancers; Stone removal; Stones; Tapeworms; Taste; Toilet training; Trichinosis; Ulcer surgery; Ulcers; Vagotomy; Weight loss and gain; Worms.

For Further Information:

Brandt, Lawrence J., ed. *The Clinical Practice of Gastroenterology*. 2 vols. Philadelphia: Current Medicine, 1999.

Cheifetz, Adam S. *Oxford American Handbook of Gastroenterology and Hepatology*. New York: Oxford University Press, 2010.

Hay, David W. *The Little Black Book of Gastroenterology*. Sudbury, Mass.: Jones & Bartlett Learning, 2011.

Heuman, Douglas M., A. Scott Mills, and Hunter H. McGuire, Jr. *Gastroenterology*. Philadelphia: W. B. Saunders, 1997.

Janowitz, Henry D. *Indigestion: Living Better with Upper Intestinal Problems, from Heartburn to Ulcers and Gallstones*. New York: Oxford University Press, 1994.

Massoni, Margaret. "Nurses' GI Handbook." *Nursing* 20 (November, 1990): 65–80.

Peikin, Steven R. *Gastrointestinal Health*. Rev. ed. New York: Quill, 2001.

Plevris, John N. *Problem-Based Approach of Gastroenterology and Hepatology*. Chichester: Wiley-Blackwell, 2011.

Steiner-Grossman, Penny, Peter A. Banks, and Daniel H. Present, eds. *The New People, Not Patients: A Source Book for Living with Inflammatory Bowel Disease*. Rev. ed. Dubuque, Iowa: Kendall/Hunt, 1997.oxy_options track_changes="on"?

GASTROINTESTINAL DISORDERS
Disease/Disorder

Anatomy or system affected: Abdomen, gastrointestinal system, intestines, stomach

Specialties and related fields: Gastroenterology, internal medicine, microbiology

Definition: The many problems that can affect the gastrointestinal tract, such as infections, injuries, dysfunctions, tumors, congenital defects, and genetic abnormalities.

Key terms:

endoscope: any of several flexible fiber-optic scopes used to examine the inside of the gut; it is equipped with tools to cauterize wounds or remove tissue or gallstones

gastroenterologist: a medical specialist in diseases of the gut

intestines: the section of the gut between the anus and the stomach, consisting of the rectum, colon, and small bowel (subdivided into the ileus, jejunum, and duodenum)

motility: the spontaneous movements of the gut during swallowing, digestion, and elimination

mucosa: the tissue lining the interior of the gastrointestinal tract, through which nutrients pass into the bloodstream

stool: the waste products excreted from the body upon defecation; feces

tumor: a mass of abnormal cells that can be cancerous

Causes and Symptoms

What and how people eat, their digestion, and their toilet habits affect their health more than any other voluntary daily activity. Breathing, circulation, and the brain's control of most bodily functions normally take place without conscious thought. The intake of nourishment, by contrast, affords a great variety of choices. Accordingly, poor or self-destructive eating and toilet habits lie behind many gastrointestinal (GI) disorders. Yet not all disorders result from an individual's habits. Many arise because of a person's cultural or physical environment, some are hereditary or congenital, and a fair amount have no known cause. All told, more than one hundred disorders may originate in the GI tract and related organs, including infections, cancer, dysfunctions, obstructions, autoimmune diseases, malabsorption of nutrients, and

---

Information on Gastrointestinal Disorders

Causes: Congenital and hereditary factors, infection, cancer, obstructions, autoimmune diseases, malabsorption of nutrients, reactions to toxins

Symptoms: Varies; can include abdominal discomfort and pain, constipation, diarrhea, fever, nausea, weight loss, fatigue, indigestion, bloating, aversion to food, difficulty swallowing

Duration: Ranges from acute to chronic

Treatments: Drug therapy, surgery, dietary regulation, lifestyle changes

---

reactions to toxins taken in during eating, drinking, or breathing. Furthermore, diseases in other organs, systemic infections such as lupus, immune suppression such as that caused by acquired immunodeficiency syndrome (AIDS), reactions to altered body conditions as during pregnancy, and psychiatric problems can all affect the gut.

The symptoms of GI disorders range from mildly uncomfortable to life-threatening, although seldom does any single symptom except massive bleeding lead quickly to death. Indigestion, bloating, and gas send more people to gastroenterologists than any other set of symptoms, and they often reflect nothing more than overeating. Pain anywhere along the gut, aversion to food (anorexia), and nausea are general symptoms common to many disorders, although noncardiac chest pain is likely to come from the esophagus while pain in the abdomen points to a stomach or intestinal problem. Red blood in the stool indicates bleeding in the intestines, black (digested) blood suggests bleeding in the upper small bowel or stomach, and vomited blood indicates injury to the stomach or esophagus—all dangerous signs that require prompt medical attention. Chronic diarrhea, fatty stool, constipation, difficulty in swallowing, hiccuping, vomiting, and cramps point to disturbances in the GI tract's orderly, wavelike contractions or absorption of nutrients and fluid. Dysentery (bloody diarrhea) usually comes from severe inflammation or lesions caused by viruses, bacteria, or other parasites. Malnourishment is a sign of badly disordered digestion, and ascites (fluid accumulation in body cavities) can result from serious disease in the liver or pancreas. Likewise, jaundice, the yellowing of the skin or eyes because of high bilirubin levels, signals problems in the liver, pancreas, or their ducts.

The large number and complexity of GI disorders do not allow a quick, comprehensive summary. Fortunately, many are uncommon, and the most frequent problems can be described through a tour of the GI tract. The GI tract is basically a tube that moves food from the mouth to the anus, extracting energy and biochemical building blocks for the body along the way. Thus, a disorder that interrupts the flow in one section of the intestines can have secondary effects on other parts of the gut. Disorders seldom affect one area alone.

The esophagus. The GI tract's first section, the esophagus, is simply a passageway from the mouth to the stomach. Although it rarely gets infected, the esophagus is the site of several common problems, usually relatively minor, if painful. Muscle dysfunctions, including slow, weak, or spasmodic muscular movement, can impair motility and make swallowing difficult, as can strictures, which usually occur at the sphincter to the stomach. The mucosal lining of the esophagus is not as hardy as in other parts of the gut. When acid backflushes from the stomach into the esophagus, it inflames tissue there and can cause burning and even bleeding, a condition popularly known as heartburn and technically called gastroesophageal reflux disease (GERD). Retching and vomiting, usually resulting from alcohol abuse or associated with a hiatal hernia, can tear the mucosa. Smokers and drinkers run the risk of esophageal cancer, which can spread down into the gut early in its development and can be deadly; however, it accounts for only about 1 percent of cancers. Most esophageal conditions can be cured or controlled if diagnosed early enough.

The stomach. To store food and prepare it for digestion lower in the gut, the stomach churns its contents into a homogenous mass and releases it in small portions into the small bowel; meanwhile, the stomach also secretes acid to kill bacteria. Bacteria that are acid-resistant, however, can multiply there. One type, *Helicobacter pylori*, is thought to be involved in the development of ulcers and perhaps cancer. Overuse of aspirins and other nonsteroidal anti-inflammatory drugs (NSAIDs) can also cause stomach ulcers. A variety of substances, including alcohol, can prompt inflammation and even hemorrhaging. Stomach cancer has been shown to strike those who have a diet high in salted, smoked, or pickled foods; the most common cancer in the world, although not in the United States, it has a low survival rate. When stomach muscle function fails, food accumulates until the stomach overstretches and rebounds, causing vomiting. Some foods can coalesce into an indigestible lump, and hair and food fibers can roll into a ball, called a bezoar; such masses can interfere with digestion.

The small intestine. The five to six meters of looped gut between the stomach and colon is called the small intestine. It secretes fluids, hormones, and enzymes into food passing through, breaking it down chemically and absorbing nutrients. Although cancers seldom develop in the small intestine itself, they frequently do so in the organs connected to it, the liver and pancreas. The major problem in the small bowel is the multitude of diseases causing diarrhea, dysentery, or ulceration: They include bacterial, viral, and parasitic disease; motility disorders; and the chronic, progressive inflammatory illness called Crohn's disease, which also ulcerates the bowel wall. Although most diarrhea is temporary, if it persists diarrhea severely weakens patients through dehydration and malnourishment. For this reason, diarrheal diseases caused by toxins in water or food are the leading cause of childhood death worldwide. An increasingly common disorder of the small bowel is celiac disease, or gluten enteropathy, an autoimmune disease that results in malabsorption. Furthermore, the small bowel can become paralyzed, twisted, or kinked, thereby obstructing the passage of food. Sometimes its contents rush through too fast, a condition called dumping syndrome. All these disorders reduce digestion, and if they are chronic, then malnutrition, vitamin deficiency, and weight loss ensue.

The large intestine. The small intestine empties into the large intestine, or colon, the last meter of the GI tract; here the water content of digestive waste matter (about a liter a day) is reabsorbed, and the waste becomes increasingly solid along the way to the rectum, forming feces. Unlike the small bowel, which is nearly sterile under normal conditions, the colon hosts a large population of bacteria that ferments the indigestible fiber in waste matter, and some of the by-products are absorbed through the colon's mucosa. Bacteria or parasites gaining access from the outside world can cause diarrhea by interfering with this absorption (a condition called malabsorption) or by irritating the mucosa and speeding up muscle action. For unknown reasons, the colon can also become chronically inflamed, resulting in cramps and bloody diarrhea, an illness known as ulcerative colitis; Crohn's disease also can affect the colon. Probably because it is so often exposed to a variety of toxins, the colon is particularly susceptible to cancer in people over fifty years old: Colorectal cancer accounts for the fourth highest number of cancer deaths worldwide, in an equal proportion of men and women. As people age, the muscles controlling the colon deteriorate, sometimes forming small pouches in the bowel wall, called diverticula, that can become infected (diverticulitis). In addition, small knobs called polyps can grow, and they may become cancerous. One of the most common lower GI disorders is constipation, which may derive from a poor diet, motility malfunction, or both.

The rectum. The last segment of the colon, the rectum collects and holds feces for defecation through the anus. The rectum is susceptible to many of the diseases affecting the colon, including cancer and chronic inflammation. The powerful anal sphincter muscle, which controls defecation, can be the site of brief but intensely painful spasms called proctalgia fugax, which strikes for unknown reasons. The tissue lining the anal canal contains a dense network of blood vessels; straining to eliminate stool because of constipation or diarrhea or simply sitting too long on a toilet can distend these blood vessels, creating hemorrhoids, which may burn, itch, bleed, and become remarkably uncomfortable. If infected, hemorrhoids or anal fissures may develop painful abscesses (sacs of pus). Extreme straining can cause the rectum to turn inside out through the anus, or prolapse.

The liver. The GI tract's organs figure prominently in many disorders. The liver is a large spongy organ that filters the blood, removing toxins and dumping them with bile into the duodenum. A number of viruses can invade the liver and inflame it, a malady called hepatitis. Acute forms of the disease have flulike symptoms and are self-limited. Some viruses, however, as well as alcohol or drug abuse and worms, cause extensive cirrhosis (the formation of abnormal, scarlike tissue) and chronic hepatitis. Although only recently common in the United States, viral hepatitis has long affected a large number of people in Southeast Asia; because hepatitis can trigger the mutation of normal cells, liver cancer is among the most common cancers worldwide. Hepatitis patients often have jaundice, as do those who, as a result of drug reactions, cancer, or stones, have blocked bile flow. Because of congenital or inherited errors of metabolism, excess fat, iron, and copper can build up in the liver, causing upper abdominal pain, skin discolorations, weakness, and behavioral changes; complications can include cirrhosis, diabetes mellitus, and heart disease.

The gallbladder. A small sac that concentrates and stores bile from the liver, the gallbladder is connected to the liver and duodenum by ducts. The concentrate often coalesces into stones, which seldom cause problems if they stay in one place. If they block the opening to the gallbladder or lodge in a duct, however, they can cause pain, fever, and jaundice. Although rare, tumors may also grow in the gallbladder or ducts, perhaps as a result of gallstone obstruction.

The pancreas. Lying just behind the stomach, the pancreas produces enzymes to break down fats and proteins for absorption and insulin to metabolize sugar; a duct joins it to the duodenum. The pancreas can become inflamed, either because of toxins (largely alcohol) or blockage of its duct, usually by gallstones. Either cause precipitates a painful condition, pancreatitis, that may last a few days, with full recovery, or turn into a life-threatening disease. If the source of inflammation is not eliminated, then chronic pancreatitis may develop and with it the gradual loss of the pancreas" ability to make enzymes and insulin. Severe abdominal pain, malnutrition, diarrhea, and diabetes may develop. Pancreatic cancer has a very poor prognosis, with five-year survival less than 5 percent in most cases. Scientists are unsure of the causes; pancreatitis, gallstones, diabetes, and alcohol have been implicated, but only smoking is well attested to increase the risk of contracting pancreatic cancer, which is very lethal and difficult to treat. It is estimated that cigarette smoking is responsible for 30 percent of pancreatic cancer cases.

Functional diseases. Finally, some disorders appear to affect several parts of the GI tract at the same time, often with no identifiable cause but with chronic or recurrent symptoms. Gastroenterologists call them functional diseases, and they afflict as much as 30 percent of the population in Western countries. People with irritable bowel syndrome (IBS) complain of abdominal pain, urgency in defecation, and bloating from intestinal gas; they often feel that they cannot empty their rectums completely, even after straining. Functional dyspepsia manifests itself as upper abdominal pain, bloating, early feelings of fullness during a meal, and nausea. Also included in this group are various motility disorders in the esophagus and stomach, whose typical symptom is vomiting, and pseudo-obstruction, a condition in which the small bowel acts as if it is blocked but no lesion can be found. Many gastroenterologists believe that emotional disturbance plays a part in some of these diseases.

Treatment and Therapy

The majority of GI disorders are transient and pose no short-term or long-term threat to life. The body's natural defenses can combat most bacterial and viral infections in the gut without help. Even potentially dangerous noninfectious conditions, such as pancreatitis, resolve on their own if the irritating agent is eliminated. Many disorders require a gastroenterologist's help, however. Regulation of diet and the use of drugs to combat infections or relieve pain are important treatments. If these fail, as is likely to happen in such serious conditions as chronic inflammatory disease and cancer, cures or palliation is possible because of gastroenterological technology, particularly endoscopy, and surgical techniques developed in the twentieth century.

While it is not true that GI disorders would necessarily disappear with improved diet, since genetic disorders would remain, gastroenterologists stress that proper nourishment is the first line of defense against GI trouble. For example, incidence of stomach cancer plummets in countries where people eat fresh foods and use refrigeration rather than salting and smoking to preserve food. Regions where fiber makes up a high percentage of the diet, such as Africa, have a far lower incidence of inflammatory bowel disease. Last, and certainly not least, groups that do not drink alcohol or smoke (such as Mormons) have far lower incidences of cancer and inflammatory disease throughout the GI tract.

—*Roger Smith, Ph.D.*

See also Abdomen; Abdominal disorders; Acid reflux disease; Anal cancer; Anus: Appendectomy; Appendicitis; Appetite loss; Bacterial infections; Bariatric surgery; Bile; Botulism; Bypass surgery; *Campylobacter* infections; Candidiasis; Celiac sprue; Cholecystitis; Cholera; Chyme; Cirrhosis; Colic; Colitis; Colon; Colon therapy; Colonoscopy and sigmoidoscopy; Colorectal cancer; Colorectal polyp removal; Colorectal surgery; Constipation; Crohn's disease; Diabetes mellitus; Diarrhea and dysentery; Digestion; Diverticulitis and diverticulosis; Enemas; Enterocolitis; Fistula repair; Food poisoning; Gallbladder; Gallbladder cancer; Gallbladder diseases; Gastrectomy; Gastroenteritis; Gastroenterology; Gastroenterology, pediatric; Gastrointestinal system; Gastrostomy; Gluten intolerance; Heartburn; Hemorrhoid banding and removal; Hemorrhoids; Hernia; Hernia repair; Hirschsprung's disease; Ileostomy and colostomy; Incontinence; Indigestion; Internal medicine; Intestinal disorders; Intestines; Irritable bowel syndrome (IBS); Jaundice; Kwashiorkor; Lactose intolerance; Liver; Liver cancer; Liver disorders; Malabsorption; Malnutrition; Metabolism; Nausea and vomiting; Nonalcoholic steatohepatitis (NASH); Noroviruses; Nutrition; Obstruction; Pancreas; Pancreatitis; Peristalsis; Peritonitis; Pinworms; Poisoning; Poisonous plants; Polyps; Proctology; Protozoan diseases; Pyloric stenosis; Rectum; Rotavirus; Roundworms; Salmonella infection; Shigellosis; Small intestine; Soiling; Stomach, intestinal, and pancreatic cancers; Tapeworms; Toilet training; Trichinosis; Tumor removal; Tumors; Typhoid fever; Typhus; Ulcer surgery; Ulcers; Vagotomy; Weight loss and gain; Worms.

For Further Information:

Feldman, Mark, Lawrence S. Friedman, and Lawrence J. Brandt, eds. *Sleisenger and Fordtran's Gastrointestinal and Liver Disease: Pathophysiology, Diagnosis, Management*. New ed. 2 vols. Philadelphia: Saunders/Elsevier, 2010.

"Gastrointestinal Disorders." *Columbia University College of Dental Medicine*, March 1, 2013.

"GI Disorders." *International Foundation for Functional Gastrointestinal Disorders*, January 17, 2013.

Heuman, Douglas M., A. Scott Mills, and Hunter H. McGuire, Jr. *Gastroenterology*. Philadephia: W. B. Saunders, 1997.

Janowitz, Henry D. *Indigestion: Living Better with Upper Intestinal Problems, from Heartburn to Ulcers and Gallstones*. New York: Oxford University Press, 1994.

Sachar, David B., Jerome D. Waye, and Blair S. Lewis, eds. *Pocket Guide to Gastroenterology*. Rev. ed. Baltimore: Williams & Wilkins, 1991.

Thompson, W. Grant. *The Angry Gut: Coping with Colitis and Crohn's Disease*. New York: Plenum Press, 1993.

GASTROINTESTINAL SYSTEM
Anatomy

Anatomy or system affected: Abdomen, gallbladder, intestines, liver, pancreas, stomach, teeth, throat

Specialties and related fields: Dentistry, gastroenterology, internal medicine, nutrition, oncology, otorhinolaryngology

Definition: A compartmentalized tube that is equipped to reduce food, both mechanically and chemically, to a state in which it is absorbed and used by the body; this system includes the mouth, esophagus, stomach, small intestine, and colon (large intestine), as well as the salivary glands, pancreas, liver, and gallbladder.

Key terms:

absorption: the movement of digested food from the small intestine into blood vessels and from blood into body cells

bolus: food that has been mixed with saliva and formed into a ball; the bolus passes from the mouth to the stomach through a process called swallowing or deglutition

chyme: the semiliquid state of food as it is found in the stomach and first part of the small intestine

digestion: the mechanical and chemical breakdown of food into physical and molecular units that can be absorbed and used by cells

enzymes: substances that aid in the chemical digestion of food; enzymes are produced and secreted by glands found in digestive organs

peristalsis: a muscular contraction that helps to move food through the digestive tube

sphincter: a circular muscle that controls the opening and closing of an orifice

villus: a fingerlike projection in the small intestine that provides a site for the absorption of digested food into the circulatory and lymph systems

Structure and Functions

The gastrointestinal system or alimentary canal exists as a tube that runs through the body from mouth to anus. The wall of the tube is composed of four layers of tissue. The outermost layer, the serosa, is part of a large tissue called the peritoneum, which covers internal organs and lines body cavities. Extensions of the peritoneum called mesenteries anchor the organs of digestion to the body wall. Fatty, apronlike structures that hang in front of the abdominal organs are also modifications of the peritoneum. They are called the lesser and the greater omentum. The muscular layer, composed of circular and longitudinal muscles, makes up the bulk of the wall of the tube. The contractions of this layer aid in moving materials through the tube. Nerves, blood vessels, and lymph vessels are found in the third layer, the submucosa. The innermost or mucous layer has glands for secretion and modifications for absorption.

The tube is compartmentalized, and each section is equipped to accomplish some part of the digestive process. The mechanical phase of digestion involves the physical reduction of food to a semiliquid state; this is accomplished by tearing, chewing, and churning the food. Chemical digestion utilizes enzymes to reduce food to simple molecules that can be absorbed and used by the body to provide energy and to build and repair tissue.

The mouth (also called the buccal or oral cavity) marks the beginning of the gastrointestinal system and the digestive process. The mouth is divided into two areas. The vestibule is the space between the lips, cheeks, gums, and teeth. Lips, or labia, are the fleshy folds that surround the opening to the mouth. The skin covers the outside, while the inside is lined with mucous membrane. The colored part of the lips, called the vermilion, is a juncture of these two tissues. Because the tissue at this point is unclouded, underlying blood vessels can be seen. A membrane called the labial frenulum attaches each lip to the gum, or gingivalum.

The oral cavity occupies the space posterior to the teeth and anterior to the fauces or opening to the throat. It is bounded on the sides by cheeks and on the roof by an anterior bony structure called the hard palate and a posterior muscular area, the soft palate. The uvula, a cone-shaped extension of the soft palate, can be seen hanging down in front of the fauces. The floor of the oral cavity is formed by the tongue and associated muscles. Taste buds are found on the surface of the tongue. The bottom of the tongue is anchored posteriorly to the hyoid bone. Anteriorly, the membranous frenulum lingua anchors the tongue to the floor of the mouth. The tongue's movement is controlled by extrinsic muscles that form the floor of the mouth and by intrinsic muscles that are part of the tongue itself. The movements of the tongue assist in speaking, swallowing, and forming food into a bolus.

Teeth, found in gum sockets, are the principal means of mechanical digestion in the mouth. Human teeth appear in two sets. The deciduous or milk teeth are the first to appear. There are usually ten in each jaw, and they are replaced by the second, permanent set during childhood. The permanent set consists of sixteen teeth in each jaw. The four incisors and two canines have sharp chiseled edges, which permit biting and tearing of food. The four premolars and six molars have flat surfaces that are used in grinding the food. Frequently, the third pair of molars or wisdom teeth do not erupt until later in adolescence. The crown of a tooth appears above the gum line while the roots are embedded in the gum socket. The small area between the crown and the root is called the neck. The crown is covered with enamel and the root with cementum. Dentin is beneath the covering in both areas and forms the bulk of the tooth. The central cavity of the tooth is filled with a soft membrane called pulp. Blood vessels and nerves are embedded in the pulp.

At the rear of the mouth, the fauces or opening leads to the pharynx. The pharynx is a common passageway for the movement of air from nasal cavity to trachea and food from mouth to esophagus. The esophagus is a tube approximately twenty-five centimeters long. Most of the esophagus is located within the thoracic cavity, although the lower end of the tube pierces the diaphragm and connects with the stomach in the abdominal cavity. Both ends of the esophagus are controlled by a circular muscle called a sphincter. The movement of food through the esophagus is assisted by gravity and the contractions of the muscularis layer. No digestion is accomplished in either the pharynx or the esophagus.

The stomach, a J-shaped organ, is divided into four areas: the cardia, fundus, body, and pyloris. The cardia lies just below the sphincter at the juncture of esophagus and stomach, while the fundus is a pouch that pushes upward and to the left of the cardia. The large central area is the body, and the lower end of the stomach is the pyloris. Here another sphincter, the pyloric valve, controls the opening between stomach and intestine. The mucosa of the stomach is arranged in folds called rugae. The rugae permit distension of the organ as it fills. Gastric and mucus glands are present in the mucosa. The gastric glands produce and secrete enzymes that are specific for protein digestion, as well as hydrochloric acid, which creates the proper acid environment for enzyme action. The muscularis of the stomach wall has three layers of muscle with a circular, longitudinal, and oblique arrangement. The muscle arrangement facilitates the churning action that reduces the food to a semiliquid called chyme. The pyloric valve relaxes under neuronal and hormonal influence, and the chyme is moved into the small intestine.

The site for the completion of digestion and the absorption of digested material is the small intestine. This tube, with a 2.5-centimeter diameter and a length of 6.4 meters, is coiled into the mid and lower abdomen. The first twenty-five centimeters of the small intestine constitute the duodenum. This is followed by the jejunum, which is 2.5 meters long. The ileum, at 3.6 meters, terminates at the ileocecal valve, which connects the small to the large intestine. The interior of the small intestine is characterized by the presence of fingerlike projections of the mucosa called villi that contain blood and lymph capillaries and circular folds of submucosa (the plicae circularis), both of which provide absorption surface for the digested food. Mucosal glands produce enzymes that contribute to the digestion of carbohydrates, lipids, and proteins. Enzymes from the pancreas and bile from the liver enter the small intestine at the duodenum and aid the chemical digestion.

The final compartment in the gastrointestinal system is the large intestine, sometimes called the bowel or colon. This tube, with a diameter of 6.5 centimeters and a length of 1.5 meters, is divided into the cecum; the ascending, transverse, and descending colon; the rectum; and the anal canal. The cecum is a blind pouch located just below the ileocecal valve. The fingerlike appendix is attached to the cecum. The ascending colon extends from the cecum up the right side of the abdomen to the underside of the liver, where it turns and runs across the body. The colon descends along the left side of the abdomen. The last few centimeters of colon form an S-shaped curve that gives the section its name, sigmoid colon. Three bands of longitudinal muscle called taeniae coli run the length of the colon. Contraction of these bands causes pouches or haustra to form in the colon, giving the tube a puckered appearance. The sigmoid colon leads into the rectum, a twenty-centimeter segment that terminates in a short anal canal. The anus is the opening from the anal canal to the exterior of the body.

Disorders and Diseases

Because the primary function performed in the gastrointestinal system is the physical and chemical preparation of food for cellular absorption and use, any malfunction of the process has implications for the overall metabolism of the body. Structural changes or abnormalities in the anatomy of the system interfere with the proper mechanical and chemical preparation of the food.

Teeth are the principal agents of mechanical digestion or mastication in the mouth. Dental caries or tooth decay involves a demineralization of the enamel through bacterial action. Disrupted enamel provides an entrance for bacteria to underlying tissues, resulting in infection and inflammation of the tissues. The resulting pain and discomfort interfere with the biting, chewing, and grinding of food. Three pairs of salivary glands secrete the water-based, enzyme-containing fluid called saliva. These glands can be the target of the virus that causes mumps. (Although the pain and swelling that are typical of this disease can prevent swallowing, the more important effect of the virus in males is the possible inflammation

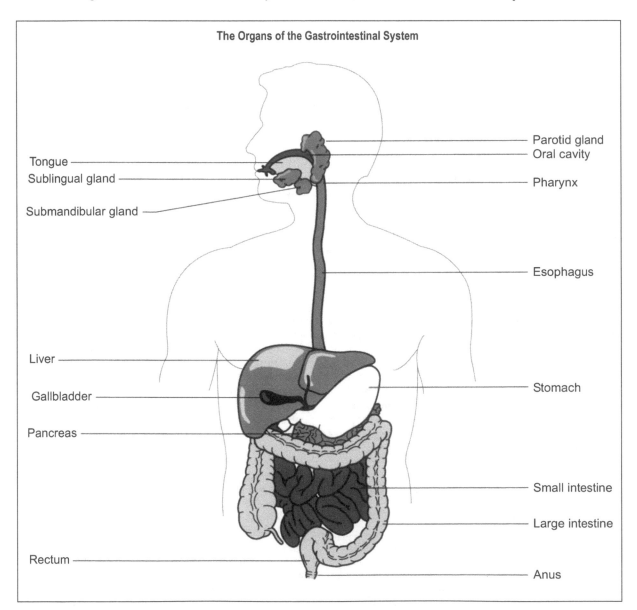

The Organs of the Gastrointestinal System

Tongue
Sublingual gland
Submandibular gland
Liver
Gallbladder
Pancreas
Rectum

Parotid gland
Oral cavity
Pharynx
Esophagus
Stomach
Small intestine
Large intestine
Anus

of the testes and subsequent sterility.)

The gastroesophageal sphincter at the lower end of the esophagus controls the movement of materials from the stomach into the esophagus. Relaxation of this sphincter allows a backflow of food (gastroesophageal reflux) to occur. The acidity of the stomach contents damages the esophageal lining, and a burning sensation is experienced. Substances such as citric fruits, chocolate, tomatoes, alcohol, and nicotine as well as body positions that increase abdominal pressure, such as bending or lying on the side, induce heartburn or indigestion. A hiatal hernia occurs when a defect of the diaphragm allows the lower portion of the esophagus and the upper portion of the stomach to enter the chest cavity; it causes heartburn and difficulty in swallowing.

Pathologies and abnormalities of the stomach and intestines are studied in the medical science called gastroenterology. The stomach is the site of both mechanical and chemical digestion. Although small amounts of digested food begin to pass into the small intestine within minutes following a meal, the chyme usually remains in the stomach for three to five hours. Relaxation of the gastroesophageal sphincter will result in reflux; and stimulation by nerves from the medulla of the brain can cause the forceful emptying of stomach contents through the mouth. This is called vomiting and may be brought about by irritation, overdistension, certain foods, or drugs. Excessive vomiting results in dehydration, which in turn upsets electrolyte and fluid balance.

Chemical digestion in the stomach requires an acidic environment. This is provided by gastric glands, which secrete hydrochloric acid. The tissue lining the stomach protects it from this acidity and prevents self-digestion. Oversecretion of the gastric juices or a breakdown of the stomach lining can cause lesions or peptic ulcers to form in the mucosal lining. Gastritis, the inflammation of the stomach mucosa brought on by the ingestion of irritants such as alcohol and aspirin or an overactive nervous stimulation of the gastric glands, may be the underlying cause of ulcer formation. Ulcers can form in the lower esophagus, stomach, and duodenum because these are the organs that come in contact with gastric juice. The terms "gastric ulcer" and "duodenal ulcer" refer to peptic ulcers located in the stomach and the first portion of the small intestine, respectively.

Gastroenteritis could involve the stomach, the small intestine, or the large intestine. It is a disorder marked by nausea, vomiting, abdominal discomfort, and diarrhea. The condition has various causes and is known by several names. Bacteria are a common cause of the condition known as food poisoning. Amoebas, parasites, and viruses can bring about the symptoms associated with intestinal influenza or travelers" diarrhea. Allergic reactions to food or drugs may cause gastroenteritis.

Although diverticulitis may be found anywhere along the gastrointestinal tract, it is most commonly found in the sigmoid colon. This disorder results from the formation of pouches or diverticula in the wall of the tract. Undigested food and bacteria collect in the diverticula and react to form a hard mass. The mass interferes with the blood supply to the area and ultimately irritates and inflames surrounding tissue. Abscess, obstruction, and hemorrhage may develop. A diet lacking in fiber appears to be the major contributor to this disorder.

Colitis, or inflammation of the bowel, is accompanied by abdominal cramps, diarrhea, and constipation. It may be brought about by psychological stress, as in irritable bowel syndrome, or may be a manifestation of such disorders as chronic ulcerative colitis and Crohn's disease.

A change in the rate of motility through the colon or large intestine results in one of two disorders: diarrhea or constipation. As food passes through the colon, water is reabsorbed by the body. If the food moves too quickly through the colon, then much of the water will remain in the feces and diarrhea results. Severe diarrhea affects electrolyte balance. Viral, bacterial, and parasitic organisms may initiate the rapid motility of substances through the colon. Another condition, called constipation, develops from sluggish motility. When the food remains for too long a time in the bowel, too much water is reabsorbed by the body. The feces then become dry and hard, and defecation is difficult. Lack of fiber in the diet and lack of exercise are the leading causes of constipation.

Hemorrhoids are varicose veins that develop in the rectum or anal canal. Varicose veins are the result of weakened venous valves. Factors such as pressure, lack of muscle tone as a result of aging, straining at defecation, pregnancy, and obesity are among the common contributors. Hemorrhoids become irritated and bleed when hard stools are passed.

Malignancies can occur at any point along the gastrointestinal tract. Cancers of the mouth are frequently associated with tobacco use. Esophageal cancer may be associated with heavy alcohol use, tobacco, or chronic reflux. Gastric cancer may be the result of chronic ulcer disease or heavy exposure to foods high in nitrites. Colon cancer is one of the leading causes of death in the United States, and it may be associated with certain genetic disorders or might arise spontaneously.

Disorders in the accessory organs contribute to the malfunctioning of the gastrointestinal system. Gallstones, cirrhosis of the liver, pancreatitis, and pancreatic cancer are among the major diseases affecting the digestive process. These disorders generally involve the obstruction of tubes or the destruction of glands, so that enzymes do not reach the intended site of digestion.

Perspective and Prospects

The proper functioning of the gastrointestinal system is dependent on the anatomical structure and health of the organs. The organs provide the site for the mechanical and chemical digestion of food, the absorption of food and water, and the elimination of waste material. Two factors play a primary role in causing anatomical abnormalities in digestion: aging and eating disorders.

The aging process gradually changes anatomical structure. For food to be chewed properly, teeth must be in good health. Dental caries, periodontal disease, and missing teeth prevent the proper mastication of food. Because of these problems, older people tend to avoid foods that require chewing. This may lead to an unbalanced diet. Another age-related change in the mouth is the atrophy of the salivary glands and other secretory glands, which interferes with chemical digestion and swallowing. A loss of muscle tone in the organ walls impedes mechanical digestion and slows down the movement of food through the system. Often, the elimination of waste material becomes difficult and constipation results.

Eating disorders such as anorexia nervosa and bulimia contribute to digestive malfunctioning. These disorders are most often associated with but are not limited to young women. Anorexia is self-imposed starvation, while bulimia is characterized by a binge-purge cycle that incorporates vomiting and/or abuse of laxatives. Both conditions induce nutrient deficiencies and upset water and electrolyte balances. The vomiting of the acid contents of the stomach damages esophageal, pharyngeal, and mouth tissue. It also destroys tooth enamel. In addition to the harm done to the gastrointestinal system, eating disorders affect several other systems, such as the reproductive system.

The field of medical science that studies and diagnoses digestive system disorders is gastroenterology. Gastroenterologists use several investigative techniques. Blood tests and stool examination are used to detect internal bleeding and deficiency disorders. For a time, X rays were the only nonsurgical means of obtaining information on the structure of internal organs. The advent of nuclear medicine in the 1950s led to the use of radioisotopes in body scanning procedures. Instruments capable of a more detailed and direct visualization were developed, such as fiber optics and the fluoroscope. Fiber optics involves the use of long, threadlike fibers of glass or plastic that transmit light into the organ and reflect the image back to the viewer; this method allows the physician to detect ulcers, lesions, neoplasms, and structural abnormalities. The fluoroscope uses X rays to permit continuous observation of motion within the organs.

The 1970s saw the development of more sophisticated scanning and imaging techniques. computed tomography (CT) scanning uses X-ray techniques to scan very thin slices of tissue and presents a defined, unobstructed view. Magnetic resonance imaging (MRI) can provide detailed information even to the molecular level; energies from powerful magnetic fields are translated into a visual representation of the structure being studied. Another technique, ultrasonography, passes sound waves through a body area, intercepts the echoes that are produced, and translates them into electrical impulses, which are recorded and interpreted by the physician.

—*Rosemary Scheirer, Ed.D.*

See also Abdomen; Acid reflux disease; Anus; Bariatric surgery; Colon; Constipation; Diarrhea and dysentery; Digestion; Endoscopy; Enzymes; Food biochemistry; Gallbladder; Gastroenterology; Gastroenterology, pediatric; Gastrointestinal disorders; Glands; Hemorrhoids; Hernia; Host-defense mechanisms; Indigestion; Internal medicine; Intestinal disorders; Intestines; Laparoscopy; Lipids; Liver; Malnutrition; Metabolism; Muscles; Nausea and vomiting; Nutrition; Obstruction; Peristalsis; Proctology; Rectum; Sense organs; Small intestine; Systems and organs; Taste; Teeth.

For Further Information:
Abrahams, Peter H., Sandy C. Marks, Jr., and Ralph Hutchings. *McMinn's Color Atlas of Human Anatomy.* 6th ed. St. Louis, Mo.: Mosby/Elsevier, 2008.
Carson-DeWitt, Rosalyn. "Ulceratuve Colitis." *Health Library*, September 10, 2012.
Keshav, Satish, and Adam Bailey. *The Gastrointestinal System at a Glance.* Malden, Mass.: Blackwell, 2013.
Moog, Florence. "The Lining of the Small Intestine." *Scientific American* 245 (November, 1981): 154–176.
Shannon, Diane W. "Viral Gastroenteritis." *Health Library*, September 26, 2012.
Tortora, Gerard J., and Bryan Derrickson. *Principles of Anatomy and Physiology.* 12th ed. Hoboken, N.J.: John Wiley & Sons, 2009.
Young, Emma. "Alimentary Thinking." *New Scientist* 2895 (December 15, 2012): 38–42.

GASTROSTOMY
Procedure
Anatomy or system affected: Abdomen, gastrointestinal system, stomach
Specialties and related fields: Gastroenterology, oncology
Definition: The creation of a hole through the wall of the abdomen into the stomach in order to feed a patient who is unable to swallow.

Indications and Procedures

Gastrostomies are carried out during situations in which a patient is unable to swallow food. This condition may result from cancer or strictures of the esophagus; when an esophageal fistula is present, causing the diversion of swallowed food; or when a patient is unconscious. In some cases, the patient is a child who has swallowed a caustic substance, causing damage to the esophagus. Under such circumstances in which a gastrostomy is warranted, an artificial opening is prepared through the abdominal wall into the stomach, and a tube is inserted through the opening.

The gastrostomy tube, which is usually made of plastic or nylon, may be permanently inserted or removed after each feeding. The development of the Barnes-Redo prosthesis has alleviated some of the problems associated with permanent gastrostomies. The device, which is permanently installed, has a cap placed over the opening between feedings. When it is time to eat, the cap is removed, and a catheter is placed through the tube into the stomach, allowing food or liquids to be fed to the patient. When the meal is finished, the catheter is removed and the cap replaced on the gastrostomy tube.

Food for gastrostomy patients cannot be solid. It is recommended that any food first be thoroughly cooked and then blended into a mushy consistency. Patients should smell and taste the food prior to feeding, both to minimize difficulty in adjustment to the situation and to stimulate gastric secretions, which will aid in digestion.

Uses and Complications

Care must be taken with gastrostomy patients to minimize the chance of infection. Any tubes that will be inserted into the stomach must be sterilized prior to use. In addition, the skin around the gastrostomy tube must be protected from gastric juices such as stomach acid, which could cause irritation. The major adjustment for these patients, however, is often psychological—particularly for those with permanent gastrostomies, since meals are often times for social gatherings.

—Richard Adler, Ph.D.

See also Cancer; Catheterization; Critical care; Critical care, pediatric; Gastroenterology; Gastroenterology, pediatric; Gastrointestinal disorders; Gastrointestinal system; Nutrition; Stomach, intestinal, and pancreatic cancers.

For Further Information:

Barrett, Catherine, ed. *Gastrostomy Care: A Guide to Practice*. San Francisco: Ausmed, 2004.
Breckman, Brigid, ed. *Stoma Care and Rehabilitation*. New York: Churchill Livingstone/Elsevier, 2005.
Broadwell, Debra C., and Bettie S. Jackson, eds. *Principles of Ostomy Care*. St. Louis, Mo.: Mosby, 1982.
Edwards-Jones, Valerie, and Anne Leahy-Gilmartin. "Gastrostomy Site Infections: Dealing with a Common Problem." *British Journal of Community Nursing*, supplement (May, 2012): S8–S13.
"Feeding Tube Insertion—Gastrostomy." *MedlinePlus*, May 16, 2012.
"Gastrostomy: Permanent and Temporary." *Health Library*, November 26, 2012.
Gauderer, Michael W. L., and Thomas A. Stellato. *Gastrostomies: Evolution, Techniques, Indications, and Complications*. Chicago: Year Book Medical, 1986.
Ponsky, Jeffrey L., ed. *Techniques of Percutaneous Gastrostomy*. New York: Igaku-Shoin, 1988.

GAUCHER'S DISEASE
Disease/Disorder

Anatomy or system affected: Abdomen, bones, cells, liver, lymphatic system, spleen
Specialties and related fields: Biochemistry, cytology, genetics, internal medicine, pediatrics, toxicology
Definition: A congenital disorder caused by a defect in lipid metabolism and characterized by cell hyperplasia in the liver, spleen, and bone marrow.

Key terms:

enzyme: a protein that catalyzes a biological reaction in the body
hyperplasia: enlargement

Causes and Symptoms

Gaucher's disease (also referred to as Gaucher disease) is an inherited disorder resulting from a mutation in the gene that encodes the enzyme glucocerebrosidase, one of a class of enzymes that functions in the breakdown (hydrolysis) of glucosyl ceramide lipids. The result is an accumulation of a class of lipids known as glucosyl ceramide sphingolipids, primarily in cells of the liver, spleen, or bone marrow. Normally, these lipids are hydrolyzed within digestive organelles called lysosomes, found within these cells. The buildup of lipids within these structures classifies Gaucher's disease as a form of lysosomal storage disease; cells in which these pathologies are presented are known as Gaucher cells.

> ### Information on Gaucher's Disease
> **Causes:** Genetic enzyme deficiency
> **Symptoms:** Varies with type; may include liver and spleen enlargement, bone marrow abnormalities, severe anemia, severe bleeding, central nervous system damage
> **Duration:** Chronic
> **Treatments:** Enzyme replacement therapy, genetically engineered drugs

Gaucher's disease is not common in the general population and affects approximately 1 in 60,000 persons, although three to four times that number probably carry one copy of the defective gene. However, in the ethnic population of Ashkenazi (Eastern European) Jews, approximately 1 in 450 persons is afflicted with the disease, making it among the most common genetic disorders in this group. In 2003, the National Gaucher Foundation, an organization that monitors the disorder, estimated that approximately 2,500 Americans had the disease.

Three different types of Gaucher's disease have been described, differing in their severity, in the presence or absence of neurological defects, and in the general demographics of the disorder. The most common form is Type I, characterized by hyperplasia of the liver and spleen and accompanied by bone marrow abnormalities; neurological problems are not observed in this form. Its symptoms include severe anemia, attributable to pathological events among the bone marrow precursors; low numbers of platelets, resulting in severe bleeding; and significant hyperplasia in the spleen and liver. The disease, when observed, is generally found in the adult population, though not all persons with this genetic mutation actually experience all, or even any, of the symptoms. Type II (infantile) disorder, a neuropathic or malignant presentation, is a significantly more severe form that affects children under the age of six months; rarely do these children survive beyond two years as a result of significant central nervous system damage, especially among the cranial nerves. The third form, Type III (juvenile), is less severe than Type II and significantly more variable in its prognosis; children can usually grow into their adult years.

Treatment and Therapy

Until the 1990s, control of Gaucher's disease involved a combination of splenectomy and repeated blood transfusions. The development of enzyme replacement therapy in 1991 provided a means of controlling the disease through the direct presentation of the missing enzyme glucocerebrosidase to the patient's system. The enzyme was obtained and purified from human placentas collected following hospital births. The initial studies using the natural form of glucocerebrosidase were disappointing, but a chemically modified product proved more successful. The modified form of the enzyme was presented intravenously to persons on an outpatient basis approximately twice each month. Though costly, the process proved effective in controlling most forms of Type I disease, the most common, but less effective for other forms of the disease. In those patients for whom therapy had proven effective, other aspects of the disorder such as cell hyperplasia were often reversed.

Treatments developed in the late 1990s included genetically engineered forms of drugs that could be taken orally. This form of treatment has proven highly effective with those expressing the Type I form and to a lesser extent the Type III form. In addition to replacement of the defective enzyme, a new class of drugs was also developed that inhibited the actual synthesis of the potentially toxic lipids by blocking the action of the enzyme glucosylceramide synthase.

No effective treatment exists for the Type II form of Gaucher's disease, and central nervous system damage is not reversible, even if the disease does respond to therapy.

Perspective and Prospects

Since the chromosomal site of Gaucher's disease is known—chromosome 1q21, or the long arm of chromosome number 1—prenatal testing is possible to determine whether the developing fetus carries the defective gene. The course, or any decision with regard to treatment, is difficult because of the variable nature of many forms of the disease. Carriers can be observed through the use of molecular techniques, such as restriction fragment length polymorphisms (RFLPs), which detect the presence of abnormal forms of the affected gene. However, even within the population affected, such as Ashkenazi Jews, multiple forms of mutations can be found. The significance of different mutations within the same gene remains confusing, in that different persons with even similar defects may manifest the disease in a variety of forms. Clearly, the role of other factors in the expression of Gaucher's disease remains to be clarified.

The disease is not manifested in every individual carrying the mutation; genetic testing of parents in at-risk groups, or the testing of normal parents who have a child with the disorder, may also provide a means of screening during pregnancy for the possibility of illness in the developing child. Given the variable nature of the disease, the issue of screening remains controversial.

Ideally, gene replacement remains the only method, which, in theory, could cure the disease. The systemic aspect of the disorder, however, means that even if possible, replacement would have to be carried out in utero. For the near future, treatment and control rest upon an increasingly effective use of oral drugs to compensate for the absent enzyme.

—*Richard Adler, Ph.D.*

See also Enzyme therapy; Enzymes; Genetic counseling; Genetic diseases; Glycogen storage diseases; Lipids; Metabolic disorders; Metabolism; Mucopolysaccharidosis (MPS); Niemann-Pick disease; Screening; Tay-Sachs disease.

For Further Information:

Bellenir, Karen, ed. *Genetic Disorders Sourcebook: Basic Consumer Information About Hereditary Diseases and Disorders*. 4th ed. Detroit: Omnigraphics, 2010.

Futerman, Anthony H., and Ari Zimran, eds. *Gaucher Disease*. Boca Ratonm, Fla.: CRC/Taylor & Francis, 2007.

Kaneshiro, Neil K. "Gaucher Disease." *MedlinePlus*, November 12, 2012.

Kliegman, R. M., ed. *Nelson Textbook of Pediatrics*. 19th ed. Philadelphia: Saunders Elsevier, 2011.

"NINDS Gaucher Disease Information Page." *National Institute of Neurological Disorders and Stroke*, April 24, 2013.

Oster, Harry. *Legacy: A Genetic History of the Jewish Population*. Oxford: Oxford University Press, 2012.

Parker, James N., and Philip M. Parker, eds. *The Official Parent's Sourcebook on Gaucher's Disease*. San Diego: Icon, 2002.

GENDER IDENTITY DISORDER
Disease/Disorder

Also known as: Transsexualism

Anatomy or system affected: Genitals, psychic-emotional system

Specialties and related fields: Endocrinology, ethics, general surgery, genetics, pediatrics, psychiatry, psychology

Definition: A psychiatric classification describing persons experiencing a strong and persistent incongruity between their anatomy and the gender with which they identify. Gender identity disorder is not concurrent with either disorders of sexual development (intersex conditions) or with homosexuality.

Key terms:

disorder of sexual development: medical terminology, also known as intersex, used to describe an individual with an atypical development of chromosomal, gonadal, or phenotypic sex

gender: a personal and socially construed concept of appropriate roles, behavior, activities, and attributes for men and for women

gender identity: self-identification as a man or woman; also, self-identification as both a man and a woman, or neither

gender reassignment surgery: also known as sex reassignment surgery; surgery aimed to alter a person's physical sexual characteristics to resemble that of the other gender

hormone replacement therapy: the process of replacing the hormones naturally occurring in a person's body with those of the other sex

transgender: a general term for persons who deviate from masculine and feminine gender norms

transvestism: cross-dressing, that is, wearing clothing deemed appropriate for a person of the gender to which one is not socially and culturally identified

Causes and Symptoms

The exact cause of gender dysphoria is not clearly understood or universally agreed upon. Many believe that the condition is not pathological. Others feel that gender dysphoria results from multiple pathways that can work alone or together. These pathways result from an individual's psychological, sociocultural, biological, and genetic factors and background. Relevant terms in any discussion of gender dysphoria include "sex," which refers to the physical characteristics associated with being either male or female, and "gender," which refers to the culturally defined roles and behaviors associated with a given sex. Concepts related to

---

Information on Gender Identity Disorder

Causes: Psychological, biological, familial, and sociocultural factors

Symptoms: Gender dysphoria, feeling trapped in body of wrong sex, repeatedly stated desire or insistence of being other sex, cross-dressing, difficulty with same-gender peer interaction, disgust toward genitals or secondary sexual characteristics, psychiatric comorbidity (depression, anxiety, bipolar disorder), behavior problems

Duration: Diagnosed in childhood or adulthood; can be temporary or chronic

Treatments: Psychological interventions, social interventions, sexual reassignment surgery (genital surgery, breast surgery), hormone replacement therapy, (puberty-delaying hormones, estrogen, testosterone), voice therapy

---

gender dysphoria include "transsexualism," which refers to people who actively identify with the opposite sex and choose to live as a member of that sex, and "transgender," a catch-all term for people whose gender identity does not match traditional expectations for their sex.

A psychiatrist or psychologist typically makes the diagnosis of gender dysphoria. Diagnostic criteria for both childhood and adult forms have been established by the American Psychological Association in the *Diagnostic and Statistical Manual of Mental Disorders* (DSM). ("Gender dysphoria" appears in the fifth edition, published in 2013, and represents a renaming of the diagnosis from previous editions, where it appeared as "gender identity disorder.") To carry a diagnosis of childhood gender dysphoria, a child must have an onset of symptoms before puberty. The majority of children resolve their gender dysphoria; others have a continuation of symptoms into adolescence or adulthood. Some people are first diagnosed as adults. Once gender dysphoria is diagnosed in adults, it tends to have a chronic course.

To meet the criteria for diagnosis, an individual must have a cross-gender identification exceeding the desire for perceived cultural advantages of being the other sex. A persistent discomfort with the person's sex or with the gender role of that sex must exist. The disturbance must cause clinically significant distress in important areas of functioning. Gender dysphoria is not necessarily concurrent with disorders of sexual development, a condition in which an individual may be born with ambiguous genitalia (intersexuality). Gender dysphoria is also independent of sexual orientation, occurring in people who identify as both homosexual and heterosexual.

Treatment and Therapy

The World Professional Association for Transgender Health (WPATH, formerly the Harry Benjamin International Gender Dysphoria Association) has a set of guidelines established for the standards of care for gender dysphoria. The *Standards of Care for the Health of Transsexual, Transgender, and Gender Nonconforming People* identifies multiple therapeutic approaches to gender dysphoria. These include changes in gender expression and role (cross-dressing and other behavioral changes, either full or part time), hormone replacement therapy (estrogen or testosterone to either feminize of masculinize the body), sex reassignment surgery, and psychotherapy. Therapy should proceed focusing on resolving any comorbid psychological disorders, promoting acceptance, and discussing further treatment options.

Hormone therapy can be given to adolescents to delay puberty. This allows time for an individual to explore gender identity and to make a gender transition more conspicuously. In the United States, estrogen or testosterone can be given to an individual who is eighteen and who demonstrates knowledge about the benefits and risks, has spent a prescribed period living in the desired role or a period of psychotherapy, and demonstrates readiness.

Sex reassignment surgery is the final step that some people with gender dysphoria choose to pursue. Genital reconstruction can occur in both males and females. An individual who is anatomically female may also desire removal of the breasts, uterus, ovaries, and Fallopian tubes, as well as liposuction and other aesthetic procedures. For someone who is anatomically male, surgery may include breast implants, facial feminization surgery, and voice surgery.

Perspective and Prospects

Gender dysphoria exists in every culture. It has been recorded as early as Hippocrates, who is credited with the first classification system for what was called Scythian disease. Magnus Hirschfeld coined the term "transvestism" in 1915, describing individuals who cross-dress. In 1949, David Caudwell coined the term "transsexual." In 1966, Harry Benjamin developed a Sex Orientation Scale to differentiate the various forms of transvestism and transsexualism. Since then, there has been extensive debate concerning the correct classification and terminology surrounding gender dysphoria and transgenderism.

The diagnosis of gender identity disorder was added to the DSM in 1987. The transgender community campaigned for many years, with eventual success, to have this classification changed, as many transgender people found it offensive and incorrect to label gender dysphoria as a disorder. People argue that concepts of gender roles are socially constructed and therefore wonder how a society can define, scientifically, what a "normal" gender identity is. Many people support the idea that transgendered people are leading the way in redefining and updating traditional concepts of gender.

—*Amber M. Mathiesen, M.S.*

See also Breast surgery; Breasts, female; Gender reassignment surgery; Genetics and inheritance; Grafts and grafting; Hermaphroditism and pseudohermaphroditism; Hormone therapy; Hormones; Hysterectomy; Men's health; Penile implant surgery; Plastic surgery; Psychiatry; Reproductive system; Sexual differentiation; Sexual dysfunction; Sexuality; Women's health.

For Further Information:

American Psychological Association. *Diagnostic and Statistical Manual of Mental Disorders: DSM-5*. Washington, D.C.: Author,

2013.

"Answers to Your Questions about Transgender People, Gender Identity, and Gender Expression." *American Psychological Association*, 2011.

Brown, Mildred L., and Ann Rounsley. *True Selves: Understanding Transsexualism—For Families, Friends, Coworkers, and Helping Professionals*. San Francisco: Jossey-Bass, 1996.

Cohen-Kettenis, Peggy T., and Friedemann Pfäfflin. *Transgenderism and Intersexuality in Childhood and Adolescence: Making Choices*. Thousand Oaks, Calif.: Sage Publications, 2003.

"Gender Identity Disorder." MedlinePlus, February 13, 2012.

"Standards of Care for the Health of Transsexual, Transgender, and Gender Nonconforming People." 7th version. *World Professional Association for Transgender Health*, 2011.

World Health Organization. *International Statistical Classification of Diseases and Related Health Problems: 10th Revision–ICD-10*. 2d ed. Geneva, Switzerland: Author, 2000.

GENDER REASSIGNMENT SURGERY

Procedure

Anatomy or system affected: Breasts, endocrine system, genitals, glands, reproductive system, uterus

Specialties and related fields: Endocrinology, general surgery, gynecology, plastic surgery, psychiatry, psychology, urology

Definition: A set of procedures designed to alter the sexual characteristics of an anatomic male to a female or of an anatomic female to a male.

Key terms:

labia: the folds of tissue along the external portion of a woman's vagina and urethra

testosterone: the male sex hormone that produces male fertility and secondary sexual characteristics, such as body hair and musculature

transsexuals: individuals who believe that their genitalia do not correspond to their gender

urethra: the tube through which urine is conducted from the bladder to the outside of the body

Indications and Procedures

Gender reassignment surgery is performed to allow an individual's anatomic sex to conform to his or her gender identity. In cases of hermaphroditism or intersexuality, in which an individual is born with ambiguous genitalia, the genitalia may not be altered upon birth to conform to chromosomal sexual identity. Anatomical changes at puberty, however, may conflict with the intersex teenager's gender identity, and thus surgery may be used to correct the discrepancy. More commonly, gender reassignment surgery is performed on an adult who feels "trapped" within the body of the wrong gender, which causes severe emotional and psychological distress. Extensive psychological tests are performed on individuals seeking to change their anatomic sex.

In male-to-female surgery, the penis, testicles, and scrotum are removed and a vagina and labia may be created. Prior to surgery, the patient has taken estrogen supplements. In the surgery itself, the surgeon removes each testicle through an incision at the base of the penis and ties off the spermatic cords. The skin and urethra are separated from the penis, and a tunnel for the vagina is created from skin at the base of the urethra. A scalpel is used to remove the base of the penis. The lower abdominal and penile skin is sutured to the pubic bone, and some of this skin is used to create a vagina. A colonic segment can also be used to create the vagina. A lubricated glass mold is inserted into the vagina to prevent shrinkage, and labia are formed from the scrotal skin.

During female-to-male surgery, breasts and hormone-secreting reproductive organs are removed and replaced with male secondary sexual characteristics. Prior to surgery, the patient undertakes a program of body-building exercises and testosterone supplements that promote body and facial hair development and suppress menstruation. Surgical procedures begin with the removal of excess breast tissue, in a procedure similar to breast reduction, and with a hysterectomy to remove the uterus, Fallopian tubes, and ovaries, along with their female sex hormones. At a later date, a penis may be constructed from abdominal-wall tissue or a skin graft, or both, and a scrotum containing plastic testicles formed from labia. An inflatable cylinder in the penis and a fluid pump within the scrotum can be used to simulate erection.

Uses and Complications

Because of the critical and irreversible nature of this type of surgery, the American Psychological Association has developed guidelines for diagnosing genuine transsexualism and for defining who should be considered for gender reassignment surgery in the United States. To be considered, transsexuals must feel a profound inappropriateness about their anatomic sex, have attempted to obtain gender reassignment surgery persistently for at least two years in spite of rejection for the procedure, have no genetic abnormalities or psychiatric disorders, and be past the age of puberty. In earlier cases, when such rigorous selection criteria were not in effect, some individuals who obtained gender reassignment surgery experienced severe social, sexual, and psychological trauma; some committed suicide.

Potential complications of male-to-female surgery include infection of incisions, closure of the urethral opening, and formation of an abnormal connection between the vagina and rectum, all of which are correctable. Long-term effects include dryness and potential shrinkage of the constructed vagina, unless the glass mold is worn the majority of the time, and an inability to achieve orgasm except through mental stimulation. Individuals may opt for breast augmentation surgery and must take female hormones for at least one year, perhaps for life, to maintain fat deposits on breasts and hips. Additional cosmetic surgery may be undertaken to achieve feminization of features.

Female-to-male surgery carries serious potential side effects from the hysterectomy, including pain, infection, and debilitation. Most individuals do not undertake penile construction and instead use a dildo or prosthetic penis. Constructed penises are usually unsatisfactory in that they are significantly shorter than the average erect penis and are incapable of transmitting sexual sensation. In some cases, pumps have become defective and required further corrective surgery. Male hormone supplements must be taken for the remainder of the individual's life.

Perspective and Prospects

For centuries, hermaphrodites—persons born with ambiguous genitalia—were subjected to severe psychological trauma as they reached adulthood and/or developed a sexual anatomy contrary to the gender identity in which they were reared. In the mid-twentieth century, when chromosome analysis became available, those born with ambiguous genitalia could be identified as to chromosomal sex, and their outward ambiguities could be surgically altered soon after birth.

Transsexuals, too, have been ostracized and humiliated throughout history; in the latter half of the twentieth century, psychologists diagnosed transsexuals as genuinely feeling as if they had been born the wrong gender. What leads one to feel this sense of "wrongness," whether the cause is biological or cultural, or both, is unknown. Theories such as exposure to large amounts of opposite-sex hormones during fetal gestation have been proven wrong.

Individuals who undergo gender reassignment surgery do not experience normal physical sensations in their new genitalia. They are also sterile and therefore unable to reproduce or become pregnant. Research into neurobiology may lead to future procedures allowing physical sensations, as well as to the possibility of transplanting functioning reproductive organs. Even in the current state of the procedure, individuals who are properly psychologically and physically prepared find peace and fulfillment in what is for them a normal gender identity.

—*Karen E. Kalumuck, Ph.D.*

See also Breast surgery; Breasts, female; Gender identity disorder; Genetics and inheritance; Grafts and grafting; Hermaphroditism and pseudohermaphroditism; Hormone therapy; Hormones; Hysterectomy; Men's health; Penile implant surgery; Plastic surgery; Psychiatry; Reproductive system; Sexual differentiation; Sexual dysfunction; Sexuality; Women's health.

For Further Information:

American Psychological Association. "Answers to Your Questions About Transgender People, Gender Identity, and Gender Expression." Author, 2011.

Bockting W. "Sexual Identity Development." In *Nelson Textbook of Pediatrics*, edited by R.M. Kliegman, et al. 19th ed. Philadelphia: Saunders Elsevier, 2011.

Boylan, Jennifer Finney. *She's Not There: A Life in Two Genders*. New York: Broadway Books, 2003.

Ettner, Randi, Stan Monstrey, and A. Evan Eyler, eds. *Principles of Transgender Medicine and Surgery*. New York: Haworth Press, 2007.

National Center for Transgender Equality and the National Gay and Lesbian Task Force. "Injustice at Every Turn." Washington, D.C.: Author, 2011.

Shrage, Laurie, ed. *"You've Changed": Sex Reassignment and Personal Identity*. New York: Oxford University Press, 2009.

Simpson, Joe Leigh. *Disorders of Sexual Differentiation: Etiology and Clinical Delineation*. New York: Academic Press, 1976.

GENE THERAPY
Treatment

Also known as: Gene transfer

Anatomy or system affected: Cells

Specialties and related fields: Biotechnology, cytology, genetics

Definition: The delivery of genetic material into a cell for the purpose of either correcting a genetic problem or giving the cell a new biochemical function.

Key terms:

gene: the deoxyribonucleic acid (DNA) instructions necessary for the manufacture of a functional protein in a cell

genome: the total genetic information found within a virus, cell, or organism

germ cells: cells involved in the process of sexual reproduction and inheritance; also called gametes

somatic cells: cells that make up the majority of the human body and that are not passed on from generation to generation

stem cells: cells that are undifferentiated, meaning that they have the potential to develop into a variety of cell and tissue types

vector: in genetics, a system (usually a virus) that is used to carry a gene into the cell for gene therapy

virus: an infectious agent that consists of a protein coat enclosing a small piece of genetic material; viruses are usually less than one-thousandth the size of the living cell

Indications and Procedures

The overall goal of gene therapy is to correct an undesirable trait or disease by introducing a modified copy of a gene into a target cell. In most cases, the purpose is not to replace a defective gene in the host cell but rather to provide a new copy so that the correct protein can be expressed and the detrimental effects of the defective gene neutralized. While technically any genetic disorder may be treated by gene therapy, currently there are some limitations. First, the precise genetic mechanism of the disorder must be known, and it must be a single-gene defect. Second, scientists must know the complete genetic sequence of the gene, including regulatory regions, so that a functional copy can be delivered to the cell. Third, there needs to be an effective *vector*, or delivery system, for administering the correct copy to the target cells.

Generally, scientists classify forms of gene therapy as belonging to one of three types. Theoretically, the most effective form of this procedure is in situ gene therapy, which means that the genetic material is administered directly to the target cells. Unfortunately, it has been difficult to ensure that only target cells receive the genetic material, but there have been some successes. A second method injects the vector containing the genetic material into the fluids of the body. In this method, called in vivo gene therapy, the vector travels throughout the body until it reaches the target cells. A third mechanism, called ex vivo gene therapy, removes cells from the body to be exposed to the vector and then reintroduced back into the body. This method works especially well with undifferentiated stem cells.

Scientists have developed several mechanisms by which the genetic information can be introduced into the target cell. The most common is the viral vector. Viruses are used because typically they are very specific in the types of cells that they infect. Furthermore, their genomes are usually very small and well understood by scientists. The viruses that are chosen are derived almost exclusively from nonpathogenic strains or have been genetically engineered so that pathogenic portions of the genome have been removed. Common viral vectors are adenoviruses, retroviruses, and herpes simplex viruses. The choice of vector depends on the target and size of gene to be replaced. In each case, after the virus infects the target cell, the DNA is either incorporated directly into the host genome or becomes extrachromosomal.

Medical researchers are also investigating the use of nonviral vectors to deliver DNA into target cells. As is the case with viral vectors, these mechanisms must not disrupt the normal metabolic machinery of the target cell. One system, called plasmid DNA, utilizes small circular pieces of DNA called plasmids to deliver the genetic material. If small enough, the plasmids can pass through the cell membrane. Although they do not integrate into the host genome in the same way as viral vectors do, they are a simple mechanism and lack the potential problems associated with viral vectors. Another mechanism being studied is the packaging of the genetic material within a lipid-based vector called a liposome to ease transport across the membrane. In trials, however, both liposomes and plasmids have displayed a low efficiency in delivering genetic material into target cells.

Uses and Complications

Since the early 1990s, numerous scientific studies have examined the potential effectiveness of gene therapy in treating diseases in mammalian model species, such as mice and monkeys. Using gene therapy, researchers have demonstrated that it may be possible to treat diseases such as Parkinson's disease, sickle cell anemia, and some forms of cancer. Weekly scientific journals such as *Gene Therapy* report the status of these tests. Gene therapy trials in humans are a relatively recent development and represent the next stage in the treatment of human diseases. Severe combined immunodeficiency syndrome (SCID) was the first human disorder for which successful gene therapy was reported, and clinical trials of gene therapy for the treatment of Canavan disease, adenosine deaminase (ADA) deficiency, and cystic fibrosis have begun. Medical researchers have suggested that, in the future, almost any genetic defect may be treatable using gene therapy.

While gene therapy may appear to be the "silver bullet" for diseases such as cancer and Parkinson's disease, the procedure is not without its risks. Since gene therapy using viral

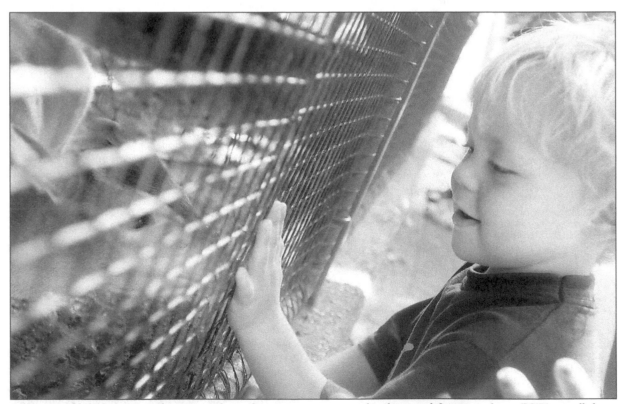

A three-year-old child who received experimental gene therapy to cure severe combined immunodeficiency syndrome (SCID), so-called bubble boy disease, visits a zoo in Amsterdam in 2002. (AP/Wide World Photos)

vectors was first proposed, scientists have recognized the inherent problems with the procedure. Since the technology does not yet exist to target the virus to insert its DNA directly into the specific gene of interest, the chances are that the viral vector will integrate the genetic information into the genome at some site other than the location of the defective gene. This means that the potential exists for the virus to insert itself into a regulatory or structural region of a gene and either render it unusable or impart a new function to the protein. Because of the size of the human genome (more than three billion bases) and the fact that less than 2 percent of the genome is believed to produce functional proteins, the odds of such an event occurring are relatively low. Given the large numbers of vectors used, however, this risk remains a real possibility.

Two cases illustrate the dangers associated with viral vectors. First was the death of a gene therapy trial volunteer at the University of Pennsylvania in 1999. The volunteer, Jesse Gelsinger, suffered from a form of liver disorder called ornithine transcarbamylase deficiency (OTC). OTC is identified as being the result of a single defective gene in a five-step metabolic pathway. Using an adenovirus, researchers sought to replace the defective gene causing OTC in Gelsinger. Shortly after the gene therapy was begun, Gelsinger developed a systemic immune response to the vector and died.

The second case is actually a story of both success and failure. A French research team at the Necker Hospital for Sick Children in Paris effectively used a retrovirus vector to treat a group of young boys with SCID. Also called "bubble boy disease," SCID is a rare disorder in which the immune system is rendered inoperative. One form of the disease has been traced to a gene on the X chromosome. Using the procedure of ex vivo gene therapy, the researchers removed stem cells from the bone marrow of the boys and, using a retrovirus vector, delivered a functional copy of the defective gene into the cells. The cells were then reinserted back into the bone marrow. The procedure was successful in that all boys were cured of the disease. Thirty months later, however, one of the boys developed leukemia, which was followed four months later by a second case. Analysis of the boys" DNA indicated that the inserted gene had disrupted a gene in which mutations had previously been shown to cause cancer.

While the number of individuals that have developed complications from gene therapy is relatively small, these cases do indicate the potential hazards of using a viral system and have accelerated the research into using nonviral systems such as liposomes and plasmids. Additional research is underway to develop a means of targeting a specific host gene for the insertion of the therapeutic DNA. Scientists are also investigating the possibility of developing a so-called suicide gene, or "off switch," for the procedure that could terminate treatment if an error in insertion were detected.

Perspective and Prospects

The process of gene therapy represents one of the more modern of advances in the life sciences. Since James Watson and Francis Crick proposed the structure of DNA in 1953, scientists have been suggesting the possibility of correcting

genetic defects in a cell. It has been only since the early 1990s, however, that advances in biotechnology have enabled the actual procedure to be conducted.

The science of gene therapy actually began as enzyme replacement therapy. For patients suffering from diseases in which an enzyme in a metabolic pathway is defective, enzyme replacement therapy provides a temporary cure. In these cases, however, the therapy must be administrated continuously since the presence of a defective gene means that the body lacks the ability to manufacture new enzymes.

In the 1980s, enzyme replacement therapy was being used to treat a number of diseases including ADA deficiency, in which an enzyme in a biochemical pathway that converts toxins in the body to uric acid is defective. As a result, the toxins accumulate and eventually render the immune system ineffective. The modern era for gene therapy began in the early 1990s as scientists began to treat ADA deficiency with gene therapy. Through a series of trials, researchers learned that ex vivo treatment of stem cells proved to be the most effective mechanism for treating ADA deficiency with gene therapy. In 1993, researchers obtained stem cells from the umbilical cords of three babies who were born with ADA deficiency. After the correct genes were inserted into these stem cells, the altered cells were inserted back into the donor babies. After years of monitoring, it appears that the process has worked and the potentially fatal effects of ADA deficiency in these children have been reversed.

Cystic fibrosis is a serious respiratory disease that results from a missing protein that forms calcium channels in the membranes of the cells lining the respiratory tract. Affected individuals collect mucus in these respiratory cells and are susceptible to life-threatening respiratory infections. Gene therapy has been used with modest success to replace the defective gene in these cases. The major problem is that these cells have a relatively short life span, so that the relief is only temporary and these expensive treatments must be repeated every few months. The targeting of the replacement gene to only those cells in the respiratory tract where it is needed has also been a considerable technological hurdle to overcome.

Another promising area of gene therapy is the treatment of cancer. Cancer treatment using gene therapy would probably not involve replacing defective genes but rather "knocking out" those genes that are causing uncontrolled cell division within cancer cells. By arresting cell division, scientists can halt the spread of the cancer. This treatment would be especially useful in areas of the body where surgery is risky, such as brain tumors. The primary challenge at this stage is the targeting of the vector. A knockout vector would need to infect only cancer cells and not the other dividing cells of the human body.

A potential area of gene therapy that has yet to be exploited is germ-line gene therapy. Germ cells are those that are responsible for the formation of gametes, or egg and sperm cells. Since a germ cell contains only half the genetic information of an adult cell, it is relatively easy to replace genes using available procedures learned from biotechnology. Furthermore, since following fertilization the genetic material in the germ cells is responsible for the formation of all the remaining more than sixty-three trillion cells in the human body, any genetic change in the germ cells has the ability to be inherited by subsequent generations. Somatic cell therapy, such as that used to treat ADA deficiency and SCID, has the ability to influence only the affected individual, since these cells are not normally part of the reproductive process. Gene therapy in germ cells is currently considered unethical, but many consider it to be the mechanism of eliminating certain diseases from the human species.

While the use of gene therapy to correct human diseases may be stalled temporarily until technical obstacles are overcome, little doubt exists in the biomedical community that gene therapy represents the procedure of the future. At a fundamental level, gene therapy has the potential to be the ultimate cure for many ailments and diseases of humankind. For most of recorded history, medicine has been confined to the treatment of symptoms. Since the start of the twentieth century, advances have enabled enhanced surgical procedures, pharmaceutical drugs that alter or interact with the biochemistry of the cell, improved diagnostic techniques, and a deeper understanding of genetic inheritance. Gene therapy represents the ultimate preventive procedure.

—*Michael Windelspecht, Ph.D.;*
updated by Jeffrey A. Knight, Ph.D.

See also Bionics and biotechnology; Cancer; Cells; Clinical trials; DNA and RNA; Enzyme therapy; Enzymes; Ethics; Genetic diseases; Genetic engineering; Genetics and inheritance; Genomics; Mutation; Severe combined immunodeficiency syndrome (SCID); Stem cells; Viral infections.

For Further Information:

"Frequently Asked Questions about Genetic and Genomic Science." *National Human Genome Research Institute*, Nov. 14, 2012.

"Genes and Gene Therapy." *MedlinePlus*, June 13, 2013.

"Gene Therapy for Diseases." *American Society of Gene & Cell Therapy*, 2011.

Goodman, Denise M., Cassio Lynm, and Edward H. Livingston. "Genomic Medicine." *Journal of the American Medical Association* 309.14 (2013): 1544.

Gorman, Jessica. "Delivering the Goods: Gene Therapy Without the Virus." *Science News* 163 (January, 2003): 43–44.

Kresina, Thomas F., ed. *An Introduction to Molecular Medicine and Gene Therapy.* New York: Wiley-Liss, 2001.

Lewis, Ricki. *Human Genetics: Concepts and Applications.* 10th ed. Dubuque, Iowa: McGraw-Hill, 2012.

National Institute of General Medical Sciences. *The New Genetics.* NIH Pub No. 10-662. Washington, DC: US Department of Health and Human Services: National Institutes of Health, Apr. 2010.

Panno, Joseph. *Gene Therapy: Treating Disease by Repairing Genes.* New York: Facts On File, 2005.

Templeton, Nancy Smyth, ed. *Gene Therapy: Therapeutic Mechanisms and Strategies.* 3d ed. Boca Raton, Fla.: CRC Press, 2009.

GENETIC COUNSELING

Specialty

Anatomy or system affected: Cells, reproductive system, uterus

Specialties and related fields: Cytology, embryology, genetics, obstetrics, preventive medicine, psychology

Definition: The scientific field that uses several biochemical and imaging techniques, as well as family histories, to provide information about genetic conditions or diseases in order to help individuals make medical and reproductive decisions.

Key terms:

chromosomal abnormality: any change to the number, shape, or appearance of the forty-six chromosomes in each human cell; the presence of many such abnormalities will prevent the normal development of an individual and lead to a miscarriage

dominant genetic disease: a disease caused by a mutation in a gene that can be inherited from only one parent

genetic screening: a program designed to determine whether individuals are carriers of or are affected by a particular genetic disease

karyotype: a photograph of the chromosomes taken from the cells of an individual; a karyotype can be used to predict the sex of a fetus or the presence of a large chromosomal abnormality

mutation: an alteration in the DNA sequence of a gene that usually leads to the production of a nonfunctional enzyme or protein and, thus, a lack of a normal metabolic function; this defect may cause a medical condition called a genetic disease

recessive genetic disease: a disease caused by a mutation in a gene that must be inherited from both parents for an individual to show the symptoms of the disease; such a disease may show up only occasionally in a family history, especially if the mutation is rare

Science and Profession

Genetic counseling is a process of communicating to a couple the medical problems associated with the occurrence of an inherited disorder or birth defect in a family. Included in this process is a discussion of the prognosis and treatment of the problem. Specific reproductive options include abortion of an ongoing pregnancy, birth control or sterilization to prevent additional pregnancies, artificial insemination, the use of surrogate mothers, embryo transplantation, and adoption.

In all cases, the role of the counselor is to provide unbiased information and options to the couple seeking advice. The counselor must not only discuss the medical implications of a condition but also help to alleviate the emotional impact of positive diagnoses and, in particular, to assuage the guilt or denial that a diagnosis may elicit in parents.

The two major categories of medical problems covered by counselors are birth defects and genetic diseases. The first group includes Down syndrome and spina bifida, while the latter includes hemophilia, sickle cell disease, and Tay-Sachs disease. Although the distinction between these two categories can sometimes blur, the key difference involves the clear pattern of inheritance shown by the genetic diseases.

Humans have between thirty thousand and thirty-five thousand genes. Genes are segments of deoxyribonucleic acid (DNA) that are arranged in linear fashion along the forty-six chromosomes. Most genes contain the information necessary for the cells to produce a specific protein, which often is involved in controlling some critical physiological function. For example, the beta globin gene produces a protein called beta globin that makes up half of the hemoglobin that carries oxygen in the red blood cells.

A genetic disease can occur when the DNA changes in structure. Such a change is also known as a mutation. A mutation can lead to the production of a defective protein that cannot carry out its normal function, thus causing a physiological defect. In the case of beta globin, changing only one of the 106 molecules that make up this protein leads to a form of hemoglobin that can produce nonfunctional protein aggregates in red blood cells. These aggregates can cause the red blood cells to collapse and take on a sickle shape. Such cells lose their function, and the tissues are starved for oxygen—a condition known as anemia. This defect, which is called sickle cell disease, is a fatal, heritable disease. As with all genetic disease, such mutations are relatively rare. Certain diseases may, however, be more prevalent within certain ethnic groups; for example, African Americans have a high incidence of sickle cell disease, and Ashkenazic Jews have a high incidence of Tay-Sachs disease.

Humans have two of each kind of chromosome; one set of twenty-three is inherited from the mother, and the other set of twenty-three is inherited from the father. Thus, each person has two copies of each gene, one located on a maternal chromosome, the other on a paternal one. Many types of defects, such as sickle cell disease, require that both genes have mutations in order for the disease to have an effect. Individuals who have one normal gene and one with a mutation are normal but carry the disease; they can pass the mutation on to the next generation in their eggs and sperm. This type of disease is called a recessive genetic disease. The only way a child can have sickle cell disease is if both parents are carriers, since it is unlikely that a person affected by the disease will live long enough to have children.

Since it is equally likely for each parent to pass on the normal gene in eggs or sperm as to pass on the mutation, the laws of probability predict that, on the average, one-fourth of such a couple's offspring should have the disease. One of the major tasks of a genetic counselor is to advise couples of these probabilities if the diagnoses and family histories suggest that they are carriers. Since the laws of genetics involve random occurrences, however, it is possible that in a family with three or four children, all the children will be normal, or that in another family, all the children will have the disease. This degree of uncertainty produces stress and anxiety in couples who seek counseling only to hear that they indeed are at risk. Discussing concepts that involve sophisticated genetic or biochemical themes or issues of probable risk with couples untrained in scientific thinking is difficult, especially considering the highly emotional atmosphere of such discussions.

Other diseases, such as Huntington's chorea, also known as Woody Guthrie's disease for the folksinger who was afflicted by it, are caused by a dominant mutation. A mutation is dominant when an individual needs to inherit only one copy of the mutation in order to have the disease. Unlike recessive diseases that can disappear from a family for generations, a dominant mutation can be inherited only from a person who has the disease. In most cases, such a person has one normal gene and one with the mutation, which means that there is a 50 percent chance that the gene will be passed on. Huntington's chorea is a particularly insidious genetic disease, because the symptoms usually begin to show only in middle age, often after childbearing decisions have been made. Thus, the children of an afflicted parent may have had children before knowing whether they have inherited the mutation from their parents.

There are no cures for the permanent physiological defects that result from genetic disease. In some cases, the disease symptoms can be controlled by supplementing the protein that is lacking. Some forms of insulin-dependent diabetes and most cases of hemophilia can be treated in this way. In other cases, as with the disease phenylketonuria (PKU), special diets can prevent the severe neurological problems that inevitably lead to childhood death if the disease is left untreated.

DNA technology and genetic engineering offer potential cures for some diseases in which the primary defect caused by the mutation is well understood. Gene therapy is a process by which an additional copy of a normal gene is inserted into the cells of an affected individual or the defective gene is replaced by a normal one. Successful experiments with animals have given scientists confidence that these techniques will provide cures for many genetic diseases. These same DNA technologies are making better diagnoses possible and, as in the case of cystic fibrosis, are helping to extend the lives and enhance the quality of life of individuals afflicted with incurable diseases.

One of the more controversial aspects of genetic counseling is the procedure of screening. In this procedure, individuals suspected to be at risk are tested for the presence of a mutation. Screening can let people know whether they have a disease as well as whether they are carriers of the disease and therefore can pass the disease on to their children. Screening can be extended to all individuals, regardless of family or ethnic history. For example, in the United States, most states require that all newborn infants undergo a PKU test. This simple test involves taking a small sample of blood by pricking the heel of the baby. Although the costs of this screening are not insignificant, the benefit is that those infants found to have the disease can be treated immediately by being placed on a special diet so as to avoid the debilitating effects of the disease.

Other screening procedures are targeted at specific groups. The screening program for Tay-Sachs disease focuses on ethnic Jewish populations. This successful, voluntary program has reduced the incidence of Tay-Sachs disease significantly in the United States. The key to the success of the program was the money spent to educate the targeted group. In addition, key members of the population played a leading role in designing the overall program. Because of the much larger size of the potential group at risk, similar efforts to screen African American populations for sickle cell disease have been much less successful. Ethical concerns about the motivations behind government-sponsored or government-encouraged screening of minority populations make these programs difficult to implement. In addition, in mandatory programs, concerns about confidentiality and information release become major obstacles.

Diagnostic and Treatment Techniques

Genetic counseling usually begins when a couple or an individual seeks the advice of a family physician or obstetrician regarding the medical risks associated with having a child. Motivating this request may be a previous birth of a child with a defect, a general uneasiness on the part of a couple worried about environmental exposure to potentially harmful agents, a family history of genetic disease, or advanced maternal age (which can be a factor in certain chromosomal abnormalities). Often, the family is referred to a genetic counseling clinic where most of the actual diagnosis and counseling will occur.

Arriving at a proper diagnosis for any obvious condition, as well as giving advice about potential risks, involves obtaining as much family history as possible with respect to the trait, as well as diagnostic information from the couple. If pregnant already, the woman may undergo a prenatal diagnostic procedure that could include ultrasound, blood tests, amniocentesis, and chorionic villus sampling.

Ultrasound is a technique that uses sound waves to visualize the exterior of the developing fetus. This widely used procedure is almost routine in many large urban hospitals. Ultrasound can be used to detect the presence of twins as well as of some profound birth defects such as hydrocephalus (water on the brain) or spina bifida. The latter defect, which involves the failure of the neural tube to close properly during development, leads to weakness, paralysis, and lack of function in lower body areas. The severity of the defect is hard to predict, and, unlike genetic disease, the incidence of recurrence is no higher than normal for subsequent children.

Supplementing ultrasound in the detection of spina bifida is a simple blood test that looks for a protein that the fetus spills into the amniotic fluid in higher quantities if the neural tube fails to close properly. The protein, which is called alpha-fetoprotein, crosses the placenta to circulate in the mother's blood. The amount of this normal protein in the mother's blood correlates with the developmental age of the fetus; therefore, an abnormal level might indicate a problem. Older-than-calculated fetuses and twins can both cause increased levels of alpha-fetoprotein, so care must be taken in this diagnosis. If abnormally high levels of the protein are found, amniocentesis would then be used to measure the protein level in the amniotic fluid, thus increasing the reliability of the diagnosis. In amniocentesis, a few teaspoonfuls of amniotic fluid are removed from the sac that surrounds and protects the developing fetus. Ultrasound is used to visualize the exterior of the fetus to allow the safe removal of this fluid, which contains some fetal cells. Biochemical tests can be performed directly on the fluid and results obtained quickly.

Tay-Sachs disease is an example of a genetic disease that can be detected in this fashion, since fetuses with the disease fail to make an enzyme that their normal counterparts do make.

Many techniques, however, require obtaining large numbers of fetal cells and/or DNA. In these cases, the cells must be cultured for one to two weeks in a laboratory in order to get enough material to test. The delay between taking the sample and discussing the results with the clients is a source of stress and anxiety for parents undergoing counseling.

Preparing a karyotype, a photograph showing the numbers and sizes of the chromosomes of the fetus, is a commonly performed procedure following amniocentesis. Normal fetuses contain forty-six chromosomes, and any change in chromosome number, shape, or size can be detected by a skilled clinician. A large percentage of miscarriages involve fetuses with chromosomal abnormalities, so this diagnosis can be critical. A relatively common type of birth defect that can be diagnosed with a karyotype is Down syndrome. Most children born with Down syndrome have forty-seven chromosomes instead of forty-six; thus, this diagnosis is very accurate. In addition, the sex of the fetus can be determined from a karyotype, since male fetuses have an X and a Y chromosome while females have two X chromosomes. This information can be valuable to couples who are at risk for carrying a sex-linked genetic disease such as hemophilia, which could not affect any female offspring. Such information could potentially be used inappropriately for sexual selection of offspring, however, and the counselor must provide this information cautiously.

Amniocentesis is usually performed in the sixteenth week of pregnancy to allow the fetus to grow to a size at which the removal of a small amount of amniotic fluid would not be harmful. Although there is little risk to mother or fetus in this procedure, the delay associated with laboratory culturing means that results are often known in the eighteenth week of pregnancy or even later. At this stage, abortion becomes a more traumatic medical procedure. Chorionic villus sampling, on the other hand, can actually sample small amounts of fetal tissue directly. Since the procedure can safely obtain enough tissue to diagnose most problems and can be performed as early as the ninth or tenth week of pregnancy, abortion becomes a medically less traumatic option.

DNA technology provides the counselor with a battery of new diagnostic procedures that can look directly for the presence of a mutation in the DNA of the fetus. These tests can be performed on parents who are worried about being carriers for a particular disease or can be used on DNA obtained from fetal cells grown in a laboratory. Such tests have very high reliability and can give information about diseases such as sickle cell disease, Huntington's chorea, muscular dystrophy, and cystic fibrosis.

The counselor's task is to take the diagnostic results and interpret them in the context of the medical history and particular family situation. The counselor must point out the options available, both for further diagnosis to confirm or rebut less sensitive preliminary tests and to discuss potential medical interventions such as the special diets available for children born with PKU. In cases in which no medical intervention is possible, the severity of the problem should be discussed honestly so that the parents can choose either to continue or to abort the pregnancy. Other options, including adoption, artificial insemination, and embryo transplants, can also be evaluated. Finally, the risk of recurrence of the problem in future pregnancies should be discussed.

Counselors need to realize that their clients are often in emotionally fragile states. They must guard against using bias or interjecting their own personal beliefs or values when counseling their clients. Full disclosure of information, both verbally and in a carefully written report, is usually provided.

Compounding the tasks of the counselor is the fact that, in many cases, exact diagnoses are not yet possible. Sometimes, only the relative risks associated with another pregnancy can be determined. Different couples will perceive risks very differently depending on their own religious and moral backgrounds, as well as on the expected severity of the defect. In the case of a genetic disease such as Tay-Sachs, which is 100 percent fatal and requires extensive hospitalization of the child, a modest risk may be considered unacceptable, while in the case of a birth defect such as Down syndrome, whose severity cannot be predicted, and in which case the child may lead a long and rich life, a modest risk may be considered quite differently.

Perspective and Prospects

The need for centers specializing in genetic counseling arose when it became clear that certain diseases and birth defects had a hereditary component. Many families request the services of counselors from these centers, and the centers are also involved in both voluntary and mandatory screening programs.

Physicians have always served as counselors to families, but the rapid advances made in genetics and molecular science during the second half of the twentieth century have clearly surpassed the abilities of most physicians to keep current with treatments and diagnoses. The first formal clinic for genetic counseling was established at the University of Michigan in the 1940s. Most clinics specializing in this field were based at large medical centers; first in major metropolitan areas, and later in smaller population centers.

Genetic counseling clinics usually employ a range of specialists, including clinicians, geneticists, laboratory personnel for performing diagnostic testing, and public health and social workers. In 1969, Sarah Lawrence College instituted a master's-level program in genetic counseling to train candidates formally in the scientific, medical, and counseling skills required for this profession. Since that time, many other programs have been established in the United States. Most large counseling programs at medical centers use these specially trained personnel. In rural areas, however, family physicians are still a primary source of counseling; thus, genetic training is an important component of basic medical education.

The sophisticated medical diagnostic tools described above allow a counselor to provide abundant information to couples requesting counseling, but the power of DNA technology has expanded and will continue to expand the scope of current practice. Soon, counselors will not have to give advice in terms of probabilities and likelihoods of risk; molecular detection techniques will make possible the absolute identification of not only individuals with a disease but also related carriers.

As these DNA tools become more widely available, counseling will become a more integral part of preventive medicine. A DNA diagnostic procedure for a heritable form of breast cancer is available that allows women who have the mutation to monitor their health closely in order to receive prompt, lifesaving medical intervention. An important ethical issue here is that some women who have been diagnosed as having the mutation are undergoing preventive mastectomies without having developed any growths in order to ensure that they will not develop cancer. This radical therapy carries with it considerable emotional stress and should be undertaken only after consultation with a physician. As DNA-based diagnostic procedures, perhaps coupled with mandatory screening, become more commonplace, concerns about the release of this information to potential employers or health insurers will become more critical.

—*Joseph G. Pelliccia, Ph.D.*

See also Abortion; Amniocentesis; Birth defects; Blood testing; Chorionic villus sampling; Diagnosis; DNA and RNA; Down syndrome; Ethics; Gene therapy; Genetic diseases; Genetic engineering; Genetics and inheritance; Hemophilia; Laboratory tests; Mutation; Niemann-Pick disease; Phenylketonuria (PKU); Screening; Sickle cell disease; Spina bifida; Tay-Sachs disease; Ultrasonography.

For Further Information:

Centers for Disease Control and Prevention. "Genetic Counseling." *CDC Pediatric Genetics*, January 20, 2011.

Davis, Dena S. *Genetic Dilemmas: Reproductive Technology, Parental Choices, and Children's Futures.* 2d ed. New York: Routledge, 2010.

Filkins, Karen, and Joseph F. Russo, eds. *Human Prenatal Diagnosis.* 2d rev. ed. New York: Marcel Dekker, 1990.

Genetics Home Reference. "Genetic Consultation." *Genetics Home Reference*, August 5, 2013.

Harper, Peter S. *Practical Genetic Counselling.* 7th ed. London: Hodder Arnold, 2010.

Jorde, Lynn B., et al. *Medical Genetics.* 4th ed. Philadelphia: Mosby/Elsevier, 2010.

King, Richard A., Jerome I. Rotter, and Arno G. Motulsky, eds. *The Genetic Basis of Common Diseases.* 2d ed. New York: Oxford University Press, 2002.

Lewis, Ricki. *Human Genetics: Concepts and Applications.* 10th ed. New York: McGraw-Hill, 2012.

Martin, Richard J., Avroy A. Fanaroff, and Michele C. Walsh, eds. *Fanaroff and Martin's Neonatal-Perinatal Medicine: Diseases of the Fetus and Infant.* St. Louis: Mosby/Elsevier, 2011.

MedlinePlus. "Genetic Counseling." *MedlinePlus*, June 21, 2013.

Moore, Keith L., and T. V. N. Persaud. *The Developing Human: Clinically Oriented Embryology.* 9th ed. Philadelphia: Saunders/Elsevier, 2013.

Pierce, Benjamin A. *The Family Genetic Sourcebook.* New York: John Wiley & Sons, 1990.

Pritchard, D. J. and Bruce R. Korf. *Medical Genetics at a Glance.* 3d ed. Chichester: John Wiley & Sons, 2013.

GENETIC DISEASES
Disease/Disorder

Anatomy or system affected: All

Specialties and related fields: Embryology, genetics, internal medicine, neonatology, obstetrics, pediatrics

Definition: A variety of disorders transmitted from parent to child through chromosomal material; most people experience disease related to genetics in some form, and research into this area is yielding greater understanding of the relationship between disease and hereditary proclivities toward disease, as well as new strategies for early detection and prevention or therapy.

Key terms:

autosomal recessive disease: a disease that is expressed only when two copies of a defective gene are inherited, one from each parent; present on non-sex-determining chromosomes

chromosomes: rod-shaped structures in each cell that contain genes, the chemical elements that determine traits

deoxyribonucleic acid (DNA): the chemical molecule that transmits hereditary information from generation to generation

dominant gene: a gene that can express its effect when an individual has only one copy of it

gene: the hereditary unit, composed of DNA, that resides on chromosomes

inheritance: the passing down of traits from generation to generation

X-linked: a term used to describe genes or traits that are located on the X chromosome; a male needs only one copy of an X-linked gene for it to be expressed

Causes and Symptoms

Hereditary units called genes determine the majority of the physical and biochemical characteristics of an organism. Genes are composed of a chemical compound called deoxyribonucleic acid (DNA) and are organized into rod-shaped structures called chromosomes that reside in each cell of the body. Each human cell carries forty-six chromosomes organized as twenty-three pairs, each composed of several thousand genes. Twenty-two of the chromosome pairs are homologous pairs; that is, similar genes are located at similar sites on each chromosome. The remaining chromosomes are the sex chromosomes. Human females bear two X chromosomes, and human males possess one X and one Y chromosome.

Human Chromosomes

Genetic diseases are caused by defects in the number of chromosomes, their structure, or the genes on the chromosome (mutation). Shown here is the human complement of chromosomes (twenty-three pairs) and three errors of chromosome number (trisomies, or three instances of a particular chromosome instead of just two) that lead to the genetic disorders Patau syndrome (trisomy no. 13), Edwards syndrome (trisomy no. 18), and the more common Down syndrome (trisomy no. 21).

During the formation of the reproductive cells, the chro-

Information on Genetic Diseases

Causes: Abnormal genes in the reproductive cells of one or both parents, environmental factors causing mutations

Symptoms: Varies widely; can include mental retardation, respiratory dysfunction, neurological deterioration, progressive muscle deterioration, cleft palate, spina bifida, anencephaly, heart abnormalities

Duration: Typically lifelong

Treatments: Typically alleviation of symptoms through surgery, drug therapy, hormone therapy, dietary regulation

mosome pairs separate, and one copy of each pair is randomly included in the egg or sperm. Each egg will contain twenty-two autosomes (non-sex chromosomes) and one X chromosome. Each sperm will contain twenty-two autosomes and either one X or one Y chromosome. The egg and sperm fuse at fertilization, which restores the proper number of chromosomes, and the genes inherited from the baby's parents will determine its sex and much of its physical appearance and future health and well-being.

Genetic diseases are inherited as a result of the presence of abnormal genes in the reproductive cells of one or both parents of an affected individual. There are two broad classifications of genetic disease: those caused by defects in chromosome number or structure and those resulting from a much smaller flaw within a gene. Within the latter category, there are four predominant mechanisms by which the disorders can be transmitted from generation to generation: autosomal dominant inheritance, in which the defective gene is inherited from one parent; autosomal recessive inheritance, in which defective genes are inherited from both parents, who themselves may show no signs of the disorder; X-linked chromosomal inheritance (often called sex-linked), in which the flawed gene has been determined to reside on the X chromosome; and multifactorial inheritance, in which genes interact with each other and/or environmental factors.

Errors in chromosome number include extra and missing chromosomes. The most common chromosomal defect observed in humans is Down syndrome, which is caused by the presence of three copies of chromosome 21, instead of the usual two. Down syndrome occurs at a frequency of about one in eight hundred live births, this frequency increasing with increasing maternal age. The symptoms of this disorder include intellectual disability, short stature, and numerous other medical problems. The most common form of Down syndrome results from the failure of the two copies of chromosome 21 to separate during reproductive cell formation, which upon fusion with a normal reproductive cell at fertilization produces an embryo containing three copies of chromosome 21.

Gross defects in chromosome structure include duplicated and deleted portions of chromosomes and broken and rearranged chromosome fragments. Prader-Willi syndrome results from the deletion of a small portion of chromosome 15.

Children affected with this disorder are prone to intellectual disability, obesity, and diabetes. Cri du chat (literally, "cat cry") syndrome is associated with a large deletion in chromosome 5. Affected infants exhibit facial abnormalities, are severely intellectually disabled, and produce a high-pitched, catlike wail.

Genetic diseases caused by defects in individual genes result when defective genes are propagated through many generations or a new genetic flaw develops in a reproductive cell. New genetic defects arise from a variety of causes, including environmental assaults such as radiation, toxins, or drugs. More than four thousand such gene disorders have been identified.

Manifestation of an autosomal dominant disorder requires the inheritance of only one defective gene from one parent who is afflicted with the disease. Inheritance of two dominant defective genes, one from each parent, is possible but generally creates such severe consequences that the child dies while still in the womb or shortly after birth. An individual who bears one copy of the gene has a 50 percent chance of transmitting that gene and the disease to his or her offspring.

Among the most common autosomal dominant diseases are hyperlipidemia and hypercholesterolemia. These disorders result in elevated levels of lipids and cholesterol in the blood, respectively, which contribute to artery and heart disease. Onset of the symptoms is usually in adulthood, frequently after the affected individual has had children and potentially transmitted the faulty gene to them.

Huntington's chorea causes untreatable neurological deterioration and death, and symptoms do not appear until affected individuals are at least in their forties. Children of parents afflicted with Huntington's chorea may have already made reproductive decisions without the knowledge that they might carry the defective gene. They risk a 50 percent chance of transmitting the disease to their offspring.

Autosomal recessive genetic diseases require that an affected individual bear two copies of a defective gene, inheriting one from each parent. Usually the parents are simply carriers of the defective gene; their one normal copy masks the effect of the one flawed copy. If two carriers have offspring, those children have a 25 percent chance of receiving two copies of the flawed gene and inheriting the disease and a 50 percent chance of being asymptomatic carriers.

Cystic fibrosis is an autosomal recessive disease that occurs at a rate of about one in two thousand live births among Caucasians. The defective gene product causes improper chloride transport in cells and results in thick mucous secretions in lungs and other organs. Sickle cell disease, another autosomal recessive disorder, is the most common genetic disease among African Americans in the United States. Abnormality in the protein hemoglobin, the component of red blood cells that carries oxygen to all the body's tissues, leads to deformed blood cells that are fragile and easily destroyed.

X-linked genetic diseases are transmitted by faulty genes located on the X chromosome. In the case of X-linked recessive diseases, which are by far the more common, females need two copies of the defective gene to acquire such a disease, and in general women carry only one flawed copy, making them asymptomatic carriers of the disorder. Males, having only a single X chromosome, need only one copy of the defective gene to express an X-linked disease. Males with X-linked disorders inherit the defective gene from their mothers, since fathers must contribute a Y chromosome to male offspring. All male offspring of a carrier female will have a 50 percent chance of inheriting the defective gene and developing the disease. In the rare case of a female with two defective X-linked genes, 100 percent of her male offspring will inherit the disease gene and, assuming that the father does not carry the defective gene, her female offspring will be carriers. There are more than 250 X-linked disorders, some of the more common being Duchenne muscular dystrophy, which results in progressive muscle deterioration and early death; hemophilia; and red-green color blindness, which affects about 8 percent of Caucasian males.

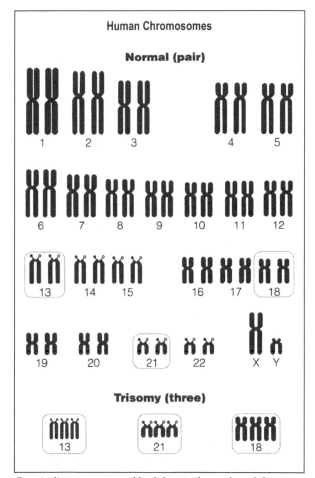

Genetic diseases are caused by defects in the number of chromosomes, in their structure, or in the genes on the chromosome (mutation). Shown here is the human complement of chromosomes (23 pairs) and three errors of chromosome number (trisomies) that lead to the genetic disorders Patau's syndrome (trisomy no. 13), Edward's syndrome (trisomy no. 18), and the more common Down syndrome (trisomy no. 21).

Multifactorial inheritance, which accounts for a number of genetic diseases, is caused by the complex interaction of one or more genes with each other and with environmental factors. This group of diseases includes many disorders that, anecdotally, "run in families." Representative disorders include cleft palate, spina bifida, anencephaly, and some inherited heart abnormalities. Other diseases appear to have a genetic component predisposing an individual to be susceptible to environmental stimuli that trigger the disease. These include cancer, hypertension, diabetes, schizophrenia, alcoholism, depression, and obesity.

Diagnosis and Detection

Most, but not all, genetic diseases manifest their symptoms immediately or soon after the birth of an affected child. Rapid recognition of such a medical condition and its accurate diagnosis are essential for the proper treatment and management of the disease by parents and medical personnel. Medical technology has developed swift and accurate diagnostic methods, in many cases allowing testing of the fetus prior to birth. In addition, tests are available that determine the carrier status of an individual for many autosomal recessive and X-linked diseases. These test results are used in conjunction with genetic counseling of individuals and couples who are at risk of transmitting a genetic disease to their offspring so that they can make informed decisions about their reproductive futures.

Errors in chromosome number and structure are detected in an individual by analyzing his or her chromosomes. A small piece of skin or a blood sample is taken, the cells in the sample are grown to a sufficient number, and the chromosomes within each cell are stained with special dyes so that they may be viewed with a microscope. A picture of the chromosomes, called a karyotype, is taken, and the patient's chromosome array is compared with that of a normal individual. Extra or missing chromosomes or alterations in chromosome structure indicate the presence of a genetic disease. The analysis of karyotypes is the method used to detect Down, Prader-Willi, and cri du chat syndromes, among others.

Defects in chromosome number and structure can also be identified in the fetus prior to birth. Samples may be collected from the fetus by amniocentesis or by chorionic villus sampling. In amniocentesis, a needle is inserted through the pregnant woman's abdomen and uterus, into the fluid-filled sac surrounding the fetus. A sample of this fluid, the amniotic fluid, is withdrawn. The amniotic fluid contains fetal cells sloughed off by the fetus. The cells are grown for several weeks until there are enough to perform chromosome analysis. This procedure is performed only after sixteen weeks' gestation, in order to ensure adequate amniotic fluid for sampling.

Chorionic villus sampling relies on a biopsy of the fetal chorion, a membrane surrounding the fetus that is composed of cells that have the same genetic constitution as the fetus. A catheter is inserted through the pregnant woman's vagina and into the uterus until it is in contact with the chorion. The small sample of this tissue that is removed contains enough cells to perform karyotyping immediately, permitting diagnosis by the next day. Chorionic villus sampling can be performed as early as the eighth or ninth week of pregnancy. This earlier testing gives the procedure an advantage over amniocentesis, since the earlier determination of whether a fetus is carrying a genetic disease allows safer pregnancy termination if the parents choose this course.

Karyotype analysis is limited to the diagnosis of genetic diseases caused by very large chromosome abnormalities. The majority of hereditary disorders are caused by gene flaws that are too small to see microscopically. For many of these diseases, diagnosis is possible through either biochemical testing or DNA analysis.

Many genetic disorders cause a lack of a specific biochemical necessary for normal metabolism. These types of disorders are frequently referred to as "inborn errors of metabolism." Many of these errors can be detected by the chemical analysis of fetal tissue. For example, galactosemia is a disease that results from the lack of galactose-1-phosphate uridyl transferase. Infants with this disorder cannot break down galactose, one of the major sugars in milk. If left untreated, galactosemia can lead to developmental disabilities, cataracts, kidney and liver failure, and death. By analyzing fetal cells obtained from amniocentesis or chorionic villus sampling, the level of this important chemical can be assessed, and, if necessary, the infant can be placed on a galactose-free diet immediately after birth.

DNA analysis can be used to determine whether a genetic disease has been inherited when either the chromosomal location of the gene, the chemical sequence of the DNA, or particular DNA sequences commonly associated with the gene in question (called markers) are known.

Genes are made up of sequences of four chemical elements of DNA: adenine (A), guanine (G), thymine (T), and cytosine (C). Sometimes the proper DNA sequence of a gene is known, as well as the changes in the sequence that cause disease. Direct analysis of the DNA of an individual suspected of carrying a certain genetic disorder is possible in these cases. For example, in sickle cell disease, it is known that a change in a single DNA chemical element leads to the disorder. To test for this disease, a tissue sample is obtained from the fetus, and the DNA is isolated from the cells and analyzed with highly specific probes that can detect the presence of the defective gene that will lead to sickle cell disease. Informed action may then be taken regarding the future of the fetus or the care of an affected child.

Occasionally a disease gene itself has not been precisely isolated or had its DNA sequence determined, but sequences very near the gene of interest have been analyzed. If specific variations within these neighboring sequences are always present when the gene of interest is flawed, these nearby sequences can then be used as markers for the presence of the defective gene. When the variant sequences are present, so is the disease gene. Prenatal testing for cystic fibrosis has been done by looking for such variant sequences.

Individuals who come from families in which genetic diseases tend to occur can be tested as carriers, so they will know the risk of passing a certain disease to their offspring. For example, individuals whose families have a history of cystic fibrosis, but who themselves are not affected, may be asymptomatic carriers. If they have children with individuals who are also cystic fibrosis carriers, they have a 25 percent chance of passing two copies of the defective gene to their offspring. DNA samples from the potential parents can be analyzed for the presence of a defective gene. If both partners are carriers, their decision about whether to have children will be made with knowledge of the possible risk to their offspring. If only one or neither of them is a carrier, their offspring will not be at risk of inheriting cystic fibrosis, as it is an autosomal recessive disease. Carrier testing is possible for many genetic diseases, as well as for disorders that appear late in life, such as Huntington's chorea.

Many of the gene flaws of multifactorial diseases, those that interact with environmental factors to produce disease, have been identified and are testable. Individuals who know they have a gene that puts them at risk for certain disorders can incorporate preventive measures into their lifestyle, thus minimizing their chances of developing the disease. For example, certain cancers, such as colon and breast cancer, have a genetic component. Individuals who test positive for the genes that predispose them to develop cancer can modify their diets to include cancer-fighting foods and receive frequent medical checkups to detect cancer development at its earliest, most treatable stage. Those with genes that contribute to arteriosclerosis and heart disease can modify their diets and increase exercise, and those with a genetic predisposition for alcoholism can avoid the consumption of alcohol.

Perspective and Prospects

The scientific study of human genetics and genetic disease is relatively new, having begun in the early twentieth century. However, there are many early historical records that recognize that certain traits are hereditarily transmitted. Ancient Greek literature is peppered with references to heredity, and the Jewish book of religious and civil laws, the Talmud, describes in detail the inheritance pattern of hemophilia and its ramifications for circumcision.

The Augustinian monk Gregor Mendel worked out many of the principles of heredity by manipulating the pollen and eggs of pea plants over many generations. His work was conducted from the 1860s to the 1870s but was unrecognized by the scientific community until 1900.

At about this time, many disorders were being recognized as genetic diseases. Pedigree analysis, a way to trace inheritance patterns through a family tree, has been used since the mid-nineteenth century to track the incidence of hemophilia in European royal families. This analysis indicates that the disease was transmitted through females (indeed, hemophilia is an X-linked disorder). In the early twentieth century, Archibald Garrod, a British physician, recognized certain biochemical disorders as genetic diseases and proposed accurate mechanisms for their transmission.

In 1953, Francis Crick and James D. Watson discovered the structure of DNA; thus began studies on the molecular biology of genes. This research resulted in the monumental discovery in 1973 that pieces of DNA from animals and bacteria could be cut and spliced together into a functional molecule. This recombinant DNA technology fostered a revolution in genetic analysis, in which pieces of human DNA can be removed and put into bacteria. The bacteria then replicate millions of copies of the human DNA, permitting detailed analysis. These recombinant molecules also produce human gene products, such as RNA and protein, thereby facilitating the analysis of normal and aberrant genes.

The recombinant DNA revolution spawned the development of DNA tests for genetic diseases and carrier status. Knowledge of what a normal gene product is and does is exceptionally helpful in the treatment of genetic diseases. For example, Duchenne muscular dystrophy is known to be caused by the lack of a protein called dystrophin. This suggests that one possible treatment is to provide functional dystrophin to an individual with this disease.

Ultimately, medical science seeks to treat genetic diseases by providing a functional copy of the flawed gene to the affected individual. While such gene therapy would not affect the reproductive cells—the introduced gene copy would not be passed down to future generations—the normal gene product would alleviate the genetic disorder in the individual.

—*Karen E. Kalumuck, Ph.D.*

See also Albinos; Amniocentesis; Batten's disease; Birth defects; Breast cancer; Cerebral palsy; Chorionic villus sampling; Colon cancer; Color blindness; Congenital heart disease; Cornelia de Lange syndrome; Cystic fibrosis; Diabetes mellitus; DiGeorge syndrome; DNA and RNA; Down syndrome; Dwarfism; Embryology; Environmental diseases; Fragile X syndrome; Fructosemia; Gaucher's disease; Gene therapy; Genetic counseling; Genetic engineering; Genetics and inheritance; Genomics; Gigantism; Glycogen storage diseases; Hemochromatosis; Hemophilia; Huntington's disease; Immunodeficiency disorders; Klinefelter syndrome; Klippel-Trenaunay syndrome; Laboratory tests; Leukodystrophy; Maple syrup urine disease (MSUD); Marfan syndrome; Metabolic disorders; Mental retardation; Mucopolysaccharidosis (MPS); Muscular dystrophy; Mutation; Neonatology; Neurofibromatosis; Niemann-Pick disease; Oncology; Pediatrics; Phenylketonuria (PKU); Polycystic kidney disease; Porphyria; Prader-Willi syndrome; Progeria; Proteomics; Rubinstein-Taybi syndrome; Screening; Severe combined immunodeficiency syndrome (SCID); Sickle cell disease; Spina bifida; Tay-Sachs disease; Thalassemia; Thrombocytopenia; Turner syndrome; Von Willebrand's disease; Wilson's disease; Wiskott-Aldrich syndrome.

For Further Information:

Cooper, Necia Grant, ed. *The Human Genome Project: Deciphering the Blueprint of Heredity.* Rev. ed. Mill Valley, Calif.: University Science Books, 1994.

GeneTests. http://www.ncbi.nlm.nih.gov/sites/GeneTests

Genetic Alliance. http://www.geneticalliance.org

Gormley, Myra Vanderpool. *Family Diseases: Are You at Risk?* Baltimore: Genealogical Publishing, 2007.

Hereditary Disease Foundation. http://www.hdfoundation.org

Jorde, Lynn B., John C. Carey, and Michael J. Bamshad. *Medical Genetics.* 4th ed. Philadelphia: Mosby/Elsevier, 2010.

Judd, Sandra J., ed. *Genetic Disorders Sourcebook: Basic Consumer Information About Hereditary Diseases and Disorders.* 4th ed. Detroit: Omnigraphics, 2010.

King, Richard A., Jerome I. Rotter, and Arno G. Motulsky, eds. *The Genetic Basis of Common Diseases*. 2d ed. New York: Oxford University Press, 2002.

Lewis, Ricki. *Human Genetics: Concepts and Applications*. 10th ed. New York: McGraw-Hill, 2012.

McCance, Kathryn L., and Sue E. Huether, eds. *Pathophysiology: The Biologic Basis for Disease in Adults and Children*. 6th ed. Saint Louis: Mosby/Elsevier, 2010.

Marshall, Elizabeth L. *The Human Genome Project: Cracking the Code Within Us*. New York: Franklin Watts, 1997.

Milunsky, Aubrey, and Jeff M. Milunsky, eds. *Genetic Disorders of the Fetus: Diagnosis, Prevention, and Treatment*. 6th ed. Hoboken, N.J.: Wiley-Blackwell, 2010.

Springhouse Corporation. *Everything You Need to Know About Diseases*. Springhouse, Pa.: Author, 1996.

Wingerson, Lois. *Mapping Our Genes: The Genome Project and the Future of Medicine*. New York: Plume, 1991.

GENETIC ENGINEERING

Procedure

Also known as: Biotechnology, gene splicing, recombinant DNA technology

Anatomy or system affected: All

Specialties and related fields: Alternative medicine, biochemistry, biotechnology, dermatology, embryology, ethics, forensic medicine, genetics, pharmacology, preventive medicine

Definition: A wide array of techniques that alter the genetic constitution of cells or individuals by selective removal, insertion, or modification of individual genes or gene sets.

Key terms:

gene cloning: the development of a line of genetically identical organisms that contain identical copies of the same gene or deoxyribonucleic acid (DNA) fragments

gene therapy: the insertion of a functional gene or genes into a cell, tissue, or organ to correct a genetic abnormality

polymerase chain reaction (PCR): an in vitro process by which specific parts of a DNA molecule or a gene can be made into millions or billions of copies within a short time

recombinant DNA: a hybrid DNA molecule created in the test tube by joining a DNA fragment of interest with a carrier DNA

southern blot: a procedure used to transfer DNA from a gel to a nylon membrane, which in turn allows the finding of genes that are complementary to particular DNA sequences called probes

Genetic Engineering and Human Health

Genetic engineering, recombinant DNA technology, and biotechnology constitute a set of techniques used to achieve one or more of three goals: to reveal the complex processes of how genes are inherited and expressed, to provide better understanding and effective treatment for various diseases (particularly genetic disorders), and to generate economic benefits, which include improved plants and animals for agriculture and the efficient production of valuable biopharmaceuticals. The characteristics of genetic engineering possess both vast promise and potential threats to humankind. It is an understatement to say that genetic engineering

has revolutionized medicine and agriculture in the twenty-first century. As this technology unleashes its power to have an impact on daily life, it has also brought challenges to ethical systems and religious beliefs.

Soon after the publication of the short essay by Francis Crick and James Watson on DNA structure in 1953, research began to uncover the way by which DNA molecules can be cut and spliced back together. With the discovery of the first restriction endonuclease by Hamilton Smith and colleagues in 1970, the real story of genetic engineering began to unfold. The creation of the first engineered DNA molecule through the splicing together of DNA fragments from two unrelated species was made public in 1972. What soon followed was an array of recombinant DNA molecules and genetically modified bacteria, viruses, fungi, plants, and animals. The debate over the issues of "tinkering with God" heated up, and public outcry over genetic engineering was widespread. In 1996, the birth of Dolly, a ewe that was the first mammal cloned from an adult body cell, elevated the debate over the impact of biological research to a new level. Furthermore, a number of genetically modified organisms (GMOs) have been released commercially since 1996. In 2006, it was estimated that more than 75 percent of food products in the United States contained some ingredients from GMOs.

Genetic engineering holds tremendous promise for medicine and human well-being. Medical applications of genetic engineering include the diagnosis of genetic and other diseases, treatment for genetic disorders, regenerative medicine using pluripotent (stem) cells, the production of safer and more effective vaccines and pharmaceuticals, and the prospect of curing genetic disorders through gene therapy. Many human diseases such as cystic fibrosis, Down syndrome, fragile X syndrome, Huntington's disease, muscular dystrophy, sickle cell anemia, and Tay-Sachs disease are inherited. There are usually no conventional treatments for these disorders because they do not respond to antibiotics or other conventional drugs. Genetic engineering is currently used successfully in the treatment of chronic lymphocytic leukemia (CLL), Parkinson's disease, and X-linked severe combined immunodeficiency (SCID). Another area in which genetic engineering is commonly used is the commercial production of vaccines and pharmaceuticals through genetic engineering, which has emerged as a rapidly developing field. The potential of embryonic stem cells to become any cell, tissue, or organ under adequate conditions holds enormous promise for regenerative medicine. Particularly large studies have focused on animal models, mostly mice, to serve as human models for genetic modifications. Also, pig to human organ transplantation is a field that is rapidly growing due to the inadequate human organ availability.

Prevention of genetic disorders. Although prevention may be achieved by avoiding any environmental factors that cause an abnormality, the most effective prevention, when possible, is to reduce the frequency of or eliminate entirely the harmful genes (mutations) from the general population. As more precise tools and procedures for manipulating individual genes are optimized, this will eventually become more commonly

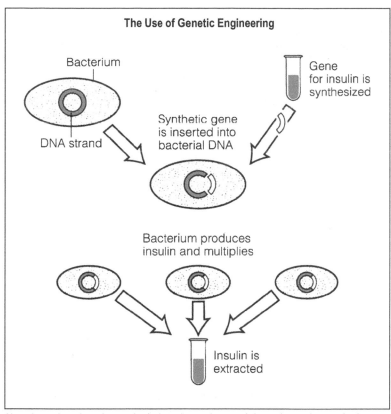

The Use of Genetic Engineering

Bacterium

Gene for insulin is synthesized

DNA strand

Synthetic gene is inserted into bacterial DNA

Bacterium produces insulin and multiplies

Insulin is extracted

Genetic engineering, the manipulation of genetic material, can be used to synthesize large quantities of drugs or hormones, such as insulin.

used. As of 2013, take-home kits for under $100 that assess individual DNA are available to the public, allowing people to gain an understanding of the genetic diseases they may have or carry. However, the prevention of genetic disorders at present is usually achieved by ascertaining those individuals in the population who are at risk for passing a serious genetic disorder to their offspring and then offering them genetic counseling and prenatal screening, followed (in some serious cases) by the option of selective abortion of affected fetuses.

Genetic counseling is the process of communicating information gained through classic genetic studies and contemporary research to those individuals who are themselves at risk or have a high likelihood of passing defects to their offspring. During counseling, information about the disease itself-its severity and prognosis, whether effective therapies exist, and the risk of recurrence-is generally presented. For those couples who find the risks unacceptably high, counseling may also include discussions of contraceptive methods, adoption, prenatal diagnosis, possible abortion, and artificial insemination by a donor. The final decision must still rest with the couple themselves, but the significant increase in the accuracy of risk assessment through genetic technology has made it easier for parents to make well-informed decisions.

For those couples who find the burden of having an affected child unbearable, prenatal diagnosis may solve their

dilemma. Prenatal screening could be performed for a variety of genetic disorders. It requires samples, acquired through either amniocentesis or chorionic villus sampling, of fetal cells or chemicals produced by the fetus. After sampling, several analyses can be performed. First, biochemical analysis is used to determine the concentration of chemicals in the sample and therefore to diagnose whether a particular fetus is deficient or low in enzymes that facilitate specific biological reactions. Next, analysis of the chromosomes of the fetal cells can show if all the chromosomes are present and whether there are structural abnormalities in any of them. Finally, the most effective means of detecting the defective genes is through recombinant DNA techniques. This has become possible with the rapid increase of DNA copies through a technique called polymerase chain reaction (PCR), which can produce virtually unlimited copies of a specific gene or DNA fragment, starting with as little as a single copy. Routine prenatal diagnosis can be performed to screen a fetus for Down syndrome, Huntington's disease, sickle cell anemia, and Tay-Sachs disease.

Treatment of diseases and genetic disorders. Genetic engineering may be used for direct treatments of diseases or genetic disorders through various means, including the production of possible vaccines for acquired immunodeficiency syndrome (AIDS), the treatment of various cancers, and the synthesis of biopharmaceuticals for a variety of metabolic, growth, and development diseases. In general, biosynthesis is a process in which the gene coding for a particular product is isolated, cloned into another organism (mostly bacteria), and later expressed in that organism (the host). By cultivating the host organism, large quantities of the gene products can be harvested and purified. A few examples can illustrate the useful features of biosynthesis.

Insulin is essential for the treatment of insulin-dependent diabetes mellitus, the most severe form of diabetes. Historically, insulin was obtained from a cow or pig pancreas. Two problems exist for this traditional supply of insulin. First, large quantities of the pancreas are needed to extract enough insulin for continuous treatment of one patient. Second, insulin so obtained is not chemically identical to human insulin; hence some patients may produce antibodies that can seriously interfere with treatment. Human insulin produced through genetic engineering is quite effective yet without any side effects. It has been produced commercially and made available to patients since 1982.

Another successful story in biosynthesis is the production of human growth hormone (HGH), which is used in the treatment of children with growth retardation called pituitary dwarfism.

The successful biosynthesis of HGH is important for several reasons. The conventional source of HGH was human pituitary glands removed at autopsy. Each child afflicted with pituitary dwarfism needs twice-a-week injections until the age of twenty. Such a treatment regime requires more than a thousand pituitary glands. The autopsy supply could hardly keep up with the demand. Furthermore, as a result of a small amount of virus contamination in the extracted HGH, many children receiving this treatment developed virus-related diseases.

Another gene therapy treatment that has recently been approved in Europe is alipogene tiparvovec, used for people with a lipoprotein lipase deficiency (LPLD). LPLD is a condition that results in high fat concentration in the bloodstream and increase the risk of pancreatitis. Alipogene tiparvovec has been shown to greatly reduce the incidence of pancreatitis and decrease fat concentrations in the blood in a few weeks. Other biopharmaceuticals under development or in preclinical or clinical trials through genetic engineering include anticancer drugs, anti-aging agents and possible vaccines for AIDS and malaria.

Broadly speaking, three types of gene therapy exist: germ line therapy, enhancement gene therapy, and somatic gene therapy. All gene therapy trials currently underway or in the pipeline are restricted to the somatic cells as targets for gene transfer. Germ line therapy involves the introduction of novel genes into germ cells, such as eggs or in early embryos. Although it has the potential for correcting defective genes completely, germ line therapy is highly controversial. Enhancement gene therapy, through which human potential might be enhanced for some desired traits, raises an even greater ethical dilemma. Both germ line and enhancement gene therapies have been banned based on the unresolved ethical issues surrounding them.

Somatic gene therapy is designed to introduce functional genes into body cells, thus enabling the body to perform normal functions and providing temporary correction for genetic abnormalities. The cloned human gene is first transferred into a viral vector, which is used to infect white blood cells removed from the patient. The transferred normal gene is then inserted into a chromosome and becomes active. After growth to enhance their numbers under sterile conditions, the cells are re-implanted into the patient, where they produce a gene product that is missing in the untreated patient, allowing the individual to function normally. Several disorders are currently being treated with this technique, including severe combined immunodeficiency disease (SCID). Individuals with SCID have no functional immune system and usually die from infections that would be minor in normal people. While several young boys with SCID remarkably showed almost complete recovery following gene therapy, a high percentage of them have subsequently developed leukemia following the introduction of genetically engineered bone marrow stem cells. Gene therapy is also being used or tested as a treatment for cystic fibrosis, skin cancer, breast cancer, brain cancer, and AIDS.

Most of these treatments are only partially successful, and they are prohibitively expensive. Over a ten-year period, from 1990 to 2000, more than four thousand people were treated through gene therapy. Unfortunately, most of these trials were failures that led to some loss of confidence in gene therapy. These failures have been attributed to inefficient vectors and the inability in many cases to specifically target the required host tissues. In the future, as more efficient vectors are engineered, gene therapy is expected to be a common method for treating a large number of genetic disorders.

Genetic Engineering in Agriculture, Forensics, and Environmental Science

As the use of genetic engineering expands rapidly, it is difficult to generate an exhaustive list of all possible applications, but three other areas are worth noting: forensic, environmental, and agricultural applications. Although these areas are not directly related to medicine, they certainly have profound impacts on human well-being. There are numerous ways that genetic engineering may be used to benefit agriculture and food production. First, the production of vaccines and the application of methods for transferring genes are likely to benefit animal husbandry, as scientists can alter commercially important traits such as milk yield, butterfat, and proportion of lean meat. For example, the bovine growth hormone produced through genetic engineering has been used since the late 1980s to boost milk production by cows. A mutant form of the myostatin gene has been identified and found to cause heavy muscling after this gene was introduced first into a mouse and later into the Belgian Blue bull. This technique marks the first step toward breeding cows and meat animals with lower fat and a higher proportion of lean meat. Other examples of using genetic engineering in animal husbandry include hormones for a faster growth rate in poultry and the production of recombinant human proteins in the milk of livestock.

Second, genetic engineering is expected to alter dramatically the conventional approaches of developing new strains of crops through breeding. The technology allows the transferring of genes for nitrogen fixation; the improvement of photosynthesis (and therefore yield); the promotion of resistance to pests, pathogens, and herbicides and tolerance to frost, drought, and increased salinity; and the improvement of nutritional value and consumer acceptability. Genetically engineered tobacco plants have been grown to produce the protein phaseolin, which is naturally synthesized by soybeans and other legume crops. The first genetically engineered potato was approved for human consumption by the U.S. government in 1995 and by Canada in 1996. This NewLeaf potato, developed by corporate giant Monsanto, carries a gene from the bacterium Bacillus thuringiensis. This gene produces a protein toxic to the Colorado potato beetle, an insect that causes substantial loss of the crop if left uncontrolled. The production of this protein by potato plants equips them with resistance to beetles, hence alleviating crop loss, saving on the cost on pesticides, and reducing the risk of environment contamination.

Antiviral genes have been successfully transferred and expressed into cotton, and the release of new cotton strains with resistance to multiple viruses is a matter of time. At least five transgenic corn strains with resistance to herbicides or pathogens had been developed and commercially produced by U.S. farmers by 2002. Some genes coding tolerance to drought and to subfreezing temperatures have been cloned and transferred into or among crop plants, some of which have already made a great impact on agriculture in developing countries. Initial effort has been made to replace chemical fertilizers with more environment-friendly biofertilizers. Secondary metabolites produced naturally by plants have also been purified and used as biopesticides. Genetically enhanced vitamin enriched food is on the rise as well. A prime example is "golden rice," rice that has been engineered to have a higher content of vitamin A. Currently, many grain, produce, milk, and meat produced by animals or plants have been genetically engineered in some manner.

Genetic engineering is also useful in forensics. DNA fingerprints from samples collected at crime scenes provide strong evidence in trials, thus helping to solve many violent crimes. DNA can be isolated easily from tissue left at a crime scene, a splattering of blood, a hair sample, or even skin left under a victim's fingernails. A variety of techniques can be used routinely to determine the probability of matching between sample DNA and that of a suspect. DNA fingerprints are also useful in paternity and property disputes and in the study of the genealogy of various species.

The metabolism of micro-organisms can be altered through genetic engineering, which enables them to absorb and degrade waste and hazardous material from the environment. The growth rate and metabolic capabilities of micro-organisms offer great potential for coping with some environmental problems. Sewage plants can use engineered bacteria to degrade many organic compounds into nontoxic substances. Microbes may be engineered to detoxify specific substances in waste dumps or oil spills. Many bacteria can extract heavy metals (such as lead and copper) from their surroundings and incorporate them into compounds that are recoverable, thus cleaning them from the environment. Many more such applications have yet to be tested or discovered.

Perspective and Prospects

Since the discovery of the double-helical structure of DNA by Francis Crick and James Watson in 1953, human curiosity regarding this amazing molecule has propelled the advancement of biological sciences in an unprecedented fashion. The first successful experiment in genetic engineering was described in 1972 when DNA fragments from two different organisms were joined together to produce a biologically functional hybrid DNA molecule. The next milestone came in 1975, when Edward Southern introduced Southern blotting, a technique that has many applications and has proved invaluable for the subsequent development of genetic engineering. This technique is used to identify a particular gene or DNA fragment from a mixture of thousands of different genes or DNA fragments. Later, the automated DNA sequencers, which can rapidly churn out letter sequences from DNA fragments, and the discovery of reverse transcriptase and PCR further improved the capabilities of scientists in studying and manipulating DNA molecules and the genes that they carry.

Using these techniques, the first prenatal diagnosis of a genetic disease was made in 1976 for alpha-thalassemia, a genetic disorder caused by the absence of globin genes. This represented a monumental step forward in the use of genetic tools in the medical field. It paved the way for the later development in which mutations in many genes could be detected in early pregnancy. Three years later, insulin was first synthesized through genetic engineering. In 1982, the commercial production of genetically engineered human insulin became a reality.

Gene therapy trials began in 1990, first with SCID. The first complete human genetic map was published in 1993, and various new techniques in DNA fingerprinting and the isolation of specific genes were developed. Also, an increasing number of pharmaceuticals have been produced through genetic engineering. Two versions of the draft copy of the human genome were published in 2001, launching the genomic revolution, and by 2006 complete DNA sequences of the genomes of over two hundred model research organisms, from bacteria to mice, were publicly available for researchers. In the twenty-first century, genetic engineering will continue to offer more benefits in medicine and in agriculture in undreamed of ways.

In retrospect, genetic engineering presents a mixed blessing of invaluable benefits and dilemmas that science and technology have always offered humankind. There are those who would like to restrict the uses of genetic engineering and who might prefer that such technology had never been developed. Others believe that the benefits far outweigh the possible risks and that any potential threat can be overcome easily through government regulation or legislation. Others do not take sides on the debate in general but are greatly concerned with some specific applications.

Obviously, the power of genetic engineering demands a new set of decisions, both ethical and economical, by individuals, government, and society. Considerable concern has been expressed by both scientists and the general public regarding possible biohazards from genetic engineering. What if engineered organisms prove resistant to all known antibiotics or carry cancer genes that might spread throughout the community? What if a genetically engineered plant becomes an uncontrollable super weed? Would these kinds of risks outweigh the potential benefits? Others argue that the risk has been exaggerated and therefore do not want to impose limits on research. Genetic engineering has also generated legal issues concerning intellectual properties and patents for different aspects of the technology.

Even more controversial are the many ethical issues. Perhaps the most obvious ethical issue surrounding genetic engineering is the objection to some applications that are considered socially undesirable and morally wrong. One example is bovine growth hormone. Some vigorously opposed its use in boosting milk production for two main reasons. First, the recombinant hormone could change the composition of the milk. However, this view was dismissed by experts from the National Institutes of Health (NIH) and the Food and Drug Administration (FDA) after a thorough study. Second, many dairy farmers feared that greater milk production per cow would drive prices down even farther and put some small farmers out of business.

Numerous aspects of the application of genetic engineering to humans also present ethical challenges. In some couples, both people carry a defective gene and have an appreciable chance of having an affected child. Should they refrain entirely from having children of their own? For genetic disorders caused by chromosomal abnormalities, such as Tay-Sachs disease, prenatal diagnosis can detect the defect in a fetus with great precision. Should the fetus be aborted if the screening result is positive? Should screening tests of infants for genetic disorders be required? If so, would such a requirement infringe the rights of the individual by the government? Perhaps the greatest concern of all is the possibility of designing or cloning a human being through genetic engineering. The debate over the ethical, legal, and social implications of genetic engineering should help in the formulation and optimization of public policy and laws regarding this technology, and genetic engineering research and its applications should proceed with caution.

—Ming Y. Zheng, Ph.D.;
updated by Sarit Sandowski, OMS-II

See also Bacteriology; Bionics and biotechnology; Cancer; Cells; Chemotherapy; Cloning; Cytology; Diabetes mellitus; DNA and RNA; Enzyme therapy; Enzymes; Ethics; Fetal tissue transplantation; Gene therapy; Genetic counseling; Genetics and inheritance; Genomics; Hormones; Immunization and vaccination; Mutation; Pharmacology; Screening; Stem cells

For Further Information:
Brungs, Robert S.J., and R.S.M. Postiglione, eds. *The Genome: Plant, Animal, Human.* St. Louis: ITEST Faith/Science Press, 2000. A collection of excellent scientific, ethical, educational, and theological papers focuses on the genomic revolution and the application of genetic engineering to plants, humans, and other animals.

Daniell, H., S.J. Streatfield, and K. Wycoff. "Medical Molecular Farming: Production of Antibodies, Biopharmaceuticals, and Edible Vaccines in Plants." *Trends in Plant Science* 6 (2001): 219-226. A contemporary review of the production of plant-based medicinal products through genetic engineering and related biotechnology.

Frankel, M.S., and A. Teich, eds. *The Genetic Frontier.* Washington, D.C.: American Association for the Advancement of Science, 1994. A wonderful collection of essays from many experts and organizations dealing with the ethics, laws, and policies of genetic engineering.

"Genetic Engineering & Biotechnology News." Mary Ann Lieber Inc., 2013. http://www.genengnews.com. A website with articles that are up to date on genetic engineering advancements.

Gerdes, Louise I., ed. *Genetic Engineering: Opposing Viewpoints.* Farmington Hills, MI: Greenhaven Press, 2004. Presents balanced and well-thought-out opposing views on genetic engineering by proponents and opponents from various angles.

Haddley, K. "Alipogene Tiparvovec for the Treatment of Lipoprotein Lipase Deficiency." *Drugs of Today* 49, no. 3 (2013): 161. http://journals.prous.com/journals/servlet/xmlxsl/pk_journals.xml_summaryn_pr?p_JournalId=4&p_RefId=1937398#. An article explaining the mechanism of how gene therapy is used to treat LPLD.

Holland, Suzanne, Karen Lebacqz, and Laurie Zoloth, eds. *The*
Human Embryonic Stem Cell Debate: Science, Ethics, and Public Policy. Cambridge, MA: MIT Press, 2001. Very thoughtful reflections on debates regarding stem cell research and potential pros and cons by a number of extraordinary people from diverse disciplines.

Kilner, John F., R.D. Pentz, and F.E. Young, eds. *Genetic Ethics: Do the Ends Justify the Genes?* Grand Rapids, MI: Wm. B. Eerdmans, 1997. An assembly of experts addresses three dimensions of the genetic challenge: perspective, information, and intervention. A wonderful collection of useful and informative guiding principles on genetic engineering.

Merino, Noël. *Genetic Engineering: Opposing Viewpoints.* Detroit: Greenhaven Press, 2013. Addresses controversial questions surrounding the issue of genetic engineering such as the benefits and risks of genetic engineering, the environmental impact of genetic engineering, and the pros and cons of regulation of genetic engineering.

Panno, Joseph. *Gene Therapy: Treating Disease by Repairing Genes.* New York: Facts on File, 2005. A well-illustrated basic introduction to the principles and possibilities of gene therapy.

Pasternak, Jack J. *An Introduction to Human Molecular Genetics.* 2nd ed. Hoboken, NJ: Wiley-Liss, 2005. An excellent primer on many technologies as applied to humans, including genetic engineering, stem cell research, cloning, and gene therapy.

Primrose, S.B., R.M. Twyman, and R.W. Old. *Principles of Genetic Manipulation: An Introduction to Genetic Engineering.* 6th ed. Palo Alto, Calif.: Blackwell Science, 2001. A resource that provides foundational knowledge on the principles and processes of genetic engineering.

Tal, J. "Adeno-Associated Virus-Based Vectors in Gene Therapy." *Journal of Biomedical Science* 7 (2000): 279-291. A good summary of gene therapy and the outlook on recent developments.

GENETIC IMPRINTING
Biology
Also known as: Genomic imprinting, parental imprinting
Anatomy or system affected: All
Specialties and related fields: Embryology, genetics, oncology
Definition: The silencing of specific genes by means of deoxyribonucleic acid (DNA) methylation that is initially established during sperm and oocyte production. Typically, gene expression is influenced by the genetic contribution from both parents. For an imprinted gene, expression in the offspring is determined by just one of the parents, the parent in whom the gene has not been silenced through methylation.

Key terms:
allele: alternative form of a gene
autosome: a nonsex chromosome of which there are 22 pairs in a normal human. Humans also have a 23rd pair of chromosomes, the sex chromosomes.
deacetylation: removal of an acetyl group

Acetyl group

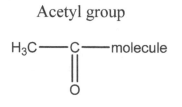

differentiation: process in which a cell becomes more specialized

gametogenesis: production of sperm in males and oocytes in females

gene expression: for genes that code for proteins, a collective term for transcription of the gene, translation of the resulting messenger ribonucleic acid (mRNA), and posttranslational modifications of the resulting protein, all of which determine the quantity and timing of appearance of the protein in the cell

histone proteins: proteins involved in forming histone octamers that package and compact chromosomal DNA

locus: physical region on a chromosome where a specific gene or genes reside

methyltransferase: a protein enzyme that catalyzes methylation, the addition of a methyl group (-CH₃) to a cytosine base of certain CpG dinucleotides in DNA

RNA polymerase: enzyme that synthesizes RNA from a DNA template in the process called transcription

Structure and Functions

In any given normal individual, the expression of most genes occurs from both of the alleles, the one inherited from the father and the one inherited from the mother. Expression of imprinted genes varies from this paradigm in that only one of the alleles is actively expressed. The active allele and the silent allele are determined during gametogenesis in the parents. At least 1 percent of mammalian genes are thought to be imprinted, and the purpose of this phenomenon is to fine-tune gene expression during differentiation and development. Mammals silence these genes and maintain this silencing through the attachment of -CH₃ or methyl groups (methylation) to cytosine bases in DNA at CpG dinucleotides (see Figure 1). During DNA replication, enzymes called maintenance methyltransferases attach methyl groups to cytosine bases in the newly formed strand of DNA in order to match the methylation pattern found on the parental DNA strand. During meiosis, a special type of cell division used to produce gametes (eggs and sperm), the DNA is reactivated

(the methylated groups are removed), and then a different set of enzymes called de novo methyltransferases establish the gender-specific imprinting pattern (sex-specific pattern of base methylation in the DNA). This mechanism is used for imprinting genes on both X chromosomes and autosomes.

Genetic imprinting can be illustrated by describing gene expression from the first chromosome locus where imprinting was observed. This locus is on human chromosome 15 and contains the gene for insulin-like growth factor 2 (Igf2) as well as a gene named H19, which encodes a regulatory RNA thought to be involved in the suppression of tumors. The Igf2 gene is silenced or imprinted on the maternal chromosome but actively expressed from the chromosome contributed by the male. The opposite imprinting pattern applies to the H19 gene. H19 is imprinted on the paternal chromosome but actively expressed from the maternal chromosome. As a result maternal Igf2 and paternal H19 gene expression is silenced while maternal H19 and paternal Igf2 gene expression is active. Normal development requires this gene expression pattern, and severe abnormalities occur in individuals who inherit disruptions of this pattern.

The details of the imprinting mechanism of the Igf2 and H19 genes are complex but provide a good example of common molecular aspects of many imprinted gene clusters. Along the Igf2/H19 locus is a region of DNA called an enhancer, which is bound by a protein factor called an activator. The activator typically recruits RNA polymerase and its associated protein transcription factors to the locus for transcription of these genes. Another DNA sequence known as an insulator is located nearby and lies between the Igf2 and H19 genes. The insulator is bound by a protein called the CCCTC-binding factor (CTCF), and CTCF binding prevents transcription of the Igf2 gene by shielding the Igf2 gene from the activator. Specifically CTCF attracts a complex of proteins that contain a histone deacetylase. Histone deacetylase catalyzes the "deacetylation" of histone proteins (the removal of acetyl groups), thus tightening the histones' grip on the DNA (see Figure 2). DNA in the tightened grip of histones is less accessible to RNA polymerase and transcriptional activators; conse-

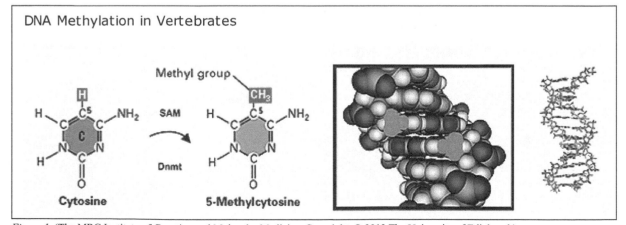

Figure 1. (The MRC Institute of Genetics and Molecular Medicine, Copyright © 2013 The University of Edinburgh)

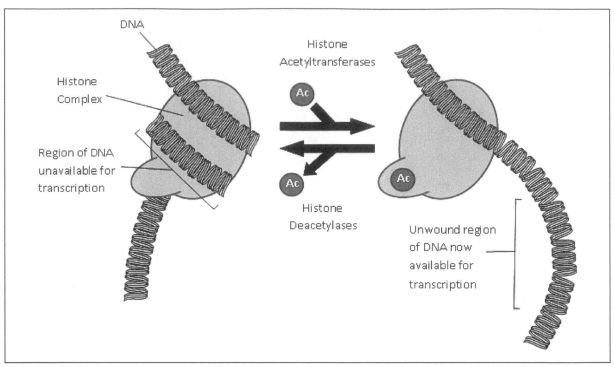

Figure 2. Role of histone acetyltransferases and histone deacetylases. (Copyright © 2014 The University of Queensland)

quently, that DNA is not transcribed and is said to be silenced. On the maternal chromosome, CTCF binds to the insulator sequence, effectively turning off Igf2 gene transcription; however, the activator is still able to stimulate H19 gene transcription nearby. On the paternal chromosome, the H19 gene and the insulator sequences are methylated, preventing the activator from turning on H19 gene transcription and preventing the binding of CTCF to the insulator sequence. Without CTCF binding to the insulator sequence, the activator is free to stimulate Igf2 gene transcription (see Figure 3).

Disorders and Diseases

Prader-Willi syndrome (PWS) occurs in 1 out of every 25,000 births, affecting 350,000-400,000 people across the world, and is the most common genetic cause of life-threatening obesity. Pedigree and molecular genetic analyses reveal that roughly 80 percent of cases involve deletion of a gene or genes on the long arm of chromosome 15 in the father that is exacerbated by genetic imprinting of the maternal chromosome 15 in the same region of the paternal deletion. Affected individuals are small at birth with feeding difficulties and retarded development, both physically and mentally. Children often exhibit self-injurious behavior such as skin picking. At 6 months of age feeding difficulties improve but transition to uncontrolled eating habits as an adolescent and adult, leading to obesity and diabetes. The major treatment is weight control through calorie restriction and the administration of recombinant human growth hormone to decrease body fat while increasing muscle mass.

A closely related disorder is Angelman syndrome (AS) in which affected individuals have seizures, jerky limb movements, marked mental retardation, a small head, and periods of inappropriate laughter. The estimated prevalence for AS is 1 in 15,000. In 50 percent of AS patients, the same region of chromosome 15 involved in PWS, which is imprinted (methylated) from the male, is deleted from the corresponding ma-

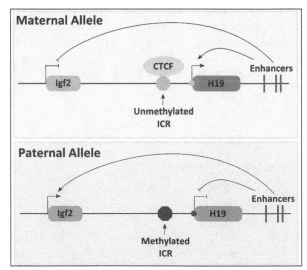

Figure 3. The Igf2-H19 imprinted gene cluster. (Copyright © 2014 Fastbleep Ltd)

ternal chromosome. The critical gene in this region required for early brain development is the ubiquitin ligase gene, UBE3A. Ubiquitin ligase enzymes are indispensable in cells because they catalyze the attachment of the small protein named ubiquitin onto proteins that are improperly folded or worn out, thus marking them for destruction.

Silver-Russell syndrome (SRS) occurs about once in every 75,000 births. These individuals have stunted growth with asymmetry of the limbs and immature bone development, especially prevalent in the head and upper trunk. Characteristically a small, triangular face with frontal bone prominence is observed. SRS is thought to be the first human pathology caused by imprinting disruptions of genetic loci on two different chromosomes, chromosomes 7 and 11.

Beckwith-Wiedemann syndrome (BWS) is characterized by several clinical features. Some of those features include craniofacial development anomalies, hypoglycemia, enlargement of the kidneys, liver, and spleen, and abdominal tumors. Consequently, regular tumor monitoring through abdominal sonograms and analysis of urine and blood tumor markers is a critical aspect of care. Hypomethylation of an imprinted region of chromosome 11 appears to be involved in 40-60 percent of BWS cases. The estimated incidence is 1 in 13,700.

Albright hereditary osteodystrophy (AHO) is due to mutation in an imprinted gene that encodes the alpha subunit of the membrane-associated trimeric G protein (GNAS). Considered a rare disorder, some estimates place the incidence at 1 in roughly 7 million. As a result of maternal gene disruption, those affected are not responsive to the parathyroid hormone as well as other hormones, especially the thyroid-stimulating hormone. Because of the parathyroid hormone insensitivity, the kidneys respond as if the parathyroid hormone is deficient; hence, the disorder is also called pseudohypoparathyroidism (PHP). The clinical features include short build, short metacarpals with a rounded face, and short neck. It is possible to observe mineralization in subcutaneous tissue and AHO patients also show low blood calcium levels (hypocalcemia) with excessively high blood levels of phosphate (hyperphosphatemia). Dental characteristics include delayed eruption of teeth and lack of tooth enamel formation. Those individuals who have these features and hormone resistance are said to have PHP type Ia, and those who lack the clinical features but still have hormone resistance are said to express the type Ib subtype. Treatment for these patients includes calcium and vitamin D doses to help maintain normal calcium and parathyroid hormone levels in the bloodstream. Individuals with the clinical features but normal hormone responsiveness are said to display pseudopseudohypoparathyroidism (pseudoPHP) resulting from disruption of the paternal copy of the GNAS gene.

Perspective and Prospects

The disorders resulting from genetic imprinting defects were studied clinically and reported beginning in the 1940s. The molecular mechanisms of genetic imprinting were approached once the advent of recombinant DNA technologies occurred in the 1980s. Scientists began to use the mouse as a model to better understand imprinting in humans. The Igf2/H19 locus imprinting phenomenon was the first elucidated, in part through studies of an Igf2 knockout mouse strain (mouse in which the Igf2 gene was removed through recombinant DNA techniques). Progeny that inherited the deletion from the female parent were normal sized, but those mice that received the deletion from the father were small. As a result it was understood that the Igf2 gene is only expressed from the paternal chromosome and hence is an imprinted gene. Genetic engineering techniques are used to create mouse strains that model imprinting disorders, like PWS. Scientists have developed some mouse strains in which genes are introduced (transgenes) to alter the dosage or expression level of those genes to mimic imprinting phenomena. Recent publication and annotation of the complete mouse genome sequence will aid scientists in their efforts to further understand imprinting.

Through computational approaches and microarray (known DNA sequences affixed to a microchip) technology, researchers have identified imprinted genes. In yet another method, scientists have extended DNA sequencing to sequencing RNA in such a way that all of the RNAs in a given cell, tissue, or organ can be sequenced and quantitated at a given time. This allows for the identification of genes that undergo tissue-specific and time-specific expression as a result of imprinting. Using an RNA sequencing approach, a group recently identified over 347 imprinted autosomal genes in the mouse cerebral cortex and hypothalamus.

Studies of the epigenome (the chemical modifications to DNA bases and histone proteins that package the DNA of a genome) are accelerating as advances in molecular biology techniques have made it possible to investigate how genes are silenced. The National Institutes of Health (NIH) initiated the Roadmap Epigenomics Program in 2008 and, as of May 2012, had compiled over 61 complete epigenomes from different cell types. These studies are adding to our knowledge of imprinting as well.

—*Daniel Jones, D.D.S., Ph.D.*

See also Angleman syndrome; Embryology; Endocrinology; Genetic counseling; Genetic engineering; Neonatology; Neurology; Obesity, childhood; Pediatrics; Perinatology

For Further Information:

Butler, Merlin G. "Genomic Imprinting Disorders in Humans: A Mini-Review." *Journal of Assisted Reproduction and Genetics,* 26 (2009): 477-486. An exhaustive review of the clinical and genetic findings of several human disorders that result from defects involving genomic imprinting.

Gregg, Christopher, et al. "Sex-Specific Parent-of-Origin Allelic Expression in the Mouse Brain." *Science* 329, no. 5992 (August, 2010): 682-685. An analysis of different mouse brain tissues through a genome-wide analysis to discover imprinted X-linked and autosomal genes.

Russell, Peter. "Regulation of Gene Expression in Eukaryotes." *iGenetics: A Molecular Approach,* edited by Beth Wilbur. San Francisco: Pearson Benjamin Cummings, 2010. The chapter has a section that clearly explains the Igf2/H19 gene locus imprinting process with a figure to make the complicated mechanism easier to understand.

Sanders, Mark. "Regulation of Gene Expression in Eukaryotes."

" *Genetic Analysis: An Integrated Approach,* edited by Beth Wilbur. Glenview, IL: Pearson Education, Inc., 2012. This chapter contains a good explanation of the erasure and then the re-establishment of imprinting during gametogenesis. A clear figure is presented to help clarify the concept.

Watson, James. "Transcriptional Regulation in Eukaryotes" and "Model Organisms." *Molecular Biology of the Gene,* edited by Beth Wilbur. Cold Spring Harbor, NY: Cold Spring Harbor Press, 2014. A current text authored by experts in the field. The transcriptional regulation chapter includes a thorough explanation of how genes can be switched off through DNA methylation and modification of histones. The model organism chapter contains a discussion of imprinting in mice and emphasizes the importance of the completed sequencing and annotation of the mouse genome to further efforts in understanding development and disease in humans.

Wood, Andrew, and Rebecca J. Oakey. "Genomic Imprinting in Mammals: Emerging Themes and Established Theories." *PLOS Genetics* 2, no. 11 (November, 2006): 1677-1685. This review article summarizes work in mice to understand the prevalence and mechanisms of imprinting, theories of the development and spread of imprinting, and the role of imprinting in the physiology of the placenta.

GENETIC SEQUENCING. *See* **GENOMICS.**

GENETICS AND INHERITANCE
Biology

Anatomy or system affected: All

Specialties and related fields: Embryology, forensic medicine, genetics, pediatrics

Definition: The passage of traits from parents to offspring in discrete units called genes.

Key terms:

allele: a version of a gene; different alleles of a gene have slightly different nucleotide sequences, resulting in differences in the protein encoded in the gene

chromosome: one of the DNA molecules of a nucleus; in humans, chromosomes occur in twenty-three pairs, with each member of a pair having the same genes but possibly having different alleles of the genes

deoxyribonucleic acid (DNA): the hereditary molecule, in which sequences of nucleic acids encode genetic information

dominant allele: the version of a gene that can produce a recognizable trait in offspring when present in only one of the two chromosomes of a pair

fertilization: the process by which chromosome pairs, separated in production of egg and sperm cells, are rejoined

gene: a sequence of nucleotides in DNA encoding a protein

meiosis: a division mechanism in which homologous chromosomes are separated and delivered singly to egg or sperm cells; as a part of meiosis, recombination generates new combinations of alleles

nucleotide: a chemical subunit of DNA; different sequences of linked nucleotides spell out instructions for the assembly of proteins

recessive allele: a version of a gene that must be present on both chromosomes of a pair in order to produce a

recognizable trait in offspring

recombination: the reciprocal exchange of segments between the two chromosomes of a pair, producing new combinations of alleles

The Rules of Inheritance

The primary genes of interest to heredity consist of a set of coded directions for making proteins. Each gene codes for a protein; distinct versions of a gene, which encode slightly different versions of the protein, may be carried in the same or different individuals. The distinct versions of a gene, called alleles, are responsible for differences in hereditary traits among individuals. Each individual receives a combination of alleles encoding proteins that directly or indirectly determine traits such as eye, skin, and hair color; height; and, to a degree, characteristics such as personality, behavior, and intelligence.

In molecular terms, genes consist of a sequence of chemical units called nucleotides, linked end to end in long, linear deoxyribonucleic acid (DNA) molecules. There are four kinds of nucleotides in DNA; each gene has its own nucleotide sequence. The alleles of a gene differ slightly in nucleotide sequence—some alleles differ in the substitution of only a single nucleotide. There are many thousands of genes arranged in tandem on the DNA molecules of a human cell; each DNA molecule is known as a chromosome. In humans, the chromosomes occur in twenty-three pairs, for a total of forty-six chromosomes. The two members of a chromosome pair contain the same genes in the same order, but different alleles of a gene may be present in the two members of a pair. One member of a chromosome pair is derived from the female parent of the individual; the other member is derived from the male parent. These are called the maternal and paternal chromosomes of the pair.

Inheritance, and the variation in traits among individuals, depends on two processes that separate and rejoin the chromosome pairs in sexual reproduction. One is a division mechanism, meiosis, which occurs in cell lines leading to egg or sperm cells. Meiosis separates the chromosome pairs and places one member of each pair in an egg or sperm cell. The particular combination of maternal and paternal chromosomes delivered to an egg or sperm cell is random. This random segregation, as it is called, is one source of the variability among offspring in a family. Because there are so many chromosomes, the possibility that two egg or sperm cells produced by the same individual could receive the same combination of maternal and paternal chromosomes is very small—equivalent to one chance in 8.4 million. Another important source of variability comes from a mechanism that occurs before the pairs are separated in meiosis. In this mechanism, called recombination, the two members of a chromosome pair line up side by side and exchange segments perfectly and reciprocally. As a result, alleles are exchanged between the pairs, generating new combinations of alleles. The variability generated by recombination adds to that produced by independent segregation of maternal and paternal chromosomes, so that it is essentially impossible for an individual to produce two egg or sperm cells that are genetically the same.

The second process underlying inheritance is fertilization, in which a sperm and an egg cell fuse, rejoining the twenty-three pairs of chromosomes. Fertilization is another random process, in which any of the millions of sperm cells ejaculated by a male and any of the hundreds of egg cells carried in a female may join. The total variability generated by independent segregation of alleles, recombination, and random union of gametes is such that each human individual, except identical twins, receives a unique combination of alleles. Thus the possibility that any individual has or will ever have a genetic double in the human population, except for an identical twin, is essentially zero. (In the case of identical twins, a single fertilized egg divides to produce two separate, genetically identical cells; instead of remaining together to produce a two-celled embryo, as is normally the case, the cells separate to create two embryos, which develop into genetically identical individuals.)

Because chromosomes occur in pairs, each individual receives two alleles of every gene of the human complement. The two alleles may be the same or different. Some alleles are dominant in their effects, so that one copy of the allele on either chromosome is sufficient to produce the trait encoded in the allele. Other alleles are recessive, so that both chromosomes of the pair must carry the allele for the trait to appear in offspring. In humans, few physical traits are determined by a single gene. Most are the result of complex interactions between several genes, as well as environmental influences. Nonetheless, some traits do tend to follow certain inheritance patterns, but there are exceptions. For example, brown eyes tend to be dominant to blue eyes. If either chromosome carries the brown eye allele, the individual will usually have brown eyes. To have blue eyes, an individual usually carries two genes for blue eyes. Human traits that tend toward dominant inheritance include nearsightedness and farsightedness, astigmatism, dark or curly hair, early balding in males, normal body pigment (as compared to albinism), supernumerary fingers or toes, short fingers or toes, and webbing between fingers and toes. Alleles that tend to be expressed in a recessive fashion include blond hair, straight hair, and congenital deafness.

Although each individual normally carries a maximum of two alleles of any gene, several or many alleles of a gene may exist in the human population as a whole. The major histocompatibility complex (MHC), for example, occurs in hundreds of different alleles throughout the human population—so many that unrelated individuals are unlikely to carry the same combination of MHC alleles. The proteins encoded in these alleles are recognized by the immune system as "self" or "foreign." Unless the same, or a very similar, combination of MHC alleles is present, cells are recognized by the immune system as foreign, and the cells are destroyed. Therefore, MHC combinations recognized as foreign are the primary factor in the rejection of tissue or organ transplants among humans. If the transplant does not come from an individual with the same or a very similar MHC combination, rejection is likely unless the immune system is suppressed by drugs such as cyclosporine. The best donor for a transplant is a close relative, who is most likely to have a similar MHC combination. Because identical twins have the same MHC combination, tissues and organs can be transplanted between them with no danger of rejection.

Sex is determined by a pair of chromosomes that is different in males and females. Females have two members of the pair, the X chromosomes, which have the same genes in the same order but which may have different alleles of the genes. One member of the XX pair was derived from the female's father, and the other from her mother. Males have only one member of this pair, a single X. In addition, males have a small, single chromosome, the Y, which is not present in females. Thus females are XX, and males are XY. During meiosis in females, the XX pair is separated, so that an egg cell may receive either member of the pair. In males, the X and Y are separated, so that a sperm cell receives either an X or a Y. In fertilization, the X chromosome carried by the egg may be joined with an X-carrying sperm, producing a female (XX), or, the egg may be fertilized by a sperm cell carrying a Y, producing a male (XY). Thus, in humans the sex of the offspring is determined by the type of sperm cell, an X or a Y, fertilizing the egg. Most genes carried on an X chromosome have no counterparts on the Y chromosome. Therefore, traits encoded in genes on the X chromosomes (almost none are carried on the Y) are inherited differently from traits carried on other chromosomes of the set, in a pattern known as sex-linked inheritance.

Disorders and Diseases

Many human diseases, involving every system in the body, depend on the presence of particular dominant or recessive alleles and are directly inherited. Only the disposition for development of other diseases is inherited—that is, some individuals inherit a combination of alleles that increases the possibility that a genetically based disease will develop during their lifetimes.

The list of diseases contracted through inheritance of a dominant allele is long and impressive. Among the more important of these diseases are achondroplasia, in which individuals are short statured; familial hypercholesterolemia, in which cholesterol concentration in the blood is abnormally high, leading to vascular disease, particularly of the coronary arteries; Huntington's disease, a disease characterized by dementia, delusion, paranoia, and abnormal movements that begins in persons between twenty and fifty years of age and progresses steadily to death in about fifteen years; Marfan syndrome, a disease of connective tissues involving the skeleton, eyes, and cardiovascular system, characterized by elongated limbs, abnormal position of the eye lens, and structural weakness of blood vessels, particularly of the aorta; neurofibromatosis, characterized by tumors dispersed throughout the body and coffee-colored skin lesions; polycystic kidney disease, in which dilated cysts grow in the kidneys and interfere with kidney function, leading to hypertension and chronic renal failure; spherocytosis, another disease in which blood cells are fragile and easily broken during

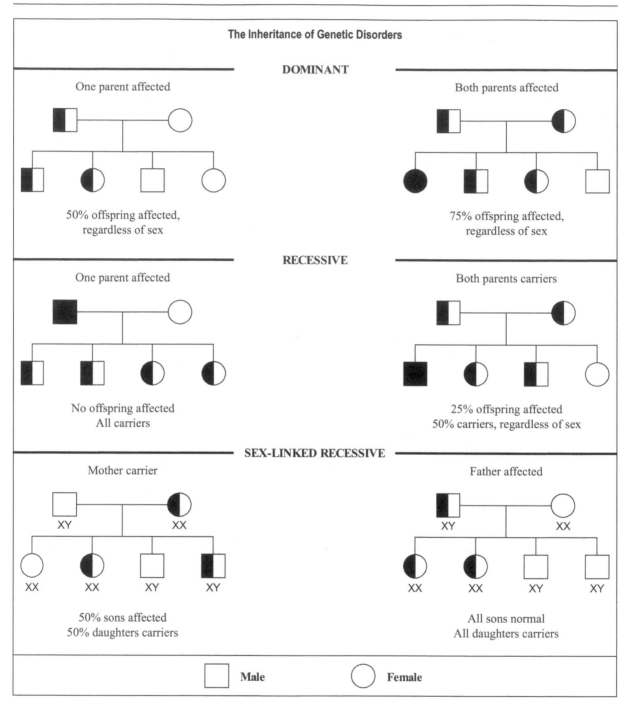

travel through the circulatory system, producing anemia and jaundice; and thalassemia, a group of diseases most common in persons of Mediterranean descent in which hemoglobin production is faulty, leading to anemias that range from mild to severe.

Diseases caused by recessive genes also appear in the human population. Although many persons are carriers for these diseases, affected persons are rare because both alleles must be present in the recessive form for the disease to develop. Diseases in this category include albinism; sickle cell disease, common in persons of African descent, in which hemoglobin is faulty, leading to fragility of red blood cells, anemia, blockage of blood vessels, and susceptibility to infection; phenylketonuria (PKU), in which the amino acid phenylalanine accumulates in excess in the bloodstream, leading to nervous system damage including mental retardation; Tay-Sachs disease, most common in persons of Jewish descent, characterized by accumulation of lipid molecules in nerve cells leading to motor incoordination, blindness, and mental deterioration; and glycogen storage diseases, with symptoms ranging from cramps to serious muscular and cardiac disease and convulsions. Sickle cell disease is recessively inherited. A person with one copy of the sickle cell gene makes sufficient normal hemoglobin that symptoms of the disease occur only under extreme low oxygen conditions. Cystic fibrosis, one of the most common of genetically determined diseases in Caucasians, is probably also attributable to a recessive allele. In this disease, sweat and mucus-secreting glands are affected; the most serious effects are caused by the secretion of unusually thick and viscid mucus, leading to blockage of ducts in the lungs, liver, pancreas, and salivary glands. Most critical to survival is blockage of passages in the lungs, producing a chronic cough and persistent pulmonary infections. The average life expectancy of persons with cystic fibrosis is twenty years of age.

A number of diseases are caused by recessive genes carried on the X chromosomes and are inherited in sex-linked patterns. Among these are one form of diabetes (diabetes insipidus) in which glucose uptake by cells is faulty, leading to the accumulation of glucose in the blood; hemophilia, in which the blood-clotting mechanism is deficient, making afflicted persons subject to uncontrolled bleeding; and some forms of muscular dystrophy, characterized by progressive muscular weakness. The Duchenne muscular dystrophy appears early in life, progresses rapidly, and leads to death in most cases by the age of twenty.

Because males receive only one copy of the X chromosome, recessive genes are fully expressed in males—there is no chance for a normal allele to compensate for the effects of the recessive gene. For a sex-linked disease to appear in females, both X chromosomes must carry the recessive allele. For these reasons, sex-linked recessive diseases are much more common in males than in females; for some, appearance of the disease is limited almost exclusively to males.

The molecular basis for some genetically based diseases is known. In familial hypercholesterolemia, for example, receptors for cholesterol on cell surfaces are faulty or not produced, preventing the normal uptake of cholesterol from the bloodstream. As a result, cholesterol accumulates and reaches a dangerously high concentration in the blood. In persons carrying dominant alleles for familial hypercholesterolemia on both chromosomes of the pair, coronary arterial disease advances so rapidly that death from heart attack by the age of twenty is frequent. The disease is among the most common of genetically based defects—about one in five hundred persons has at least one allele for hypercholesterolemia and develops premature coronary artery disease. In PKU, individuals lack an enzyme normally produced in the liver. The enzyme, phenylalanine hydroxylase, converts excess phenylalanine into another amino acid, tyrosine. Without the enzyme, phenylalanine taken in the diet accumulates to dangerously high levels in the body. Some forms of PKU are treatable by restricting dietary intake of phenylalanine from infancy onward.

Some persons have a genetically determined predisposition to develop certain cancers with greater frequency than the average in the population. About 5 percent of cancers are strongly predisposed—that is, individuals inherit a marked tendency to develop the cancer. Among these are familial retinoblastoma, in which retinal tumors develop; familial adenomatous polyps of the colon; and multiple endocrine neoplasia, in which tumors develop in the thyroid, adrenal medulla, and parathyroid glands. Often underlying these strongly predisposed cancers is the inheritance of a faulty gene (called an oncogene) that promotes uncontrolled cell division, or the opposite—inheritance of a faulty gene that in its normal form suppresses cell division (called a tumor suppressor gene). Typically, oncogenes are inherited as dominant genes, and tumor suppressor genes as recessives. In addition, some cancers, including breast, ovarian, and colon cancers other than familial adenomatous polyps, show a degree of predisposition in family lines.

Perspective and Prospects

The primary features of meiosis and fertilization, random segregation of chromosome pairs in meiosis and random rejoining of pairs in fertilization, makes heredity subject to analysis by mathematical techniques. In fact, mathematical analysis of heredity was carried out successfully before there was any understanding concerning meiosis or DNA. The groundwork for this analysis was laid down in the 1860s by an Austrian monk, Gregor Mendel. Mendel's research approach and his conclusions were so advanced that they were misunderstood and unappreciated during his lifetime.

Mendel chose garden peas for his research because they could be grown easily and they possessed several hereditary traits that were known to breed true—that is, to appear dependably in offspring. Mendel crossed pea plants with different traits in various combinations. On analyzing the results of his crosses, Mendel realized that the numbers of offspring exhibiting different traits could be explained mathematically if he assumed that parents contain a pair of factors governing the inheritance of each trait. Furthermore, he concluded that the factors separate, or segregate, independently as gametes are formed and are reunited randomly at fertilization. He also discovered that some traits are inherited as dominant and some as recessive. Mendel's factors were later called genes.

Until Mendel's time, inheritance was commonly believed to occur through a blending of maternal and paternal characteristics. Mendel's work showed instead that traits are passed on as units; depending on whether a trait is dominant or recessive, it may appear in all offspring or only in a definite, predictable percentage. Some time after Mendel's discoveries, in the early twentieth century, meiosis was discovered. At this time, Walter Sutton pointed out that Mendel's genes and chromosomes behave similarly in meiosis and fertilization: Both genes and chromosomes occur in pairs that separate randomly in meiosis and are rejoined at fertilization. Genes were therefore concluded to be carried on the chromosomes. Further genetic research confirmed that Mendel's findings with plant genes also apply to animals, including humans, and worked out many additional features of inheritance, including genetic recombination and sex linkage. Later, in the 1950s, almost one hundred years after Mendel's findings, James D. Watson and Francis Crick discovered the structure of DNA and deduced the fact that hereditary information is encoded in the sequence of nucleotides in DNA.

Research in human genetics differs from genetic investigation in other organisms because, for obvious reasons, it is impossible to set up experimental crosses to test whether particular diseases are inherited. Instead, human family lines are analyzed carefully in pedigrees to trace the appearance of disease over several generations. If a disease is genetically determined, it shows up in definite patterns as dominant, recessive, or sex-linked among parents and offspring in the pedigrees. On this basis, prospective parents can be counseled on the chances that their offspring will develop a hereditary disease.

In June of 2000, Francis Collins, director of the National Human Genome Research Initiative, and J. Craig Venter, of Celera Genomics, announced that they had jointly sequenced the entire human genome and that the first working draft was available. In 2003, researchers with the Human Genome Project reported that they had identified close to twenty-five thousand genes in human DNA and sequenced the three billion chemical base pairs of which it is made up. Sequencing the human genome allowed scientists to directly compare healthy DNA to DNA harboring disease genes. By 2013 researchers had discovered the genetic basis for close to five thousand diseases and developed genetic tests for nearly two thousand conditions or diseases. Additionally, genetic testing became faster and less expensive to conduct as sequencing technology became more sophisticated. Although these advances have led to a greater understanding of certain disease processes, as well as the development of some diagnostic procedures and potential therapy and cures, scientists have cautioned that the human genome is larger and more complex than initially thought. More research will be required before treatments can be developed to target illnesses such as those caused by not just one gene but several gene variants.

—*Stephen L. Wolfe, Ph.D.;*
updated by Karen E. Kalumuck, Ph.D.

See also Aging; Amniocentesis; Bioinformatics; Biostatistics; Birth defects; Chorionic villus sampling; Cloning; DNA and RNA; Embryology; Environmental diseases; Gene therapy; Genetic counseling; Genetic diseases; Genetic engineering; Genomics; Laboratory tests; Metabolic disorders; Multiple births; Mutation; Neonatology; Obstetrics; Oncology; Pediatrics; Pregnancy and gestation; Preventive medicine; Proteomics; Screening; Sexual differentiation; Sexuality.

For Further Information:
Campbell, Neil A., et al. *Biology: Concepts and Connections*. 6th ed. San Francisco: Pearson/Benjamin Cummings, 2008.
Kaneshiro, Neil K. "Genetics." *MedlinePlus*, May 16, 2012.
Lewin, Benjamin. *Genes X*. 10th ed. Burlington, Mass.: Jones and Bartlett Learning, 2011.
Lewis, Ricki. *Human Genetics: Concepts and Applications*. 10th ed.
New York: McGraw-Hill, 2012.
Marieb, Elaine N. *Essentials of Human Anatomy and Physiology*. 10th ed. Harlow: Pearson Education, 2012.
MedlinePlus. "Genes and Gene Therapy." *MedlinePlus*, July 8, 2013.
MedlinePlus. "HealthDay: 10 Years On, Still Much to Be Learned from Human Genome." *MedlinePlus*, April 12, 2013.
Moore, Keith L., and T. V. N. Persaud. *The Developing Human: Clinically Oriented Embryology*. 9th ed. Philadelphia: Saunders/Elsevier, 2013.
NIH National Institute of General Medical Sciences. "The New Genetics." *NIH National Institute of General Medical Sciences*, January 8, 2012.
Ridley, Matt. *Nature via Nurture: Genes, Experience, and What Makes Us Human*. New York: HarperCollins, 2003.
Wolfe, Stephen L. *Molecular and Cellular Biology*. Belmont, Calif.: Wadsworth, 1993.

GENITAL DISORDERS, FEMALE
Disease/Disorder

Anatomy or system affected: Genitals, reproductive system, uterus

Specialties and related fields: Family medicine, gynecology, obstetrics, oncology, urology

Definition: All maladies affecting the reproductive organs of women.

Key terms:

cervix: the narrow portion of the uterus situated at the upper end of the vagina

cyst: a closed sac having a distinct border that develops abnormally within a body space or structure

estrogen: the hormone responsible for female sexual characteristics, produced primarily by the ovaries

Fallopian tubes: tiny tubes that connect the ovaries to the uterus; after ovulation, the egg travels through these tubes, and its fertilization by sperm occurs here

hormone: a chemical compound produced at one site in the body which travels to other parts of the body to exert its effect

hysterectomy: the surgical removal of the uterus; in a total hysterectomy, the uterus, ovaries, and Fallopian tubes are removed

laparoscopy: a surgical procedure in which an instrument is inserted into the body through tiny incisions; usually performed without hospitalization

Causes and Symptoms

Diseases and disorders of the female genitals and related internal organs encompass a huge number of different types of conditions that can range in severity from merely physically annoying to life-threatening. These disorders affect the vulva, vagina, uterus, ovaries, and Fallopian tubes. Many develop from unknown causes, and others have clear-cut origins, such as sexually transmitted diseases. Some have immediately recognizable symptoms, while others are silent until the disease has progressed to a serious stage. Early recognition of symptoms or abnormalities and proper treatment can alleviate pain and save lives.

Endometriosis is a chronic, recurring disease in which the

tissue that lines the uterus may be found growing in sites outside the uterus. The endometrial tissue, frequently called endometrial implants, may be found in a variety of extrauterine sites. Endometrial tissue is hormonally responsive, and the symptoms of endometriosis are cyclic. The endometrial tissue responds to the same hormonal cues that signal the sloughing off of the uterine lining during menstruation; however, the blood from the endometrial tissue cannot leave the abdominal cavity, leading to inflammation. As the inflammation subsides, it is replaced with scar tissue. This process will repeat with each menstrual cycle, and the scarring can result in infertility, organ malfunction, or adhesions that bind organs together. Some women with endometriosis experience no symptoms, while many experience severe abdominal pain before, during, and after their menstrual periods. Endometrial tissue can be definitively diagnosed only with laparoscopy. The cause of endometriosis is unknown, but some evidence suggests an inherited tendency to develop endometriosis.

Vaginitis is a general term for infections of the vagina. The three most common vaginal infections are yeast infections, usually caused by the fungus *Candida albicans*; trichomonaisis, caused by a small parasite, *Trichomonas vaginalis*; and bacterial vaginosis, which is caused by an imbalance of the normal bacteria in the vagina. Diagnosis of the causative organism is critical in choosing the correct treatment, and also for addressing issues of sexual transmission. Yeast vaginitis is not sexually transmitted. Bacterial vaginosis is not transmitted by a partner but may have some sexual association based on pH changes that can occur with sexual activity. Trichomoniasis is sexually transmitted, and partners must be treated to eradicate the infection.

Uterine fibroids are benign tumors made mainly of muscle tissue that can grow inside the uterus or along its outer surface. They grow slowly and are dependent on the hormone estrogen for continued growth. They are usually not problematic, but if they become very large they may cause extremely heavy bleeding during menstruation and can interfere with pregnancy and childbirth. Their cause is unknown, but they will shrink or disappear after menopause.

Uterine prolapse occurs when the pelvic muscles lose tone and are no longer able to support the pelvic organs, causing the uterus to "fall" into the vagina. Prolapse may occur only inside the vagina with straining, such that the uterus "drops" from its position high in the vagina; may occur within the vagina without straining; or may be a rare condition in which the cervix and even the uterus protrudes outside the vagina. This disorder is most common in women of older age and is often precipitated by one or more difficult births. Obesity is also implicated as a risk factor.

Ovarian cysts form when an egg developing inside a follicle within the ovary does not ovulate but instead keeps growing. Small cysts will be painless, but larger ones (up to 7.5 centimeters in diameter) may cause abdominal pain. Most cysts will go away on their own, but some can rupture and cause severe pain.

The hallmark of cancer is uncontrolled cell growth. Cancer may prove fatal by causing destruction of a particular or-

---

Information on Female Genital Disorders

Causes: Endometriosis, hormonal imbalances, infection, disease, uterine fibroids, sexually transmitted diseases

Symptoms: Vary; can include abdominal pain, pain during menstruation or sexual intercourse, vaginal itching, vaginal discharge, burning upon urination

Duration: Acute or chronic, often with recurrent episodes

Treatments: Depends on cause; may include oral contraceptives, corticosteroids, hormone therapy, anti-inflammatory drugs, surgery, radiation therapy, chemotherapy, immunotherapy

---

gan at the site of origin or by spreading throughout the body and damaging other organs and systems. All the organs of the female reproductive system can be affected by cancer. Cervical cancer begins in superficial layers of the cervix but may spread rapidly through the vagina and throughout the body. Cervical cancer can be detected in its early, most curable stages by a Pap test. Endometrial cancer affects the glands that line the uterus. It can occur at any age, but the most common age of onset is sixty. Abnormal bleeding accompanies this disorder, which is diagnosed by examination of a biopsy of uterine tissue. Sarcomas of the uterus are malignant tumors of muscle tissue frequently confused with benign fibroids. This rare cancer is aggressive and difficult to treat. Ovarian cancer constitutes about 25 percent of female reproductive tract cancers, is difficult to detect and cure, and therefore has a high mortality rate. There are no early symptoms, and the cancer seems to occur frequently in those with a family history of the disease. Cancers of the Fallopian tubes and vagina are very rare, but vaginal cancer occurs with greater frequency in women whose mothers were treated with the synthetic estrogen diethylstilbestrol (DES) during the 1940s through the 1960s with the intent of preventing miscarriages. Cancer of the vulva, a form of skin cancer, is relatively easy to treat and has a high cure rate.

Sexually transmitted diseases (STDs), now more properly referred to as sexually transmitted infections (STIs), can involve any part of the female genital system. Common STIs of bacterial origin include gonorrhea and chlamydia, which are major precursors to pelvic inflammatory disease (PID) and syphilis. Untreated, these diseases can lead to serious complications. Common STDs with a viral cause include genital herpes, genital warts, and acquired immunodeficiency syndrome (AIDS). The causative agent of trichomoniasis vaginalis is a protozoan. STIs are transmitted through direct sexual contact with an infected person, and each has its own set of symptoms and diagnostic criteria.

Treatment and Therapy

A variety of treatments are available for endometriosis, depending on the severity of the disorder. Over-the-counter or prescription anti-inflammatory drugs may give immediate relief from pain, but the condition itself is frequently treated

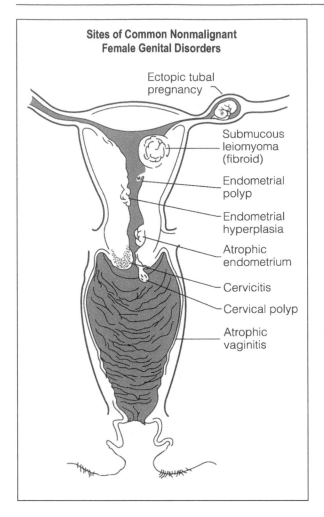

Sites of Common Nonmalignant Female Genital Disorders

Ectopic tubal pregnancy

Submucous leiomyoma (fibroid)

Endometrial polyp

Endometrial hyperplasia

Atrophic endometrium

Cervicitis

Cervical polyp

Atrophic vaginitis

with hormone therapy. Birth control pills that are high in the hormone progestin and low in estrogen can help shrink endometriosis. Danazol, a synthetic male hormone, suppresses the production of estrogen by the ovaries, thereby helping to eliminate the condition, but it has undesirable side effects. In some cases, surgical removal of the tissue is necessary. In laparoscopy, an instrument is inserted through tiny abdominal incisions and used to remove the tissue. In the most severe cases, a complete hysterectomy (removal of the uterus and ovaries) is performed.

Vaginitis needs to be diagnosed either by direct microscopic visualization through a wet prep along with a test of pH of the discharge, or by other serologic laboratory technologies. Culture is rarely employed. Medications for vaginal yeast infection are available over the counter as vaginal creams or suppositories or by prescription as vaginal creams or as a one-dose antifungal oral medication. Medication for *Trichomonas vaginalis* is generally with oral metronidazole (Flagyl), and partners must be treated as well. Medication for bacterial vaginosis can be oral or intravaginal with metronidazole or clindamycin, or with oral tinidazole.

If no major discomfort is experienced by the woman when uterine fibroids are first detected, usually no treatment beyond regular observation is necessary. For those experiencing pain or difficulty in conception or pregnancy, the fibroids may be surgically removed in an operation called a myomectomy; in severe cases, a hysterectomy is performed. A laparoscope can be used to remove tumors on the outside of the uterus, or a hysteroscope can be inserted through the cervix, which uses a laser to burn away internal fibroids. Uterine artery embolization, in which the arteries that supply the fibroids are blocked, is another surgical option; this is less invasive than a hysterectomy and has similar success rates. Various medications are also available to treat the symptoms of uterine fibroids as well as block their growth. For example, synthetic hormones called gonadotropin-releasing hormone analogs block the ovaries" production of estrogen, which leads to shrinking of the fibroids and the possible avoidance of surgery. .

A prolapsed uterus is frequently treated by hysterectomy, but other therapies are possible. Kegel exercises, designed to strengthen the muscles of the pelvic floor, are effective if done regularly for an extended period of time. A pessary, a ring-shaped device that fits around the cervix and props up the uterus, is another alternative, though an inconvenient one. Major surgery to resuspend the uterus is a surgical alternative to hysterectomy.

Ovarian cysts will usually be resorbed into the ovary within one to three menstrual cycles. Proper monitoring by a physician is needed to determine if the cysts have cleared. If the cyst does not disappear within three months, or if it increases in size, ultrasound and/or laparoscopy will be used to determine if a different type of ovarian tumor is present, which would necessitate surgical removal.

Cancer treatment is highly specialized for the particular variety of the disease, its severity, and consideration of the affected individual. Typical treatments include surgical removal of the tumor and/or affected organ, radiation therapy, chemotherapy, and immunotherapy (the reinforcement of the immune system, generally administered after radiation or chemotherapy). When diagnosed in premalignant stages, cervical abnormalities may be treated by cryosurgery (freezing and killing the abnormal cells) or laser destruction of the abnormal cells. Advanced cervical cancer is treated by hysterectomy. Endometrial cancer is treated with total hysterectomy, including the uterus, ovaries, and Fallopian tubes, and if the cancer has spread, radiation and/or chemotherapy. The only known cure for uterine sarcoma is total hysterectomy, and removal of both the ovaries and the Fallopian tubes is performed for ovarian cancer. The tumors of vaginal cancer are eliminated surgically or with laser treatment.

Sexually transmitted diseases of bacterial origin can be treated successfully with antibiotics. Drug therapy can also eliminate trichomoniasis. There are no cures for the virally transmitted STDs. Certain drugs can reduce the frequency of outbreaks of genital herpes, and genital warts may be removed by freezing, burning, or surgery. No cure exists for AIDS, although drugs are available to prolong life.

Perspective and Prospects

The diagnosis and treatment of female genital disorders and diseases have evolved from a state of some being considered psychosomatic to being the focus of a field that spurs the continued development and improvement of diagnostic and treatment technologies. It is also a field that has been a major force in the mass screening of diseases and in public health issues. Many conditions, such as endometriosis, have historically been misdiagnosed and the associated pain dismissed as imagined—to the dismay of the suffering woman. This and other conditions, such as prolapsed uterus and fibroids, were typically treated with the drastic surgery of hysterectomy. Women have demanded that more research into the causes of these disorders, and alternatives to hysterectomy, be developed. Laparoscopy has replaced hysterectomy in many cases, preserving the uterus and childbearing capacity.

The treatment of all female cancers has benefited from research into the cause and treatment of these disorders. For decades, the Pap test has been routinely used with American women on an annual basis, and it has been responsible for saving thousands of lives through early detection of abnormal cervical cells that may progress to a cancerous state. Public education about the necessity of early cancer detection has helped to improve the survival chances of individuals with cancer, and sensitive blood tests can detect some cancers at their most treatable stages, long before any symptoms occur. Discovery of the hereditary nature of female genital cancers has established routine monitoring of those at risk for the disease, again resulting in early detection. New, better radiation and chemotherapy treatments, as well as improved immune system support, benefit all cancer patients. The connection between certain "cancer-fighting" foods and good health has led to a revision of Americans" eating habits.

While some sexually transmitted diseases are easily cured with antibiotics if caught early, those of viral origin are not and may have fatal consequences. Information provided through such diverse means as television and grade-school programs has educated people about this problem and the best ways to protect themselves from becoming victims of an incurable STD. Continuing research into diagnostic methods and treatment regimes in this area will lead to improved health for everyone.

—*Clair Kaplan, A.P.R.N./M.S.N.; additional material by Karen E. Kalumuck, Ph.D.*

See also Amenorrhea; Aphrodisiacs; Behçet's disease; Candidiasis; Cervical, ovarian, and uterine cancers; Cervical procedures; Childbirth; Childbirth complications; Chlamydia; Circumcision, female, and genital mutilation; Conception; Contraception; Culdocentesis; Cystitis; Dysmenorrhea; Ectopic pregnancy; Electrocauterization; Endometrial biopsy; Endometriosis; Episiotomy; Gonorrhea; Gynecology; Herpes; Infertility, female; Menopause; Menorrhagia; Menstruation; Miscarriage; Ovarian cysts; Ovaries; Pap test; Pelvic inflammatory disease (PID); Pregnancy and gestation; Premature birth; Premenstrual syndrome (PMS); Reproductive system; Sexual dysfunction; Sexuality; Sexually transmitted diseases (STDs); Sterilization; Stillbirth; Syphilis; Urology; Urology, pediatric; Uterus; Warts; Women's health.

For Further Information:

Berek, Jonathan S., ed. *Berek and Novak's Gynecology.* 14th ed. Philadelphia: Lippincott Williams & Wilkins, 2007.

Boston Women's Health Book Collective. *Our Bodies, Ourselves.* 40th anniversary ed. New York: Simon & Schuster, 2011.

Carlson, Karen J., Stephanie A. Eisenstat, and Terra Ziporyn. *The New Harvard Guide to Women's Health.* Cambridge, Mass.: Harvard University Press, 2004.

"Disorders of the Vulva." *American College of Obstetricians and Gynecologists*, May, 2011.

Foley, Denise, and Eileen Nechas. *Women's Encyclopedia of Health and Emotional Healing: Top Women Doctors Share Their Unique Self-Help Advice on Your Body, Your Feelings, and Your Life.* New York: Bantam Books, 1995.

Henderson, Gregory, and Batya Swift Yasgur. *Women at Risk: The HPV Epidemic and Your Cervical Health.* New York: Putnam, 2002.

Rushing, Lynda, and Nancy Joste. *Abnormal Pap Smears: What Every Woman Needs to Know.* Rev. ed. Amherst, N.Y.: Prometheus Books, 2008.

Shaw, Michael, ed. *Everything You Need to Know About Diseases.* Springhouse, Pa.: Springhouse Press, 1996.

Stewart, Elizabeth Gunther, and Paula Spencer. *The V Book: A Doctor's Guide to Complete Vulvovaginal Health.* New York: Bantam Books, 2002.

"Vagina: What's Normal, What's Not." *Mayo Clinic*, February 25, 2012.

GENITAL DISORDERS, MALE

Disease/Disorder

Anatomy or system affected: Genitals, reproductive system

Specialties and related fields: Family medicine, oncology, proctology, urology

Definition: Disorders and diseases of the male reproductive system, including sexual dysfunction, infertility, genital cancer, and sexually transmitted diseases.

Key terms:

autonomic nervous system: the part of the vertebrate nervous system that controls involuntary actions

dysfunction: the disordered or impaired function of a body system or organ

endocrine: relating to the production or action of a hormone

hormone: a substance that creates a specific effect in an organ distant from its site of production

impotence: the inability to have or maintain an erection satisfactory for sexual intercourse

organic: pertaining to, arising from, or affecting a body organ

parasympathetic nervous system: the part of the autonomic nervous system that stimulates digestion, slows the heart, and dilates blood vessels, acting in opposition to sympathetic nerves

psychogenic: originating in the mind or in mental conditions and activities

spermatogonia: cells of the testes that become sperm during spermatogenesis

sphincter: a ringlike muscle that constricts or relaxes to close or open a body orifice or passage, as required by normal body function

sympathetic nervous system: the part of the autonomic nervous system that represses digestion, speeds up the heart, and constricts blood vessels, acting in opposition to parasympathetic nerves

Process and Effects

Before discussion of male genital disorders and diseases, it is useful to describe the male reproductive system, which is composed of the scrotum, testes, epididymis, vas deferens, prostate and bulbourethral glands, seminal vesicles, penis, and urethra. The scrotum, composed of skin and underlying muscle, encloses the two testes and protects these sperm-making organs.

Each human testis is an ovoid structure about 5 centimeters long and 3.3 centimeters in width. A testis is composed of seminiferous tubules, a structure that surrounds the sperm-producing tubules, and accessory cells (the Leydig cells). The production of sperm, spermatogenesis, is controlled by hormones from the brain's hypothalamus and pituitary glands. It begins with the secretion of testosterone, the main male sex hormone, by Leydig cells. Brain hormone and testosterone actions cause the metamorphosis of cells called spermatogonia into sperm during a two-month passage through the seminiferous tubules.

The highly coiled seminiferous tubules, tiny in diameter and more than 200 meters long, coalesce into the efferent tubules, which release sperm into the epididymis. In a twelve-day trip through the highly coiled, 4.5-meter-long epididymis, sperm attain the ability to move (motility) and to fertilize a human egg cell, or ovum. Next, they enter the vas deferens, paired structures that connect the epididymis of each testis to its ejaculatory duct and the urethra. The only known vas function is to transport sperm, as a result of the action of nearby nerves and muscles, into the latter structures. The vas are cut in bilateral vasectomy surgery, which is often used for male sterilization.

The prostate, seminal vesicles, and bulbourethral glands produce the secretions that constitute most sperm-containing semen, which is ejaculated during intercourse. The prostate gland is situated immediately below the urinary bladder and surrounds the portion of the urethra closest to the bladder. It is a fibromuscular gland that empties into the male urethra on ejaculation. Prostate secretions contain important enzymes and make up a quarter of the seminal fluid.

The seminal vesicles are 7.5 centimeters long and empty into the ejaculatory ducts. They produce more than half of the liquid portion of semen, contributing fluid rich in fructose, the main nutrition source of sperm. The tiny, paired bulbourethral (or Cowper's) glands are located below the prostate. They secrete lubricants into the male urethra that ease semen passage.

The male urethra passes from the urinary bladder, through the prostate, and then through the penis. At the end of the penis, it reaches outside the body, to pass semen and urine. The penis, a cylindrical erectile organ, surrounds most of the male urethra and contains three cavernous regions. One, the corpus spongiosum, is found around the urethra. The others, the paired corpora cavernosa, are erectile tissues that fill with blood to produce an erection upon male sexual arousal. Erection is a complex reflex that involves both the sympathetic and parasympathetic portions of the human nervous system.

At the time of erection, nerve impulses dilate blood vessels

Information on Male Genital Disorders

Causes: Psychological factors, genital cancer, sexually transmitted diseases, anatomic dysfunction, various diseases, certain medications
Symptoms: Sexual dysfunction, infertility, impotence
Duration: Acute or chronic
Treatments: Depends on cause; may include psychotherapy, counseling, hormone therapy, discontinuation of medications or addictive drugs, corrective surgery (e.g., penile implants), drug therapy, surgery, radiation, chemotherapy

---

that communicate with the corpora cavernosa and allow them to fill with blood. Sphincters then close off the portion of the urethra closest to the urinary bladder. At the same time, sperm, prostate secretions, bulbourethral gland secretions, and seminal vesicle secretions enter the urethra. Next, upon stimulation sufficient to achieve orgasm, muscle contractions propel the ejaculate out of the urethra. The blood then leaves the corpora cavernosa, and the penis resumes its flaccid state.

Complications and Disorders

Proper male sexual function involves several closely coordinated hormonal, nervous, and chemical processes. After a discussion of the male reproductive system, it thus becomes clear that many factors can cause male genital problems and diseases. Male infertility, for example, can be attributable to inadequate sperm production; undersecretion by the seminal vesicles, Cowper's glands, and/or prostate; malfunction of other endocrine glands or of the nervous system; and dysfunction or lack of the epididymis. Impotence, the inability to have or maintain a satisfactory erection for intercourse, is another frequent male genital problem. It may be psychogenic or caused by anatomic dysfunction, disease, or medications used to treat health problems.

The male sexual response cycle is mediated by the complex interplay of parasympathetic and sympathetic nerves. For example, penis erection is mostly parasympathetic, while ejaculation is largely attributable to sympathetic enervation. Dysfunction disorders include low sexual desire, impotence (erectile dysfunction), and lost orgiastic control (premature ejaculation). Impotence is the most frequent of these problems.

Erectile dysfunction is said to occur when the failure to complete successful intercourse occurs at least 25 to 30 percent of the time. Most often, it is short term (secondary impotence) and related to individual partners or to temporary damage to male self-esteem. Secondary impotence may also be caused by diseases such as diabetes mellitus, medications such as tranquilizers and amphetamines, alcoholism and other psychoactive drug addictions, and minor genital abnormalities. Aging is not necessarily a cause of impotence, even in octogenarians. Effective medications called phosphodiesterase type 5 inhibitors have been developed for treating erectile dysfunction; the main ones include sildenafil (Viagra), vardenafil (Levitra), and tadalafil (Cialis).

Long-lasting (or primary) impotence that occurs despite corrective medical treatment is generally attributable to severe psychopathology and must be treated by psychotherapy and counseling. Psychogenic impotence is implicated when an erection can be achieved by masturbation. The treatment of impotence caused by organic problems may include testosterone administration, the discontinuation of drug therapy or addictive drugs, or corrective surgery, which may include inflatable penis implants.

Male infertility is a problem found in about a third of all cases in which American couples are unable to have children. The problem is thus estimated to occur in 4 to 5 percent of American men. There are a wide number of causes for male infertility, which is always characterized by the failure to deliver adequate numbers of mature sperm into the female reproductive tract as a result of organic problems. Impaired spermatogenesis, a frequent cause of male infertility, may have numerous causes. Examples include severe childhood mumps, brain and/or testicular hormone imbalances, drug abuse, obstruction or anatomic malformation of the seminal tract (especially the seminiferous tubules and epididymis), and a defective prostate gland.

Diagnosis includes careful physical examination by a urologist and evaluation of ejaculated semen to identify the number, activity, and potential for fertilization of its sperm. Blood tests will identify hormone imbalances and other possible causative agents. Many treatments are possible for male infertility, ranging from medications to corrective surgery to artificial insemination with sperm collected and frozen until enough are on hand to effect fertilization.

Cancer of the male genital organs may occur in the prostate, urethra, penis, or testis. The most important of these is prostate cancer. Urethral cancer is rare. More common is carcinoma of the penis, which occurs most often in uncircumcised men who practice poor genital hygiene. It is very often located beneath the foreskin and does not spread quickly. Total or partial removal of the penis is often required in advanced cases that have been ignored for long periods. Testicular cancers account for most solid genital malignancies in young men. These cancers appear as painful scrotal masses which increase rapidly in size. Any large, firm mass arising from a testis is suspicious and should be examined immediately by x-ray, computed tomography (CT) scan, and tests for various tumor markers seen in the blood. Treatment of these tumors includes surgery, radiation, and chemotherapy. Survival rates vary greatly and depend upon the cancer type. Cancer of the prostate and other male genital organs is not clearly understood and may have hormonal and chemical bases. It is believed that periodic self-examination is the most valuable preventive methodology.

Common disorders of the male genital organs include priapism, hydrocele and spermatocele, testicular torsion, and varicocele. Priapism is persistent, painful erection not accompanied by sexual arousal. It is caused by a poorly understood mechanism and is characterized by both pain and much-thickened blood in the corpora cavernosa. Priapism often occurs after prolonged sexual activity and may accom-

pany prostate problems, genital infections such as syphilis, and addictive drug use. Treatment of priapism includes draining blood from the penis following local anesthetic, administration of a medication called an alpha-adrenergic sympathomimetic, and surgery. In the absence of prompt, effective treatment, priapism may end male sexual function permanently.

A hydrocele is a swelling of the scrotum. The problem is caused by fluid accumulation resulting from testis inflammation. A hydrocele is not painful and is removed surgically only if excessive in size. Closely related in appearance is a spermatocele, which contains sperm and occurs adjacent to the epididymis. Testicular torsion is a twisting of the vas deferens, which causes pain and swelling; surgery is required to return blood flow to the testis. Varicocele describes varicose veins of the testis, which is common and usually harmless.

Sexually transmitted diseases can also affect the male genitals. These diseases include herpes, gonorrhea, syphilis, chlamydia, and genital warts. For the prevention of sexually transmitted diseases, abstention, the careful choice of sexual partners, and the use of male or female condoms are useful.

Perspective and Prospects

Treatment of the various types of male genital disorders and diseases has evolved greatly. Particularly valuable are the strides made in the treatment of impotence. It has been realized that such sexual dysfunction is often a consequence of organic problems that may be remedied by the cessation of causative medication use or by minor surgery. In addition, the utilization of inflatable penis implants in the cases where insoluble psychogenic or organic problems occur has been a milestone in the treatment of this emotionally devastating male genital problem.

Wide examination of the entire spectrum of male genital problems has led to numerous advantageous treatments and to an understanding that withholding unneeded medical treatments can be beneficial. For example, information regarding spermatoceles, hydroceles, and many related nonacute male genital problems has decreased the incidence of unnecessary male genital surgery, and its related risks, for patients.

Another important concept is that of frequent self-examination of the male genitals. This practice has led to a shortening of the time lag between the appearance of a suspicious mass in the scrotum, testes, or other male sex organ and medical attention from professionals (such as urologists) trained both to evaluate their seriousness and to treat them. Early detection has diminished the severity of many genital cancers and facilitated their treatment. Moreover, several clinical tests for such lesions have become more available and more widely used by the public.

It is hoped that these avenues and others, as well as further advances in both diagnostic techniques and treatment possibilities, will eventually eradicate male genital diseases and disorders. Two areas in need of advancements are priapism and prostate cancer, which is an effective killer.

—Sanford S. Singer, Ph.D.

See also Aphrodisiacs; Behçet's disease; Candidiasis; Chlamydia; Circumcision, male; Erectile dysfunction; Gonorrhea; Herpes; Hydroceles; Hypospadias repair and urethroplasty; Infertility, male; Men's health; Orchitis; Penile implant surgery; Prostate cancer; Prostate enlargement; Prostate gland; Prostate gland removal; Reproductive system; Semen; Sexual dysfunction; Sexuality; Sexually transmitted diseases (STDs); Sterilization; Stones; Syphilis; Testicles, undescended; Testicular cancer; Testicular surgery; Testicular torsion; Urology; Urology, pediatric; Vas deferens; Vasectomy; Warts.

For Further Information:

American Psychiatric Association. *Diagnostic and Statistical Manual of Mental Disorders: DSM-5.* Arlington, Va.: Author, 2013.

Beers, Mark H., et al., eds. *The Merck Manual of Diagnosis and Therapy.* 18th ed. Whitehouse Station, N.J.: Merck Research Laboratories, 2006.

Ellsworth, Pamela. *One Hundred Questions and Answers About Men's Health: Keeping You Happy and Healthy Below the Belt.* Sudbury, Mass.: Jones and Bartlett, 2011.

Ellsworth, Pamela, and Bob Stanley. *One Hundred Questions and Answers About Erectile Dysfunction.* 2d ed. Sudbury, Mass.: Jones and Bartlett, 2008.

Milsten, Richard, and Julian Slowinski. *The Sexual Male: Problems and Solutions.* New York: W. W. Norton, 2001.

Montague, Drogo K. *Disorders of Male Sexual Function.* Chicago: Year Book Medical, 1988.

Parker, James N., and Philip M. Parker, eds. *The Official Patient's Sourcebook on Impotence.* San Diego, Calif.: Icon Health, 2002.

Parker, James N., and Philip M. Parker, eds. *The Official Patient's Sourcebook on Testicular Cancer.* Rev. ed. San Diego, Calif.: Icon Health, 2002.

Sherwood, Lauralee. *Human Physiology: From Cells to Systems.* 8th ed. Pacific Grove, Calif.: Brooks/Cole, 2013.

Taguchi, Yosh, and Merrily Weisbord, eds. *Private Parts: An Owner's Guide to the Male Anatomy.* 3d ed. Toronto, Ont.: McClelland & Stewart, 2003.

Genomics
Specialty
Anatomy or system affected: All

Specialties and related fields: Bacteriology, biochemistry, biotechnology, cytology, embryology, ethics, genetics, microbiology, pharmacology

Definition: The study of whole genomes; a genome is the complete set of genetic information found in a particular organism.

Key terms:

bioinformatics: a computational discipline that provides the tools needed to study whole genomes and proteomes

DNA microarrays: solid supports which contain many or all genes from a given genome, enabling the expression of these genes to be monitored simultaneously

DNA sequencing: determining the order of deoxyribonucleic acid (DNA) bases in a particular unit of genetic information

orthologues: similar genes from different species that are thought to be related by evolution

proteomics: the study of proteomes; a proteome is the complete set of proteins in a particular cell type

synteny: when whole regions of chromosomes from different species are similar in structure

A New Scientific Discipline

Genomics grew out of the field of genetics, the study of heredity. Until the late twentieth century, it had not been possible to study the complete set of hereditary information in a living organism. Thus, while the field of genetics traces its roots to the 1860s, when the Austrian monk Gregor Mendel performed experiments on the mechanism of heredity in pea plants, the field of genomics is much younger, dating from the 1980s. It was in this decade that American geneticist Thomas Roderick used the term *genomics* to name a new scientific journal that dealt with the analysis of genomic information. In Mendel's time, while organisms were seen to exhibit certain traits, it was not known how these traits were determined. By the early twentieth century, it was recognized that traits are inherited in units of information called genes, although the chemical nature of the gene was still unknown. It took until the middle of that century to recognize that genes were made up of deoxyribonucleic acid (DNA), the structure of which was first identified by American biologist James Watson and British biophysicist Francis Crick in 1953.

DNA is made up of four different deoxyribonucleotides, commonly referred to as bases: adenine (A), cytosine (C), guanine (G), and thymine (T). Together, they spell out a chemical code that is used by the cell to make proteins. Since it is the set of proteins contained within a cell that gives that cell its unique properties, determining the order of DNA bases in a given genetic unit will reveal what types of proteins are encoded by this information, a procedure known as DNA sequencing. While a gene has been defined as the amount of DNA needed to encode one protein, a genome is the entire set of genes found in an organism, including any noncoding DNA found between genes. The number of genes that have been found to be present in an organism varies from fewer than two hundred in some obligately parasitic bacteria to about twenty-three thousand (in the simple flowering plant *Arabidopsis*); humans were found to have slightly fewer than this number.

During the 1980s, a public consortium, the International Human Genome Sequencing Consortium, was formed with the goal of sequencing the human genome by 2005. The Human Genome Project, as this effort was called, also had the goal of sequencing the genomes of a number of model organisms that have been used by scientists to help understand biological complexity. These model organisms, which included the *Escherichia coli* bacterium, yeast, *Caenorhabditis elegans* (a roundworm), *Drosophila* (the fruit fly), and the mouse, also served as steps by which the efficiency of DNA sequencing could be improved over time. *E. coli*, like most bacteria, has a genome that numbers in the millions of bases—usually abbreviated bp (for base pair), since each base in DNA is paired with its complementary base, A to T and G to C—while yeast has a genome of approximately ten million bp and the next three organisms have genomes that number in the hundreds of millions of bp. Mice, like humans, have genomes that are three billion bp in size. Around the turn of the twentieth century, steady progress was made on the genome efforts described above as the sequence of each respec-

In the News:
Last Human Chromosome Sequenced

In May, 2006, British molecular biologist Simon G. Gregory, along with more than 160 of his colleagues, published in the journal *Nature* the sequence of human chromosome 1, the last human chromosome to have its deoxyribonucleic acid (DNA) sequenced. This event, although largely ignored in the popular press, officially brought the Human Genome Project to an end. Perhaps the lack of fanfare can be linked to the fact that the project had already celebrated a few widely publicized conclusions. In June, 2000, U.S. president Bill Clinton and British prime minister Tony Blair announced the completion of a "rough draft" of the human genome sequence. This meant that 90 percent of the genome had been completed, with an error rate of 1 in 1,000 base pairs, despite the fact that more than 150,000 gaps in the sequence were still present. This rough draft was published in *Nature* as well as in the journal *Science* about six months after this announcement. The publication of the "final" sequence followed in these same journals in April, 2003. In this case, "final" meant that 99 percent of the genome had been completed, with an error rate of 1 in 10,000 base pairs, and fewer that 400 gaps were left.

Raw DNA sequence, however, is not as useful to scientists as a fully annotated sequence. Annotation involves the identification of potential genes as well as making an educated guess at their function. The first annotated sequence of a human chromosome (number 22) was published in *Nature* in December, 1999. The number of human chromosomes had originally been established using cytology. At that time, the twenty-two pairs of autosomal (nonsex) chromosomes had been numbered from 1 to 22, based on their apparent size from largest to smallest. Modern techniques have since shown that it is actually the two penultimately numbered chromosomes that are the largest and smallest chromosomes, namely chromosomes 2 and 21, respectively. Although chromosome 1 was ultimately not the largest human chromosome, it does contain the greatest number of genes (3,141) and has the most known genetic diseases associated with it, including Alzheimer's and Parkinson's diseases, certain forms of autism and mental retardation, and a number of cancers. With the publication of "The DNA Sequence and Biological Annotation of Human Chromosome 1" by Gregory and colleagues, the Human Genome Project was (once again) brought to completion.

—James S. Godde, Ph.D.

tive genome was determined and made publicly available via computer databases. The completion of the human genome was announced in April, 2003, the month of the fiftieth anniversary of Watson and Crick's first description of the structure of DNA.

Does the field of genomics represent a new scientific discipline in and of itself, or is it just another extension of genetics? Other than the sheer size of hereditary information being analyzed in genomics, another major difference would support the former possibility. Ever since Mendel's time, genetics has taken a reductionist approach. Since Mendel could not have dreamed of understanding the pea plant as a whole, he limited his investigation to a number of easily characterized traits, such as plant height and seed color. Since that time, many scientists have sought to understand complex biological processes by breaking them into manageable pieces. Genomics attempts a different, expansionist approach. In the postgenomics era (as the twenty-first century has been called by some scientists), the questions being posed are holistic in nature: they attempt for the first time to understand an organism as a whole using its complete set of genetic information as a guide. In fact, genomics has spawned a new set of fields that end in "-omics," denoting the fact that they attempt to study the complete set of particular molecules in an organism

or cell type. Proteomics is the study of the complete set of proteins in a cell type, while metabolomics is the study of the complete set of metabolic reactions in a cell.

New approaches to science call for new tools as well. The tools on which geneticists have relied over the years have largely proved to be insufficient for studying entire genomes. Bioinformatics is a subdiscipline of computational biology that has arisen to provide such tools. Bioinformatics includes the computational methods required to find patterns in the huge genomic databases that have been produced, to track the expression of genes using DNA microarrays, to identify all the proteins in a cell, and to model the protein interactions involved in cell metabolism, among other things.

Divisions within the Field
In addition to producing the "-omics" disciplines, the field of genomics can itself be subdivided. Although these divisions are somewhat artificial, they do help illustrate the different goals of genomics research. The main divisions of genomics are structural genomics, functional genomics, and comparative genomics.

Structural genomics is concerned with the structure of hereditary information. The determination of the number, location, and order of genes on a particular chromosome is one pursuit of this field. While bacterial genomes are typically contained within a single circular chromosome, humans have twenty-three pairs of chromosomes and some organisms have even more. Studying regions of DNA between genes, or intergenic regions, is also the realm of structural genomics. Intergenic regions are often composed of a highly repetitive DNA sequence that does not code for any type of protein. In the early twenty-first century, the precise function of these regions still eluded scientists. Although noncoding sequence is relatively rare in bacteria, it makes up a major portion of many multicellular organisms, including about 98 percent of the human genome. A separate goal of structural biology is the determination of the three-dimensional structure of all the proteins encoded by a genome, an endeavor called structural proteomics.

Functional genomics is less concerned with the structure of a genome and more concerned with its function. This division of genomics tends to be of more interest to pharmaceutical companies and the medical community as a whole. Functional genomics asks questions such as, "What do the products of individual genes do?" and "How does the perturbation of gene function lead to disease states?" Determining the function of a gene, however, is not as straightforward as it might appear. By the early twenty-first century, determining the structure of a given genome was the relatively easy part, but the function of up to half the genes in a typical sequenced genome remained undetermined. Even the determination of the three-dimensional structure of a protein that is produced by a specific gene does not guarantee that its function can be discerned, but scientists are always hopeful that this will lead to conjecture concerning its function.

Another clue concerning gene function can be derived by the determination of where and when a particular gene is expressed (activated to produce its corresponding protein). While gene expression has traditionally been monitored one gene at a time using molecular genetic techniques, around the turn of the twenty-first century researchers began experimenting with DNA microarrays., or "gene chips," which include copies of many, if not all, genes from a given genome attached to a solid support such as a glass slide. The expression of these genes can be monitored at any given time by binding fluorescently tagged sequences of DNA that are complementary to the genes in question. An automated scanner then measures the fluorescence of each spot and records the data into a computer.

The final division of genomics, comparative genomics, encompasses the goals of the other two divisions but achieves these goals by making comparisons between two or more different genomes. For example, the structure of a given genome, by itself, may not appear significant until the same basic structure is detected in another species. Regions of chromosomes from two different species that are similar in structure are said to display synteny. Comparative genomics as a discipline was not possible until the mid-1990s, when computing technology had developed to the point where huge databases of genomic information could be stored and compared quickly and accurately. Comparative genomics has also aided in the quest to determine gene function. One of the most common techniques of determining gene function is by looking for orthologues in related species. Orthologues are genes from different species that are thought to be related by evolution; they often encode similar, but not identical, proteins with related functions.

Perspective and Prospects

Genomics can trace its origins to the development of techniques used to determine the sequence of DNA. In 1977, British biochemist Frederick Sanger and colleagues published a sequencing method based on the principle of chain termination. In this method, the sequence of target DNA is determined by enzymatically producing a complementary strand of DNA. In Sanger sequencing, as it is now called, a molecular "poison" is included in a given reaction mixture so that the newly synthesized complementary chain is terminated at specific bases. Sanger's method was then modified in the 1990s to include fluorescent dyes on the chain-terminating bases so that the DNA sequence could be read using a scanner and recorded directly into a computer. Some have claimed that

Sanger and colleagues were actually the first group to sequence a genome, since they published the sequence of a viral genome in the same year that they described their revolutionary technique. Viruses, however, are not free-living organisms, and their genomes are thousands of times smaller than the typical bacterial genome.

The Human Genome Project was first proposed in 1986 and was funded two years later at an expected cost of three billion dollars. The project officially got under way in 1990 as sequencing began in earnest on some of the smaller model genomes. In 1995, as some of these sequencing efforts were nearing completion, American pharmacologist Craig Venter and his colleagues at a private not-for-profit institute, the Institute for Genome Research, published the genome sequence of the bacterium *Haemophilus influenzae*, the first free-living organism to have its genome sequenced.

While the public consortium had been working on sequences using established techniques, Venter and colleagues had developed a faster technique for determining the sequence of whole genomes. While this technique still used the basic Sanger-style chain termination procedure, it simplified an earlier step in the process in which large numbers of clones of genomic fragments were made before sequencing could begin. Venter had circumvented this cloning step; he called his approach whole-genome shotgun sequencing. During the next two years, the public consortium published the sequences of yeast and *E. coli*, respectively, and in 1998 announced that the sequence of *C. elegans* was complete. That same year, Venter announced that he was starting a for-profit company, Celera Genomics, which would complete the human genome within three years using shotgun sequencing. Up until this time, however, Venter had only demonstrated this approach using bacterial genomes. To demonstrate the validity of the shotgun approach on large genomes, and to gear up for sequencing the human genome, Celera sequenced the 170 million bp genome of the fruit fly in 2000, at that time the largest genome ever sequenced.

During the final years of the twentieth century, spurred on by the competition from the private sector, the public consortium had redoubled its efforts on the human genome. In February, 2001, the race to sequence the human genome ended in a tie. Both sequencing efforts, public and private, published their draft sequence of the human genome at this time, and in April, 2003, the two efforts together announced the final completed sequence. The mouse genome sequence was also published in 2003. In fact, by mid-2003, about 150 genomic sequences had been determined (the vast majority of which were bacterial genomes) and almost 600 more were underway, including many more multicellular organisms.

Are the time, effort, and money that have been spent on various genome-sequencing projects really worth it? One promise that genomics may hold for the future is the identification of all human disease genes. While this has been one of the main justifications for the Human Genome Project, one should keep in mind that identifying the gene that causes a particular disease is not always equivalent to finding a cure for that disease. Another potential benefit of genomic research is the development of better treatments for bacterial and parasitic infections. A number of disease-causing bacteria have already been the subject of genome sequencing efforts, including the causative agents of bubonic plague, anthrax, and tuberculosis, to name a few. Some indirect benefits of genomics (which may, in time, prove just as valuable) include a better understanding of evolutionary relationships between species as well as a firmer grasp on basic cellular function. In all, the field of genomics promises to be a powerful means of scientific inquiry well into the future.

—James S. Godde, Ph.D.;
updated by Jeffrey A. Knight, Ph.D.

See also Bioinformatics; Biostatistics; Cloning; DNA and RNA; Gene therapy; Genetic counseling; Genetic diseases; Genetic engineering; Genetics and inheritance; Laboratory tests; Mutation; Screening.

For Further Information:

Brown, Terence A. *Genomes*. 3d ed. New York: Garland Science, 2007.

Campbell, A. Malcolm, and Laurie J. Heyer. *Discovering Genomics, Proteomics, and Bioinformatics*. 2d ed. San Francisco: CSHL Press, 2009.

Centers for Disease Control. "Genomics & Health Impact Update: August 6, 2013." *CDC Public Health Genomics*, August 1–August 8, 2013.

Clark, M. S. "Comparative Genomics: The Key to Understanding the Human Genome Project." *BioEssays* 21 (1999): 121–130.

Collins, Francis S., et al. "A Vision for the Future of Genomics Research." *Nature* 422 (April, 2003): 835–847.

DeRisi, Joseph L., and Vishwanath R. Iyer. "Genomics and Array Technology." *Current Opinion in Oncology* 11 (1999): 76–79.

Goodman, Denise M., et al. "Genomic Medicine." *JAMA: The Journal of the American Medical Association*, April 10, 2013.

Klug, William S., and Michael R. Cummings. "Genomics, Bioinformatics, and Proteomics." In *Concepts of Genetics*. 8th ed. Upper Saddle River, N.J.: Prentice Hall, 2007.

Olson, Steve, and Institute of Medicine (US). *Integrating Large-Scale Genomic Information into Clinical Practice: Workshop Summary*. Washington, D.C.: National Academies Press, 2012.

Snustad, D. Peter, and Michael J. Simmons. "Genomics." In *Principles of Genetics*. 5th ed. Hoboken, N.J.: John Wiley & Sons, 2009.

Urbano, Kevin V. *Advances in Genetics Research*. New York: Nova Science, 2011.

Wei, Liping, et al. "Comparative Genomics Approaches to Study Organism Similarities and Differences." *Journal of Biomedical Informatics* 35 (2002). 142–150.

GERIATRIC ASSESSMENT
Procedure
Anatomy or system affected: All

Specialties and related fields: Gerontology, internal medicine, family medicine

Definition: A tool used to gather information about an older adult.

Key term:
assessment: the process of documenting knowledge, evidence, skills, attitudes, beliefs, or other pertinent information so as to elucidate a phenomenon or contribute to understanding

Description and Background Information

Geriatric assessment investigates many different aspects of an older person's life: medical issues, psychological issues, social issues, functional capabilities, and limitations; activities like driving, cooking meals, practicing adequate hygiene, and paying bills. It is an instrument that can be incorporated in a variety of clinical practice settings, from home care to hospital care, and everywhere in between.

Health care providers from all disciplines-including but not limited to doctors, nurse practitioners, social workers, case managers, and nurses-can use the information gathered from a geriatric assessment to create a treatment plan, establishing short-term goals, long-term goals, and a plan for follow-up, and generally make the best use of the health care resources available to the older adult. These efforts are ideally discussed and agreed upon by the health care provider(s) and older adult; however, family and caregiver input are valuable and often essential in the case of the older adult with cognitive impairment or other debilitating disease.

A truly comprehensive geriatric assessment may involve several encounters with an older adult (or caregivers, loved ones) initially over a period of time determined by the health care provider(s) and individual/family, and again at mutually agreed-upon intervals. The comprehensive assessment encompasses a wide variety of domains. Areas that may be investigated by geriatric specialists include:

- A full, head-to-toe physical examination
- Current symptoms, illnesses, or other stressors that may be impacting the older adult's life
- Medications taken: what they are for, when they are taken, how are they being tolerated, are they affordable
- Past and current illnesses: diagnoses, hospitalizations (if any), surgeries (if any)
- Other major life events: marriage(s), deaths, personal successes, failures
- Social health: involvement with neighborhood, community, region; includes presence of family, availability of family, and who the older person defines as family. Who is looking after this person, if anyone?
- An objective measure of cognitive status
- An objective assessment of mobility and balance
- An assessment of the older adult's environment: neighborhood safety, home safety, adequate resources to maintain living situation
- Emotional health; history of or current substance abuse
- Nutritional status and needs; ability to prepare meals, food preferences and eating routines, any difficulties with chewing, swallowing, or obtaining food
- Risk factors for disease, immunizations; health promotion activities

Geriatric assessment differs from a traditional medical evaluation in three important ways: (1) It focuses on elderly individuals whom often have complex, interconnected issues; (2) It emphasizes quality of life, and (3) It may be administered effectively through the collaboration of many different health care providers or just one health care provider. If several health care providers are involved in administering this assessment, one person (regardless of discipline) is often the coordinator. The coordinator facilitates group meetings or communiqués so that the multidisciplinary group can operate effectively and efficiently. The older adult is always the center of the mutually agreed-upon goals of care.

—*Christopher J. Norman, B.A., B.S.N., R.N.-B.C., B.C.*

See also Allied health; Alternative medicine; Anatomy; Aging; Geriatrics; Gerontology; Holistic medicine; Medicare; Nursing; Physical examination; Safety issues for the elderly; Signs and symptoms; Telemedicine; Women's health

For Further Information:

Boltz, M., et al. *Evidence-based Geriatric Nursing Protocols for Best Practice.* 4th ed. New York: Springer, 2012.

Foreman, M.D., et al. *Critical Care Nursing of Older Adults: Best Practices.* 3rd ed. New York: Springer, 2010.

Geriatrics at Your Fingertips: http://geriatricscareonline.org

Halter, J., et. al. *Hazzard's Geriatric Medicine and Gerontology.* 6th ed. New York: McGraw-Hill, 2009.

Ham, R.J., et al. *Primary Care Geriatrics: A Case-based Approach.* 5th ed. New York: Mosby, 2007.

Hartford Institute for Geriatric Nursing: http://consultgerirn.org

GERIATRICS AND GERONTOLOGY

Specialty

Anatomy or system affected: All

Specialties and related fields: All

Definition: Geriatrics refers to the social and health care of the elderly; gerontology is the study of the aging process.

Key terms:

decubitus ulcer: ulceration of the skin and subcutaneous tissues, resulting from protein deficiency and prolonged, unrelieved pressure on bony prominences

dementia: a deterioration or loss of intellectual faculties, reasoning power, memory, and will that is caused by organic brain disease

glaucoma: an eye disease characterized by increased intraocular pressure, which can lead to degeneration of the optic nerve and ultimately blindness if left untreated

Medicare: the popular designation for 1965 amendments to the U.S. Social Security Act, providing hospitalization and certain other benefits to people over the age of sixty-five

polypharmacy: the prescription of many drugs at one time, often resulting in excessive use of medications and adverse drug interactions

prostate: in men, the organ surrounding the neck of the urinary bladder and beginning of the urethra; its secretions make up about 40 percent of semen

The Study of Aging

The field of geriatrics deals with the care of the elderly. The U.S. government's definition of elderly includes persons sixty-five years of age or older. Geriatricians are physicians with specialized training in geriatric medicine who restrict their practices to caring for persons seventy-five years of age or older. These patients are most likely to suffer from specific geriatric syndromes, including dementia, delirium, urinary incontinence, malnutrition, osteoporosis, falls and immobility, decubitus ulcers, polypharmacy, and sleep disorders.

The majority of older persons in the United States live in family settings with their spouses or children. Approximately 30 percent of older persons live alone, the majority of them being women. According to the U.S. Census Bureau, in 2000 the proportion of older persons (those over sixty-five) who lived in nursing homes was about 4.5 percent. Those aged eighty-five and over had a higher proportion, at 18.2 percent, thus indicating that the number of elderly people residing in nursing homes increases strikingly with age. However, the overall percentage of the elderly living in nursing homes is declining. While one may attribute this change to improvements in health care, it may also be attributable to the use of home health aides who provide assisted living services to seniors.

The focus of geriatric medicine is on improving functional disability and treating chronic disease conditions that impair a person's ability to perform such activities of daily living as bathing and dressing, maintaining urinary and bowel continence, and eating. A more objective measure of an older person's ability to live independently is the instrumental activities of daily living scale. This scale measures an individual's ability to use the telephone, obtain transportation, go shopping, prepare meals, do housework and laundry, self-administer medicines, and manage money.

The maximum life span of an organism is the theoretical longest duration of that organism's life, excluding premature, unnatural death. The maximum life span of humans is unknown, although most experts believe it to be approximately 120 years. Most people will die of disease or accident, however, before they reach this biological limit. Attempts to understand why this occurs have led to the development of several theories of aging. The aging process is controlled, in large part, by genetic mechanisms. Aging is a biologic process characterized by a progressive development and maturation leading to senescence and death. There are profound changes in cells, tissues, and organs as well as in physiological, cognitive, and psychological processes. Aging is not the acquisition of disease, although aging and disease can be related. In the absence of disease, normal aging is a slow process. It involves the steady decline of organ reserves and homeostatic control mechanisms, which is often not apparent unless there is maximal exertion or stress on an individual system or on the total organism.

Numerous changes in the body occur as people age. For example, one can expect to lose two inches in height from age forty to age eighty. This shrinkage results from a decrease in vertebral bone mass and in the thickness of intervertebral disks, as well as from postural alterations with increased flexion or bending at the hips and knees. Total body fat increases as one ages, accompanied by decreases in muscle mass and total body water. Such changes in body composition have important implications for drug treatments and nutritional plans. For example, fat-soluble medications exhibit a longer duration of action in the elderly. Older persons also experience a thinning of the dermal layer of the skin, with thinner blood vessels, decreased collagen, and less skin elasticity. Sun damage can accelerate these changes. Graying of the hair reflects a progressive loss of functional melanocytes from the hair bulbs. The number of hair follicles of the scalp decreases, as does the growth rate of remaining follicles. The brain also alters with age: The weight of the brain declines, blood flow to the brain decreases, and there is a loss of neurons in specific areas of the brain. These changes in brain structure are highly variable and do not necessarily affect thinking and behavior.

Many changes occur in the vision of the older person. Loss of elasticity in the lens leads to presbyopia, the most common visual problem associated with aging. Presbyopia is a condition in which the distance that is needed to focus on near objects increases. Cataracts increase in prevalence with age, although unprotected exposure of the eyes to ultraviolet rays has been implicated in the pathogenesis as well. Glaucoma also occurs more often in the elderly.

Older persons often experience hearing loss from degenerative processes, including atrophy of the external auditory canal and thickening of the tympanic membrane. The result is presbycusis, a bilateral hearing loss for pure tones. Higher frequencies are more affected than lower ones, and the condition is more severe in men than in women. Pitch discrimination also declines with age, which may account for an increased difficulty in speech discrimination.

The heart alters with age, although the significance of these changes is unclear in the absence of disease. There are declines in intrinsic contractile function and electrical activity. The resting heart rate and cardiac output do not change, but the maximum heart rate decreases in a linear fashion and may be estimated by subtracting a person's age from 220. There are also modest increases in systolic blood pressure.

Minor changes occur in the gastrointestinal system. The liver and pancreas maintain adequate function throughout life, although the metabolism of specific drugs is prolonged in older people. Kidney function declines with age, with a 30 percent loss in renal mass and a decrease in renal blood flow. A linear decline in the ability of the kidneys to filter blood after the age of forty can lead to a decrease in the clearance of some drugs from the body.

In the endocrine system, the blood glucose level before meals changes minimally after the age of forty, although the level of blood glucose after meals increases. These changes may be related to decreases in muscle mass and a decreased insulin secretion rate. Glucose intolerance with aging must be distinguished from the hyperglycemia that can accompany diabetes mellitus; the latter requires treatment. No clinically significant alterations in the levels of the thyroid hormone occur, although the end organ response to thyroid hormones may be decreased. The hypothalamic-pituitary-adrenal axis remains intact. Plasma basal and stimulated norepinephrine levels are higher in healthy elderly individuals than in the young. The secretion of hormones such as androgens and estrogens falls sharply as a result of the loss of endocrine cells.

Diseases Affecting the Elderly

One of the chronic diseases frequently seen in elderly people is osteoporosis. Osteoporosis is defined as a decreased amount of bone per unit of volume; mineralization of the bone remains normal. Many studies have shown that bone mass decreases with age. Vertebral fractures resulting from osteoporosis cause deformity of the spine, loss in height, and pain. The absolute number of vertebral fractures that occur in older persons has been difficult to estimate, as some of these fractures go undiagnosed. The approximately 300,000 hip fractures that the elderly in the United States suffer annually have much more serious consequences. The lifetime risk of hip fracture by the age of eighty is approximately 15 percent for white women and 7 percent for white men. The risk of hip fracture by this age is significantly less in African Americans, with a 6 percent risk for women and a 3 percent risk for men.

One approach to preventing osteoporosis is to maximize the amount of bone that is formed during adolescence. Under normal circumstances, people begin to experience a net bone loss after the age of thirty-five. In women, the onset of menopause accelerates bone loss because of the decline in estrogen levels. Relative calcium deficiency has also been implicated in age-related osteoporosis. By definition, age-related osteoporosis is a diagnosis of exclusion. An older patient who has suffered a fracture first should be evaluated for other causes of osteoporosis, including hyperparathyroidism, hyperthyroidism, diabetes, glucocorticoid excess, or, in men, hypogonadism. Other secondary causes of osteoporosis include malignancy, such as multiple myeloma, leukemia, or lymphoma, and the drug-related effects of alcohol or steroids. Any identifiable causes should be corrected.

People at increased risk for age-related osteoporosis include those with a family history of the disease; light hair, skin, and eyes; and a small body frame. Bone densitometry or quantitative computed tomography (CT) scanning can be performed to provide the most accurate estimates of the risk of an initial fracture. There are a number of prevention and treatment strategies for patients. One should ensure an adequate calcium intake; the current recommendation is a daily intake of 1,200 milligrams of calcium for postmenopausal women. Weight-bearing exercise should be performed throughout the life span. After menopause when estrogen levels decrease, the bone breakdown process accelerates. In postmenopausal women, two types of treatment options are available, estrogen treatment and bisphosphonates. Bisphosphonates are the most common medications prescribed. Bisphosphonates slow the bone breakdown process. While estrogen has not been shown conclusively to increase bone density, it does prevent further bone loss. However, estrogen replacement therapy may increase the risk of heart attacks and some types of cancer. In patients who cannot take estrogen, an alternative treatment is the hormone calcitonin. Calcitonin works by inhibiting osteoclast function, thereby halting the otherwise normal breakdown of bone.

A disorder that is commonly seen in elderly men is benign prostatic hyperplasia (BPH), or prostate enlargement. The incidence of this disease increases in a progressive fashion, with approximately 90 percent of men aged eighty affected by this condition. The pathogenesis of BPH is hormonal, caused by increased levels of dihydrotestosterone formed from the testosterone within the gland itself. The usual symptoms are those of urinary obstruction, which include hesitancy, straining, and decreased force and dimension of the urinary stream. Screening for benign prostatic hypertrophy includes two parts. The first is a blood test for prostate-specific antigens. The second is a digital rectal exam to inspect the prostate gland. Patients with positive findings will require further evaluation. A significant increase in prostatic tissue may need to be removed surgically. In patients with minimal disease, drug treatment may be used. Finesteride is an inhibitor of the enzyme 5-alpha reductase that is responsible for the conversion of testosterone to dihydrotestosterone. It slows the rate of increase in prostate tissue mass.

Depression is a common problem in both men and women as they get older. The elderly can experience transient mood changes that are the result of an identifiable stress or loss. In older persons, however, depression may be related to some medical condition, particularly dementia, which is associated with multiple strokes or Parkinson's disease. Major depression is more common in hospital and long-term care settings, where the prevalence is about 13 percent. The symptoms of depression include significant weight change, insomnia or hypersomnia, psychomotor agitation or retardation, decreased energy and easy fatigability, feelings of worthlessness or excessive guilt, decreased ability to think or concentrate, and recurrent thoughts of death or suicide. The diagnosis of major depression can be made if at least five of these symptoms are present for at least two weeks. Depressive symptoms must be taken seriously in the elderly. The rate of suicide in older persons is higher than for other groups, with older white males having the highest rates of any age, racial, or ethnic group.

Another depressive disorder experienced by the elderly is dysthymia. Dysthymic disorders are characterized by less severe symptoms than those associated with major depression and by a duration of at least two years. The symptoms generally include at least two of the following: poor appetite or overeating, insomnia or hypersomnia, low energy and fatigue, low self-esteem, poor concentration or difficulty in making decisions, and feelings of hopelessness. Dysthymia may be primary or secondary to a preexisting chronic psychiatric or medical illness, with accompanying loss of function and debilitation.

Adjustment disorders with depressed mood are also seen in older persons. Such disorders occur within three months of a stressful situation and last up to six months. The prototypical situation is the depressive reaction that follows an acute medical illness. In the elderly, the four most common stressors are physical illness, reactions to the death of family and friends, retirement, and moving to an institutional setting. In dealing with depressive symptoms, however, it is important to consider other diagnoses, such as underlying medical illnesses, drug reactions to prescribed or over-the-counter medicines, hypochondriasis, alcohol abuse, and dementias.

In older patients, the disorder most often associated with depression is dementia.

Incontinence affects a vast number of elders yet is often unaddressed during a clinic visit because of either lack of the patient's knowledge about potential treatments or embarrassment regarding the issue. Incontinence has a major impact on an elder's quality of life, and, as it is often a treatable condition, it should be discussed by patients with their physicians.

Another topic frequently not discussed involves the issue of remaining sexually active as an elder. Over half of married elders continue to have sex, although sometimes this activity is complicated by fears such as having a heart attack or stroke as a result of the exertion. In addition, medical problems and medication side effects can affect the elder's sexual abilities. Some potential treatments for sexual dysfunction include phosphodiesterase inhibitors and, in the case of low testosterone or low estrogen, hormone therapies, which can aid in increasing the sexual satisfaction of elders.

A thorough diagnostic evaluation can help in the diagnosis of a depressive disorder and can rule out other complicating problems. A careful history is elicited from the patient and from a family member or caretaker. A formal mental status examination is conducted to uncover abnormalities in concentration, speech, psychomotor skills, cognitive ability, and memory. Laboratory blood tests often include a complete blood count, chemical analysis, and thyroid function tests. Abbreviated neuropsychological tests can differentiate between patients with dementia and those with depression alone. The treatment of depression includes psychotherapy and pharmacotherapy. Behavioral interventions, such as special weekly activities and assignments, can be helpful. Most often, some kind of antidepressant medication is effective.

Perspective and Prospects

In the United States, there has been increasing interest in the fields of geriatrics and gerontology because of the country's changing demographics. In 2000, 35 million Americans were sixty-five years of age or older. Because of the very large numbers in the baby-boom age group-that is, people born between 1946 and 1964-it was expected that the number of elderly people would increase dramatically by the year 2030 to 71.5 million, more than doubling the amount of elderly people in 2000. By 2050, it is expected that this number will reach 86.7 million. Those individuals aged sixty-five and over made up approximately 12.5 percent of the U.S. population in 2000. In 2030, this percentage could increase to 19.5 percent.

Another reason for the increase in the size of the older population in the United States is an increase in life expectancy. Life expectancy is defined as the average number of years a person is expected to live, given population mortality rates. It can be calculated for any age category but is usually given as life expectancy from birth. The life expectancy in the United States is much higher than in undeveloped countries and in most other developed countries as well. This figure rose steadily throughout the twentieth century. A child born in 2000 could expect to live seventy-five years, while someone born in 1900 could expect to live only fifty years. Most of this increase in life expectancy is attributable to a decreased death rate for infants and children resulting from improvements in sanitation, active immunization against childhood diseases, and advances in medical treatments. For persons aged sixty-five, there was an increase in life expectancy over that same time period of only five years, probably the result of improved medical therapies. While the geriatric population is dramatically increasing, the availability of geriatricians is not. As the population continues to grow, the shortage will increase.

Making healthy lifestyle modifications, receiving appropriate medical screening exams, and partaking in numerous prevention strategies may improve the quality of life of the elderly. These actions may also lead to preventing serious accidents and disabling conditions. Lifestyle modifications that should be attempted include alcohol and smoking cessation, as well as diet and exercise programs. With the increasing awareness of obesity as a major problem in society, it is important to keep the geriatric population at a healthy weight that will not lead to adverse health effects.

With the decline in vision and hearing that may be experienced by the older population, audio/visual screening should be performed and proper corrective measures taken. This may help avoid accidents around the home and while driving. Vaccinations should be up to date to help prevent disease. Unless contraindicated, the elderly should consider obtaining the annual flu vaccine. The pneumococcal vaccine should also be considered. In addition, screening tests are available to assess some of the common conditions affecting the elderly. Those preventive services covered by Medicare as of 2006 include a "Welcome to Medicare Physical Exam" once during the first six months of enrollment, serum cholesterol levels every five years, annual mammograms in women aged forty and over, biannual Pap tests and pelvic exams, fecal occult blood tests starting at age fifty and then annually, a flexible sigmoidoscopy at age fifty and then every four years, a colonoscopy at age fifty and then every ten years, serum prostate specific antigen levels and digital rectal exams starting at age fifty and then annually, glaucoma screening if over fifty and then annually, and bone densitometry testing in women over fifty or at high risk and then biannually. Medicare will also cover the following vaccines: pneumococcal one time, hepatitis B vaccine series one time, and influenza vaccines annually.

Because elders may be taking multiple medications, it is important that they occasionally review these medications with their doctors. By doing so, side effects can be discussed and any drug interactions may be avoided. All dosages and correct use should be reviewed to make sure that the appropriate medications are taken daily and that accidental overdose may be avoided. Pillboxes are an excellent tool to make sure that medications are taken correctly. In addition, it is advisable that elders keep a list of all medications and allergies on their person should an emergency arise.

With the popularity of herbal supplements, it is essential that the elderly discuss their use with a physician. Some of these regimens may have adverse effects of which patients are unaware. In addition, herbal supplements may interact with some of the medications that their physicians have prescribed.

As Americans live longer, the length of time that older persons will rely on society for their care increases as well. This situation places a greater burden on those persons who are working, as they must support greater numbers of people receiving Social Security and Medicare benefits, and requires a rethinking of the age requirements to be eligible for these programs. In 1997, while older persons represented 13 percent of the population, they accounted for 38 percent of the total costs for health care. Other factors adding to the cost of health care include such new technologies as specialized imaging equipment, complex laboratory procedures, and new therapeutic drugs. The goal of much research in geriatric medicine is to prevent or slow down the effects of aging so that the elderly may live in good health. Further research to understand better the mechanisms involved in human aging will help to design preventive and treatment strategies.

—RoseMarie Pasmantier, M.D. and
L. Fleming Fallon, Jr., M.D., Ph.D., M.P.H.;
updated by Christie Leal, D.O.

See also Aging; Aging: Extended care; Alzheimer's disease; Appetite loss; Arthritis; Assisted living facilities; Bedsores; Bed-wetting; Blindness; Bone disorders; Brain disorders; Cardiac arrest; Cataract surgery; Cataracts; Critical care; Deafness; Death and dying; Dementias; Depression; Domestic violence; Emergency medicine; Endocrinology; Euthanasia; Family medicine; Fatigue; Hearing; Hearing loss; Hip fracture repair; Home care; Hormone therapy; Hospitals; Incontinence; Living will; Memory loss; Nursing; Nutrition; Ophthalmology; Orthopedics; Osteoporosis; Pain management; Paramedics; Parkinson's disease; Pharmacology; Physician assistants; Pick's disease; Polypharmacy; Prostate enlargement; Psychiatry; Psychiatry, geriatric; Rheumatology; Sleep; Sleep disorders; Spinal cord disorders; Spine, vertebrae, and disks; Suicide; Vision; Vision disorders

For Further Information:

Beerman, Susan, and Judith Rappaport-Musson. *Eldercare 911: The Caregiver's Complete Handbook for Making Decisions.* Rev. ed. Amherst, NY: Prometheus Books, 2008. A practical guide for elder care. Includes topics such as locating services, managing medications, understanding benefits, choosing a nursing home, coping with memory loss, hiring and handling in-home help, helping a parent who refuses help, and recognizing signs of elder abuse.

Beers, Mark H., and Robert Berkow, eds. *The Merck Manual of Geriatrics.* 3rd ed. Whitehouse Station, NJ: Merck Research Laboratories, 2000. Addresses the challenges of geriatric care. Provides diagnosis and treatment information specific to aging patients.

Birren, James E., and K. Warner Schaie, eds. *Handbook of the Psychology of Aging.* 6th ed. Boston: Academic Press/Elsevier, 2007. Twenty-four contributions from international researchers explore topics such as the genetics of behavioral aging, environmental influences on aging, gender roles, mental health, declining motor control, wisdom, and technological change and the older worker.

Centers for Disease Control and Prevention. Injury Center. http://www.cdc.gov/HomeandRecreationalSafety/Falls/index.html. This site includes a suggestion of all precautions that can be implemented by the elderly population to help reduce the risk of fracture.

Coni, Nicholas, et al. *Lecture Notes on Geriatrics.* 6th ed. Malden,

MA: Blackwell Science, 2003. Easy-to-read study notes on geriatric medicine. Discusses the different changes that occur in the patient during the aging process and characterizes the different diseases seen in the elderly.

Ferri, Fred F., Marsha Fretwell, and Tom J. Wachtel. *Practical Guide to the Care of the Geriatric Patient.* 3rd ed. St. Louis: Mosby/Elsevier, 2007. An excellent resource. The text is clearly written, and the index is especially useful. Nonprofessional readers will have no trouble understanding this book.

Hampton, Roy, and Charles Russell. *The Encyclopedia of Aging and the Elderly.* New York: Facts On File, 1992. Includes much well-stated information. The scope of this work is broad-lifestyle, myths and misconceptions, medical and legal concerns, death and dying. Includes statistical information in charts and tables, a list of organizations, and a useful bibliography.

He, Wan, et al. *65+ in the United States: 2005.* Washington, DC: Government Printing Office, 2005. A special report that is also available at http://www.census.gov/prod/2006pubs/p23-209.pdf.

Hooyman, Nancy, and H. Asuman Kiyak. *Social Gerontology: A Multidisciplinary Perspective.* New York: Prentice Hall, 2010. Contributions from social workers, psychologists, gerontology professionals, and professors examine the ways in which age-related changes in the biological, functional, and psychological domains can influence the older person's interactions with his or her social and physical environment.

Hoyer, William J., and Paul A. Roodin. *Adult Development and Aging.* 6th ed. Boston: McGraw-Hill, 2009. An interdisciplinary exploration of the biological, social, and cultural contexts in which change occurs during the adult years.

Isaacs, Bernard. *The Challenge of Geriatric Medicine.* London: Oxford Medical, 1992. This volume presents the issues associated with geriatric medicine and the care of older citizens. It is well written and should be of interest to most readers who want additional information on this subject.

Margolis, Simeon. *The Johns Hopkins Medical Guide to Health after 50.* New York: Rebus, 2002. This may well be the best authoritative consumer guide for those over 50 who are interested in prevention of diseases and conditions that are part of normal aging; it also includes focused reviews of pathologies and illnesses that typically occur in the elderly. A good read for those who want to enter their senior years in good health and for those who develop problems after they get there.

Margolis, Simeon, and Hamilton Moses III, eds. *The Johns Hopkins Medical Handbook: The One Hundred Major Medical Disorders of People over the Age of Fifty.* Rev. ed. Garden City, NY: Random House, 1999. Though a 1999 publication, this remains the definitive home medical reference for adults. It offers an in-depth review of the most common medical problems occurring in adults over fifty. The directory of hospitals and other health care resources, from support groups to treatment centers, is comprehensive.

Masoro, Edward J., and Steven N. Austad, eds. *Handbook of the Biology of Aging.* 6th ed. Boston: Academic Press/Elsevier, 2007. Part of a three-volume series that includes the biological, psychological, and social aspects of aging. Focuses on research approaches to understanding aging, including genetic studies, cellular and molecular biology, neurobiology, and nutrition.

Stenchever, Morton A. *Health Care for the Older Woman.* New York: Chapman and Hall, 1996. A reference that provides medical practitioners and students with comprehensive, current information specific to the care of middle-aged and advanced-aged women. It covers health maintenance issues, including diet, exercise, safety, psychological and psychosocial problems, social problems, and grief and loss.

GESTATIONAL DIABETES
Disease/Disorder

Anatomy or system affected: Endocrine system, reproductive system

Specialties and related fields: Endocrinology, nutrition, obstetrics

Definition: A medical condition in which diabetes, or unregulated blood glucose, first occurs during pregnancy.

Key terms:

diabetes: a group of disorders characterized by hyperglycemia caused by a lack of insulin secretion or ineffective insulin action

hyperglycemia: high blood glucose

insulin: a hormone secreted by the pancreas whose primary function is to maintain blood glucose levels within a normal range

Causes and Symptoms

Gestational diabetes mellitus (GDM) is the medical term describing a type of diabetes mellitus that is first diagnosed during a woman's pregnancy. Diabetes is a condition in which blood glucose is not kept within a normal range. Normally, insulin is a key regulator of blood glucose. In diabetes, insulin may be absent, be present in insufficient amounts, or be ineffective. Gestational diabetes occurs in 1 to 14 percent of all pregnancies. There is variance in incidence rates as a result of race or ethnicity, advanced age, and genetic predisposition. In general, women with a family history of diabetes are more likely to develop gestational diabetes, as are women who were overweight or obese prior to pregnancy, are carrying multiple fetuses, or have previously had unexplained miscarriage or stillbirth. Women with gestational diabetes often experience no symptoms themselves; when symptoms do present in the mother, they may include increased hunger, thirst, and urination, along with weight loss and fatigue.

Gestational diabetes generally develops midway through pregnancy. Testing is typically scheduled for between twenty-four and twenty-eight weeks into the pregnancy. A two-step approach is used to screen women who are not at high risk for diabetes. The first step is the 50-gram oral glucose tolerance test. For this test, the woman is given 50 grams of glucose in solution after having fasted overnight. Her blood glucose is tested one hour after drinking the solution. If her blood glucose is above a normal range, the next step is a 100-gram three-hour oral glucose tolerance test. Normally, a person's insulin would react to the ingested glucose to keep the blood glucose within a normal range. If that does not occur, and blood glucose remains high, then a diagnosis of gestational diabetes is made.

As maternal blood glucose rises, so does the risk of fetal complications. The most common complication is fetal macrosomia, or having a birth weight greater than or equal to 4.5 kilograms. Fetal macrosomia is associated with an increased risk of birth trauma, especially shoulder dystocia. Infants this large may require a cesarean section for birth, which itself has greater health risks than a vaginal birth. Addition-

Information on Gestational Diabetes

Causes: Unknown; risk increases with family history of diabetes

Symptoms: Often none for mother; excessive fetal size; hypoglycemia, heart and lung problems, sometimes coma or death in newborn

Duration: Gestational period and shortly after birth

Treatments: Diet restriction in mother to achieve stable blood glucose levels, insulin use if necessary

ally, higher maternal glucose levels lead to poorer placental functioning at an earlier point in pregnancy. While the placenta is designed to work as a filtering mechanism for thirty-eight to forty-two weeks, in gestational diabetics, the placenta often begins to malfunction by thirty-seven weeks. Therefore, infants of diabetic mothers are delivered early (at thirty-seven weeks) to avoid placental malfunction. Preeclampsia, or high blood pressure, in the mother can also develop and may lead to preterm birth.

When maternal blood glucose levels are elevated above normal, the fetus is stimulated to increase production of insulin. Although this manages the problem of the increased blood glucose for the fetus, it also has negative consequences. If the mother's blood glucose has been elevated just prior to delivery, then the infant's insulin level will be elevated. After delivery, the infant's insulin level may remain elevated, although there is no longer a need for it. This can lead to hypoglycemia, or low blood glucose. Continued hypoglycemia can lead to coma or death for the newborn. In addition, high insulin levels and poor control of the mother's blood glucose is associated with problems with the infant's heart and lung function. Other potential complications include respiratory distress and jaundice (yellowing of the skin).

Treatment and Therapy

Diet is the primary treatment for gestational diabetes. Depending on the meal planning approach, a certain number of calories and/or a certain amount of carbohydrates is prescribed. The total carbohydrates to be eaten is about 40 to 45 percent of total daily calories. Calories should be prescribed to allow for recommended weight gain during pregnancy and to prevent blood glucose from being either too high or too low. If caloric intake is too high, then the blood glucose level will rise, which is detrimental to the fetus. If caloric intake is too low, then the body will break down the mother's body fat or protein reserves to supply the needed energy. When this occurs, breakdown products called "ketones" are produced. Ketones in the mother's blood are also detrimental to the fetus.

Consistency, in the form of eating the same amount of food at the same time each day, is important. This is most likely to occur if the individual eats small, frequent meals throughout the day. The diet must support three outcomes: blood glucose levels within a target range, adequate nutrient intake to support the pregnancy, and appropriate weight gain for pregnancy. If these three outcomes cannot be achieved by diet alone, then insulin will be used to achieve the desired blood glucose level. Oral hypoglycemic medications such as sulfonylureas, either alone or in combination with insulin, may be helpful in blood glucose regulation; patients should discuss the potential risks and benefits of these medications with their physicians.

Because achieving a normal or near-normal blood glucose level is so critical, the woman will monitor her blood glucose at home using a fingerstick blood sample and a home glucometer. Blood glucose levels are usually tested three to four times a day, although some women will need to test their blood glucose six times each day. Decisions about adjustments in diet and insulin will be based on blood glucose levels.

Regular exercise is also recommended as a means of regulating blood glucose levels. Patients should consult with their physicians about what types of exercise are safe and appropriate during the various stages of pregnancy.

Usually blood glucose levels normalize postpartum, and continued diet or medication therapy is not needed. However, women who develop gestational diabetes have a higher likelihood of developing type 2 diabetes mellitus later in life. For women who have developed gestational diabetes, an oral glucose tolerance test is administered six to eight weeks postpartum and then at three-year intervals. These women should maintain an optimal weight, since obesity is strongly associated with onset of type 2 diabetes.

Perspective and Prospects

Observations in the 1950s and 1960s that infants born to mothers who had an elevated blood glucose level had a higher rate of morbidity and mortality led to the screening, diagnosis, and treatment guidelines used today. Adherence to these guidelines has greatly improved the health of infants born to mothers with gestational diabetes. However, these infants do have a greater risk of becoming obese and/or developing diabetes in adolescence. Additionally, daughters of mothers who have had gestational diabetes have a greater likelihood of developing gestational diabetes themselves.

—*Karen Chapman-Novakofski, R.D., L.D.N., Ph.D.;*
updated by Robin Kamienny Montvilo, R.N., Ph.D.

See also Cesarean section; Childbirth; Childbirth complications; Diabetes mellitus; Endocrine disorders; Endocrinology; Endocrinology, pediatric; Hormones; Hypoglycemia; Insulin resistance syndrome; Neonatology; Obesity; Perinatology; Pregnancy and gestation; Women's health.

For Further Information:

American Diabetes Association. "Diagnosis and Classification of Diabetes Mellitus." *Diabetes Care* 30, suppl. 1 (January, 2007): S42–S47.

A.D.A.M. Medical Encyclopedia. "Gestational Diabetes." *MedlinePlus*, August 8, 2012.

Gestational Diabetes: What to Expect. 5th ed. Alexandria, Va.: American Diabetes Association, 2005.

Jovanovic-Peterson, Lois. *Managing Your Gestational Diabetes: A Guide for You and Your Baby's Good Health.* New York: John Wiley & Sons, 1998.

Langer, Oded. "Oral Antidiabetic Drugs in Pregnancy: The Other Alternative." *Diabetes Spectrum* 20, no. 2 (April, 2007): 101–105.

National Diabetes Information Clearinghouse. "What I Need to Know about Gestational Diabetes." *National Institute of Diabetes and Digestive and Kidney Diseases*, January 22, 2013.

Nicholson, W. K., et al. "Maternal Race, Procedures, and Infant Birth Weight in Type 2 and Gestational Diabetes." *Obstetrics and Gynecology* 108, no. 3 (2006): 626–634.

Ross, Tami, Jackie Boucher, and Belinda O'Connell, eds. *American Dietetic Association Guide to Diabetes Medical Nutrition Therapy and Education*. Chicago: American Dietetic Association, 2005.

Wood, Debra, and Andrea Chisholm. "Gestational Diabetes." *Health Library*, September 10, 2012.

GIARDIASIS
Disease/Disorder

Anatomy or system affected: Gastrointestinal system

Specialties and related fields: Family medicine, gastroenterology, pediatrics

Definition: An acute or chronic parasitic infection of the gastrointestinal system.

Causes and Symptoms

The parasite *Giardia lamblia*, which causes giardiasis, is a protozoan acquired through the ingestion of contaminated food or water. This organism can also be spread by person-to-person contact involving fecal contamination. It is the most frequent parasite acquired by children in day care centers and preschools.

After exposure, the incubation period before the onset of symptoms is one to two weeks. After infection, only 25 to 50 percent of affected individuals become symptomatic. The disease is characterized by abdominal pain, cramps, flatulence, weight loss, and diarrhea, which in many cases may be chronic (of a duration longer than fifteen days).

Treatment and Therapy

Some cases of giardiasis are self-limited. The treatment of choice for giardiasis in the United States is a single oral dose of tinidazole. Metronidazole and nitazoxanide are alternative oral medications, but require multiple doses over several days. Furazolidone and metronidazole are equally efficacious; the first may be more practical in children because of its availability in liquid form.

Giardiasis can be prevented by strict hand-washing, especially in those individuals who are in close contact with patients with diarrhea or children in diapers at day care centers. Another important consideration in the prevention of giardiasis resides in the purification of drinking water, which can be achieved through boiling or chemical decontamination. It has been demonstrated that breast-feeding protects infants against symptomatic infection.

Perspective and Prospects

G. lamblia was first observed by microscopist Antoni van Leeuwenhoek in 1675. It was once considered a harmless organism, but its pathogenic role was clearly established in the 1960s. This parasite is one of the most common protozoans able to infect humans.

—*Benjamin Estrada, M.D.*

Information on Giardiasis

Causes: Parasitic infection

Symptoms: Often asymptomatic; can include abdominal pain, cramps, flatulence, weight loss, diarrhea

Duration: One to two weeks; occasionally chronic

Treatments: Medication (furazolidone, metronidazole, paromomycin)

See also Diarrhea and dysentery; Food poisoning; Gastroenteritis; Gastroenterology; Gastroenterology, pediatric; Gastrointestinal disorders; Gastrointestinal system; Parasitic diseases; Protozoan diseases.

For Further Information:

Alan, Rick, and Michael Woods. "Giardiasis." *Health Library*, November 2012.

Berger, Stephen A., and John S. Marr. *Human Parasitic Diseases Sourcebook*. Sudbury, Mass.: Jones and Bartlett, 2006.

Despommier, Dickson D., et al. *Parasitic Diseases*. 5th ed. New York: Apple Tree, 2006.

"Giardia Infection (Giardiasis)." *Mayo Clinic*, November 14, 2012.

"Giardiasis Frequently Asked Questions." *Centers for Disease Control and Prevention*, July 11, 2012.

Hill, David R., and Theodore E. Nash. "*Giardia lamblia*." In *Mandell, Douglas, and Bennett's Principles and Practice of Infectious Diseases*, edited by Gerald L. Mandell, John F. Bennett, and Raphael Dolin. 7th ed. New York: Churchill Livingstone/Elsevier, 2010.

Roberts, Larry S., and John Janovy, Jr., eds. *Gerald D. Schmidt and Larry S. Roberts" Foundations of Parasitology*. 7th ed. Boston: McGraw-Hill Higher Education, 2005.

GIGANTISM
Disease/Disorder

Also known as: Acromegaly

Anatomy or system affected: Arms, bones, brain, circulatory system, endocrine system, eyes, hair, hands, legs, musculoskeletal system, reproductive system

Specialties and related fields: Biochemistry, cardiology, endocrinology, family medicine, general surgery, internal medicine, neurology

Definition: A rare congenital disease that begins in children with pituitary gland tumors that make too much growth hormone, which yields pituitary giants who often die at relatively young ages. After adolescence, the disease is manifested as acromegaly, which is quite serious over the long term.

Key terms:

acromegaly: a disease of adults initially characterized by pathological enlargement of bones of the hands, feet, and face; caused by chronic pituitary gland overproduction of growth hormone by tumors

congenital: referring to a condition (such as a health problem) present or occurring at birth

growth hormone: a hormone produced by the pituitary gland that mediates overall growth

pituitary gland: a peanut-sized gland at the base of the vertebrate brain; its hormone secretions control many other hormone-producing (endocrine) glands and hence control growth, gender maturation, and many other life processes

Causes and Symptoms

Gigantism is a rare disease most often caused by the presence of tumors of the peanut-sized pituitary gland, located at the base of the brain. Such tumors produce an excess of growth hormone, the biomolecule responsible for overall growth. In children or adolescents who have these tumors, excess growth hormone results in overgrowth of all parts of the body. Gigantism occurs because the bones of the arms and legs have not yet calcified and can grow much longer than usual. Hence, an afflicted child becomes very large in size and very tall, often reaching a height of more than 6 feet, 6 inches.

A young child afflicted with pituitary gigantism grows in height as much as six inches per year. Thus, an important symptom that identifies the problem is that such children are much taller and larger than others of the same age. In many cases, this great size difference may lead to individuals who are more than twice the height of their playmates. Excessive growth of this sort should lead parents to seek the immediate advice of their family physician, who can aid in the selection of a specialist to identify the problem and develop an appropriate treatment.

As gigantism proceeds, pituitary tumors often invade and replace the rest of the pituitary gland. This is unfortunate, because the pituitary gland produces several other hormones—called "trophic hormones"—that control mental processes, sexual maturation, and healthy overall growth. Consequently, prolonged, untreated gigantism may yield a huge individual who suffers from mental illness, is sexually immature, and becomes quite unhealthy. In addition, the human musculoskeletal system is not designed to accommodate individuals attaining the great heights of many postadolescent pituitary giants. Hence, it is fairly common that affected individuals have great difficulty standing and walking; some can do so only with the aid of canes. Moreover, the average life expectancy of an individual with untreated gigantism or acromegaly is shorter than that of individuals of normal stature.

In cases where pituitary tumors that oversecrete growth hormone occur after calcification of the long bones is complete—after adolescence—gigantism will not occur. Such individuals develop acromegaly. This often-fatal disease, progressive throughout life, thickens bones and causes the overgrowth of all body organs. Hands and feet grow larger, and the lower jaw, brow ridges, nose, and ears enlarge, coarsening the features. More damaging is the development of headaches, high blood pressure, high cholesterol levels, arthritis, type 2 diabetes, sleep apnea, and even colon cancer over the long run. It should be noted that these disabilities are rarely seen in pediatric patients and most often begin in the third or fourth decade of life. Many medical scientists believe that pituitary gigantism and acromegaly are the basis for the legends about giants and ogres.

Information on Gigantism

Causes: Congenital endocrine disorder resulting in pituitary gland tumors
Symptoms: Enlargement of bones of hands, feet, and face; excessive growth and height; sometimes mental illness; sexual immaturity; difficulty walking and standing
Duration: Lifelong
Treatments: Chemotherapy, antigrowth hormone drugs, surgery, radiation therapy

---

Treatment and Therapy

If a diagnosis of gigantism or acromegaly seems probable, the physician or specialist involved will order a blood test to identify the amount of growth hormone present in the body. Computed tomography (CT) and magnetic resonance imaging (MRI) scans will also be carried out, especially in those suspected of having acromegaly, to identify possible organ changes away from normal size.

In cases where growth hormone levels are high and cannot be reduced by chemotherapy—for example, with antigrowth hormone drugs such as somatostatin analogs, dopamine agonists, and growth hormone receptor antagonists—and/or the presence of a clearly defined tumor is identified via CT and MRI, surgery to excise the tumor will be attempted. Radiation therapy is associated with a number of detrimental effects and with a slower response time; thus, chemotherapeutic and surgical interventions are preferred over radiation in most cases.

Perspective and Prospects

It must be recognized that the success of any therapeutic regimens or their combination will prevent additional gigantism or symptoms of acromegaly from occurring. It is not possible, however, to reverse existing consequences of the pituitary tumors on young children and adolescents with gigantism or on adults with acromegaly.

For this reason, it is essential for worried parents or adult patients to visit an appropriate physician as quickly as possible. Such foresight will usually minimize problems associated with either manifestation of pituitary tumors and enable an afflicted individual to have the best possible future life. In addition to extirpating causative tumors, it will then become possible, after additional blood tests and the thorough examination of CT and MRI data, to identify which body organs need to be treated and to arrest or minimize health complications, such as those associated with the reproductive, cardiovascular, and musculoskeletal systems.

—*Sanford S. Singer, Ph.D.*

See also Birth defects; Bones and the skeleton; Congenital heart disease; Dwarfism; Endocrine disorders; Endocrine system; Endocrinology; Endocrinology, pediatric; Growth; Hormones; Orthopedics, pediatric.

For Further Information:
A.D.A.M. Medical Encyclopedia. "Acromegaly." *MedlinePlus*, December 11, 2011.

A.D.A. M. Medical Encyclopedia. "Gigantism." *MedlinePlus*, December 11, 2011.

Alan, Rick, and Kari Kassir. "Acromegaly." *Health Library*, October 30, 2012.

Bar, Robert S., ed. *Early Diagnosis and Treatment of Endocrine Disorders*. Totowa, N.J.: Humana Press, 2003.

Beers, Mark H., et al., eds. *The Merck Manual of Diagnosis and Therapy*. 19th ed. Whitehouse Station, N.J.: Merck Research Laboratories, 2011.

Griffin, James E., and Sergio R. Ojeda, eds. *Textbook of Endocrine Physiology*. 6th ed. New York: Oxford University Press, 2011.

Henry, Helen L., and Anthony W. Norman, eds. *Encyclopedia of Hormones*. 3 vols. San Diego, Calif.: Academic Press, 2003.

Hormone Health Network. "Growth Disorders." *The Endocrine Society*, 2013.

Imura, Hiroo, ed. *The Pituitary Gland*. 2d ed. New York: Raven Press, 1994.

Landau, Elaine. *Standing Tall: Unusually Tall People*. New York: Franklin Watts, 1997.

Melmed, Schlomo, ed. *The Pituitary*. 3d ed. London: Academic Press, 2010.

National Endocrine and Metabolic Diseases Information Service. "Acromegaly." *National Institute of Diabetes and Digestive and Kidney Diseases*, April 6, 2012.

GINGIVITIS

Disease/Disorder

Anatomy or system affected: Gums, mouth, teeth

Specialties and related fields: Bacteriology, biochemistry, dentistry

Definition: A gum disease that begins when plaque and calculus cause gum inflammation and bleeding. It can lead to periodontitis, which is associated with tooth loss, cardiovascular disease, and diabetes.

Key terms:

collagen: a fibrous protein of bone, cartilage, and connective tissue

epithelium: a tissue made of closely arranged cells that covers most internal surfaces and organs

gingiva: tissue surrounding the teeth

periodontitis: gum disease that causes bone and tooth loss

Causes and Symptoms

Healthy pink gingiva (gums) end at tooth bases in epithelium-covered connective tissue, detached from teeth for 0.15 to 0.30 millimeter. This free gingiva is demarcated from the next gum portion, attached gingiva, by a gingival groove. The space between free gingiva and a tooth is the gingival sulcus. Attached gingiva is bound to the bone that it covers and is 3 to 6 millimeters deep. Free gingiva between teeth, interdental papillae, extend upward in the front of teeth and make the gums look scalloped. All gingival epithelium covers connective tissue holding collagen fibers. Gingival sulcus epithelium holds oral crevicular and junctional epithelium (JE). JE forms a tooth collar, which is joined to tooth surfaces. Each collar girdles the neck of a tooth and prevents marginal gingivitis and periodontitis.

Gingivitis begins when plaque and calculus irritate free gingiva, causing inflammation and bleeding. Unchecked, it leads to the more serious periodontitis, which can result in tooth loss, cardiovascular disease, and diabetes. Plaque starts as aggregates of bacteria and their capsules on tooth surfaces. It forms in a protein film deposited on the surfaces and thickens as bacteria become established in a growing matrix of protein and capsule polysaccharide, extending into attached gingiva. Plaque and bacterial toxins damage tissue, producing gingivitis by irritating free gingiva, loosening collars around teeth, and causing the detachment of attached gingiva. Plaque is best identified via disclosing solutions of dyes (such as erythrosin). Many view it as the main factor in initial gingival inflammation. Plaque calcification produces calculus, which is most problematic when it causes irritation if gingiva push up against it.

Acute gingivitis of several types is short term and of minor interest. Nonspecific acute gingivitis occurs with colds and influenza. It causes diffuse redness, swelling, and discomfort but resolves quickly upon recovery. Localized acute gingivitis arises from gingival trauma (such as hard food). Removing its causes promotes rapid healing. Ulcerative acute gingivitis, called trench mouth, occurs widely, mostly in one's teens or twenties. Patients report soreness, difficulty eating, facile gum bleeds, and headache. It also occurs in heavy smokers as a result of chemical and thermal irritation.

Chronic marginal gingivitis, which accounts for most cases, begins with the reddening and swelling of interdental papilla and/or the gingival margin. Attempts to explore a sulcus cause bleeding. Enlargement, as a result of edema or hyperplasia, may be extensive and followed, after years of disease, by chronic periodontitis where supporting bone is lost. The initial symptoms of chronic marginal gingivitis reported most often are gingival bleeding, either spontaneous or caused by brushing or chewing; gingival margin recession; gums coming away from teeth; gingival enlargement; and color change to red or reddish-purple.

Three types of chronic marginal gingivitis are associated with sex hormones in people who do not practice good oral hygiene: chronic marginal gingivitis of puberty, pregnancy, and menopause. In the puberty type, the hormone changes that come with approaching adulthood are causative. Puberty gingivitis is often accompanied by hyperplasia of interdental papillae. Pregnancy gingivitis occurs in women whose chronic marginal gingivitis worsens after the first trimester. The culprits here, changed blood-vessel permeability and increased inflammation, are the result of hormone changes. The condition produces severe inflammation, marked edema, gingival enlargement, and loose teeth. With good oral hygiene, these problems disappear by the third trimester or birth. Menopausal

---

Information on Gingivitis

Causes: Irritation of the gums by dental plaque and tartar; sometimes occurs with colds and influenza or with hormonal changes

Symptoms: Inflammation and bleeding of gums, which become red or reddish-purple

Duration: Chronic; sometimes acute

Treatments: Removal of plaque and tartar

chronic marginal gingivitis, which can occur at and after the menopause, causes blotchy, reddened attached gingiva, starting as blisters. It may be immunological, the result of patients developing antibodies to their own epithelia.

Treatment and Therapy

Trench mouth is treated with bacteria-killing penicillin or peroxide. The key to treating chronic marginal gingivitis begins by determining gum health from gingival sulcus depth. To obtain this measurement, a metal probe is inserted into the gingiva at several mouth sites until slight resistance is felt. Sulcus depths under 0.30 millimeter indicate healthy gums. Greater depths indicate chronic marginal gingivitis. The deeper the sulcus, the more serious is the gingivitis. The first gingivitis-related dental visit begins with sulcus examination.

When chronic marginal gingivitis is apparent, most plaque and calculus is removed, and the patient is quizzed on oral hygiene habits. The information gained is used to plan several more visits to prove that the patient practices good oral hygiene and to remove any remaining plaque and calculus. The larger and deeper the deposits and the longer exposure to poor hygiene, the more visits required.

Most chronic marginal gingivitis disappears after dental cleaning and ensuing good oral hygiene. Calculus and plaque removal eliminates the source of irritation and causes healing. Gums become healthy in a few weeks. Mild periodontitis requires more extensive treatment: Bacterial pockets are cleaned out, and antiseptic mouthwash or toothpaste is prescribed. Severe periodontitis may require surgery.

Perspective and Prospects

The best current way to treat gingivitis is preventing it via good oral hygiene, which consists of regular brushing and periodic dental cleaning to prevent plaque and calculus buildup. It is best to brush all teeth and gums with a soft-bristled brush and fluoride toothpaste. Brushing should be done at least twice daily, in the morning and at bedtime. Daily flossing is also recommended. Floss is used to scrape the underside of each tooth, just below the gum line, to remove interdental plaque and to massage the gums. In addition to good daily oral hygiene, annual or semiannual dental visits for cleaning and checkup are valuable.

Curing chronic marginal gingivitis and preventing periodontitis are now thought to diminish the risk of heart disease and stroke, as research has found a relationship between oral bacteria and clogged arteries. A relationship also exists between diabetes mellitus and chronic marginal gingivitis or periodontitis: Diabetes increases the risk of developing

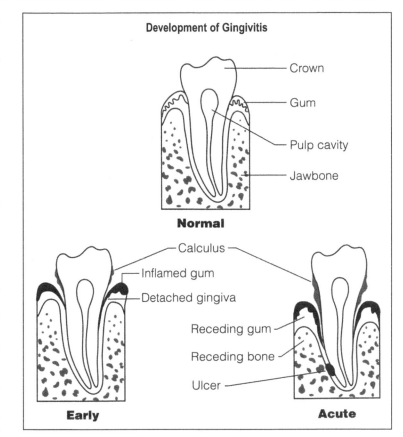

Development of Gingivitis

Crown
Gum
Pulp cavity
Jawbone

Normal

Calculus
Inflamed gum
Detached gingiva
Receding gum
Receding bone
Ulcer

Early　　　　**Acute**

periodontitis, and oral infection makes blood glucose harder to control. People having serious periodontitis and lung problems may inhale mouth bacteria and develop pneumonia. It is believed that susceptibility to gingivitis differs between individuals.

—Sanford S. Singer, Ph.D.

See also Cavities; Dental diseases; Dentistry; Endodontic disease; Gum disease; Periodontal surgery; Periodontitis; Plaque, dental; Root canal treatment; Teeth; Tooth extraction; Toothache.

For Further Information:

Cook, Allan R., ed. *Oral Health Sourcebook: Basic Information About Diseases and Conditions Affecting Oral Health.* Detroit: Omnigraphics, 1998.

Fotek, Paul. "Gingivitis." *MedlinePlus*, February 22, 2012.

Cross, William G. *Gingivitis.* 2d ed. Bristol, England: J. Wright, 1977.

"Gingivitis." *Mayo Clinic*, November 18, 2010.

Icon Health. *Gingivitis: A Medical Dictionary, Bibliography, and Annotated Research Guide to Internet References.* San Diego: Author, 2004.

Wilson, Thomas G., and Kenneth S. Kornman, eds. *Fundamentals of Periodontics.* 2d ed. Chicago: Quintessence, 2003.

Wood, Debra. "Gingivitis (Gum Disease)." *Health Library*, September 10, 2012.

Your Dental Health: A Guide for Patients and Families. Farmington: Conn., Consumer Health Information Network, University of Connecticut Health Center, 2008.

GLANDS

Anatomy

Anatomy or system affected: Breasts, endocrine system, gastrointestinal system, genitals, nervous system, pancreas, reproductive system, skin

Specialties and related fields: Biochemistry, dermatology, endocrinology, gastroenterology, gynecology, vascular medicine

Definition: Cells, organs or tissues that produce, store, and secrete fluids.

Key terms:

endocrine system: the system of glands located throughout the body that produces hormones and secretes them directly into the blood for delivery by the circulatory system

exocrine gland: a gland that secretes fluid into a duct

hormone: a product of the endocrine glands transported throughout the bloodstream that controls and regulates other glands or organs by chemical stimulation

pancreas: the gland located under the stomach that produces insulin and glucagon, the hormones responsible for control of the body's blood sugar level; it also produces enzyme-containing digestive juices

pituitary gland: a tiny gland located under the brain that controls the thyroid, adrenal, and sex glands

thyroid gland: an endocrine gland located in the neck, which regulates the rate of energy production throughout the body

Structure and Functions

A gland is formed from a group of specialized cells that together produce and secrete substances necessary for optimal bodily function. Some release fluid into a duct or tube that ultimately empties into a body cavity or an area outside the body. These glands are known as exocrine glands, meaning "externally secreting." Other glands, known as endocrine, or "internally secreting," glands pass their secretions directly into closely associated blood vessels. Endocrine glands secrete a certain type of molecule called a hormone. Hormones act as chemical messages that regulate almost every important function in the body.

Major endocrine glands include the pituitary, pineal gland, and hypothalamus in the brain; the thyroid and parathyroid glands in the neck; the adrenal glands and pancreas in the abdomen; the female ovaries in the pelvic cavity; and the male testes in the scrotum.

There are many exocrine glands spread throughout the human body. How they are classified depends on the method by which they produce their secreted product, and by the composition of the secretion. The cells of merocrine glands remain intact; their product is secreted by a process called exocytosis. In exocytosis, the substance to be secreted is surrounded by a membrane inside the cell, forming a structure called a secretory vesicle. At the time of release, the vesicle membrane fuses with the cell membrane, releasing the vesicle contents to the extracellular space. Examples of merocrine glands include salivary glands, which produce saliva; lacrimal glands, which produce tears; and sweat glands.

In apocrine glands, such as the milk-producing mammary gland, part of the cell is pinched off and shed to release cytoplasm, which contains the secretory product, into the duct; the remaining portion of the cell then regenerates. The last class of exocrine gland is the holocrine gland. The cells within these glands collect their secretory product internally and then rupture, releasing the product and cell debris into the duct; the cell is then replaced. Sebaceous (oil-producing) glands in the skin are an example of this type of gland.

Unlike endocrine glands, which secrete only hormones, exocrine glands produce a more diverse range of substances. Mucous glands produce mucins, sugar-bound proteins that, when mixed with water, form mucus, a sticky gelatinous substance. Mucus has a lubricative role; for example, it protects reproductive and digestive tracts from friction forces. In addition, it forms a protective barrier that traps foreign particles and bacteria that may cause irritation or infection, and protects the cells of the digestive tract from digestive enzymes and acid.

Serous glands produce serous fluid which has a more watery consistency than mucus. Examples of serous glands include mammary glands, tear glands, and the pancreas.

Salivary glands are mixed glands. The largest salivary glands, the parotids, secrete purely serous fluid; however, the submaxillary and sublingual glands secrete saliva containing mucin.

The function of exocrine glands is not necessarily discrete from that of the endocrine system: Exocrine secretion and hormones from the endocrine system work together in concert. For example, hormones regulate the complex process of digestion, absorption, and usage of nutrients started by exocrine secretions.

The pancreas, found behind the stomach, is both an exocrine gland, producing digestive enzymes for the intestine, and an important endocrine gland. The exocrine part makes up a majority of the pancreas mass. It consists of acinar cells which secrete pancreatic juice, containing digestive enzymes such as trypsin, chymotrypsin, lipase and amylase, and the pancreatic ductal system which delivers the pancreatic juice to the duodenum of the small intestine. Secretion of pancreatic juice is induced by the release of the hormones secretin and cholecystokinin, produced by the duodenum in response to signals brought about by the presence of food. Cells in the lining of the pancreatic ducts release an alkaline secretion containing bicarbonate ions, which serves to neutralize the acidic juices traveling down to the duodenum from the stomach.

Scattered within the exocrine pancreas are structures known as islets of Langerhans which comprise the endocrine portion of the pancreas. The major hormones secreted by the islets of Langerhans, insulin and glucagon, are the major regulators of the blood sugar level. Soon after a meal is digested, insulin is released, enabling cells to take excess sugar out of the blood at a rapid rate. Sugar, mainly stored in the liver as glycogen, is then released steadily into the blood between meals because of glucagon production in the pancreas. The careful balancing of these two hormones enables the body to have just the right sugar content in the blood at all times. Defects in insulin production or usage result in elevated blood glucose levels and diabetes mellitus. The long-term effects of the high blood sugar level of diabetics include heart disease and high blood pressure, unhealed wounds which become gangrenous, kidney failure, endless infections, nerve damage, and possible coma.

The thyroid is wrapped around the windpipe in the throat. By means of the two iodine-containing hormones that it produces, called thyroxine (T_4) and triiodothyronine (T_3), this gland controls the rate of the body's metabolism.

The four parathyroid glands on the back of the thyroid supply parathyroid hormone, which maintains the proper balance of calcium in the body. If there is not enough calcium, parathyroid hormone instructs the intestine to absorb more calcium and the kidneys to retain more. If the blood still has an insufficient level of calcium, parathyroid hormone causes it to be released from storage in the bones.

The hormones that bring about the most striking changes in both anatomy and behavior are known as the sex hor-

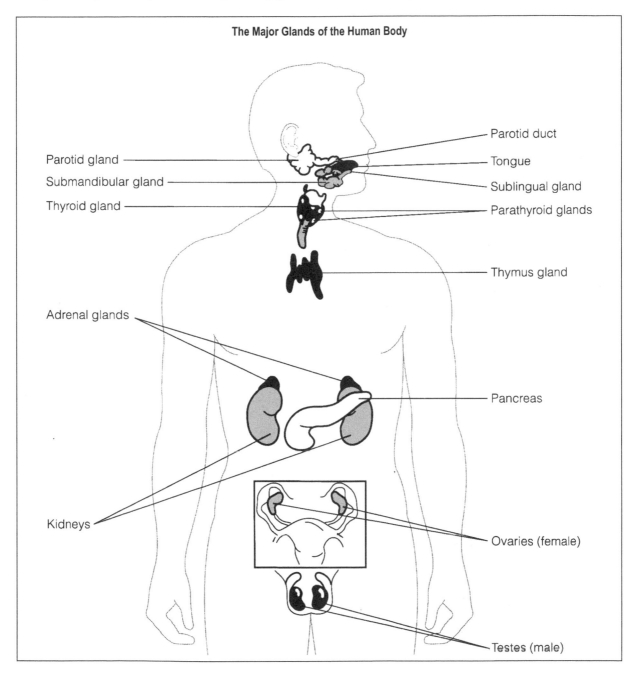

The Major Glands of the Human Body

mones. Because sex hormone levels are high in the fetus, they directly influence the development of its sex organs. In females, puberty is caused by an increase in hormones, produced by the two ovaries (located in the pelvic cavity), causes breast development, the growth of pubic and underarm hair, and the broadening of hips and thighs. Each month, the levels of estrogens and progesterones rise and fall, controlling the release of an egg from the ovary.

In addition, estrogen controls exocrine function in the female reproductive tract. Increasing levels of estrogen as ovulation approaches cause cervical crypt glands in the cervix to secrete mucus that is more conducive to sperm survival and movement. After ovulation has taken place, progesterone takes over as the main female hormone, and cervical mucus reverts to an inhospitable consistency or even dries up altogether.

In women, the mammary gland, or breast, undergoes changes throughout life. This is another example in which endocrine hormones influence exocrine function. Before birth, the nipple and some of the milk ducts are formed. At puberty, the ovaries secrete an increased level of estrogens, which leads to the formation of a more elaborate milk duct system along with connective tissue and fat deposition. This results in enlargement and rounding of the breast. At the onset of ovulation and menstruation, the milk ducts are fully mature, with the presence of alveolar cells at the terminal ends of the milk ducts. It is these cells that produce and secrete the milk.

If pregnancy occurs, then increased secretion of estrogen and progesterone from the placenta causes further development of the ductal system; by the time the baby is born most of the fat is replaced by milk ducts. Pregnancy also induces secretion of prolactin that stimulates milk production by the alveolar cells. During pregnancy, high levels of progesterone inhibit the release of milk from the milk duct. At birth, the placenta is expelled and the level of progesterone decreases dramatically so the milk can be released. The event of the infant suckling causes yet another hormone, oxytocin, to be released, which causes contraction of the milk duct near to the alveolar cells, squeezing the milk toward the nipple. Finally, at or just prior to menopause, the ductal system undergoes a process called involution as a result of decreased estrogen levels.

In males, two testes are located in the scrotal sac. They bring about puberty by their production of testosterone and other androgen hormones. These hormones are responsible for male secondary sex characteristics such as facial hair, deepening of the voice, and heavier muscles and bones.

The adrenal glands, perched on top of the kidneys, are responsible for regulating the body's response to stress. One of the major hormones of the adrenal cortex is cortisol. Cortisol helps maintain blood pressure, regulates fluid levels, directs protein and sugar metabolism, increases or decreases body fat reserves, and affects the immune system. A second area of the cortex secretes aldosterone, which directs the kidney to retain sodium and excrete potassium, controlling their levels in the blood. The third cortex area produces some testosterone and estrogen in both males and females.

The adrenal medulla responds to sudden stress by pouring epinephrine, formerly called adrenaline, into the blood. Dramatic changes in the working of the heart, lungs, liver, muscles, and many other organs then enable the body to cope with sudden emergencies.

The pineal gland is embedded close to the very center of the brain. Although the exact function structure is a mystery, it appears to be the only gland producing the hormone melatonin.

The careful and precise control of most of these glands is the work of the pituitary, causing it to be called "the master gland." This small gland has three distinct parts: the front or anterior pituitary, the back or posterior pituitary, and a tiny middle section.

The anterior pituitary sends thyroid-stimulating hormone (TSH) to the thyroid, causing it to release T_3 and T_4. It also secretes adrenocorticotropic hormone (ACTH), which causes the adrenal cortex to give off its many secretions. In the female, the follicle-stimulating hormone (FSH) that the anterior pituitary sends to the ovary causes an egg to mature, while in the male it fosters sperm development. Luteinizing hormone (LH), from the anterior pituitary, triggers the monthly release of an egg. The male's LH causes clusters of cells in the testes, called interstitial cells, to produce testosterone. The anterior pituitary also secretes growth hormone (GH), which stimulates body growth until maturity, and secretes prolactin hormone to cause the female breast to produce milk for a nursing baby.

The posterior pituitary secretes only two hormones: oxytocin, which brings about labor and birth, and antidiuretic hormone (ADH), which is also known as vasopressin. ADH causes the kidney to reabsorb the proper amount of water needed by the body.

The hypothalamus is a small area of tissue below the brain that relays messages from the brain and the rest of the body to the pituitary. It produces a number of releasing and inhibiting hormones which, in turn, carefully control the anterior pituitary's secretion of FSH, LH, TSH, ACTH, prolactin, and growth hormone.

Many endocrine glands pathways are regulated by negative feedback. For example, an increase in thyrotropin-releasing hormone (TRH) from the hypothalamus causes the pituitary to release TSH. This in turn triggers the production of T_3 and T_4. Increased levels of T_3 and T_4 stop the hypothalamus from releasing TRH, dampening the pathway.

Disorders and Diseases

Complex interactions in the endocrine system involving the concept of feedback have made many treatments possible for defective glands. Appropriate medical treatment of thyroid disease, for example, requires careful understanding of its feedback mechanism.

Hypothyroidism arises when insufficient thyroid hormones are produced. It is quite common, with one in every one thousand men and two in every one hundred women afflicted at some time during life. Symptoms include sensitivity to cold temperatures, weight gain, high blood pressure, yellowed skin, and loss of hair. It is often caused by an inability of the thyroid gland to produce enough hormones, the result of a disease of the pituitary that prevents it from producing TSH, or a disease of the hypothalamus that prevents it from producing TRH. Surprisingly, an underactive thyroid is often enlarged but still unable to produce enough T_3 or T_4. This enlargement is called a goiter. In the type called Hashimoto's thyroiditis, the hypothyroidism develops because the body mistakenly produces antibodies that destroy the thyroid tissue.

In addition, the thyroid can oversecrete as well as undersecrete. Hypersecretion is also quite common, with three or four out of one thousand people having this disease, the majority being women. The resulting excessive rate of metabolism causes many possible symptoms including intolerance to heat, irritability, excessive perspiration, heart palpitations, rapid weight loss, weakness, shortness of breath, and sore, bulging eyes.

There are two main types of hyperthyroidism. By far the most common is called Graves' disease. It is brought about when the patient's own immune system creates antibodies that cause continuous excess hormone production by the thyroid even though the pituitary is sending the normal amount of TSH. The less common cases of hyperthyroidism involve lumps or nodules that form in the thyroid and oversecrete T_3 and T_4 for no apparent reason. One of three treatments is usually used to cure hyperthyroidism: Radioactive iodine is given to destroy part of the overactive gland, surgery is used to remove part of the gland, or certain drugs are prescribed that prevent the thyroid from producing its hormones.

Although no one objects to attempts to aid sufferers of thyroid disorders or diabetes mellitus, ethical questions have arisen concerning defects in some endocrine glands. A striking example involves a lack of growth hormone from the pituitary. Doctors, parents, and youngsters often disagree over whether GH therapy should be given to a child who is noticeably shorter than peers at a given age. Because GH, like any hormone, may produce many unwanted side effects, there is much controversy over this particular medical application of endocrine gland research.

It is estimated that one in two thousand children are born with cystic fibrosis, a disorder which affects many exocrine glands. This disease is caused by mutations in the cystic fibrosis transmembrane conductance regulator (CFTR) gene. The protein product of this gene is critical for the transport of salts into secretory cells of the lungs, intestine, pancreas, liver, reproductive tract, and skin. In individuals with cystic fibrosis, salt imbalance in these cells results in thick, sticky mucus that cannot be cleared by cilia. This means that blockages occur and secretory products cannot function, leading to problems such as breathing difficulty, inadequate digestion, and infertility. In addition, the thick mucus is an ideal site for bacteria to thrive, resulting in chronic infections in cystic fibrosis patients. Due to the complications resulting from cystic fibrosis, as of 2007 the median life expectancy in the United States for individuals with this disease was under forty years old. Cystic fibrosis is diagnosed by testing the salt content of sweat and by genetic analysis. Treatment consists of a strict diet that is supplemented with enzymes, vitamins, and bile salts to replace those deficient in the patient; physical therapy and medication to reduce the mucus buildup in the lungs; and antibiotics to treat bacterial infection.

Sjögren's syndrome is an autoimmune disease in which certain types of exocrine cells are destroyed by white blood cells. In 2011, the US National Library of Medicine reported that the disease affected between one and four million Americans. The great majority of people with the syndrome are women. Most commonly, the lacrimal and salivary glands are affected and, without sufficient tears and saliva, the patient experiences dry eyes and mouth accompanied by recurring eye and mouth infections, difficulty swallowing certain foods, and discomfort of the eyes (such as a gritty feeling). Additionally, secretory cells in the skin, respiratory passages, and vaginal tissues can be affected, causing dryness in these tissues. The symptoms of dry eyes and mouth are treated using medications that stimulate saliva production and artificial tears applied as drops or as an ointment.

Perspective and Prospects

Glands, together with the nervous system, are the body's means of control and coordination. Given this fact, the discovery of each gland's functions had ramifications for medical science as a whole.

Although the ancient Greeks, Romans, and Chinese suspected the importance of some glands, it was only in the seventeenth century that scientists began to acquire useful knowledge of them. At that time, the Englishman Thomas Wharton first recognized the difference between duct and ductless glands. In the 1660s, Théophile Bordeu, a Frenchman regarded by many as the founder of endocrinology, declared that some parts of the body gave off "emanations" that had dramatic effects on other parts of the body. Following Bordeu's lead, the Dutchman Fredrik Ruysch claimed in the 1690s that the thyroid poured important substances into the bloodstream.

Two major breakthroughs occurred in the late 1800s when Paul Langerhans found the actual pancreas cell clusters, called islets, that produce insulin and when Charles-Edouard Brown-Séquard developed a technique to use extracts from glands to determine their function.

The year 1900 brought three major discoveries: William Bayliss and Ernest Starling found that a chemical messenger from the intestine causes the pancreas to excrete digestive juice; Jokichi Takamine discovered that adrenaline increases heart rate and blood pressure; and Alfred Frölich described dwarfed individuals who had suffered previous pituitary damage.

In 1914, in Minnesota, Edward Kendall obtained the chemical he named thyroxine from animal thyroids. Similarly, in 1921, Frederick Banting and Charles Best isolated insulin from the pancreases of animals. By the mid-1970s, Rosalind Yalow and her colleagues had perfected a technique called radioimmunoassay, which uses radioactive materials to measure minute quantities of hormones. This enables physicians to measure the circulating level of nearly every hormone and diagnose anyone with an excess or deficiency. Many hormones such as insulin, growth hormone, and estrogen can then be given to supplement what the body is underproducing; they have been very expensive and hard to obtain in quantity from animals or deceased humans. By the 1980s, however,recombinant DNA technology and the polymerase chain reaction (PCR) offered unlimited, pure, and readily accessible hormones.

—*Grace D. Matzen;*
revised by Claire L. Standen, Ph.D.

See also Abscess drainage; Abscesses; Addison's disease; Adrenalectomy; Brain; Breasts, female; Corticosteroids; Cyst removal; Cystic fibrosis; Cysts; Diabetes mellitus; Dwarfism; Endocrine disorders; Endocrine glands; Endocrinology; Endocrinology, pediatric; Gigantism; Goiter; Hashimoto's thyroiditis; Hormone therapy; Hormones; Hyperparathyroidism and hypoparathyroidism; Hypoglycemia; Hypothalamus; Mastectomy and lumpectomy; Mumps; Pancreas; Parathyroidectomy; Pituitary gland; Prostate enlargement; Prostate gland; Prostate gland removal; Sjögren's syndrome; Systems and organs; Testicular cancer; Testicular surgery; Thymus gland; Thyroid disorders; Thyroid gland; Thyroidectomy.

For Further Information:

Akers, R. Michael. *Lactation and the Mammary Gland.* Ames: Iowa State University Press, 2002.
Brook, Charles G. D., and Nicholas J. Marshall. *Essential Endocrinology.* 4th ed. Malden, Mass.: Blackwell Science, 2003.
Goodman, H. Maurice. *Basic Medical Endocrinology.* 4th ed. Boston: Academic Press, 2008.
Health Library. "Sjogren's Syndrome." *Health Library,* December 30, 2011.
Henry, Helen L., and Anthony W. Norman, eds. *Encyclopedia of Hormones.* 3 vols. San Diego, Calif.: Academic Press, 2003.
Melmed, Shlomo, and Robert Hardin Williams, eds. *Williams Textbook of Endocrinology.* 12th ed. Philadelphia: Elsevier/Saunders, 2011.
MedlinePlus. "Hormones." *MedlinePlus,* June 26, 2013.
Ruggieri, Paul, and Scott Isaacs. *A Simple Guide to Thyroid Disorders: From Diagnosis to Treatment.* Omaha, Nebr.: Addicus Books, 2010.
Scanlon, Valerie, and Tina Sanders. *Essentials of Anatomy and Physiology.* 6th ed. Philadelphia: F. A. Davis, 2012.
Thomson, Anne H., and Ann Harris. *Cystic Fibrosis.* Oxford, England: Oxford University Press, 2008.
Vorvick, Linda J. "Endocrine Glands." *MedlinePlus,* May 1, 2011.

GLASGOW COMA SCALE

Anatomy or system affected: Neurological and brain systems
Specialties and related fields: Neurology, neuroethics, neuroscience
Definition: The Glasgow Coma Scale is a neurological tool for assessing the level of consciousness of a patient suffering from a brain injury.

Key terms:

abnormal flexion response: an involuntary extension of the arms or legs that indicates severe brain injury

brain trauma: any kind of injury sustained to the brain due to trauma (hitting one's head on the ground after a fall) or nontraumatic event such as brain swelling due to a virus

minimally conscious state: a condition of severely altered consciousness in which minimal, but definite, behavioral evidence of self or environmental awareness is demonstrated

persistent vegetative state: a severely altered state of consciousness that occurs several weeks after a coma, which results in very limited self-awareness or response to outside stimulation

Description and Background Information

The Glasgow Coma Scale (GCS) was created out of a need for a standardized assessment of consciousness to track the severity of brain trauma after head injury. Prior to its creation in 1974 by Graham Teasdale and Bryan Jennett, both from the University of Glasgow's Institute of Neurological Sciences, individual doctors assessed consciousness subjectively. The GCS provided the first objective method of assessment for tracking symptoms over the course of days, weeks, and months during the recovery process. The GCS has three sections: eye opening, verbal response, and motor response. Eye opening is used to assess visual response to speech, pain, and the surrounding environment. Eyes that open spontaneously receive the highest score (4), while no eye opening receives the lowest score (1). Verbal response assesses the degree to which a patient can intelligently respond to a question such as: What year is it? If the response indicates that the person is aware of his environment, time and situation, then he will receive a score of 5. If the person does not respond at all, then a score of 1 will be assessed. Motor responses assess the ability of the patient to respond physically to commands, shown in arm movement and shoulder abduction. Correctly obeying a simple command to the request "Show me two fingers" will result in the highest score (6) and a flaccid response will produce the lowest score (1).

Patients are given a GCS score of 3 to 15. (Note: Older versions of GCS use a 14 score system, in which abnormal flexion under motor response is omitted.) A score of 13-15 indicates mild trauma, a score of 9-12 moderate trauma, and a score of 3-8 severe trauma. In medical records, a GCS recording will usually appear using the following symbols: GCS 11 = E3 V6 M2, often followed by the hour and minute in which the evaluation was administered. The equation provides the total score of the patient and secondary scores broken into the three subsections. GCS is the total score.

Deficiencies of the Glasgow Coma Scale

The Glasgow Coma Scale measures symptoms that can supplement additional medical data that will aid a physician in coming to a diagnosis. It is a behavioral assessment to give us a glimpse into the biological explanation for what is occurring in the brain. Because the scale results are reliant upon the observations of medical personnel, as with other behaviorally oriented assessments, a margin for error does exist. Therefore, the scale is useful in giving rough estimations of severity of symptoms, but it is inadequate in identifying the cause of unresponsiveness. Employing additional medical testing, such as an MRI (magnetic resonance imaging) or CT (

computed tomography) scan, can significantly contribute to a more definitive diagnosis for what might have caused problems related to awareness and consciousness.

The scale has proven to be reliable but not valid in many cases. It is simple and short to read and apply. Therefore, most medical personnel can use it to record symptom progress with consistency and ease. However, the symptoms that are being tracked may have no connection to the cause of the injury. For example, if dealing with a patient with eye impairment, their eye opening scores will be inadequate, not because of a diminishment of consciousness levels but because of deficiencies in the ability to control eye movement. If a patient has a lesion on his brainstem, the patient's scores could misrepresent the level of brain trauma since the lesion is in an area that could compromise his ability to display awareness.

To compensate for GCS deficiencies, additional scales have been developed, the most prominent being the Pediatric Glasgow Coma Scale (PGCS). PGCS has the same 3-15 score rating scale as the GCS but changes the criteria for specific scores so that it is appropriate for a child younger than 36 months who has undeveloped motor and verbal response skills. Instead of speech, inconsolable crying or moaning is assessed; and instead of motor response, bodily posture is assessed.

Science and Profession

Because of its universality, multiple specialists within the medical profession use the GCS. Neurologists, emergency room doctors, and nurses utilize the scale to measure levels of consciousness within a hospital setting. Emergency medical technicians use it upon arrival at the scene of a consciousness-related trauma. GCS training is taught in medical schools and emergency medical services (EMS) courses.

Perspective and Prospects

For decades, the GCS has been regarded as the "gold standard" for a simple-to-use behavioral assessment tool to assess the level of consciousness. However, in 2004, Giacino and colleagues introduced the Coma Recovery Scale-Revised (CRS-R), which includes several additional subscales to the GCS. In addition, there are more standardized procedures to follow in order to improve upon the variability that can come from different assessors. The CRS-R has been helpful to differentiate patients considered to be in a persistent vegetative state from those who are in a minimally conscious state. Additional assessment methods are being investigated that use the electroencephalogram (EEG) as a means to determine the degree to which conscious brain activity is present in someone who cannot verbalize their thoughts.

—*Bryan C. Auday, Ph.D. and Allee Keener*

See also Coma; Minimally conscious state

For Further Information:

Bruno, Marie-Aurelie, and Steven Laureys. "Uncovering Awareness: Medical and Ethical Challenges in Diagnosing and Treating the Minimally Conscious State." Cerebrum (June, 2010): 12.

Giacino, Joseph, and Kathleen Kalmar. "Coma Recovery Scale-Revised 2006." The Center for Outcome Measurement in Brain Injury. http://www.tbims.org/combi/crs/crsref.html

Teasdale, Graham, and Bryan Jennett. "Assessment of Coma and Impaired Consciousness: A Practical Scale." *The Lancet* 13, no. 7872 (1974): 81-84.

GLAUCOMA

Disease/Disorder

Anatomy or system affected: Eyes

Specialties and related fields: Ophthalmology, optometry

Definition: A group of eye diseases characterized by an increase in the eye's intraocular pressure; early diagnosis through regular eye examinations can manage the effects of the disease, while late diagnosis may result in impaired vision or blindness.

Key terms:

aqueous humor: the liquid filling the space between the lens and the cornea of the eye, which nourishes and lubricates them

ciliary body: a structure built of muscle and blood vessels which produces the aqueous humor

cornea: the curved, transparent membrane forming the front of the outer coat of the eyeball that serves primarily as protection and focuses light onto the lens

intraocular pressure: the degree of firmness of the eyeball, as controlled by the proper secretion and drainage of the aqueous humor

lens: a transparent, flexible structure, convex on both surfaces and lying directly behind the iris of the eye; it focuses light rays onto the retina

ophthalmic laser: a high-intensity beam of light that permits a surgeon to cut tissue precisely in the treatment of eye diseases

optic disc: the portion of the optic nerve at its point of entrance into the rear of the eye

peripheral vision: side vision, or the visual perception to all sides of the central object being viewed

retina: the thin, delicate, and transparent sheet of nerve tissue that receives visual stimuli and transmits them to the brain through the optic nerve

tonometer: an instrument used to measure the eye's intraocular pressure, thus checking for the presence of glaucoma

Causes and Symptoms

Glaucoma is an eye disease caused by higher-than-normal pressure inside the eye. The intraocular pressure can increase slowly or suddenly for various reasons but always with detrimental results. Of all the causes of blindness, glaucoma is among the most common, but it is also the most preventable. If diagnosed early, it can be controlled and the loss of sight avoided. What complicates the problem is that the most common form of glaucoma shows no symptoms until extensive, irreversible damage has occurred. There is no pain, and the first sign that something is amiss may be that peripheral vision and seeing out of the corner of the eye is diminished, while frontal vision remains clear.

Information on Glaucoma

Causes: Congenital or hereditary factors
Symptoms: Often asymptomatic; eye pressure; slow progression toward blindness; at times, terrible pain, nausea, vomiting, severe headaches
Duration: Ranges from acute to chronic
Treatments: Eyedrops, ointments, pills, surgery

To understand this disease, it is necessary to know what occurs within the eye when the intraocular pressure increases. The inner surface of the cornea is nourished by the aqueous humor, which is also called the aqueous fluid. This secretion from the ciliary body flows into the space behind the iris and then through the pupil into the space in front of the iris. Where the front of the iris joins the back of the cornea is a point called the venous sinus, at the anterior drainage angle. Here the aqueous humor is reabsorbed and transported to the bloodstream. In a normal eye, this drainage process works correctly and the balance between the amount secreted and the amount reabsorbed maintains a constant intraocular pressure. In glaucoma, the drainage part of the process works inefficiently. For a variety of reasons, some of which are not fully understood, the drainage mechanism is defective. The upset balance in secretion drainage causes the unwanted increase in intraocular pressure in one eye or, more commonly, in both. The iris is pushed forward, further inhibiting drainage of the aqueous fluid.

Even a very small elevation in intraocular pressure will affect the eye adversely, causing damage to its most delicate parts. Although the eye as a whole is quite tough, the optic nerve is vulnerable to increased pressure. This vital connection between the eye and the brain is damaged by the stress within the harder eyeball. The delicate nerve fibers and blood vessels of the optic disc, as the beginning of the optic nerve is called, then die. Once they die, they can never be regenerated or replaced, and blindness is the result. The destruction of the optic disc causes a condition called cupping. A normal optic disc is quite level with the retina. Glaucoma causes it to collapse, creating a genuine indentation. Thus, cupping is a definite sign of glaucoma.

The damage that glaucoma inflicts is progressive. The defect in drainage does not necessarily worsen, and the pressure, once elevated, does not necessarily continue to increase. Once begun, however, the killing of the optic nerve cells continues until the resulting loss of vision progresses to total blindness. The first nerve fibers to die are the ones near the outer edge of the optic disc, which originates near the periphery of the retina. The first decrease in vision, therefore, is in one's peripheral vision. Then, as each layer of nerve fibers dies, the visual field narrows and narrows.

This slow, progressive route to blindness is typical of chronic simple glaucoma, or primary open-angle glaucoma (POAG), which accounts for more than 90 percent of glaucoma cases. It is called "simple" because the rise in intraocular pressure does not result from any known underlying reason. Although individuals with a family history of glaucoma are more prone to the disease, it is not directly hereditary. Moreover, not everyone with a family history of glaucoma will develop the disease. For reasons that are not well understood, people of African ancestry have glaucoma in much greater numbers than those of European ancestry. In the United States, the incidence of glaucoma among African Americans is three times that of Caucasians.

In persons of all races, chronic simple glaucoma usually begins after the age of forty; however, the aging process does not seem to be a direct cause of glaucoma. Unlike the formation of senile cataracts, which result from inevitable eye changes as one grows older, glaucoma's development is not explained by the aging process. It can safely be said that glaucoma seems to occur in persons who have a tendency toward inadequate aqueous fluid drainage. As those persons grow older and their bodies lose their resiliency in general, the drainage problem reaches a point where it begins to raise the intraocular pressure beyond the normal range. Those with untreated chronic simple glaucoma are seldom aware of the disease before considerable damage has been done. The progressive death of nerve fibers is ordinarily very slow because the elevation of pressure is slight and causes no pain or blurriness of sight.

Chronic simple glaucoma makes up about 95 percent of all cases of the disease. Several other rare types together make up the other 5 percent. In chronic secondary glaucoma, the drainage defect is caused by some complication of a different eye problem. The causes of chronic secondary glaucoma include inflammation from an eye infection, an allergic reaction, trauma to the eye, a tumor, or even the presence of a cataract. Medications such as corticosteroids can sometimes cause this type of glaucoma to develop. Whatever the cause, chronic secondary glaucoma exhibits the same increased pressure, slow nerve destruction, and ultimate loss of vision as chronic simple glaucoma.

A third variety, acute glaucoma, is both rare and dramatic in its onset. The increase in intraocular pressure is many times higher than that in chronic glaucoma. It also occurs very rapidly, sometimes within hours. The anterior drainage angle where drainage is accomplished is almost totally blocked. The eyeball becomes so hard that the elevated pressure can often be felt simply by touching the front of the eye. The great pressure causes terrible pain and immediate damage to the eye. When nausea, vomiting, and severe headaches accompany eye pressure, acute glaucoma should be suspected. Immediate treatment is required to prevent blindness. Acute glaucoma can be either simple or secondary. It is termed simple when a drainage area that has always been abnormally narrow suddenly becomes totally blocked. It is called secondary when it is precipitated by some other eye condition.

The rarest type of glaucoma, congenital glaucoma, is present at birth or develops during early infancy. It results from the incorrect formation of drainage canals while the eye is developing. Because a baby's eyeball is much smaller and softer than an adult's, this glaucoma is often recognized by

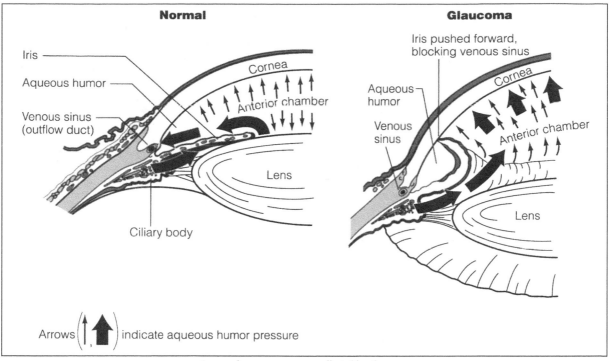

Normal

Iris

Aqueous humor

Venous sinus
(outflow duct)

Cornea

Anterior chamber

Lens

Ciliary body

Glaucoma

Iris pushed forward,
blocking venous sinus

Aqueous
humor

Cornea

Venous
sinus

Anterior chamber

Lens

Arrows (↑ , ⬆) indicate aqueous humor pressure

A normal eye versus an eye affected by glaucoma.

the bulging of the eyes.

It is quite easy for an eye doctor to detect even the apparently symptomless chronic glaucoma, and the rate of successful treatment is high. It is unfortunate, then, that glaucoma is responsible for innumerable cases of permanent loss of vision. In the vast majority of these patients, the destruction of the eye could have been prevented had it been detected and treated earlier. If everyone over the age of forty had an annual eye examination, blindness caused by glaucoma could essentially be eliminated.

Treatment and Therapy

The treatments available for glaucoma include eyedrops, ointments, pills, and surgery, using both scalpels and lasers. In both acute and congenital glaucoma, there is no time for the use of medications. Patients need to be admitted to the hospital and operated on immediately if their eyesight is to be saved. For open-angle glaucoma, medications may be topical—eye drops or ointments, or inserts, thin medicated strips put in to the corner of the eye—or oral (pills and tablets). Some of the more recent medications are unoprostone isopropyl/ophthalmic solution, brinzolamide ophthalmic suspension, dorzamide hydrochloride-timolo meleate ophthalmic solution, and brimonidine tartrate ophthalmic solution.

If diagnosed early, cases of both chronic simple and chronic secondary glaucoma can often be effectively treated by medications. The first drug given in the form of eyedrops was discovered in the nineteenth century. Called pilocarpine,

it is obtained from the leaves or roots of a South American bush. The drug is classified as a miotic because it constricts the pupil of the eye. Constriction of the pupil draws it away from the drainage angle, automatically increasing the drainage of aqueous fluid and therefore decreasing the pressure. To be effective, it is generally used four times a day. Other glaucoma drugs act to decrease the secretion of the fluid, which also decreases the intraocular pressure. Timolol maleate works in this fashion. It usually needs to be used twice a day. Some ophthalmologists prefer to use some of both types of drops for the same patient, decreasing pressure by both mechanisms. Others prescribe one medication that produces both effects. Dipivefrin is one such medication.

In either case, to avoid possible unpleasant side effects, the most dilute concentration, to be used the fewest times each day, is prescribed first. If this does not control the pressure, more concentrated drops, to be used more times daily, must then be prescribed. The medications in these eyedrops can often be used more easily by elderly patients in the form of a gel, an ointment, or a tiny disc which is placed on the cornea. Although considerably more costly than frequent drops, these methods are less of a nuisance. The gels and ointments need only be used once a day, while the discs are time-released over an entire week.

If drops or gels do not produce the desired reduction in pressure, pills can be used, not to replace the drops but to supplement them. These tablets are essentially diuretics that decrease the production of aqueous humor. Taken once a day, or less frequently in a time-release capsule, acetazolamide is the drug most often prescribed.

There are also several fast-acting drugs that can be injected into a vein to lower pressure by rapidly pulling some aqueous fluid into blood vessels in the eye, bypassing the drainage angle. These are not used in the treatment of chronic glaucoma except as preparation for a planned surgery. They are, however, often used when patients are admitted to the hospital for acute glaucoma to prevent damage until emergency surgery can be performed.

In the great number of patients, chronic glaucoma can be controlled by one of these medications. In those rare cases when it cannot, surgery must be performed. Although initially successful, such surgeries must often be repeated in the future. As with the above medications, glaucoma surgery aims to decrease the intraocular pressure by decreasing secretion or increasing effective drainage.

Although surgery can never reverse the optic nerve damage that has already occurred, it is often effective in preventing further destruction. The first of these surgical procedures was developed in the mid-nineteenth century. Called an iridectomy or iridotomy, it attempts to provide a better access to the patient's drainage angle by removing part of the iris. A second type of surgical procedure, known as a trabeculectomy or filtering operation, attempts to control intraocular pressure by creating a new, wider drainage outlet for the aqueous humor. Until the use of lasers, both of these operations were performed manually by a surgeon with steady hands using sharp blades on a tiny part of the eye.

To perform an iridectomy, the surgeon must cut a tiny hole into the edge of the iris with surgical scissors, allowing aqueous fluid to flow into the space between the iris and the cornea. Covered by the upper eyelid, this small hole is visible only by close examination and should not let in unwanted extra light or cause any discomfort to the patient.

The filtering operation, or trabeculectomy, can be performed in several different ways, but each involves the eye surgeon's use of a scalpel to create an artificial canal through the outer wall of the patient's eye. The passageway created, known as a fistula or filtering bleb, permits the aqueous humor to drain properly from the inner eye. By removing a part of the abnormal tissue from the drainage angle, the surgeon unclogs the drainage mechanism.

A different approach to glaucoma control does not involve cutting. It attempts to help the patient by destroying part of the source of the excess fluid, the oversecreting ciliary body. When a cold probe is applied to the ciliary body, the procedure is termed cryotherapy; when a hot probe is used, the method is called cyclodiathermy. No incision is required in either case because the probes are applied externally. A very common side effect of these two procedures, however, is fairly severe inflammation. Even when inflammation does not occur, the desired result may be only partially achieved. Both cryotherapy and cyclodiathermy are less commonly used than either iridectomy or trabeculectomy, and the procedures are usually performed only on older patients.

Many of these manual procedures are being replaced by several types of laser therapy. A laser is a precisely directed beam of high-intensity light that can function as a surgical knife. Laser surgery is generally safer than the older methods because it is less invasive to the body, as no incision is made in the eye. It can be done on an outpatient basis with only a local anesthetic. Recovery time, the likelihood of complications, and postoperative discomfort are all lessened. Patients with acute glaucoma, chronic simple glaucoma, and certain types of secondary glaucoma (depending on the cause) can be successfully treated with lasers.

Both iridotomy and trabeculectomy can be performed using an instrument called the argon laser. This particular laser is relatively low-powered, but it is efficient. After a drop of anesthetic is placed in the eye, the surgeon aims the highly focused argon beam at a precise location within the affected eye. The beam need only be directed into the eye for one-tenth of a second to achieve its effect. In an iridotomy, the laser simply drills a tiny hole in the iris for the fluid to circulate freely, while in a trabeculectomy several laser cuts are made on the clogged drainage angle to open it. A more sophisticated ophthalmic laser is the YAG laser. After a drop of anesthetic is placed on the eye, a weak "aiming beam" of helium-neon laser light is shone directly into the afflicted eye to pinpoint the area to be treated. This is followed by two to five bursts of the YAG laser, which drills a hole for better drainage.

All the above treatments for glaucoma, whether pharmaceutical or surgical, have the potential for serious side effects and complications. Consequently, research continues to seek therapies with better rates of success and fewer complications. Some of the possible complications include infection, bleeding, undesirable changes in the intraocular pressure, and loss of vision. Side effects include stinging or redness of the eyes, blurred vision, headache, changes in heart rate, mood changes, tingling of the fingers and toes, drowsiness, and loss of appetite.

Perspective and Prospects

In 1851, the German doctor Hermann von Helmholtz invented the ophthalmoscope, which enables one to study the interior of the eye. His instrument focuses a beam of light into the patient's eye and then magnifies its reflection. If this test reveals early signs of cupping of the optic disc, glaucoma can be diagnosed long before other symptoms have appeared.

Intraocular pressure can be measured with an instrument called a tonometer. The two basic varieties are called Schiötz tonometry and applanation tonometry. Both became possible only after biochemists developed anesthetic drops to put in the eye so that the patient would not feel the device touching the very sensitive cornea. The earlier of the two devices, developed in 1905 by the Norwegian physician Hjalmar Schiötz, is a very simple device that is still the most widely used tonometer in the world. With the patient lying down and looking upward, the physician places the hand-sized instrument directly on the cornea. A simple lever is moved by the pressure within the eye to indicate whether that pressure is within the normal range or dangerously high. The Goldman applanation tonometer is considered even more accurate and is often used to confirm the results of the simpler Schiötz device. An orange dye called fluorescein is added to the anesthetic. The patient, in a sitting position, rests the head against a bar to steady it. The doctor uses a tonometer to touch the cornea while simultaneously peering into it with a well-illuminated microscope.

More specialized glaucoma examination may require gonioscopy, visual field tests, or tonography. The gonioscope has mirrors and facets to provide an illuminated view of the drainage angle, a normally dark corner at a 90 degree angle from the examiner. Excessive narrowing of the angle is an indication of glaucoma. There are many kinds of visual field tests, but all give a map of the central area where vision is sharp and more acute, versus the peripheral area where it is weaker. Since damage to the optic nerve always causes a narrowing of the visual field, this mapping is very important. The ability to measure the field has grown from oculokinetic perimetry—using an inexpensive test chart, pencil, record sheet, and human examiner—to the sophisticated automated perimetry, which generates a computer analysis. Tonography does not measure the visual field but addresses the problem by measuring the intraocular pressure. Unlike the ordinary use of tonometry, which involves momentary contact with the cornea, tonography uses the tonometer for four minutes to massage the eye. In a normal eye, pressure will drop; in a glaucoma patient, it will not.

All these tests, developed through years of ophthalmic research, have given medical science invaluable tools to diagnose glaucoma and prevent blindness.

—*Grace D. Matzen;*
updated by Victoria Price, Ph.D.

See also Blindness; Cataract surgery; Cataracts; Eye infections and disorders; Eye surgery; Eyes; Laser use in surgery; Ophthalmology; Optometry; Sense organs; Vision; Vision disorders.

For Further Information:

Buettner, Helmut, ed. *Mayo Clinic on Vision and Eye Health: Practical Answers on Glaucoma, Cataracts, Macular Degeneration, and Other Conditions*. Rochester, Minn.: Mayo Foundation for Medical Education and Research, 2002.

Eden, John. *The Physician's Guide to Cataracts, Glaucoma, and Other Eye Problems*. Yonkers, N.Y.: Consumer Reports Books, 1992.

Epstein, David L., et al., eds. *Chandler and Grant's Glaucoma*. 4th ed. Baltimore: Williams & Wilkins, 1997.

Galloway, N. R., et al. *Common Eye Diseases and Their Management*. 3d ed. London: Springer, 2006.

LaRusso, Laurie. "Glaucoma." *Health Library*, September 1, 2011.

Lusby, Franklin W., Linda J. Vorvick, and David Zieve. "Glaucoma." *Medline Plus*, September 14, 2011.

Marks, Edith. *Coping with Glaucoma*. Garden City Park, N.Y.: Avery, 1997.

Morrison, John C., and Irvin P. Pollack. *Glaucoma: Science and Practice*. New York: Thieme, 2003.

Samz, Jane. *Vision*. New York: Chelsea House, 1990.

Sutton, Amy L., ed. *Eye Care Sourcebook: Basic Consumer Health Information About Eye Care and Eye Disorders*. 3d ed. Detroit, Mich.: Omnigraphics, 2008.

GLOMERULONEPHRITIS. *See* **NEPHRITIS.**

GLIOMA
Disease/Disorder
Anatomy or system affected: Brain
Specialties and related fields: Endocrinology, histology, neurology, oncology
Definition: An excessive reproduction of glial cells that leads to tumor formation in the central nervous system that can cause damage to nervous tissue.

Key terms:

benign tumor: a group of cells that slowly divides and differentiates into a mass that serves no significant function; it does not metastasize or infiltrate and is often encapsulated by a fibrous sheath

cancer: a pathogenic tumor that grows uncontrollably and has the potential to invade other tissues and cause significant damage

glial cell: cellular connective tissue of the nervous system; supports metabolic processes of neurons

hyperosmotic agents: drugs that can reduce intracranial pressure

malignant tumor: a group of cells that infiltrate surrounding tissues and cause damage; a tumor that tends to spread and kills surrounding cells

metastasis: growth of cancerous cells in different parts of the body due to detachment from the original tumor and movement through the bloodstream

tumor: an abnormal growth of cells in response to a genetic mutation; can be benign or malignant

Causes and Symptoms

The central nervous system is comprised of two major categories of cells-neuron and glial cells. Within the human brain, glial cells outnumber neurons ten-to-one. While neurons are outnumbered by glia, they perform the critical function of producing and transmitting an electrical impulse from one place to another, allowing for a person to interact with the environment. Neurons, however, cannot do much other than signal transmission. They rely on glial cells to do the majority of their metabolism and regulation. Because glial cells are responsible for metabolism and waste management for multiple cells, they divide and reproduce more frequently than most cells. This makes them a prime candidate for tumor formation.

A tumor is a mass of similar cells that reproduces independently and has no normal function. Tumors arise from cell types that replicate often, and can be caused by a simple genetic mutation that allows the mass to grow unchecked. In the brain, tumors arise from glial cells. There are three major kinds of glial cells-astrocytes, oligodendrocytes, and ependymal cells-and each can form tumors with different characteristics. A tumor originating from glial cells is most commonly referred to as a glioma.

Gliomas have a variety of symptoms, dependent on the kind of cell forming the tumor and its location, but there are several general symptoms common to nearly all brain tumors. These symptoms result from increased intracranial pressure, and include headaches, vomiting, slowing of the heart rate (bradycardia), double vision, and mental dullness. There can also be significant damage to the tissue around the site of the tumor.

Gliomas are commonly categorized by two factors, and graded on a scale from 1-4 based on severity. Tumors can be either infiltrative or encapsulated, malignant or benign. Malignant tumors are tumors that invade surrounding tissues, destroy normal cells, and commonly regrow or spread. Benign tumors are surrounded by a fibrous capsule that prevents them from spreading. Infiltrative tumors are almost always malignant, because they take over and destroy surrounding tissue. Encapsulated tumors are areas of excessive cell growth differentiated from brain tissue. These tumors cause damage by pushing on surrounding tissue in order to find room to grow, but are most often benign.

Tumors are graded according to a system established by the World Health Organization. This system assesses the malignancy of tumors, as determined by the rate at which it grows, and its potential to cause damage. Grade 1 tumors are slow growing and rarely show any neurological side effects. Grade 2 and 3 tumors are more intermediate, and usually grow but do not metastasize and show some neurological defects. Grade 4 tumors are much more dangerous, and contribute to a poor prognosis. They commonly metastasize, grow very rapidly, and can cause significant neurological damage.

Because of the variety of symptoms and severity, properly diagnosing a glioma is not only critical to patient care, but very difficult. The development of new imaging technology has had a significant impact on tumor diagnosis. A CT (computed tomography) scan or an MRI (magnetic resonance imaging) is the best way to diagnose a patient with neurological symptoms. The fMRI (functional MRI) has become an invaluable tool in both diagnosis and proper surgical treatment. If routine imaging techniques prove inconclusive, a spinal tap is often the next course of action. Analysis of the cerebrospinal fluid can reveal either elevated protein levels secondary to increased cellular reproduction, or neoplastic cells that can be used to determine specific tumor types.

Treatment and Therapy

Once diagnosed, tumors can be difficult to treat. The prognosis for a glioma is rarely positive, often limiting patients to months of quality life. Glioma treatment can take on two different forms-palliative or curative. The most straightforward treatment is surgical removal followed by intensive radiation therapy. This is the only form of curative therapy, but is limited to easily accessible, often encapsulated tumors, and is only successful if the surgeon is capable of removing every cancerous cell.

Most gliomas do not fall into this category, and must be treated using palliative measures. Chemotherapy can be effective against new, small, and rapidly dividing tumors, but it can take a greater toll on glioma patients than other cancer patients. Gliomas require higher doses of the chemotherapy drugs than other cancers due to the filtering effects of the blood brain barrier, a protective boundary formed by nor-

mally functioning glial cells that naturally keeps drugs from directly effecting central nervous tissues. Some hyperosmotic agents can be used in conjunction with surgical decompression to reduce edema and damage caused by swelling, but this is rarely more than a comfort measure towards the end of a terminal illness.

Perspective and Prospects

Cancer research does have a bright future, however. Because it has become such a common and deadly condition, oncological research has rapidly expanded, and technology is being developed to help counter the intricate defenses that cancerous tissues have developed. The most promising long-term solution comes from research being done to completely understand the mechanisms of tumor immunity. Tumors are capable of producing a self-vaccine that tricks the host immune system into viewing the cancerous cells as noninvasive, allowing them to grow free of inhibition. Research is being done to develop a potential method to deactivate this mechanism and cause immune cells to attack cancerous tissues, destroying the growth with no medical intervention.

Surgical advances have been made, allowing surgeons to increase the percentage of tumor removal during resection, in turn increasing the rate of surgical cure. Sophisticated surgical microscopy and laser scalpels have become standard in tumor removal. Fluorescent resection-infusing the cancerous cells with a radioactive tag that fluoresces during surgery-has also shown much better results. Between these newer methods used to treat patients now and the promising research being done into the nature of cancers, there is great potential for reducing cancer incidence in the years to come.

—Bryan C. Auday, Ph.D., and David Parr

See also Brain tumors; Brains; Computed tomography (CT) scanning; Cancer; Glia cell; Glioma; Hospice; Imaging and radiology; National Cancer Institute; Neuroimaging; Neurology; Neurosurgery

For Further Information:
Kolb, Bryan, and Ian Q. Whishaw. *Fundamentals of Human Neuropsychology.* 6th ed. New York: Worth Publishers, 2009.
Koob, Andrew. *The Root of Thought: Unlocking Glia-The Brain Cell That Will Help Us Sharpen Our Wits, Heal Injury, and Treat Brain Disease.* Upper Saddle River, NJ: Pearson Education, Inc., 2009.
McKinnell, Robert G., Ralph E. Parchment, Alon O. Perantoni, and G. Barry Pierce. *The Biological Basis of Cancer.* Cambridge, UK: The Press Syndicate of the University of Cambridge, 1998.
Swenson, Rand. "Disorders of the Nervous System." Hanover, NH: Dartmouth Medical School. 2008. http://www.dartmouth.edu/~dons/part_3/chapter_28.html#chapter_28_glioma.
Zillmer, Eric A., Mary V. Spiers, and William C. Culbertson. *Principles of Neuropsychology.* 2nd ed. Belmont, CA: Thomson Wadsworth, 2008.

GLUTEN INTOLERANCE
Disease/Disorder

Also known as: Non-celiac gluten sensitivity, dermatitis herpetiformis

Anatomy or system affected: Gastrointestinal system, immune system, skin

Specialties and related fields: Dermatology, gastroenterology, immunology, nutrition

Definition: A chronic, immune-mediated condition of progressive, itchy skin lesions triggered by the ingestion of gluten.

Key terms:

autoimmune: referring to an immune system response to something in the body that should not be considered a foreign or dangerous object

chronic: long-lasting or indefinite and often incurable when referring to a disease or condition

gluten: a protein found in wheat, barley, and rye grains

gluten-free diet: a diet that removes all-obvious and hidden-sources of gluten from ingestion

immunoglobulin: an antibody protein developed by the body to attack a foreign object in an immune system reaction

prodromal: sensation before an event occurs

tissue transglutaminase: an enzyme in the body that breaks down major components of gluten in grains, and a primary trigger for an antibody response to gluten

Causes and Symptoms

Gluten, a protein found in wheat, rye, and barley grains, is a common part of the twenty-first century diet. However, in people who develop gluten intolerance—which most commonly develops between the ages of twenty and forty—gluten triggers a specific immune system response. Gluten intolerance, or gluten sensitivity, comprises celiac disease, which is a gastric reaction, and dermatitis herpetiformis (DH), which is primarily a skin-based reaction. Unlike the majority of food allergies that are mediated by immunoglobulin (Ig) E antibodies, gluten ingestion in patients with DH signals the body to develop an immune response that is mediated by IgA instead. IgA antibodies build up and attack tissue transglutaminase (tTG) and epidermal transglutaminase, enzymes that break down gliadin, a component of wheat gluten. Gliadin, and related substances in rye and barley grains, appears to be the antigen, or trigger, of the immune response that leads to the characteristic symptom of DH—an intensely itchy and progressive skin rash. Indeed, instead of relying on only a dietary challenge for diagnosis of DH, this gluten sensitivity may be diagnosed by immunofluorescence to identify IgA deposits in skin lesions or by screening for the disease-specific presence of a tTG attack.

Symptoms of gluten intolerance in DH begin slowly as small, itchy areas on the skin but progress rapidly to extremely blistered, burning, and itchy lesions that appear in groups, often symmetrically. Affected areas are most often found on the knees, elbows, buttocks, and back. In severe skin disease, prodromal irritation may occur at sites of new lesions. Gastrointestinal discomfort, ranging from stomach pain to oral ulcers, has been reported infrequently along with the primarily dermal symptoms of DH.

Even without gastric symptoms, gastrointestinal biopsies of people with DH reveal abnormal changes to parts of the gastrointestinal wall and IgA deposits in parts of the gastroin-

---

Information on Gluten Intolerance

Causes: Immune system overreaction to gluten (protein in wheat, barley, rye grains)

Symptoms: Blistered skin lesions that often appear symmetrically or in groups on arms, legs, back, or buttocks, accompanied by extreme itch; possibly mild gastrointestinal distress, oral dryness, ulcers

Duration: Chronic

Treatments: Oral sulfone medications to reduce immunoglobulin A and heal lesions; strict gluten-free diet for long-term remission

---

testinal wall. Increased tTG reactivity appears proportional to the likelihood of this gastric involvement. Because of this gastric link, some researchers consider DH to be a precursor to the development of celiac disease and related malabsorption problems if the skin condition remains untreated.

Treatment and Therapy

Treatment of DH is twofold. First, symptomatic relief is provided by oral sulfones—dapsone and sulfasalazine—to reduce lesions. Sulfones work by unknown mechanisms, possibly related to enzyme stabilization, and they quickly reduce the severity and number of skin lesions, often within only two days. Dapsone, 150 to 200 milligrams daily, is the first-line agent, and the dose can be reduced to 50 to 100 milligrams daily after severe lesions have healed. Because dapsone in particular is associated with high rates of peripheral neuropathy, at times with sensory loss, sulfasalazine is a secondary sulfone choice. Potential side effects of any sulfone treatment include blood-related problems, such as anemia and decreased leukocyte counts. When an alternative to symptomatic sulfone treatment is required because of such side effects, tetracycline or minocycline may be used successfully but with less dramatic rates of improvement.

Gluten removal from the diet is the only treatment known to induce disease remission, to reduce the IgA accumulation to nearly zero, to heal existing lesions, and to prevent eruption of new lesions. In severe disease occurrences, full improvement of symptoms may take as long as two years; most often, six months of a gluten-free diet will allow a patient to discontinue sulfone treatment without a disease flare. A diet without wheat, rye, or barley must be continued indefinitely for successful disease control, because dermal symptoms return as soon as gluten is reintroduced. Rice, corn, and pure oats are recommended replacement grains. Consultation with a dietician is often suggested to ensure that the gluten-free diet provides adequate nutritional needs and to learn about ways to avoid hidden sources of gluten.

Perspective and Prospects

As early as the 1930s, dentist Weston Price associated greater amounts of processed foods in American diets with increasingly poor oral, digestive, and overall health. During the 1940s and 1950s, Willem Dicke of the Netherlands noted that children with nonspecific health complaints, including gastric pain, experienced improvement during food rations, when most grains were unavailable. Dicke expanded this observation with extensive research, presentations, and publications that pointed to early identification of DH and celiac disease.

In the second half of the twentieth century, more research evolved to identify biopsy results and immune responses in patients with skin lesions as similar to those in patients with gastric symptoms of celiac disease; the term "nonceliac gluten syndrome" was coined to identify patients whose skin and mild gastric symptoms improved despite negative test results for celiac disease, and the differentiation of DH and celiac disease began.

As research about the abnormal immune system response to gluten continues, potential links to other autoimmune disorders, such as autoimmune thyroid disease, multiple sclerosis, and irritable bowel syndrome, have been identified. Additionally, researchers are trying to determine how closely linked celiac disease and DH may be and whether lack of disease control in either gluten sensitivity may lead to progressive gastric disease, malabsorption, and even lymphoma.

Awareness of gluten sensitivity increased greatly in the twentieth century and into the twenty-first, which has made identification of gluten-free foods simpler. Still, gluten is a common filler ingredient and may be hidden in foods such as gravy, beer, or soy sauce; medications such as vitamin supplements; and even makeup such as lip balm. As with many chronic conditions, patient education is key to reducing symptoms and improving quality of life.

Researchers at the Mayo Clinic indicated that cases of celaic disease rose considerable in the first decade of the twenty-first century, plateauing in 2004. The increase is the effect of several factors, including changes in the environment and society's increased consumption of food high in gluten, such as pizza. Interestingly, a 2013 Swedish report stated that infants, beginning at four months, can bolster their defenses against celiac disease by consuming small doses of grain-based foods in tandem with breastfeeding.

—*Nicole M. Van Hoey, Pharm.D.*

See also Allergies; Autoimmune disorders; Celiac sprue; Food allergies; Food poisoning; Gastroenterology; Gastroenterology, pediatric; Gastrointestinal disorders; Gastrointestinal system; Immune system; Immunology; Lactose intolerance; Nutrition; Rashes.

For Further Information:

Boettcher E., S. E. Crowe. "Dietary Proteins and Functional Gastrointestinal Disorders." *American Journal of Gastroenterology* 108, no. 5 (May 2013): 728–736.

Feldman, M., L. S. Friedman, and L. J. Brandt. *Sleisenger and Fordtran's Gastrointestinal and Liver Disease*. 9th ed. Maryland Heights, Mo.: Saunders/Elsevier, 2010.

Gluten Intolerance Group of North America. *GIG Newsletter Education Bulletin: Dermatitis Herpetiformis*. Auburn, Wash.: Author, 2009.

Habif, T. P. "Vesicular and Bullous Diseases." In *Clinical Dermatology*. 5th ed. Rockville, Md.: Mosby, 2009.

Humbert, P., F. Pelletier, and B. Dreno, et al. "Gluten Intolerance and Skin Diseases." *European Journal of Dermatology* 16, no. 1 (2006): 4–11.

Ivarsson A. "Prevalence of Childhood Celiac Disease and Changes in Infant Feeding." *Pediatrics* 131, no. 3 (March, 2013): 687–694.

Love, H. W. "Dermatitis Herpetiformis and a Gluten-Free Diet." *American Family Physician* 67, no. 3 (2003): 470.

Sampson, H. A., and A. W. Burks. "Adverse Reactions to Food: Non-IgE-Mediated Food Hypersensitivity." In *Middleton's Allergy: Principles and Practice*, edited by N. F. Adkinson et al. 7th ed. Rockville, Md.: Mosby/Elsevier, 2008.

Stuart, Shelly. *Gluten Toxicity: The Mysterious Symptoms of Celiac Disease, Dermatitis Herpetiformis and Non-Celiac Gluten Intolerance*. South Surrey, B.C.: Create Space, 2010.

Turchin, I., and B. Barankin. "Dermatitis Herpetiformis and Gluten-Free Diet." *Dermatology Online Journal* 11, no. 1 (2005).

Wangen, Stephen. *Healthier Without Wheat: A New Understanding of Wheat Allergies, Celiac Disease, and Non-Celiac Gluten Intolerance*. Seattle: Innate Health, 2009.

GLYCOGEN STORAGE DISEASES

Disease/Disorder

Anatomy or system affected: Heart, liver, muscles

Specialties and related fields: Biochemistry, biotechnology, nutrition, pediatrics, perinatology

Definition: Inherited metabolic disorders that lead to the accumulation of an abnormal amount or type of glycogen in the liver, muscles, and heart.

Key terms:

autosomal recessive trait: a genetic trait coded on an autosomal chromosome (not an X or Y chromosome) that is expressed only when two copies are inherited, one from each parent

cirrhosis: the abnormal formation of connective tissue in an organ, resulting in loss of function; usually refers to the liver

enzyme: a protein that catalyzes a biological reaction in the body

glycogen: the storage form of carbohydrate in the body; a polymer of glucose units that has a highly branched, tree-like structure

lysosome: an organelle inside cells that contains a variety of enzymes for breaking down cellular constituents

nasogastric tube: a tube fed through the nose to the stomach

X-linked trait: a genetic trait coded on the X chromosome; predominantly affects males, who have only one X chromosome

---

Information on Glycogen Storage Diseases

Causes: Genetic enzyme defects

Symptoms: In liver diseases, may include seizures, coma, growth retardation, kidney problems, and liver cancer; in muscle diseases, may include exercise intolerance, susceptibility to fatigue, heart enlargement, and heart failure

Duration: Lifelong

Treatments: Varies by type; includes continuous glucose intake

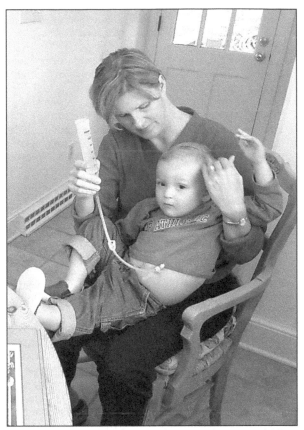

A mother pours liquid cornstarch solution into her young child's feeding tube. He has a rare glycogen storage disease and must have cornstarch every four hours in order to avoid seizures. (AP/Wide World Photos)

Causes and Symptoms

Glycogen storage diseases are caused by inherited defects in the enzymes involved in the synthesis or breakdown of glycogen and are characterized by the accumulation of an abnormal type or amount of glycogen. At least twelve such diseases have been identified; they can be diagnosed by enzymatic analysis of a biopsy tissue sample. Prenatal diagnosis of most of these conditions is possible but, because their overall frequency is estimated at 1 in 20,000 to 25,000 live births, is generally not performed unless warranted. Most of these diseases are inherited as autosomal recessive traits, although phosphorylase kinase deficiency is X-linked. In many cases, the causative deoxyribonucleic acid (DNA) mutations have been identified. These diseases primarily affect the liver and muscles, which normally contain most of the glycogen in the body.

Maintaining normal blood glucose levels is essential for the function of various tissues and particularly the brain, which depends on blood glucose as a source of energy. In the fed state, when dietary carbohydrate is digested, blood glucose levels rise and are used to replenish liver glycogen. In the fasting state, when blood glucose levels otherwise fall, liver glycogen is broken down and used to maintain normal blood glucose levels. This cycling in the storage and breakdown of liver glycogen is essential to permit the body to survive periods without meals, especially overnight.

In liver glycogen storage diseases, this cycling is disrupted. Most cases are attributed to defects in four enzymes: glucose-6-phosphatase, glycogen branching enzyme, glycogen debrancher enzyme, and glycogen phosphorylase (or phosphorylase kinase). Because glucose-6-phosphatase is responsible for converting the breakdown product of glycogen (glucose-6-phosphate) to free glucose for release into the blood, its deficiency does not allow stored liver glycogen to restore depleted blood glucose, as during an overnight fast. If untreated, this condition, also known as von Gierke's disease, results in seizures, coma, and death. Inadequately treated patients may survive but are more likely to experience growth retardation and to develop kidney problems and liver cancer.

Muscle glycogen is also synthesized in the fed state, but it is broken down to provide energy for muscle contraction. Glycogen storage diseases of muscle usually cause intolerance to exercise and susceptibility to fatigue. Most of these cases are attributed to defects in three enzymes: lysosomal glucosidase, glycogen phosphorylase, and phosphofructokinase. The glucosidase found in lysosomes is responsible for breaking down any glycogen that accumulates in these intracellular organelles. When this enzyme is missing, the lysosomes become engorged with glycogen, disrupting their normal function and other cellular metabolism. In the most severe cases, glycogen accumulation in the heart is pronounced, resulting in an enlarged heart and death from heart failure before age two. Glycogen phosphorylase in muscle breaks down glycogen for its use in contraction. When this enzyme is deficient, muscle tissues lack the fuel to provide for extensive exercise, resulting in cramping. Phosphofructokinase is a crucial enzyme in the metabolism of glucose; in the muscle, its deficiency has a consequence much like that of glycogen phosphorylase, namely the inability to engage in strenuous exercise.

When glycogen is synthesized, the branching enzyme inserts branchpoints to give it a treelike structure. A defect in this enzyme leads to an abnormal, long, unbranched glycogen. Because it folds back on itself in a way that makes it difficult for glycogen-breakdown enzymes to act on it, it is not broken down. While this condition generally does not lead to low fasting blood glucose, as alternative pathways are available, the accumulated abnormal glycogen, apparently considered a foreign object, leads to liver cirrhosis and death by age five; no treatment is available other than liver transplantation. A defect in the debranching enzyme that removes the branchpoints during the breakdown of glycogen severely restricts the yield of glucose to those units beyond a branchpoint. Glycogen phosphorylase is the main enzyme that breaks down glycogen to monomeric units, and its deficiency or that of an enzyme controlling its activity (phosphorylase kinase) results in variable manifestation, depending on the severity of the condition. Most patients with the latter diseases usually require no specific treatment.

Treatment and Therapy

A defect in glucose-6-phosphatase can be treated by providing continuous sources of glucose during the day (snacks between meals) and especially overnight (nightly nasogastric infusions of glucose or eating slowly digested carbohydrate, such as uncooked cornstarch, before sleep). If this condition is detected early and treated properly, then normal growth and development are observed. A liver transplant surgery may be necessary in certain cases. Medications such as alglucosidase alfa may help to replace the enzymes needed for proper muscle function.

Perspective and Prospects

The first observation of a defect in glycogen metabolism was made in 1928. In 1929, Edgar von Gierke first noted glucose-6-phosphatase deficiency, and in 1932, J. C. Pompe first reported the lysosomal glucosidase deficiency; their names remain associated with these conditions. As normal glycogen metabolism came to be understood, the enzymatic basis for at least twelve glycogen storage disorders were identified. Each is a candidate for enzyme replacement therapy or gene replacement therapy.

—*James L. Robinson, Ph.D.*

See also Enzyme therapy; Enzymes; Fatty acid oxidation disorders; Food biochemistry; Metabolic disorders; Metabolism; Niemann-Pick disease.

For Further Information:

Badash, Michelle. "Glycogen Storage Diseases." *Health Library,* September 12, 2012.

Chen, Y.-T. "Glycogen Storage Diseases." In *The Metabolic and Molecular Bases of Inherited Disease,* edited by Charles R. Scriver et al. 8th ed. New York: McGraw-Hill, 2001.

Hirschhorn, R., and A. J. J. Reuser. "Glycogen Storage Disease Type II: Acid-Glucosidase (Acid Maltase) Deficiency." In *The Metabolic and Molecular Bases of Inherited Disease,* edited by Charles R. Scriver et al. 8th ed. New York: McGraw-Hill, 2001.

Maheshwari, Anurag, et al. "Outcomes of Liver Transplantation for Glycogen Storage Disease: A Matched-Control Study and Review of Literature." Clinical Transplantation 26, no. 3 (2012): 432–436.

Professional Guide to Diseases. 10th ed. Philadelphia: Lippincott Williams & Wilkins, 2012.

GLYCOLYSIS

Biology

Anatomy or system affected: Blood, cells, muscles, musculoskeletal system

Specialties and related fields: Biochemistry, cytology, exercise physiology, pharmacology, sports medicine

Definition: The chemical process of splitting a molecule of glucose in order to obtain energy for other cellular processes; at times of intense activity, glycolysis produces most of the energy used by muscles.

Key terms:

adenosine triphosphate (ATP): an important biological molecule that represents the energy currency of the cell; the energy in a special high-energy bond in ATP is used to drive almost all cellular processes that require energy

aerobic: occurring in the presence of oxygen

anaerobic: occurring in the absence of oxygen

cellular respiration: a complex series of chemical reactions by which chemical energy stored in the bonds of food molecules is released and used to form ATP

chemical energy: the energy locked up in the chemical bonds that hold the atoms of a molecule together; food molecules, such as glucose, contain much energy in their bonds

creatine phosphate: an energy-containing molecule present in significant quantities in muscle tissue; energy is stored in a high-energy bond similar to that of ATP

enzyme: a biological catalyst that speeds up a chemical reaction without itself being used up; enzymes are made of protein, and a single enzyme can usually only catalyze a single chemical reaction

nicotinamide adenine dinucleotide (NAD): a molecule used to hold pairs of electrons when they have been removed from a molecule by some biological process; the empty molecule is denoted by NAD+, while it is denoted as NADH when it is carrying electrons

Structure and Functions

Glycolysis is the first step in the process that cells use to extract energy from food molecules. Although energy can be extracted from most types of food molecule, glycolysis is usually considered to begin with glucose. In fact, the term "glycolysis" actually means the splitting (*lysis*) of glucose (*glyco*). This is a good description for the process, since the glucose molecule is split into two halves. The glucose molecule consists of a backbone of six carbon atoms to which are attached, in various ways, twelve hydrogen atoms and six oxygen atoms. The glucose molecule is inherently stable and unlikely to split spontaneously at any appreciable rate.

When the energy is extracted from a glucose molecule, it is stored, for the short term, in a much less stable molecule called adenosine triphosphate (ATP). The ATP molecule consists of a complex organic molecule (adenosine) to which are attached three simple phosphate groups (see figure).

ATP consists of a five-carbon sugar called ribose, linked on one side to the nitrogenous base adenine and on the other side to a linear chain of phosphate groups. The molecule formed by the attachment of adenine to ribose is called adenosine, and the linkage of three phosphates generates adenosine triphosphate. The first phosphate is attached to the ribose sugar by means of a chemical bond whose energy is no greater than those bonds found anywhere else in the molecule. While the first phosphate is attached by what one could call a "normal" chemical bond, the second and third phosphates are attached by high-energy bonds. These are chemical bonds that require a considerable amount of energy to create. Thus ATP is an ideal energy storage molecule that provides readily available energy for the biosynthetic reactions of the cell and other energy-requiring processes.

When one of the high-energy bonds of ATP is broken, a large amount of energy is released. Usually, only the bond holding the last phosphate is broken, producing a molecule of adenosine diphosphate (ADP) and a free phosphate group. The phosphate group is only split from ATP at the precise moment when energy is required by some other process in the cell. This breaking of ATP provides the energy to drive cellular processes. The processes include activities such as the synthesis of molecules, the movement of molecules, and the contraction of muscle. The third phosphate can be reattached to ADP using energy released from glycolysis, or by other components of cellular respiration. The production of ATP can be diagrammed as follows: "energy from glycolysis + ADP + phosphate " ATP." Similarly, the breakdown of ATP can be diagrammed as "ATP " ADP + phosphate + usable energy." With this understanding of how ATP works, one can look at how it is generated in the cell by glycolysis.

The first step in the production of energy from sugar is really an energy-consuming process. Since glucose is inherently a stable molecule, it must be activated before it will split. It is activated by attaching a phosphate group to each end of the six-carbon backbone. These phosphate groups are supplied by ATP. Therefore, glycolysis begins by using the energy from two ATP molecules. The atoms of the glucose molecule are also rearranged during the activation process so that it is changed into a very similar sugar, fructose. A fructose molecule with a phosphate group on either end is called fructose 1,6-diphosphate. Thus one can summarize the activation process as "glucose + 2 ATP " fructose 1,6-diphosphate + 2 ADP."

Fructose 1,6-diphosphate is a much more reactive molecule and can be readily split by an enzyme called aldolase into two three-carbon compounds called dihydroxyacetone phosphate (DHAP) and glyceraldehyde 3-phosphate (G3P). DHAP is converted into G3P by an enzyme called triose phosphate isomerase, which makes G3P the starting point for all the following steps of glycolysis.

Each G3P undergoes several reactions, but only the more consequential reactions will be mentioned. G3P undergoes an oxidation reaction, catalyzed by an enzyme called glyceraldehyde 3-phosphate dehydrogenase. Oxidation reactions involve the loss of high-energy electrons. Electrons are highly energetic and have a negative electrical charge. They are picked up and carried by molecules specially designed for this purpose.

These energy-carrying molecules are called nicotinamide adenine dinucleotide (NAD). Biologists have agreed on a conventional notation for this molecule to allow the reader to know whether the molecule is carrying electrons or is empty. Since the empty molecule has a net positive charge, it is denoted as NAD+. When full, it holds a pair of electrons. One

electron would neutralize the positive charge, while two result in a negative charge. The negative charge attracts one of the many hydrogen ions (H+) in the cell. Thus when carrying electrons the molecule is denoted NADH. G3P surrenders two high-energy electrons to NAD+. The G3P molecule also picks up a free phosphate group at the end opposite from where one is already attached to form 1,3-bisphosphoglycerate. One can summarize the reaction as "2 Glyceraldehyde 3-phosphate + 2 NAD$^+$ + 2 inorganic phosphates " ? 2 1,3-bisphosphoglycerate + NADH + H$^+$." The following reactions merely transfer the energy in these chemical bonds to high-energy bonds by transferring these phosphate groups to ADP molecules to produce ATP. Since each G3P eventually produces two ATPs, and two G3Ps are produced from each original glucose molecule, glycolysis produces four ATP molecules all together. However since two ATPs were used to activate the glucose, the cell has a net gain of two ATP molecules for each glucose molecule used.

The rearrangement of the atoms leaves them in a form called pyruvate. Pyruvate still contains much energy locked up in its chemical bonds. In most of the cells of the body and most of the time, pyruvate will be further broken down and all of its energy released. This further breakdown of pyruvate requires oxygen and is beyond the scope of this topic. It should be pointed out, however, that the complete breakdown of two molecules of pyruvate can produce more than thirty additional ATP molecules. With the addition of oxygen, the end products are the simple molecules of carbon dioxide and water.

The oxidative pathways that completely break down pyruvate are limited by the lack of oxygen in very active muscles. The ability to deal with electrons from NADH is also drastically reduced. Glycolysis can continue even in the ab-

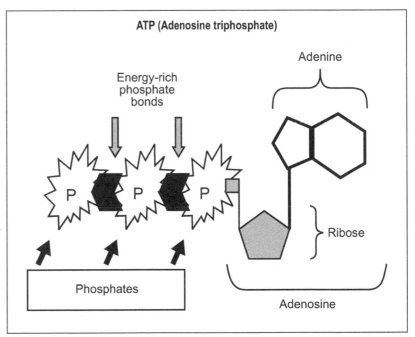

ATP (Adenosine triphosphate)

Energy-rich phosphate bonds

Adenine

P P P

Ribose

Phosphates

Adenosine

sence of oxygen, but the electrons produced by glycolysis must be dealt with.

There is a very limited amount of NAD+ in each cell. NAD+ is designed to hold electrons briefly, while they are transferred to some other system. In the absence of oxygen, the electrons are transferred to pyruvate. Since pyruvate cannot be broken down without oxygen, there is an ample supply. Transferring electrons from NADH to pyruvate allows the empty NAD+ to pick up more electrons produced by glycolysis. Therefore, glycolysis can continue producing two ATP molecules from each glucose molecule used. While two ATPs per glucose molecule is a small amount compared to the more than thirty ATPs produced by oxidative metabolism, it is better than none at all.

The process of generating energy (ATPs) in the absence of oxygen is referred to as fermentation. Most people are familiar with the fermentation of grapes to produce wine. Yeast has the enzymes to transfer electrons from NADH to a derivative of pyruvate and to convert the resulting molecule into alcohol and carbon dioxide. No further energy is obtained from this process. Alcohol still contains much of the energy that was in glucose. Humans and other mammals have different enzymes than yeast cells. These enzymes transfer the electrons from NADH to pyruvate, producing lactate.

Glycolysis and Muscle Activity

When yeast is fermented anaerobically (without oxygen), it will continue producing alcohol until it poisons itself. Most yeast cannot tolerate more than about 12 percent alcohol, the concentration found in most wine. The lactate produced by fermentation in humans is also poisonous. People, however, do not respire completely anaerobically. The two ATPs produced per glucose molecule used are simply not enough to supply the energy needs of most human cells. Muscle cells have to be somewhat of an exception. There are times when one asks the muscle cells to use energy much faster than one can supply them with oxygen. One may consider a muscle working under various levels of physical activity and examine its oxygen requirements and waste products.

At rest, a muscle requires very little ATP energy. For an individual sitting on the couch watching television, energy demands are minimal. The lungs inhale and exhale slowly and take in enough oxygen to keep its concentration in the blood high. A relatively slow heart rate can pump enough of this oxygen-rich blood to the muscles to supply their very minimal needs. As soon as one uses a muscle, however, its ATP consumption increases dramatically. Even if an individual simply walks as far as the refrigerator, large quantities of ATP are required to cause the leg muscles to contract. Muscle cells maintain a constant level of ATP so that, as soon as one asks a muscle to contract, it can do so. The ATP that is broken down is almost instantly regenerated from an additional energy store peculiar to muscle cells. Creatine phosphate is a molecule similar to ATP, in that the phosphate group is attached by a high-energy bond. There is more creatine phosphate in muscle cells than ATP. As soon as ATP is broken down, phosphates, and their high-energy bonds, are transferred from

creatine phosphate. Within the first few seconds of activity, the ATP concentration in a muscle cell remains almost constant, but the creatine phosphate level begins to drop.

As soon as the creatine phosphate concentration drops, the aerobic (oxygen-requiring) respiratory processes speed up. These processes break down glucose all the way to carbon dioxide and water and release plenty of ATP. This ATP can then be used for muscle contraction. If the muscle has now stopped contracting, the new ATP produced will be used to rebuild the store of creatine phosphate.

Within the first minute or so of muscle contraction, the use of oxygen can be quite high. The circulatory system has not yet responded to this increased oxygen demand. Muscle tissue, however, has a reserve of oxygen. The red color of most mammalian muscles is attributable to the presence of myoglobin, which is similar to hemoglobin in that it has a strong affinity for oxygen. The myoglobin stores oxygen directly in the muscle, so that the muscle can operate aerobically while the circulatory and respiratory systems adjust to the increased oxygen demand.

At low or moderate muscle activity, the carbon dioxide produced by aerobic respiration in muscles will trigger an increase in the activity of both the circulatory and the respiratory systems. The increased demand for oxygen by the muscles is supplied by an increased blood flow. Jogging around a track or participating in aerobic exercises would be considered low to moderate muscular activity. Respiration rate and pulse rate both increase with jogging. This increase in oxygen supply to the muscles provides all that they need. The level of creatine phosphate will be lower than that in resting muscles, but it will soon be replenished when the activity is stopped. The muscle cells have a good supply of food molecules in the form of glycogen. Glycogen is simply a long string of glucose molecules connected together for convenient storage. At a rate of activity such as that created by jogging, the glycogen supply can last for hours. Even after it is used up, glycogen stored in the liver can be broken down to glucose and carried to the muscles by the blood. An individual will probably want to stop jogging before his or her muscles will want to quit.

High levels of muscular activity pose a different set of problems. After more than about a minute of vigorous exercise, the muscles begin to use ATP faster than oxygen can be supplied to regenerate it. The additional ATP is supplied by lactic acid fermentation. Glucose is only broken down as far as pyruvate, then converted to lactate by the addition of electrons from NADH. Lactate begins to accumulate in the muscle tissue. Since the body is still using large amounts of ATP but not taking in enough oxygen, it is said to enter a state of oxygen debt. When the muscular activity ends, the oxygen debt is repaid.

One can use an example of someone running to catch a bus, sprinting for fifty yards at full speed. That is not enough time for the circulation and lungs to respond to the increased demand for oxygen. The muscles have made up the difference between supply and demand with lactic acid fermentation. The individual now sits down in the bus and pants—to repay his or her oxygen debt.

Some of the oxygen will go to replenish the store in muscle myoglobin. Some of it will be used in oxidative metabolism in the muscle to replenish the reserves of creatine phosphate. The rest will be used to deal with the accumulated lactate. The lactate is not all dealt with in the muscle where it was produced. Being a small molecule, it easily enters the bloodstream. In muscles throughout the body, it can be converted back to pyruvate. Pyruvate can then reenter the oxidative pathway and be used to generate ATP, with the use of oxygen. The lactate, then, is being used as a food molecule to supply the needs of resting muscle. Much of the lactate is metabolized in the liver. Some of it will be metabolized with oxygen to produce the energy to convert the rest of it back to glucose. The glucose can then be circulated in the blood or stored in the liver or muscles as glycogen. A minimal amount of lactate is excreted in the urine or in sweat.

If the subject of the preceding example kept running at full speed, having missed the bus and run all the way to the office, lactate would build up in the muscles and in the blood. If the office was far enough away, the subject would eventually reach the point of exhaustion and stop running. At that point, the level of lactate in the leg muscles would be high enough to inhibit the enzymes of glycolysis. Glycolysis would slow down so that lactate would not become any more concentrated. The muscles" supply of creatine phosphate would be almost exhausted, but the ATP supply would be only slightly lower than in a resting muscle. The body is protected from damaging itself: Too much lactate would lower the pH to dangerous levels, and the absolute lack of ATP causes muscles to lock, as in rigor mortis. The body's self-protection mechanisms force one to stop before either of these conditions exists. Once the subject stops running, and pants long enough, he or she can continue. The additional oxygen taken in by increased respiration will have metabolized a sufficient amount of lactate to allow the muscles to start working again.

In cases where an individual has an inherited deficiency of particular enzymes of glycolysis, the consequences for muscle tissue are rather dire. Muscles, which depend heavily on glycolysis when operating under conditions of oxygen debt, fail to perform well if any of the glycolytic enzymes are defective. Symptoms include frequent muscle cramps, easy fatigability, and evidence of heavy muscle damage after strenuous exertion.

Glycolysis and Red Blood Cell Function

Red blood cells are the oxygen-ferrying units of the bloodstream and are filled with an iron-containing protein called hemoglobin. Hemoglobin binds oxygen tightly when oxygen concentrations are high and releases oxygen when oxygen concentrations are low. To perform their task successfully, red blood cells must maintain the health and functionality of their hemoglobin stores, and glycolysis helps them do that. In red blood cells, approximately 90 to 95 percent of the glucose that enters the cell is metabolized to lactate by means of glycolysis and lactate dehydrogenase. The ATP generated by glycolysis is used to bring charged atoms into the cell such as calcium, potassium, and others. The NADH generated by

glycolysis is also used to maintain the iron found in hemoglobin in a state that allows it to bind oxygen. Glycolysis is also used to form the metabolite 2,3-DPG (2,3-Diphosphoglycerate). 2,3-DPG binds to hemoglobin and forces it to release oxygen more readily when oxygen concentrations are low. Thus 2,3-DPG aids hemoglobin delivery of oxygen to the tissues.

Abnormalities in the enzymes that catalyze the reactions of glycolysis are inherited. Individuals who inherit two copies of a gene that encodes a mutant form of a glycolytic enzyme experience uncontrolled destruction of red blood cells (hemolysis). The red blood cell destruction that results from defects in glycolytic enzymes is chronic and not ameliorated by drugs. An enlarged spleen is a typical symptom of glycolytic enzyme abnormalities, as the spleen tends to fill with dying red blood cells. The red blood cell destruction can be so severe that blood transfusions might be necessary. Removal of the spleen reduces red blood cell destruction.

Insulin, Diabetes, and Glycolysis

Glycolysis is heavily regulated by the hormones insulin and glucagon. Insulin, a hormone made and released by the beta cells of the pancreatic islets, stimulates the insertion of the GLUT4 glucose transporter into the membranes of cells. People with type 1 diabetes mellitus, who are incapable of making sufficient quantities of insulin, tend to have very high blood sugar readings, since their cells cannot receive the signal to insert the glucose transporter into their membranes and take up glucose from the blood. This prevents the removal of glucose from the blood, and in type 1 diabetics the blood glucose level climbs to abnormally high levels. GLUT4 allows the uptake of glucose without the input of energy. Therefore, glycolysis occurs as fast as the cells can take up glucose.

Insulin also stimulates the synthesis of a metabolite called fructose 2,6-bisphosphate. Fructose 2,6-bisphosphate is a potent activator of phosphofructokinase, and activation of this enzyme ensures the activation of glycolysis. Insulin also activates the expression of genes that encode the protein involved in glycolysis. During uncontrolled diabetes, reduced glucose transport in muscle inhibits muscle cell glycolysis. In liver cells, reduced glycolytic gene expression and attenuation of the levels of fructose 2,6-bisphosphate reduce glycolysis. This contributes to the voluntary muscle weakness, liver dysfunction, and heart problems that are sometimes observed in diabetics.

Glycolysis and Cancer

The uptake of glucose and its degradation by glycolysis occurs ten times faster in tumor cells than in nontumor cells. This phenomenon, called the Warburg effect, seems to benefit tumor cells, since they lack an extensive capillary network to feed them oxygen and must rely on anaerobic glycolysis to generate ATP.

Oxygen-poor conditions also induce the synthesis of a protein called hypoxia-inducible factor (HIF). HIF is a transcription factor that helps turn on the expression of specific genes that help cells survive oxygen-poor conditions. The synthesis of at least eight glycolytic enzymes are activated by HIF. These fundamental observations of cancer cells have shown that glycolytic enzymes are excellent potential drug targets for anticancer agents.

Perspective and Prospects

Cellular respiration is the process by which organisms harvest usable energy in the form of ATP molecules from food molecules. Lactic acid fermentation is the form of respiration used by human muscles when oxygen is in limited supply. Glycolysis is the energy-producing component of lactic acid fermentation, which is much less efficient than aerobic cellular respiration. Fermentation harvests only two molecules of ATP for every glucose molecule used, while aerobic respiration produces a yield of more than thirty molecules of ATP. Most forms of life will resort to fermentation only when oxygen is absent or in short supply. While higher forms of life such as humans can obtain energy by fermentation for short periods, they incur an oxygen debt that must eventually be repaid. The yield of two molecules of ATP for each glucose molecule used is simply not enough to sustain their high demand for energy.

Nevertheless, lactic acid fermentation is an important source of ATP for humans during strenuous physical exercise. Even though it is an inefficient use of glucose, it can provide enough ATP for a short burst of activity. After the activity is over, the lactate produced must be dealt with, which usually requires the use of oxygen.

Most popular exercise programs focus on aerobic activity. Aerobic exercises do not place stress on muscles to the point where the blood cannot supply enough oxygen. These exercises are designed to improve the efficiency of the oxygen delivery system so that there is less need for anaerobic metabolism. Training programs in general attempt to tune the body so that the need for lactic acid fermentation is reduced. They concentrate on improving the delivery of oxygen to the muscles, storing oxygen in the muscles, or increasing the efficiency of muscular contraction.

Insulin signaling activates glycolysis whereas another pancreatic peptide hormone, glucagon, inhibits glycolysis. Diabetics can suffer from inadequate glycolytic activity in particular organs, which can result in organ dysfunction. Expression of mutant forms of various glycolytic enzymes or supporting enzymes in transgenic mice has elucidated the link between abnormalities in glycolysis and the pathology of diabetes mellitus.

In the 1920s the German biochemist Otto Warburg demonstrated that cancer cells voraciously take up glucose and metabolize to lactate. Glycolysis is very active in cancer cells and helps them flourish under low-oxygen conditions. The development of new glycolytic inhibitors may constitute a new class of anticancer drugs that have wide-ranging therapeutic applications.

—*James Waddell, Ph.D.;*
updated by Michael A. Buratovich, Ph.D.

See also Cells; Enzymes; Exercise physiology; Food biochemistry; Metabolism; Muscles; Sports medicine.

For Further Information:

Alberts, Bruce, et al. *Essential Cell Biology*. 3d ed. New York: Garland Science, 2010.

Campbell, Neil A., et al. *Biology: Concepts and Connections*. 6th ed. San Francisco: Pearson/Benjamin Cummings, 2009.

Fox, Stuart Ira. *Human Physiology*. 13th ed. Boston: McGraw-Hill, 2013.

Nelson, David L., and Michael A. Cox. *Lehninger Principles of Biochemistry*. 5th ed. New York: W. H. Freeman, 2009.

Sackheim, George I., and Dennis D. Lehman. *Chemistry for the Health Sciences*. 8th ed. Upper Saddle River, N.J.: Pearson/Prentice Hall, 2009.

Shephard, Roy J. *Biochemistry of Physical Activity*. Springfield, Ill.: Charles C Thomas, 1984.

Wu, Chaodong, et al. "Regulation of Glycolysis: The Role of Insulin." *Experimental Gerontology* 40 (2005): 894–899.

GOITER

Disease/Disorder

Anatomy or system affected: Endocrine system, glands, neck
Specialties and related fields: Endocrinology
Definition: An enlargement of the thyroid gland that is noncancerous and not caused by a temporary condition such as inflammation.
Key terms:

goitrogenic: referring to a factor (typically food or chemicals) that produces goiter

hypersecretion: the excess production and secretion of a hormone or other chemical

Causes and Symptoms

Goiter is often a painless medical condition. Its only visible symptoms may be a slight but visible enlargement of the thyroid that creates a swelling at the base of the neck. In severe cases, the swelling becomes massive and the patient experiences difficulty breathing or swallowing as the enlarged thyroid compresses against the windpipe or esophagus. Other symptoms that may indicate goiter include weight loss, increased heart rate, elevated blood pressure, hair loss, and tremors. Goiter can be confirmed by ultrasound scan of the thyroid, blood tests for abnormal levels of thyroxine or thyroid-stimulating hormone, or low rates of iodine excretion in the urine.

The several types of medical goiter fall into two broad categories: simple goiter and toxic goiter. Simple goiter is caused by a dietary deficiency of iodine. In response, one or

---

Information on Goiter

Causes: Of simple goiter, iodine deficiency or hormonal changes (adolescence, pregnancy); of toxic goiter, excessive production of thyroxine from oversecretion of thyroid-stimulating hormone by pituitary

Symptoms: Thyroid enlargement ranging from slight to massive, with difficulty breathing or swallowing

Duration: Acute or chronic

Treatments: Iodine tablets, sometimes surgical removal of all or part of thyroid

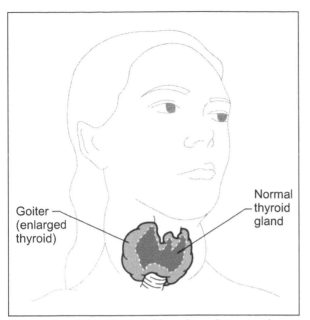

Goiter (enlarged thyroid); dashed lines show relative size of normal thyroid.

both lobes of the thyroid gland enlarge in an attempt to produce more of the iodine-containing hormone thyroxine. Two types of simple goiter are recognized: endemic goiter and sporadic goiter.

Endemic goiter typically occurs in landlocked geographic regions or in areas where farm soils are iodine-depleted. Simple goiter was once common in areas of central Asia, central Africa, and the so-called Goiter Belt of the United States, which extended from the Great Lakes to the Intermountain West (between the Rockies and the Sierras).

Simple goiter most often appears in adolescence, but it may sometimes occur during pregnancy. This condition should be corrected in pregnant women to ensure the healthy development of the fetus and the birth of a healthy infant. Simple goiter readily responds to treatment via iodine tablets, but in some patients surgical removal of all or part of the enlarged thyroid may be necessary. Public health measures undertaken to eliminate or prevent simple goiter include the addition of iodine to table salt and to water reservoirs in certain areas.

Sporadic goiter occurs in some individuals because of an excessive consumption of goitrogenic (goiter-causing) foods such as cabbage, soybeans, spinach, and radishes. Sporadic goiter has also been linked with exposure to certain medications, such as aminoglutethimide or lithium. Although this type of goiter is considered nontoxic, it does produce impaired thyroid activity. Sporadic goiter can be treated by limiting the consumption of goitrogenic foods.

Toxic goiter is caused by an excessive production of thyroxine hormone by the thyroid gland. This type of goiter is also called hyperthyroid goiter, exopthalmic goiter, or Graves' disease. Toxic goiter results from an oversecretion (hypersecretion) of thyroid-stimulating hormone by the pituitary. In turn, the thyroid gland responds by enlarging and secreting excess amounts of thyroxine, resulting in goiter. Symptoms of Graves" disease include elevated metabolic rate, higher body temperature, rapid weight loss, nervousness, and irritability. In some patients, this type of goiter results in protrusive eyeballs and the appearance of staring.

Euthyroid goiter occurs when dietary levels of iodine are only slightly below normal. The pituitary gland responds to lowered thyroxine levels in the blood by producing additional thyroid-stimulating hormone. The thyroid gland responds to the elevated thyroid-stimulating hormone by enlarging in an effort to increase thyroxine production.

Treatment and Therapy

Most goiters can be treated effectively through dietary supplements of iodine. The administration of iodine supplements must be very carefully regulated, however, to prevent a so-called thyroxin storm resulting from excess thyroxine production by the enlarged thyroid gland. Some patients may choose alternative natural herbal therapies taken in tablet form, but these substances should be used only in consultation with a physician.

—Dwight G. Smith, Ph.D.

See also Endocrine disorders; Endocrine gland; Endocrinology; Endocrinology, pediatric; Glands; Hyperparathyroidism and Hypoparathyroidism; Malnutrition; Thyroid disorders; Thyroid gland; Thyroidectomy.

For Further Information:
Cakir, Mehtap. *Differential Diagnosis of Hyperthyroidism.* New York: Nova Science, 2010.
DeMaeyer, E. M. *The Control of Endemic Goiter.* Washington, D.C.: World Health Organization, 1988.
Gaitan, Eduardo, ed. *Environmental Goitrogenesis.* Boca Raton, Fla.: CRC, 1989.
Hall, R., and J. Köbberling, eds. *Thyroid Disorders Associated with Iodine Deficiency and Excess.* New York: Raven Press, 1985.
Hamburger, J. I. *Nontoxic Goiter: Concept and Controversy.* Springfield, Ill.: Charles C. Thomas, 1973.
Icon Health. *Goiter: A Medical Dictionary, Bibliography, and Annotated Research Guide to Internet References.* San Diego, Calif.: Author, 2004.
Jameson, J. Larry, and DeGroot, Leslie J. *Endocrinology: Adult and Pediatric.* Philadelphia: Elsevier Saunders, 2010.
McDermott, Michael T. *Endocrine Secrets.* 6th ed. Philadelphia: Elsevier Saunders, 2013.
"Thyroid Disorders Overview." *Hormone,* 2013.

GONORRHEA
Disease/Disorder

Anatomy or system affected: Eyes, genitals, reproductive system, throat, urinary system

Specialties and related fields: Gynecology, microbiology

Definition: A common treatable sexually transmitted disease that primarily infects the reproductive tract and which is caused by the bacterium *Neisseria gonorrhea.*

Key terms:

contact tracing: also known as partner referral; a process that consists of identifying the sexual partners of infected patients, informing these partners of their exposure to disease, and offering resources for counseling and treatment

screening procedures: tests that are carried out in populations which are usually asymptomatic and at high risk for a disease in order to identify those in need of treatment

sexually transmitted disease: an infection caused by organisms transferred through sexual contact (genital-genital, oral-genital, oral-anal, or anal-genital); the transmission of infection occurs through exposure to lesions or secretions that contain the organisms

Causes and Symptoms

Gonorrhea is the second most common bacterial sexually transmitted infection (STI) in the United States, the most common being chlamydia. In the United States, the incidence of gonorrhea has fallen. In 1995, the incidence was about 150 cases out of every 100,000 persons, down from the mid-1970s of more than 400 cases per 100,000 persons. After 1997, the percentage of infections increased slightly, but by 2009, the rate per 100,000 reached an all-time low of 98.1. The following two years saw a slight increase in the rate of infection, reaching 104.2 in 2011. However, overall, from 2007 to 2011, the rate of infection decreased by nearly 12 percent. The highest incidence of gonorrhea is in sexually active men and women under twenty-five years of age; since 2002, the rate of infection for women of any age group has been higher than for men (108.9 cases per 100,000 compared with 98.7 for men).

Gonorrhea is caused by the bacterium *Neisseria gonorrhea*, a gram-negative diplococcus. The bacterium infects the mucous membranes with which it comes in contact, most commonly the urethra and the cervix but also the throat, rectum, and eyes. Some men will be asymptomatic, but most will experience urinary discomfort and a purulent urethral discharge. Long-term complications of this infection in men include epididymitis, prostatitis, and urethral strictures (scarring). In women, the disease is more likely to be asymptomatic.

Women with symptoms may have purulent vaginal discharge, urinary discomfort, urethral discharge, lower abdominal discomfort, or pain with intercourse. Pelvic inflammatory disease (PID) and its consequences may occur if gonorrheal infection ascends past the cervix into the upper genital tract (uterus, Fallopian tubes, ovaries, and pelvic cavity) in women. Complications of PID include infertility and an increased risk of ectopic pregnancy.

In rare cases, gonorrhea can enter the bloodstream and disseminate throughout the body, causing fever, joint pain, and skin lesions. Gonorrhea can infect the heart valves, pericardium, and meninges as well. When it infects the joints, a condition known as septic arthritis occurs, characterized by pain and swelling of the joints and potential destruction of the joints.

Gonorrhea can be transmitted to infants through the birth canal, leading to an eye infection that can damage the eye and impair vision. Fortunately, erythromycin eye drops are rou-

---

> ### Information on Gonorrhea
>
> **Causes:** Bacterial infection through intercourse
> **Symptoms:** In men, sometimes urinary discomfort and discharge, with long-term complications of epididymitis, prostatitis, and urethral scarring; in women, sometimes vaginal discharge, urinary discomfort, urethral discharge, lower abdominal discomfort, and pain with intercourse, with possible pelvic inflammatory disease, infertility, and increased risk of ectopic pregnancy
> **Duration:** Acute
> **Treatments:** Antibiotics, counseling regarding safe sex

---

tinely given to newborns to prevent eye infection. These eyedrops are effective against *Neisseria gonorrhea* as well as *Chlamydia trachomatis*.

Treatment and Therapy

Treatment for gonorrhea consists of the use of antibiotics. With the development of penicillin-resistant strains of gonorrhea, effective therapy relies on antibiotics, such as ceftriaxone, to which gonorrhea remains susceptible. In uncomplicated cases of gonorrheal infection, such as cervicitis or urethritis, a single dose is given.

A patient who has risk factors for STIs (primarily contact with a suspected infected partner) or a clinical picture suggestive of gonorrhea, or both, may receive treatment presumptively, before confirmatory laboratory test results for gonorrhea are available. Because a large number of patients with gonorrhea also have chlamydia, patients are treated concomitantly with an antibiotic directed against chlamydia, such as azithromycin. Occasional doxycycline may be used as well. Once laboratory test results confirm the diagnosis of gonorrhea, patients should be advised that it is recommended that they be tested for other STIs, such as human immunodeficiency virus (HIV), hepatitis B and C, and syphilis.

As with all STIs, a key component of therapy includes counseling regarding safer sex. This includes the use of barrier contraceptives, such as condoms, and the avoidance of high-risk sexual behaviors. Contact tracing is another important element to STI treatment. It notifies the patient's sexual partners of their exposure to gonorrhea or other STIs. Contact tracing also involves offering resources to these partners for medical attention. Contact tracing can prevent both reinfection of the patient through subsequent sexual encounters and can prevent the spread of STIs from the patient's partner to his or her subsequent sexual partners.

Perspective and Prospects

The symptoms of gonorrhea have been described in numerous cultures in the past, including those dating back to the ancient Chinese, Egyptians, and Romans. The actual gonorrhea bacterium was first identified by Albert Neisser in the 1870s, and it was one of the first bacteria ever discovered. *Neisseria gonorrhea* has continued to be well-studied on both the molecular and the epidemiological level.

Antibiotic therapy, in the form of sulfanilamide, was first used to combat *N. gonorrhea* in the 1930s. By the 1940s, however, gonococcal strains resistant to this antibiotic appeared, and the therapy of choice became penicillin. Over the next several decades, *N. gonorrhea* evolved the ability to resist penicillin, forcing clinicians to use other drugs to combat the bacterium, such as ceftriaxone and ciprofloxacin. In the 1980s, the Centers for Disease Control instituted surveillance programs to monitor antibiotic resistance patterns in different US cities. Continued success in combating *N. gonorrhea* will depend on the ability to minimize the development of antibiotic resistance.

Finally, since many patients with gonorrhea infection have no symptoms, screening programs of asymptomatic patients who are in high-risk groups (those younger than twenty-five and/or with multiple sexual partners) play a vital role in decreasing the incidence of *N. gonorrhea* infections.

—*Anne Lynn S. Chang, M.D.*

See also Bacterial infections; Blindness; Conjunctivitis; Eyes; Genital disorders, female; Genital disorders, male; Gynecology; Pelvic inflammatory disease (PID); Reproductive system; Sexually transmitted diseases (STDs); Urology.

For Further Information:

Armed Forces Health Surveillance Center. "Predictive Value of Reportable Medical Events for *Neisseria gonorrhoeae* and *Chlamydia trachomatis*. *MSMR* 20, no. 2 (February, 2013): 11–14.

Beharry, M. S., T. Shafii, G. R. Burstein. "Agnosis and Treatment of Chlamydia, Gonorrhea, and Trichomonas in Adolescents." *Pediatric Annals* 42, no. 2 (February, 2013): 26–33.

Centers for Disease Control and Prevention. *Sexually Transmitted Diseases Treatment Guidelines 2010*. Atlanta: Author, 2010.

Shmaefsky Brian R. *Gonorrhea*. 2d ed. New York: Chelsea House, 2011.

Holmes, King K., et al., eds. *Sexually Transmitted Diseases*. 4th ed. New York: McGraw-Hill Medical, 2008.

Kasper, Dennis L., et al., eds. *Harrison's Principles of Internal Medicine*. 18th ed. New York: McGraw-Hill, 2012.

Ryan, Kenneth J., and C. George Ray, eds. *Sherris Medical Microbiology: An Introduction to Infectious Diseases*. 4th ed. New York: McGraw-Hill, 2004.

Sutton, Amy L., ed. *Sexually Transmitted Diseases Sourcebook*. 5th ed. Detroit, Mich.: Omnigraphics, 2013.

GOUT
Disease/Disorder
Also known as: Gouty arthritis
Anatomy or system affected: Feet, joints
Specialties and related fields: Internal medicine, podiatry, rheumatology
Definition: A form of arthritis of the peripheral joints, often characterized by painful, recurrent acute attacks and resulting from deposits of uric acid in joint spaces.
Key terms:
acute gout: a very painful gout attack, most common in the left big toe; usually the first indicator of occurrence of the disease
arthritis: any of more than a hundred related diseases,

including gout, that are characterized by joint inflammation
cartilage: a tough, white, fibrous connective tissue attached to the bone surfaces that is involved in movement
corticosteroid: a fatlike steroid hormone made by the adrenal glands, or similar synthetic chemicals manufactured by pharmaceutical companies
gene: a piece of the hereditary material deoxyribonucleic acid (DNA) that carries the information needed to produce an inheritable characteristic
genetic engineering: also called recombinant DNA research; a group of scientific techniques that allow scientists to alter genes
hyperuricemia: the presence of abnormally high uric acid levels, which usually leads to gout symptoms
rheumatologist: a physician who studies rheumatoid arthritis and related diseases
secondary gout: gout symptoms caused by other diseases and by therapeutic drugs
synovial fluid: the thick, clear, lubricating fluid that bathes joints and helps them to move smoothly
tophaceous gout: chronic gout that may be characterized by tophi, severe joint degeneration, and/or serious kidney problems
tophi: lumps in the cartilage and joints of chronic gout sufferers, caused by crystals of uric acid

Causes and Symptoms

Gout, once called the "affliction of kings," is a hereditary disease that causes inflammation of the peripheral joints. It is also called gouty arthritis because arthritis means joint inflammation and describes a number of related diseases. Gout has afflicted humans since antiquity, and it was first described by Hippocrates in the fifth century BCE. It usually first presents itself as an extremely painful swelling of the big toe of the left foot in men over the age of forty. Gout attacks, termed acute gout, are quite rare in premenopausal women. In fact, more than 90 percent of all gout sufferers are men. The prevalence of gout is extremely high in Pacific Islanders, with nearly 7 percent of adult males afflicted. One characteristic portrayal of gout sufferers, which may come from the "affliction of kings" concept, is of obese and obviously affluent individuals. This is partly a misconception because gout can affect anyone. Nevertheless, acute gout attacks are often brought on by very rich meals or by drinking sprees, so obesity is accurately portrayed as a contributing factor. Gout is caused by high levels of uric acid in the body, which builds up

---

Information on Gout

Causes: Heredity, female hormones, disease, medications (chemotherapy, diuretics, some antibiotics)
Symptoms: Joint inflammation (particularly the big toe), scarring, and deformity
Duration: Chronic with acute episodes
Treatments: Drugs, surgery, dietary changes

during the metabolism of substances called purines. If a person eats a too many purine-rich foods or if the kidneys do not remove uric acid quickly enough, gout can occur.

An acute gout attack may occur in almost any joint, with the most common sites after the big toe being the ankles, fingers, feet, wrists, elbows, and knees. Such attacks are not often seen in the shoulders, hips, or spine and, if they do occur, appear only after a gout sufferer has had many previous attacks in other joints. Acute gout of the big toe occurs so often that it has been given its own name, podagra. Common explanations for the frequent occurrence of podagra are that considerable pressure is placed on the big toe in the process of walking and that most people are right-handed and are therefore "left-footed," putting more pressure on the left foot than on the right one in walking or in sports.

An acute gout attack is preceded by feelings of weakness, nausea, chills, and excessive urination. Then, the area that is affected becomes red to purple, swollen, and so tender that the slightest touch is very painful. This pain is so severe that many sufferers describe it as being crushing, burning, or even excruciating. Acute gout attacks come on suddenly, and many victims report suddenly being jolted awake by pain in the night. Fortunately, such attacks are few and far between and usually last only from a few days to a week. In addition, many patients who have one attack of podagra will never have another gout attack.

The problems associated with acute gout are attributable to a chemical called uric acid. Uric acid does not dissolve well in the blood and other biological fluids, such as the synovial fluid in joints. When overproduced by the body or excreted too slowly in urine, undissolved uric acid forms sharp crystals. These crystals and their interactions with other joint components cause the pain felt by gout sufferers. It is interesting to note that gout is caused by the overproduction of uric acid in some individuals and by uric acid underexcretion in others. Many of the foods that seem to cause gout are rich in chemicals called purines, which are converted to uric acid in the course of preparation for excretion by the kidneys.

Much more dangerous to gout victims than the acute attacks is leaving the disease untreated. When this happens, crystals of uric acid produce lumps or masses in the joints throughout the body and in the kidneys. In the joints, the masses, called tophi, lead to inflammation, scarring, and deformity that can produce an irreversible degenerative process. Tophi are most common in the fingers and the cartilage of various parts of the body, and external tophi are found in the cartilage of the ears of gout sufferers. The visible tophi, however, are only representative, and undetected uric acid masses may be widely spread throughout the body. Such untreated gout is called chronic or tophaceous gout.

Tophaceous gout is another disease with a long history. It was first described by the Greek physician Galen in the second century CE. Another extremely dangerous aspect of tophaceous gout is unseen kidney stones, which will cause great pain on urination, produce high blood pressure, and even cause fatal liver failure if left untreated.

The prime indicator of gout is high blood levels of uric acid, called hyperuricemia; however, this condition, without other symptoms, does not always signal existent, symptomatic gout. Therefore, the best indicator of the presence of the disease is a combination of hyperuricemia, acute attacks, and observed uric acid in the synovial fluid of all troublesome, gouty joints.

Some investigators propose that gout sufferers are highly intelligent because such famous individuals as Michelangelo, Leonardo da Vinci, Martin Luther, Charles Darwin, and Benjamin Franklin were afflicted with the disease. This trend, however, may indicate that famous people are usually able to afford a lifestyle that causes the predilection to high uric acid levels (for example, the eating of purine-rich foods and high alcohol consumption). Rheumatologists who have studied gout would argue that alcoholism is a better predictor for the disease because gout is common in heavy drinkers. In fact, studies in which gout patients were given purine-rich diets or purine-rich diets plus alcoholic beverages showed that alcohol increased the number and severity of gout attacks.

Gout is also associated with a number of other diseases, including Down syndrome, lead poisoning, some types of diabetes, psoriasis, and kidney disease. Furthermore, a number of therapeutic drugs used in chemotherapy for cancer, diuretics, and some antibiotics can cause acute gout symptoms. These types of gout are differentiated from the hereditary disease already described—so-called primary gout—by the term "secondary gout." Drug-induced secondary gout goes away quickly when the administration of the offending drug is stopped.

Another group of diseases that have symptoms somewhat

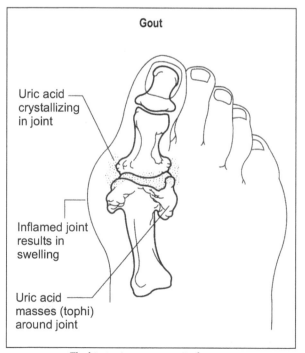

Gout

Uric acid crystallizing in joint

Inflamed joint results in swelling

Uric acid masses (tophi) around joint

The big toe is a common site for gout.

similar to gout are called pseudogout. They have an entirely different cause (mineral crystals in the joints), occur in men and women with equal frequency, usually begin in extreme old age, and are treated quite differently.

It is also interesting that while premenopausal women are nearly gout-free, the disease becomes increasingly common after menopause. This fact supports a role for female hormones in preventing the disease. Primary gout in women is usually much more severe and destructive than gout in men. In those families in which maternal gout is observed, it is likely that occurrence of the disease in male offspring will occur earlier than is usual, such as near the age of thirty.

Treatment and Therapy

Once primary gout has been diagnosed, three methods are available for treating it: therapeutic drugs, surgery, and special diets. Most often, gout treatment uses therapeutic drugs, with the drug of choice being colchicine. Colchicine treatment can be traced back for thousands of years, to Egypt in 1500 BCE. Originally, it was given as an extract of the meadow saffron plant, *Colchicum autumnale*. In modern times, the pure chemical has been isolated for medicinal use.

Colchicine is reportedly a specific remedy for gout and has no effect on any other type of arthritis. In fact, the reversal of severe joint pain with colchicine is often used as a diagnostic tool that tells physicians that the joint disease being treated is indeed gout. Colchicine can be utilized to treat acute gout attacks or can be taken routinely for long periods of time. Its actions in the handling of acute attacks are quick and profound. In some cases, however, colchicine will have side effects, including severe stomach cramps, nausea, and diarrhea. When these effects occur, colchicine use is discontinued until they disappear, and then its use is reinstituted.

Most of the basis for colchicine action is its decrease of the inflammation that causes the pain of gout attacks. This action is believed to be attributable to colchicine's interaction with white blood cells that destroy uric acid crystals and subsequent prevention of the cells from releasing inflammatory factors. Other drugs that work in this way are nonsteroidal anti-inflammatory drugs (NSAIDs) such as aspirin, ibuprofen, indomethacin, naproxen, and phenylbutazone. Colchicine and NSAIDs are usually given by mouth. In some cases, anti-inflammatory steroid hormones called corticosteroids, such as prednisone and prednisolone, are used to treat acute gout. The corticosteroids are given by injection into the gouty joint. Despite the rapid, almost miraculous effects of these steroids, they are best avoided unless absolutely necessary because they can lead to serious medical problems.

Another group of antigout medications consists of the uricosuric drugs. Two favored examples of such drugs are probenecid (Benemid) and sulfinpyrazone (Anturane). These medications are given to patients whose kidneys underexcrete uric acid. The uricosuric drugs prevent the occurrence of hyperuricemia and eventual tophaceous gout by increasing uric acid excretion in the urine, therefore lowering the uric acid levels in the blood. This lowering has two ef-

fects: the prevention of the attainment of uric acid levels in the blood and joints that lead to crystal or tophus formation and the eventual dissolution of crystals and tophi as blood levels of uric acid drop.

Uricosuric drugs have no effect, however, on an acute gout attack and can sometimes make such attacks even more painful. For this reason, uricosuric drug therapy is always started after all acute gout attack symptoms have subsided. Aspirin blocks the effects of the uricosuric drugs and should be replaced with acetaminophen (for example, Tylenol). Side effects of excessive doses of uricosuric drugs can include headache, nausea and vomiting, itching, and dizziness. Their use should be discontinued immediately when such symptoms occur. Later reuse of the uricosuric drugs is usually possible.

The third category of antigout drugs is a single chemical, allopurinol (usually, Lopurin or Zyloprim). This drug lowers the body's ability to produce uric acid. It is highly recommended for all gout-afflicted people who have kidney disease that is severe enough for kidney stones to form. It has undesired side effects, however, that include skin rashes, drowsiness, a diminished blood count, and severe allergic reactions. As a result, the use of allopurinol is disqualified for many patients. One advantage of allopurinol chemotherapy over the use of uricosuric agents is the fact that it can be taken along with aspirin.

The end result of a chemotherapeutic regimen with uricosuric drugs and/or allopurinol is the lowering of the blood and urinary uric acid levels so that crystals and tophi do not form or, where formed, redissolve. Often, their combination with colchicine is useful for preventing the occurrence of gout attacks during the initial chemotherapy period.

While surgery is not a common treatment for gout, people who have large tophi that have opened up, become infected, or interfere with joint mobility may elect to have them removed in this fashion. In some cases, severe disability or joint pain caused by the degenerative effects of long-term tophaceous gout is also corrected surgically. Care should be taken, however, to evaluate the consequences of such surgery carefully because the postoperative healing process is often quite slow and many other problems can be encountered.

Media sources often praise special diets in treating gout, without firm proof of their effectiveness. The finding that gout is usually a hereditary disease resulting from metabolic defects that either prevent uric acid excretion or cause its accumulation has underscored that most dietary factors have a relatively small effect on the disease. Consequently, chemotherapy is much more effective than dietary intervention for diminishing gout symptoms. Nevertheless, there are several incontestable dietary aspects essential to the well-being of persons afflicted with gout.

First, dieting is quite useful, and overweight gout sufferers should lose weight. Such action is best taken slowly and under medical supervision. In fact, excessively fast weight loss can temporarily worsen gout symptoms by elevating blood uric acid levels. In addition, gout sufferers should limit their intake of a number of foods because they are overly rich in the purines that give rise to uric acid when the body processes them. Some examples are the organ meats (liver, kidneys, and sweetbreads), mushrooms, anchovies, sardines, caviar, gravy and meat extracts, shellfish, wine, and beer. Modest intake of these foods is allowable. For example, the daily intake of one can of beer, a glass of wine, or an ounce or two of hard liquor is permissible. The gout sufferer should remember that excessive alcohol intake often brings on acute gout attacks and, even worse, will contribute to worsening tophus and kidney stone formation.

Another adjunct to the prevention or diminution of gout symptoms is the daily intake of at least a half gallon of water or other nonalcoholic beverages. This will help to flush uric acid out of the body in the urine, and may help to dissipate both tophi and kidney stones. Plain water is best, as it contains no calories that will increase body weight, potentially aggravating gout and leading to other health problems.

Perspective and Prospects

Many sources agree that if primary gout is under the control of afflicted patients, they can look forward to a normal life without permanent adverse effects from the disease. Those individuals who seek medical treatment at the first appearance of gout symptoms may combine chemotherapy, an appropriate diet regimen, and alcohol avoidance to prevent all but a few acute attacks of the disease. In addition, they will not develop tophi or kidney problems.

Even those afflicted persons who put off treatment until kidney stones or tophi appear can be helped easily. Again, an appropriate diet and chemotherapy agents will make up the principal treatment. Only the patients who neglect all gout treatment until excessive joint damage and severe kidney disease occur are at serious risk, yet even with these individuals, remission of most severe symptoms is usually possible. The long-term neglect of gout symptoms is unwise, however, because severe tophaceous gout can be both deforming and fatal.

Currently, the eradication of most primary gout, not gout treatment, is seen as the desired goal of research. It is believed that a prime methodology for the eradication of gout will be the use of genetic engineering for gene replacement therapy. Primary gout sufferers are victims of gene lesion diseases: Their bodies lack the ability, because of defective genes, to control either the production or the excretion of uric acid. It is hoped that gene replacement technology will enable medical science to add the missing genes back into their bodies. Other research aspects viewed worthy of exploration in the attempts to vanquish primary gout are the understanding of how to cause white blood cells to destroy uric acid crystals in the joints more effectively and safely and to decode the basis for the gout-preventing effects of female hormones related to their presence in premenopausal women.

—*Sanford S. Singer, Ph.D.*

See also Alcoholism; Arthritis; Down syndrome; Feet; Foot disorders; Inflammation; Joints; Lead poisoning; Obesity; Podiatry; Rheumatology; Urinary disorders.

For Further Information:

Devlin, Thomas M., ed. *Textbook of Biochemistry: With Clinical Correlations.* 7th ed. Hoboken, N.J.: Wiley-Liss, 2010.
Fries, James F. *Arthritis: A Take-Care-of-Yourself Health Guide for Understanding Your Arthritis.* 5th ed. Reading, Mass.: Addison-Wesley, 1999.
Hollenstein, Jenna. "Gout." *Health Library*, September 1, 2011.
Parker, James N., and Philip M. Parker, eds. *The Official Patient's Sourcebook on Gout.* Rev ed. San Diego, Calif.: Icon Health, 2005.
Porter, Robert S., and Justin L. Kaplan, eds. *The Merck Manual of Diagnosis and Therapy.* 19th ed. Whitehouse Station, N.J.: Merck, 2011.
Schumacher, H. Ralph. "Gout." *American College of Rheumatology*, September 2012.
Scriver, Charles R., et al., eds. *The Metabolic and Molecular Basis of Inherited Disease.* 8th ed. New York: McGraw-Hill, 2001.
"What Is Gout?" *National Institute of Arthritis and Musculoskeletal and Skin Diseases*, July 2010.

GRAFTS AND GRAFTING
Procedure
Anatomy or system affected: All
Specialties and related fields: Critical care, dermatology, emergency medicine, general surgery, genetics, immunology, neurology, physical therapy, plastic surgery
Definition: The transplantation of tissue from one part of the body to another or from one individual to another in order to treat disease or injury; such surgery requires careful genetic matching in order to avoid a harmful immune response.

Key terms:

allograft: a graft of tissue from one individual to another individual (usually between close relatives)

autograft: a graft of tissue from one part of an individual's body to another part

graft-versus-host disease (GVHD): a genetic incompatibility between tissues in which immune system cells from the grafted tissue attack host tissue

histocompatibility: tissue compatibility, as determined by histocompatibility protein antigens present on the cell membranes of all tissue cells

histology: the study of tissues and their development, roles, and locations within the body

host-versus-graft disease (HVGD): a tissue rejection in which the immune system cells of the graft recipient attack the grafted tissue from a donor individual

immune response: the reaction of an intricate system of cells that identify, attack, immobilize, and remove foreign tissue from the body through chemical signals

leukocytes: white blood cells, immune system cells which either produce antibodies or phagocytically consume cells and tissues that are genetically foreign in nature

tissue: a specialized region of cells that forms organs within the body; the four principal types are epithelial, connective, nervous, and muscular

totipotence: the capacity for cells of a given tissue type to regenerate and replace killed or damaged cells within a given body region

Indications and Procedures

In medicine, a graft is a tissue region which is transferred from one part of the body to another body part (autograft) or from one individual to another individual (allograft). Grafts between individuals of differing species (xenografts) also are possible. The actual transfer of tissue is called a transplant. The identification and matching of appropriate tissue types and the surgical connection of the tissue constitute grafting.

Examples of autografts include the use of leg veins to reconstruct the coronary arteries during heart bypass surgery, skin transplants during reconstructive facial surgery, and thumb/big toe interposable transplants following the loss of a hand or foot digit. Examples of allografts include major organ transplantations (including that of the heart, liver, and kidney), bone marrow transplantation, and blood transfusions between two genetically matched individuals. Xenograft examples include the grafting of animal tissue such as skin or stomach epithelia to the equivalent body parts in humans.

Genetic matching of donor and recipient tissues in grafting and transplantation is critical to the success of the tissue graft. Thus, tissue compatibility, termed histocompatibility, is of primary importance for successful grafting. Autografts are the most successful grafts because they occur on the same individual, and consequently there is no genetic difference between donor and recipient cells. As the genetic difference between donors and graft recipients increases, however, the probability decreases that a graft will be successful.

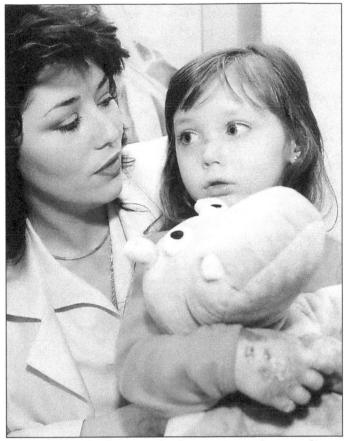

A four-year-old girl with a genetic skin disease waits to undergo a grafting procedure using laboratory-grown skin. (AP/Wide World Photos)

For example, grafts between identical twins are highly successful because the donor and recipient are genetically identical; hence, the situation is the same as an autograft. Grafts between siblings are likely to succeed. Allografts between people having distinct genetic differences, however, are less likely to succeed. Xenografts are extremely difficult except for basic mammalian tissues, such as epithelial tissue.

Histology is the study of tissues and their development within the human body. The four principal tissue types within the human body and within other mammalian species are epithelial tissue, which lines the inside and outside surfaces of organs throughout the body; connective tissue (such as cartilage, bone, fat, and blood), which provides structure or transport throughout the body; nervous tissue, which conducts electrical impulses as information networks throughout the body; and muscular tissue, which provides contractility and movement for various body parts. All organs consist of a specific pattern of these four tissues: Epithelial tissue provides cover and protection, connective tissue provides support, nervous tissue provides information from the central control regions of the brain, and muscular tissue allows responses to localized change in the organ. In addition, the cells of tissues subspecialize for unique roles within the tissue of which they

are a part. For example, nervous system cells may specialize to form receiving sensory neurons or transmitting motor neurons.

Regardless of tissue type, each of the thousand trillion cells in an individual possesses the same basic genes as the others, and therefore many of the same proteins are expressed throughout the body. All cells within an individual have proteins located within the lipid bilayers of their cell membranes. Several of these proteins are located on every single cell of the individual and thus serve as genetic identification markers for the individual's immune system. These cell surface identification proteins are called histocompatibility proteins.

The histocompatibility proteins, of which there are many, are encoded by a battery of human genes called the major histocompatibility complex (MHC). These proteins ensure tissue compatibility for all cells in an individual with respect to that individual's immune system. The cells of the immune system recognize the specific histocompatibility proteins of one's own cells as "self" markers. Foreign cells, which are missing a few or many of the individual's specific set of histocompatibility proteins, are recognized by the immune system as "nonself" and are attacked. This self-versus-nonself reaction is how the immune system distinguishes its own cells from any invading foreign cells and tissues. Therefore, the histocompatibility proteins play a critical role in the successful identification of one's own cells and the destruction of infections, such as those caused by bacterial or fungal cells.

An immune response occurs when immune system cells called leukocytes (white blood cells) cannot locate the specific "self" histocompatibility proteins on a sampled cell. A type of leukocyte called a T lymphocyte will release a protein called immunoglobulin to immobilize the foreign "nonself" cell lacking the correct histocompatibility antigens (the proteins on the cell membranes). Immunoglobulins, also called antibodies, are proteins secreted by T lymphocytes to immobilize foreign antigens.

After the T lymphocyte antibodies have immobilized the antigens on the foreign cells, another type of leukocyte called a B lymphocyte produces antibodies that attack the foreign antigens. Furthermore, the B lymphocytes will multiply themselves, creating millions of copies to produce a clone army of B lymphocytes, all of which make the same antibodies targeted at the same foreign antigens. These specialized clones constitute a memory cell line, which will attack these antigens again if the organism is exposed to them in the future. This reaction is the basis of immunization.

Furthermore, after the T and B lymphocyte antibodies immobilize the foreign antigens, phagocytic leukocytes such as neutrophils and macrophages migrate to the region to ingest and completely destroy the foreign cells. This process will continue until either the foreign cells are vanquished or the immune system is exhausted.

The immune response just described may appear simple, but it is very complicated. In addition to the complex chemical identification of histocompatibility proteins on all of an individual's cells, the production of specific antibodies by T and B lymphocytes involves an extraordinary rearrangement of genes within these immune cells that is still poorly understood.

The immune response directly affects grafts and grafting. For transplants performed between two individuals, most tissues require a close genetic match between the donor and the recipient. They should be as closely related to each other as possible so that they share a common genetic heritage and, therefore, a high probability that their respective cells have most, if not all, of the same histocompatibility proteins. A close genetic relationship between the graft donor and recipient maximizes the chance that a graft will succeed and that an immune response against nonself tissues will not occur.

Uses and Complications

Grafts, grafting, and transplants between individuals are extremely important in the treatment of maiming or disfiguring accidents and life-threatening diseases. A huge demand exists for grafted tissue, not merely organ transplants, for use in a variety of medical conditions and procedures.

The most common and successful types of grafts are autografts from one part of an individual's body to another part, or from one identical twin to her or his sibling. In autograft cases, there is a perfect match for the histocompatibility proteins on all the cells and tissues. Thus, an immune response will not occur unless the immune system is abnormal in some way, as with such autoimmune diseases as lupus erythematosus and rheumatoid arthritis.

An example of an autograft is the transfer of a vein from the leg to the heart in a patient suffering from coronary artery disease; the grafted vein serves as a replacement coronary artery, supplying blood, nutrients, and oxygen to the heart muscle. Another type of autograft is the transfer of skin from the abdomen or pelvic region to the face as part of reconstructive plastic surgery. A severed thumb can be replaced by the big toe, its equivalent digit on the foot.

Allografts, those between different individuals, can be successful if there is careful genetic matching between the donor and recipient tissues. Because of the specificity of matching for certain tissue and cell types, donor-recipient matching may mean an average of any two people out of a thousand or, with more critical tissue lines such as stem cells, two people out of ten million. Often, siblings will serve as tissue donors. Otherwise, the lengthy process of finding possible tissue donors and determining their specific histocompatibility profiles must be conducted before the graft can take place between a recipient and a matched tissue donor.

Grafts are simple between generalized surface tissue such as epithelial and connective tissues. Pig epithelial tissue has been used for skin and stomach tissue grafts on human recipients. Bone marrow transplants for aplastic anemia and leukemia patients, however, require more difficult histocompatibility matching. The use of fetal nervous tissue grafts into the brain tissue of Alzheimer's disease patients has yielded promising results in regenerating brain tissue and slowing the acceleration of this debilitating disease, which generally strikes the elderly.

Grafts are useful for tissue lines lacking totipotence, the ability to regenerate damaged or dead cells. The example cited above of fetal tissue being used to treat Alzheimer's disease is a clear illustration of such tissue-grafting applications. Mature brain tissue in adult humans cannot regenerate. Fetal tissue grafts, however, have facilitated the regenerative capacity of some brain tissue in these patients.

Likewise, stem cell lines such as the red bone marrow of flat bones, where white blood cells (leukocytes) and red blood cells (erythrocytes) are manufactured, are important targets for tissue grafting. In leukemia, a patient's bone marrow is rapidly producing malignant leukocytes. It is clear that the stem cell line producing these cells is aberrant in such patients. Consequently, a small graft of bone marrow tissue from a histocompatible donor's bone marrow may lead to the establishment of a healthy stem cell line in the patient to stop the overproduction of aberrant cells.

In any grafting process, the donor tissue is surgically inserted and secured into the recipient's tissue site. There, the tissue, if the graft is successful, can grow and expand into the localized organ region to perform its correct function in the individual's body. In the event that there is not a histocompatible match between the donor tissue within the recipient's body, two possible rejection mechanisms can ensue. In host-versus-graft disease (HVGD), which is the most common type, the recipient's immune system releases antibodies and eventually destroys the donor tissue. In graft-versus-host disease (GVHD), immune system cells transplanted with the donor tissue into the recipient migrate into the recipient's tissues and attack the cells; the recipient will become ill and may die. The grafted tissue has rejected the entire body into which it has been transferred.

Perspective and Prospects

In 1990, the Nobel Prize in Physiology or Medicine was awarded to American medical researchers Joseph E. Murray of the Harvard Medical School and E. Donnall Thomas of Seattle's Fred Hutchinson Cancer Research Center. These two scientists were pioneers in the use of grafts, grafting, and tissue transplants to save people's lives. Murray performed the first successful kidney transplant, between two identical twins, in 1954. Murray teamed with Thomas at Harvard to study methods for preventing host-versus-graft rejections. During the 1960s at the University of Washington, Thomas developed the technique of destroying a potential bone marrow recipient's immune system using radiation, followed by the grafting of donor bone marrow tissue into the patient, thereby increasing the chances that the transplant will succeed before the patient's immune system can become active again. Both scientists also made important discoveries concerning the major histocompatibility proteins.

Grafts and grafting play a vital role in medicine. Grafts can save the lives of people with such diseases as leukemia, anemia, and cancer. Grafts also can be useful in reconstructing damaged organs and skin, especially for burn victims. Still, much research is needed to understand histocompatibility better and to reduce the chance of tissue rejection.

—*David Wason Hollar, Jr., Ph.D.*

See also Alzheimer's disease; Amputation; Blood vessels; Bone grafting; Bone marrow transplantation; Breast surgery; Burns and scalds; Cleft lip and palate repair; Corneal transplantation; Critical care; Critical care, pediatric; Dermatology; Dermatopathology; Emergency medicine; Facial transplantation; Fetal tissue transplantation; Hair transplantation; Heart transplantation; Heart valve replacement; Immune system; Kidney transplantation; Laceration repair; Lesions; Leukemia; Liver transplantation; Pigmentation; Plastic surgery; Skin; Skin lesion removal; Transplantation; Xenotransplantation.

For Further Information:

Adelman, Daniel C., et al., eds. *Manual of Allergy and Immunology.* 4th ed. Philadelphia: Lippincott Williams & Wilkins, 2002.

Alberts, Bruce, et al. *Molecular Biology of the Cell.* 5th ed. New York: Garland, 2008.

Beck, William S., Karel F. Liem, and George Gaylord Simpson. *Life: An Introduction to Biology.* 3d ed. New York: HarperCollins, 1991.

"Bone Marrow Transplant." *MedlinePlus,* February 7, 2012.

Cohen, Barbara J. *Memmler's The Human Body in Health and Disease.* 11th ed. Philadelphia: Wolters Kluwer Health/Lippincott Williams & Wilkins, 2009.

Eisen, Herman N. *General Immunology: An Introduction to Molecular and Cellular Principles of the Immune Response.* 3d ed. Philadelphia: J. B. Lippincott, 1990.

Kindt, Thomas J., Richard A. Goldsby, and Barbara A. Osborne. *Kuby Immunology.* 6th ed. New York: W. H. Freeman, 2007.

Palca, Joseph. "Overcoming Rejection to Win a Nobel Prize." *Science* 250 (October 19, 1990): 378.

"Skin Graft." *Health Library,* November 26, 2012.

Wood, Debra. "Bone Graft." *Health Library,* December 21, 2011.

GRAM STAINING

Procedure

Anatomy or system affected: Cells, immune system

Specialties and related fields: Bacteriology, biochemistry, cytology, microbiology

Definition: A staining process used as a means of differentiating microorganisms, which are classified as either gram-positive or gram-negative.

Key terms:

cell wall: a structure outside the cell membrane of most bacteria, composed of varying amounts of carbohydrates, lipids, and amino acids

gram-negative: referring to microorganisms that appear pink following the Gram-staining procedure

gram-positive: referring to microorganisms that appear violet following the Gram-staining procedure

Gram's stain: a method of staining bacteria as a primary means of differentiation and identification

lipopolysaccharide (LPS): a major component of the cell wall of gram-negative bacteria; the toxicity of LPS is associated with illnesses caused by gram-negative organisms

mordant: a chemical that acts to fix a stain within a physical structure; the role played by iodine in Gram's stain

peptidoglycans: repeating units of sugar derivatives that make up a rigid layer of bacterial cell walls; found in both gram-positive and gram-negative cells

Indications and Procedures

The observation and identification of bacteria are of obvious primary importance in the study of microorganisms. Even with the use of powerful microscopes, direct observation of unstained bacteria is difficult. The use of stains to increase their contrast with the background allows bacteria to be observed more easily.

As a result of resident acidic groups—polysaccharides or nucleic acids—the surfaces of bacteria tend to be negatively charged. Conversely, the dye portion of common stains such as methylene blue or crystal violet consists of positively charged ions. For staining purposes, a sample of bacteria is placed on a glass slide and allowed to dry. The solution of stain is flooded over the bacterial "smear" for about a minute, and the slide is then rinsed. The main purpose of such simple stains is to allow the cells to be observed.

In contrast with simple stains, differential staining methods do not stain all cells in the same manner. Bacteria grown under different environmental conditions, or bacteria that may differ from one another in their physical structure, will exhibit different staining properties when treated with differential stains. Gram staining (also called Gram's stain) is an example of a differential stain.

Gram staining is a relatively simple procedure and is among the first practices learned by students in microbiology laboratories. The process begins with the preparation of a bacterial smear on the slide. A stain, crystal violet, is allowed to flood the dried smear. The slide is rinsed, and a solution of iodine is dropped over the smear. The iodine functions as a mordant, fixing the crystal violet into a complex insoluble in water. Following another rinse, the smear is covered with either an alcohol or an acetone "destaining" solution for several seconds, rinsed again, and counterstained with the red dye safranin. After a last wash, the bacteria are observed with a microscope. If they were not destained by the alcohol step, retaining the blue or violet color, they are considered gram-positive; if they have stained pink because of the counterstain safranin, they are considered gram-negative.

The precise means by which gram staining works is not entirely clear. The cell wall structure of gram-positive bacteria either prevents the alcohol/acetone solution from removing the crystal violet-iodine complex from the cell or prevents the solution from having access to the complex. Though the question remains whether the cell wall structure is the sole determining factor in the differential procedure, there is no doubt that the cell wall features are primary factors in the determination of gram-staining results. Therefore, the structure of the cell wall in most bacteria reflects the gram-staining characteristics.

The cell wall structure found in gram-positive bacteria differs significantly from that in gram-negative cells. While both contain a rigid layer called the peptidoglycan, the peptidoglycan layer is much thicker and makes up a significantly larger portion of the cell wall in gram-positive bacteria. In contrast, a significant portion of the cell wall found in gram-negative bacteria is composed of lipid derivatives.

The peptidoglycan portion of the cell is composed of repeating units of two sugar derivatives: N-acetylglucosamine and N-acetylmuramic acid. The peptidoglycan within the wall is in the form of sheets, layered on top of one another. In gram-positive bacteria, approximately 90 percent of the cell wall material consists of peptidoglycan; among gram-negative bacteria, about 10 percent of the wall is represented by this rigid layer.

These cell wall structures are stabilized by short chains of amino acids that cross-link the layers of peptidoglycan. Formation of the cross bridges is an enzymatic process called transpeptidation. The antibiotic penicillin inhibits the enzyme that carries out the formation of such cross-links. The result is a weakening in the cell wall, and possibly cell death. Since the peptidoglycan layer of gram-negative bacteria represents a much smaller proportion of the cell wall, such microorganisms are often more resistant to the action of penicillin than are gram-positive bacteria.

During the gram-staining procedure, decolorization of the cell is carried out during the wash with alcohol or acetone. The thick peptidoglycan layer found in gram-positive bacteria, however, prevents movement of the crystal violet-iodine complex from the cell. Thus, the cells do not decolorize; they retain their violet appearance.

The peptidoglycan layer is a small proportion of the gram-negative cell wall. Much of the outer wall in these bacteria is a layer of lipopolysaccharide (LPS), which acts as a physical barrier but also contains pharmacological properties. The LPS layer is a complex structure containing a lipid portion (lipid A), a core polysaccharide consisting of a variety of sugars, and an outer layer of branched sugars called the O-region (O-polysaccharide). The LPS layer is anchored to the thin peptidoglycan portion of the cell wall through a lipoprotein complex. The LPS portion of gram-negative cell walls is often termed the endotoxin because of its pharmacological activity. Release of LPS as a result of cell death during certain types of infection can result in high fever or shock.

Since the cell wall of gram-negative bacteria contains proportionately little peptidoglycan, the crystal violet-iodine complex is easily removed during the gram-staining procedure. Following the alcohol step, the cells again appear colorless. Therefore, when they are counterstained with the safranin, the bacteria will appear pink.

An evaluation of gram-staining characteristics is generally the first step in the identification of newly isolated bacteria. Most bacteria can be classified as either gram-positive or gram-negative, and this step, along with characterization of the shape of the organism, is of immense importance in narrowing down the possible identities of an isolate.

Further means of identification generally involve the use of selective or differential types of media. These processes use the biochemical properties of bacteria for their identification. A selective medium is one in which chemical compounds have been added that inhibit the growth of certain forms of bacteria but allow the growth of others. For example, the chemical dye eosin-methylene blue (EMB) inhibits the growth of gram-positive bacteria while allowing gram-negative bacteria to grow. If a mixed culture of bacteria is inoculated onto EMB medium, only the gram-negative microorganisms will grow. A differential medium will allow a variety of bacteria to grow, but different types of bacteria may produce different reactions on the medium. Since EMB agar contains lactose as a carbon source, it is also a differential medium. Bacteria that ferment lactose produce a green metallic color of colony on EMB; bacteria that do not ferment lactose produce a pink colony.

Biochemical tests are more useful for the identification of organisms that are gram-negative than for those that are gram-positive. Biochemical variations among both genera and species of gram-positive bacteria tend to be too variable for effective identification of these organisms. By contrast, such biochemical results among gram-negative bacteria generally do not vary significantly within the species and hence are useful means of further identification.

The biochemical tests used for identification of gram-negative bacteria can be summarized in the form of a flowchart. Such charts represent the series of tests that divide bacteria into smaller and smaller groups. For example, following a determination of morphological and gram-staining characteristics, differential tests may be carried out to observe the ability of the bacteria to ferment various types of carbohydrates. A series of broths containing such sugars as glucose, lactose, or sucrose are inoculated. Generally, a pH indicator such as the chemical phenol red is included, as is an inverted glass tube (Durham tube) for observation of gas production. If the organism can ferment lactose and produces acid and gas, the broth tube of lactose will appear yellow and there will be a gas bubble in the Durham tube. If the organism does not ferment lactose, no growth or change from the red color of the broth will be observed in that tube.

Further differentiation of either lactose-positive or lactose-negative organisms, to continue with this particular example, can be carried out with other biochemical tests. Certain species of bacteria are capable of removing a molecule of carbon dioxide from amino acids; others are not. In some cases, multiple tests can be run at the same time. For example, a common differential test for gram-negative bacteria uses a medium called triple sugar iron (TSI) agar. TSI agar contains a small amount of glucose and larger amounts of lactose and sucrose, hence the designation of triple sugar. Iron is also contained in the medium. The agar is prepared in a test tube and allowed to harden on a slant. Organisms are inoculated onto the surface of the slant and stabbed into the butt of the slant. If glucose alone is fermented, only enough acid is produced to turn the butt yellow. If either lactose or sucrose is fermented, both the slant and butt of the agar will turn yellow. Production of hydrogen sulfide gas is indicated by a black precipitate from iron sulfide; other gas production is indicated by bubble formation in the region of the stab. In this manner, inoculation of a single type of medium can provide multiple tests for identification.

At one time, each of these differential tests had to be carried out individually. Beginning in the 1970s, however, a variety of media kits became available that allow fifteen to twenty tests to be run simultaneously. These kits consist of strips of miniaturized versions of biochemical tests that permit the rapid identification of gram-negative bacteria.

Even though some biochemical tests are less helpful in the identification of gram-positive bacteria, some characteristics of these organisms can be used. These organisms may be round (cocci) or rod-shaped (bacilli). If bacilli, they may be aerobic (they utilize oxygen) or anaerobic (they do not utilize oxygen). By testing for coagulase, an enzyme that will cause the coagulation of plasma, cocci can be further differentiated.

Finally, serological methods can be used in the identification of either gram-positive or gram-negative organisms. In these tests, a fluorescent dye is attached to molecules of antibodies, proteins directed against the surface molecules of specific bacteria. The ability of the antibodies to attach to bacteria is indicative of the species.

Uses and Complications

The use of gram-staining methodology is arguably the single most important step in the identification of microorganisms; its applications are far-ranging. Most diseases of humans and other animals, as well as of plants, are caused by microorganisms. Isolation and identification of disease-causing bacteria are key aspects in understanding the etiology of such diseases. Many aspects of technology, from the discovery or development of new antibiotics to the development of new strains of microbes, utilize such methodologies as gram's stain in the identification of fresh isolates.

Clinical methods for the identification of infectious agents follow a series of defined steps. The particular material involved depends on the type and site of infection and can include such fluids as blood, urine, pus, or saliva. The specific symptoms of the illness may also provide clues as to the particular agents involved.

For example, among the most common infections are those of the urinary tract. These are particularly common nosocomial, or hospital-acquired, infections. A clean-voided or catheter-collected urine specimen is inoculated onto a plate containing selective or differential agar media using a calibrated loop. The number of bacterial colonies that grow after incubation can then be counted to estimate the concentration of bacteria present in the urine. This helps determine if an infection is present. Generally speaking, such infections are usually associated with gram-negative bacteria. The majority of these infections, about 90 percent, are caused by *Escherichia coli* (*E. coli*), a common intestinal organism. To a lesser extent, such infections may be associated with other genera such as *Klebsiella*, *Pseudomonas*, *Proteus*, or *Streptococcus*. All but *Streptococcus* are gram-negative bacilli.

Confirmation of the gram morphology follows growth on selective media. The media of choice in this example are those selective for gram-negative bacteria: either eosin-methylene blue or MacConkey agars. Both inhibit the replication of bacteria such as *Staphylococcus*, commonly found on the surface of the skin and a possible contaminant during the swabbing of the site of infection.

The presence of the sugar lactose in either MacConkey or EMB agar allows these media to be differential in addition to being selective. Lactose fermenters such as *Escherichia*, *Klebsiella*, or *Enterobacter* will produce pink colonies on MacConkey agar, while gram-negative organisms such as *Proteus*, *Pseudomonas*, or *Salmonella*, which do not ferment lactose, will produce colorless colonies on this medium. Analogous results can be seen with other differential enteric agars. More detailed types of analysis using other forms of media or utilizing immunological methods may be necessary to fine-tune the diagnosis, or antibiotic susceptibility tests may simply be conducted to determine the treatment of choice.

In some instances, gram morphology may be sufficient for the identification of a microorganism. For example, the presence of gram-negative cocci in a cervical smear from a patient suspected of having contracted a sexually transmitted disease is indicative of a *Neisseria gonorrhea* infection. The identification can be confirmed using immunological methods or through growth on selective media such as Thayer-Martin agar, which contains antibiotics inhibitory to most other gram-negative bacteria.

If the clinical sample consists of blood or cerebrospinal fluid, both of which are normally sterile, either gram-negative or gram-positive organisms may be involved. The initial step toward identification is a gram stain of the material. Gram-negative bacteria can be identified using methods already described. Generally speaking, the bacterial content of blood during bacteremia will be too low for ready observation. For this reason, blood samples are inoculated into bottles of nonselective growth media, one of which is grown under aerobic conditions and one under anaerobic conditions. If and when growth becomes apparent, smears are prepared for gram staining.

Gram-positive cocci will almost always be members of either of two genera: *Staphylococcus* or *Streptococcus*. The two can be differentiated on the basis of catalase production, an enzyme which degrades hydrogen peroxide; staphylococci produce the enzyme, while streptococci do not. A variety of commercial kits are available for rapid identification of species. These contain a battery of tests based on biochemical properties of the organisms, including tolerance of high salt, fermentation of unusual sugars, and growth characteristics on blood agar plates (nutrient agar containing sheep red blood cells).

The identification of gram-positive bacilli is more difficult, given their biochemical variation even within the genus. The major subdivisions of this group are based on their tolerance of oxygen. Obligate gram-positive anaerobes, organisms that cannot tolerate oxygen, include the genus *Clostridium*, members of which cause tetanus, gangrene, and food poisoning. Aerobes and facultative anaerobes, which are oxygen-tolerant, include the genera *Bacillus*, *Corynebacterium*, and *Listeria*. Further identification often requires immunological means.

The gram-negative bacillus *E. coli* is frequently used as a marker for sewage contamination of water supplies. Since it is a common intestinal organism and rarely found in soil, its presence in water samples is indicative of possible fecal contamination of that water. Testing for the presence and level of *E. coli* utilizes the biochemical properties of the microbe. Various quantities of the water sample are placed in tubes of lactose broth; growth is indicative of a lactose fermenter and is presumptive for the presence of *E. coli*. A sample of the lactose culture is then streaked on EMB agar. The development of metallic green-colored colonies of gram-negative bacilli confirms the presence of *E. coli*. The smaller the volume of the water sample that produced growth in lactose, the higher the level of *E. coli* in that sample. In a sense, *E. coli* serves as a surrogate marker in these tests. It may not itself be a pathogen (though some strains of *E. coli* may indeed cause severe intestinal infections), but other gram-negative intestinal pathogens such as *Salmonella*, *Shigella*, or *Vibrio*, even if present in water supplies, may be in a concentration too low for ready detection. Therefore, the presence of *E. coli* suggests possible fecal contamination, allowing for proper sewage treatment. Conversely, the absence of *E. coli* in the water sample indicates that fecal contamination, and therefore the presence of other intestinal pathogens, is unlikely.

Perspective and Prospects

During the latter portion of the nineteenth century, the role of bacteria as etiological agents of disease became apparent. Eventually the experimental observations linking the presence of bacteria with various illnesses coalesced in the so-called germ theory of disease. During the early 1880s, the German physician Robert Koch, along with his colleagues and students, developed an experimental method that could be applied to associate a particular organism with a specific disease. These procedures eventually became known as Koch's postulates. Inherent in Koch's postulates was the necessity to observe the microbial agent, either in tissue or following growth in the laboratory. Staining methods, however, were often crude or imprecise. The best one might hope for was to be able to at least observe the organism.

Hans Christian Gram, a Danish physician working with C. Friedlander in Berlin during the early 1880s, was able to introduce a highly effective method of staining bacteria. Gram's method was a modification of that developed earlier by Paul Ehrlich. The procedure began by first staining the sample with Gentian Violet in aniline water, followed by treatment with iodine in a potassium iodide solution. Gram found that when tissue sections or smears treated in such a manner were washed with dilute alcohol, certain types of bacteria (or schizomycetes, as they were then known) became decolorized (gram-negative), while other forms of bacteria retained their violet appearance (gram-positive). The procedure, published in 1884, was shown to be applicable for most types of bacteria. As a result, a process for differentiation between various types of bacteria became available. In addition, the ability to detect smaller quantities of bacteria in tissue increased significantly.

—*Richard Adler, Ph.D.*

See also Bacterial infections; Bacteriology; Cells; Cytology; Diagnosis; *E. coli* infection; Laboratory tests; Microbiology; Salmonella infection; Shigellosis; Staphylococcal infections; Streptococcal infections.

For Further Information:

Alcamo, I. Edward. *Microbes and Society: An Introduction to Microbiology*. 2d ed. Sudbury, Mass.: Jones and Bartlett, 2008.

Alcamo, I. Edward, and Lawrence M. Elson. *Microbiology Coloring Book*. New York: HarperCollins, 1996.

Goodsell, David. *The Machinery of Life*. New York: Springer, 1993.

Lab Tests Online. "Gram Stain." *American Association for Clinical Chemistry*, September 6, 2011.

Madigan, Michael T., and John M. Martinko. *Brock Biology of Microorganisms*. 12th ed. San Francisco: Pearson/Benjamin Cummings, 2009.

MedlinePlus. "Bacterial Infections." *MedlinePlus*, June 10, 2013.

Oregon Health and Science University. "Gram Stain." *Oregon Health and Science University*, 2013.

Singleton, Paul. *Bacteria in Biology, Biotechnology, and Medicine*. 6th ed. Hoboken, N.J.: John Wiley & Sons, 2005.

Snyder, Larry, and Wendy Champness. *Molecular Genetics of Bacteria*. 3d ed. Washington, D.C.: ASM Press, 2007.

Wilson, Michael, Brian Henderson, and Rod McNab. *Bacterial Disease Mechanisms: An Introduction to Cellular Microbiology*. New York: Cambridge University Press, 2002.

Winn, Washington C., Jr., et al. *Koneman's Color Atlas and Textbook of Diagnostic Microbiology*. 6th ed. Philadelphia: Lippincott Williams & Wilkins, 2006.

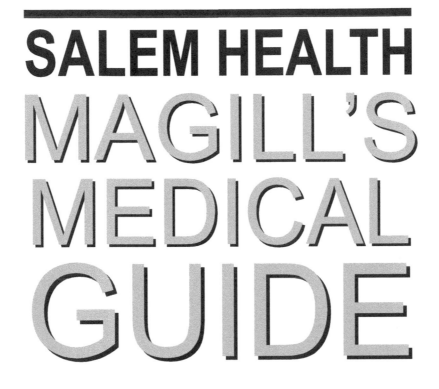

SALEM HEALTH

MAGILL'S MEDICAL GUIDE

ENTRIES BY ANATOMY OR SYSTEM AFFECTED

ALL
Abscesses
Abuse of the elderly
Accidents
Acupuncture
Adrenal glands
Aging
Aging: Extended care
Alternative medicine
Anatomy
Antibiotic resistance
Antibiotics
Antihypertensives
Anti-inflammatory drugs
Antioxidants
Autoimmune disorders
Autopsy
Bionics and biotechnology
Birth defects
Burkitt's lymphoma
Cancer
Carcinogens
Carcinoma
Chemotherapy
Chronic granulomatous disease
Clinical trials
Club drugs
Coccidioidomycosis
Cockayne Disease
Collagen
Congenital disorders
Critical care
Cryosurgery
Cysts
Death and dying
Diagnosis
Dietary reference intakes (DRIs)
Disease
Embryology
Emergency medicine
Emergency rooms
Emerging infectious diseases
Environmental diseases
Enzyme therapy
Epidemics and pandemics
Epidemiology
Epidermal nevus syndromes
Family medicine
Fascia
Fatigue
Fever
First aid

First responder
Food guide plate
Forensic pathology
Genetic diseases
Genetic engineering
Genetic Imprinting
Genetics and inheritance
Genomics
Geriatric assessment
Geriatrics and gerontology
Grafts and grafting
Growth
Healing
Herbal medicine
Histology
Homeopathy
Hydrotherapy
Hyperadiposis
Hyperthermia and hypothermia
Hypertrophy
Hypochondriasis
Iatrogenic disorders
Imaging and radiology
Immunopathology
Infection
Inflammation
Insect-borne diseases
Internet medicine
Interpartner violence
Invasive tests
Leptin
Lesions
Longevity
Macronutrients
Magnetic resonance imaging (MRI)
Malignancy and metastasis
Malnutrition
Massage
Medical home
Meditation
Men's health
Metabolic disorders
Metabolic syndrome
Mucopolysaccharidosis (MPS)
Multiple births
Münchausen syndrome by proxy
Neonatology
Noninvasive tests
Nursing
Nutrition
Occupational health
Oncology

Opportunistic infections
Ovaries
Over-the-counter medications
Pain
Pain management
Palliative care
Palliative medicine
Paramedics
Parasitic diseases
Pathology
Pediatrics
Perinatology
Physical examination
Physician assistants
Physiology
Phytochemicals
Plastic surgery
Positron emission tomography (PET) scanning
Preventive medicine
Progeria
Prognosis
Prostheses
Protein
Proteomics
Psychiatry
Psychosomatic disorders
Puberty and adolescence
Radiation therapy
Radiopharmaceuticals
Retroviruses
Safety issues for children
Safety issues for the elderly
Screening
Self-medication
Shock
Signs and symptoms
Stem cells
Stress
Stress reduction
Substance abuse
Sudden infant death syndrome (SIDS)
Suicide
Supplements
Surgical procedures
Surgical technologists
Syndrome
Systemic lupus erythematosus (SLE)
Systemic sclerosis
Systems and organs
Teratogens
Terminally ill: Extended care

Toxic shock syndrome
Toxicology
Transitional care
Tumor removal
Tumors
Viral hemorrhagic fevers
Viral infections
Vitamin D deficiency
Vitamins and minerals
Well-baby examinations
Wounds
Xenotransplantation
Zoonoses

ABDOMEN
Abdominal disorders
Adrenalectomy
Amebiasis
Amniocentesis
Aneurysmectomy
Appendectomy
Appendicitis
Back pain
Bariatric surgery
Bladder removal
Bypass surgery
Campylobacter infections
Candidiasis
Cesarean section
Cholecystectomy
Cholecystitis
Colitis
Colon
Colon therapy
Colorectal cancer
Colorectal polyp removal
Colorectal surgery
Constipation
Culdocentesis
Cushing's syndrome
Diabetes mellitus
Dialysis
Diarrhea and dysentery
Digestion
Diverticulitis and diverticulosis
Eating disorders
Endoscopic retrograde
    cholangiopancreatography (ERCP)
Endoscopy
Enemas
Fistula repair
Gallbladder
Gallbladder diseases
Gastrectomy
Gastroenteritis
Gastroenterology
Gastrointestinal disorders

Gastrointestinal system
Gastrostomy
Gaucher's disease
Hernia
Hernia repair
Ileostomy and colostomy
Incontinence
Internal medicine
Intestinal disorders
Intestines
Irritable bowel syndrome (IBS)
Kidney transplantation
Kidneys
Laparoscopy
Liposuction
Lithotripsy
Liver
Liver transplantation
Mesothelioma
Nephrectomy
Nephrology
Obesity
Pancreas
Pancreatitis
Peristalsis
Peritonitis
Polyps
Pregnancy and gestation
Prostate cancer
Reproductive system
Roseola
Shunts
Small intestine
Splenectomy
Stents
Sterilization
Stevens-Johnson syndrome
Stone removal
Stones
Tubal ligation
Tularemia
Ulcerative colitis
Ultrasonography
Urinary disorders
Urinary system
Urology
Vasculitis

ANUS
Amebiasis
Anal cancer
Colon therapy
Colorectal cancer
Colorectal polyp removal
Colorectal surgery
Endoscopy
Enemas

Episiotomy
Fistula repair
Hemorrhoid banding and removal
Hemorrhoids
Hirschsprung's disease
Human papillomavirus (HPV)
Intestinal disorders
Intestines
Irritable bowel syndrome (IBS)
Polyps
Rape and sexual assault
Rectum
Soiling
Sphincterectomy
Syphilis
Ulcerative colitis

ARMS
Amputation
Arthroplasty
Auras
Carpal tunnel syndrome
Casts and splints
Charcot-Marie-Tooth Disease
Cornelia de Lange syndrome
Cutis marmorata telangiectatica
    congenita
Dyskinesia
Fracture and dislocation
Fracture repair
Gigantism
Hemiplegia
Liposuction
Mesenchymal stem cells
Muscles
Neonatal brachial plexus palsy
Phlebotomy
Pityriasis alba
Quadriplegia
Roseola
Rotator cuff surgery
Sarcoma
Skin lesion removal
Slipped disk
Spinocerebellar ataxia
Streptococcal infections
Tendinitis
Thalidomide
Tremors
Upper extremities

BACK
Ankylosing spondylitis
Back pain
Bone disorders
Bone marrow transplantation
Bones and the skeleton

Chiropractic
Cushing's syndrome
Disk removal
Dwarfism
Juvenile rheumatoid arthritis
Kyphosis
Laminectomy and spinal fusion
Neuroimaging
Osteoporosis
Pityriasis alba
Pityriasis rosea
Sarcoma
Sciatica
Scoliosis
Slipped disk
Stevens-Johnson syndrome
Streptococcal infections
Sympathectomy
Tendon disorders

BLADDER
Abdomen
Abdominal disorders
Bed-wetting
Bladder cancer
Bladder removal
Candidiasis
Catheterization
Cystitis
Cystoscopy
Diuretics
Endoscopy
Fetal surgery
Fistula repair
Hematuria
Incontinence
Internal medicine
Lithotripsy
Polyps
Pyelonephritis
Schistosomiasis
Smoking
Sphincterectomy
Stone removal
Stones
Toilet training
Ultrasonography
Uremia
Urethritis
Urinalysis
Urinary disorders
Urinary system
Urology
Williams syndrome

BLOOD
Acquired immunodeficiency

syndrome (AIDS)
Anemia
Angiography
Antibodies
Aspergillosis
Avian influenza
Babesiosis
Biological therapies
Bleeding
Blood pressure
Blood testing
Blood vessels
Bone marrow transplantation
Bulimia
Candidiasis
Carbohydrates
Circulation
Cold agglutinin disease
Connective tissue
Cushing's syndrome
Cyanosis
Cytomegalovirus (CMV)
Deep vein thrombosis
Defibrillation
Dialysis
Disseminated intravascular
    coagulation (DIC)
Diuretics
E. coli infection
Ebola virus
End-stage renal disease
Epstein-Barr virus
Ergogenic aids
Fetal surgery
Fetal tissue transplantation
Fistula repair
Fluids and electrolytes
Glycolysis
Gulf War syndrome
Heart
Hematology
Hematomas
Hematuria
Hemolytic disease of the newborn
Hemolytic uremic syndrome
Hemophilia
Histiocytosis
Host-defense mechanisms
Hyperbaric oxygen therapy
Hypercholesterolemia
Hyperlipidemia
Hypoglycemia
Immune system
Immunization and vaccination
Jaundice
Laboratory tests
Leukemia

Liver
Lymph
Malaria
Menorrhagia
Methicillin-resistant staphylococcus
    aureus (MRSA) infection
Nephrology
Pharmacology
Phenylketonuria (PKU)
Phlebotomy
Plasma
Pulse rate
Rh factor
Salmonella infection
Schistosomiasis
Septicemia
Serology
Sickle cell disease
Single photon emission computed
    tomography (SPECT)
Snakebites
Staphylococcal infections
Sturge-Weber syndrome
Subdural hematoma
Thalassemia
Thrombocytopenia
Thrombolytic therapy and TPA
Thrombosis and thrombus
Thymus gland
Transfusion
Transplantation
Ultrasonography
Uremia
Von Willebrand's disease
Wiskott-Aldrich syndrome
Yellow fever

BLOOD VESSELS
Aneurysms
Angiography
Angioplasty
Arteriosclerosis
Avian influenza
Bedsores
Bile
Bleeding
Blood and blood disorders
Blood pressure
Blood testing
Blood vessels
Bruises
Bypass surgery
Caffeine
Carotid arteries
Catheterization
Cholesterol
Circulation

Claudication
Cluster headaches
Cold agglutinin disease
Cutis marmorata telangiectatica
    congenita
Deep vein thrombosis
Defibrillation
Diabetes mellitus
Disseminated intravascular
    coagulation (DIC)
Diuretics
Dizziness and fainting
Edema
Electrocauterization
Embolism
Embolization
End-stage renal disease
Endarterectomy
Erectile dysfunction
Eye infections and disorders
Facial transplantation
Hammertoe correction
Heart
Heart disease
Heat exhaustion and heatstroke
Hematomas
Hemorrhoid banding and removal
Hemorrhoids
Hormone therapy
Hypercholesterolemia
Hypertension
Hypotension
Infarction
Intravenous (IV) therapy
Ischemia
Kawasaki disease
Klippel-Trenaunay syndrome
Leptospirosis
Methicillin-resistant staphylococcus
    aureus (MRSA) infection
Necrotizing fasciitis
Nephritis
Neuroimaging
Obesity
Phlebitis
Phlebotomy
Plasma
Polycystic kidney disease
Polydactyly and syndactyly
Pulse rate
Raynaud's phenomenon
Rocky Mountain spotted fever
Roundworms
Schistosomiasis
Scleroderma
Scurvy
Single photon emission computed

tomography (SPECT)
Stenosis
Stents
Strokes
Sturge-Weber syndrome
Temporal arteritis
Thalidomide
Thrombolytic therapy and TPA
Thrombosis and thrombus
Toxemia
Transient ischemic attacks (TIAs)
Umbilical cord
Varicose vein removal
Varicose veins
Vascular medicine
Vascular system
Vasculitis
Venous insufficiency
Von Willebrand's disease

BONES

Amputation
Ankylosing spondylitis
Arthritis
Arthroplasty
Aspergillosis
Back pain
Bone cancer
Bone disorders
Bone grafting
Bone marrow transplantation
Bowlegs
Bunions
Cartilage
Casts and splints
Cells
Chiropractic
Cleft lip and palate
Cleft lip and palate repair
Connective tissue
Craniosynostosis
Cushing's syndrome
Dengue fever
Disk removal
Dwarfism
Ear surgery
Ears
Eating disorders
Ewing's sarcoma
Facial transplantation
Failure to thrive
Feet
Foot disorders
Fracture and dislocation
Fracture repair
Gaucher's disease
Gigantism

Hammertoe correction
Head and neck disorders
Hearing
Heel spur removal
Hip fracture repair
Hip replacement
Histiocytosis
Hormone therapy
Jaw wiring
Joints
Kneecap removal
Kyphosis
Laminectomy and spinal fusion
Leishmaniasis
Lower extremities
Marfan syndrome
Mesenchymal stem cells
Methicillin-resistant staphylococcus
    aureus (MRSA) infection
Motor skill development
Necrosis
Neurofibromatosis
Neurosurgery
Niemann-Pick disease
Nuclear medicine
Nuclear radiology
Orthopedic surgery
Orthopedics
Osteochondritis juvenilis
Osteogenesis imperfecta
Osteomyelitis
Osteonecrosis
Osteopathic medicine
Osteoporosis
Paget's disease
Periodontitis
Physical rehabilitation
Pigeon toes
Podiatry
Polydactyly and syndactyly
Prader-Willi syndrome
Rheumatology
Rickets
Rubinstein-Taybi syndrome
Sarcoma
Scoliosis
Spina bifida
Spinal cord disorders
Sports medicine
Syphilis
Teeth
Temporomandibular joint (TMJ)
    syndrome
Tendon disorders
Tendon repair
Upper extremities

BRAIN

Abscess drainage
Acidosis
Acquired immunodeficiency
   syndrome (AIDS)
Addiction
Adrenoleukodystrophy
Agnosia
Alcoholism
Altitude sickness
Alzheimer's disease
Amnesia
Anesthesia
Anesthesiology
Aneurysmectomy
Aneurysms
Angelman syndrome
Angiography
Anorexia nervosa
Anosmia
Antianxiety drugs
Antidepressants
Aortic stenosis
Aphasia and dysphasia
Apnea
Aromatherapy
Aspergillosis
Ataxia
Attention-deficit disorder (ADD)
Auras
Autism
Batten's disease
Biofeedback
Body dysmorphic disorder
Brain damage
Brain disorders
Brain tumors
Brucellosis
Bulimia
Caffeine
Carbohydrates
Carotid arteries
Cerebral palsy
Chiari malformations
Chronic wasting disease (CWD)
Cluster headaches
Cognitive development
Cognitive enhancement
Concussion
Cornelia de Lange syndrome
Craniotomy
Creutzfeldt-Jakob disease (CJD)
Cutis marmorata telangiectatica
   congenita
Cytomegalovirus (CMV)
Defibrillation
Dehydration

Dementias
Depression
Developmental stages
Dizziness and fainting
Down syndrome
Drowning
Dwarfism
Dyskinesia
Dyslexia
Electroencephalography (EEG)
Embolism
Embolization
Encephalitis
Endocrine glands
Endocrinology
Enteroviruses
Epilepsy
Ergogenic aids
Eye infections and disorders
Failure to thrive
Fetal alcohol syndrome
Fetal surgery
Fetal tissue transplantation
Fibromyalgia
Fragile X syndrome
Frontal lobe syndrome
Frontotemporal dementia (FTD)
Gigantism
Glioma
Gulf War syndrome
Head and neck disorders
Headaches
Hearing
Hearing loss
Hemiplegia
Hemolytic disease of the newborn
Hormone therapy
Huntington's disease
Hydrocephalus
Hypertension
Hypnosis
Hypotension
Hypothalamus
Infarction
Intraventricular hemorrhage
Ischemia
Kawasaki disease
Kinesiology
Kluver-Bucy syndrome
Korsakoff's syndrome
Lead poisoning
Learning disabilities
Leptospirosis
Leukodystrophy
Light therapy
Listeria infections
Lumbar puncture

Melatonin
Memory loss
Meningitis
Mental retardation
Mental status exam
Mirror neurons
Narcolepsy
Narcotics
Nausea and vomiting
Neuroimaging
Neurology
Neuropsychology
Neuroscience
Neurosis
Neurosurgery
Niemann-Pick disease
Nuclear radiology
Pharmacology
Phenylketonuria (PKU)
Phrenology
Pick's disease
Pituitary gland
Poliomyelitis
Polycystic kidney disease
Prader-Willi syndrome
Prion diseases
Psychiatric disorders
Rabies
Restless legs syndrome
Resuscitation
Reye's syndrome
Rocky Mountain spotted fever
Roseola
Sarcoidosis
Schizophrenia
Seizures
Shock therapy
Shunts
Single photon emission computed
   tomography (SPECT)
Sleep
Sleep disorders
Sleeping sickness
Sleepwalking
Spina bifida
Spinocerebellar ataxia
Split-brain
Strokes
Sturge-Weber syndrome
Subdural hematoma
Synesthesia
Syphilis
Teeth
Tetanus
Thrombosis and thrombus
Tics
Tinnitus

Carotid arteries
Catheterization
Chest
Cholera
Cholesterol
Circulation
Claudication
Cold agglutinin disease
Computed tomography (CT) scanning
Congenital heart disease
Coronary artery bypass graft
Cutis marmorata telangiectatica
  congenita
Decongestants
Deep vein thrombosis
Defibrillation
Dehydration
Diabetes mellitus
Dialysis
Disseminated intravascular
  coagulation (DIC)
Diuretics
Dizziness and fainting
Drowning
Ebola virus
Echocardiography
Edema
Electrocardiography (ECG or EKG)
Electrocauterization
Embolism
Encephalitis
End-stage renal disease
Endarterectomy
Endocarditis
Ergogenic aids
Exercise physiology
Facial transplantation
Food allergies
Gigantism
Heart
Heart attack
Heart disease
Heart failure
Heart transplantation
Heart valve replacement
Heat exhaustion and heatstroke
Hematology
Hemolytic uremic syndrome
Hemorrhoid banding and removal
Hemorrhoids
Hormone therapy
Hormones
Hyperbaric oxygen therapy
Hypercholesterolemia
Hypertension
Hypotension
Immune system

Intravenous (IV) therapy
Ischemia
Juvenile rheumatoid arthritis
Kawasaki disease
Kidneys
Kinesiology
Klippel-Trenaunay syndrome
Lead poisoning
Liver
Lymph
Lymphatic system
Mesenchymal stem cells
Methicillin-resistant staphylococcus
  aureus (MRSA) infection
Mitral valve prolapse
Motor skill development
Obesity
Osteochondritis juvenilis
Oxygen therapy
Pacemaker implantation
Palpitations
Phlebitis
Phlebotomy
Placenta
Plasma
Preeclampsia and eclampsia
Pulmonary edema
Pulse rate
Resuscitation
Reye's syndrome
Rocky Mountain spotted fever
Roundworms
Sarcoidosis
Schistosomiasis
Scleroderma
Septicemia
Shunts
Single photon emission computed
  tomography (SPECT)
Smoking
Snakebites
Sports medicine
Staphylococcal infections
Stenosis
Stents
Steroid abuse
Streptococcal infections
Strokes
Sturge-Weber syndrome
Temporal arteritis
Testicular torsion
Thrombocytopenia
Thrombolytic therapy and TPA
Thrombosis and thrombus
Toxemia
Transfusion
Transient ischemic attacks (TIAs)

Transplantation
Typhoid fever
Typhus
Uremia
Varicose vein removal
Varicose veins
Vascular medicine
Vascular system
Vasculitis
Venous insufficiency
Yellow fever

EARS
Adenoids
Adrenoleukodystrophy
Agnosia
Altitude sickness
Antihistamines
Aspergillosis
Audiology
Auras
Bell's palsy
Cartilage
Charcot-Marie-Tooth Disease
Cold agglutinin disease
Cornelia de Lange syndrome
Cytomegalovirus (CMV)
Deafness
Decongestants
Dyslexia
Ear infections and disorders
Ear surgery
Earwax
Facial transplantation
Fetal alcohol syndrome
Fragile X syndrome
Hearing
Hearing aids
Hearing loss
Hearing tests
Histiocytosis
Leukodystrophy
Measles
Ménière's disease
Motion sickness
Myringotomy
Nervous system
Neurology
Osteogenesis imperfecta
Otoplasty
Otorhinolaryngology
Pharynx
Raynaud's phenomenon
Rubinstein-Taybi syndrome
Sense organs
Speech disorders
Streptococcal infections

Tinnitus
Tonsillitis
Vasculitis
Vertigo
Williams syndrome
Wiskott-Aldrich syndrome

ENDOCRINE SYSTEM
Addison's disease
Adrenalectomy
Adrenoleukodystrophy
Amenorrhea
Anorexia nervosa
Assisted reproductive technologies
Bariatric surgery
Biofeedback
Carbohydrates
Computed tomography (CT) scanning
Congenital adrenal hyperplasia
Congenital hypothyroidism
Corticosteroids
Cushing's syndrome
Diabetes mellitus
Dwarfism
End-stage renal disease
Endocrine disorders
Endocrine glands
Endocrinology
Ergogenic aids
Failure to thrive
Fibrocystic breast condition
Gender reassignment surgery
Gestational diabetes
Gigantism
Glands
Goiter
Gynecomastia
Hashimoto's thyroiditis
Hormones
Hyperparathyroidism and
    hypoparathyroidism
Hypoglycemia
Hypothalamus
Klinefelter syndrome
Lead poisoning
Liver
Melatonin
Nonalcoholic steatohepatitis (NASH)
Obesity
Overtraining syndrome
Pancreas
Pancreatitis
Parathyroidectomy
Pituitary gland
Placenta
Plasma
Polycystic ovary syndrome

Postpartum depression
Prader-Willi syndrome
Preeclampsia and eclampsia
Prostate gland
Prostate gland removal
Sexual differentiation
Small intestine
Steroid abuse
Steroids
Testicular cancer
Testicular surgery
Thymus gland
Thyroid disorders
Thyroid gland
Thyroidectomy
Turner syndrome
Weight loss medications
Williams syndrome

EYES
Acquired immunodeficiency
    syndrome (AIDS)
Adenoviruses
Adrenoleukodystrophy
Agnosia
Angelman syndrome
Ankylosing spondylitis
Antihistamines
Aspergillosis
Astigmatism
Auras
Batten's disease
Behçet's disease
Bell's palsy
Blindness
Blurred vision
Botox
Cataract surgery
Cataracts
Chlamydia
Color blindness
Conjunctivitis
Corneal transplantation
Cornelia de Lange syndrome
Cutis marmorata telangiectatica
    congenita
Cytomegalovirus (CMV)
Dengue fever
Diabetes mellitus
Dry eye
Dyslexia
Enteroviruses
Eye infections and disorders
Eye surgery
Face lift and blepharoplasty
Facial transplantation
Fetal alcohol syndrome

Fetal tissue transplantation
Galactosemia
Gigantism
Glaucoma
Gonorrhea
Gulf War syndrome
Hay fever
Juvenile rheumatoid arthritis
Keratitis
Kluver-Bucy syndrome
Laser use in surgery
Leptospirosis
Leukodystrophy
Lyme disease
Macular degeneration
Marfan syndrome
Motor skill development
Multiple chemical sensitivity
    syndrome
Myopia
Ophthalmology
Optometry
Pigmentation
Pterygium/Pinguecula
Ptosis
Refractive eye surgery
Reiter's syndrome
Rubinstein-Taybi syndrome
Sarcoidosis
Scurvy
Sense organs
Sjögren's syndrome
Sphincterectomy
Spinocerebellar ataxia
Stevens-Johnson syndrome
Strabismus
Sturge-Weber syndrome
Styes
Syphilis
Tears and tear ducts
Trachoma
Transplantation
Vasculitis
Vision
Vision disorders
Williams syndrome

FEET
Athlete's foot
Bones and the skeleton
Bowlegs
Bunions
Charcot-Marie-Tooth Disease
Cold agglutinin disease
Cornelia de Lange syndrome
Corns and calluses
Dyskinesia

Pharynx
Pinworms
Poisoning
Polycystic kidney disease
Polyps
Proctology
Protozoan diseases
Pyloric stenosis
Radiation sickness
Rectum
Reiter's syndrome
Rotavirus
Roundworms
Salmonella infection
Scleroderma
Sense organs
Shigellosis
Shunts
Small intestine
Smallpox
Smoking
Soiling
Staphylococcal infections
Stenosis
Stevens-Johnson syndrome
Tapeworms
Taste
Teeth
Toilet training
Toxoplasmosis
Trichinosis
Tumor removal
Typhoid fever
Ulcer surgery
Ulcerative colitis
Ulcers
Vagotomy
Vasculitis
Weaning
Weight loss and gain

GENITALS
Adrenoleukodystrophy
Aphrodisiacs
Assisted reproductive technologies
Behçet's disease
Candidiasis
Catheterization
Cervical procedures
Chlamydia
Congenital adrenal hyperplasia
Contraception
Cyst removal
Embolization
Endometrial biopsy
Episiotomy
Erectile dysfunction

Ergogenic aids
Fragile X syndrome
Gender identity disorder
Gender reassignment surgery
Glands
Gonorrhea
Gynecology
Hemochromatosis
Hermaphroditism and
    pseudohermaphroditism
Herpes
Hormone therapy
Human papillomavirus (HPV)
Hydroceles
Hyperplasia
Hypospadias repair and urethroplasty
Klinefelter syndrome
Kluver-Bucy syndrome
Masturbation
Mumps
Orchitis
Pap test
Pelvic inflammatory disease (PID)
Penile implant surgery
Prader-Willi syndrome
Rape and sexual assault
Reproductive system
Rubinstein-Taybi syndrome
Semen
Sexual differentiation
Sexual dysfunction
Sexuality
Sexually transmitted diseases (STDs)
Sperm banks
Sterilization
Stevens-Johnson syndrome
Streptococcal infections
Syphilis
Testicular cancer
Testicular surgery
Testicular torsion
Toilet training
Trichomoniasis
Urethritis
Urology
Uterus
Vas deferens
Vasectomy

GLANDS
Abscess drainage
Addison's disease
Adrenalectomy
Adrenoleukodystrophy
Assisted reproductive technologies
Biofeedback
Breast cancer

Breast disorders
Breast-feeding
Breast surgery
Cushing's syndrome
Cyst removal
Dengue fever
Diabetes mellitus
DiGeorge syndrome
Dwarfism
Endocrine disorders
Endocrine glands
Endocrinology
Epstein-Barr virus
Ergogenic aids
Eye infections and disorders
Gender reassignment surgery
Goiter
Gynecomastia
Hashimoto's thyroiditis
Hormones
Hyperhidrosis
Hyperparathyroidism and
    hypoparathyroidism
Hypoglycemia
Hypothalamus
Immune system
Internal medicine
Liver
Mastitis
Melatonin
Mumps
Neurosurgery
Nuclear medicine
Nuclear radiology
Pancreas
Parathyroidectomy
Pituitary gland
Prader-Willi syndrome
Prostate gland
Prostate gland removal
Quinsy
Semen
Sexual differentiation
Sleep
Steroids
Sweating
Testicular cancer
Testicular surgery
Thymus gland
Thyroid disorders
Thyroid gland
Thyroidectomy

GUMS
Abscess drainage
Bulimia
Cavities

Cleft lip and palate repair
Dengue fever
Dental diseases
Dentistry
Dentures
Fluoride treatments
Gingivitis
Gulf War syndrome
Gum disease
Jaw wiring
Mouth and throat cancer
Oral and maxillofacial surgery
Orthodontics
Periodontal surgery
Periodontitis
Root canal treatment
Scurvy
Teeth
Teething
Tooth extraction
Wisdom teeth

HAIR
Alopecia
Angelman syndrome
Anorexia nervosa
Collodion baby
Cornelia de Lange syndrome
Cushing's syndrome
Dermatitis
Dermatology
Gigantism
Gulf War syndrome
Hair
Hair transplantation
Klinefelter syndrome
Pigmentation
Radiation sickness

HANDS
Amputation
Arthritis
Arthroplasty
Bursitis
Carpal tunnel syndrome
Casts and splints
Charcot-Marie-Tooth Disease
Cold agglutinin disease
Cornelia de Lange syndrome
Corns and calluses
Dyskinesia
Fetal alcohol syndrome
Fracture and dislocation
Fragile X syndrome
Frostbite
Ganglion removal
Gigantism

Mesenchymal stem cells
Methicillin-resistant staphylococcus
    aureus (MRSA) infection
Nail removal
Nails
Neurology
Orthopedic surgery
Orthopedics
Polydactyly and syndactyly
Raynaud's phenomenon
Rheumatology
Rubinstein-Taybi syndrome
Scleroderma
Skin lesion removal
Spinocerebellar ataxia
Sports medicine
Stevens-Johnson syndrome
Streptococcal infections
Tendinitis
Tendon repair
Thalidomide
Tremors
Upper extremities
Vasculitis

HEAD
Alopecia
Altitude sickness
Aneurysms
Angelman syndrome
Angiography
Antihistamines
Bell's palsy
Botox
Brain
Brain disorders
Brain tumors
Cluster headaches
Concussion
Cornelia de Lange syndrome
Craniosynostosis
Craniotomy
Dengue fever
Dizziness and fainting
Dyskinesia
Electroencephalography (EEG)
Epilepsy
Eye infections and disorders
Facial transplantation
Fetal alcohol syndrome
Fibromyalgia
Hair transplantation
Head and neck disorders
Headaches
Hemiplegia
Hydrocephalus
Meningitis

Motion sickness
Nasal polyp removal
Neuroimaging
Neurology
Neurosurgery
Oral and maxillofacial surgery
Paget's disease
Pharynx
Rubinstein-Taybi syndrome
Seizures
Shunts
Single photon emission computed
    tomography (SPECT)
Spinocerebellar ataxia
Sports medicine
Stevens-Johnson syndrome
Strokes
Sturge-Weber syndrome
Tears and tear ducts
Temporomandibular joint (TMJ)
    syndrome
Thrombosis and thrombus
Tinnitus
Tremors
Whiplash

HEART
Acidosis
Anemia
Aneurysmectomy
Aneurysms
Angina
Angiography
Angioplasty
Anorexia nervosa
Anxiety
Aortic stenosis
Apgar score
Arrhythmias
Arteriosclerosis
Aspergillosis
Atrial fibrillation
Avian influenza
Beriberi
Biofeedback
Bites and stings
Blood pressure
Blood vessels
Blue baby syndrome
Brucellosis
Bulimia
Bypass surgery
Caffeine
Cardiac arrest
Cardiac rehabilitation
Cardiac surgery
Cardiology

Cardiopulmonary resuscitation (CPR)
Carotid arteries
Catheterization
Congenital heart disease
Cornelia de Lange syndrome
Coronary artery bypass graft
Defibrillation
Depression
Diabetes mellitus
DiGeorge syndrome
Diphtheria
Diuretics
Drowning
Echocardiography
Electrical shock
Electrocardiography (ECG or EKG)
End-stage renal disease
Endocarditis
Enteroviruses
Ergogenic aids
Exercise physiology
Fatty acid oxidation disorders
Fetal alcohol syndrome
Gangrene
Glycogen storage diseases
Heart attack
Heart disease
Heart failure
Heart transplantation
Heart valve replacement
Hemochromatosis
Hormone therapy
Hypercholesterolemia
Hypertension
Hypotension
Infarction
Internal medicine
Interstitial pulmonary fibrosis (IPF)
Intravenous (IV) therapy
Juvenile rheumatoid arthritis
Kawasaki disease
Kinesiology
Lyme disease
Marfan syndrome
Methicillin-resistant staphylococcus
  aureus (MRSA) infection
Mitral valve prolapse
Mononucleosis
Obesity
Oxygen therapy
Pacemaker implantation
Palpitations
Plasma
Prader-Willi syndrome
Pulmonary edema
Pulse rate
Renal failure

Respiratory distress syndrome
Resuscitation
Reye's syndrome
Rheumatic fever
Rheumatoid arthritis
Rubinstein-Taybi syndrome
Sarcoidosis
Scleroderma
Single photon emission computed
  tomography (SPECT)
Sleeping sickness
Sports medicine
Stenosis
Stents
Steroid abuse
Streptococcal infections
Strokes
Syphilis
Teeth
Thoracic surgery
Thrombolytic therapy and TPA
Thrombosis and thrombus
Transplantation
Ultrasonography
Uremia
Whooping cough
Williams syndrome

HIPS

Ankylosing spondylitis
Arthritis
Arthroplasty
Arthroscopy
Back pain
Bones and the skeleton
Bowlegs
Chiropractic
Dwarfism
Fracture and dislocation
Fracture repair
Hip fracture repair
Hip replacement
Liposuction
Lower extremities
Orthopedic surgery
Orthopedics
Osteochondritis juvenilis
Osteonecrosis
Osteoporosis
Paget's disease
Physical rehabilitation
Pigeon toes
Rheumatology
Sciatica

IMMUNE SYSTEM

Acquired immunodeficiency

  syndrome (AIDS)
Adenoids
Adenoviruses
Allergies
Ankylosing spondylitis
Anorexia nervosa
Anthrax
Antibodies
Antihistamines
Arthritis
Asthma
Bacillus Calmette-Guérin (BCG)
Bacterial infections
Bacteriology
Bedsores
Bile
Biological therapies
Bites and stings
Blood and blood disorders
Bone grafting
Bone marrow transplantation
Candidiasis
Cells
Chagas' disease
Childhood infectious diseases
Chronic fatigue syndrome
Cold agglutinin disease
Conjunctivitis
Cornelia de Lange syndrome
Coronaviruses
Corticosteroids
Coughing
Cytology
Cytomegalovirus (CMV)
Cytopathology
Dermatology
Dermatopathology
DiGeorge syndrome
Disseminated intravascular
  coagulation (DIC)
Ehrlichiosis
Endocrinology
Epstein-Barr virus
Facial transplantation
Fetal tissue transplantation
Food allergies
Fungal infections
Gluten intolerance
Gram staining
Guillain-Barré syndrome
Gulf War syndrome
Hashimoto's thyroiditis
Hay fever
Hematology
Histiocytosis
Hives
Host-defense mechanisms

Human immunodeficiency virus (HIV)
Immunization and vaccination
Immunodeficiency disorders
Impetigo
Juvenile rheumatoid arthritis
Kawasaki disease
Leishmaniasis
Leprosy
Lymph
Lymphatic system
Magnetic field therapy
Malaria
Marburg virus
Mesenchymal stem cells
Microbiology
Mold and mildew
Monkeypox
Multiple chemical sensitivity syndrome
Mutation
Myasthenia gravis
Nephritis
Noroviruses
Pancreas
Pharmacology
Pharynx
Plasma
Poisoning
Polymyalgia rheumatica
Pulmonary diseases
Pulmonary medicine
Renal failure
Rh factor
Rheumatoid arthritis
Rheumatology
Roseola
Sarcoidosis
Scarlet fever
Scleroderma
Serology
Severe acute respiratory syndrome (SARS)
Severe combined immunodeficiency syndrome (SCID)
Sjögren's syndrome
Small intestine
Stevens-Johnson syndrome
Temporal arteritis
Thalidomide
Thymus gland
Tonsils
Toxoplasmosis
Transfusion
Transplantation
Ulcerative colitis
Vasculitis

Vitiligo
Wiskott-Aldrich syndrome

INTESTINES
Abdomen
Abdominal disorders
Acidosis
Acquired immunodeficiency syndrome (AIDS)
Adenoviruses
Amebiasis
Anus
Appendectomy
Appendicitis
Avian influenza
Bacterial infections
Bariatric surgery
Bulimia
Bypass surgery
Campylobacter infections
Carbohydrates
Celiac sprue
Cholera
Chyme
Colic
Colitis
Colon
Colon therapy
Colonoscopy and sigmoidoscopy
Colorectal cancer
Colorectal polyp removal
Colorectal surgery
Constipation
Crohn's disease
Diarrhea and dysentery
Digestion
Diverticulitis and diverticulosis
E. coli infection
Eating disorders
Endoscopy
Enemas
Enterocolitis
Fiber
Fistula repair
Food poisoning
Fructosemia
Gastroenteritis
Gastroenterology
Gastrointestinal disorders
Gastrointestinal system
Hemorrhoid banding and removal
Hemorrhoids
Hernia
Hernia repair
Hirschsprung's disease
Ileostomy and colostomy
Infarction

Internal medicine
Intestinal disorders
Irritable bowel syndrome (IBS)
Kaposi's sarcoma
Lactose intolerance
Laparoscopy
Malabsorption
Malnutrition
Meckel's diverticulum
Metabolism
Obesity
Peristalsis
Peritonitis
Pinworms
Polyps
Proctology
Rectum
Roundworms
Small intestine
Soiling
Sphincterectomy
Tapeworms
Toilet training
Trichinosis
Tumor removal
Typhoid fever
Ulcer surgery
Ulcerative colitis
Vasculitis

JOINTS
Amputation
Angelman syndrome
Ankylosing spondylitis
Arthritis
Arthroplasty
Arthroscopy
Back pain
Bowlegs
Brucellosis
Bursitis
Carpal tunnel syndrome
Cartilage
Casts and splints
Celiac sprue
Charcot-Marie-Tooth Disease
Cyst removal
Electrocauterization
Endoscopy
Ergogenic aids
Exercise physiology
Fracture and dislocation
Fragile X syndrome
Gout
Gulf War syndrome
Hemiplegia
Hip fracture repair

Juvenile rheumatoid arthritis
Klippel-Trenaunay syndrome
Kneecap removal
Ligaments
Lyme disease
Mesenchymal stem cells
Methicillin-resistant staphylococcus
  aureus (MRSA) infection
Motor skill development
Obesity
Orthopedic surgery
Orthopedics
Osteoarthritis
Osteochondritis juvenilis
Osteomyelitis
Osteonecrosis
Physical rehabilitation
Pigeon toes
Polymyalgia rheumatica
Reiter's syndrome
Rheumatology
Rotator cuff surgery
Rubella
Sarcoidosis
Sarcoma
Scleroderma
Spondylitis
Sports medicine
Streptococcal infections
Syphilis
Temporomandibular joint (TMJ)
  syndrome
Tendinitis
Tendon repair
Tularemia
Von Willebrand's disease

KIDNEYS
Abdomen
Abdominal disorders
Abscess drainage
Addison's disease
Adrenalectomy
Anemia
Anorexia nervosa
Aspergillosis
Avian influenza
Babesiosis
Carbohydrates
Cholera
Diabetes mellitus
Dialysis
Diuretics
Drowning
End-stage renal disease
Ergogenic aids
Fructosemia

Hantavirus
Hematuria
Hemolytic uremic syndrome
Hypertension
Hypotension
Infarction
Internal medicine
Intravenous (IV) therapy
Kidney cancer
Kidney disorders
Kidney transplantation
Laparoscopy
Leptospirosis
Lithotripsy
Metabolism
Methicillin-resistant staphylococcus
  aureus (MRSA) infection
Nephrectomy
Nephritis
Nephrology
Nuclear medicine
Nuclear radiology
Polycystic kidney disease
Polyps
Preeclampsia and eclampsia
Proteinuria
Pyelonephritis
Renal failure
Reye's syndrome
Rocky Mountain spotted fever
Sarcoidosis
Scleroderma
Scurvy
Sickle cell disease
Stone removal
Stones
Syphilis
Toilet training
Transplantation
Typhoid fever
Typhus
Ultrasonography
Uremia
Urinalysis
Urinary disorders
Urinary system
Urology
Vasculitis
Williams syndrome

KNEES
Amputation
Angelman syndrome
Arthritis
Arthroplasty
Arthroscopy
Bowlegs

Bursitis
Cartilage
Casts and splints
Endoscopy
Exercise physiology
Fracture and dislocation
Joints
Kneecap removal
Liposuction
Lower extremities
Lyme disease
Mesenchymal stem cells
Orthopedic surgery
Orthopedics
Osgood-Schlatter disease
Osteonecrosis
Physical rehabilitation
Pigeon toes
Rheumatology
Sports medicine
Stevens-Johnson syndrome
Tendinitis
Tendon repair

LEGS
Amputation
Arthritis
Arthroscopy
Auras
Back pain
Bone disorders
Bones and the skeleton
Bowlegs
Bursitis
Bypass surgery
Casts and splints
Charcot-Marie-Tooth Disease
Claudication
Cornelia de Lange syndrome
Cutis marmorata telangiectatica
  congenita
Deep vein thrombosis
Dwarfism
Dyskinesia
Fracture and dislocation
Fracture repair
Gigantism
Hemiplegia
Hip fracture repair
Kneecap removal
Liposuction
Lower extremities
Mesenchymal stem cells
Methicillin-resistant staphylococcus
  aureus (MRSA) infection
Muscles
Muscular dystrophy

Numbness and tingling
Orthopedic surgery
Orthopedics
Osteoporosis
Paget's disease
Paralysis
Paraplegia
Physical rehabilitation
Pigeon toes
Poliomyelitis
Quadriplegia
Rheumatology
Roseola
Sarcoma
Sciatica
Slipped disk
Spinocerebellar ataxia
Sports medicine
Stevens-Johnson syndrome
Streptococcal infections
Tendinitis
Tendon disorders
Tendon repair
Thalidomide
Tremors
Varicose vein removal
Vascular system
Vasculitis
Venous insufficiency

LIGAMENTS
Ankylosing spondylitis
Back pain
Bowlegs
Casts and splints
Collagen
Connective tissue
Electrocauterization
Eye infections and disorders
Flat feet
Joints
Mesenchymal stem cells
Muscles
Orthopedic surgery
Orthopedics
Osteogenesis imperfecta
Physical rehabilitation
Pigeon toes
Sports medicine
Tendon disorders
Tendon repair
Whiplash

LIVER
Abdomen
Abdominal disorders
Abscess drainage

Acquired immunodeficiency
    syndrome (AIDS)
Alcoholism
Amebiasis
Aspergillosis
Babesiosis
Bile
Blood and blood disorders
Brucellosis
Cholecystitis
Chyme
Circulation
Cirrhosis
Cold agglutinin disease
Cytomegalovirus (CMV)
Edema
Embolization
Endoscopic retrograde
    cholangiopancreatography (ERCP)
Ergogenic aids
Fatty acid oxidation disorders
Fetal surgery
Fructosemia
Galactosemia
Gastroenterology
Gastrointestinal system
Gaucher's disease
Glycogen storage diseases
Hematology
Hemochromatosis
Hemolytic disease of the newborn
Hepatitis
Histiocytosis
Hypercholesterolemia
Immune system
Internal medicine
Jaundice
Kaposi's sarcoma
Leptospirosis
Liver cancer
Liver disorders
Liver transplantation
Malabsorption
Malaria
Metabolism
Methicillin-resistant staphylococcus
    aureus (MRSA) infection
Niemann-Pick disease
Nonalcoholic steatohepatitis (NASH)
Phenylketonuria (PKU)
Polycystic kidney disease
Reye's syndrome
Shunts
Thrombocytopenia
Transplantation
Typhoid fever
Wilson's disease

Yellow fever

LUNGS
Abscess drainage
Acquired immunodeficiency
    syndrome (AIDS)
Acute respiratory distress syndrome
    (ARDS)
Adenoviruses
Allergies
Altitude sickness
Antihistamines
Apgar score
Apnea
Asbestos exposure
Aspergillosis
Asphyxiation
Asthma
Avian influenza
Bacterial infections
Bronchi
Bronchiolitis
Bronchitis
Cardiopulmonary resuscitation (CPR)
Chest
Childhood infectious diseases
Chlamydia
Choking
Chronic obstructive pulmonary
    disease (COPD)
Cold agglutinin disease
Common cold
Coronaviruses
Coughing
Croup
Cystic fibrosis
Cytomegalovirus (CMV)
Diaphragm
Drowning
Edema
Embolism
Emphysema
Endoscopy
Exercise physiology
Fetal surgery
Hantavirus
Hay fever
Heart transplantation
Heimlich maneuver
Hiccups
Histiocytosis
H1N1 influenza
Hyperbaric oxygen therapy
Hyperventilation
Hypoxia
Infarction
Influenza

Internal medicine
Interstitial pulmonary fibrosis (IPF)
Intravenous (IV) therapy
Kaposi's sarcoma
Kinesiology
Legionnaires' disease
Leptospirosis
Lung cancer
Lung surgery
Measles
Mesothelioma
Mold and mildew
Multiple chemical sensitivity
    syndrome
Niemann-Pick disease
Oxygen therapy
Plague
Pleurisy
Pneumocystis jirovecii
Pneumonia
Pneumothorax
Pulmonary diseases
Pulmonary edema
Pulmonary hypertension
Pulmonary medicine
Quinsy
Respiration
Respiratory distress syndrome
Resuscitation
Rhinoviruses
Roundworms
Sarcoidosis
Schistosomiasis
Scleroderma
Severe acute respiratory syndrome
    (SARS)
Sickle cell disease
Stevens-Johnson syndrome
Thoracic surgery
Thrombolytic therapy and TPA
Thrombosis and thrombus
Transplantation
Tuberculosis
Tumor removal
Vasculitis
Wiskott-Aldrich syndrome

LYMPHATIC SYSTEM
Acquired immunodeficiency
    syndrome (AIDS)
Adenoids
Antibodies
Bacillus Calmette-Guérin (BCG)
Bacterial infections
Biological therapies
Blood and blood disorders
Blood vessels

Breast cancer
Breast disorders
Bruises
Chlamydia
Cold agglutinin disease
Colorectal cancer
Coronaviruses
DiGeorge syndrome
Edema
Elephantiasis
Embolism
Epstein-Barr virus
Gaucher's disease
Hay fever
Hodgkin's disease
Immune system
Kawasaki disease
Klippel-Trenaunay syndrome
Leishmaniasis
Leptospirosis
Lower extremities
Lung cancer
Lymph
Lymphadenopathy and lymphoma
Mononucleosis
Overtraining syndrome
Prostate cancer
Roundworms
Rubella
Sarcoidosis
Skin cancer
Sleeping sickness
Small intestine
Splenectomy
Thymus gland
Tonsillectomy and adenoid removal
Tonsillitis
Tonsils
Tularemia
Upper extremities
Vascular medicine

MOUTH
Acid reflux disease
Acquired immunodeficiency
    syndrome (AIDS)
Adenoids
Angelman syndrome
Auras
Behçet's disease
Bell's palsy
Candidiasis
Canker sores
Chickenpox
Cleft lip and palate repair
Cold sores
Cornelia de Lange syndrome

Crowns and bridges
Dengue fever
Dental diseases
Dentistry
Dentures
DiGeorge syndrome
Dyskinesia
Eating disorders
Endodontic disease
Epstein-Barr virus
Esophagus
Facial transplantation
Fetal alcohol syndrome
Fluoride treatments
Gingivitis
Gum disease
Hand-foot-and-mouth disease
Heimlich maneuver
Herpes
Jaw wiring
Kawasaki disease
Lisping
Measles
Mouth and throat cancer
Oral and maxillofacial surgery
Orthodontics
Periodontal surgery
Pharynx
Quinsy
Rape and sexual assault
Raynaud's phenomenon
Reiter's syndrome
Root canal treatment
Rubinstein-Taybi syndrome
Sense organs
Sjögren's syndrome
Taste
Teething
Temporomandibular joint (TMJ)
    syndrome
Thumb sucking
Tooth extraction
Ulcers
Wisdom teeth

MUSCLES
Acidosis
Acupressure
Amputation
Anesthesia
Anesthesiology
Apgar score
Avian influenza
Back pain
Bed-wetting
Bedsores
Bell's palsy

Beriberi
Bile
Biofeedback
Botox
Bowlegs
Carbohydrates
Charcot-Marie-Tooth Disease
Chest
Chiari malformations
Childhood infectious diseases
Chronic fatigue syndrome
Cushing's syndrome
Diaphragm
Ebola virus
Electrocauterization
Electromyography
Epstein-Barr virus
Exercise physiology
Eye infections and disorders
Facial transplantation
Fatty acid oxidation disorders
Fibromyalgia
Flat feet
Foot disorders
Gangrene
Glycogen storage diseases
Glycolysis
Guillain-Barré syndrome
Gulf War syndrome
Head and neck disorders
Hemiplegia
Hiccups
Kinesiology
Kwashiorkor
Leukodystrophy
Mesenchymal stem cells
Methicillin-resistant staphylococcus
    aureus (MRSA) infection
Motor neuron diseases
Motor skill development
Multiple chemical sensitivity
    syndrome
Multiple sclerosis
Muscular dystrophy
Necrotizing fasciitis
Neurology
Numbness and tingling
Orthopedic surgery
Orthopedics
Osteopathic medicine
Overtraining syndrome
Palpitations
Palsy
Paralysis
Parkinson's disease
Physical rehabilitation
Pigeon toes

Poisoning
Poliomyelitis
Ptosis
Rabies
Respiration
Restless legs syndrome
Rotator cuff surgery
Sarcoma
Scurvy
Seizures
Smallpox
Speech disorders
Sphincterectomy
Spinocerebellar ataxia
Sports medicine
Steroid abuse
Strabismus
Streptococcal infections
Tattoos and body piercing
Temporomandibular joint (TMJ)
    syndrome
Tendon disorders
Tendon repair
Tetanus
Tics
Torticollis
Tourette's syndrome
Tremors
Trichinosis
Tularemia
Upper extremities
Weight loss and gain
Williams syndrome
Yoga

MUSCULOSKELETAL SYSTEM
Acupressure
Amputation
Amyotrophic lateral sclerosis
Anesthesia
Anesthesiology
Ankylosing spondylitis
Anorexia nervosa
Arthritis
Ataxia
Atrophy
Avian influenza
Back pain
Bed-wetting
Biofeedback
Bone cancer
Bone disorders
Bone grafting
Bone marrow transplantation
Bones and the skeleton
Brucellosis
Bulimia

Cartilage
Casts and splints
Cells
Charcot-Marie-Tooth Disease
Chest
Childhood infectious diseases
Chiropractic
Chronic fatigue syndrome
Cleft lip and palate
Cleft lip and palate repair
Collagen
Computed tomography (CT) scanning
Congenital hypothyroidism
Connective tissue
Dengue fever
Depression
Diaphragm
Dwarfism
Ear surgery
Ears
Ehrlichiosis
Ergogenic aids
Ewing's sarcoma
Exercise physiology
Feet
Fibromyalgia
Flat feet
Foot disorders
Fracture and dislocation
Fracture repair
Gigantism
Glycolysis
Guillain-Barré syndrome
Hammertoe correction
Head and neck disorders
Heel spur removal
Hematology
Hematomas
Hemiplegia
Hip fracture repair
Hyperparathyroidism and
    hypoparathyroidism
Jaw wiring
Joints
Juvenile rheumatoid arthritis
Kinesiology
Kneecap removal
Lead poisoning
Ligaments
Lower extremities
Marfan syndrome
Mesenchymal stem cells
Methicillin-resistant staphylococcus
    aureus (MRSA) infection
Motor neuron diseases
Motor skill development
Multiple sclerosis

Muscles
Muscular dystrophy
Myasthenia gravis
Neurology
Nuclear medicine
Nuclear radiology
Numbness and tingling
Orthopedic surgery
Orthopedics
Osgood-Schlatter disease
Osteoarthritis
Osteochondritis juvenilis
Osteogenesis imperfecta
Osteomyelitis
Osteonecrosis
Osteopathic medicine
Paget's disease
Palsy
Paralysis
Parkinson's disease
Physical rehabilitation
Poisoning
Poliomyelitis
Prader-Willi syndrome
Precocious puberty
Rabies
Radiculopathy
Respiration
Restless legs syndrome
Rheumatoid arthritis
Rheumatology
Rickets
Scoliosis
Seizures
Sleepwalking
Slipped disk
Speech disorders
Sphincterectomy
Spinal cord disorders
Spinocerebellar ataxia
Sports medicine
Staphylococcal infections
Teeth
Tendinitis
Tendon disorders
Tendon repair
Tetanus
Tics
Tourette's syndrome
Trichinosis
Upper extremities
Weight loss and gain

NAILS
Anorexia nervosa
Athlete's foot
Collodion baby

Dermatology
Fungal infections
Malnutrition
Nail removal
Podiatry

NECK
Botox
Carotid arteries
Casts and splints
Chiari malformations
Choking
Congenital hypothyroidism
Dyskinesia
Encephalitis
Endarterectomy
Facial transplantation
Goiter
Hashimoto's thyroiditis
Head and neck disorders
Heimlich maneuver
Hyperparathyroidism and
    hypoparathyroidism
Mouth and throat cancer
Neuroimaging
Paralysis
Parathyroidectomy
Pharynx
Pityriasis alba
Slipped disk
Stevens-Johnson syndrome
Streptococcal infections
Sympathectomy
Thyroid disorders
Thyroid gland
Thyroidectomy
Torticollis
Trachea
Tracheostomy
Vagus nerve
Whiplash
Whooping cough

NERVES
Agnosia
Alzheimer's disease
Anesthesia
Anesthesiology
Angelman syndrome
Avian influenza
Back pain
Bell's palsy
Biofeedback
Brain
Bulimia
Carpal tunnel syndrome
Cells

Cluster headaches
Concussion
Dyskinesia
Electromyography
Encephalitis
Epilepsy
Eye infections and disorders
Facial transplantation
Fibromyalgia
Guillain-Barré syndrome
Hearing
Herpes
Hirschsprung's disease
Huntington's disease
Leprosy
Leukodystrophy
Listeria infections
Local anesthesia
Lower extremities
Lumbar puncture
Lyme disease
Motor neuron diseases
Motor skill development
Multiple chemical sensitivity
    syndrome
Multiple sclerosis
Neonatal brachial plexus palsy
Nervous system
Neuroimaging
Neurology
Neurosis
Neurosurgery
Numbness and tingling
Palsy
Paralysis
Parkinson's disease
Physical rehabilitation
Poliomyelitis
Postherpetic neuralgia
Ptosis
Radiculopathy
Sarcoidosis
Sciatica
Seizures
Sense organs
Shock therapy
Skin
Slipped disk
Spinal cord disorders
Spinocerebellar ataxia
Sturge-Weber syndrome
Sympathectomy
Tics
Tinnitus
Touch
Tourette's syndrome
Tremors

Upper extremities
Vagotomy
Vasculitis

NERVOUS SYSTEM
Abscess drainage
Acupressure
Addiction
Adenoviruses
Adrenoleukodystrophy
Agnosia
Alcoholism
Altitude sickness
Alzheimer's disease
Amnesia
Amputation
Amyotrophic lateral sclerosis
Anesthesia
Anesthesiology
Aneurysms
Angelman syndrome
Anorexia nervosa
Anosmia
Anthrax
Antidepressants
Anxiety
Apgar score
Aphasia and dysphasia
Apnea
Aromatherapy
Ataxia
Atrophy
Attention-deficit disorder (ADD)
Auras
Avian influenza
Back pain
Balance disorders
Batten's disease
Behçet's disease
Beriberi
Biofeedback
Botulism
Brain
Brain damage
Brain disorders
Brain tumors
Brucellosis
Caffeine
Cells
Chagas' disease
Charcot-Marie-Tooth Disease
Chiari malformations
Chiropractic
Chronic wasting disease (CWD)
Cluster headaches
Cognitive development
Colon

Computed tomography (CT) scanning
Concussion
Congenital hypothyroidism
Creutzfeldt-Jakob disease (CJD)
Cutis marmorata telangiectatica
    congenita
Deafness
Defibrillation
Dementias
Developmental disorders
Developmental stages
Diabetes mellitus
Diphtheria
Disk removal
Dizziness and fainting
Down syndrome
Drowning
Dwarfism
Dyskinesia
Dyslexia
E. coli infection
Ear surgery
Ears
Ehrlichiosis
Electrical shock
Electroencephalography (EEG)
Electromyography
Encephalitis
Endocrinology
Enteroviruses
Epilepsy
Eyes
Facial transplantation
Fetal tissue transplantation
Fibromyalgia
Frontotemporal dementia (FTD)
Glands
Glasgow coma scale
Guillain-Barré syndrome
Hammertoe correction
Head and neck disorders
Headaches
Hearing tests
Heart transplantation
Hemiplegia
Hemolytic uremic syndrome
Histiocytosis
Huntington's disease
Hydrocephalus
Hypnosis
Hypothalamus
Intraventricular hemorrhage
Irritable bowel syndrome (IBS)
Kinesiology
Lead poisoning
Learning disabilities
Leprosy

Leptospirosis
Light therapy
Listeria infections
Local anesthesia
Lower extremities
Lumbar puncture
Lyme disease
Maple syrup urine disease (MSUD)
Measles
Memory loss
Ménière's disease
Meningitis
Mental retardation
Mental status exam
Mercury poisoning
Motion sickness
Motor neuron diseases
Motor skill development
Multiple chemical sensitivity
    syndrome
Multiple sclerosis
Mumps
Myasthenia gravis
Narcolepsy
Nausea and vomiting
Neurofibromatosis
Neuroimaging
Neurology
Neurosis
Neurosurgery
Niemann-Pick disease
Nuclear radiology
Numbness and tingling
Orthopedic surgery
Orthopedics
Overtraining syndrome
Palsy
Paralysis
Paraplegia
Parkinson's disease
Pharmacology
Phenylketonuria (PKU)
Physical rehabilitation
Pick's disease
Poisoning
Poliomyelitis
Porphyria
Precocious puberty
Preeclampsia and eclampsia
Prion diseases
Quadriplegia
Rabies
Radiculopathy
Restless legs syndrome
Reye's syndrome
Rocky Mountain spotted fever
Rubella

Factitious disorders
Failure to thrive
Fibromyalgia
Frontotemporal dementia (FTD)
Gender identity disorder
Gulf War syndrome
Headaches
Hormone therapy
Hormones
Hydrocephalus
Hypnosis
Hypochondriasis
Hypothalamus
Interpartner violence
Kinesiology
Klinefelter syndrome
Learning disabilities
Light therapy
Memory loss
Menopause
Mental retardation
Miscarriage
Morgellons disease
Motor skill development
Narcolepsy
Neurology
Neurosis
Neurosurgery
Obesity
Obsessive-compulsive disorder
Overtraining syndrome
Paranoia
Pharmacology
Phobias
Pick's disease
Postpartum depression
Post-traumatic stress disorder
Prader-Willi syndrome
Precocious puberty
Premenstrual syndrome (PMS)
Psychiatric disorders
Psychoanalysis
Psychosis
Rabies
Rape and sexual assault
Restless legs syndrome
Schizophrenia
Seasonal affective disorder
Separation anxiety
Sexual dysfunction
Sexuality
Shock therapy
Sleep
Sleep disorders
Sleeping sickness
Sleepwalking
Soiling

Speech disorders
Sperm banks
Steroid abuse
Strokes
Suicide
Synesthesia
Tics
Tinnitus
Toilet training
Tourette's syndrome
Weight loss and gain
West Nile virus
Wilson's disease
Yoga

REPRODUCTIVE SYSTEM
Abdomen
Abortion
Acquired immunodeficiency
    syndrome (AIDS)
Adrenoleukodystrophy
Amenorrhea
Amniocentesis
Anorexia nervosa
Assisted reproductive technologies
Avian influenza
Breast-feeding
Brucellosis
Candidiasis
Catheterization
Cervical procedures
Cesarean section
Childbirth
Childbirth complications
Chlamydia
Chorionic villus sampling
Computed tomography (CT) scanning
Conception
Congenital adrenal hyperplasia
Contraception
Culdocentesis
Cyst removal
Cystoscopy
Dysmenorrhea
Eating disorders
Ectopic pregnancy
Endocrine glands
Endocrinology
Endometrial biopsy
Endometriosis
Episiotomy
Erectile dysfunction
Fistula repair
Gamete intrafallopian transfer (GIFT)
Gender reassignment surgery
Genetic counseling
Gestational diabetes

Gigantism
Glands
Gonorrhea
Gynecology
Hermaphroditism and
    pseudohermaphroditism
Hernia
Herpes
Hormone therapy
Human papillomavirus (HPV)
Hydroceles
Hypospadias repair and urethroplasty
Hysterectomy
In vitro fertilization
Internal medicine
Klinefelter syndrome
Laparoscopy
Lead poisoning
Ligaments
Menopause
Menorrhagia
Menstruation
Miscarriage
Myomectomy
Obstetrics
Orchiectomy
Orchitis
Ovarian cysts
Pap test
Pelvic inflammatory disease (PID)
Penile implant surgery
Placenta
Polycystic ovary syndrome
Polyps
Precocious puberty
Preeclampsia and eclampsia
Pregnancy and gestation
Premature birth
Premenstrual syndrome (PMS)
Prostate cancer
Prostate enlargement
Prostate gland
Semen
Sexual differentiation
Sexual dysfunction
Sexuality
Sexually transmitted diseases (STDs)
Sperm banks
Sterilization
Steroid abuse
Stevens-Johnson syndrome
Stillbirth
Syphilis
Testicular surgery
Testicular torsion
Toxemia
Trichomoniasis

Tubal ligation
Turner syndrome
Ultrasonography
Urology
Uterus
Vas deferens
Vasectomy
Von Willebrand's disease

RESPIRATORY SYSTEM
Abscess drainage
Acidosis
Acquired immunodeficiency
    syndrome (AIDS)
Acute respiratory distress syndrome
    (ARDS)
Adenoviruses
Adrenoleukodystrophy
Altitude sickness
Amyotrophic lateral sclerosis
Anthrax
Antihistamines
Apgar score
Apnea
Asbestos exposure
Asphyxiation
Asthma
Avian influenza
Babesiosis
Bacterial infections
Bronchi
Bronchiolitis
Bronchitis
Cardiopulmonary resuscitation (CPR)
Chest
Childhood infectious diseases
Choking
Chronic obstructive pulmonary
    disease (COPD)
Cold agglutinin disease
Common cold
Computed tomography (CT) scanning
Coronaviruses
Coughing
Croup
Cystic fibrosis
Decongestants
Defibrillation
Diaphragm
Drowning
Dwarfism
Edema
Emphysema
Epiglottitis
Exercise physiology
Fetal surgery
Fluids and electrolytes

Food allergies
Fungal infections
Hantavirus
Hay fever
Head and neck disorders
Heart transplantation
Heimlich maneuver
Hiccups
H1N1 influenza
Hyperbaric oxygen therapy
Hyperventilation
Hypoxia
Influenza
Internal medicine
Kinesiology
Laryngectomy
Legionnaires' disease
Lung cancer
Lung surgery
Lungs
Measles
Mesothelioma
Methicillin-resistant staphylococcus
    aureus (MRSA) infection
Mold and mildew
Monkeypox
Multiple chemical sensitivity
    syndrome
Nasopharyngeal disorders
Niemann-Pick disease
Obesity
Otorhinolaryngology
Oxygen therapy
Pharynx
Plague
Plasma
Pneumocystis jirovecii
Pneumonia
Pneumothorax
Poisoning
Pulmonary diseases
Pulmonary edema
Pulmonary hypertension
Pulmonary medicine
Respiration
Resuscitation
Rheumatoid arthritis
Rhinitis
Rhinoviruses
Sarcoidosis
Severe acute respiratory syndrome
    (SARS)
Sinusitis
Sleep apnea
Smoking
Sore throat
Staphylococcal infections

Stevens-Johnson syndrome
Thoracic surgery
Thrombolytic therapy and TPA
Thrombosis and thrombus
Tonsillectomy and adenoid removal
Trachea
Tracheostomy
Transplantation
Tuberculosis
Tularemia
Tumor removal
Typhus
Vasculitis
Voice and vocal cord disorders
Whooping cough

SKIN
Abscess drainage
Acne
Acquired immunodeficiency
    syndrome (AIDS)
Acupressure
Adenoviruses
Adrenoleukodystrophy
Allergies
Amputation
Anesthesia
Anesthesiology
Angelman syndrome
Anorexia nervosa
Anthrax
Anxiety
Athlete's foot
Auras
Bacillus Calmette-Guérin (BCG)
Bariatric surgery
Batten's disease
Bedsores
Behçet's disease
Bites and stings
Blisters
Blood testing
Body dysmorphic disorder
Bruises
Burns and scalds
Candidiasis
Canker sores
Casts and splints
Cells
Chagas' disease
Chickenpox
Cleft lip and palate repair
Cold agglutinin disease
Cold sores
Collagen
Collodion baby
Corns and calluses

Cushing's syndrome
Cutis marmorata telangiectatica
  congenita
Cyanosis
Cyst removal
Dengue fever
Dermatitis
Dermatology
Dermatopathology
Ebola virus
Eczema
Edema
Electrical shock
Electrocauterization
Enteroviruses
Face lift and blepharoplasty
Facial transplantation
Fibrocystic breast condition
Fifth disease
Food allergies
Frostbite
Fungal infections
Gangrene
Glands
Gluten intolerance
Gulf War syndrome
Hair
Hair transplantation
Hand-foot-and-mouth disease
Heat exhaustion and heatstroke
Hematomas
Hemolytic disease of the newborn
Herpes
Histiocytosis
Hives
Hormone therapy
Host-defense mechanisms
Human papillomavirus (HPV)
Hyperhidrosis
Impetigo
Intravenous (IV) therapy
Jaundice
Kaposi's sarcoma
Kawasaki disease
Kwashiorkor
Laceration repair
Laser use in surgery
Leishmaniasis
Leprosy
Light therapy
Lower extremities
Lyme disease
Measles
Melanoma
Methicillin-resistant staphylococcus
  aureus (MRSA) infection
Mold and mildew

Moles
Monkeypox
Morgellons disease
Multiple chemical sensitivity
  syndrome
Nails
Necrotizing fasciitis
Neurofibromatosis
Numbness and tingling
Otoplasty
Pigmentation
Pinworms
Pityriasis alba
Pityriasis rosea
Polycystic ovary syndrome
Polydactyly and syndactyly
Porphyria
Psoriasis
Radiation sickness
Reiter's syndrome
Ringworm
Rocky Mountain spotted fever
Rosacea
Roseola
Rubella
Sarcoidosis
Scabies
Scarlet fever
Sense organs
Shingles
Skin cancer
Skin disorders
Skin lesion removal
Smallpox
Streptococcal infections
Sturge-Weber syndrome
Styes
Sweating
Tattoo removal
Tattoos and body piercing
Touch
Toxoplasmosis
Tularemia
Typhoid fever
Typhus
Umbilical cord
Upper extremities
Vasculitis
Vitiligo
Von Willebrand's disease
Williams syndrome
Wiskott-Aldrich syndrome

SPINE
Anesthesia
Anesthesiology
Ankylosing spondylitis

Atrophy
Back pain
Brain tumors
Brucellosis
Charcot-Marie-Tooth Disease
Chiari malformations
Chiropractic
Diaphragm
Disk removal
Fetal tissue transplantation
Head and neck disorders
Kinesiology
Laminectomy and spinal fusion
Lumbar puncture
Marfan syndrome
Meningitis
Mesenchymal stem cells
Methicillin-resistant staphylococcus
  aureus (MRSA) infection
Motor neuron diseases
Multiple sclerosis
Nervous system
Neuroimaging
Neurology
Neurosurgery
Orthopedic surgery
Orthopedics
Osteogenesis imperfecta
Osteoporosis
Paget's disease
Paralysis
Paraplegia
Physical rehabilitation
Poliomyelitis
Quadriplegia
Radiculopathy
Sciatica
Scoliosis
Slipped disk
Spina bifida
Spinal cord disorders
Spondylitis
Sports medicine
Stenosis
Sympathectomy
Whiplash
Williams syndrome

SPLEEN
Abscess drainage
Aspergillosis
Brucellosis
Cold agglutinin disease
Gaucher's disease
Hematology
Immune system
Internal medicine

Entries by Specialties and Related Fields

ALL
Abscesses
Accidents
Anatomy
Autoimmune disorders
Biostatistics
Carcinogens
Clinical trials
Cysts
Diagnosis
Disease
Emergency rooms
Emerging infectious diseases
Environmental diseases
Epidermal nevus syndromes
Fetal alcohol syndrome
First aid
Geriatrics and gerontology
Herbal medicine
Iatrogenic disorders
Internet medicine
Invasive tests
Medical home
Men's health
Neuroimaging
Physical examination
Physiology
Preventive medicine
Prognosis
Proteomics
Self-medication
Signs and symptoms
Substance abuse
Syndrome
Systemic sclerosis
Systems and organs
Terminally ill: Extended care
Toxicology
Transitional care

ALTERNATIVE MEDICINE
Acidosis
Acupressure
Acupuncture
Amyotrophic lateral sclerosis
Antioxidants
Aphrodisiacs
Aromatherapy
Back pain
Biofeedback
Biological therapies
Chemotherapy

Club drugs
Colon
Colon therapy
Enzyme therapy
Fiber
Genetic engineering
Healing
Hydrotherapy
Hypnosis
Irritable bowel syndrome (IBS)
Magnetic field therapy
Marijuana
Massage
Meditation
Melatonin
Pain management
Small intestine
Stress reduction
Supplements
Yoga

ANESTHESIOLOGY
Acidosis
Acupuncture
Anesthesia
Anesthesiology
Aneurysmectomy
Arthroplasty
Back pain
Catheterization
Cesarean section
Critical care
Defibrillation
Dentistry
Hyperbaric oxygen therapy
Hyperthermia and hypothermia
Hypnosis
Hypoxia
Intravenous (IV) therapy
Local anesthesia
Lumbar puncture
Mesenchymal stem cells
Oral and maxillofacial surgery
Oxygen therapy
Pain
Pain management
Palliative medicine
Pharmacology
Pulse rate
Surgical procedures
Surgical technologists

AUDIOLOGY
Adrenoleukodystrophy
Aging: Extended care
Charcot-Marie-Tooth Disease
Cockayne Disease
Deafness
Dyslexia
Ear infections and disorders
Ear surgery
Ears
Earwax
Hearing
Hearing aids
Hearing loss
Hearing tests
Ménière's disease
Neurology
Otoplasty
Otorhinolaryngology
Sense organs
Speech disorders
Tinnitus
Vertigo
Williams syndrome

BACTERIOLOGY
Acquired immunodeficiency
  syndrome (AIDS)
Amebiasis
Anthrax
Antibiotic resistance
Antibiotics
Antibodies
Bacillus Calmette-Guérin (BCG)
Bacterial infections
Botulism
Brucellosis
Campylobacter infections
Cells
Childhood infectious diseases
Chronic granulomatous disease
Cold agglutinin disease
Conjunctivitis
Cystitis
Cytology
Cytopathology
Diphtheria
E. coli infection
Encephalitis
Endocarditis
Epidemics and pandemics
Epiglottitis

Eye infections and disorders
Fluoride treatments
Gangrene
Gastroenteritis
Genomics
Gingivitis
Gram staining
Impetigo
Infection
Insect-borne diseases
Laboratory tests
Legionnaires' disease
Leprosy
Leptospirosis
Listeria infections
Lyme disease
Mastitis
Methicillin-resistant staphylococcus
   aureus (MRSA) infection
Microbiology
Microscopy
Necrotizing fasciitis
Opportunistic infections
Osteomyelitis
Peritonitis
Plague
Salmonella infection
Sarcoidosis
Scarlet fever
Serology
Shigellosis
Staphylococcal infections
Streptococcal infections
Styes
Syphilis
Tetanus
Tuberculosis
Tularemia
Typhoid fever
Typhus
Urethritis
Whooping cough
Zoonoses

BIOCHEMISTRY
Acid-base chemistry
Acidosis
Amyotrophic lateral sclerosis
Antibodies
Antidepressants
Autopsy
Avian influenza
Bacteriology
Bulimia
Caffeine
Carbohydrates
Cholesterol

Collagen
Colon
Connective tissue
Corticosteroids
Digestion
Endocrine glands
Endocrinology
Enzyme therapy
Ergogenic aids
Fatty acid oxidation disorders
Fluids and electrolytes
Fluoride treatments
Food biochemistry
Food guide plate
Fructosemia
Galactosemia
Gaucher's disease
Genetic engineering
Genomics
Gigantism
Gingivitis
Glands
Glycogen storage diseases
Glycolysis
Gram staining
Gulf War syndrome
Histology
Hormones
Hyperadiposis
Hypothalamus
Insect-borne diseases
Leptin
Leukodystrophy
Lipids
Lumbar puncture
Macronutrients
Malabsorption
Malaria
Metabolic disorders
Metabolism
Nephrology
Niemann-Pick disease
Nutrition
Osteogenesis imperfecta
Ovaries
Pathology
Pharmacology
Phenylketonuria (PKU)
Pituitary gland
Plasma
Protein
Respiration
Retroviruses
Rhinoviruses
Sleep
Small intestine
Stem cells

Steroids
Thymus gland
Tourette's syndrome
Urinalysis
Wilson's disease

BIOTECHNOLOGY
Antibodies
Assisted reproductive technologies
Biological therapies
Bionics and biotechnology
Cloning
Computed tomography (CT) scanning
Defibrillation
Dialysis
Electrocardiography (ECG or EKG)
Electroencephalography (EEG)
Fatty acid oxidation disorders
Gene therapy
Genetic engineering
Genomics
Glycogen storage diseases
Huntington's disease
Hyperbaric oxygen therapy
Insect-borne diseases
Magnetic resonance imaging (MRI)
Malabsorption
Mesenchymal stem cells
Nephrology
Pacemaker implantation
Positron emission tomography (PET)
   scanning
Prostheses
Rhinoviruses
Severe combined immunodeficiency
   syndrome (SCID)
Sperm banks
Stem cells
Xenotransplantation

CARDIOLOGY
Acute respiratory distress syndrome
   (ARDS)
Aging: Extended care
Anemia
Aneurysms
Angina
Angiography
Angioplasty
Antihypertensives
Anxiety
Aortic aneurysm
Aortic stenosis
Arrhythmias
Arteriosclerosis
Aspergillosis
Atrial fibrillation

Biofeedback
Blood pressure
Blood vessels
Blue baby syndrome
Brucellosis
Bypass surgery
Cardiac arrest
Cardiac rehabilitation
Cardiac surgery
Cardiopulmonary resuscitation (CPR)
Carotid arteries
Catheterization
Chest
Circulation
Computed tomography (CT) scanning
Congenital heart disease
Coronary artery bypass graft
Critical care
Defibrillation
DiGeorge syndrome
Diphtheria
Diuretics
Dizziness and fainting
Echocardiography
Electrocardiography (ECG or EKG)
Electrocauterization
Embolism
Emergency medicine
End-stage renal disease
Endocarditis
Enteroviruses
Exercise physiology
Fetal surgery
Gigantism
Heart
Heart attack
Heart disease
Heart failure
Heart transplantation
Heart valve replacement
Hematology
Hemochromatosis
Hormone therapy
Hypercholesterolemia
Hypertension
Hypotension
Infarction
Internal medicine
Ischemia
Kawasaki disease
Kinesiology
Leptin
Lesions
Lyme disease
Marfan syndrome
Metabolic syndrome
Methicillin-resistant staphylococcus

aureus (MRSA) infection
Mitral valve prolapse
Mucopolysaccharidosis (MPS)
Muscles
Neonatology
Noninvasive tests
Nuclear medicine
Oxygen therapy
Pacemaker implantation
Palliative care
Palpitations
Paramedics
Plasma
Polycystic kidney disease
Prader-Willi syndrome
Progeria
Prostheses
Pulmonary edema
Pulmonary hypertension
Pulse rate
Rheumatic fever
Rubinstein-Taybi syndrome
Sarcoidosis
Single photon emission computed
    tomography (SPECT)
Spondylitis
Sports medicine
Staphylococcal infections
Stem cells
Stenosis
Stents
Systemic lupus erythematosus (SLE)
Thoracic surgery
Thrombolytic therapy and TPA
Thrombosis and thrombus
Transplantation
Ultrasonography
Uremia
Varicose veins
Vascular medicine
Vascular system
Vasculitis
Venous insufficiency
Williams syndrome

CRITICAL CARE
Acidosis
Aging: Extended care
Amputation
Anesthesia
Anesthesiology
Aneurysmectomy
Anthrax
Apgar score
Botulism
Burns and scalds
Carotid arteries

Catheterization
Chronic granulomatous disease
Club drugs
Concussion
Craniotomy
Defibrillation
Diuretics
Drowning
Echocardiography
Electrical shock
Electrocardiography (ECG or EKG)
Electrocauterization
Electroencephalography (EEG)
Embolization
Emergency medicine
Epidemics and pandemics
Grafts and grafting
Hantavirus
Heart attack
Heart transplantation
Heat exhaustion and heatstroke
Hydrocephalus
Hyperbaric oxygen therapy
Hyperthermia and hypothermia
Hypotension
Hypoxia
Infarction
Insect-borne diseases
Intravenous (IV) therapy
Ischemia
Lumbar puncture
Methicillin-resistant staphylococcus
    aureus (MRSA) infection
Necrotizing fasciitis
Neonatology
Nursing
Oncology
Osteopathic medicine
Oxygen therapy
Pain management
Paramedics
Peritonitis
Psychiatry
Pulmonary medicine
Pulse rate
Radiation sickness
Resuscitation
Safety issues for children
Safety issues for the elderly
Severe acute respiratory syndrome
    (SARS)
Shock
Stevens-Johnson syndrome
Streptococcal infections
Thrombolytic therapy and TPA
Toxic shock syndrome
Tracheostomy

Reiter's syndrome
Ringworm
Rocky Mountain spotted fever
Rosacea
Sarcoidosis
Scabies
Scleroderma
Sense organs
Shingles
Skin
Skin cancer
Skin disorders
Skin lesion removal
Smallpox
Staphylococcal infections
Stevens-Johnson syndrome
Streptococcal infections
Stress
Sturge-Weber syndrome
Styes
Sweating
Systemic lupus erythematosus (SLE)
Tattoo removal
Tattoos and body piercing
Touch
Vasculitis
Vitiligo
Von Willebrand's disease
Wiskott-Aldrich syndrome

EMBRYOLOGY
Amniocentesis
Assisted reproductive technologies
Birth defects
Blue baby syndrome
Brain disorders
Chorionic villus sampling
Cloning
Conception
Down syndrome
Ectopic pregnancy
Fetal tissue transplantation
Gamete intrafallopian transfer (GIFT)
Genetic counseling
Genetic diseases
Genetic engineering
Genetic Imprinting
Genetics and inheritance
Genomics
Growth
Hermaphroditism and
    pseudohermaphroditism
In vitro fertilization
Karyotyping
Klinefelter syndrome
Meckel's diverticulum
Miscarriage

Mucopolysaccharidosis (MPS)
Multiple births
Neonatology
Obstetrics
Ovaries
Perinatology
Phenylketonuria (PKU)
Placenta
Pregnancy and gestation
Premature birth
Reproductive system
Rh factor
Sexual differentiation
Spina bifida
Stem cells
Syphilis
Teratogens
Ultrasonography
Uterus

EMERGENCY MEDICINE
Abdominal disorders
Abscess drainage
Acidosis
Adrenoleukodystrophy
Advance directives
Altitude sickness
Amputation
Anesthesia
Anesthesiology
Aneurysmectomy
Aneurysms
Angiography
Anthrax
Appendectomy
Appendicitis
Asphyxiation
Atrial fibrillation
Back pain
Bites and stings
Bleeding
Blurred vision
Botulism
Bruises
Burns and scalds
Cardiac arrest
Cardiology
Cardiopulmonary resuscitation (CPR)
Carotid arteries
Casts and splints
Catheterization
Cesarean section
Choking
Cholecystitis
Chronic granulomatous disease
Club drugs
Cold agglutinin disease

Computed tomography (CT) scanning
Concussion
Critical care
Croup
Defibrillation
Dizziness and fainting
Drowning
Echocardiography
Electrical shock
Electrocardiography (ECG or EKG)
Electrocauterization
Electroencephalography (EEG)
Embolization
Epiglottitis
First responder
Fracture and dislocation
Frostbite
Gangrene
Grafts and grafting
Head and neck disorders
Heart attack
Heart transplantation
Heat exhaustion and heatstroke
Heimlich maneuver
H1N1 influenza
Hyperbaric oxygen therapy
Hyperthermia and hypothermia
Hyperventilation
Hypotension
Hypoxia
Impetigo
Infarction
Influenza
Interpartner violence
Interstitial pulmonary fibrosis (IPF)
Intravenous (IV) therapy
Jaw wiring
Laceration repair
Local anesthesia
Lung surgery
Meningitis
Mental status exam
Monkeypox
Nail removal
Necrotizing fasciitis
Noninvasive tests
Nursing
Osteopathic medicine
Oxygen therapy
Pain management
Palliative medicine
Paramedics
Peritonitis
Physician assistants
Plague
Plastic surgery
Pleurisy

Pneumonia
Pneumothorax
Poisoning
Pulmonary medicine
Pulse rate
Pyelonephritis
Radiation sickness
Rape and sexual assault
Resuscitation
Reye's syndrome
Rocky Mountain spotted fever
Safety issues for children
Safety issues for the elderly
Severe acute respiratory syndrome
  (SARS)
Shock
Snakebites
Spinal cord disorders
Splenectomy
Sports medicine
Stevens-Johnson syndrome
Streptococcal infections
Strokes
Surgical technologists
Thrombolytic therapy and TPA
Toxic shock syndrome
Tracheostomy
Transfusion
Transplantation
Tularemia
Wounds

ENDOCRINOLOGY
Addison's disease
Adrenalectomy
Adrenoleukodystrophy
Amenorrhea
Anti-inflammatory drugs
Assisted reproductive technologies
Bariatric surgery
Carbohydrates
Computed tomography (CT) scanning
Congenital adrenal hyperplasia
Congenital hypothyroidism
Corticosteroids
Cushing's syndrome
Diabetes mellitus
Dwarfism
End-stage renal disease
Endocrine disorders
Endocrine glands
Ergogenic aids
Failure to thrive
Gamete intrafallopian transfer (GIFT)
Gender identity disorder
Gender reassignment surgery
Gestational diabetes

Gigantism
Glands
Glioma
Goiter
Growth
Gynecology
Gynecomastia
Hashimoto's thyroiditis
Hemochromatosis
Hermaphroditism and
  pseudohermaphroditism
Hormone therapy
Hormones
Hyperadiposis
Hyperparathyroidism and
  hypoparathyroidism
Hyperplasia
Hypertrophy
Hypoglycemia
Hypothalamus
Hysterectomy
Internal medicine
Klinefelter syndrome
Laboratory tests
Laparoscopy
Leptin
Liver
Melatonin
Menopause
Menstruation
Metabolic disorders
Metabolic syndrome
Nephrology
Neurology
Niemann-Pick disease
Nonalcoholic steatohepatitis (NASH)
Nuclear medicine
Obesity
Ovaries
Pancreas
Pancreatitis
Parathyroidectomy
Pharmacology
Pituitary gland
Plasma
Polycystic ovary syndrome
Precocious puberty
Prostate enlargement
Prostate gland
Puberty and adolescence
Pulse rate
Radiopharmaceuticals
Sexual differentiation
Sexual dysfunction
Sleep
Small intestine
Stem cells

Steroids
Systemic lupus erythematosus (SLE)
Testicular cancer
Thymus gland
Thyroid disorders
Thyroid gland
Thyroidectomy
Tumors
Turner syndrome
Vitamins and minerals
Vitiligo
Weight loss and gain
Weight loss medications
Williams syndrome

ENVIRONMENTAL HEALTH
Acidosis
Asbestos exposure
Asthma
Babesiosis
Blurred vision
Cholera
Cognitive development
Coronaviruses
Creutzfeldt-Jakob disease (CJD)
Drowning
Elephantiasis
Enteroviruses
Food poisoning
Frostbite
Gastroenteritis
Gulf War syndrome
Hantavirus
Hyperthermia and hypothermia
Insect-borne diseases
Lead poisoning
Legionnaires' disease
Lung cancer
Lungs
Mercury poisoning
Microbiology
Mold and mildew
Multiple chemical sensitivity
  syndrome
Occupational health
Parasitic diseases
Pigmentation
Plague
Poisoning
Pulmonary diseases
Pulmonary medicine
Roundworms
Schistosomiasis
Skin cancer
Sleeping sickness
Smallpox
Stress

Stress reduction
Trachoma
Tularemia
Typhoid fever
Typhus
West Nile virus
Yellow fever

EPIDEMIOLOGY
Acquired immunodeficiency
    syndrome (AIDS)
Amebiasis
Avian influenza
Bacillus Calmette-Guérin (BCG)
Bacterial infections
Bacteriology
Brucellosis
Candidiasis
Cerebral palsy
Chickenpox
Childhood infectious diseases
Cholera
Coronaviruses
Creutzfeldt-Jakob disease (CJD)
Diphtheria
E. coli infection
Ebola virus
Elephantiasis
Encephalitis
Epidemics and pandemics
Food poisoning
Forensic pathology
Gulf War syndrome
Hantavirus
Hepatitis
H1N1 influenza
Human papillomavirus (HPV)
Influenza
Insect-borne diseases
Laboratory tests
Legionnaires' disease
Leprosy
Leptospirosis
Lyme disease
Marburg virus
Mercury poisoning
Methicillin-resistant staphylococcus
    aureus (MRSA) infection
Microbiology
Multiple chemical sensitivity
    syndrome
Necrotizing fasciitis
Occupational health
Parasitic diseases
Phenylketonuria (PKU)
Plague
Pneumonia

Poisoning
Poliomyelitis
Prion diseases
Pulmonary diseases
Rabies
Rhinoviruses
Rocky Mountain spotted fever
Rotavirus
Roundworms
Screening
Severe acute respiratory syndrome
    (SARS)
Sexually transmitted diseases (STDs)
Sleeping sickness
Smallpox
Staphylococcal infections
Stress
Syphilis
Trichomoniasis
Tularemia
Typhoid fever
Typhus
Viral hemorrhagic fevers
Viral infections
West Nile virus
Yellow fever
Zoonoses

ETHICS
Abortion
Advance directives
Assisted reproductive technologies
Cloning
Defibrillation
Ergogenic aids
Facial transplantation
Fetal surgery
Fetal tissue transplantation
Gender identity disorder
Genetic engineering
Genomics
Gulf War syndrome
Longevity
Marijuana
Münchausen syndrome by proxy
Neurosis
Sperm banks
Stem cells
Xenotransplantation

EXERCISE PHYSIOLOGY
Acidosis
Ataxia
Biofeedback
Blood pressure
Bones and the skeleton
Cardiac rehabilitation

Carotid arteries
Defibrillation
Dehydration
Electrocardiography (ECG or EKG)
Ergogenic aids
Fascia
Glycolysis
Heart
Hemiplegia
Hypotension
Hypoxia
Juvenile rheumatoid arthritis
Kinesiology
Ligaments
Lungs
Massage
Metabolism
Motor skill development
Muscles
Osteoarthritis
Overtraining syndrome
Physical rehabilitation
Pulmonary medicine
Pulse rate
Respiration
Slipped disk
Sports medicine
Stenosis
Steroid abuse
Sweating
Tendinitis
Vascular system

FAMILY MEDICINE
Abdominal disorders
Abscess drainage
Acne
Advance directives
Alcoholism
Allergies
Amenorrhea
Amyotrophic lateral sclerosis
Anemia
Angelman syndrome
Angina
Anorexia nervosa
Anosmia
Antianxiety drugs
Antidepressants
Antihistamines
Antihypertensives
Anti-inflammatory drugs
Antioxidants
Aspergillosis
Ataxia
Atrophy
Attention-deficit disorder (ADD)

Autism
Bed-wetting
Bell's palsy
Beriberi
Biofeedback
Bleeding
Blisters
Blood pressure
Blurred vision
Body dysmorphic disorder
Bronchiolitis
Bronchitis
Bruises
Bulimia
Bunions
Burkitt's lymphoma
Caffeine
Candidiasis
Canker sores
Carotid arteries
Casts and splints
Cerebral palsy
Chagas' disease
Chickenpox
Childhood infectious diseases
Cholecystitis
Cholesterol
Chronic fatigue syndrome
Chronic granulomatous disease
Cirrhosis
Clostridium difficile infection
Coccidioidomycosis
Cold sores
Common cold
Conjunctivitis
Constipation
Corticosteroids
Coughing
Cryosurgery
Cushing's syndrome
Cytomegalovirus (CMV)
Death and dying
Decongestants
Deep vein thrombosis
Defibrillation
Dehydration
Dengue fever
Depression
Diabetes mellitus
Diarrhea and dysentery
Digestion
Diphtheria
Dizziness and fainting
E. coli infection
Earwax
Eating disorders
Echocardiography

Ehrlichiosis
Electrocauterization
Enterocolitis
Epiglottitis
Ergogenic aids
Exercise physiology
Factitious disorders
Failure to thrive
Fatigue
Fever
Fiber
Fifth disease
Fungal infections
Ganglion removal
Geriatric assessment
Giardiasis
Gigantism
Gynecology
Headaches
Healing
Heart disease
Heat exhaustion and heatstroke
Hemiplegia
Hemolytic uremic syndrome
Hemorrhoid banding and removal
Hemorrhoids
Herpes
Hiccups
Hirschsprung's disease
Hives
H1N1 influenza
Hormone therapy
Hyperadiposis
Hyperlipidemia
Hypertension
Hypertrophy
Hypoglycemia
Hypoxia
Impetigo
Incontinence
Infarction
Infection
Inflammation
Influenza
Interpartner violence
Intestinal disorders
Juvenile rheumatoid arthritis
Kawasaki disease
Keratitis
Kluver-Bucy syndrome
Kwashiorkor
Leishmaniasis
Leukodystrophy
Malabsorption
Maple syrup urine disease (MSUD)
Mastitis
Measles

Methicillin-resistant staphylococcus
  aureus (MRSA) infection
Mitral valve prolapse
Moles
Mononucleosis
Motion sickness
Mumps
Münchausen syndrome by proxy
Myringotomy
Nail removal
Nasal polyp removal
Nasopharyngeal disorders
Neurosis
Niemann-Pick disease
Nonalcoholic steatohepatitis (NASH)
Obesity
Orchitis
Osteopathic medicine
Otoplasty
Over-the-counter medications
Palliative medicine
Parasitic diseases
Pediatrics
Pharmacology
Physician assistants
Pick's disease
Pinworms
Pituitary gland
Pityriasis alba
Pityriasis rosea
Pleurisy
Pneumonia
Polycystic ovary syndrome
Polyps
Prader-Willi syndrome
Precocious puberty
Premenstrual syndrome (PMS)
Psychiatry
Ptosis
Puberty and adolescence
Pulse rate
Pyelonephritis
Raynaud's phenomenon
Reiter's syndrome
Rheumatic fever
Rhinitis
Ringworm
Rocky Mountain spotted fever
Roseola
Rubella
Safety issues for children
Safety issues for the elderly
Salmonella infection
Scabies
Scarlet fever
Sciatica
Sexuality

Shingles
Shock
Sinusitis
Sjögren's syndrome
Skin disorders
Sleep
Slipped disk
Sore throat
Sports medicine
Sterilization
Stevens-Johnson syndrome
Streptococcal infections
Stress
Stuttering
Styes
Supplements
Systemic lupus erythematosus (SLE)
Temporomandibular joint (TMJ)
    syndrome
Tendinitis
Testicular torsion
Tetanus
Thalassemia
Tinnitus
Toilet training
Tonsillitis
Tonsils
Tourette's syndrome
Toxoplasmosis
Trachoma
Ulcers
Urethritis
Urology
Vascular medicine
Vasectomy
Viral infections
Vitamins and minerals
Von Willebrand's disease
Weaning
Weight loss medications
Whooping cough
Wounds

FORENSIC MEDICINE
Antianxiety drugs
Autopsy
Blood testing
Cytopathology
Defibrillation
Dermatopathology
Genetic engineering
Genetics and inheritance
Hematology
Laboratory tests
Pathology

GASTROENTEROLOGY
Abdomen
Abdominal disorders
Achalasia
Acid reflux disease
Acidosis
Acquired immunodeficiency
    syndrome (AIDS)
Adenoviruses
Amebiasis
Amyotrophic lateral sclerosis
Anal cancer
Anus
Appendicitis
Bariatric surgery
Bile
Bulimia
Bypass surgery
Campylobacter infections
Celiac sprue
Cholecystitis
Cholera
Chronic granulomatous disease
Chyme
Clostridium difficile infection
Colic
Colitis
Colon
Colonoscopy and sigmoidoscopy
Colorectal cancer
Colorectal polyp removal
Colorectal surgery
Computed tomography (CT) scanning
Constipation
Critical care
Crohn's disease
Cytomegalovirus (CMV)
Diarrhea and dysentery
Digestion
Diverticulitis and diverticulosis
E. coli infection
Emergency medicine
Endoscopic retrograde
    cholangiopancreatography (ERCP)
Endoscopy
Enemas
Enterocolitis
Epidemics and pandemics
Esophagus
Failure to thrive
Fiber
Fistula repair
Food allergies
Food biochemistry
Food poisoning
Gallbladder
Gallbladder cancer

Gallbladder diseases
Gastrectomy
Gastroenteritis
Gastrointestinal disorders
Gastrointestinal system
Gastrostomy
Giardiasis
Glands
Gluten intolerance
Hemochromatosis
Hemolytic uremic syndrome
Hemorrhoid banding and removal
Hemorrhoids
Hernia
Hernia repair
Hiccups
Ileostomy and colostomy
Infarction
Internal medicine
Intestinal disorders
Intestines
Irritable bowel syndrome (IBS)
Jaundice
Lactose intolerance
Laparoscopy
Lesions
Liver
Liver cancer
Liver disorders
Liver transplantation
Malabsorption
Malnutrition
Meckel's diverticulum
Metabolism
Nausea and vomiting
Nonalcoholic steatohepatitis (NASH)
Noroviruses
Pancreas
Pancreatitis
Peristalsis
Peritonitis
Polycystic kidney disease
Polyps
Proctology
Pyloric stenosis
Rectum
Rotavirus
Salmonella infection
Scleroderma
Shigellosis
Small intestine
Soiling
Stenosis
Stevens-Johnson syndrome
Stone removal
Stones
Tapeworms

Cells
Cold agglutinin disease
Colon
Cytology
Cytopathology
Dermatology
Dermatopathology
Endometrial biopsy
Eye infections and disorders
Fluids and electrolytes
Forensic pathology
Glioma
Healing
Laboratory tests
Microscopy
Nails
Necrotizing fasciitis
Pathology
Pityriasis alba
Rhinoviruses
Sarcoma
Small intestine
Smallpox
Tumor removal
Tumors

IMMUNOLOGY
Acquired immunodeficiency
    syndrome (AIDS)
Adenoids
Adenoviruses
Allergies
Ankylosing spondylitis
Antibiotics
Antibodies
Antihistamines
Aspergillosis
Asthma
Avian influenza
Bacillus Calmette-Guérin (BCG)
Bacterial infections
Biological therapies
Bionics and biotechnology
Bites and stings
Blood and blood disorders
Bone cancer
Bone grafting
Bone marrow transplantation
Cancer
Candidiasis
Carcinoma
Chickenpox
Childhood infectious diseases
Chronic fatigue syndrome
Chronic granulomatous disease
Cold agglutinin disease
Colorectal cancer

Coronaviruses
Corticosteroids
Crohn's disease
Cushing's syndrome
Cytology
Cytomegalovirus (CMV)
Dermatology
Dermatopathology
DiGeorge syndrome
Endocrinology
Epidemics and pandemics
Epstein-Barr virus
Fetal tissue transplantation
Food allergies
Fungal infections
Gluten intolerance
Grafts and grafting
Hay fever
Healing
Hematology
Histiocytosis
Hives
Homeopathy
Host-defense mechanisms
Human immunodeficiency virus
    (HIV)
Hypnosis
Immune system
Immunization and vaccination
Immunodeficiency disorders
Immunopathology
Juvenile rheumatoid arthritis
Kawasaki disease
Laboratory tests
Leprosy
Liver cancer
Lung cancer
Lymph
Lymphatic system
Malaria
Microbiology
Multiple chemical sensitivity
    syndrome
Multiple sclerosis
Myasthenia gravis
Nephritis
Noroviruses
Oncology
Opportunistic infections
Pancreas
Prostate cancer
Pulmonary diseases
Pulmonary medicine
Renal failure
Rheumatic fever
Rheumatoid arthritis
Rheumatology

Rhinitis
Rhinoviruses
Sarcoidosis
Scleroderma
Serology
Severe combined immunodeficiency
    syndrome (SCID)
Skin cancer
Small intestine
Smallpox
Stem cells
Stevens-Johnson syndrome
Stress
Stress reduction
Thalidomide
Thymus gland
Transfusion
Transplantation
Tularemia
Wiskott-Aldrich syndrome
Xenotransplantation

INTERNAL MEDICINE
Abdomen
Abdominal disorders
Acidosis
Acquired immunodeficiency
    syndrome (AIDS)
Adenoids
Alcoholism
Allergies
Alzheimer's disease
Amebiasis
Amyotrophic lateral sclerosis
Anemia
Angina
Anthrax
Antianxiety drugs
Antibodies
Anti-inflammatory drugs
Antioxidants
Anus
Anxiety
Aortic stenosis
Apnea
Arteriosclerosis
Arthritis
Aspergillosis
Ataxia
Auras
Babesiosis
Bacillus Calmette-Guérin (BCG)
Bacterial infections
Bariatric surgery
Bedsores
Behçet's disease
Bile

Rectum
Renal failure
Reye's syndrome
Rocky Mountain spotted fever
Sarcoidosis
Scarlet fever
Schistosomiasis
Sciatica
Septicemia
Severe acute respiratory syndrome (SARS)
Sexuality
Sexually transmitted diseases (STDs)
Shingles
Shock
Sinusitis
Sleep
Sleeping sickness
Small intestine
Sports medicine
Staphylococcal infections
Stevens-Johnson syndrome
Stones
Stress
Supplements
Syphilis
Tetanus
Thrombosis and thrombus
Toxic shock syndrome
Tremors
Tumors
Typhoid fever
Typhus
Ulcers
Ultrasonography
Urethritis
Viral infections
Vitamins and minerals
Weight loss medications
Wilson's disease
Wounds

MICROBIOLOGY
Acquired immunodeficiency syndrome (AIDS)
Amebiasis
Anthrax
Antibiotic resistance
Antibiotics
Antibodies
Aspergillosis
Autopsy
Bacillus Calmette-Guérin (BCG)
Bacterial infections
Bacteriology
Bionics and biotechnology
Brucellosis

Campylobacter infections
Chemotherapy
Chlamydia
Cholera
Chronic granulomatous disease
Coccidioidomycosis
Conjunctivitis
Creutzfeldt-Jakob disease (CJD)
Dengue fever
Diphtheria
E. coli infection
Enteroviruses
Epidemics and pandemics
Epstein-Barr virus
Fluoride treatments
Fungal infections
Gastroenteritis
Gastroenterology
Gastrointestinal disorders
Genomics
Gonorrhea
Gram staining
Hematuria
Human immunodeficiency virus (HIV)
Immune system
Immunization and vaccination
Impetigo
Insect-borne diseases
Laboratory tests
Leptospirosis
Methicillin-resistant staphylococcus aureus (MRSA) infection
Microscopy
Mold and mildew
Opportunistic infections
Pathology
Pelvic inflammatory disease (PID)
Peritonitis
Pharmacology
Plasma
Pneumocystis jirovecii
Protozoan diseases
Serology
Severe acute respiratory syndrome (SARS)
Sleeping sickness
Staphylococcal infections
Streptococcal infections
Syphilis
Toxic shock syndrome
Trichinosis
Tuberculosis
Urinalysis
Urology

NEONATOLOGY
Angelman syndrome

Apgar score
Apnea
Birth defects
Blue baby syndrome
Bonding
Breast disorders
Cesarean section
Childbirth
Childbirth complications
Cleft lip and palate
Cleft lip and palate repair
Collodion baby
Congenital disorders
Congenital heart disease
Cutis marmorata telangiectatica congenita
Cystic fibrosis
Disseminated intravascular coagulation (DIC)
E. coli infection
Embryology
Failure to thrive
Fetal surgery
Genetic diseases
Hemolytic disease of the newborn
Hydrocephalus
Intraventricular hemorrhage
Karyotyping
Malabsorption
Maple syrup urine disease (MSUD)
Motor skill development
Multiple births
Neonatal brachial plexus palsy
Nursing
Obstetrics
Pediatrics
Perinatology
Phenylketonuria (PKU)
Physician assistants
Premature birth
Pulse rate
Respiratory distress syndrome
Rh factor
Shunts
Spina bifida
Sudden infant death syndrome (SIDS)
Syphilis
Tay-Sachs disease
Transfusion
Trichomoniasis
Umbilical cord
Well-baby examinations

NEPHROLOGY
Abdomen
Addison's disease
Anemia

Aspergillosis
Chronic granulomatous disease
Diabetes mellitus
Dialysis
Diuretics
E. coli infection
Edema
End-stage renal disease
Ergogenic aids
Hematuria
Hemolytic uremic syndrome
Internal medicine
Kidney cancer
Kidney disorders
Kidney transplantation
Kidneys
Leptospirosis
Lesions
Lithotripsy
Nephrectomy
Nephritis
Palliative care
Polycystic kidney disease
Polyps
Preeclampsia and eclampsia
Proteinuria
Pyelonephritis
Renal failure
Sarcoidosis
Stenosis
Stone removal
Stones
Transplantation
Uremia
Urinalysis
Urinary disorders
Urinary system
Urology
Vasculitis
Williams syndrome

NEUROLOGY
Acquired immunodeficiency
    syndrome (AIDS)
Adrenoleukodystrophy
Aging: Extended care
Agnosia
Altitude sickness
Alzheimer's disease
Amnesia
Amyotrophic lateral sclerosis
Anesthesia
Anesthesiology
Aneurysms
Angelman syndrome
Anorexia nervosa
Anosmia

Antidepressants
Aphasia and dysphasia
Apnea
Ataxia
Atrophy
Attention-deficit disorder (ADD)
Audiology
Auras
Balance disorders
Batten's disease
Bell's palsy
Biofeedback
Blindsight
Botox
Brain
Brain damage
Brain disorders
Brain tumors
Brucellosis
Caffeine
Capgras syndrome
Carotid arteries
Carpal tunnel syndrome
Cerebral palsy
Charcot-Marie-Tooth Disease
Chiari malformations
Chiropractic
Chronic wasting disease (CWD)
Cluster headaches
Cockayne Disease
Cognitive enhancement
Concussion
Cornelia de Lange syndrome
Craniotomy
Creutzfeldt-Jakob disease (CJD)
Critical care
Cryosurgery
Cutis marmorata telangiectatica
    congenita
Delirium
Dementias
Developmental stages
Diabetes mellitus
Disk removal
Dizziness and fainting
Dyskinesia
Dyslexia
Ear infections and disorders
Ears
Electrical shock
Electroencephalography (EEG)
Electromyography
Embolism
Emergency medicine
Encephalitis
Enteroviruses
Epilepsy

Eye infections and disorders
Fascia
Fetal tissue transplantation
Frontal lobe syndrome
Frontotemporal dementia (FTD)
Gigantism
Glasgow coma scale
Glioma
Grafts and grafting
Guillain-Barré syndrome
Head and neck disorders
Headaches
Hearing
Hearing tests
Hematomas
Hemiplegia
Hemolytic disease of the newborn
Hiccups
Huntington's disease
Hydrocephalus
Hyperhidrosis
Hypothalamus
Hypoxia
Infarction
Intraventricular hemorrhage
Ischemia
Korsakoff's syndrome
Learning disabilities
Lesions
Leukodystrophy
Lower extremities
Lumbar puncture
Lyme disease
Marijuana
Melatonin
Memory loss
Meningitis
Mercury poisoning
Minimally conscious state
Morgellons disease
Motion sickness
Motor neuron diseases
Motor skill development
Multiple chemical sensitivity
    syndrome
Multiple sclerosis
Myasthenia gravis
Narcolepsy
Neonatal brachial plexus palsy
Nervous system
Neurofibromatosis
Neuropsychology
Neuroscience
Neurosis
Neurosurgery
Niemann-Pick disease
Numbness and tingling

Otorhinolaryngology
Pain
Palsy
Paralysis
Paraplegia
Parkinson's disease
Phenylketonuria (PKU)
Phrenology
Pick's disease
Poliomyelitis
Porphyria
Postherpetic neuralgia
Prader-Willi syndrome
Precocious puberty
Preeclampsia and eclampsia
Prion diseases
Psychiatry
Quadriplegia
Rabies
Radiculopathy
Restless legs syndrome
Reye's syndrome
Rubinstein-Taybi syndrome
Sarcoidosis
Sciatica
Seizures
Sense organs
Shingles
Shock therapy
Skin
Sleep
Sleep disorders
Sleeping sickness
Sleepwalking
Smell
Spinal cord disorders
Split-brain
Stem cells
Stenosis
Strokes
Sturge-Weber syndrome
Stuttering
Subdural hematoma
Sympathectomy
Synesthesia
Syphilis
Tardive dyskinesia
Taste
Tay-Sachs disease
Tetanus
Tics
Tinnitus
Torticollis
Touch
Tourette's syndrome
Transient ischemic attacks (TIAs)
Traumatic brain injury

Tremors
Upper extremities
Vagotomy
Vagus nerve
Vasculitis
Vertigo
Vision
Wernicke's aphasia
West Nile virus
Williams syndrome
Wilson's disease

NEUROPSYCHOLOGY
Capgras syndrome
Frontal lobe syndrome
Minimally conscious state
Neuroscience
Traumatic brain injury
Wernicke's aphasia
Williams syndrome

NEUROSCIENCE
Blindsight
Frontal lobe syndrome
Glasgow coma scale
Mirror neurons
Neuroethics
Neuropsychology
Phrenology
Split-brain
Traumatic brain injury
Wernicke's aphasia

NEUROSURGERY
Chiari malformations
Minimally conscious state
Wernicke's aphasia

NUCLEAR MEDICINE
Chemotherapy
Imaging and radiology
Magnetic resonance imaging (MRI)
Noninvasive tests
Nuclear radiology
Pneumocystis jirovecii
Positron emission tomography (PET)
    scanning
Radiation therapy
Single photon emission computed
    tomography (SPECT)

NURSING
Acidosis
Aging: Extended care
Alzheimer's disease
Ataxia
Atrophy

Bedsores
Cardiac rehabilitation
Carotid arteries
Casts and splints
Critical care
Diuretics
Drowning
Emergency medicine
Epidemics and pandemics
Eye infections and disorders
Fiber
Home care
H1N1 influenza
Hypoxia
Infarction
Influenza
Intravenous (IV) therapy
Methicillin-resistant staphylococcus
    aureus (MRSA) infection
Minimally conscious state
Palliative care
Pediatrics
Physician assistants
Polycystic ovary syndrome
Pulse rate
Radiculopathy
Surgical procedures
Surgical technologists
Well-baby examinations

NUTRITION
Aging: Extended care
Anorexia nervosa
Antioxidants
Bariatric surgery
Bedsores
Bell's palsy
Bile
Breast-feeding
Bulimia
Carbohydrates
Cardiac rehabilitation
Celiac sprue
Cholesterol
Colon
Crohn's disease
Cushing's syndrome
Dietary reference intakes (DRIs)
Digestion
Exercise physiology
Eye infections and disorders
Fatty acid oxidation disorders
Fiber
Food allergies
Food biochemistry
Food guide plate
Fructosemia

Galactosemia
Gastroenterology
Gastrointestinal system
Gestational diabetes
Gluten intolerance
Glycogen storage diseases
Hemolytic uremic syndrome
Hyperadiposis
Hypercholesterolemia
Irritable bowel syndrome (IBS)
Jaw wiring
Korsakoff's syndrome
Kwashiorkor
Lactose intolerance
Leptin
Leukodystrophy
Lipids
Macronutrients
Malabsorption
Malnutrition
Mastitis
Metabolic disorders
Metabolic syndrome
Metabolism
Nursing
Obesity
Osteoporosis
Phenylketonuria (PKU)
Phytochemicals
Pituitary gland
Plasma
Polycystic ovary syndrome
Protein
Rickets
Scurvy
Small intestine
Sports medicine
Supplements
Taste
Ulcer surgery
Ulcers
Vagotomy
Vitamin D deficiency
Vitamins and minerals
Weaning
Weight loss and gain
Weight loss medications

OBSTETRICS
Amniocentesis
Apgar score
Assisted reproductive technologies
Birth defects
Breast-feeding
Cerebral palsy
Cesarean section
Childbirth

Childbirth complications
Chorionic villus sampling
Conception
Congenital disorders
Contraception
Critical care
Cytomegalovirus (CMV)
Disseminated intravascular
  coagulation (DIC)
Down syndrome
Embryology
Emergency medicine
Endometrial biopsy
Endoscopy
Episiotomy
Family medicine
Fetal surgery
Gamete intrafallopian transfer (GIFT)
Genetic counseling
Genetic diseases
Gestational diabetes
Growth
Gynecology
Hirschsprung's disease
Incontinence
Intravenous (IV) therapy
Karyotyping
Listeria infections
Mastitis
Miscarriage
Multiple births
Neonatal brachial plexus palsy
Neonatology
Noninvasive tests
Ovaries
Perinatology
Pituitary gland
Placenta
Polycystic ovary syndrome
Postpartum depression
Preeclampsia and eclampsia
Pregnancy and gestation
Premature birth
Pyelonephritis
Reproductive system
Rh factor
Sexuality
Sperm banks
Stillbirth
Streptococcal infections
Teratogens
Toxemia
Trichomoniasis
Tubal ligation
Turner syndrome
Ultrasonography
Urology

Uterus

OCCUPATIONAL HEALTH
Acidosis
Agnosia
Altitude sickness
Angelman syndrome
Asbestos exposure
Asphyxiation
Ataxia
Bacillus Calmette-Guérin (BCG)
Biofeedback
Blurred vision
Brucellosis
Cardiac rehabilitation
Carpal tunnel syndrome
Charcot-Marie-Tooth Disease
Gulf War syndrome
Hearing tests
Leptospirosis
Leukodystrophy
Lung cancer
Mercury poisoning
Mesothelioma
Multiple chemical sensitivity
  syndrome
Nasopharyngeal disorders
Pneumonia
Prostheses
Pulmonary diseases
Pulmonary medicine
Radiation sickness
Skin disorders
Slipped disk
Spinocerebellar ataxia
Stress reduction
Tendinitis
Tendon disorders
Tendon repair

OCCUPATIONAL THERAPY
Home care
Minimally conscious state
Williams syndrome

ONCOLOGY
Acquired immunodeficiency
  syndrome (AIDS)
Aging: Extended care
Amputation
Anal cancer
Anemia
Antibodies
Antioxidants
Anus
Asbestos exposure
Assisted suicide

Biological therapies
Biopsy
Bladder cancer
Bone cancer
Bone disorders
Bone marrow transplantation
Brain tumors
Breast cancer
Burkitt's lymphoma
Cancer
Carcinoma
Chemotherapy
Cold agglutinin disease
Colon
Colorectal cancer
Computed tomography (CT) scanning
Cryosurgery
Cystoscopy
Cytology
Cytopathology
Dermatology
Dermatopathology
Disseminated intravascular
    coagulation (DIC)
Embolization
Epstein-Barr virus
Ewing's sarcoma
Fibrocystic breast condition
Gallbladder cancer
Gastrectomy
Gastroenterology
Gastrointestinal system
Gastrostomy
Genetic Imprinting
Glioma
Gynecology
Hematology
Histology
Hodgkin's disease
Hormone therapy
Human papillomavirus (HPV)
Hysterectomy
Intravenous (IV) therapy
Kaposi's sarcoma
Karyotyping
Kidney cancer
Laboratory tests
Laryngectomy
Laser use in surgery
Lesions
Light therapy
Liver cancer
Lumbar puncture
Lung cancer
Lungs
Lymph
Lymphadenopathy and lymphoma

Malignancy and metastasis
Mammography
Massage
Mastectomy and lumpectomy
Meckel's diverticulum
Mesothelioma
Mouth and throat cancer
Necrosis
Nephrectomy
Oral and maxillofacial surgery
Pain
Pain management
Palliative care
Pap test
Pathology
Pharmacology
Plastic surgery
Proctology
Prostate cancer
Prostate gland
Prostate gland removal
Prostheses
Pulmonary diseases
Radiation sickness
Radiation therapy
Radiopharmaceuticals
Rectum
Retroviruses
Sarcoma
Serology
Skin
Skin cancer
Skin lesion removal
Small intestine
Smoking
Stem cells
Stenosis
Stress
Testicular cancer
Thalidomide
Thymus gland
Tonsils
Transplantation
Tumor removal
Tumors
Uterus
Wiskott-Aldrich syndrome

OPHTHALMOLOGY

Acquired immunodeficiency
    syndrome (AIDS)
Adrenoleukodystrophy
Aging: Extended care
Anesthesia
Anesthesiology
Anti-inflammatory drugs
Aspergillosis

Astigmatism
Batten's disease
Behçet's disease
Blindness
Blindsight
Blurred vision
Botox
Cataract surgery
Cataracts
Cockayne Disease
Conjunctivitis
Corneal transplantation
Cutis marmorata telangiectatica
    congenita
Dry eye
Eye infections and disorders
Eye surgery
Eyes
Glaucoma
Juvenile rheumatoid arthritis
Keratitis
Kluver-Bucy syndrome
Laser use in surgery
Lesions
Light therapy
Lyme disease
Macular degeneration
Marfan syndrome
Myopia
Optometry
Prostheses
Pterygium/Pinguecula
Ptosis
Refractive eye surgery
Reiter's syndrome
Rubinstein-Taybi syndrome
Sarcoidosis
Sense organs
Sphincterectomy
Spinocerebellar ataxia
Spondylitis
Stevens-Johnson syndrome
Strabismus
Sturge-Weber syndrome
Subdural hematoma
Tears and tear ducts
Trachoma
Vasculitis
Vision
Vision disorders
Williams syndrome

OPTOMETRY
Aging: Extended care
Astigmatism
Blindsight
Blurred vision

Cataract surgery
Cataracts
Cockayne Disease
Color blindness
Conjunctivitis
Eye infections and disorders
Eye surgery
Eyes
Glaucoma
Keratitis
Myopia
Ophthalmology
Pterygium/Pinguecula
Ptosis
Sarcoidosis
Sense organs
Spinocerebellar ataxia
Tears and tear ducts
Vision disorders
Williams syndrome

ORTHODONTICS

Bones and the skeleton
Dentistry
Jaw wiring
Periodontal surgery
Periodontitis
Teeth
Teething
Tooth extraction
Williams syndrome

ORTHOPEDICS

Amputation
Anti-inflammatory drugs
Arthritis
Arthroplasty
Arthroscopy
Ataxia
Atrophy
Bariatric surgery
Bone cancer
Bone disorders
Bone grafting
Bones and the skeleton
Bowlegs
Bunions
Cancer
Cartilage
Casts and splints
Cerebral palsy
Charcot-Marie-Tooth Disease
Chiropractic
Connective tissue
Craniosynostosis
Cutis marmorata telangiectatica
    congenita

Disk removal
Dwarfism
Endoscopy
Ergogenic aids
Ewing's sarcoma
Fascia
Feet
Flat feet
Foot disorders
Fracture and dislocation
Fracture repair
Growth
Hammertoe correction
Hammertoes
Heel spur removal
Hemiplegia
Hip fracture repair
Hip replacement
Hormone therapy
Joints
Juvenile rheumatoid arthritis
Kinesiology
Kneecap removal
Knock-knees
Kyphosis
Laminectomy and spinal fusion
Ligaments
Lower extremities
Marfan syndrome
Mesenchymal stem cells
Methicillin-resistant staphylococcus
    aureus (MRSA) infection
Motor skill development
Muscles
Necrosis
Neonatal brachial plexus palsy
Neurofibromatosis
Orthopedic surgery
Osgood-Schlatter disease
Osteoarthritis
Osteochondritis juvenilis
Osteogenesis imperfecta
Osteomyelitis
Osteonecrosis
Osteoporosis
Paget's disease
Physical rehabilitation
Pigeon toes
Podiatry
Prostheses
Radiculopathy
Reiter's syndrome
Rheumatology
Rickets
Rotator cuff surgery
Rubinstein-Taybi syndrome
Scoliosis

Slipped disk
Spondylitis
Sports medicine
Staphylococcal infections
Stenosis
Tendinitis
Tendon disorders
Tendon repair
Upper extremities
Whiplash

OSTEOPATHIC MEDICINE

Acidosis
Acquired immunodeficiency
    syndrome (AIDS)
Alternative medicine
Atrophy
Bones and the skeleton
Colon
Family medicine
Fascia
Ligaments
Muscles
Physical rehabilitation
Pituitary gland
Radiculopathy
Rickets
Slipped disk
Small intestine

OTOLARYNGOLOGY

Head and neck disorders
Ménière's disease
Vasculitis

OTORHINOLARYNGOLOGY

Acquired immunodeficiency
    syndrome (AIDS)
Adenoids
Allergies
Anosmia
Antihistamines
Anti-inflammatory drugs
Aromatherapy
Aspergillosis
Audiology
Cartilage
Cleft lip and palate
Cleft lip and palate repair
Cockayne Disease
Common cold
Croup
Cryosurgery
Decongestants
Ear infections and disorders
Ear surgery
Ears

Earwax
Epidemics and pandemics
Esophagus
Gastrointestinal system
Hay fever
Hearing aids
Hearing tests
Laryngectomy
Laryngitis
Lesions
Ménière's disease
Motion sickness
Myringotomy
Nasal polyp removal
Nasopharyngeal disorders
Nausea and vomiting
Oral and maxillofacial surgery
Pharyngitis
Pharynx
Polyps
Pulmonary medicine
Quinsy
Respiration
Rhinitis
Rhinoplasty and submucous resection
Rhinoviruses
Sense organs
Sinusitis
Sleep apnea
Smell
Sore throat
Taste
Tinnitus
Tonsillectomy and adenoid removal
Tonsillitis
Tonsils
Trachea
Vertigo
Voice and vocal cord disorders
Whooping cough

PATHOLOGY
Acquired immunodeficiency
    syndrome (AIDS)
Adrenoleukodystrophy
Anthrax
Antibodies
Atrophy
Autopsy
Avian influenza
Bacteriology
Biological therapies
Biopsy
Blood testing
Breast cancer
Cholecystitis
Chronic granulomatous disease

Cold agglutinin disease
Colon
Cytology
Cytopathology
Dermatopathology
Electroencephalography (EEG)
Embolization
Epidemics and pandemics
Epstein-Barr virus
Eye infections and disorders
Forensic pathology
Frontotemporal dementia (FTD)
Hematology
Histology
Homeopathy
Immunopathology
Inflammation
Karyotyping
Laboratory tests
Ligaments
Lumbar puncture
Malaria
Malignancy and metastasis
Mastectomy and lumpectomy
Melanoma
Mesothelioma
Microbiology
Microscopy
Motor skill development
Mutation
Niemann-Pick disease
Noninvasive tests
Oncology
Pityriasis rosea
Polycystic ovary syndrome
Prion diseases
Radiculopathy
Renal failure
Retroviruses
Rhinoviruses
Sarcoma
Serology
Small intestine
Smallpox
West Nile virus

PEDIATRICS
Acne
Adrenoleukodystrophy
Allergies
Angelman syndrome
Appendicitis
Ataxia
Attention-deficit disorder (ADD)
Autism
Batten's disease
Bed-wetting

Beriberi
Birth defects
Blisters
Blurred vision
Bowlegs
Bronchiolitis
Bruises
Burkitt's lymphoma
Casts and splints
Celiac sprue
Cerebral palsy
Charcot-Marie-Tooth Disease
Chickenpox
Childhood infectious diseases
Chronic granulomatous disease
Cleft lip and palate
Cleft lip and palate repair
Cockayne Disease
Cognitive development
Cold agglutinin disease
Colic
Collodion baby
Colon
Congenital disorders
Congenital heart disease
Cornelia de Lange syndrome
Crohn's disease
Croup
Cutis marmorata telangiectatica
    congenita
Cystic fibrosis
Cytomegalovirus (CMV)
Diabetes mellitus
Diarrhea and dysentery
DiGeorge syndrome
Diphtheria
Down syndrome
Dwarfism
E. coli infection
Eating disorders
Eczema
Ehrlichiosis
Emergency medicine
Enterocolitis
Epiglottitis
Epstein-Barr virus
Ewing's sarcoma
Eye infections and disorders
Failure to thrive
Family medicine
Fatty acid oxidation disorders
Fetal surgery
Fever
Fifth disease
Fistula repair
Fructosemia
Galactosemia

Gaucher's disease
Gender identity disorder
Genetic diseases
Genetics and inheritance
Giardiasis
Glycogen storage diseases
Growth
Hand-foot-and-mouth disease
Hearing tests
Hemolytic uremic syndrome
Hirschsprung's disease
Hives
H1N1 influenza
Impetigo
Incontinence
Influenza
Interpartner violence
Intravenous (IV) therapy
Juvenile rheumatoid arthritis
Kawasaki disease
Klippel-Trenaunay syndrome
Kluver-Bucy syndrome
Knock-knees
Kwashiorkor
Lead poisoning
Learning disabilities
Leukodystrophy
Listeria infections
Malabsorption
Malnutrition
Maple syrup urine disease (MSUD)
Massage
Measles
Menstruation
Mercury poisoning
Metabolic disorders
Methicillin-resistant staphylococcus
    aureus (MRSA) infection
Mold and mildew
Mononucleosis
Motor skill development
Mucopolysaccharidosis (MPS)
Multiple births
Multiple sclerosis
Mumps
Münchausen syndrome by proxy
Muscular dystrophy
Nail removal
Neonatal brachial plexus palsy
Neonatology
Neuroscience
Niemann-Pick disease
Nonalcoholic steatohepatitis (NASH)
Nursing
Osgood-Schlatter disease
Osteogenesis imperfecta
Otoplasty

Otorhinolaryngology
Palliative medicine
Perinatology
Phenylketonuria (PKU)
Pigeon toes
Pinworms
Pituitary gland
Pityriasis alba
Poliomyelitis
Polycystic ovary syndrome
Polydactyly and syndactyly
Porphyria
Prader-Willi syndrome
Precocious puberty
Premature birth
Progeria
Puberty and adolescence
Pulse rate
Pyloric stenosis
Respiratory distress syndrome
Reye's syndrome
Rheumatic fever
Rhinitis
Rickets
Roseola
Rotavirus
Rubella
Rubinstein-Taybi syndrome
Safety issues for children
Salmonella infection
Scarlet fever
Seizures
Severe combined immunodeficiency
    syndrome (SCID)
Sexuality
Small intestine
Soiling
Sore throat
Steroids
Stevens-Johnson syndrome
Streptococcal infections
Sturge-Weber syndrome
Stuttering
Sudden infant death syndrome (SIDS)
Syphilis
Tay-Sachs disease
Teething
Testicular torsion
Thalassemia
Thumb sucking
Toilet training
Tonsillectomy and adenoid removal
Tonsillitis
Tonsils
Toxoplasmosis
Trachoma
Weaning

Well-baby examinations
Whooping cough
Wiskott-Aldrich syndrome

PERINATOLOGY
Amniocentesis
Assisted reproductive technologies
Birth defects
Breast-feeding
Cesarean section
Childbirth
Chorionic villus sampling
Congenital hypothyroidism
Embryology
Fatty acid oxidation disorders
Glycogen storage diseases
Hydrocephalus
Karyotyping
Metabolic disorders
Miscarriage
Motor skill development
Neonatal brachial plexus palsy
Neonatology
Nursing
Obstetrics
Pediatrics
Premature birth
Shunts
Spina bifida
Trichomoniasis
Umbilical cord
Uterus
Well-baby examinations

PHARMACOLOGY
Acid-base chemistry
Acidosis
Acquired immunodeficiency
    syndrome (AIDS)
Aging: Extended care
Allergies
Antianxiety drugs
Antibiotic resistance
Antibiotics
Antibodies
Antihistamines
Antihypertensives
Assisted suicide
Autism
Bacteriology
Blurred vision
Chemotherapy
Chronic granulomatous disease
Club drugs
Colon
Critical care
Digestion

Diuretics
Dyskinesia
Emergency medicine
Epidemics and pandemics
Ergogenic aids
Fluids and electrolytes
Food biochemistry
Genetic engineering
Genomics
Glycolysis
Homeopathy
Hormones
Hypercholesterolemia
Hypotension
Laboratory tests
Marijuana
Melatonin
Mesothelioma
Metabolism
Methicillin-resistant staphylococcus
   aureus (MRSA) infection
Narcotics
Neuropsychology
Neuroscience
Oncology
Over-the-counter medications
Pain management
Polycystic ovary syndrome
Prader-Willi syndrome
Psychiatry
Rheumatology
Sleep
Small intestine
Sports medicine
Steroids
Tardive dyskinesia
Thrombolytic therapy and TPA
Tremors

PHYSICAL THERAPY
Aging: Extended care
Amputation
Amyotrophic lateral sclerosis
Angelman syndrome
Arthritis
Ataxia
Atrophy
Biofeedback
Bowlegs
Burns and scalds
Cardiac rehabilitation
Casts and splints
Cerebral palsy
Charcot-Marie-Tooth Disease
Cornelia de Lange syndrome
Disk removal
Dyskinesia

Electromyography
Exercise physiology
Facial transplantation
Fascia
Grafts and grafting
Hemiplegia
Home care
Hydrotherapy
Kinesiology
Knock-knees
Leukodystrophy
Ligaments
Lower extremities
Massage
Minimally conscious state
Motor skill development
Muscles
Muscular dystrophy
Neonatal brachial plexus palsy
Neurology
Numbness and tingling
Orthopedic surgery
Orthopedics
Osteopathic medicine
Osteoporosis
Pain
Pain management
Palsy
Paralysis
Parkinson's disease
Physical rehabilitation
Pigeon toes
Plastic surgery
Prostheses
Pulse rate
Radiculopathy
Scoliosis
Slipped disk
Spinal cord disorders
Spinocerebellar ataxia
Sports medicine
Tendinitis
Tendon disorders
Torticollis
Upper extremities
Whiplash
Williams syndrome

PLASTIC SURGERY
Amputation
Bariatric surgery
Body dysmorphic disorder
Botox
Breast surgery
Burns and scalds
Cleft lip and palate
Cleft lip and palate repair

Craniosynostosis
Cryosurgery
Cyst removal
DiGeorge syndrome
Face lift and blepharoplasty
Facial transplantation
Gender reassignment surgery
Grafts and grafting
Hair transplantation
Healing
Jaw wiring
Laceration repair
Liposuction
Malignancy and metastasis
Mastectomy and lumpectomy
Mesenchymal stem cells
Moles
Necrotizing fasciitis
Neonatal brachial plexus palsy
Neurofibromatosis
Oral and maxillofacial surgery
Otoplasty
Otorhinolaryngology
Prostheses
Ptosis
Rhinoplasty and submucous resection
Skin
Skin lesion removal
Spina bifida
Sturge-Weber syndrome
Surgical procedures
Tattoos and body piercing
Varicose vein removal
Varicose veins
Vision

PODIATRY
Athlete's foot
Bones and the skeleton
Bunions
Cartilage
Cerebral palsy
Corns and calluses
Feet
Flat feet
Foot disorders
Gout
Hammertoe correction
Hammertoes
Heel spur removal
Joints
Lesions
Lower extremities
Methicillin-resistant staphylococcus
   aureus (MRSA) infection
Nail removal
Orthopedic surgery

Orthopedics
Polydactyly and syndactyly
Tendon disorders
Tendon repair

PREVENTIVE MEDICINE
Acidosis
Acupressure
Acupuncture
Alternative medicine
Anemia
Aneurysmectomy
Antibodies
Antihistamines
Antihypertensives
Aromatherapy
Assisted living facilities
Bacillus Calmette-Guérin (BCG)
Biofeedback
Blurred vision
Breast cancer
Brucellosis
Caffeine
Cardiac surgery
Cardiology
Cerebral palsy
Chemotherapy
Chiropractic
Cholesterol
Club drugs
Computed tomography (CT) scanning
Congenital hypothyroidism
Croup
Electrocardiography (ECG or EKG)
Endometrial biopsy
Exercise physiology
Family medicine
Fiber
Food guide plate
Genetic counseling
Genetic engineering
Hormone therapy
Host-defense mechanisms
Immune system
Immunization and vaccination
Insect-borne diseases
Lead poisoning
Mammography
Massage
Meditation
Melatonin
Mesothelioma
Noninvasive tests
Nursing
Nutrition
Occupational health
Osteopathic medicine

Over-the-counter medications
Oxygen therapy
Pharmacology
Phytochemicals
Polycystic ovary syndrome
Psychiatry
Rhinoviruses
Screening
Scurvy
Serology
Sleep
Slipped disk
Smallpox
Sports medicine
Stress reduction
Tendinitis
Vitamin D deficiency
Yoga

PROCTOLOGY
Acquired immunodeficiency
    syndrome (AIDS)
Anal cancer
Anus
Bladder removal
Chronic granulomatous disease
Colorectal cancer
Colorectal polyp removal
Colorectal surgery
Diverticulitis and diverticulosis
Endoscopy
Fistula repair
Hemorrhoid banding and removal
Hemorrhoids
Hirschsprung's disease
Internal medicine
Polyps
Prostate gland removal
Rectum
Reproductive system
Urology

PSYCHIATRY
Acquired immunodeficiency
    syndrome (AIDS)
Addiction
Adrenoleukodystrophy
Aging: Extended care
Alcoholism
Alzheimer's disease
Amnesia
Amyotrophic lateral sclerosis
Angelman syndrome
Anorexia nervosa
Antianxiety drugs
Antidepressants
Anxiety

Asperger's syndrome
Attention-deficit disorder (ADD)
Auras
Autism
Bariatric surgery
Bipolar disorders
Body dysmorphic disorder
Bonding
Brain
Brain damage
Brain disorders
Breast surgery
Bulimia
Chronic fatigue syndrome
Club drugs
Cognitive enhancement
Computed tomography (CT) scanning
Dementias
Depression
Developmental disorders
Developmental stages
Dyskinesia
Eating disorders
Electroencephalography (EEG)
Emergency medicine
Factitious disorders
Failure to thrive
Family medicine
Fatigue
Frontotemporal dementia (FTD)
Gender identity disorder
Gender reassignment surgery
Gynecology
Havening touch
Huntington's disease
Hypnosis
Hypochondriasis
Hypothalamus
Incontinence
Interpartner violence
Kluver-Bucy syndrome
Korsakoff's syndrome
Light therapy
Marijuana
Masturbation
Memory loss
Mental retardation
Mental status exam
Morgellons disease
Münchausen syndrome by proxy
Neuropsychology
Neuroscience
Neurosis
Neurosurgery
Obesity
Obsessive-compulsive disorder
Pain

Pain management
Paranoia
Penile implant surgery
Phobias
Phrenology
Pick's disease
Postpartum depression
Post-traumatic stress disorder
Prader-Willi syndrome
Premenstrual syndrome (PMS)
Psychiatric disorders
Psychoanalysis
Psychosis
Psychosomatic disorders
Rape and sexual assault
Restless legs syndrome
Schizophrenia
Seasonal affective disorder
Separation anxiety
Sexual dysfunction
Sexuality
Shock therapy
Single photon emission computed
    tomography (SPECT)
Sleep
Sleep disorders
Speech disorders
Split-brain
Steroid abuse
Stress
Stress reduction
Sudden infant death syndrome (SIDS)
Suicide
Synesthesia
Tardive dyskinesia
Tinnitus
Toilet training
Tourette's syndrome
Traumatic brain injury
Tremors

PSYCHOLOGY
Abuse of the elderly
Addiction
Aging
Aging: Extended care
Alcoholism
Amnesia
Amyotrophic lateral sclerosis
Angelman syndrome
Anorexia nervosa
Antidepressants
Anxiety
Aromatherapy
Asperger's syndrome
Attention-deficit disorder (ADD)
Auras

Bariatric surgery
Bed-wetting
Biofeedback
Bipolar disorders
Blindsight
Bonding
Brain
Brain damage
Bulimia
Capgras syndrome
Cardiac rehabilitation
Cerebral palsy
Cirrhosis
Club drugs
Cognitive development
Death and dying
Depression
Developmental disorders
Developmental stages
Dyslexia
Eating disorders
Electroencephalography (EEG)
Ergogenic aids
Facial transplantation
Factitious disorders
Failure to thrive
Family medicine
Forensic pathology
Frontal lobe syndrome
Gender identity disorder
Gender reassignment surgery
Genetic counseling
Gulf War syndrome
Gynecology
Huntington's disease
Hypnosis
Hypochondriasis
Hypothalamus
Interpartner violence
Juvenile rheumatoid arthritis
Kinesiology
Klinefelter syndrome
Kluver-Bucy syndrome
Korsakoff's syndrome
Learning disabilities
Light therapy
Marijuana
Memory loss
Mental retardation
Mental status exam
Mirror neurons
Miscarriage
Motor skill development
Münchausen syndrome by proxy
Neonatal brachial plexus palsy
Neuropsychology
Neurosis

Obesity
Obsessive-compulsive disorder
Occupational health
Overtraining syndrome
Pain management
Palliative care
Palliative medicine
Paranoia
Phobias
Phrenology
Pick's disease
Plastic surgery
Polycystic ovary syndrome
Postpartum depression
Post-traumatic stress disorder
Premenstrual syndrome (PMS)
Psychosomatic disorders
Puberty and adolescence
Restless legs syndrome
Separation anxiety
Sexual dysfunction
Sexuality
Sleep
Sleep disorders
Sleepwalking
Speech disorders
Split-brain
Sports medicine
Steroid abuse
Stress
Stress reduction
Sturge-Weber syndrome
Sudden infant death syndrome (SIDS)
Suicide
Synesthesia
Temporomandibular joint (TMJ)
    syndrome
Tics
Toilet training
Tourette's syndrome
Traumatic brain injury
Weight loss and gain
Wernicke's aphasia
Williams syndrome

PUBLIC HEALTH
Acquired immunodeficiency
    syndrome (AIDS)
Acute respiratory distress syndrome
    (ARDS)
Adenoviruses
Advance directives
Aging: Extended care
Alternative medicine
Amebiasis
Antibiotic resistance
Antibodies

Assisted living facilities
Babesiosis
Bacillus Calmette-Guérin (BCG)
Bacteriology
Blood testing
Brucellosis
Cerebral palsy
Chagas' disease
Chickenpox
Childhood infectious diseases
Cholera
Chronic obstructive pulmonary
   disease (COPD)
Club drugs
Common cold
Coronaviruses
Creutzfeldt-Jakob disease (CJD)
Dengue fever
Dermatology
Diarrhea and dysentery
E. coli infection
Ebola virus
Elephantiasis
Emergency medicine
Encephalitis
Epidemics and pandemics
Epidemiology
Food guide plate
Food poisoning
Forensic pathology
Gulf War syndrome
Hantavirus
H1N1 influenza
Human papillomavirus (HPV)
Immunization and vaccination
Influenza
Insect-borne diseases
Interpartner violence
Legionnaires' disease
Leishmaniasis
Leprosy
Leptospirosis
Macronutrients
Malaria
Malnutrition
Managed care
Marijuana
Measles
Meningitis
Methicillin-resistant staphylococcus
   aureus (MRSA) infection
Microbiology
Monkeypox
Multiple chemical sensitivity
   syndrome
Neurosis
Niemann-Pick disease

Nursing
Nutrition
Obesity
Occupational health
Osteopathic medicine
Parasitic diseases
Pharmacology
Physician assistants
Pinworms
Plague
Pneumonia
Poliomyelitis
Polycystic ovary syndrome
Prion diseases
Protozoan diseases
Psychiatry
Rabies
Radiation sickness
Rape and sexual assault
Retroviruses
Rhinoviruses
Roundworms
Salmonella infection
Schistosomiasis
Screening
Serology
Severe acute respiratory syndrome
   (SARS)
Sexually transmitted diseases (STDs)
Shigellosis
Sleeping sickness
Smallpox
Syphilis
Tapeworms
Tattoos and body piercing
Tetanus
Trichinosis
Trichomoniasis
Tuberculosis
Tularemia
Typhoid fever
Typhus
West Nile virus
Yellow fever
Zoonoses

PULMONARY MEDICINE
Acquired immunodeficiency
   syndrome (AIDS)
Acute respiratory distress syndrome
   (ARDS)
Adrenoleukodystrophy
Amyotrophic lateral sclerosis
Antihistamines
Apnea
Aspergillosis
Asthma

Bronchi
Bronchiolitis
Bronchitis
Catheterization
Chest
Chronic granulomatous disease
Chronic obstructive pulmonary
   disease (COPD)
Coccidioidomycosis
Cold agglutinin disease
Coronaviruses
Coughing
Critical care
Cyanosis
Cystic fibrosis
Diaphragm
Drowning
Edema
Emergency medicine
Emphysema
Endoscopy
Epidemics and pandemics
Fluids and electrolytes
Forensic pathology
Fungal infections
Hantavirus
Hyperbaric oxygen therapy
Hyperventilation
Hypoxia
Internal medicine
Interstitial pulmonary fibrosis (IPF)
Leptospirosis
Lesions
Lung cancer
Lung surgery
Lungs
Mesothelioma
Methicillin-resistant staphylococcus
   aureus (MRSA) infection
Mold and mildew
Occupational health
Oxygen therapy
Palliative care
Paramedics
Pediatrics
Pharynx
Pleurisy
Pneumocystis jirovecii
Pneumonia
Pneumothorax
Polyps
Prader-Willi syndrome
Pulmonary diseases
Pulmonary edema
Pulmonary hypertension
Respiration
Respiratory distress syndrome

Sarcoidosis
Severe acute respiratory syndrome (SARS)
Single photon emission computed tomography (SPECT)
Sleep apnea
Smoking
Stem cells
Stevens-Johnson syndrome
Thoracic surgery
Thrombolytic therapy and TPA
Trachea
Tuberculosis
Tumors
Vasculitis

RADIOLOGY
Achalasia
Angiography
Aspergillosis
Atrophy
Biopsy
Bone cancer
Brain tumors
Breast cancer
Cancer
Cartilage
Catheterization
Chronic granulomatous disease
Cold agglutinin disease
Computed tomography (CT) scanning
Critical care
Cushing's syndrome
Embolization
Emergency medicine
Endoscopic retrograde cholangiopancreatography (ERCP)
Ewing's sarcoma
Eye infections and disorders
Gallbladder cancer
Imaging and radiology
Joints
Liver cancer
Lung cancer
Magnetic resonance imaging (MRI)
Mammography
Mastectomy and lumpectomy
Meckel's diverticulum
Mesothelioma
Methicillin-resistant staphylococcus aureus (MRSA) infection
Mouth and throat cancer
Neonatal brachial plexus palsy
Noninvasive tests
Nuclear medicine
Nuclear radiology
Oncology

Palliative care
Palliative medicine
Pneumocystis jirovecii
Positron emission tomography (PET) scanning
Prostate cancer
Radiation sickness
Radiation therapy
Radiculopathy
Radiopharmaceuticals
Sarcoidosis
Single photon emission computed tomography (SPECT)
Stents
Testicular cancer
Ultrasonography

REHABILITATION
Neuropsychology
Traumatic brain injury

RHEUMATOLOGY
Aging: Extended care
Ankylosing spondylitis
Anti-inflammatory drugs
Arthritis
Arthroplasty
Arthroscopy
Atrophy
Behçet's disease
Bone disorders
Brucellosis
Bursitis
Cartilage
Cold agglutinin disease
Collagen
Connective tissue
Fibromyalgia
Gout
Hip replacement
Hydrotherapy
Inflammation
Joints
Ligaments
Lyme disease
Mesenchymal stem cells
Methicillin-resistant staphylococcus aureus (MRSA) infection
Orthopedic surgery
Orthopedics
Osteonecrosis
Paget's disease
Pain
Polymyalgia rheumatica
Radiculopathy
Rheumatoid arthritis
Rotator cuff surgery

Sarcoidosis
Scleroderma
Sjögren's syndrome
Sports medicine
Syphilis
Temporal arteritis
Vasculitis

SEROLOGY
Babesiosis
Blood and blood disorders
Blood testing
Chronic granulomatous disease
Cold agglutinin disease
Cytology
Cytopathology
Dialysis
Epidemics and pandemics
Fluids and electrolytes
Forensic pathology
Hematology
Hemophilia
Hodgkin's disease
Host-defense mechanisms
Hyperbaric oxygen therapy
Hyperlipidemia
Hypoglycemia
Immune system
Immunopathology
Laboratory tests
Leukemia
Lymph
Plasma
Rh factor
Rhinoviruses
Sarcoidosis
Septicemia
Snakebites
Transfusion
Tremors

SPEECH PATHOLOGY
Adenoids
Agnosia
Amyotrophic lateral sclerosis
Angelman syndrome
Aphasia and dysphasia
Ataxia
Audiology
Autism
Cerebral palsy
Cleft lip and palate
Deafness
Dyslexia
Ear surgery
Ears
Electroencephalography (EEG)

Hearing loss
Hearing tests
Home care
Jaw wiring
Laryngitis
Lisping
Minimally conscious state
Pharynx
Rubinstein-Taybi syndrome
Speech disorders
Spinocerebellar ataxia
Strokes
Stuttering
Subdural hematoma
Thumb sucking
Voice and vocal cord disorders
Wernicke's aphasia

SPORTS MEDICINE
Acidosis
Acupressure
Arthroplasty
Atrophy
Biofeedback
Blurred vision
Bones and the skeleton
Cartilage
Casts and splints
Concussion
Critical care
Dehydration
Emergency medicine
Ergogenic aids
Exercise physiology
Fiber
Fracture and dislocation
Glycolysis
Head and neck disorders
Heat exhaustion and heatstroke
Hematomas
Hydrotherapy
Impetigo
Joints
Kinesiology
Ligaments
Macronutrients
Massage
Mesenchymal stem cells
Methicillin-resistant staphylococcus
  aureus (MRSA) infection
Motor skill development
Muscles
Nail removal
Orthopedic surgery
Orthopedics
Overtraining syndrome
Pain

Physical rehabilitation
Pigeon toes
Pulse rate
Radiculopathy
Rotator cuff surgery
Safety issues for children
Slipped disk
Steroid abuse
Steroids
Tendinitis
Tendon disorders
Tendon repair

TOXICOLOGY
Acidosis
Bites and stings
Blood testing
Chemotherapy
Club drugs
Critical care
Cyanosis
Diphtheria
Emergency medicine
Ergogenic aids
Food poisoning
Forensic pathology
Gaucher's disease
Hepatitis
Laboratory tests
Lead poisoning
Leukemia
Liver
Mold and mildew
Multiple chemical sensitivity
  syndrome
Neuroscience
Occupational health
Pharmacology
Poisoning
Sarcoidosis
Tremors
Urinalysis

UROLOGY
Abdomen
Adenoviruses
Bed-wetting
Bladder cancer
Bladder removal
Catheterization
Chronic granulomatous disease
Cold agglutinin disease
Congenital adrenal hyperplasia
Contraception
Cryosurgery
Cushing's syndrome
Cystitis

Cystoscopy
Dialysis
Diuretics
E. coli infection
Endoscopy
Erectile dysfunction
Fetal surgery
Fluids and electrolytes
Gender reassignment surgery
Hemolytic uremic syndrome
Hermaphroditism and
  pseudohermaphroditism
Herpes
Hydroceles
Hyperplasia
Hypospadias repair and urethroplasty
Incontinence
Kidney cancer
Kidney disorders
Kidneys
Laser use in surgery
Leptospirosis
Lesions
Lithotripsy
Nephrectomy
Nephrology
Orchiectomy
Pediatrics
Penile implant surgery
Polycystic kidney disease
Polyps
Prostate cancer
Prostate enlargement
Prostate gland
Prostate gland removal
Proteinuria
Pyelonephritis
Reiter's syndrome
Reproductive system
Semen
Sexual differentiation
Sexual dysfunction
Sexually transmitted diseases (STDs)
Sperm banks
Staphylococcal infections
Sterilization
Stevens-Johnson syndrome
Stone removal
Stones
Testicular cancer
Testicular surgery
Testicular torsion
Toilet training
Transplantation
Trichomoniasis
Ultrasonography
Uremia

Urethritis
Urinalysis
Urinary disorders
Urinary system
Vas deferens
Vasectomy

VASCULAR MEDICINE
Acidosis
Amputation
Aneurysms
Angiography
Angioplasty
Antihypertensives
Anti-inflammatory drugs
Aortic aneurysm
Arteriosclerosis
Biofeedback
Bleeding
Blood pressure
Blood vessels
Bruises
Cardiac surgery
Cardiology
Carotid arteries
Cholesterol
Circulation
Claudication
Cold agglutinin disease
Computed tomography (CT) scanning
Congenital heart disease
Cutis marmorata telangiectatica
   congenita
Dehydration
Diabetes mellitus
Electrocauterization
Embolism
Embolization
End-stage renal disease
Endarterectomy
Endocarditis
Glands
Healing
Heart failure
Hematology
Histology
Hormone therapy
Hypercholesterolemia

Hyperlipidemia
Infarction
Ischemia
Klippel-Trenaunay syndrome
Lesions
Lipids
Lungs
Lymphadenopathy and lymphoma
Lymphatic system
Mitral valve prolapse
Necrotizing fasciitis
Osteochondritis juvenilis
Phlebitis
Plasma
Podiatry
Preeclampsia and eclampsia
Progeria
Pulse rate
Raynaud's phenomenon
Respiration
Shunts
Smoking
Stem cells
Stents
Strokes
Sturge-Weber syndrome
Thrombolytic therapy and TPA
Thrombosis and thrombus
Transfusion
Transient ischemic attacks (TIAs)
Ultrasonography
Varicose vein removal
Varicose veins
Vascular system
Venous insufficiency
Von Willebrand's disease

VIROLOGY
Avian influenza
Chickenpox
Childhood infectious diseases
Cold agglutinin disease
Common cold
Conjunctivitis
Coronaviruses
Creutzfeldt-Jakob disease (CJD)
Croup
Cytomegalovirus (CMV)

Dengue fever
Ebola virus
Encephalitis
Enteroviruses
Epidemics and pandemics
Epstein-Barr virus
Eye infections and disorders
Fever
Gastroenteritis
Hand-foot-and-mouth disease
Hantavirus
Hepatitis
Herpes
H1N1 influenza
Human immunodeficiency virus (HIV)
Human papillomavirus (HPV)
Infection
Influenza
Laboratory tests
Marburg virus
Measles
Microbiology
Microscopy
Monkeypox
Mononucleosis
Noroviruses
Opportunistic infections
Orchitis
Paget's disease
Parasitic diseases
Poliomyelitis
Pulmonary diseases
Rabies
Retroviruses
Rhinoviruses
Rotavirus
Sarcoidosis
Serology
Severe acute respiratory syndrome
   (SARS)
Sexually transmitted diseases (STDs)
Shingles
Smallpox
Viral hemorrhagic fevers
Viral infections
West Nile virus
Yellow fever
Zoonoses